SAMPLE NURSING CARE PLANS

MATERNITY NURSING

JANICE HOLMES, R.N., M.S.
Assistant Professor
Olivet Nazarene University
Kankakee, Illinois

LANA MAGIERA, R.N., M.H.S.
Nursing Instructor
Kankakee Community College
Kankakee, Illinois

MATERNITY NURSING

Macmillan Publishing Company
New York

Collier Macmillan Canada, Inc.
Toronto

Collier Macmillan Publishers
London

Printed in the United States of America

Macmillan Publishing Company
866 Third Avenue, New York, New York 10022

Collier Macmillan Canada, Inc.
Collier Macmillan Publishers, London

Library of Congress Cataloging-in-Publication Data

Holmes, Janice.
Maternity nursing.

Includes index.
1. Obstetrical nursing. 2. Perinatology. 3. Family—Psychological aspects. I. Magiera, Lana. II. Title.
[DNLM: 1. Family—nurses' instruction. 2. Obstetrical Nursing—methods. 3. Perinatology—nurses' instruction.
WY 157.3 H751m]
RG951.H64 1987 618.92'01 86-31068
ISBN 0-02-356480-6

Printing: 1 2 3 4 5 6 7 8 Year: 7 8 9 0 1 2 3 4 5

DEDICATION

TO OUR FAMILIES

Glenn Holmes
Emory, Lillian, and Marilynn Netzel
Lisa Varboncoeur
Tom Holmes
Mike Magiera
Edwin and Mickie Leuck
Marc Magiera
Lisa Magiera
Matthew Magiera

Without their help and support, this project would not have been possible.

PREFACE

PURPOSE OF THE TEXT

Meeting the needs of the family throughout the childbearing experience continues to be one of the most demanding and rewarding challenges in contemporary nursing practice. While mastering increasingly complex "high-tech" interventions, nursing has set new standards for promoting emotional well-being in the entire family experiencing the birth of a new child.

The purpose of this textbook is to help nursing students become equipped to provide care that fully addresses physiologic aspects as well as psychosocial needs. In every chapter, our goal has been to introduce the student to the essentials of maternity care while building awareness of the diversity now seen in childbearing experiences with respect to physical needs, cultural background, age, family configuration, and many other variables.

INNOVATIVE APPROACH TO NURSING DIAGNOSIS IN MATERNITY CARE

The nursing process is the framework underlying our discussion of maternity care throughout the textbook. Special emphasis has been given to nursing diagnosis. Content and sample care plans have been organized to help students quickly learn how to formulate nursing diagnoses as well as how to plan, implement, and evaluate maternal-newborn care.

Unique sample care plans demonstrate how specific nursing diagnoses are linked to specific goals and nursing interventions. For each nursing diagnosis, goal, and intervention, corresponding rationales and evaluation criteria are provided.

CONTENT OVERVIEW

To facilitate the learning process, the content has been organized to provide learning across the span of the reproductive process. However, independent use of individual units may accommodate specific learning needs. Within chapters, essential physiologic and psychosocial content is presented in basic form. This content is then expanded to include more advanced applications.

Unit I presents an overview of the family during the childbearing years. Included in this unit are historical perspectives related to childbearing and maternity nursing care in contemporary society. The heritage of maternity nursing serves as a background for the understanding of current clinical trends. Family members are viewed as active participants in the entire childbearing cycle. Cultural aspects and societal influences on childbearing are presented as dynamic forces influencing the role of the nurse in the maternity cycle.

More specific physiologic dimensions are presented in Unit II which progresses to a review of the reproductive system. Normal physiology of the female and male reproductive systems, genetics, family planning, and fundamentals of fetal development are discussed.

Humanism in the delivery of health care during the antepartal period is emphasized in Unit III. Preparations for pregnancy and care during the antepartal period embody this concept. All members of the family are included in health care and education during this period. The role of the nurse is seen as a facilitator for the achievement of a successful childbearing family experience.

Nursing assessment and management of the family during the labor and delivery process is the focus of Unit IV. The learner progresses from a basic understanding of the normal anatomy and physiology to the more advanced concepts of maternal and family adaptations to the birthing process.

Unit V centers on the participation of both the client and the nurse in the three areas of decision making during the puerperium. Responsibilities involved in nurse-centered decisions, shared decisions, and family-centered decisions, are discussed. The normal newborn is introduced in this unit. The newborn's impact on family adaptations and responsibilities are explored.

Interruptions in maternal and newborn health are addressed in Units VI and VII. Implicit in the discussion of the content is an understanding of the "normal" aspects of childbearing and fetal development. These units are organized to present deviations from normal which influence the health and welfare of the entire family.

LEARNING AIDS WITHIN THE TEXT

To facilitate learning and emphasize priorities, the following are featured in the text:

Objectives open each chapter.

Key Terms are listed at the beginning of each chapter to alert students to essential vocabulary.

A comprehensive *Glossary* appears at the end of the book for quick reference and review.

Sample Nursing Care Plans corresponding to individual case studies clarify nursing diagnosis formulation and care planning.

Highlighted *Nursing Responsibilities* emphasize crucial nursing actions and precautions.

COMPREHENSIVE TEACHING-LEARNING PACKAGE

In addition to the learning aids supplied within the text, the following instructional supplements are offered:

The *Workbook in Maternity Nursing* provides questions that reinforce factual recall and mastery of concepts, and it offers exercises in applying information to clinical situations.

A detailed *Instructor's Manual* provides a content outline with corresponding lecture notes, extended bibliographies, lists of audiovisual resources, additional suggested activities, and masters for producing your own overhead transparencies.

An extensive *Test Bank* of approximately 2,000 items is available on disks for all IBM PC and Apple II computers as well as in printed form.

A selection of acetate *Overhead Transparencies* is provided for immediate classroom use.

ACKNOWLEDGMENTS

Many are the hearts and souls which embraced the writing of this book. Each contributed a special effort and offered a special expertise, yet all collectively friends and supporters in every sense of the word. To these gracious, talented individuals, we are truly appreciative and indebted.

First and foremost are our families, whose patience and understanding were elixirs to our productivity. To the nurses and friends who read, reread, and critiqued the manuscript, we are grateful. A special thanks to Glenn Holmes and Susan Shearer who meticulously proofread each manuscript page. To Carol Reams, Lisa Varboncoeur, Marilynn Netzel, and Mickie Leuck, we give our thanks for typing endless pages. To Cathy Gray, Perinatal Outreach Coordinator at the University of Chicago, a special thanks for her review of the chapter on the high-risk neonate. Robert Witham and Robert Bott took endless pictures to enhance the manuscript. The support of our colleagues at Olivet Nazarene University, Kankakee Community College, Riverside Medical Center, and St. Mary's Hospital was invaluable. Last, but not least, we would like to thank Carol Wolfe, Senior Editor of Nursing at Macmillan, for her assistance and guidance in bringing this dream to reality.

CONTENTS IN BRIEF

UNIT IV

UNIT V

UNIT VI

UNIT VII

EXPANDED TABLE OF CONTENTS

APPENDIX

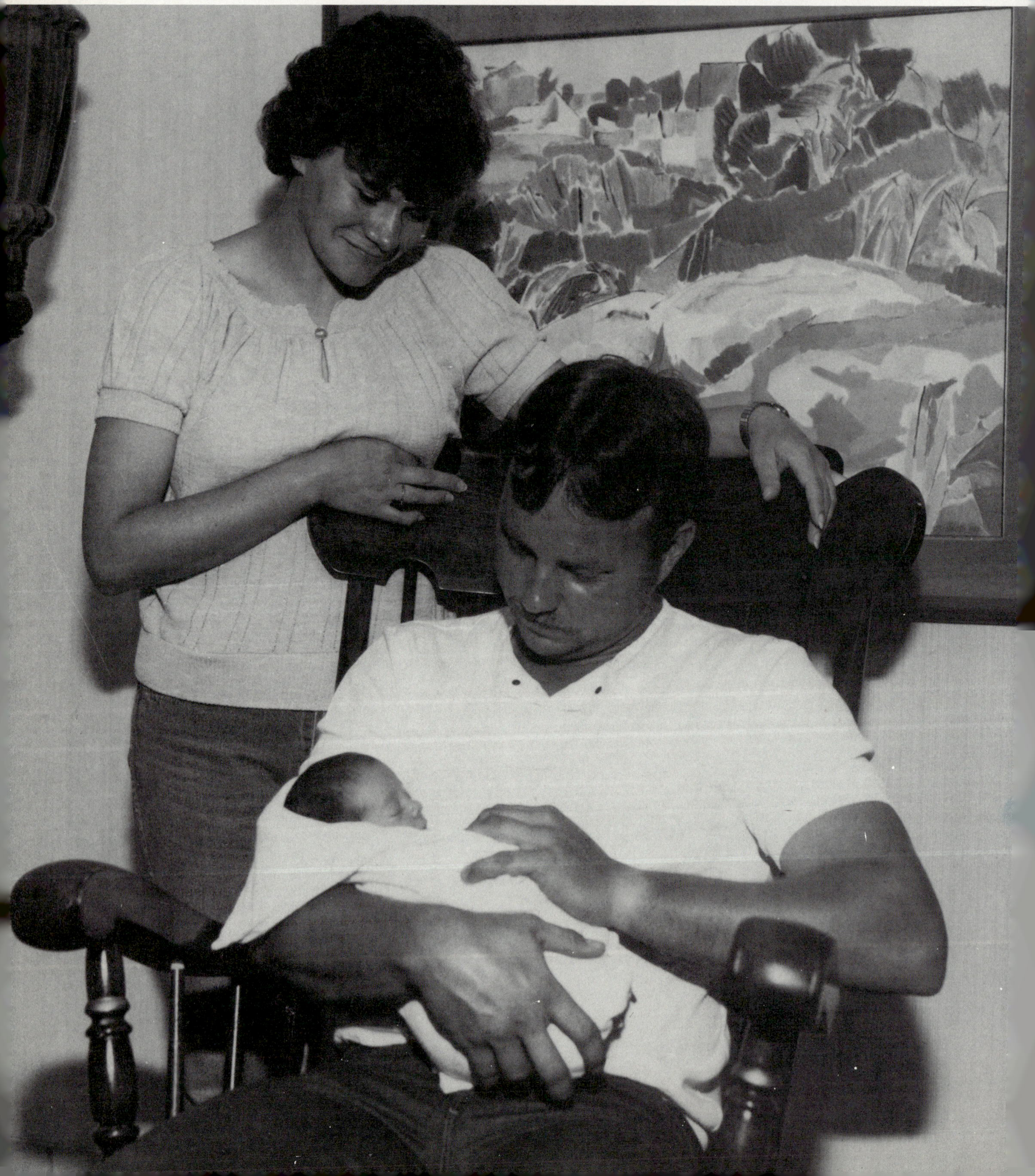

UNIT I

THE FAMILY DURING THE CHILDBEARING YEARS

UNIT 1

THE FAMILY DURING THE CHILDBEARING YEARS

chapter 1

MATERNITY NURSING TODAY

OBJECTIVES

Upon completion of this chapter, the reader will be able to:

1. Define family-centered maternity nursing.
2. Discuss the growth of maternity care and the contributions of nursing and midwifery to maternal and infant care.
3. Define the role of the maternity nurse in family-centered maternity care.
4. Cite examples of the expanded role of the maternity nurse.
5. Discuss influences that have had an effect on the developing trends in maternity nursing.
6. Discuss classifications used when referring to statistical data applicable to maternity nursing.
7. Identify government influences in the development of maternity care.
8. Cite influences that will affect the future of maternity nursing.

KEY TERMS

Birthrate
Childbearing family
Family-centered maternity nursing
Fertility rate
Fetal mortality
Infant mortality
Maternal mortality
Maternity clinical specialist
Maternity nurse practitioner
Midwifery
Neonatal mortality
Nurse midwife
Nursing process
Perinatal mortality rate
Postneonatal mortality rate

INTRODUCTION

Maternity nursing is the provision of knowledge-based, quality care to the pregnant woman and her family during the childbearing experience. The scope of this care is not limited to physical dimensions alone but includes the physiologic, psychological, developmental, and social-cultural-spiritual dimensions that affect the well-being of the childbearing family. Emphasis is no longer on only the events occurring at birth, but includes the influencing factors present from conception, during life in the womb, and the period of adaptation as the newborn becomes acquainted with his or her environment.

Nurses with expertise in this area formerly described themselves as obstetric nurses. This term, although widely used, describes only the medical and surgical management of pregnancy, labor, and delivery and the care following delivery. Maternity nursing, however, places an emphasis on the delivery of nursing care not only to the mother and neonate, but to the family as well.

How can we, as nurses, provide care that can truly be called maternity nursing and not just an extension of obstetric care? The answer lies in the nursing process, which provides the pathway to effective nursing management. Each step of the process, including assessment, analysis, planning, implementation, and evaluation, forms the framework for competent nursing care. Using critical analysis and decision-making skills, we formulate nursing diagnoses for organizing and implementing nursing care and management. Throughout the entire process, the maternity nurse consults and interacts with the client, providing an opportunity to share in the management of client care. Our nursing efforts are not singular in their direction but must be made in collaboration with other members of the health team providing family-centered maternity care.

The Growth of Maternity Care

Maternity nursing has a rich heritage, based in the contributions of medicine, nursing, and midwifery. A glimpse into the history of maternity care reveals a complex of contributing factors—some based on scientific knowledge and some the result of superstitions and customs inherent in the various cultures of society. The evolution of childbearing practices has proceeded from tribal customs and traditions to family-centered care strengthened by the application of sound knowledge-based principles.

The scientific practice of medicine developed from the early societies of the Egyptians, Romans, and Greeks. Following the decline of medicine in Medieval times, the Renaissance witnessed a surge in medical knowledge and scientific applications. Contributions to maternity care included anatomical drawings, descriptions of blood circulation and pelvic anatomy, performance of cesarean sections, and the invention of forceps.

Societal influences have continually affected childbearing practices throughout history. For example, the role of women in the birthing process can be seen as a thread interwoven through the fabric of society in every century. In early societies, birth was viewed as solely the responsibility of women. The early colonists of America depended on female family members and friends to provide support during childbearing. Traditionally, these women were the primary attendants at the birth. All births occurred within the confines of the homes, and birthing was viewed as a natural event. The knowledge of the women performing deliveries was passed from generation to generation and served as the beginning for maternity nursing.

In the eighteenth century, the practice of medicine began to include childbearing. Physicians were called on by the more affluent in both Western Europe and America, whereas midwives attended those in lower economic groups. Nurses were, for the most part, untrained and their care was often delivered in unsanitary conditions in hospitals for the poor and indigent.

As industrialization occurred in America, an influx of immigrants arrived from Europe, and maternity care acquired the complexion of many different ethnic and cultural influences. The practice of midwifery became an important component of childbearing in a rapidly growing nation. Although many midwives were well trained, others were not. The poor and the immigrant often fell victim to untrained, frequently dishonest, midwives. Trained midwives who had immigrated from Europe were mistrusted and often not allowed to practice owing to the reputations of their unscrupulous counterparts.

During the nineteenth century, nursing was given legitimacy by Florence Nightingale, the founder of modern nursing, and the first school of nursing, St. Thomas School of Nursing, was founded in London in 1860. By the late 1890s, schools of nursing were opened in America, and in 1898, Sloane Maternity Hospital in New York offered affiliations in maternity nursing to smaller hospitals, where these services were not available.

Legislation enacted in the early twentieth century in America regulating the practice of midwifery provided the impetus for the development of schools of midwifery and programs for nurse midwives. A leader in the development of these programs was Mary Breckenridge, a nurse who recognized the need for maternity care in areas not adequately served by the medical community. Through her efforts and the efforts of the Maternity Center Association, the Frontier Graduate School of Midwifery was founded. Its goals focused on the preparation of nurse midwives qualified to provide maternity care in rural America. In 1910, 50 percent of all baby deliveries in the nation were performed by midwives. By 1940, however, the percentage was down to 9.0 percent and further, to 0.5 percent in the 1970s.

Programs protecting the health of mothers and infants were developed in the latter half of the twentieth century, and significant legislation contributed to the advancement of maternity care (see Table 1–1).

TABLE 1–1
SIGNIFICANT INFLUENCES OF GOVERNMENT IN MATERNITY CARE

Year	Event
1909	The first White House Conference on children • Recommended the formation of a Federal Children's Bureau
1912	Establishment of the Federal Children's Bureau • Focused activities on the study of economic and rural factors and their relationship to infant and maternal mortality
1919	Second White House Conference • Proposed standards for child welfare and maternal health
1921	Sheppard-Towner Act • Provided federal grants to states for the development of maternal and child health services
1935	Social Security Act • Provision for maternal and infant health services, crippled children services, and children welfare services were included in the Act
1950	The Fourth White House Conference • Appropriations were made for the study of mental retardation
1963	Maternal and Child Health and Mental Retardation Planning • Amendment added to Title V of the Social Security Act authorized programs on maternity and infant care and provided for appropriations of monies for nursing research in the areas of maternal health improvements, nutrition and well child care
1967	Child Health Act • Made provisions for the funding of family planning service
1973	Legalization of abortions
1974	National Health Planning and Resources Development Act • Made possible the establishment of regionalized perinatal centers
1975	Establishment of the Women, Infants and Children supplemental food program (WIC) • Provided low income families with supplementary nutrition
1981	Authorization of Medicare payments to nurse midwives for the delivery of maternity care.

MATERNITY NURSING ROLES

What is the role of the maternity nurse? Is it teacher, health manager, client advocate, care provider, consultant, or change agent? Indeed, all of these roles are integral to the delivery of holistic care to the childbearing family. Implicit in the implementation of these roles is a blending of interpersonal, intellectual, and technical skills used by the nurse. A sound knowledge base is not adequate if the nurse is not capable of implementing techniques necessary for the administration of care. Likewise, the nurse who functions purely on a technical level without knowledge is unsafe and ineffective. Interpersonal skills enable the nurse to bring together all aspects of care for interpretation to the client. Family-centered care demands that clients not only are instructed in care, but that they also understand the implications and decisions necessary for good health care management during the childbearing experience.

Respect for individuals and their beliefs must not be ignored when providing maternity care. Tradition, culture, ethics, and values all contribute to the individual's personal philosophy and, thus, to attitudes regarding the delivery of health care. The nurse must be aware of her own personal philosophy of maternity nursing practice. She may identify with a specific nursing model based on a theory developed by a leading nursing theorist, or she may choose to develop her own nursing model consistent with the concepts basic to the implementation of her philosophy of nursing. It is essential, however, that the nurse does not use her own philosophy to control client decisions, but instead, to foster client participation in the childbearing process.

The nurse as client advocate is an essential element in the delivery of family-centered care. Although nurses are seldom called upon to plead the causes of their clients, they are often influential in securing the rights of clients. All nurses delivering maternity care should be aware of *The Pregnant Patient's Bill of Rights and Responsibilities* (Appendix A), prepared by Haire and published by the International Childbirth Education Association. The nurse must respect these rights and help clients to interpret them.

Coordination and continuity of care describes the responsibility of the maternity nurse as health care manager. She not only provides care in the prenatal setting, but also in cooperation with the client and other health care personnel develops an individualized care program for the client throughout her pregnancy.

Teaching-learning activities of the maternity nurse are not confined to prenatal education classes but are important components of nursing assessments made at every visit. The nursing diagnosis of knowledge deficit commonly appears on nursing care plans during the *antepartal* (before delivery), *intrapartal* (labor and delivery), and *postpartal* (after delivery) periods. Primary prevention is one of the most important functions of the maternity nurse and the teaching role promotes this function. Pregnancy, although a normal occurrence in the well individual and family, is a formidable experience and in some circumstances may be viewed as a crisis. Without doubt, comprehensive maternity care must include a teaching-learning component.

What do we mean when we say the maternity nurse functions as a change agent? Change does and will occur, even if we choose to ignore it. This change may or may not be productive and, in fact, may be counterproductive to the health of the childbearing family. The maternity nurse facilitates change that is deliberate and goal-oriented.

An understanding of the client's environment, both internal and external, and the stresses within that environment contributes to the decision-making process used to effect change. The nurse is able to identify the need for change within the client's environment and to implement appropriate interventions. Concomitantly, the nurse uses well-developed communication skills to begin the teaching-learning process necessary for realizing change (see Fig. 1–1).

The role of the maternity nurse as change

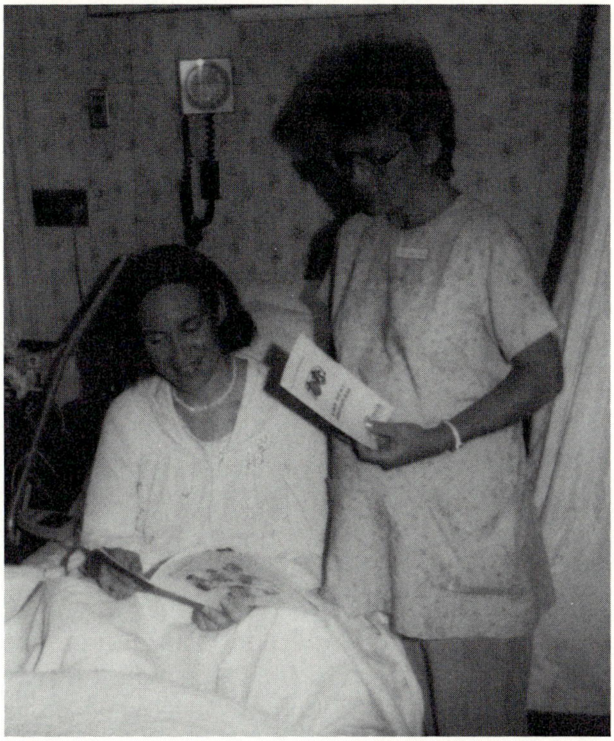

FIGURE 1-1. Maternity nurse assuming the teaching role.

agent is not limited to management of the childbearing family, but also applies to change in the health care system. With a sound understanding of the dynamics of change, the maternity nurse enters into the political, social, and technological arena of change in the health care system. Planned change in any of these areas is based on research. For years, nurses have been told to be more assertive in order to effect change. This alone is not the answer. To be assertive, the maternity nurse will not only need a sound knowledge base but will need to make a critical analysis of each issue to be addressed. Nursing research serves as the basis for analyses and conclusions that are supportive of change. As problems are identified, the nurse in her role as scientific investigator, critiques and applies research findings to her practice and to the delivery of health care. She not only takes advantage of research provided by her colleagues and other disciplines, but, when appropriate, initiates and undertakes the nursing research.

Expanded roles in maternity nursing now include those of nurse practitioners, clinicians, clinical specialists, and nurse midwives. Various practice settings, such as clinics, hospitals, home health care agencies, and private practices, are used to implement these roles. The maternity nurse practitioner (see Fig. 1–2) is a registered nurse with advanced assessment skills and education in the delivery of care to childbearing families. She is qualified to perform physical and psychological assessments in an ambulatory maternity setting and to provide basic care to the childbearing family. Her role may also include genetic and family planning counseling. The role of the clinical specialist requires a master's degree in nursing and advanced education and skills in the delivery of maternity care.

The nurse midwife is a registered nurse prepared in advanced theories and skills of midwifery. Certification is possible through the American College of Nurse Midwives (ACNM). Certified midwives have been an important addition to the delivery of quality care to the childbearing family. They provide comprehensive quality and cost-effective care to women experiencing an uncomplicated pregnancy and delivery. Nurse midwives are qualified to perform deliveries and to establish autonomous practices. Collaboration and consultation with, and referral to a physician may

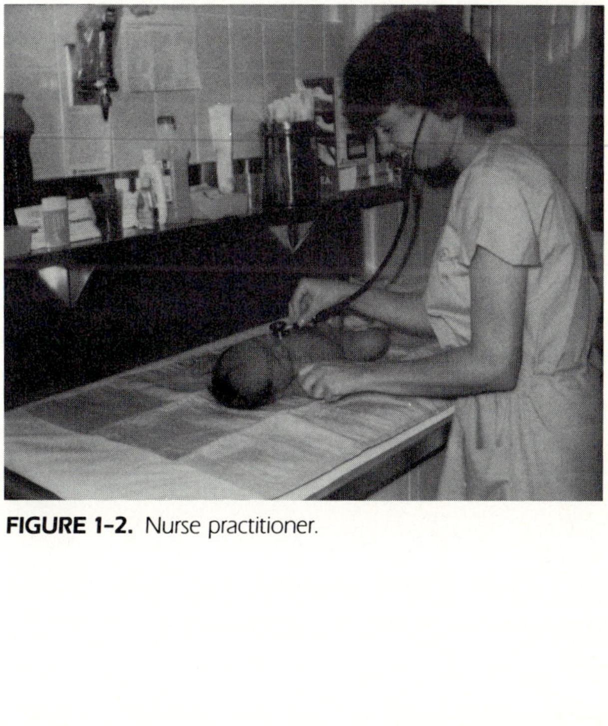

FIGURE 1-2. Nurse practitioner.

occur in management of high-risk pregnancies. Unfortunately, midwifery has not been acknowledged in the practice laws of every state.

Voluntary certification is recommended for nurses practicing in obstetric, gynecologic, and neonatal nursing specialties. Certification may be achieved through examination by the NAACOG Certification Corporation of the Nurse's Association of the American College of Obstetrics and Gynecology and/or the American Nurses' Association. Candidates for each of the examinations must be registered nurses and must meet eligibility requirements specific to the specialty area. The purpose of certification is to promote quality care through the documentation of achievement of a special body of knowledge applicable to the certified specialty area. There are no special rights to licensure or practice associated with certification.

MATERNITY NURSING TRENDS

Trends in maternity care today are the result of combined efforts of health care consumers and providers. Consumers have chosen to become more involved in decisions regarding the delivery of maternity care, making family-centered nursing care a reality in almost all areas of the country. Birthing rooms are available in most hospitals, and it is now possible for the childbearing family to manage their delivery in the manner most suited to their individual needs. Decisions regarding the use of medications during labor and delivery are now made by expectant parents who have been informed of the effects drugs may have on the fetus as well as on the expectant mother. Birthing centers are available, as are programs for early hospital discharge. Active participation of the father in all aspects of the pregnancy, including prenatal care, prenatal education, and the labor and delivery process, is encouraged. His supportive role during pregnancy is well established and adds immeasurably to the psychological and physiologic welfare of the pregnant woman.

Consumer knowledge now enables the family and individual clients to make choices regarding family planning. Contraception information is available for individuals to make informed decisions. Nurses participate in family planning clinics, teaching, counseling, and providing care.

The shifting roles of women have altered attitudes toward marriage and childrearing. Single parenting is not only common among the divorced but may be a choice of those who do not wish to enter into marriage. The rate of pregnancy among adolescents has decreased, yet more than 500,000 babies are born every year to mothers under age 20. At the other end of the spectrum, career-oriented women often choose to delay parenting. The woman expecting her first baby when she is 35 or older is not uncommon. Childbearing in later reproductive years (32 to 40 years) has increased by approximately 60 percent within the last five years. Changes in the birthrate have been realized from these societal influences. Statistical references to birth and fertility rates are determined as follows:

Birthrate: The number of live births per 1000 population.

Fertility Rate: The number of births per 1000 women of ages 15 to 44.

Within the last 30 years, the highest birth rate was experienced in 1955, at 25 per 1000 population. The ensuing years brought a drop in the birth rate, most likely resulting from newer and better forms of contraception, with the lowest level in 1976, of 14.6 per 1000 population. Today the birth rate is again increasing, in part because of the increased number of women in the childbearing age group. In 1983, an estimated 3,614,000 babies were born in the United States, with a rate of 15.5 per 1000 population. The greatest number of births occurred in women between the ages of 20 and 24.

Development of the specialty of perinatology has improved the identification, diagnosis, and treatment of high-risk pregnancies. Care of these clients may now be provided during the perinatal period from the 28th week of gestation through the 28th day following birth) at regionalized perinatal centers. The focus of care at these centers is not only on the expectant mother, but on the fetus as well, and has resulted in a reduction in infant, neonatal, and perinatal mortality. The following classification is used when referring to mortality rates:

Maternal mortality: The number of maternal deaths per 100,000 live births.

Fetal mortality: The number of neonatal deaths per 1000 live births.

Neonatal mortality: The number of fetal deaths per 1000 live births during the first 28 days of life.

Infant mortality: The number of deaths per 1000 children one year of age or younger.

Perinatal mortality: The number of fetal deaths at 28 weeks or more of gestation plus the number of neonatal deaths.

Postneonatal mortality: The number of deaths per 1000 live births from 28 days of life up to but not including one year of age.

Table 1–2 indicates the United States infant, neonatal, and postneonatal mortality rates for 1960, 1970, and 1980.

TABLE 1–2
NEONATAL, POSTNATAL AND INFANT MORTALITY RATES PER 1000 LIVE BIRTHS IN 1960, 1970, AND 1980

	Infant Mortality*	Neonatal Mortality*	Postnatal Mortality*
1960	26.0	18.7	7.3
1970	20.0	15.1	4.9
1980	12.6	8.5	4.1

*Deaths per 1000 live births
Source: National Center for Health Statistics

Other factors important to the reduction of infant and maternal mortality are prenatal care and education. Prenatal education is available in most areas of the country; however, not all socioeconomic groups have equal accessibility to prenatal classes or to adequate care facilities. In an effort to address this problem, prenatal education campaigns have been conducted to provide all expectant parents with information regarding important aspects of pregnancy such as nutrition, health care, environmental factors, and the hazards to the fetus from prenatal use of alcohol, drugs, and tobacco. Population groups at increased risk due to ethnic, medical, socioeconomic, genetic, and age-related influences have been especially targetted.

Early prenatal care is an important contributor to maternal and fetal well being. During the 1970s, the number of women receiving prenatal care in the first trimester of pregnancy increased. This increase was seen in both black and white women. According to the National Center for Health Statistics, there was an increase from 72 to 79 percent of white women receiving prenatal care in the first trimester; in black women the increase was from 44 to 62 percent. Although the percentage increase in blacks was higher than whites, the total percentage of white women receiving early prenatal care was higher (see Fig. 1–3). Early and continued prenatal care has influenced maternal mortality with a decrease from 40 maternal deaths per 100,000 live births in 1961 to 7.7 in 1981.

There has also been a steady decline in infant mortality for the past ten years. The infant mortality rate for blacks still remains almost twice the rate for whites (see Fig. 1–4). Organizations such as the Healthy Mothers, Healthy Babies Coalition have been formed to provide prenatal information to all expectant women but with a special emphasis on high-risk mothers and those in high-risk ethnic groups. This organization, composed of members from federal, professional, and voluntary

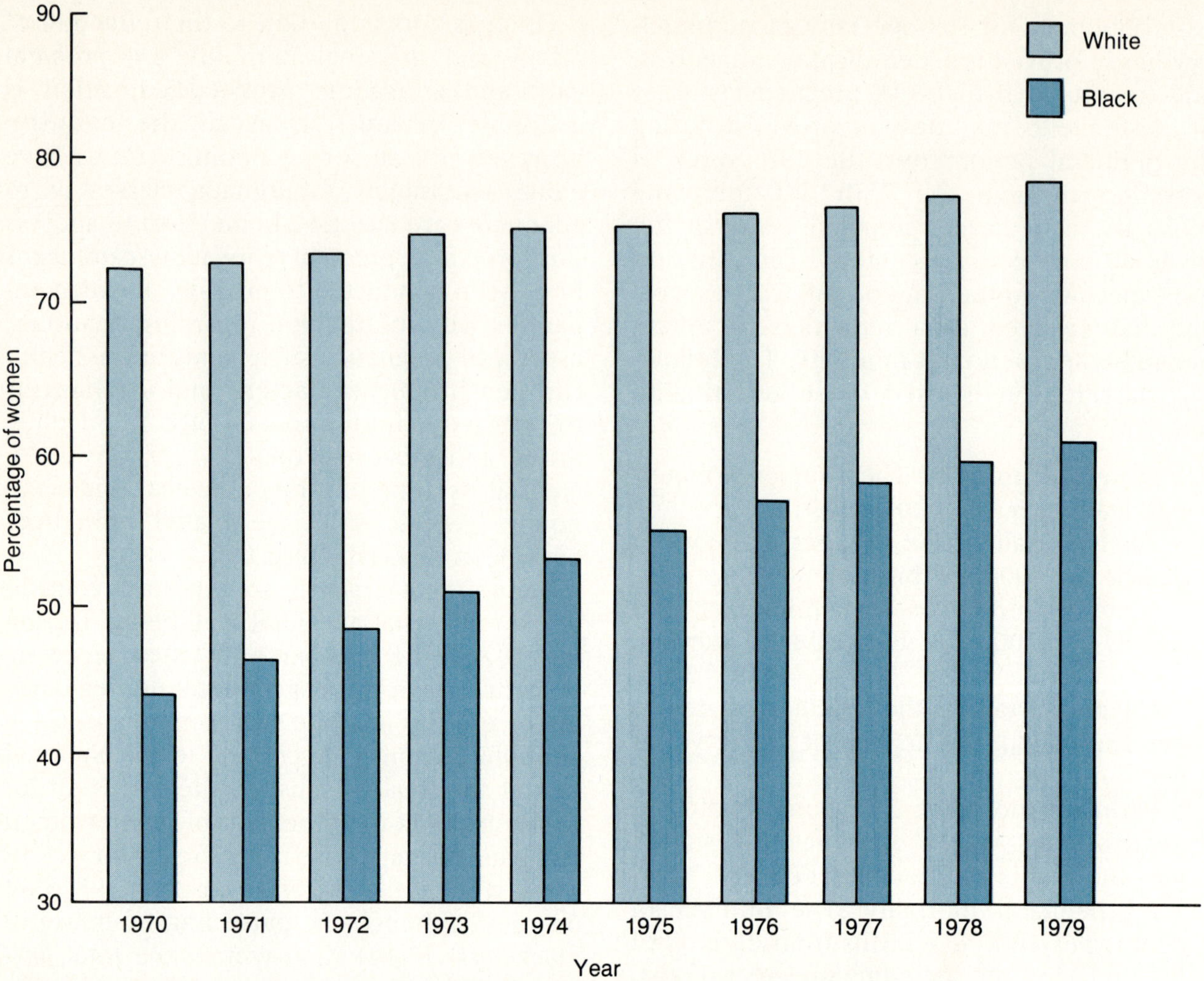

FIGURE 1-3. Percentages of women beginning prenatal care in the 1st trimester of pregnancy according to race, from 1970–1979 in the United States. Reprinted with permission. National Center for Health Statistics: Health, United States, 1982. DHHS Pub. No. (PHS) 83-1232. Public Health Service. Washington. U.S. Government Printing Office, Dec. 1982.

organizations, is now establishing a network of chapters throughout the United States.

MATERNITY CARE IN THE FUTURE

Maternity nursing in the future will continue to focus on the holistic care of the childbearing family. With the advent of new technology and advances in science, the role of the nurse will become more complex and challenging. Societal influences will continue to demand high-quality and cost-effective care. The role of the nurse practitioner will acquire new dimensions as health care delivery to the childbearing family becomes a part of the national emphasis on improved health for all. Public health measures and legislation for maternal-child health care will look to the maternity nurse for input in determining health policies.

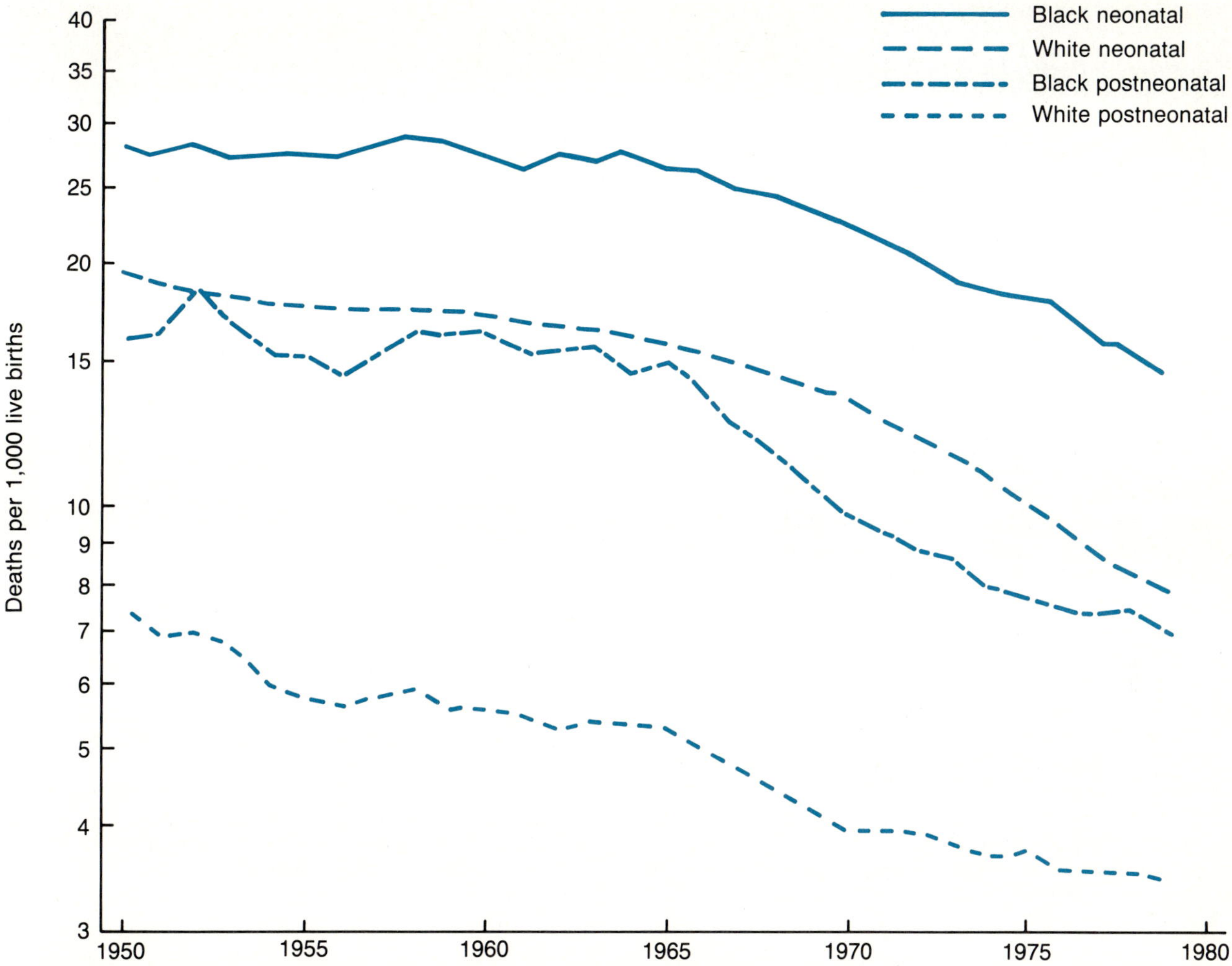

FIGURE 1-4. Infant mortality rate as reflected in neonatal and postneonatal mortality rate according to race, from 1950–1979 in the United States. Reprinted with permission. National Center for Health Statistics: Health, United States, 1982. DHHS Pub. No. (PHS) 83-1232. Public Health Service. Washington. U.S. Government Printing Office, Dec. 1982.

Maternity nurses will likely provide access to health care for childbearing families who are among the uneducated and culturally, economically, or geographically disadvantaged. Maternity nurses will serve as well-informed educators for clients and will be paramount in the fostering of optimal health education. They will be leaders in the promotion of wellness and advocates of the self-help movement in health care.

New technology will demand an increased knowledge base and competency for maternity nursing practice. Critical decision making will be essential, as will a philosophical and ethical application of the use of technology.

Maternity nursing is on the brink of an exciting future. The groundwork has been well laid. We invite you, through the pages of this text, to learn and become a part of the future of maternity nursing.

BIBLIOGRAPHY

American Nurses' Association. *Nursing: a social policy statement.* Task Force on the Nature and Scope of Nursing Practice and Characteristics of Specialization in Nursing, Kansas City, Missouri, 1980.

Annual summary of births, deaths, marriages and divorces: United States—1982. Hyattsville, Maryland, National Center for Health Statistics, 1983; *DHHS* publication no. (PHS) 83-1120. (Vital and health statistics; series 31; no. 13)

Atkinson, L. & Murray, M.E. *Fundamentals of nursing.* New York: Macmillan, 1985.

Bartkowski, J.J. & Swandby, J.M. Charting nursing's course through megatrends. *Nursing and Health Care,* 1985, **6**(7), 375–377.

David, R.J. & Siegel, E. Decline in neonatal mortality, 1968 to 1977: better babies or better care? *Pediatrics,* 1983, **71,** 531-540.

Diers, D. Nurse-Midwifery as a system of care: provider process and patient outcome. In Aiken, L. *Health policy and nursing practice,* New York: McGraw-Hill, 1981, pp. 73-89.

Kalish, B. & Kalish, P. Anatomy of the image of the nurse: Dissonant and ideal model. In Williams, C.A. (Ed.), *Image-making in nursing,* American Academy of Nursing, papers of the Scientific Session, 1983.

Kalish, P. & Kalish, B.: *The advance of American nursing*. Boston: Little, Brown, 1978.

Lee, K.S., et al.: Neonatal mortality: an analysis of the recent improvement in the United States. *American Journal of Public Health,* 1980, **70,** 15–21.

National Center for Health Statistics: Advance report of final natality statistics. 1980 Monthly Vital Statistics Report, 1982, **31,** (8, suppl.). 1982.

Reinhardt, U.E.: Health care for America's poor: the economics of a hot potato. *Princeton Alumni Weekly,* 1985, February 27, 23.

Sandelowski, M. Perinatal nursing: whose specialty is it anyway? *MCN,* 1983, **8** (5), 317–318, 321–322.

Speert, H. *Obstetrics and gynecology in America, a history.* Baltimore: Waverly Press, 1980.

Interprofessional Task Force on Health Care of Women and Children. The Development of Family-Centered Maternity/Newborn Care in Hospitals, Joint Position Statement, 1978.

U.S. Department of Commerce, Bureau of Census. *Statistical Abstracts of the United States* (105th ed.) Washington, D.C.: U.S. Government Printing Office, 1985.

U.S. Department of Health and Human Services. Public Health Service. *Health United States*. Hyattsville, Md.: National Center for Health Statistics, 1982.

U.S. Government Printing Office: *Women's Health: Report of the Public Health Service Task Force on Womens Health Issues*. 1985, **100** (1), 73-106.

Wallace, H., Gold. E., & Oglesby, A. *Maternal and child health practices*. (2nd ed.). New York: Wiley, 1982.

Wilson, F. & Neuhauser, D. *Health services in the United States*. Cambridge, Mass.: Ballinger, 1976.

chapter 2

TODAY'S FAMILY AND SOCIETY

OBJECTIVES

Upon completion of this chapter, the reader will be able to:

1. Define family.
2. State three characteristics of the family.
3. List universal functions of the family.
4. Identify the importance of assessing family strengths and weaknesses.
5. Discuss traditional family structure.
6. Describe at least two alternate family structures.
7. Define culture.
8. Given a specific cultural group, identify ways that their beliefs affect their perception of medical or nursing care.

KEY TERMS

Acculturation
Culture
Curanderos
Extended family
Familismo
Family
Machismo
Matrifocal family
Nuclear family
Pica
Subculture
Spiritualist

THE FAMILY

Nursing care of the childbearing family is family centered in nature. It focuses on the impact of pregnancy and birth on the entire family unit, not just on the mother and infant.

What Is The Family?

The family is considered the natural and fundamental unit of our society. Traditionally, the family refers to the nuclear family, consisting of husband, wife, and children. The extended family includes a group of relatives who form relationships—they may inhabit more than one household but share a common body of domestic, social, cultural, and economic activities. In the matrifocal family, the adult male is an in-and-out member.

Families are also defined as extended kin networks, in which there is a social system of grandparents, adult children, grandchildren, and other relatives.

Today our society is rapidly changing. People's needs and ideas are changing and the concept of family has also been redefined. According to sociological theory, the family is a group of two or more persons that are related by blood, marriage, or adoption, who reside in a common household and interact and communicate with each other in the respective family roles. For simplicity, an even looser definition is sometimes used. A family is two or more persons living together or in separate families, who feel bound together for mutual caring, sharing, comforting, support, companionship, and pleasure.

Regardless of the definition of family used, the family as a group generates, tolerates, prevents, and corrects health problems within its defined membership. It is a fluid, ever-changing mixture of old and new traditions, as well as future dreams.

The social system of the family is related to the functions performed by family members. Each member assumes a role to which the culture dictates behavioral expectations. In turn, the way family members view each role may vary greatly from culture to culture.

From some value perspectives, the family may be considered an outdated structural unit. Yet defined in terms of commitment and responsibility, the family remains a necessity for the continuation of humanity.

Before looking at some of the different family structures, the characteristics and functions of families, as well as the motivations for parenthood, should be examined.

FAMILY CHARACTERISTICS

Family characteristics have been influenced by many factors:

- change in the structure of society
- industrialization, with its change in the source of income from farms to industry
- change in industry itself to a level of high technology
- division of the large nuclear family by relocation
- decrease in access to kinship groups
- increase in blending of cultures
- decrease in marriage rate accompanied by increase in divorce rate
- increase in single parent families
- decrease in fertility among married women
- change in and deemphasis of sex roles
- increase in the number of married women in the work force
- decrease in availability of psychological support for parenting within the family and society
- increase in the importance of the role of friends to young parents

Some characteristics of the family have special significance for the nurse and are needed for effective use of the nursing process. The family is dynamic and constantly changing. The family is also made up of individuals. When considering the family, therefore, individual tasks involved in the functioning of that specific family should be identified. The family is a special kind of small group wherein each of its members has a deep emotional involvement with the other members.

Events that occur within a family can be viewed as a long chain of cause and effect, with each link of the chain representing an event, and each event depending upon the events before, and helping to form the events that will follow.

FAMILY FUNCTIONS

There are five universal functions of the family: reproduction, status placement, biological and emotional maintenance, socialization and care of children, and social control.

The family provides the introduction and socialization of new members. It develops a protocol for problem solving within the family unit. It helps to develop channels and patterns of communication. It concerns itself with certain key activities within the unit: definition of boundaries, providing for the health and welfare of its members, and support of an environment that permits personal growth.

MOTIVATIONS FOR PARENTHOOD

Motivations for parenthood can be divided into two basic groups: immature and mature. Immature motivations include holding together a poor or degenerating relationship, avoiding loneliness, realizing unfulfilled goals, and attaining of security. Mature motivations are those that view the child as an individual and not as the means to a parental end.

FAMILY STRENGTHS AND WEAKNESSES

Family strengths are defined as those forces or factors that contribute to solidarity and unity of the unit and help to develop potentials within the unit.

The American family system is seen by some individuals as consisting of isolated households with little help from relatives. If this description is true, then the strengths of each individual family must be assessed to determine coping abilities. Strengths that may be noted include (1) ability to provide for all needs within the family unit, (2) communication skills, (3) maintenance of constructive and responsible relationships within the family and within the community, (4) growth ability of all members, (5) family role flexibility, and (6) concern for the family members as individuals and as members of a unit.

Factors that tend to weaken a family include: (1) Loss of function within the family. In some situations, active family membership is considered optional and members may change functions. (2) Increased mobility within society. With increased mobility comes an increase in the number of adjustments that need to be made by each family member. The support of friends is sometimes lost as mobility within the system is increased. (3) An increase in the importance of materialistic values. As mobility spirals upward, the value of "things" to the individual family member may increase. (4) Urban living. The city may not give community support for the family and its maintenance. (5) The decline in the importance of the family as an economic unit. With increasing technology, the family need no longer be self-sufficient in meeting the material demands of its members.

TRADITIONAL FAMILY STRUCTURES

Traditional family structures take a number of forms in the United States today, including

> The traditional extended family, composed of a cluster of individual nuclear units who live in their own homes, usually located near the original household that is inhabited by the grandparents. Large families are encouraged and the burdens of parenthood are significantly reduced.
>
> The nuclear family, in which a husband, wife, and children live in a common household. The husband is the breadwinner, and the wife stays at home.

The dyadic nuclear family, in which there is a childless husband and wife, with one or both employed.

The dual work family, in which both partners are employed from the onset of the marriage. There may or may not be children.

The single parent family with children, in which there is one parent as a consequence of divorce, death, abandonment, or personal choice.

The two- or three-generation family, in which two or three generations live in a single household.

The middle-aged or older family, in which the husband is the provider, the wife stays at home, and the children have moved away from home.

Remarriage families, in which there is a husband and wife, children from previous marriages, and children from the present marriage.

The second career family, in which the wife enters the work force when the children are no longer at home.

Each of the traditional family types has its own characteristics and needs. As a group, the traditional family units function for reproduction, care and protection of children, socialization of children, economic production of family goods and services, love, and emotional support.

Nuclear families may experience high mobility, changing values and attitudes, communication gaps, high divorce rates, role reversal, and role blurring between the sexes. They occupy separate dwellings that are not shared with members of the extended family. They are usually economically independent. Parents give emotional support to each other and to the children to accomplish goals within the family unit. Strong social bonds tend to hold them together.

ALTERNATE FAMILY STRUCTURES

In addition to traditional family structures, there are several other forms of family structures. These include:

The monogamous commune, which includes a household of more than one monogamous couple with children. The couples share common facilities and experiences; child socialization is often a group activity.

The group marriage commune, in which a household of adults and children is known as one family. All individuals consider themselves married to each other and all are parents to the children.

The unmarried couple with a child or children. Children present in this family structure may be natural or adopted members of the family.

There were 1.89 million unmarried households in the United States in 1983, an increase of three times the number in 1970. In 1983, about 1 in 24 couples living together was not married. In addition, the number of young adults that still live at home with their parents increased by 85 percent between 1970 and 1983. The number of children under 28 who lived with only one parent increased from 11.9 percent in 1970 to 22 percent in 1983 (U.S. Bureau of the Census, 1984).

These families represent a very vulnerable group socially and economically. As society changes, single parent families and unmarried couple families become more acceptable methods of parenting. Depending on whether or not this lifestyle is entered into voluntarily, it may provide an unstable and deprived environment for growth potential of children, or it may provide a free and open system for growth and development of all family members.

WORKING WITH FAMILIES

When working with families, it must be remembered that the health care consumer of today is more knowledgeable, more sophisticated, and more critical of the health care system than ever before. New family needs are emerging, in part because of client dissatisfaction, less defined masculine and feminine roles, and lack of preparation for parenthood.

Nursing care during the childbearing years involves support of family strengths and identification of family weaknesses. It is impossible to provide adequate support and care without considering the entire family's needs and how these needs interact to influence the needs of other family members. The type of support and guidance given will influence the ability of the family to cope with pregnancy stresses and to be prepared emotionally and physically to provide a healthy environment for its newest member. Emotional stresses as well as economic, cultural, sociological, and environmental situations influence the coping ability of the family.

CULTURE

Throughout the world, society translates customs and the meanings of customs into its own terms. All cultures have explanatory models for health and illness. Today, there is heightened awareness of the importance of culture in health care, especially in the care of the childbearing family.

The United States has traditionally been known as a "melting pot" for all races, all ethnic groups, and all cultures. As these different groups continue to interact, some blending of mores (customs) will occur, owing to acculturation, but many of the "old ways" still remain. These "old ways" will influence functioning of the health care system.

Culture may be defined as the general characteristics of a society in regard to beliefs, values, attitudes, and modes of behavior that are transmitted from generation to generation. Four components of a cultural system are especially important in childbearing: the moral and value system, the kinship system, the knowledge and belief system, and the ceremonial and ritual system (Griffith, 1982). Subcultures within the various cultures also should be taken into account.

Health care in the United States is considered the best in the world; yet, it is inaccessible to large segments of the population. For a nurse to plan sensitive care that meets the needs of the individual family, a basic knowledge of different cultural groups and how they perceive medical care in our society is needed. Even when care is available and accessible, especially during the childbearing cycle, the care may not be utilized by the consumer. This nonutilization may be due to cultural variances in the perception of pregnancy as a normal event in the life cycle.

Native Americans

Native Americans comprise 1 percent of the total population of the United States. Of this number, approximately 350,000 live in urban areas, with the majority of the remainder living on reservations. Unemployment is high, and hunger, malnutrition and poor health are common. Lack of accessible transportation is often a major barrier to obtaining adequate medical and nursing care, especially on the reservations. The maternal mortality rate among Indians is higher than the overall rate in the United States.

Tradition is important to Native Americans and there is a wide range of acceptable behavior according to tribal affiliation. Generalizations about acceptable behavior and customs are made cautiously, if at all.

Native Americans live in harmony with nature and with each other. Religion plays an important part in their lives. The family is the basic unit of society, with the extended family common. Matrilineal clans and female ownership of houses is common in some communities (Higgins, 1983). Indian women are often very influential in tribal affairs and make all the major household decisions.

Pregnancy is considered a natural process, and the prenatal period is kept as harmonious as possible. Numerous myths are attached to this period. A pregnant woman is warned against looking at deformed, injured, or blind people to prevent her baby from having those defects (Neithammer, 1977). There are taboos on certain foods during pregnancy. Herbs and teas are used to relieve discomforts of pregnancy and enhance health.

The medicine man plays a very important role in pregnancy or illness within the family or tribal unit. Pueblo women go to him before labor for special blessings so that labor will proceed well.

Health problems prevalent in Native Americans influence the outcome of pregnancy. Obesity, malnutrition, and diabetes mellitus are three major health problems common in Native Americans that can influence perinatal mortality.

For labor and delivery, the attendance of tribal midwives is often preferred to that of health professionals. The father seldom becomes an active participant in birth, although this is changing somewhat in urban settings. Women generally do not cry out during labor and will not ask for medication to relieve pain. All tribes have remedies to induce contractions. Traditionally, Zuni belief maintains that a nap during labor will change the sex of the fetus. Other beliefs state that movement of the fetus on the right side indicates a girl or hard labor indicates a boy.

Position for delivery varies. A Pueblo woman gives birth on her knees holding a rope or a post (Hodge, 1983). A Zuni woman will kneel or squat while the midwife presses on her abdomen.

During the postpartum period, the new mother most commonly remains on bedrest for a week, while her chores are completed by neighbors. The newborn is dressed warmly and his head is kept covered for the first week of life.

Even though most Native American women deliver in the hospital today, traditions and customs are important. Every attempt should be made to incorporate cultural values and beliefs into the hospital setting.

The Native American woman is usually shy and will not discuss her problems or concerns with strange men. She will give answers that she thinks you want to hear. A female relative should stay with the women during any examinations.

Traditions and customs can often be accommodated without difficulty. Female relatives can be allowed and encouraged to be supportive during labor. The infant can be kept with the mother for extended periods of time.

Arab Americans

The term Arab American refers to "persons who speak Arabic and share the values and beliefs of the Arab culture" (Patai, 1973). There are approximately 3 million Arab immigrants in the United States. Regardless of their place of origin, they share many social mores and beliefs.

The need for affiliation with others is frequently an intensive and central need of the Arab American. An extensive social network is required to cope with everyday events. Arab Americans have daily gatherings and visits to console the sick or just to visit. They rely on other people to give advice and guidance in crisis situations. Often they do not actively seek advice, since Arab etiquette says advice should be offered without a specific request. Exchange of information is enhanced by body movements, posture, and eye contact. Touch is allowed only between members of the same sex (Meleis, 1981).

Disease affects the individual as a whole. The Arab American often gives a vague description of illness, owing to a lack of descriptive framework. It is believed that illness has three major causes: the evil eye, hot or cold shifts and dampness, and food deprivation.

Western medicine is sought by Arab Americans. The more intrusive the procedure or treatment, the better they feel it is. They may be suspicious of over-the-counter medications. Arab Americans do not easily disclose personal information. They respect and do not openly question authority figures. Arab Americans do not expect personalized care from health care providers, but they do expect an effective cure.

The birth experience is not glorified or cherished by the Arab American. Pregnancy, however, is considered an opportunity for an Arab women to increase her self-esteem and status. The ability to conceive, carry a pregnancy to term, and bring a healthy child (preferably a male) into the world helps to give her status and social acceptance. Time is of little importance; everything happens if Allah (God) wills. Planning ahead may be a concept foreign to the Arab American. Traditionally, if you plan ahead, you risk the "evil eye." It isn't uncommon for no layette to be ready for the newborn.

Labor and delivery are female affairs. The Arab woman is extremely modest. She surrounds herself with female friends and relatives. Even though her husband is involved extensively in all aspects of health care for his wife, he is usually a nonparticipant in the labor and delivery process.

The Arab woman is often very vocal during labor and may not accept assistance with breathing and relaxation techniques. Even though pain tolerance seems low, she usually will not accept regional anesthesia during labor. She may, however, tend to overuse pain medication during the postpartum period (Meleis and Sorrell, 1981).

If the infant is stillborn or dies, the Arab American may be expressive in grief. They will want to touch the body to permit a final farewell. Usually they will not allow autopsies.

When working with the Arab American family, each family must be assessed individually. If interpreters are needed to obtain information, use those within the individual kin network if at all possible. Use the husband to enhance compliance of the family in health care options.

Mexican Americans and Puerto Ricans

Mexican American and Puerto Rican (Hispanics) people constitute the second largest minority group in America. In this cultural community, familismo—the respect for a dedication to the family (Lasater and Montalbo, 1982)—is of prime importance. It is the strongest surviving value along with patriarchism and machismo (the cultural ideal of masculinity that equates maleness with sexual prowess).

There is often an incongruity between health care expectations and Hispanic cultural practices. The physician is often consulted only as a last resort. The Mexican American will often first consult a curanderos (native healer); the Puerto Rican may first consult a spiritualist.

Diseases are thought to be related to an imbalance between hot and cold. The healthy body is considered warm. Illnesses, medications, and foods are classified as frio (cold) or caliente (hot). Cold illnesses such as arthritis, colds, empacho, muscular spasms, and upset stomach can be caused supposedly by chills or by moving from hot to cold places. Treatment for cold illnesses is from the hot classification of medications, which includes anise, aspirin, castor oil, iron tablets, penicillin, and vitamins.

Conversely, hot illnesses such as constipation, diarrhea, rashes, tenesmus, and ulcers may be treated with medication and herbs from the cool (fresco) classification. Fresco medications and herbs include bicarbonate of soda, mastic bark, milk of magnesia, orange flower water, and sage.

Foods are also classified as hot, cool, or cold. Hot foods include alcoholic beverages, chili peppers, chocolate, coffee, corn meal, garlic, kidney beans, onions, peas, and tobacco. Cool foods include barley water, bottled milk, chicken, fruits, watercress, and raisins. Cold foods include avocado, bananas, coconut, white beans, and lima beans.

This hot-cold concept has implications in caring for the childbearing family. A pregnant woman often refuses to take iron or vitamin supplements to prevent her infant from being born with a rash.

There is often a delay in seeking prenatal care, owing to the modesty of the woman and the normalcy of pregnancy in the culture. Special diets may be difficult to follow because the normal diet is high in carbohydrates and high in sodium.

The Mexican American woman is often vocal with pain during labor and delivery. The father is not usually an active participant and her mother will often be the support person. Traditionally, boys are not circumcised. A boy is desirable for the first child; if the child is a girl, the mother may be considered at fault.

During the postpartum period, the custom of "la cuarantine" may be observed for 40 days (Clark, 1980). The mother stays in bed for several days and keeps warm by wearing warm clothing and staying totally covered with blankets in bed. Air is considered cold whatever its temperature, so windows are kept closed and no fans or air conditioners are used. Water is considered cold, so no bathing after delivery is a strongly held belief. The woman will give the appearance of agreeing and will not directly refuse the nurse's requests. Numerous visitors who all want to hold the newborn are customary. Everyone participates in the care of the newborn.

The newborn may wear an amulet to ward off evil. This amulet should not be removed. Nutritionally, the mother is not likely to change her customary diet. The nurse must compromise, not push. Contraception is poorly accepted. Umbilical binders are used to prevent hernia development and are removed by the mother and not the nurse.

MIGRANT WORKERS

Another group of Mexican Americans with whom the nurse comes in contact is migrant workers. These people make seasonal trips from Texas to Washington and back to earn a living. Families usually work as a team, with the children working alongside the adults.

Income and housing are often inadequate. Religion is central to life. The general state of health of the migrant worker is poor. Water supplies are often contaminated. Treatment for illness is often sporadic because of mobility. Common health problems include obesity, malnutrition, diabetes mellitus, and dental caries.

The cause and treatment of many illnesses is guided by folk beliefs. Native healers (curanderos) treat minor illnesses. If treatment by the curandero is unsuccessful, the professional health care system is approached for care. With mobile life style of migrant workers, only immediate health needs can be met, and followup is virtually impossible (O'Brien, 1983).

Black Americans

There are cultural similarities among black Americans that exist regardless of economics, education, or place of residence: a sense of family, a faith based on a religious foundation, and a strong will to survive. The family is an important unit economically, politically, and religiously.

Pregnancy is considered a state of wellness. This fact is one of the reasons many black women delay getting prenatal care. Once pregnancy is acknowledged and accepted, certain activities are avoided. Craving of special foods during pregnancy is considered natural by many blacks. If the craving is for a nutritionally acceptable food, no problems result; however, the craving may be for unacceptable or potentially harmful substances, such as laundry starch, clay, or dirt. Ingestion of these substances is called *pica* and is noted particularly among southern black women.

Complaints of a "cold" need further investigation. The term "cold" is used to describe symptoms of upper respiratory infection as well as to describe pain or increased mucous secretions.

Self-treatment of discomforts of pregnancy is common, with patent medicines, herb medicines, and household products. During labor and delivery, black women tend to suppress vocal reactions. They often arrive for delivery in far advanced labor. Women commonly provide emotional support during labor and delivery, and many gravidas in labor will designate their mother as support person. Many new black mothers pay so much attention to providing and caring for the newborn that they overlook simple enjoyment and emotional stimulation. Traditionally, the new mother depends upon her own mother, other female relatives, her husband, and her older children to help with duties when she goes home.

Filipino Americans

Many native traditions and customs are brought with Filipinos when moving to the United States. Natural and supernatural beliefs about health and illness are blended with the American health care system.

Many Filipino Americans practice folk medicine. Disease is associated with the total life situation and with both supernatural and natural causes. Home remedies are used to treat illnesses with a supposed natural cause. Supernatural causes of illness include spirits and environmental forces. Amulets and prayer may be used for protection.

The native healer is called a quackdoctor and is consulted before and after a medical doctor. He is sought when the health care system is too slow or fails to cure a patient.

The health care beliefs of Filipino Americans fall into three basic categories: flushing, heating, and protection. Flushing keeps the body free of debris. It stimulates perspiration, vomiting, flatus, or bleeding to remove evil forces. Vinegar is commonly used for flushing, as are ginger and lemons. Rituals may accompany flushing. Following delivery, new mothers are traditionally confined to bed for two weeks with the head of the bed elevated. Reading and sewing are discouraged. Traditionally, unhealthiness is associated with either too much heat or too much cold. Childbirth practices often involve the use of heat to maintain internal body temperature. A new mother may sit in a slotted chair over hot coals for one hour each day for nine days to restore reproductive organs. After nine days a special bath is given to remove dirty substances from the body. Protection guards from outside influences. Evil spirits and witches are believed to victimize Filipino Americans. Eye contact is important to the Filipino; if it is not established, illness and misfortune are thought to result.

To provide nursing care for Filipino Americans, a basic knowledge of beliefs and customs is necessary. Home remedies should not be shunned randomly, since many of them are very successful. If the nurse expresses a genuine interest, folk medicine and scientific medicine can blend, to give the patient comprehensive care that fits into her belief system.

Asian Americans

According to Asian beliefs, the human person is healthy when his or her life forces are in harmony, and ill when this harmony is disturbed (Gordon et al., 1980). Two polar concepts interact for health and harmony: (1) yin, which is cold, dark, and wet; and (2) yang, which is heat, bright, and dry. The Asian American depends upon the extended family for support during pregnancy. Traditional practices vary, usually in important foods, customary foods, and appropriate activities. They prefer female physicians for labor and delivery, with men usually involved.

Foods that are traditionally eaten frequently during pregnancy include those high in hotness quality such as rice, eggs, chicken, and soup. Ice water is forbidden. Certain other practices are followed after delivery that will help to regain the heat lost during the labor and delivery process.

THE INDOCHINESE

The Indochinese tend to be reticent about emotional concerns. The indirect approach often works best when dealing with the Indochinese, since their culture dictates that they should not be pressed to express their feelings. The family unit is taken into account in all health matters (Santopietro and Lynch, 1980). Barriers to communication include eye contact, beckoning gestures, and a hearty manner (Santopietro, 1980) since these denote a direct approach. A low-key informal approach is best, but a casual attitude is best avoided. Traditionally, the head is not to be touched, since the soul rests there. If talking to the family, it may be appropriate to address the husband or oldest male first. The legs are not to be crossed while sitting, since pointing with the toe may be considered rude.

The Vietnamese

An individual is defined as a family member in the Vietnamese culture. The family is the basic unit of society and is responsible for decisions and individual actions (Dobbins at al., 1981). Women extend their loyalty to the husband's family. A communal existence is led with sex-based division of labor. The elderly are respected and ancestor worship is common. The senior male in the family acts as the head of the household and must be consulted in all family dealings (Moore et al., 1983).

Buddhism is the major religion and is intertwined with Confucianism and Taoist teachings, including the value of harmony and the avoidance of excess. In Taoism, there is belief in numerous gods, with equilibrium between Yin (negative) and Yang (positive) elements needed (Stringfellow et al., 1981). Confucianism's beliefs are Jen (benevolence) and Shu (tolerance). In tradition, social and family order is attained by involvement with music, adherence to social rites, and respect for authority (Vuong, 1976). Approximately 10 percent of the people are Roman Catholic, although they still honor ancestors and pay alms to Buddhist monks (Dobbins et al., 1981).

Social status is sharply demarcated. The husband heads the family, earns the income, makes decisions, and has the highest status. The wife, with her lower status, obeys her father, is submissive to her husband, and if widowed listens to adult sons. Children are strictly disciplined and are expected to help.

Education is not accessible to the general population and there is a high illiteracy rate. Three principles govern education: humanism, nationalism, and openmindedness. Rote learning is emphasized. Students are taught to observe. Teachers have the ultimate authority and parents are not involved in education.

Everyone takes the responsibility for self-cure, and professional medical care is sought only when home remedies fail. Health depends upon an Aml Duong balance (Wadd, 1983). Two major factors that disturb his balance are strong emotions and improper diet.

During childbearing, a traditional woman thinks she must consume or avoid certain foods to maintain optimum health. The first trimester is considered "cold"; therefore, "hot" foods must be eaten. During the second trimester "cold" foods are to be eaten. "Cold" foods may also be eaten in the third trimester. "Cold" foods include gourd-type plants and most fruits. Meats, condiments, alcohol, and fatty foods are "hot." In labor, a woman believes she must not cry out to avoid embarassment. Customarily, the newborn in a Vietnamese village is bathed in tepid water and swaddled in old clothes (to avoid making the spirits jealous) before allowing the father to see his newborn. Circumcision is traditionally unacceptable. During the postpartum period, a woman is not to bathe or shampoo her hair, as it is thought that too much water leads her to lose nutrients and causes illnesses in later life (Hollingsworth et al., 1980). Proper foods for the postpartum period include salty, "hot" foods such as meat, fish, rice, and pepper. No sour foods are to be eaten and no cold liquid can be consumed for six months.

When working with the Vietnamese family, interpreters are essential. It is helpful to learn frequently used words and phrases. Family members should be encouraged to participate in care. Warm water is provided for drinking, and some dietary adjustments should be made.

THE CHINESE

The concept of family is important to the Chinese, with the father being the head of the household and having ultimate authority. Parental authority and veneration of elders are dominant in Chinese culture.

Harmony and moderation aid in maintaining good health. Herbal medicines are commonly used to treat a variety of ailments. Pregnancy is a time when there is "happiness in the body." All members of the family look forward to birth, especially the birth of a son.

THE JAPANESE

The traditional head of the family is the father. The wife devotes herself completely to the children and limits social activities to those within the neighborhood or to school. Pregnancy is an expected part of a woman's life and is a totally natural process. The only dietary restrictions are avoidance of spicy or hot foods. Regular prenatal care is desirable.

During labor, minimal medications for pain relief are used. The emphasis during labor is to think positively and use relaxation and breathing techniques as well as frequent position changes.

Cultural Implications for Nursing

Why be aware of other cultures? The main benefit to nursing from studying various cultural groups is to "help us see more clearly the effects of society on our own behavior" (Newton, 1981). Awareness of our own cultural orientation and the relationship of this orientation on individual health practices is important. Learning about other cultural groups through reading or attending seminars or workshops will aid in the identification of cultural orientations of patients.

People who are culturally different from the American mainstream are not going to disappear into the "melting pot"; they will retain their identities as Native Americans, blacks, Hispanics, or people of other ethnic origins (Farris, 1976). Patients have a right to have their sociocultural backgrounds understood in the same way they expect their physical and psychosocial needs to be recognized and understood.

An open attitude about individual cultures is one of the goals of nursing. Each person is seen as an individual with values, beliefs, and practices peculiar to their particular group. Cultural differences are to be respected and recognized for their importance to the patient and the patient's family.

BIBLIOGRAPHY

Clark, M. *Health practices in the Mexican American community*. Berkeley: University of California Press, 1980.

Dobbins, E., et al.: A beginner's guide to Vietnamese culture. *RN*, 1981, **35**, 46.

Duong, T.N. Understanding Asian families: a Vietnamese perspective. *Child Today*, 1984, **7**, 61.

Farris, L.S. Approaches to caring for the American Indian maternity patient. *MCN*, 1976, **1**, 81-87.

Gordon, V.C., Matousek, I.M., & Lang, T.A. Southeast Asian refugees: life in America. *American Journal of Nursing*, 1984, **71**, 19-21.

Green, H.G. A view of childbirth in the People's Republic of China. *Perinatal Press*, 1984, **8**(2): 19-21.

Griffith, S. Childbearing and the concept of culture. *Journal of Gynecological and Neonatal Nursing*, 1982, **11**, 181.

Higgins, P.G. Pueblo women of New Mexico: their background, culture, and childbearing practices. *Topics in Clinical Nursing*, 1983, **4**, January, 69–78.

Hodge, R.W. (ed.) *Handbook of American Indians north of New Mexico*. New York: Greenwood Press, 1983.

Hollingsworth, A.O., et al. Indochina moves to main street. The refugees childbearing: what to expect. *RN*, 1980, **34**, 45.

______, Brown, L.P., Brooten, D.: The refugees and childbearing. *RN*, 1980, **34**, 47.

Iorio, J. & Nelson, M.A. China. Caring is the same. *Nursing Outlook*, 1983, **31**, 100-104.

Jordan, B. *Birth in four cultures*. Montreal: Eden Press Woman's Publication, 1980.

Lasater, T.T., & Montalvo, F.F.: Understanding Mexican American culture; a training program. *Child Today*, 1982, **11**, May/June, 23–35.

Liu, Y.C. China: health care transition. *Nursing Outlook*, 1983, **31**, 94-99.

Meleis, A.I. The Arab American in the health care system. *American Journal of Nursing*, 1981, **81**(6), 1174.

———, & Sorrell, L. Arab American women and their birth experiences. *MCN*, 1981, **6**, 171.

Moore, M., et al. Cultural considerations in the care of a critically ill Vietnamese child and family. In K. Stahler-Miller, K. (ed.), *Neonatal and pediatric critical care nursing*. New York: Churchill Livingstone, 1983.

McKenzie, J.L. & Christman, N.J. Healing herbs, gods, and magic. *Nursing Outlook*, 1977, **25**(5), 326.

Murillo-Rohde, I. Health care for the Hispanic patient. *Critical Care Update*, 1980, **7**, 29-36.

Newton, N. Cross-cultural perspectives. In A.L. Clark, D.D. Affonso, & T.R. Harris (Eds.), *Childbearing: A nursing perspective* (2nd ed.). Philadelphia: F.A. Davis, 1981, pp. 97-106.

Niethammer, C. *Daughters of the earth*. New York: Collier Books, 1977.

O'Brien, M.E. Reaching the migrant worker. *American Journal of Nursing*, 1983, **83**, 895.

Patai, R. *The Arab mind*. New York: Scribner's, 1973.

Pillsbury, B.L.K. Doing the month: confinement and convalescence of Chinese women after childbirth. *Social Science of Medicine*, 1978, **12**, 11.

Ruiz, M.C.J. Open-closed mindedness, intolerance of ambiguity, and nursing faculty's attitudes toward culturally different patients. *Nursing Outlook*, 1981, **30**, 177-181.

Santopietro, M-C.S. Indochina moves to main street. How to get through to a refugee patient. *RN*, 1981, **35**, 43.

———, & Lynch, B.A.: Indochina moves to main street. What's behind that 'inscrutable' mask? *RN*, 1980, **34**, 40.

Snow, L.F., et al. Behavioral implications of some old wives tales. *Obstetrics & Gynecology*, 1978, **51**, 727-732.

Stringfellow, L., Nguyen, D.L., & Diepleim, L. The Vietnamese in America. In A.L. Clark (ed.), *Culture and childbearing*. Philadelphia: F.A. Davis, 1981.

United States Bureau of the Census. *Current population reports*. Washington, D.C.: U.S. Government Printing Office, 1984.

Vuong, G.T. *Getting to know the Vietnamese and their culture*. New York: Frederick Unger Publishers, 1976.

Wadd, L. Vietnamese postpartum practices: implications for nursing in the hospital setting. *Journal of Gynecological and Neonatal Nursing*, 1983, **12**, 252.

Zepeda, M. Selected maternal-infant care practices of Spanish-speaking women. *Journal of Gynecological and Neonatal Nursing*, 1982, **11**, 371-374.

chapter 3

LEGAL AND ETHICAL ISSUES IN MATERNITY CARE

OBJECTIVES

Upon completion of this chapter, the reader will be able to:

1. Explain the legal meaning and significance of a nurse-patient relationship in the delivery of family-centered maternity care.
2. Discuss standards upon which maternity nursing care may be legally measured.
3. Discuss the legal rights of a woman seeking an abortion.
4. Discuss the rights of the fetus in an abortion issue.
5. Explain the nurse's legal responsibilities involved in providing a safe environment for the maternity client.
6. Explain the concept of abandonment as it applies to maternity nursing.
7. Discuss documentation of nursing care and its relationship to malpractice claims in maternity nursing.
8. Explain the relationship between moral and ethical decision making.
9. Identify and discuss ethical dilemmas associated with artificial insemination and in vitro fertilization.
10. Identify the responsibilities of the nurse involved in ethical decision making when caring for a handicapped neonate.
11. Discuss and explore your own feelings regarding the ethical issues involved in abortion.

KEY TERMS

Abandonment
Artificial insemination
Common law
Conscience clauses
Emancipated minors
Ethics
Good Samaritan Act
Informed consent
In vitro fertilization
Malpractice
Morals
Negligence
Statutory law
Tort

LEGAL ACCOUNTABILITY IN MATERNITY NURSING

Every practicing nurse has a legal responsibility to the client. When the nurse enters into a nurse-client relationship, she has a special duty of care to the client. Using knowledge and skills, the nurse has a legal duty to exercise reasonable and ordinary care in the performance of nursing responsibilities. From the moment that she enters into a nurse-client relationship, any nursing actions performed for the client are expected to be equal to the nursing actions of other reasonably prudent nurses in the same or similar circumstances.

What does this mean to the practice of maternity nursing? Simply stated, maternity nurses are responsible for the delivery of safe, competent care to their clients that is comparable to care given by their peers in like situations. The client has the right to expect a reasonable standard of professional care.

When a nurse-client relationship has been established, the place or circumstance of delivery of care does not alter the nurse's legal liability. Care given in a hospital or clinic, or by a nurse practitioner in autonomous practice, assumes the same burden of legal liability. Even maternity nurses who enter a teaching-learning relationship with the client are responsible for their nursing involvement in that relationship. If there is no nurse-client relationship, there are no legal responsibilities apart from those which stem from the responsibilities of one human being to another.

It is important to realize that the standard of care that a nurse gives may be legally judged in accordance with the care expected of any nurse with similar education, qualifications, and experience. Nurses giving care in the maternity department of a hospital would not be judged on the same standard of care applicable to the nurse midwife in a clinical situation. Both the American Nurses Association (*ANA*), in *Standards of Maternal & Child Health Nursing Practice* (1983), and the Nurses' Association of the American College of Obstetrics and Gynecology (*NAACOG*), in *Standards for Obstetric, Gynecologic, and Neonatal Nursing* (1986), have developed standards of care for maternity nurses.

The practice of nursing is defined by the *nurse practice act* of each state. Although these acts may vary, they generally establish educational and licensure requirements for nurses and provide a broad definition of the practice of nursing. Maternity nurses, as well as all nurses, must practice within the boundaries of the nurse practice act in the state in which they are employed in whatever role they assume, whether it be that of a clinician or in an expanded role.

LEGAL ISSUES IN FAMILY-CENTERED MATERNITY NURSING

Laws that govern legal issues are derived from two sources: (1) *statutory law* (laws such as nurse practice acts, which require legislative process and enactment by a city, county, state or federal legislative body), and (2) *common law* (judicial decisions made in the settlement of disputes between two parties).

Legal issues involving liability that nurses most frequently encounter are in the realm of common law disputes. Generally, these are unintentional *torts* (wrongful acts) involving *negligence*. Negligence is viewed as the failure of a person to act as a reasonably prudent person in a specific circumstance. When a specially trained person is negligent in the performance of his or her job, the term *malpractice* is used.

Certain legal issues have specific or expanded significance when applied to the delivery of family-centered maternity care.

These issues, although not limited to maternity nursing, are within the scope of maternity nursing practice and warrant consideration in that context.

Informed Consent

Each of us, as an individual, has the right to make decisions about our personal welfare. This right extends into the realm of health care, giving us the right to consent to or deny treatment. This very basic concept is an integral part of all medical and nursing services performed for a client. Unauthorized treatment, whether given by a physician, nurse, or student nurse, is subject to liability. Hospitals routinely use consent forms for authorization of medical and surgical procedures. Although these forms may contain the signature of the client, they are not valid if the client did not know what was being signed, what it meant, or why it was necessary. Consent given by a client must be a voluntary, informed consent, whether it is verbal or written. Those giving consent must be legally competent and of legal age.

An issue that may be raised in maternity nursing regarding consent is that given by a minor when she is receiving maternity care. Pregnant adolescents of 13 and 14 are certainly not considered of legal age. In these instances, some state statutes designate minors who live apart from their parents as "emancipated minors," legally capable of giving their own consent. In some states it is legal for minors to obtain birth control information and material and to give consent for treatment of venereal disease and obstetrical procedures without the consent of their parents. Every nurse should be aware of the state statutes regarding these matters.

Informed consent is not necessary in emergency situations, as these cases are in most circumstances covered by the *good samaritan acts*. These acts, although not enacted in every state, exempt individuals from liability of ordinary negligence when rendering care in emergency situations. The definition of emergency care may vary according to the statutes of the individual state, as may the scope of coverage. For instance, the delivery of a baby in an emergency situation may be covered by the good samaritan act in some states and considered outside the nurse's legal practice in other states.

Abortion

The Supreme Court decision in *Roe v. Wade*, 1973, made abortion a legal medical procedure. Although this decision established the legality of the procedure, it did not end the controversy concerning the issue. Time and again the decision has been challenged in amendments introduced in legislative sessions. Many legal questions remain unanswered. The decision did establish the following rights:

> A state may not prohibit the right of a woman to seek and obtain an abortion during the first trimester of pregnancy (12 weeks).
>
> Consent from the husband for an abortion is not required during the first trimester of pregnancy.
>
> During the second trimester of pregnancy, the state may regulate the conditions under which the abortion is performed (types of abortion facilities, and licensure of abortionist and facility).
>
> The state has the right to prohibit abortions in the third trimester, except when it is deemed necessary by appropriate medical judgment for the protection of the health and life of the mother.

The state is under no legal obligation to provide services to an individual seeking an abortion, to establish abortion facilities, or to enact laws that facilitate abortions. Many states have *conscience clauses* that allow physicians, nurses, and nonpublic hospitals and clinics to refuse to perform or participate in abortion procedures on moral, religious, or ethical grounds. Moreover, those refusing to participate cannot be discriminated against in occupational professional, educational, or civil matters.

According to the Supreme Court decision, minors may have abortions without parental consent. This issue has been addressed by individual states with varying results. Some states do require the physician to inform the parents of a minor seeking an abortion, but parental consent is still not necessary.

According to the Hyde Amendment of 1976, federal funds may not be used for abortions unless the pregnancy is proven to be the result of a reported rape or incest, is fatally endangering the life of the mother, and if continuing the pregnancy would, in the opinion of the two qualified physicians, severely affect the physical welfare of the woman. Medicaid payments will only be made for abortions under these circumstances.

LEGAL RIGHTS OF THE FETUS

Roe v. Wade spoke to the private rights and personal liberty of women, as stated in the Fourteenth Amendment. The Supreme Court decision was, therefore, directly concerned with the rights of the individual. It would seem that, as the court addressed the rights of the individual, they would also include the individual rights of the fetus. However, the Court did not view the fetus as a "legal person" and consequently did not support fetal rights in abortions. The Court did recognize the state's rights in protecting fetal life from the time of viability. They did not fix the exact time of viability, but considered it to be at the time when the fetus has the right to the protection of the state. Viability was described in *Danforth v. Planned Parenthood*, 1976, as "that stage of fetal development when the life of the unborn child may be continued indefinitely outside the womb by natural or artificial life-supportive systems" (Fromer, 1983).

Sterilization

Sterilization as a means of permanent contraception is becoming increasingly popular in the United States, with approximately one in five couples choosing this method. Some medical reasons may necessitate sterilization, but for the most part, sterilization is an elective procedure. Since sterilization is usually intended to be permanent, clients must be counseled before a final decision is made. This counseling requires an explanation of the sterilization procedure, its benefits and risks, physiologic and psychological concerns, and alternatives to the procedure. Decisions regarding sterilization rest with the individual, but counseling of both husband and wife is recommended. Individuals seeking sterilization must be over 21 and mentally competent, and the decision must be voluntary. Informed written consent must be obtained before the procedure is undertaken; the consent of the other partner is not necessary. A waiting period is often required following the initial counseling.

Invasion of Privacy and Disclosure of Medical Information

Client information of any nature is considered private unless consent is given by the client for the release of information to a third party. Information such as birth announcements can not be released to the media unless the client gives her permission. If a client specifically requests that a member of her family not be given any information about her condition or circumstances, it would be an invasion of her privacy if the information was released. Nurses should be aware of the policies of their institution regarding disclosure of client information.

Confidentiality of all information on the client's chart is protected by law and only those directly involved in the care of the client, or the client herself, are privileged to information on the chart. Written consent must be given by the client for disclosure of her medical records to any other source.

Client Safety

A nurse involved in a nurse-client relationship has the responsibility to protect her client from any reasonably foreseeable or known harm. Safety issues are not confined to protection from bodily harm but are encountered in nursing care involving medications, procedures, and client environment. In maternity nursing, client safety must be expanded to include the safety of both mother and fetus.

MEDICATIONS

Errors in the preparation and administration of medications are related to incorrect dosages, incorrect medication, incorrect route and/or time of administration, and incorrect patient identification. Every practicing nurse must take precautions to avoid these errors. Knowledge of medication includes awareness of maternal and fetal effects. It is imperative that nurses realize that medications which are safe and therapeutic for the mother may not be safe for the fetus. Fetal toxicity, fetal drug interactions, fetal metabolism of drugs, and fetal responses to drugs must be considered when administering medications to a pregnant woman.

Consent for administration of medication to a client is obtained either orally or in writing. The pregnant woman is informed of the fetal and maternal effects of the medication and has the right to refuse it. For example, a standing order for pain medication during labor does not mean that the medication is given without the consent of the client. If the client refuses the medication, it is not given, and the refusal is noted on the client's chart.

Nurses involved in the care of the mother following delivery should also be aware of medications which may pass through the milk of the mother to the breastfed infant. It is the responsibility of the nurse to caution the mother to check with the physician or a nurse before using any medications while breastfeeding.

ANESTHESIA

Maternity nurses, unless specially schooled, are not usually involved in the administration of anesthesia. They are, however, responsible for the safety of the client while under the influence of an anesthetic that alters mental or physical competency. Regional anesthesia may be used during labor and cause a loss of sensation in the lower extremities. Clients who try to get out of bed and walk while the anesthesia is still in effect are in danger of falling. Similar circumstances may arise when the client is recovering from effects of inhalation and general anesthesia.

Clients have the right to refuse anesthesia, as they do medications. Again, the choice of whether or not to use anesthesia is that of the client in consultation with her husband or partner, the physician, and the anesthesiologist or anesthetist.

Consent forms may not be signed while the client is under the influence of anesthesia.

PROCEDURES

All procedures undertaken in the delivery of maternity care are primarily concerned with the safety of the client and her fetus. Procedures such as amniocentesis, amniotomy, chorionic villi sampling, fetal scalp blood sampling and amniofetography all carry a risk factor for the fetus. These risk factors must be explained to the client before the procedure is undertaken, and the benefits must justify use of the procedure.

A thorough knowledge of the procedures and techniques necessary for data collection and therapeutic intervention is needed by the nurse. Knowledgeable decision making requires the ability to interpret information gathered during testing and to analyze the results. The nurse who uses fetal monitoring as a diagnostic technique but is unable to assess and evaluate monitor strips does not help to provide a safe environment for the fetus.

Neonates are particularly vulnerable to accidents or unsafe environments. Care measures found in neonatal nurseries may also present potential risks to the neonate. Temperature settings on infant warmers or within isolettes can cause extreme harm if used improperly. Improper grounding of electrical equipment can cause currents to be transmitted to the neonate and subsequent injury. Sophisticated monitoring equipment has enabled nurses to provide care to high-risk neonates, but at the same time, an accurate understanding of the monitored indices is necessary. This equipment should not be used as the sole basis for evaluation but as a tool to enhance assessment skills.

ABANDONMENT

Abandonment in a nurse-client relationship indicates a failure to properly attend to the client. The essence of the claim of client abandonment implies that the nurse left the client improperly cared for, either by absence or failure to advise the proper authority when circumstances warranted it. An obvious example of this claim would be if the nurse leaves a newborn nursery unattended and a neonate chokes on mucus and develops respiratory failure. Another less direct example may be seen if the nurse fails to report to the physician signs of respiratory difficulties in a neonate and the baby dies. The nurse's awareness and experience should enable her to recognize when the condition of a client is deteriorating and medical consultation is needed.

Nurses are legally responsible for implementing physicians' orders. If the nurse is not capable of executing the necessary procedures, owing to lack of knowledge or experience, she is responsible for consulting with physicians or colleagues to have the orders fulfilled. To ignore procedures because of her incapabilities constitutes abandonment. Equally important is the nurse's responsibility when she feels the order is detrimental or inappropriate for the welfare of the client. In this circumstance, the nurse is also legally responsible for consulting with the physician and her supervisor, and then documenting her reasons for failure to comply with the order.

Documentation

The client's medical records serve as documentation for the care and treatment received while in the health care facility. The client's chart is the document most often subpoenaed for use in malpractice claims. The prudent nurse will document on the chart all of her nursing activities and the assessments substantiating her nursing interventions. The chart should provide a clear, concise account of the client's care, stated in a factual manner and indicating a reasonable standard of care. When an assessment is charted, there should also be a corresponding intervention followed by documentation of the client's response. Remember, if it wasn't charted, it wasn't assessed or done.

When a fetal monitor is being used, notations are made of the monitor strips documenting the following: types of monitoring (external or internal), paper speed (1 cm/min or 3 cm/min), patient information, date and time of each entry, procedures performed, FHR tracing (baseline variability, periodic changes interventions), and uterine contraction tracing (frequency, duration, and intensity of contraction). Monitor strips are legal documents and may be used in court decisions regarding malpractice.

ETHICAL ISSUES IN MATERNITY NURSING

Ethical decision making is an issue confronted by nurses throughout their careers. Moral philosophy, as ethics has been defined, deals with the moral ideals and goals of human action. Both terms, ethics and morals, are derived from the word "ethos" meaning a customary mode of conduct. Yet, in the practice of nursing, differentiation between morals and ethics is needed. Moral reasoning is based on the principles of right and wrong behavior according to an individual's beliefs. Ethics examines the science of moral behavior or the reason we subscribe to a moral belief. Thus, ethics develops as a system of moral principles. To illustrate, when an issue presents a moral dilemma, what is the ethical response? Suppose a nurse does not believe in abortions; morally she believes abortion to be wrong. How does she handle a situation when a teenage girl asks for help with an unwanted pregnancy? Because of her beliefs, does she simply not tell the client of the abortion option? Does she tell the client all abortions are wrong? Or does she present all options including abortion in an unbiased manner? The decision is an ethical one. Although she morally believes abortion to be wrong, the nurse is ethically responsible to refer the client to another resource person or explain all options and allow the client to make her own decision.

Ethical foundations provide the guidelines for the nurse's decision. The profession of nursing, in its commitment to the delivery of quality health care, has developed a code of ethics by which nurses may guide their practices. These guidelines are published by the American Nurses Association, (1985), the International Council of Nurses, and the Canadian Nurses' Association. The framework of these codes provides guidelines but does not establish rules or absolutes for the nurse's responsibility to the individual or to the profession of nursing.

Influencing factors affect the way nurses view moral and ethical decision making. Societal, religious, cultural, technological, scientific, legislative, and judicial factors are but a few aspects of decision making, at times operating singularly, and at other times interfacing with one another. The world we live in is constantly changing, and nurses must be aware of those changing issues that affect the ethical practice of nursing. It is not within the intent of this discussion to mention all ethical issues with which the nurse is confronted; however, some of the key issues in maternity nursing are worthy of examination.

Artificial Insemination

Male sperm introduced into the female vagina by artificial means is called *artificial insemination*. The sperm are either from the husband (AIH, artificial insemination husband) or a donor (AID, artificial insemination donor).

Two key issues generate ethical concerns: the justification of the process and the responsibilities to the conceptus created by artificial insemination. To some, justification of the process is inextricably involved with religious and moral principles. These individuals feel artificial insemination is a violation of a marriage bond which mandates the creation of life only by a sexual act between a man and a woman, and any other act utilized for this purpose is unnatural and against the laws of God and nature. Conversely, others feel that justification of the process is clearly visible with the reality of the creation of a new life, and the manner of conception gives credence to the advancement of man toward the betterment of the human race.

Arguments have also arisen over limitations on the use of artificial insemination. Should it be limited to insemination of a woman by her husband's sperm, or is donor sperm acceptable? If the husband has viable sperm, yet is a carrier of an undesirable genetic trait, is it ethical to impregnate his wife with another man's sperm? Would it be better for the couple to take a chance and produce their own child or should they remain childless? Does the use of donor sperm apply only to conditions where the husband's views oppose masturbation for the retrieval of the sperm? How are these sperm to be obtained—are these men expected to subject themselves to needle aspiration of the sperm from the testes? Does the woman commit adultery when she is inseminated without the informed consent of her husband?

Proponents of women's rights will also defend the right of the single woman to choose to have a baby conceived by AID. Does artificial insemination include this segment of society or is it only confined to marriage relationships?

Once conceived, what are the rights of the fetus? Supposing a fetus was conceived and early in the pregnancy it was found to be defective. Could we justifiably abort this fetus, especially if it were conceived by AID? Is it possible we would have to obtain consent of the sperm donor? If the defective fetus were not aborted and later the parents were divorced, what responsibilities does the husband have to the child who was conceived by AID—must he pay child support and does he have any visiting rights?

As AID becomes more widely accepted, concerns are expressed over the quality of the donor semen. The selection process used to choose donors must be considered. Who is entitled to make the selection and, in fact, are not those choosing the donors determining the genetics of the future? Is the sperm of the man with a low IQ, who is in perfect health and with many physical attributes, as acceptable as the man with a superior IQ? Is it ethical for only the woman to choose the man from whom donor sperm will be available? Is it not possible that the semen of several donors may be mixed, playing Russian roulette with the genetics of the fetus?

Record keeping also becomes an issue in donor insemination. If accurate records are not kept, it is possible that relatives of the next generation could marry without an awareness of their relationship to one another. Is it possible for a woman to conceive another pregnancy by the same donor upon request or is it limited to one donor? To take that thought one step further, does the donor have any rights in deciding who receives his semen and can he receive increased payment if his semen is in demand? Is it fair not to allow the child conceived by artificial insemination to know his heritage—are his genes not a combination of both the donor's and the mother's genes.

These are but a few of the many ethical issues confronting the use of artificial insemination (see Chapter 6 for a discussion of the techniques of artificial insemination). As the process becomes more widely used, still other concerns will emerge—each a responsibility for society, as well as medicine and nursing, to address.

In Vitro Fertilization

The acceptance of in vitro fertilization as a method of conception has rapidly increased within the last five to eight years. In 1978, the first baby, Louise Brown, was born from the result of in vitro fertilization performed in England by Drs. Patrick Steptoe and Robert Edwards. Since that time, other equally successful conceptions have been reported in the United States. In 1983, Heather and Todd Tilton became the first-born American twins to be conceived by in vitro fertilization. With improvement in techniques, this method of conception is becoming a realistic choice for many childless couples.

The technique is most frequently employed when infertility exists owing to damage or malfunctioning of the fallopian tubes. In vitro fertilization has also been employed when there is a deficiency of male sperm. Studies are being conducted to establish its validity when endometriosis (aberrant endometrial tissue in the pelvic cavity) and immunologic disorders are responsible for infertility.

The process of in vitro fertilization involves the stimulation of the ovaries to produce more than one egg at ovulation. The eggs are surgically retrieved and fertilized in the laboratory. In the event of fertilization, the developing embryo is transplanted into the uterus of the woman, where growth and development of the fetus continues until the time of birth (see Chapter 6 for a complete discussion).

In vitro fertilization is still very much in the experimental stages, even though the results have been encouraging. Ethical considerations must address the issue in this context. Among the questions to be considered are: What is to be done with the conceptus if the process results in a defective embryo? Should every fertilized embryo be implanted in the uterus, or should some be discarded? If the developing embryos are to be discarded, could they be sold, donated to another couple or individual, or preserved for future use if desired? What would happen if the parents of the preserved embryo died? Who would gain custody of the embryo or, in fact, would they be destroyed, or do they become legal heirs, necessitating their implantation in another woman? Does she then have rights to their inheritance?

In anticipation of some of the ethical dilemmas associated with in vitro fertilization, guidelines have been established by the American Fertility Society. These guidelines attempt to answer many of these questions and present direction for future development of the standards for in vitro fertilization.

Similar to in vitro fertilization but different in the process are embryo transplants, undertaken when a woman has nonfunctioning ovaries. Since it is impossible to retrieve eggs from the woman's ovaries, an ovum from another woman is substituted and the husband's sperm are used to fertilize the egg. The resulting embryo is transplanted into the uterus of the infertile woman.

Surrogate impregnation is still another artificial method of childbearing. Another woman is chosen by the childless couple to be artificially inseminated with the husband's sperm. The surrogate mother then carries the child to term and after birth releases the infant to their custody.

Again, many questions can be posed regarding the ethical and legal rights of all the individual's involved in both embryo transplant and surrogate pregnancies. Custody problems are easily generated when decisions are changed by any of the parties. Consider what would happen if the parents didn't want the baby, if it were born handicapped, or if the surrogate mother refused to give up the baby.

Neonatal Life Issues

Difficult issues faced by maternity nurses are the moral, social, legal, and ethical decisions involved in the care of handicapped neonates. These infants sent into the world with all the hopes and dreams of the future, when defective, create ethical problems that touch the core of parents, physicians, and nurses.

How should decisions regarding the welfare of handicapped neonates be made? Are these decisions exclusively the rights of the parents, who may be emotionally vulnerable at this time? Are physicians better qualified to make these decisions because of their medical knowledge? Are nurses, because of their patient advocate roles, more capable of determining the quality of life for handicapped neonates? There are no absolutes when presented with these questions, only guidelines from which we may draw.

The order for a "no code" (do not resuscitate) for handicapped neonates is ultimately the responsibility of the physician. This order is ideally the result of his discussions with the parents, informing them of the nature and scope of the neonates conditions and the ramifications for the infant's future. The nurse is legally responsible for carrying out the orders of the physician, unless she can provide justification for a contrary action. If there is no written "no code" order, it is the responsibility of the nurse to initiate resuscitation of the neonate whenever conditions warrant it. She may not, of her own volition, choose not to resuscitate a neonate when such action is needed.

When a conflict exists between the choice of the parents and the physician, who is responsible for making decisions regarding the welfare of the neonate? Should parents be allowed to make the decision to withhold surgery for their baby who has Down's syndrome plus a tracheosphageal fistula? If an agreement cannot be reached, is it the right of the state to intervene? When the state exercises the right to make these decisions, what is the protocol for future cases of a similar nature?

On the other hand, when parents prefer to continue extreme measures of treatment, even though the health care provider feels the effort is futile, and the parents have been informed of the neonate's condition, it remains the responsibility of the nurse to continue to provide treatment.

Today's neonatal intensive care nurseries are capable of sustaining the life of even the most severely affected infants. When decisions are made to sustain life at all cost, the direct care giver—the nurse—must be prepared to examine her own feelings and moral philosophies regarding these decisions. The miracle baby, as viewed by the physician and parents, who is six months old and still dependent on life supportive measures and experiencing daily seizures with minimal brain functioning, presents an ethical dilemma to nurses. Often, in the nurse's opinion, the quality of life appears minimal and watching the baby's daily struggle for life becomes painful for care providers. How does the nurse provide quality care to this infant, who she may feel deserves the right to die? How does she relate to the parents of the infant and to the physician, who regard the mere fact that the baby has lived so long as a miracle?

Over the past years, it has not been unusual for care providers, with parental consent, to withhold nourishment and treatment from handicapped neonates (passive euthanasia). In a few extreme instances, neonates were allowed to die from starvation. Although morally this would be a difficult situation to comprehend, those who withheld nutrition and treatment felt they did so on behalf of the neonate. Concerned nurses in some instances were the "whistle blowers," and a federal law was enacted to prevent abuse to handicapped neonates. Section 504 of the Rehabilitation Act of 1973 was determined by the government to be applicable to a handicapped neonate. This law prohibits discrimination on the basis of a handicap. Interpretation of the law includes that the "withholding of nourishment and medically beneficial treatment (as determined with regard for reasonable medical judgment) from handicapped infants solely on the basis of their present or anticipated mental or physical impairment" is illegal. In June of 1986 the United States Supreme Court reversed the "Baby Doe" ruling, stating that the federal government cannot force hospitals to treat severely handicapped infants when there is an objection by the parents; however, the state may assume authority to appoint a guardian when parental decisions are in conflict with the best interest of the infant. Does not this law also then infringe on the rights of the parents to make a decision regarding the welfare of their handicapped child, or does it protect the rights of a helpless infant?

Given consideration of the individual rights, another question is posed regarding the responsibilities of society to the handicapped individual. Does the right of life for the neonate supercede all consideration for the quality of that life and the cost of maintaining pure survival? Who judges what the quality of life is—and who determines when it becomes too costly for society to sustain life or care for a handicapped individual? In a world where malnutrition and illness take the lives of hundreds of infants every day, is it ethical to burden society with the cost of sustaining the life of a neonate at all cost?

Many health care associations and institutions have become concerned with ethical decisions regarding handicapped neonates and infants. The National Perinatal Association has proposed that institutions form Infant Bioethical Review Committees to review all cases associated with the withholding of life-sustaining treatments from handicapped neonates. These decisions would then be instrumental in providing guidelines for decision making involving parents and health care providers.

Abortion

Essentially, in the first 12 weeks following conception, society, being composed of individuals, has the right to grant life or death to a fetus. The law has given us this right, and so by legal standards it is a choice we are free to make. In spite of this right, there remain deep moral convictions clouding clear ethical decision making. Implicit in any decision regarding abortion is the moral principle of right and wrong. There are those who believe abortion is morally wrong and those who believe it is morally right. Even for an individual to take a middle of the road position—believing it to be neither right nor wrong—is difficult, since the abortion decision is a decree of life or death for the fetus and not just a maybe life or maybe death decision.

Those who believe abortion to be morally and ethically justified, will proclaim the rights of the individual as the basis for their belief. They believe the individual is entitled to make decisions regarding their own physical, mental, social, and economic welfare. Therefore, if the pregnancy will impinge on any of these aspects of their life, they have a right to rectify the situation. They also believe that the fetus is not an individual and consequently does not have rights. Proponents of this thought will recall examples of individuals who, through amniocentesis, find their child to be defective. They feel these individuals have the right to decide the fate of the fetus who otherwise would be born into a world incompatible with his existence or quality of life.

Those who favor a prolife point of view believe abortion to be morally wrong. Most of their rationale is derived from religious philosophy. Their concept of life begins at the moment of conception and, therefore, anything that intentionally destroys life after conception is paramount to murder. The distinction of viable fetal life does not enter into this viewpoint, since they believe life begins at conception.

New technology now provides us with methods to sustain life in even the smallest of neonates. Ethical issues arise when a live fetus is born following an abortion. Questions here involve the decisions necessary to determine what to do with this live, aborted fetus. Are nurses responsible for maintaining the life of this fetus or should the fetus be allowed to die without any special care?

Yet another question arises concerning the rights of a child who was prenatally diagnosed as having a deformity, but whose parents refused to have the defective fetus aborted. Does the resulting defective child have a right somewhere in the future to take legal action against the parents for allowing him or her to be born handicapped and, therefore, altering the quality of his or her life? Farfetched perhaps, but it is a realistic possibility.

Since the Supreme Court has denied the use of Medicaid funds for payment of abortion, does this perhaps burden society with the responsibility of dealing with unwanted children? If the only reason a woman does not have an abortion is lack of money, then how successful will she be at parenting an unwanted child? What will be the quality of life for the unwanted child? Can society afford to add this responsibility to its already heavily burdened welfare programs?

The issue of abortion will continue to present ethical dilemmas. As society changes so will the issues, political influence, and legislative aspects surrounding abortion. The nurse must be an active contributor toward the resolution of these issues—she must be concerned and informed.

Nursing Responsibilities

When facing ethical decisions, the nurse must examine her own values before addressing those of another. If these values are contradictory to those of the client, the nurse must direct her attention to focusing on the needs and values of the client before her own. In instances where this is not possible, the nurse should refer the client to another qualified member of the health care team.

Ethical decision making for both the client and nurse is based on a sound understanding of the issues, the conflicting principles involved, the alternatives available, the consequences of each alternative, the personal values involved and their relationship to the consequences, and the long-range effects of the decision on the client and other significant individuals in her life.

Not all ethical issues involved in maternity nursing have been explored in the preceding discussions, nor has every aspect of concern been viewed. However, the nurse must be aware of the need for ethical decision making and its importance in the delivery of nursing care.

BIBLIOGRAPHY

American Fertility Society. Ethical statement on in vitro fertilization. *Fertility & Sterility*, 1983, **40**, 289.

American Nurses' Association. *Code for nurses with interpretive statements*, Publ. No. G-56 Kansas City, Mo., 1985.

———, Division of Maternal and Child Health Nursing Practice. *Standards of maternal and child health nursing practice*, Publ. No. MCH-3, Kansas City, Mo., 1983.

Beebe, J., & Thompson, H. A paradigm of ethics for the maternal child nurse. *MCN*, 1979, **4**, 141.

Blank, J. Electronic fetal monitoring: nursing management defined. *Journal of Gynecological & Neonatal Nursing*, 1985, **14**, 463-467.

Broody, H. *Ethical decisions in medicine* (2nd ed.). Boston: Little, Brown, 1981.

Cushing, M. Expanding the meaning of accountability, *American Journal of Nursing*, 1983, **83**, 1202-1203.

Drane, J. The defective child: ethical guidelines for painful dilemmas, *Journal of Gynecological Nursing*, 1984, **13**, 42–48.

Elsea, S. Ethics in maternal-child nursing, *MCN*, 1985, **10**, 303.

Edgil, A. Moral problems in nursing practice. *Journal of Gynecological & Neonatal Nursing*, 1983, **12**, 210-212.

Fromer, M. *Ethical issues in sexuality and reproduction*. St. Louis: C.V. Mosby, 1983.

Gaffney, S.E. Intrauterine fetal surgery: the ramifications for nurses. *MCN*, 1985, **10**, 250-254.

Groff, B. Anatomy of a malpractice trial. *American Journal of Nursing*, 1985, **85**, 248-250.

Hodgson, J. *Abortion and sterilization: Medical and social aspects*. London: Academic Press, 1981.

Jameton, A. *Nursing practice: The ethical issues*. Englewood Cliffs, N.J.: Prentice Hall, 1984.

McCloskey, J. & Grace, H. *Current issues in nursing*. Boston: Blackwell, 1981.

Murchison, I., Nichols, T. & Hanson, R. *Legal accountability in the nursing process*. St. Louis: C. V. Mosby, 1982.

Muyskens, J. *Moral problems in nursing*. Totowa, N.J.: Roiuman and Littlefield, 1982.

NAACOG. *Standards for obstetric, gynecologic and neonatal nursing* (3rd ed.). Nurse's Association of the American College of Obstetrics and Gynecology, 1986.

Northrop, C. Telling it like it is. *Nursing 85*, 1985, **15**, 47.

Ramsey, P. *Ethics at the edges of life*. New Haven: Yale University Press, 1978.

Thompson, J. & Thompson, H. *Ethics in nursing*. New York: Macmillan, 1981.

UNIT II

REPRODUCTION IN THE FAMILY

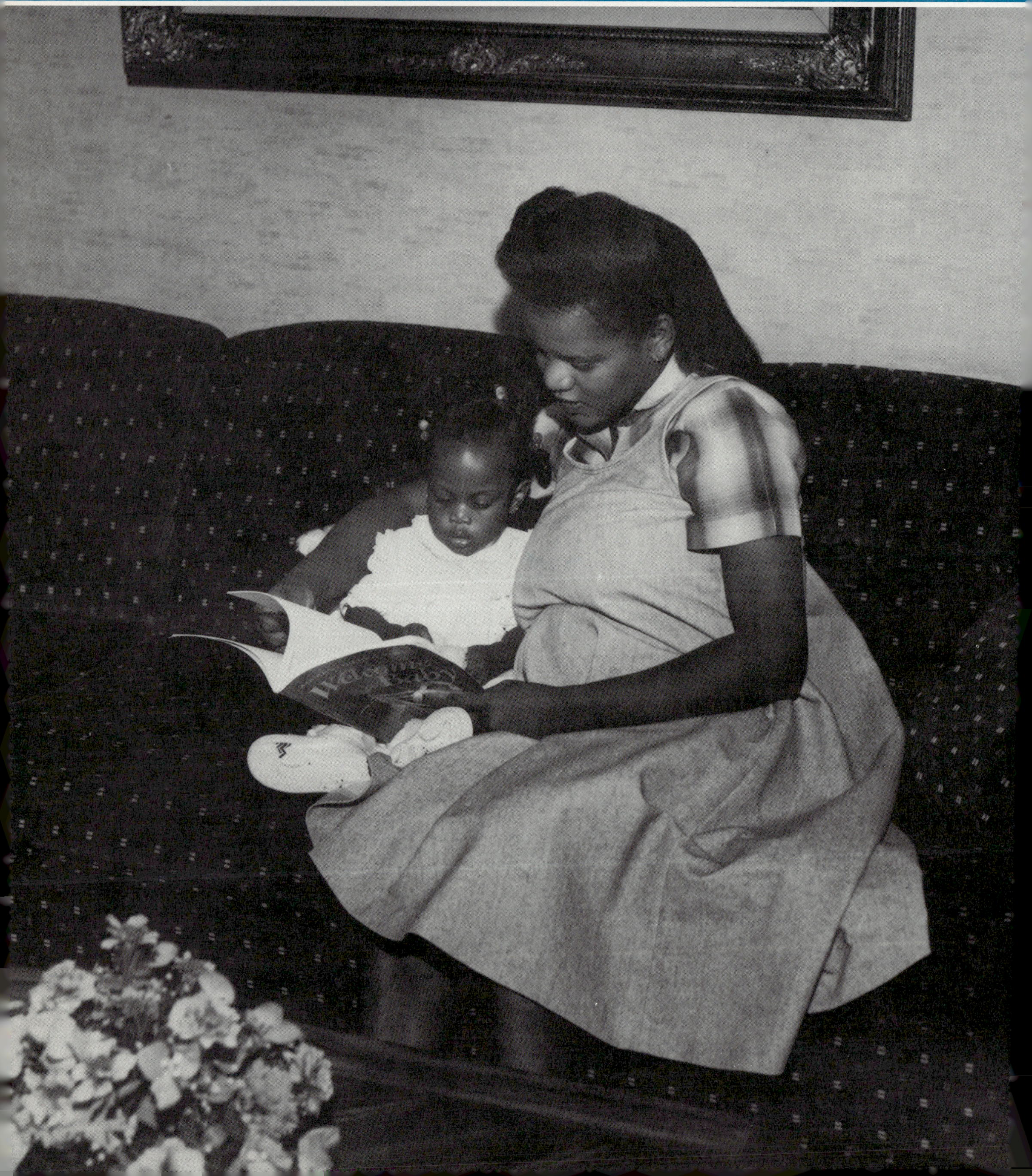

UNIT II

REPRODUCTION IN THE FAMILY

UNIT II

REPRODUCTION IN THE FAMILY

CHAPTER 4 THE SYSTEMS OF REPRODUCTION

The Female Reproductive System
Physiology of the Female Reproductive System
The Male Reproductive System

CHAPTER 5 THE GENETICS OF REPRODUCTION

Chromosomes and Genes
Cell Division
Gametogenesis
Chromosome Defects
Single Gene Defects
Polygenic Defects
Genetic Counseling

CHAPTER 6 PREPARING FOR REPRODUCTION

Preparing for Reproduction
Sexual Development
Sexual Response
Nursing Responsibilities Involving Sexuality
Family Planning
Unplanned Parenthood
Infertility

CHAPTER 7 FETAL DEVELOPMENT

Developmental Phases
Environmental Factors that Influence Development
Week 1: Fertilization and Implantation
Week 2: Bilaminar Embryo Formation
Week 3: Trilaminar Embryo Formation
Weeks 4 to 8: The Embryonic Period
The Fetal Period
Embryonic and Fetal Development
Fetal Circulation

CHAPTER 8 THE PLACENTA AND FETAL SUPPORT

Placental Development
The Umbilical Cord
Fetal Membranes
Maternal Placental Circulation
Fetal Placental Circulation
Placental Transfer of Substances
Placental Abnormalities and Dysfunctions

chapter 4

THE SYSTEMS OF REPRODUCTION

OBJECTIVES

Upon completion of this chapter, the reader will be able to:

1. Name, identify, and describe the functions of the male and female external and internal organs of reproduction.
2. Name and describe the layers of the uterine wall.
3. Name the uterine supporting muscles and ligaments.
4. Name and describe two common variations of uterine attitude.
5. Name and describe the divisions of the fallopian tube.
6. Describe the development of the primary oocyte, graafian follicle, and corpus luteum.
7. Name and describe the functions of the hormones influencing the menstrual cycle and ovulation.
8. Explain the relationship of the hypothalamus and anterior pituitary gland to the menstrual cycle.
9. Describe the functions of prostaglandins during reproduction.
10. Name the two primary functions of the testes.
11. Describe the pathway of the sperm from the testes to the urethra.
12. Name and describe the functions of the male hormones of the hypothalamus, anterior pituitary, and testes.

KEY TERMS

Anteflexion
Anteversion
Antrum
Cervix
Clitoris
Ejaculatory duct
Endometrium
Estrogen
External cervical os
Fallopian Tube
Ferning
Follicle stimulating hormone
Fundus
Hymenal sheath
Internal cervical os
Menarche
Menopause
Ovulation
Perineum
Primary follicles
Progesterone
Prostaglandin
Prostate gland
Retroflexion
Scrotum
Sperm
Testes
Testosterone
Uterine isthmus
Vagina
Vaginal introitus

The framework of maternity nursing is built on a comprehensive understanding of the reproductive systems of the male and female. With this foundation, the nurse is able to understand not only the anatomic and physiologic properties of reproduction, but also the entire spectrum of reproductive events involved in maternity nursing.

The circle of life revolves around the ability to propagate. Each generation receives a part of that which preceeded it, and each passes to the next those biologic, physiologic, and sociologic, properties involved in creation. Reproduction becomes the key element linking the past with the future. It is no surprise that reproduction is interlaced with sexuality. Reproduction results not only from the biological functions involved, but from the emotional involvement as well. To that end, reproduction is viewed by the nurse as serving two purposes, reproduction and sexuality.

THE FEMALE REPRODUCTIVE SYSTEM

The reproductive system of the female is composed of the external and internal genitalia. The external genitalia consist of the vulva and related structures. The internal genitalia include the vagina, uterus, fallopian tubes, and ovaries. Accessory structures such as the breast, pelvic bones, ligaments, and muscles, are also important contributors. The ligaments and muscles will be reviewed in this chapter, and the pelvic bones will be reviewed in Chapter 13 as part of the basis for an understanding of the labor process. The breast is discussed in Chapter 23.

Female External Genitalia

THE VULVA

Structures of the vulva are the mons pubis, labia majora, labia minora, clitoris, vestibule containing the vaginal and urinary orifices, and the Bartholin's glands and Skene's ducts (see Fig. 4–1).

Mons Pubis

The *mons pubis* is a fatty tissue pad which extends over the symphysis pubis and is covered with pubic hair. It develops at puberty and remains until old age, at which time the pubic hair becomes scanty and the fatty adipose tissue diminishes. Its function is both sexual and protective.

Labia Majora

The outer lips of the vulva (*labia majora*) are composed of fatty tissue, covered with pubic hair, and extend from the mons pubis to the perineum. They are supplied on the outer

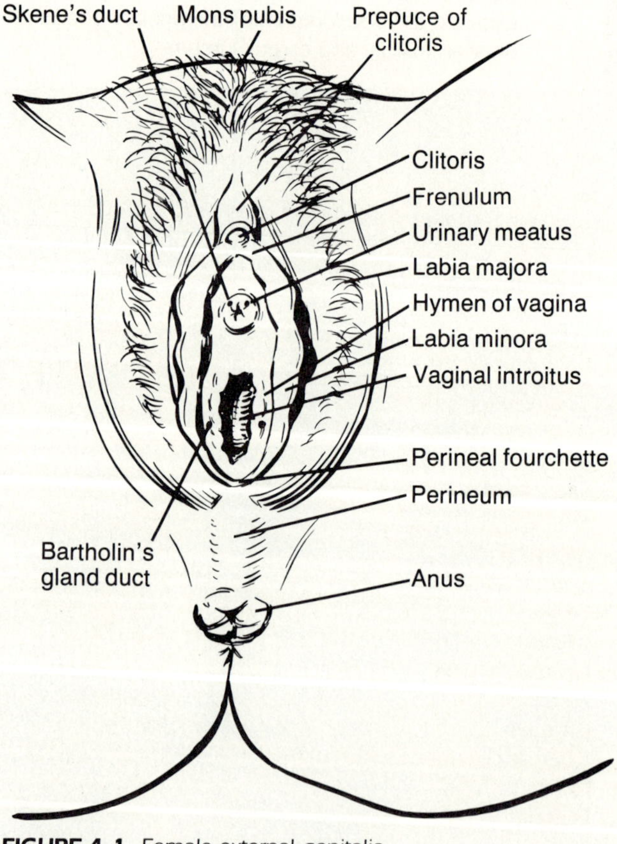

FIGURE 4–1. Female external genitalia.

surface with sebaceous glands, a complexity of nerves, and many blood vessels. The inner surfaces of the labia majora are without hair and appear to be somewhat shiny. The labia majora serve as a protection for the vaginal structures.

Labia Minora

The *labia minora* are the inner lips of the vulva and are smaller and thinner than the labia majora. They do not have a covering of pubic hair. The labia minora are located between the folds of the labia majora. Anteriorly, each labia minor subdivides into two sections, the outer and inner layers. The outer section extends to merge into the *prepuce* or hood of the clitoris. The inner sections also extend and merge with the clitoris to form a fold called the *frenulum*. Posteriorly, the labia minora merge into a junction called the *perineal fourchette*. The inner lips are well supplied with nerves and blood vessels, making them receptive to sexual stimulation. During sexual arousal they also have a lubricative function.

Clitoris

The most sexually sensitive structure of the female genitalia is the *clitoris*. It is the female sexual counterpart of the male penis, but it does not contain a urinary meatus. The clitoris is located between the folds of the labia minora, which form the prepuce and frenulum. It is erectile when stimulated, owing to venous congestion during sexual stimulation. Because of its highly sensitive nature, its main function is sexual stimulation.

Vestibule

Within the folds of the labia minora is a smooth, flat area located between the clitoris and fourchette called the *vestibule*. The vestibule contains the urethral opening, the vaginal opening, the Skene's ducts, and the Bartholin's glands. The urethral opening is called the urinary meatus and is not considered a part of the reproductive genitalia. Its proximity to the vaginal opening does, however, justify its consideration at this time. During sexual contact it often becomes the portal of entry for organisms associated with bladder infections. The urinary and vaginal openings are also often confused when catheterizations are done, and contamination of the urinary tract may occur. This is of particular significance during labor, delivery, and postpartum periods, when the genital structures may be edematous and difficult to identify.

The vaginal opening is also located in the vestibular area. It is posterior to the urinary meatus and between the labia minora. The vaginal introitus provides the entrance to the internal reproductive tract. A membranous sheath called the *hymen* may partially cover the vaginal opening. This hymenal sheath first appears in the newborn as a membranous tag protruding from the vagina. As the female matures, the membrane extends over the vaginal orifice and becomes elastic. In some individuals it will almost completely cover the vaginal opening and in others only slightly. A "tight hymen" does not indicate that a girl is a virgin. It may be stretched from the use of tampons or may simply be more elastic in one individual than another. Following intercourse and childbirth the hymenal membrane disappears, however; in some individuals remnants of the hymen may be seen as hymenal tags called *carunculae myrtiformes.*

Bartholin's Glands

Located laterally to the vaginal opening are the vulvovaginal glands called the *Bartholin's glands*. Anatomically, they are not external, but they do open onto the surface of the labia minora. Their exact function is not known, although they secrete a small amount of mucus during sexual arousal. On occasion they become infected and are then a source of discomfort. They are only palpable when infected or enlarged.

Skene's Ducts

The *Skene's ducts* are located within the vestibule, laterally and somewhat posteriorly to the urinary meatus. These ducts are inconsistent in their placement and function. They are the homologues of the male prostate gland, but they do not serve any real purpose. However, during episodes of infection, such as gonorrhea, they may become painful and are, at that time, palpable.

Perineum

Located posteriorly to the vestibule is an area designated as the *perineum*. In maternity nursing, the term perineum is used to designate the area between the vulva and the rectum. The more inclusive term, *perineal body*, refers to the perineum and the fibromuscular tissue extending into the urogenital and pelvic diaphragms. Interspaced within the center of the perineal body are the muscles of the sphincter ani, levator ani, bulbocavernosus, ischiocavernosus, and transverse perineal muscles as well as elastic and connective tissue (see Fig. 4–2). These muscles and tissue support the pelvic organs and allow the extreme stretching of the perineum needed during childbirth. Occasionally during the delivery process, deep lacerations may occur into the perineum and the external sphincter of the anus.

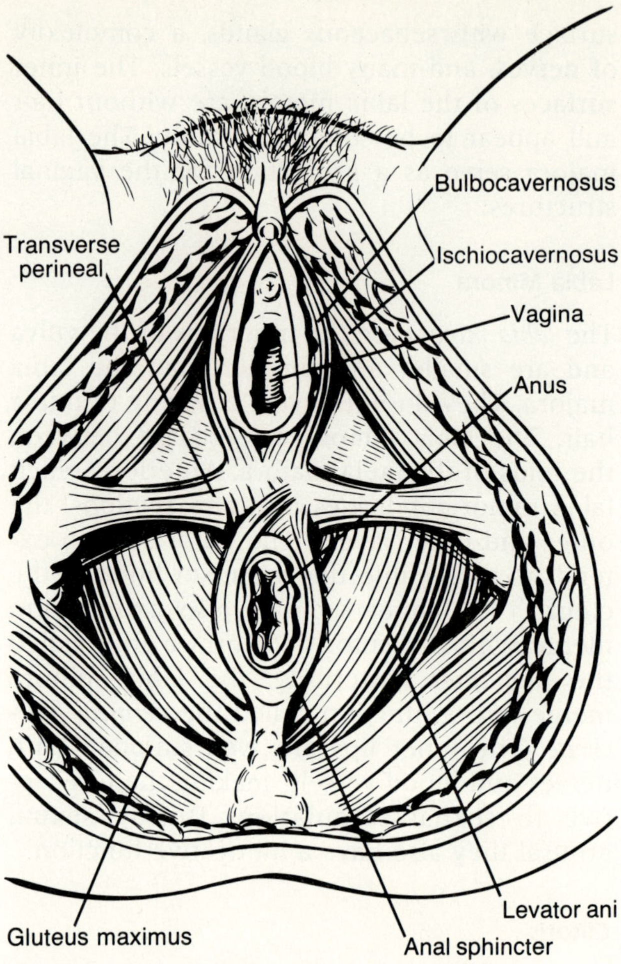

FIGURE 4–2. Muscles of the female pelvic floor.

Female Internal Genitalia

THE VAGINA

The *vagina* is a 4 to 6 inch tubular canal that is directed upward and backward in the pelvis (see Fig. 4–3). It extends from the vestibule to the uterus. Its anatomical location is between the bladder and the rectum (see Fig. 4–4). The internal wall of the vagina is made up of membranous stratified squamous epithelium, which forms thick transverse folds called *rugae*. These rugae are capable of stretching to accommodate the delivery of the baby. The vaginal mucosa is attached to the underlying musculofascial layer, which progresses from smooth muscle to deeper layers of connective tissue. The muscular layers also aid in dilatation and contraction of the vagina.

The relationship of the uterine cervix to the vagina is of clinical importance. The projecting uterine cervix attaches to the anterior wall of the vagina at a right angle, making the anterior wall shorter than the extended posterior wall. This difference may amount to as much as 2 to 3 cm. Because of the protruding cervix into the vagina, recesses form anteriorly, posteriorly, and laterally to the cervix. These surrounding recesses are called the *fornices*. Since the posterior wall of the vagina is longer than the anterior wall, the posterior fornix is deeper than the anterior fornix. This accommodates pooling of the semen during intercourse, increasing the possibility of conception. Physical examination of the fornices of the vagina allows for palpation of the pelvic structures such as the ovaries, rectum, and bladder.

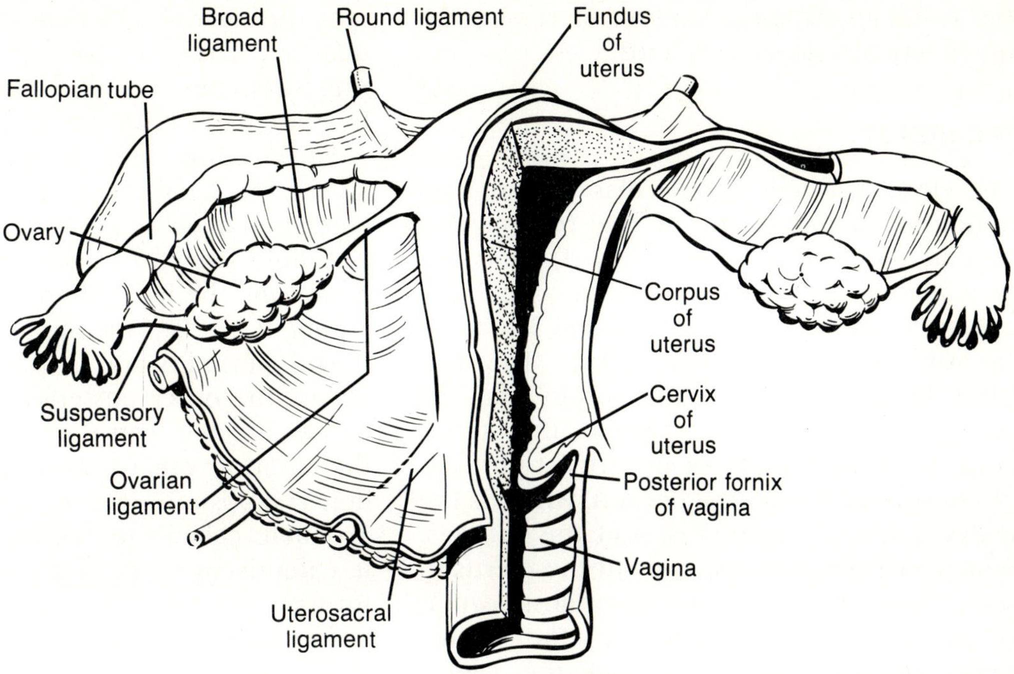

FIGURE 4-3. Female internal reproductive organs.

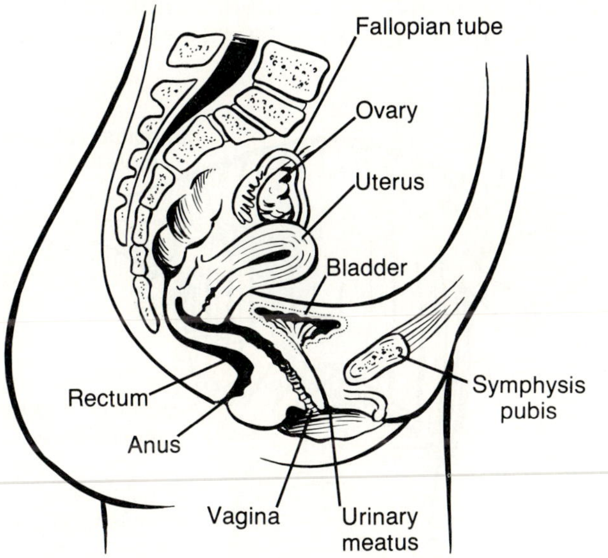

FIGURE 4-4. Relationship of female reproductive organs to bladder and rectum.

Support for the vagina is facilitated by the perineal body, the urogenital diaphragm, the levator ani muscle, and the pubocervical, transverse cervical, and sacrocervical ligaments. Surrounding the vaginal opening is the bulbocavernous muscle. During vaginal examinations, this muscle may be voluntarily contracted and relaxed to facilitate relaxation.

The blood supply to the vagina is derived from the descending branch of the cervicovaginal branch of the uterine artery, the inferior vesical arteries, the internal pudendal arteries, and the rectal (middle hemorrhoidal) arteries. Venous drainage is provided by the pudendal, uterine, and external hemorrhoidal veins. Lymphatic drainage is accomplished via the superficial inguinal nodes of the lower vagina and the presacral, hypogastric, and superficial inguinal nodes of the upper vagina.

The secretions present in the vagina are derived from two sources, the alkaline cervical secretions and the acid-producing organisms inhabiting the vagina. In spite of the alkaline cervical secretions, the pH of the vagina is acidic, with a pH of 4.0 to 5.0. This is caused by the bacterial action on the glycogen content of the epithelial cells of the vagina, resulting in the formation of lactic acid. The bacteria responsible for this reaction are thought to be the Döderlein's bacilli, which are considered normal inhabitants of the vagina. A disturbance of the inhabitation of these bacilli will cause an alkaline secretion, increasing the possibility of vaginal infections.

THE UTERUS

The *uterus* is a hollow, muscular, pear-shaped organ located in front of the rectum and behind the bladder (see Fig. 4–4). It is approximately the size of the clenched fist, averaging about 6 to 8 cm long and 3 to 5 cm in width in the nonpregnant state. The divisions of the uterus are the corpus and the cervix. The *corpus*, or the body of the uterus, consists of the fundus, or uppermost portions of the uterus; the central portion, which is the actual body of the uterus; and the isthmus, which extends from the body of the uterus to the cervix. The *cervix* is the lowermost portion of the uterus and extends into the vagina. There are two cervical openings: the *internal os*, which is the opening from the uterus to the cervix, and the *external os*, which is the opening from the cervix to the vagina.

Measurements and assessments of both the fundus of the uterus and the cervix are important throughout pregnancy and during labor, delivery, and the postpartal periods. These measurements and assessments are discussed in subsequent chapters.

The uterine wall is composed of three layers: the *perimetrium*, or the outermost layer composed of pelvic peritoneum; the *myometrium*, a middle layer of muscle fibers; and the *endometrium*, the inner lining of the uterus, consisting of mucous membranous tissue.

The perimetrium is a serosal layer that covers the outer posterior wall of the uterus and is directed over the uppermost portion of the anterior wall, continuing on over the bladder. The posterior perimetrium covering forms a pouch, called the cul-de-sac of Douglas, as it extends over the surface of the posterior fornix.

The middle myometrial layer of the uterus is a complexity of involuntary muscle fibers (see Fig. 4–5). These muscles are distributed in layers corresponding to the outer, middle, and inner parts of the uterine wall. Each layer shows a distinct distribution of muscle fibers specific to its function. The outer layer dis-

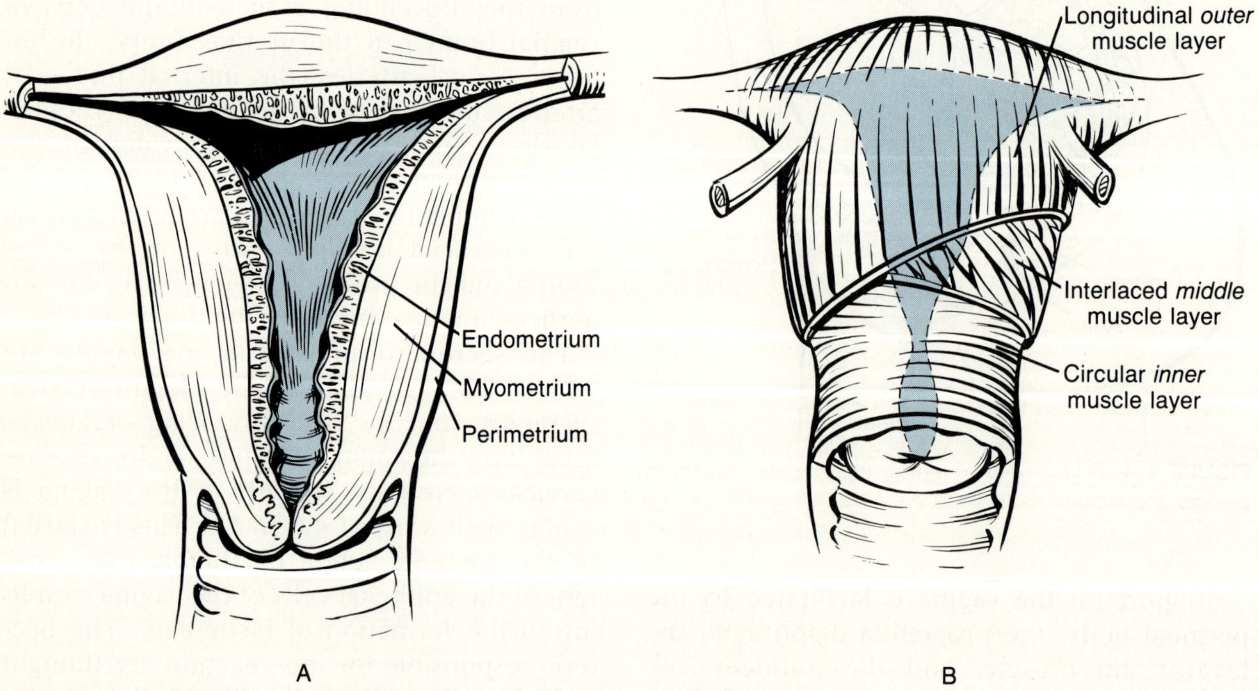

FIGURE 4-5. A. Uterine layers. **B.** Arrangement of muscle fibers of myometrium.

plays a longitudinal distribution of muscle fibers, enabling these muscles to exert a strong forceful expulsive action. In the middle layer, muscle fibers are arranged in a pattern resembling a figure-eight. Within these muscle fibers are interspaced many blood vessels. When contracted, the middle layer muscles compress the blood vessels, facilitating hemostasis. Circular inner muscle fibers are concentrated in the areas of the internal os, forming the internal sphincter. This sphincter prevents the expulsion of the fetus before labor.

Endometrial tissue covers the inner lining of the uterine cavity and cervix. This lining, within the body of the uterus, is a vascular mucous membrane containing glands that respond to hormonal cyclic changes. Essentially, this mucous membrane is shed and regenerated each month during the reproductive years. This process is known as the *menstrual cycle*.

The endometrial lining of the cervix is thin and made up of columnar epithelial tissue containing mucus-secreting glands. Responsiveness to the hormonal cyclic changes is demonstrated throughout the monthly cycle. In the first part of the cycle, prior to ovulation, the cervical mucous is slight and opaque. Immediately preceding ovulation, the cervical secretions become clear, thin, increased in amount, and alkaline, and they have a stretchable consistency. All these characteristics facilitate sperm migration and survival. Following ovulation, under the influence of progesterone, the cervical mucus becomes thick and decreased in amount, making it hostile to sperm migration and survival.

The lowermost portion of the cervix is lined with squamous epithelial endometrial tissue. The junction of the columnar epithelium and the squamous epithelium is designated as the *squamocolumnar junction.* This area is the site from which cells are obtained for Papanicolaou smears used to detect cervical carcinoma. With age the location of this site will shift.

There are two important cavities within the uterus. The corpus of the uterus contains the main uterine cavity. It is widest at the fundal section and extends to communicate laterally with the insertion of the fallopian tubes at the upper outer aspects of the uterus. The uterine cavity narrows considerably as it reaches the isthmus. It is within the uterine cavity that the endometrial tissue forms. Here the fertilized ovum implants, grows, and matures to a full-term pregnancy.

Entrance to the cervical cavity is provided by the internal os from the isthmus and vaginally by the external cervical os. The cervical cavity appears more as a canal of about 3 cm in length. Because of the elasticity of the cervix, the canal is capable of increasing from a 1-inch diameter canal to an area large enough to accommodate the passage of the full-term babies. Before childbirth the external os appears as a rounded opening. Following pregnancy the external os remains somewhat dilated and appears more as a transverse slit.

Uterine Blood Supply

Uterine blood supply is derived from the uterine and ovarian arteries that extend from the internal iliac arteries and the aorta (see Fig. 4–6). The increased demands of pregnancy necessitate a rich supply of blood to the uterus. New, larger blood vessels develop to accommodate the need of the growing uterus. Both the arteries and veins become torturous and distended. Venous circulation is accomplished via the internal iliac and common iliac vein. Lymphatic drainage is into the internal iliac glands.

Uterine Nerves

The nerves supplying the uterus are controlled by the autonomic nervous system and are involuntary. The two divisions, sympathetic and parasympathetic, both share in the control of uterine function. The sympathetic effect promotes uterine muscular contractions and vasoconstriction needed during labor and delivery. The opposite effect of vasodilation

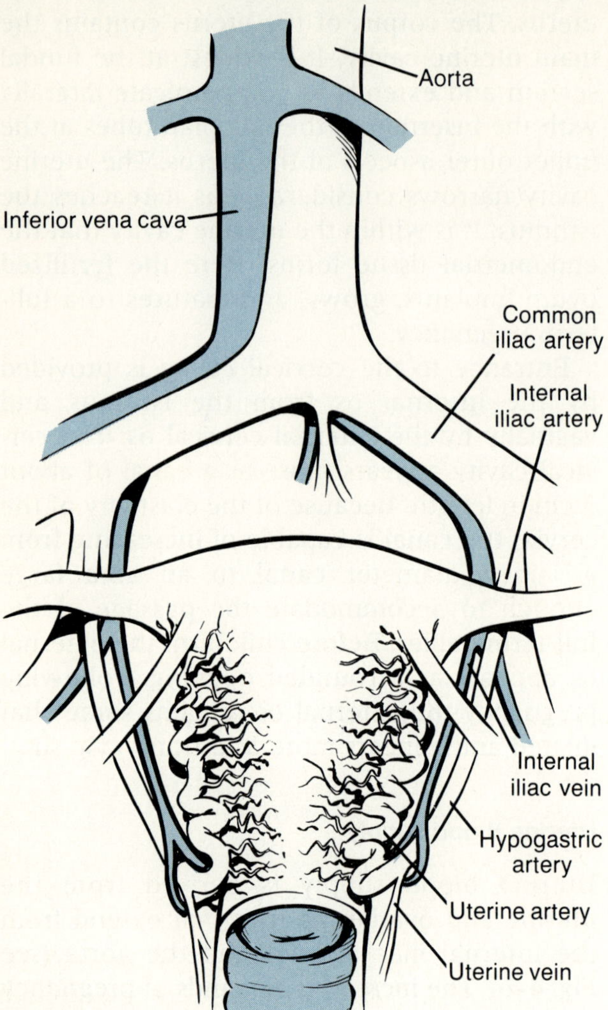

FIGURE 4-6. Uterine blood supply.

and relaxation of the musculature is accomplished by the parasympathetic system.

Uterine Support

Essential to the support of the uterus are the muscles of the pelvic diaphragm and the supporting ligaments. The pelvic diaphragm consists of the levator ani and coccygeus muscle, along with the support from the muscles interspaced within the perineal body—the sphincter ani, the bulbocavernosus, the ischiocavernosus, and the transverse perineal muscle. This slinglike support is reinforced by the more direct support of the ligaments and fascial sheaths. The fascial sheaths form investments for the pelvic organs and condense into fibrous bands, forming ligaments. Major pelvic ligaments are: the broad ligaments, the round ligaments and the uterosacral ligaments (Figure 4–3).

The *broad ligaments* are an extension of the abdominal peritoneal lining and are not composed of fascial sheaths, as are the other ligaments. These enveloping folds of peritoneum extend laterally to both pelvic walls and surround the fallopian tubes, ovaries and ligaments. They attach to the outer aspects of the uterus. Their location divides the pelvic cavity into anterior and posterior sections. The posterior segments of the broad ligament are attached to the cervical portion of the uterus and are referred to as the *cardinal ligaments*. Although they are considered part of the broad ligaments, they are thicker and consist of connective tissue.

At the cornua of the uterus are the *round ligaments* composed of bands of fibromuscular fascia. They proceed upward and outward and then pass downward as they progress through the broad ligament into the inguinal canals and end in the labia majora.

The *uterosacral ligaments* extend upward and backward from the posterior cervix. They pass on either side of the rectum and connect with the periosteum of the sacrum.

Uterine Attitude

The uterus assumes an attitude (posture) of slight anteversion in its placement between the bladder and the rectum. That is, in its normal position the fundus is tipped forward slightly over the bladder with the cervix projecting backward toward the rectum. The uterus is secured in this position mainly by the uterosacral ligaments and the round ligaments. However, this position may be altered by pregnancy, posture, fullness of the bladder and rectum, and by variations of anatomic positions. Common variations of anatomic positions are (1) *anteflexion:* The corpus of the uterus is tipped sharply forward at the cervical junction, and (2) *retroflexion:* The corpus of the uterus is tipped sharply backward toward the rectum.

FALLOPIAN TUBES

Extending from either side of the uterus are the cilia-lined peristaltic muscular *fallopian tubes*. Each pencil-shaped, 4.5 inch (10 to 12 cm) tube provides a route from the ovary to the uterus. It is within these tubes that fertilization of the ovum by the sperm occurs. The fallopian tube opens into the abdominal cavity and does not come in direct contact with the ovary.

The fallopian tubes are divided into four sections: the *interstitial segment* that is inserted into the myometrium of the uterus; the *isthmus*, 1 to 2 cm in length, that extends outward from the uterine wall; the 6 to 8 cm *ampulla*, which extends laterally and is where fertilization usually occurs; and the distal fimbriated *infundibulum* of the tube, which opens into the abdominal cavity (see Fig. 4–7). The fimbriated ends of the fallopian tubes simulate beckoning fingers extending from the armlike fallopian tubes of the uterus. These fingerlike projections (*fimbriae*) lie near the ovary, which is embedded in the broad ligament. Once the ovum is released from the ovary, the moving ciliated fimbrae encourage the ovum to enter the fallopian tube. Upon entry into the tube, enzymes secreted by the mucous membrane of the tube and by the sperm loosen the follicle cells surrounding the ovum. This enables the ovum to be fertilized by the sperm. The fertilized ovum is then propelled by the muscular peristalsis of the fallopian tube through the tube and into the awaiting uterus. (A more detailed description of fertilization is found in Chapter 7).

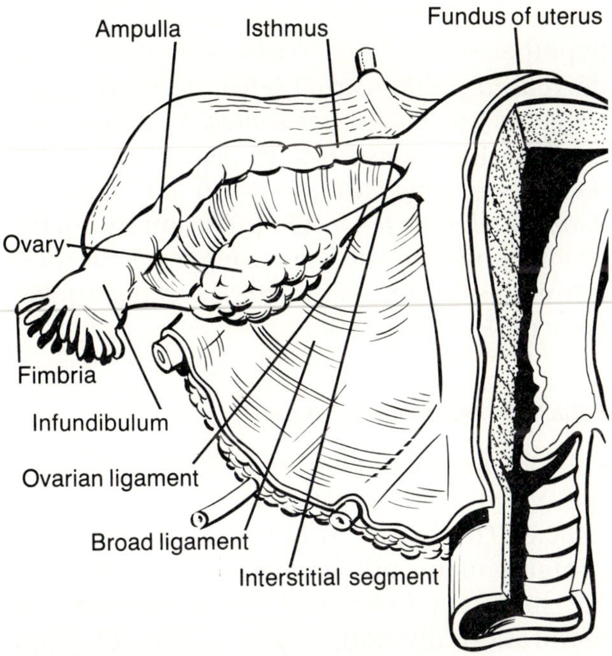

FIGURE 4–7. Divisions of the fallopian tube.

OVARIES

The *ovaries* are the female gonads comparable to the male testes. The two almond shaped ovaries are located on either side of the uterus, approximating the posterior surface of the broad ligament. They are attached to the uterus by means of the suspensory ligament (see Fig. 4–3). Each ovary varies in size, ranging from 1 to 3 cm in thickness, 3 to 5 cm in length, and 2 to 3 cm in width. Variance in ovarian size is attributed to hormonal influences experienced during the monthly cycle. Following menopause, the ovaries decrease somewhat in size.

The ovary displays two divisional areas: the cortex and the medulla. The inner area, or *medulla*, takes up approximately half of the entire ovary. It is made up of fibrous tissue, nerves, blood vessels and lymphatics. The more functional division of the ovary is the *outer cortex*, which contains the developing *primary follicles* and the mature *graafian follicle*. At birth, the full compliment of follicles (4 million or more) is present in the ovaries of the newborn. They may decrease in number during childhood but no more are produced following birth. Once puberty is reached, one of the follicles, influenced by hormones, will mature each month. The mature follicle, containing the ovum, ruptures from the surface of the cortex and releases the ovum into the abdominal cavity. It is then swept into the fallopian tube beginning its journey to possible life. (The complete process is explained in Chapter 7.)

PHYSIOLOGY OF THE FEMALE REPRODUCTIVE SYSTEM

The anatomy of the female compliments and accommodates the creation of life. Each organ is part of a harmonious system centered on the goal of creation. At puberty, when the reproductive system reaches maturity, it becomes functional, and the summit of reproductive readiness is reached.

Physiologically, the onset of puberty initiates the interaction of the endocrine glands, hormones, ovaries, and uterus. Through their mutual efforts the female reproductive cycle begins and, under normal conditions, will repeat itself every month for the remaining reproductive years—a period of about 30 to 35 years. The only normal exception to the fulfillment of the cycle is pregnancy.

The Monthly Female Reproductive Cycle

Menarche (menstruation onset) is one of the first noticeable signs the young girl experiences indicating she has entered the reproductive years. Menstruation may occur in some girls as early as ten years of age; in others, it may not occur until 16 years of age. Factors such as heredity, climate, environment, nutrition, and race may influence the onset of menstruation. It is well known that within the last decade the average age for the onset of menstruation has dropped owing to better health practices and nutrition. Likewise, the onset of *menopause* (the cessation of menstruation) in many women has been delayed beyond the normal age of 40 to 50 years of age, due, in part, to better health care.

The monthly female reproductive cycle, consisting of an ovulatory and uterine phase, is dominated by controlling hormonal influences. Synergistic efforts of the hypothalamus of the brain, the anterior pituitary gland, the ovaries, and the uterus are responsible for stimulation, release, and inhibition of these hormones. Although the monthly reproductive cycle is a continuous, ongoing process with no actual beginning or end, the normal cycle is considered to be 28 days.

The onset of the menstrual flow is designated as day 1 of the cycle. On approximately day 5 the follicular phase begins, during which the ovarian follicle is stimulated to grow and develop and the endometrial lining of the uterus begins to regenerate and becomes proliferative. *Ovulation* (release of the mature ovum) occurs at midcycle (about the 10th to the 14th day). During days 14 to 28 the endometrial lining of the uterus becomes secretory in anticipation of implantation of the fertilized ovum in the uterine cavity. If fertilization has not occurred, the endometrial lining is sloughed off and the menstrual period again begins.

DEVELOPMENT OF THE OVARIAN FOLLICLE

Even as menstruation is occurring, hormonal influences are preparing for the development of the ovarian follicles. The nerve cells of the hypothalamus of the brain, stimulated by a decreased premenstrual level of estrogen, are triggered to release *gonadotrophic releasing factors* (Gn-RF) consisting of *follicle stimulating hormone releasing factor* (FSH-RF) and *luteinizing hormone releasing factor* (LRF). The anterior pituitary responds to the increasing levels of these hormones by releasing *follicle stimulating hormone* (FSH) (see Fig. 4–8).

Follicle Stimulating Hormone

Follicle stimulating hormone (FSH) influences the growth and development of the ovarian follicle. The cortex (outer layer) of the ovary contains many primary *oocytes* (egg cells that are maturing but have not completed first maturation division). Only a few of these primary oocytes are stimulated by FSH to develop; and only one, in most cases, will

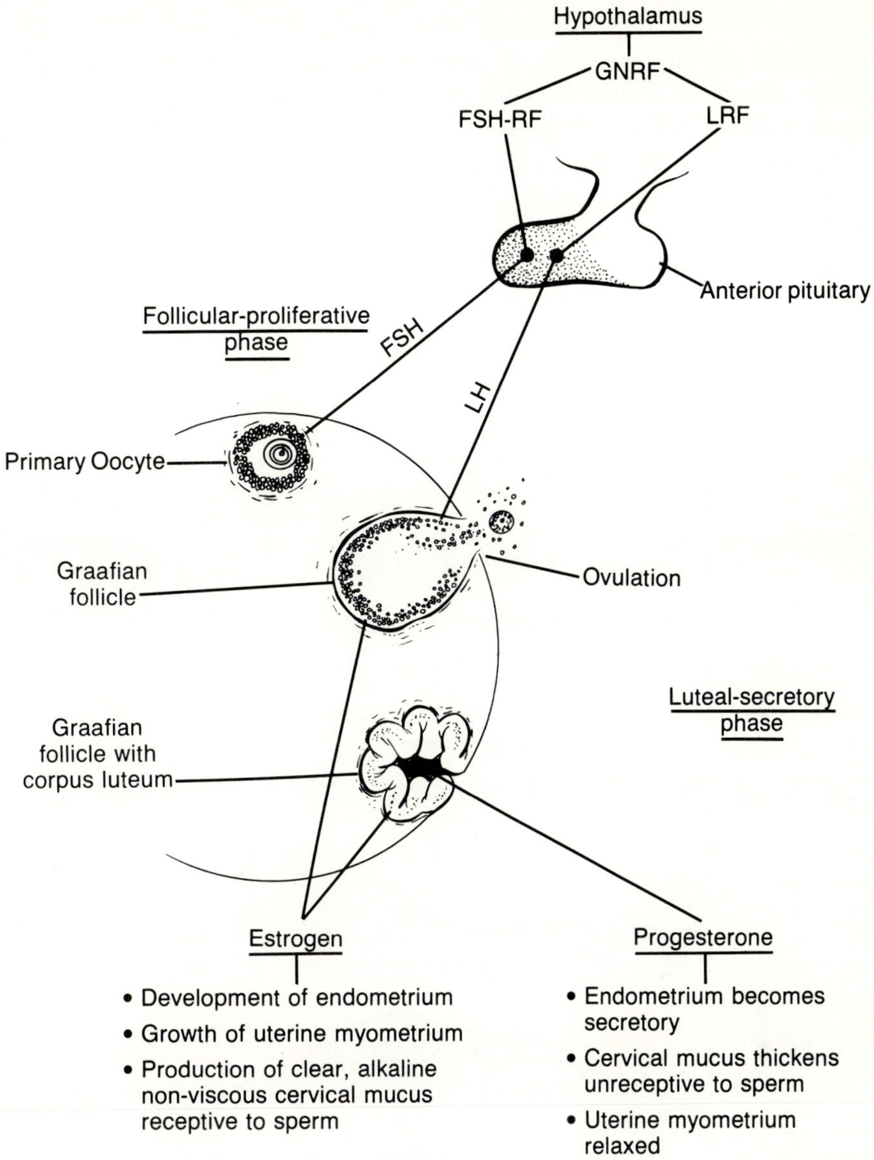

FIGURE 4–8. Hormonal influences on the menstrual cycle.

mature to become the graafian follicle (ripe egg cell). If more than one matures there is a possibility that both can be fertilized, resulting in the birth of fraternal (nonidentical) twins.

Development of the targeted primary oocyte is characterized by an enlargement of the oocyte itself as well as an enlargement and multiplication of the cells surrounding the oocyte. A fluid-filled space, called the *antrum,* develops in the center of the follicle, and at maturity a thick mucoid membrane, called the *zona pellucida,* encapsulates the follicle. The graafian follicle is quite large, measuring about 4 to 10 mm, and at this time *theca* cells of the follicle are producing estrogen. The mature follicle is larger than the 20 or so other developing oocytes and exerts a negative influence on them, eventually resulting in their degeneration. This negative influence is not clearly understood but may be the result of the production of estrogen.

Luteinizing Hormone

Participating in the final growth of the follicle is the luteinizing hormone (LH). The production of LH by the anterior pituitary is stimulated by the LRF from the hypothalamus. Although LH has been present during most of the follicular phase in small amounts, at mid-cycle (about the 10th to 14th day), there is a large surge of LH (see Fig. 4–9).

The graafian follicle is now mature, it has undergone the first *meiotic division* (reduction division of the chromosomes), and it has developed nutritive granules in its cytoplasm. The antrum occupies most of the follicle, with the oocyte and surrounding theca and granulosa cells migrated to the periphery of the follicle. Building pressure, caused by the increased fluid-filled antrum, results in a bulging of the outer surface of the follicle. Although it has not been substantiated, it is thought that LH has stimulated the synthesis of enzymes which result in a weakening of the follicle wall. The ovum, surrounded by the zona pellucida and a thin layer of granulosa cells called the *corona radiata*, is prepared for ovulation.

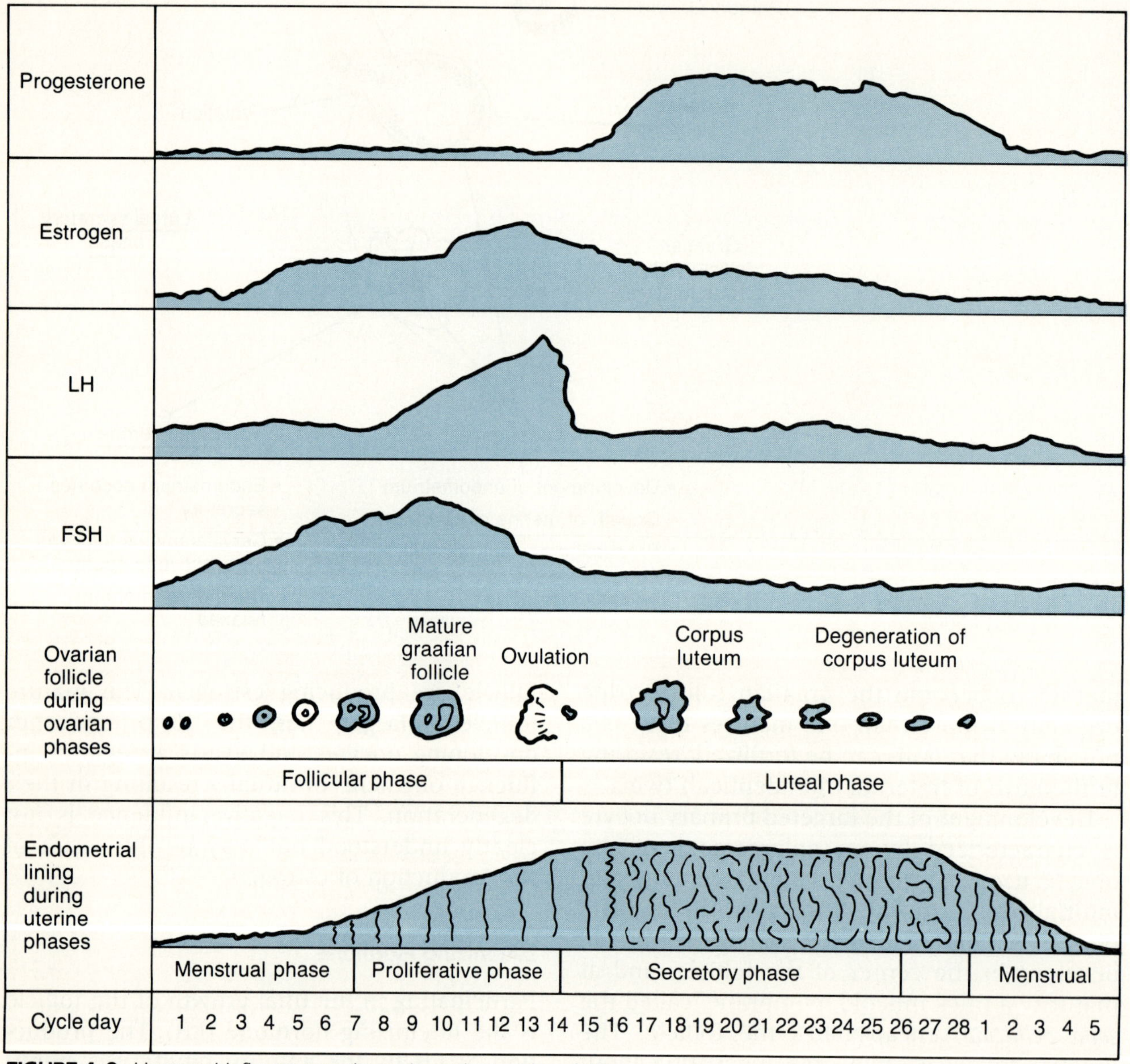

FIGURE 4–9. Hormonal influences on the endometrium and ovulation.

OVULATION

At the time of ovulation (midcycle) the graafian follicle ruptures (see Fig. 4-10) and releases the ovum and follicular fluid into the abdominal cavity near the fallopian tube. The cells of the graafian follicle now become filled with a lipidlike substance, giving the follicle a yellow color. The follicle is now known as the *corpus luteum* (yellow body). The corpus luteum will participate in the secretion of a small amount of estrogen and increasing amounts of progesterone. This phase of the ovarian cycle is designated as the luteal phase.

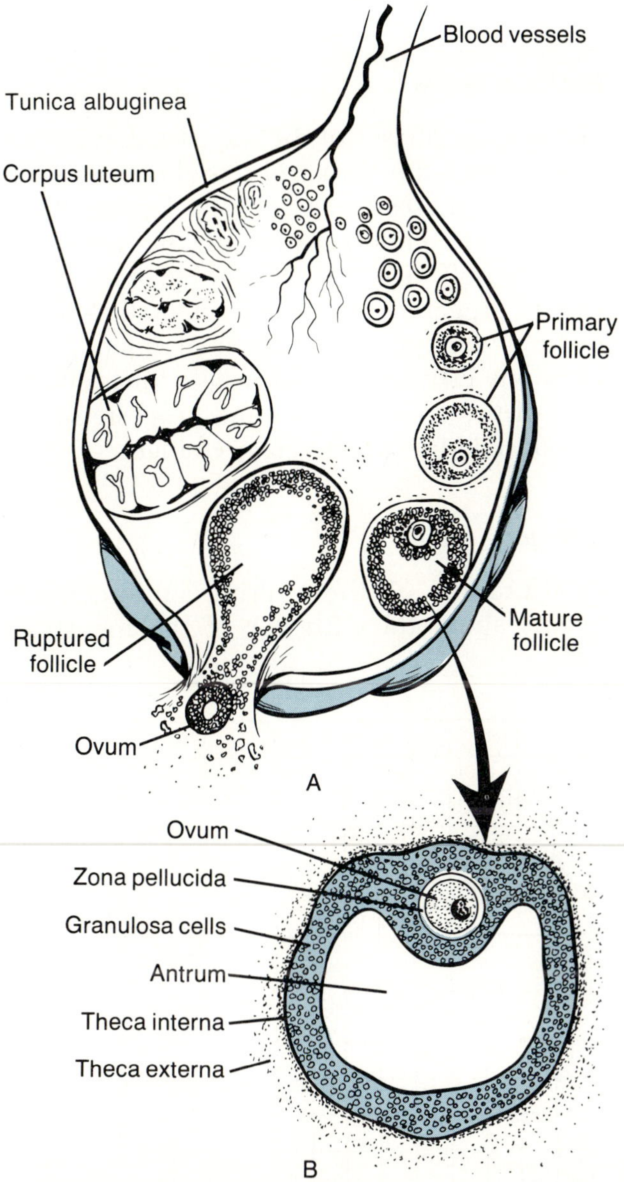

FIGURE 4-10. A. Stages of follicular development within ovary. **B.** Structure of mature follicle.

When ovulation occurs, the endometrium is prepared for reception of the fertilized ovum, and the cervical mucus, influenced by estrogen, is favorable to spermatozoan mobility. A favorable cervical environment enables the sperm to remain viable for a period of 48 hours following intercourse. The ovum, once released from the ovary, remains viable for about 24 hours. Therefore, the maximum length of time in which fertilization can occur is 72 hours. That is, intercourse occurring as much as 48 hours before ovulation or 24 hours following ovulation could result in fertilization of the ovum.

Ovulation may be manifested by certain observable characteristics. The presence of a sharp pain felt in the abdomen at the time of ovulation is noticed by some women. It is called *mittelschmerz*, meaning the middle of the cycle.

The clear alkaline cervical mucus will also demonstrate a characteristic known as *Spinnbarkeit* (stretchability of the cervical mucus) (see Fig. 4-11). Spinnbarkeit is measured by placing a small amount of cervical mucus on a glass slide and covering it with another glass slide. The mucus is drawn between the slides, producing an elastic, elongated thread. A definite Spinnbarkeit pattern is observable during the follicular phase. Measuring the Spinnbarkeit properly will result in a thread of about 4 to 6 cm on day 10 and 10 to 12 cm on day 14, when ovulation occurs. Following ovulation the cervical mucus thread may only be stretched to 3 cm on day 18 and 2 cm on day 24, when the level of estrogen is low.

Microscopic examination of the cervical mucus just prior to and at the time of ovulation will produce a ferning pattern created by the presence of sodium chloride. This increase in sodium chloride is due to the influence of increasing levels of estrogen. When progesterone increases following ovulation, sodium chloride content drops and ferning is not observable.

Basal body temperature is also affected by ovulation. While under the influence of estrogen, the basal body temperature remains low and may even drop slightly just before ovulation. Following ovulation, the temperature, influenced by progesterone, will rise (0.5 to 1.0°F) and remain elevated for the rest of the cycle (see Fig. 4–12).

It must be noted that although ovulation is considered to occur at midcycle in a 28-day cycle, not all women have regular cycles and ovulation may occur as early as the 10th day or as late as the 18th day of the cycle. Factors such as stress, illness, poor nutrition, climate changes, lack of sleep, and medications may alter the cycle.

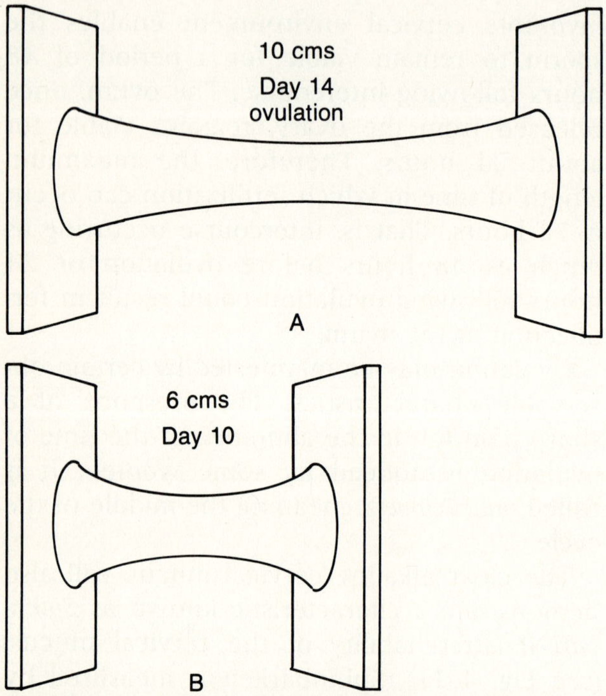

FIGURE 4–11. Spinnbarkeit—Stretchability of cervical mucus during menstrual cycle. **A.** Day 14. **B.** Day 10.

DEVELOPMENT OF THE UTERINE ENDOMETRIUM

The uterine phases of the menstrual cycle are divided into the menstrual, proliferative, and secretory phases (see Fig. 4–9). During these phases, the endometrium of the uterus is sloughed off, regenerates, and becomes secretory in preparation for the implantation of the ovum and maintenance of the pregnancy. The hormone estrogen is responsible for proliferation of the endometrium and progesterone is responsible for the secretory changes.

Estrogen

Proliferation of the uterine endometrium begins about the fifth day of the menstrual

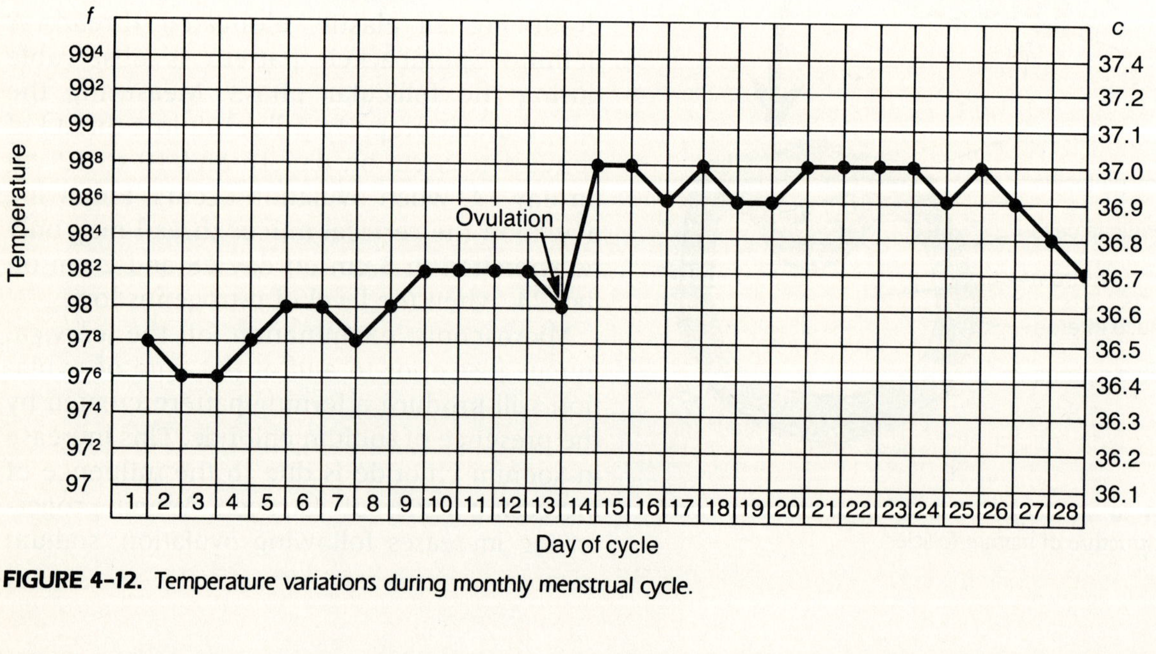

FIGURE 4–12. Temperature variations during monthly menstrual cycle.

cycle. Under the influence of estrogen the denuded endometrium is stimulated to regenerate the superficial layer lost during menstruation. This is accomplished by an increase in the number and the density of the epithelial and stromal cells and an elongation and expansion of the endometrial glands. Consequently, the endometrium thickens to a depth of about 3 to 4 mm and is prepared to receive the fertilized egg.

The effects of estrogen are not limited to the endometrium. As early as the onset of puberty, estrogen is responsible for the development of secondary sex characteristics and other effects including:

Production of clear nonviscous cervical mucus
Growth of the uterine myometrium
Growth of the breast
Deposition of fat with resulting broadening of the buttocks, hips, and thighs
Uterine size increase
Increase in scalp hair
Increased layering of the vaginal epithelial cells
Increased sexual awareness
Increased skeletal growth followed by early convergence of the epiphysis of the long bones
Stimulation of muscular peristalsis of the fallopian tubes favoring passage of the ovum

Levels of estrogen are highest in the first half of the menstrual cycle. At midcycle there is a surge of estrogen followed by a decrease during the secretory and luteal phases. The large increase of estrogen at midcycle stimulates the hypothalamus and triggers a surge of LH, which in turn stimulates ovulation.

Progesterone

Progesterone, produced by the corpus luteum, influences the proliferated endometrium to become secretory, very vascular, and abundant in tissue glycogen. The vessels become more tortuous and the glands widen and dilate. A functional layer of stromal cells develops over the dilated glands, giving the endometrium a typical spongy appearance. All the changes during the 14-day secretory phase occur in order to provide a rich nutritive bed for the fertilized ovum.

If fertilization occurs, the corpus luteum continues to secrete progesterone. The endometrium remains secretory and provides a receptive nourishing environment for the *zygote* (fertilized ovum). To further secure the pregnancy, progesterone will also have a relaxing effect on the uterine myometrium, preventing uterine contractions that could disrupt implantation.

When fertilization does not occur, the progesterone and estrogen levels diminish. The corpus luteum degenerates and endometrial changes begin. Reduction of the hormone levels brought about by the degenerating corpus luteum produces a constrictive effect on the spiral arteries, resulting in vasospasms of these vessels. The vasospasms encourage the development of necrotic areas in the endometrium. As the process continues, hemorrhagic areas develop surrounding the necrotic areas. This ischemic state results in a separation of the endometrial layers from the uterus and menstruation begins.

The menstrual flow consists of endometrial tissue, fibrolysin—to prevent clotting, and leukocytes—to prevent infection of the endometrial surface (Guyton, 1981). The normal amount of menstrual flow is about 70 to 80 ml.

Other effects of progesterone, excluding effects during pregnancy, are:

Provides secretory changes in fallopian tubes which nourish the ovum
Thickens cervical mucus discouraging sperm mobility
Stimulates breast lobule development
Elevates basal body temperature
Favors mood changes such as depression or listlessness
Relaxes uterine myometrium and other smooth muscles
Stimulates respiratory efforts

PROSTAGLANDINS

A classification of fatty acids, known as *prostaglandins*, has been identified as a contributor to the menstrual cycle. Although these fatty acids have been found in almost all tissues of the body in varying concentrations, this discussion will be limited to their reproductive activities. In the male, they are found in large concentrations in the seminal fluid. Sperm motility through the uterine passages is apparently enhanced by the prostaglandins in the seminal fluid. In the female, concentrations have been found in the ovarian follicle, in the endometrium, and in menstrual fluid. It is postulated that rupture of the ovum from the follicle is dependent on an increased follicular concentration of prostaglandins stimulated by LH. Before menstruation there is a large increase in prostaglandin production which appears to have the effect of reducing levels of progesterone and promoting degeneration of the corpus luteum. Large concentrations of prostaglandins in the endometrium have been associated with *dysmenorrhea* (painful menstruation).

THE MALE REPRODUCTIVE SYSTEM

The structural plan of the male reproductive system is divided into the external genitalia, consisting of the penis and scrotum, and the internal testes, glands, and ducts.

Testes

The main sex glands of the male are the two *testes*. Each oval-shaped testis is approximately 1.5 inches in length and 1 inch in width. They are encased in a fibrous sheath called the *tunica albuginea*. This is a tight protective sheath that does not allow for expansion when the testicles are inflamed. This is of particular importance when the male has mumps and the testicles do become inflamed. In many such cases sterility results from the adverse effect of increased heat production on spermatogenesis.

Within each testicle is an expanse of elongated convoluted loops called *seminiferous*

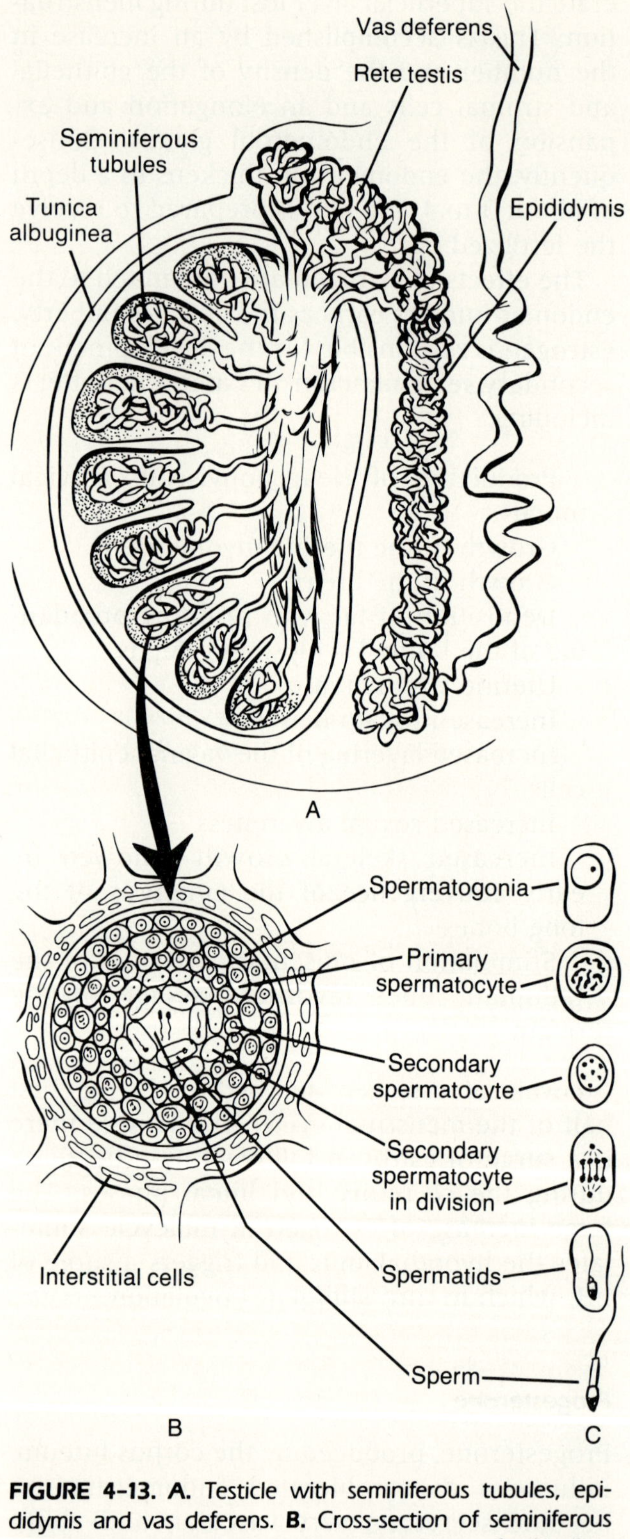

FIGURE 4-13. A. Testicle with seminiferous tubules, epididymis and vas deferens. **B.** Cross-section of seminiferous tubules showing interstitial cells, germinal layer of epithelium depicting various stages of spermatogenesis and sperm within lumen of the tube. **C.** Corresponding stages of spermatogenesis.

tubules (see Fig. 4–13). They are several hundred feet in length but are completely enclosed within the testicles. Seminiferous tubules participate in *spermatogenesis* (sperm production). Between the seminiferous tubules are clusters of cells termed *interstitial cells* (see Fig. 4–13). These cells secrete the male hormone *testosterone.*

The testes are considered internal organs. They are, however, contained within the external scrotal sac. The scrotum is divided into two compartments by a median septum. Outwardly, they are covered with rugated skin and lined on the inner surface with peritoneum. During early fetal life the testes are abdominal organs. Before birth, at about the eighth month, they descend through the inguinal canal into the scrotum. Failure of the testes to descend into the scrotum is called *cryptorchidism*. Because of the increased body heat, the sperm are destroyed and sterility may result if the condition is not corrected before puberty. The testes are not symmetrical in shape, with one being somewhat larger than the other. It appears in the normal male as if one is descended lower in the scrotal sac than the other.

EPIDIDYMIS AND VAS DEFERENS

Located on the lateral and anterior aspects of each testis is the *epididymis* (see Fig. 4–13). This narrow, tightly coiled tube, measuring 20 to 25 feet in length, serves as the passageway for the sperm from the seminiferous tubules to the vas deferens. Millions of sperm are produced daily in the seminiferous tubules and then undergo their final maturation process under the influence of secretions from the epithelium of the epididymis. The sperm are propelled through the epididymis by the peristaltic actions of the contractile tissue in the tubule walls. Upon arrival at the vas deferens, the sperm are mature and capable of motility.

The *vas deferens* (see Fig. 4–13) is a duct that transports the sperm from the epididymis through the inguinal canal to the urethra. A vas deferens extends from each testicle. Near the terminal end of the vas deferens it widens to form an area called the *ampulla* (see Fig. 4–14). Here, the vas deferens joins the seminal vesicle. Sperm is stored in the ampulla of the vas deferens. The united vas deferens and the seminal vesicle duct form the *ejaculatory duct*. The ejaculatory ducts traverse the prostate gland and terminate in the urethra.

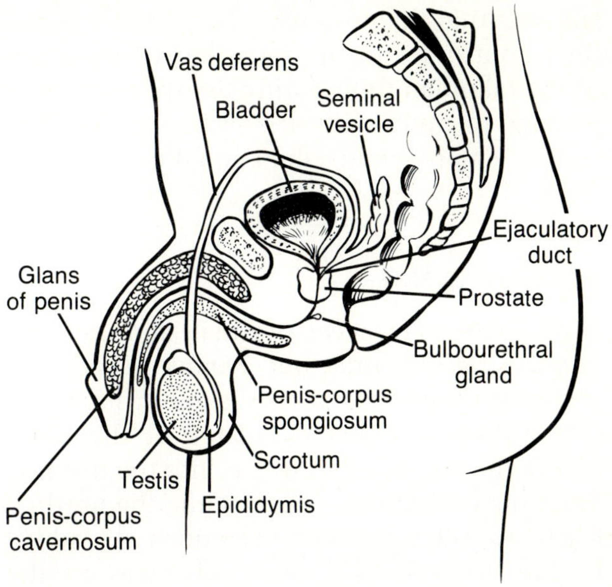

FIGURE 4–14. Internal male reproductive organs.

URETHRA

The urethra serves as the canal for the passage of both sperm and urine. It originates in the bladder, passes through the prostate (prostatic portion), and becomes the membranous urethra. It then enters the penis (penile urethra), where it descends through the corpus spongiosum.

SEMINAL VESICLES

The two *seminal vesicle glands* (see Fig. 4–14), located adjacent to the ampulla of the vas deferens, are lined with secretory columnar epithelium. They continually secrete seminal fluid, which is alkaline and composed of compounds such as fructrose, ascorbic acid, and proteins necessary for sperm survival. Seminal fluid, which is the major component of semen, aids in the dilution of the sperm, facilitating sperm motility. Prostaglandins constitute an important part of the seminal fluid. Research suggests that the prostaglandins in the seminal fluid contribute to the muscular contractions of the fallopian tube, aiding the sperm in their passage to unite with the ovum. The seminal vesicles empty seminal fluid into the ejaculatory duct.

PROSTATE GLAND

Unlike the other accessory male reproductive glands, there is only one *prostate gland*. This chestnut-shaped gland consisting of muscular and glandular tissue is located at the point where the vas deferens opens into the urethra. The prostate gland also opens into the urethra. The thin milky prostate secretions are added to the seminal fluid as it advances to the urethra. They enhance sperm motility by participating in the neutralization of the vaginal secretions. As the male ages, the prostate gland often enlarges, constricting the urethra and causing urinary retention. If this occurs, surgical removal of the prostate gland may be necessary.

BULBOURETHRAL GLAND (Cowper's glands)

Just below the prostate gland and bilateral to the urethra are located the two pea-sized *bulbourethral glands*. They add their contents to the seminal fluid before ejaculation and assist in lubrication of the urethra.

PENIS

The penis consists of a shaft composed of three cylindrical columns of erectile tissue. They are the two *corpora cavernosa* and the *corpus spongiosum* containing the urethra (see Fig. 4–14). The corpus spongiosum terminates to become the very sensitive *glans penis*. The glans penis is analogous to the female clitoris in its sensitivity. In uncircumcised males, the glans penis is covered by the *prepuce* (foreskin). Normally, the foreskin is completely retractable by one year of age; however, in some children, the foreskin will not retract and may occlude the urethral opening. This condition is called *phimosis*. Frequent cleaning under the foreskin is necessary to remove the accumulation of *smegma*, a cheesy odorous secretion, from the glands surrounding the frenulum of the penis. Circumcision is the operation used to remove the foreskin.

The penis is the organ of copulation, which, when stimulated by parasympathetic impulses, is capable of erection and enlargement. During sexual stimulation, there is dilatation of the arterioles, resulting in vasocongestion and erection of the penis. When not stimulated, the arterioles are constricted and the penis is flaccid.

During the height of sexual stimulation the sympathetic nervous system exerts its influence, conveying messages to the muscle cells of the genital ducts. The ducts respond, emitting their contents into the urethra and causing rhythmical contractions of the penis. Orgasm and ejaculation of the semen occur, followed by relaxation of the penis. Each ejaculation contains 2 to 4 ml of fluid and approximately 50 to 125 million sperm with 20 million/ml as the lower limit of normal. Repeated ejaculations during a given sexual episode will result in a decreased volume of semen and sperm.

When initially deposited in the female vagina, the semen coagulates. Fibrinolysin in the seminal fluid will cause the coagulation to dissolve and liquify in about 15 to 20 minutes. The sperm is capable of traveling 3mm/min through the uterus and fallopian tubes.

SPERM

The sperm of the human male resembles a tadpole, consisting of a head, a middle piece, and a tail (see Fig. 4–15). The head contains the nucleus of the sperm with a complete compliment of genetic material. In the frontal section of the head is the *acrosome*. Hydrolytic enzymes present in the acrosomes aid in the penetration of the zona pellicuda of the ovum. The middle portion of the sperm contains the *mitochondrial sheath*. Within this sheath, is produced the impetus necessary for propelling

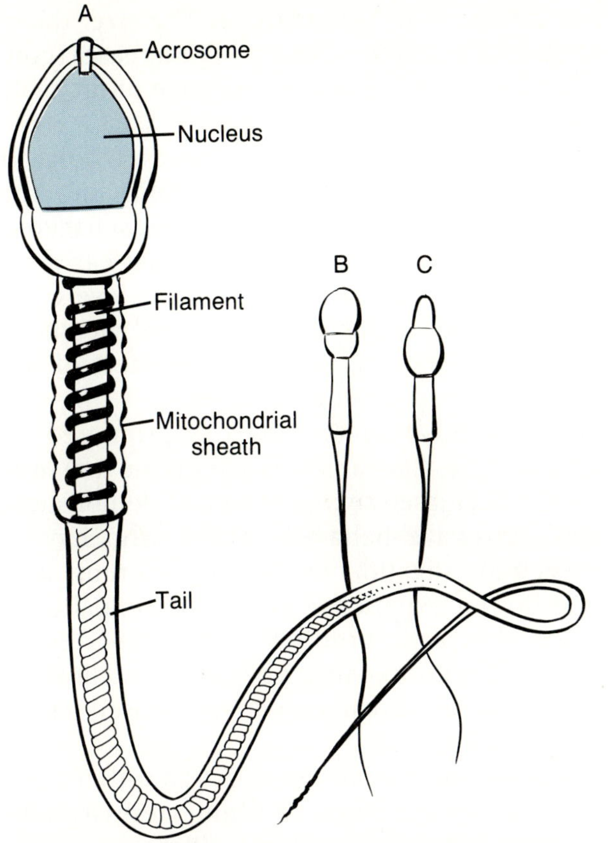

FIGURE 4-15. Mature human spermatozoan. **A.** Internal structure of spermatozoan. **B.** Front view. **C.** Side view.

the tail of the sperm. The undulating tail whips from side to side and propels the sperm on its journey through the genital tract.

Not all sperm that are ejaculated are normal. As many as one in five sperm in an ejaculation may be abnormal and incapable of motility or fertilization. Fertility may be directly altered if more than one in five abnormal sperm are found in an ejaculation.

Hormonal Influences

Puberty in the male initiates the onset of hormonal secretions necessary for reproduction. At this time, anterior pituitary hormones and testosterone exert their influence on the sex organs. The anterior pituitary hormones, FSH and LH are essentially the same as those in the female. However, their actions stimulate the testes rather than the ovaries. The testosterone is secreted by the testes and produces a wide spectrum of effects.

FOLLICLE STIMULATING AND LUTEINIZING HORMONE

Both the FSH and LH, secreted by the anterior pituitary in response to stimuli from the hypothalamus, are essential for spermatogenesis. The FSH is responsible for the transformation of the primary spermatocytes into secondary spermatocytes within the seminiferous tubules. The LH in turn will stimulate the interstitial cells of the testes to secrete testosterone. For this reason, LH is often referred to as ICSH (interstitial cell-stimulating hormone). Under the influence of testosterone, spermatogenesis proceeds to completion.

A negative feedback to the hypothalamus results when testosterone levels are high. This effect appears to be more pronounced for LH than FSH. This feedback control maintains the secretion of testosterone at a constant level.

Spermatogenesis exerts an inhibitory effect on FSH. The exact mechanism of this effect is not known. An unidentified hormone secreted by the testicles may be responsible.

TESTOSTERONE

Testosterone, secreted by the interstitial cells of the testes, is the most profound of all the androgens. It affects spermatogenesis, male growth, and the development of male secondary sexual characteristics. Even in embryonic life, testosterone has an effect on the development of male or female genital organs (see Chapter 6). During childhood little or no testosterone is secreted. It remains at a constant level during most of the mature male's life; however, it does decline steadily after age 40 but remains adequate for spermatogenesis well into later maturity for many men. Mature male production of testosterone is 6 to 8 mg/day. (Kolodny et al., 1979).

At puberty, when testosterone exerts its influence, the male penis, testes, scrotum, prostate, and seminal vesicles demonstrate changes. The penis enlargens and grows to a mature length of 4 to 6 inches when erect. The testicles enlargen and the scrotum darkens in color. The prostate and seminal vesicles produce their secretions and the young male may experience nocturnal emissions (wet dreams).

During this same period of adolescence, distinct patterns of hair distribution will develop. Hair growth develops on the face, back, chest, axillary area, and pubic area. Hair on the arms and legs becomes coarser. Scalp hair is not as directly attributed to large production of testosterone. This is not to say that the male with a full head of hair is not as masculine as the bald man. It merely indicates that because of a genetic predisposition, high levels of testosterone will decrease the growth of scalp hair in some men.

The typically deep male voice is another effect of testosterone. The boy soprano develops into a tenor. This change is brought about by the growth of the larynx.

Bone growth in the male increases owing to the influence of testosterone. The size, thickness, and strength of the bone increases, contributing to the typical appearance of the male frame.

Skeletal muscle mass increases owing to inclusion of nitrogen from protein into the muscle. The skin thickens and the sebaceous glands become more active. During early adjustments to increased testosterone levels, the male often develops acne. The basal metabolic rate also increases owing to the effect of testosterone on protein anabolism.

Sexual drive in the male is promoted by testosterone. Castrated (testicles removed) men have a decreased sexual drive and demonstrate less aggressive behavior. Males who have a vasectomy (ligation of the vas deferens) as a rule do not experience decreased sexual drive since they still produce and utilize testosterone. Homosexuality has not been clinically proven to be associated with decreased testosterone levels.

Support of spermatogenesis is another function of testosterone. Without testosterone, sperm will be produced but will not mature.

BIBLIOGRAPHY

Guyton, A. *Textbook of medical physiology*. Philadelphia: Saunders, 1981.

Kolodny, R., Masters, W., Johnson, V., & Biggs, M. *Textbook of human sexuality for nurses*. Boston: Little, Brown, 1979.

MacLaughlin, S. & Taubenheim, A. Epidural anesthesia for obstetric patients. *Journal of Gynecological & Neonatal Nursing*, 1981, **10**, 9-14.

Vander, A., Sherman, J. & Luciano, D. *Human physiology*. New York: McGraw-Hill, 1975.

chapter 5

THE GENETICS OF REPRODUCTION

OBJECTIVES

Upon completion of this chapter, the reader will be able to:

1. Define genetics.
2. State the normal diploid number of chromosomes in the human.
3. Differentiate between genotype and phenotype.
4. Describe protein synthesis.
5. Briefly describe events that occur during prophase, metaphase, anaphase, telophase, and interphase.
6. State what occurs during the first meiotic division and during the second meiotic division.
7. Define primary oocyte, primordial follicle, spermatocyte, and spermatogonia.
8. List the four mechanisms that lead to nonmultiple chromosomal abnormalities.
9. Define deletion, translocation, and ring formation.
10. State three common trisomies.
11. Briefly describe the four main patterns of single gene defects.
12. List three examples of polygenic defects.
13. Define genetic counseling.
14. List the five main goals of genetic counseling.
15. Discuss the role of the nurse in genetic counseling.
16. Describe four tests that may be ordered to aid in diagnosis of genetic disorders.

KEY TERMS

Alleles
Alpha-fetoprotein
Amniocentesis
Amniography
Autosome
Chromosome
Chromosome lag
Deletion
Deoxyribonucleic acid
Fetoscopy
Gene
Genetic counseling
Genetics
Genotype
Heterozygous
Homozygous
Maple syrup urine disease
Meiosis
Mitosis
Monosomy
Mosaicism
Neural tube defects
Oogenesis
Phenotype
Phenylketonuria
Polygenic inheritance
Primary follicle
Ribonucleic acid
Ring formation
Spermatogenesis
Spermatogonia
Translocation
Trisomy
Ultrasound

Genetics is defined as the study of heredity. At conception, each human has a set genetic inheritance that determines his or her potential for development. Life continues because of the ability of human cells to divide, replicate, and transfer characteristics to new cells.

The number of requests for genetic diagnosis during pregnancy has increased dramatically during the last decade. These requests may come from individuals with a family history of genetic anomaly or from referrals by a health care professional. A basic knowledge of genetics is needed by the nurse to help guide and support the childbearing family that may be at risk for producing an infant with a birth defect.

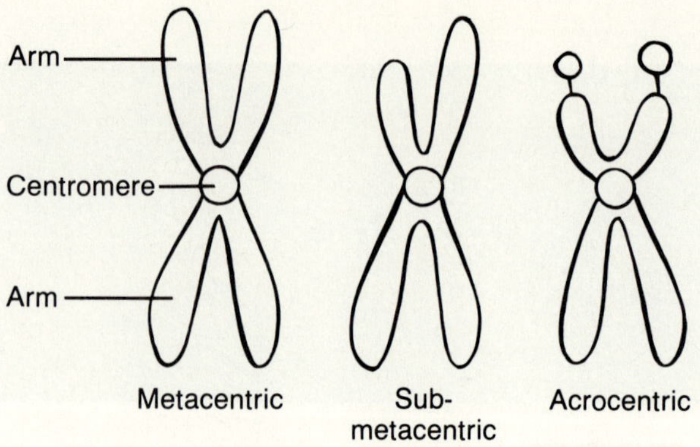

FIGURE 5-1. Chromosome morphology.

TABLE 5-1
CLASSIFICATION OF CHROMOSOMES

Group	Chromosomes by Pairs
A	1, 2, 3
B	4, 5
C	6, 7, 8, 9, 10, 11, 12, X
D	13, 14, 15
E	16, 17, 18
F	19, 20
G	21, 22, Y

CHROMOSOMES AND GENES

Chromosomes

Chromosomes are elongated, dark-staining bodies contained within the nucleus of each cell they consist of a central thread (*chromonema*), a series of beadlike structures (*chromomeres*) that lie along the chromonema, and a small circular zone (*centromere*) present at a fixed point along its length.

Chromosomes usually occur in pairs. The normal diploid chromosome number in the human is 46, of which there are 44 autosomes and two sex chromosomes. The sex chromosome constitution of the male is labeled XY and of the female XX. Chromosomes that are not sex chromosomes are called autosomes.

At the time of cell division, chromosomes are most visible; at other times they appear as very long fine strands (*chromatin*). They are classified according to total length, position of the centromere, and the length of the arms on the side of the centromere. All chromosomes are one of three shapes (see Fig. 5-1): (1) *metacentric*, with the centromere approximately in the center; (2) *submetacentric*, with the centromere closer to one end than to the other; and (3) *acrocentric*, with the centromere near one end of the chromosome.

Chromosomes are organized into seven groups identified by the letters A through G, arranged in order of descending length. Like chromosomes are matched according to their shape and size and assigned into groups (see Table 5-1). A systematically arranged set of chromosomes is called a *karyotype* (see Figs. 5-2 and 5-3) and gives the genetic picture of an individual when all the chromosomes are arranged.

Genes

Genes are points or regions on chromosomes, made up of molecules of deoxyribonucleic

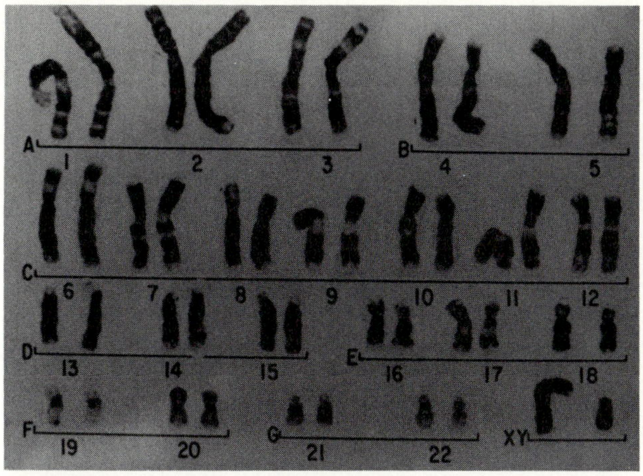

FIGURE 5-2. Normal male karotype. There are 46 chromosomes present. Note the one X and one Y chromosome. (Photo courtesy of Alexander P. vonRothe, M.D.)

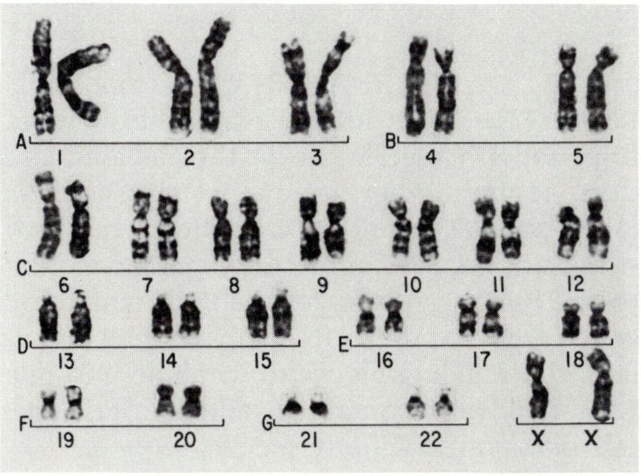

FIGURE 5-3. Normal female karotype. There are 46 chromosomes present. Note the two X chromosomes. (Photo courtesy of Alexander P. vonRothe, M.D.)

acid (DNA) and arranged in a linear order. They carry the genetic information that determines the characteristics of a given individual.

In any pair of genes, there are contrasting forms or states of the gene, known as *alleles*. Some genes have multiple alleles; for example, there are three alleles for blood types. If an individual has the same alleles for a trait on each gene of a pair, the person is said to be *homozygous* for that trait. One of the two alleles may be different; this individual is *heterozygous* for that trait. One of the two alleles may be dominant and will manifest itself in the physical characteristics of that individual. The other gene of the pair is recessive and will not be noticed physically.

A description of the genetic constitution of an individual is called a *genotype*. Genotypes are constant and are fixed at the time of fertilization. A *phenotype* is the result of interactions between the genotype and its nongenetic environment and is seen in the external appearance of an individual.

Deoxyribonucleic Acid (DNA)

Genes consist of a long double stranded helical molecule of *deoxyribonucleic acid* (*DNA*) (see Fig. 5–4). The DNA molecule is composed of smaller units called *nucleotides*. The nucleotides are made up of two very long strands of alternating deoxyribose (sugar) and phosphoric acid. Attached to each deoxyribose molecule is one of four nitrogenous bases. The four bases are the purines, adenine and guanine, and the pyramidines, thymine and cytosine. These bases are represented by the letters A, G, T, and C, respectively.

The nitrogenous bases of each strand face each other and are loosely bound by hydrogen bonds in opposite matching pairs. The deoxyribose and phosphoric acid sequences serve as the sides of the ladderlike structure and twist to form a double spiral or helix. The pairing of the bases is specific and determines the genetic code. Exact replication is needed for new daughter cells to be produced from mitosis.

Ribonucleic Acid (RNA)

A group of molecules found mostly in the cytoplasm that function to organize and coordinate the activities of DNA are called *ribonucleic acid* (*RNA*). RNA reads the information in DNA, interprets it, takes the message to the ribosomes, and supervises the making

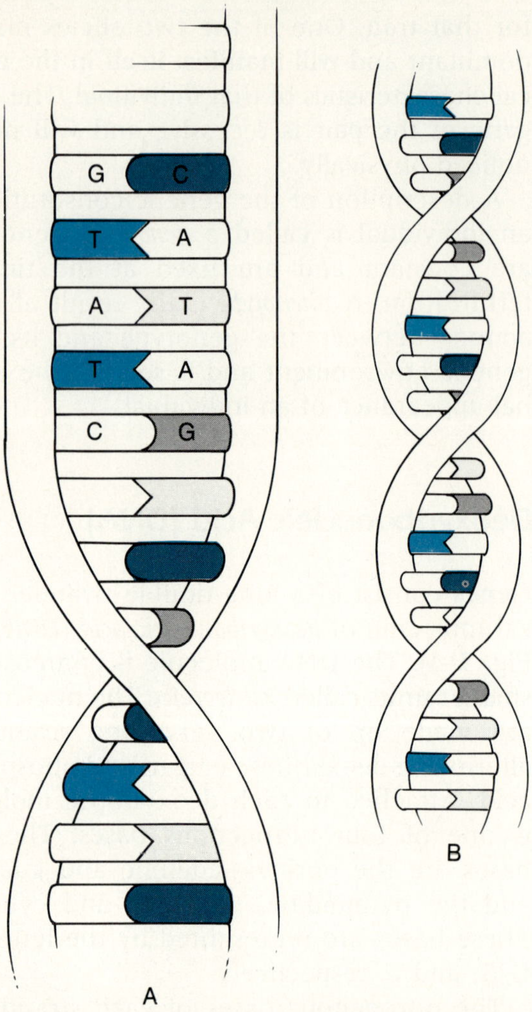

FIGURE 5-4. Deoxyribonucleic acid (DNA): A. Structure of DNA. B. DNA with 2 nucleotide chains linked with a double helix.

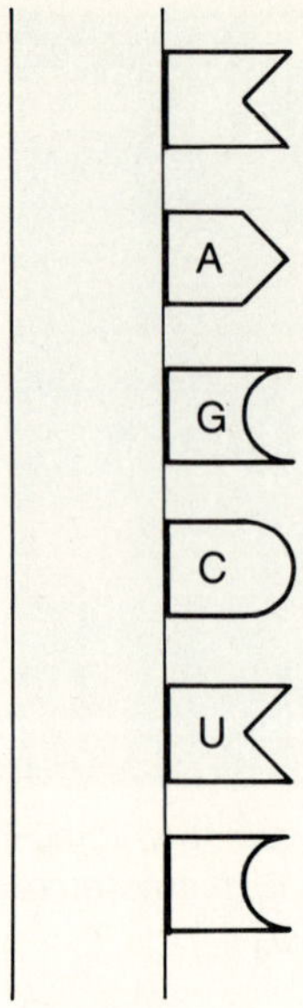

FIGURE 5-5. Structure of ribonucleic acid (RNA).

of the proteins in the proper manner (see Figure 5-5).

RNA is single stranded and contains the sugar ribose and the base uracil. One strand of DNA acts in the synthesis of each type of RNA molecule. For RNA to be synthesized, four stages must occur: (1) formation of RNA nucleotides, (2) activation of the nucleotides, (3) combination of activated nucleotides with a DNA strand, and (4) polymerization of the RNA chain.

After RNA is formed it is transported into the cytoplasm, where three separate types control protein synthesis: messenger RNA (mRNA), transfer RNA (tRNA), and ribosomal RNA (rRNA). The mRNA reads the message from the DNA molecule in the nucleus into the cytoplasm where actual protein synthesis takes place. The mRNA is formed when two strands of the DNA molecule separate and the paired building blocks for the RNA match the code of the exposed DNA. An enzyme stimulates the building blocks to combine into one RNA molecule, containing adenine, guanine, cytosine, and uracil in a specific sequence.

After matching with DNA, the RNA bases, working together as triplets or codons, are ready to read the DNA message. There are 84 codons, with each codon specifying the message for starting or stopping production of amino acids. The sequence of amino acids along a protein chain determines the nature of a protein molecule. The mRNA that contains the information in the gene of the DNA then moves to the cytoplasm.

The tRNA circulates around the cytoplasm, where it captures stray amino acids and transfers these amino acid molecules to protein molecules as the protein is being synthesized. There is a separate type of tRNA for each of the 20 amino acids that are incorporated into proteins.

The site of actual protein synthesis is at the ribosomes, which are made up of rRNA and special ribosomal proteins. The rRNA is a very stable molecule of high molecular weight that determines the alignment of the mRNA when it reaches the ribosome from the nucleus.

The tRNA, and its attached amino acid, first binds with one of the ribosomal particles. As mRNA passes through the ribosome, the amino acid is released to the forming protein while the tRNA is released back into the cytoplasm to combine with another amino acid molecule of the same type.

Protein Synthesis

Protein synthesis begins with the uncoiling of a specific DNA molecule in the nucleus. RNA parts move to line up along the code strand of the uncoiled DNA molecule, according to the base-pair rule.

The mRNA is formed and migrates out of the nucleus to the ribosomes in the cytoplasm. In the meantime, the tRNA has collected the amino acids and carried them to the ribosomes for synthesis of the protein molecule.

As the mRNA arrives at the ribosomes, it is sequentially translated and the amino acids are properly lined up, ready for protein formation. The ribosome stimulates the properly arranged amino acids to form the specific protein (see Fig. 5–6).

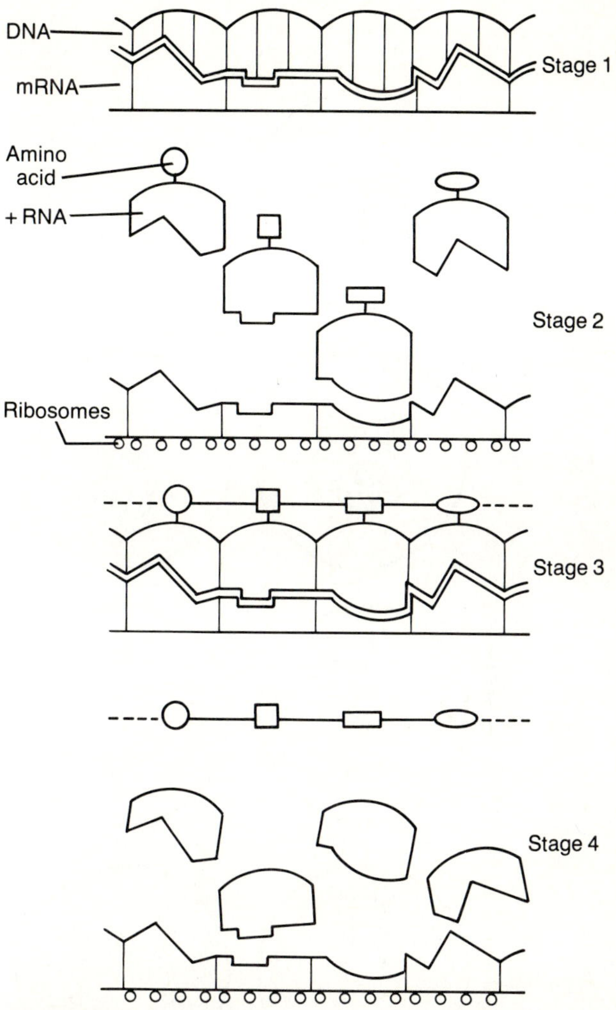

FIGURE 5–6. Protein synthesis: Stage 1. Cell nucleus preparation. DNA transfers the protein pattern to mRNA. Stage 2. The amino acids in the cell cytoplasm attach to tRNA. Stage 3. tRNA carries amino acids into position, forming the peptide linkage. Stage 4. Polypeptide chain breaks free; tRNA is released.

CELL DIVISION

Mitosis

The process by which all cells divide, with the exception of those cells that produce ova and sperm, is called *mitosis*. The result is two cells from one. The entire process occurs in four stages: prophase, metaphase, anaphase, and telophase; and interphase, the period between mitoses (see Fig. 5–7).

INTERPHASE

During *interphase*, replication of DNA and duplication of chromatin occurs. The two pairs of centrioles lie close to each other near one pole of the nucleus and at right angles to each other. Cells remain in interphase for varying periods of time.

Shortly before mitosis is to take place, the two pairs begin to move apart. Microtubules of protein (the spindle) begin to grow between

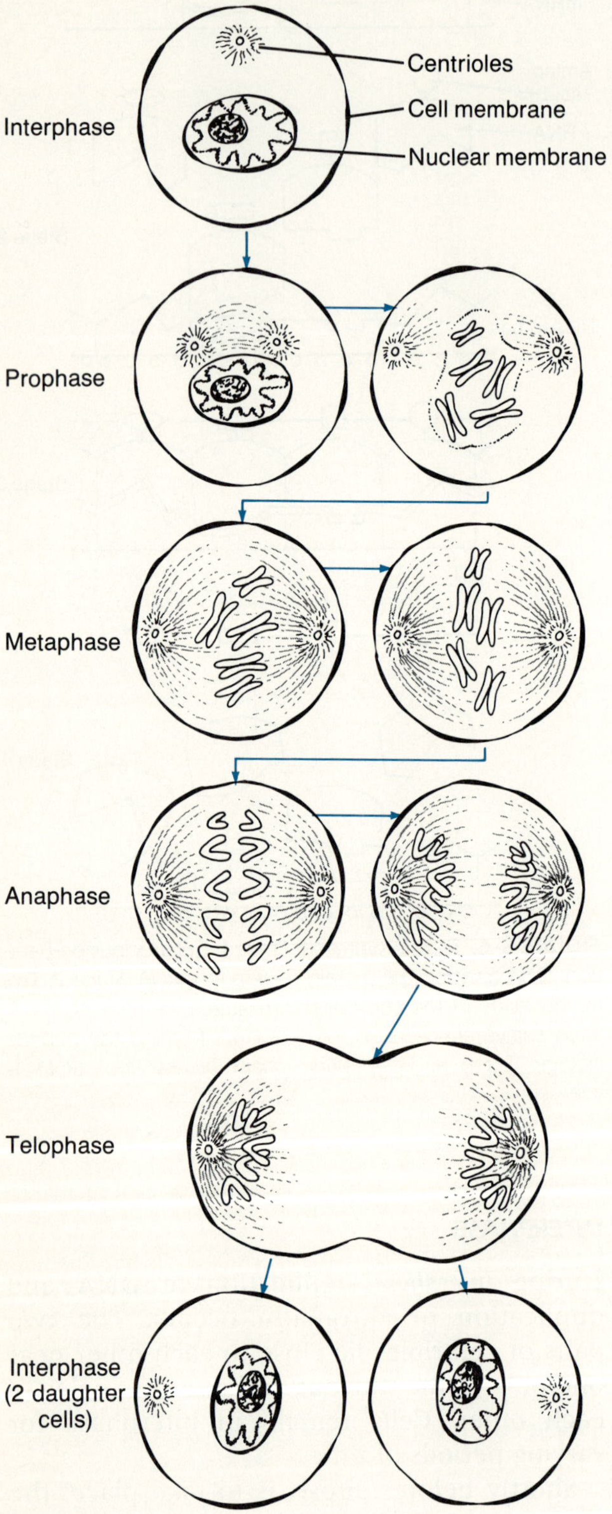

FIGURE 5-7. Mitosis.

them and then away from the centrioles. The entire set of microtubules plus the centriole is called the *mitotic apparatus*. While the spindle is forming, the chromatin material of the nucleus becomes condensed into well-defined chromosomes.

PROPHASE

Prophase begins when the chromatin threads begin to condense and chromosomes appear as thickening threads within the nucleus. As they grow thicker and shorter, they are held together at the centromere. The two daughter centrioles move to opposite sides of the cell and an achromatic spindle forms. Prophase lasts 30 to 60 minutes.

METAPHASE

When the spindle formation is complete the chromosomes line up across the spindle. The centromeres divide, begin to move apart, and the two chromatids become completely separate daughter chromosomes. *Metaphase* lasts 2 to 6 minutes.

ANAPHASE

During *anaphase*, which lasts 3 to 15 minutes, the chromosomes move to opposite poles. All 46 pairs of chromatids are separated, forming 46 daughter cells pulled to one end of the spindle, and 46 daughter cells pulled to the opposite end.

TELOPHASE

The last stage, telophase, lasts 30 to 60 minutes. During this stage the chromosomes elongate and return to their resting state, in which only the chromatin threads are visible. A new nuclear membrane forms around each set of chromosomes and the mitotic apparatus undergoes dissolution.

Meiosis

Meiosis is a pair of cell divisions during which the chromosome number is reduced by half. Each male or female germ cell receives only one of each kind of chromosome. The two cell divisions occur in succession, and each includes a prophase, metaphase, anaphase, and telophase.

FIRST MEIOTIC DIVISION (see Fig. 5-8)

Prophase

There are four stages within this phase: leptotene, zygotene, pachytene, and diplotene. In the *leptotene stage*, the chromosomes that were long thin strands become shorter and thicker. The homologous chromosomes undergo synapsis while the chromosomes are still long and thin. In the *zygotene stage*, the homologous chromosomes lie side by side and twist around each other. Each chromosome becomes visibly double and is called *bivalent*. Female sex chromosomes (XX) are alike and can pair, while the male sex chromosomes (XY) can only join together at the tip of the arms. During the *pachytene stage*, the chromosomes continue to thicken. There are two chromatids for each chromosome with four strands of genetic material. The pairs begin to separate. In the fourth or *diplotene stage*, there is a longitudinal separation of part of each chromosome. The chromatids remain joined at the centromere, creating an X-shaped junction. At the end of prophase, the double chromosomes have undergone synapsis, yielding a bundle of four homologous chromosomes called a *tetrad*.

While the chromosomes are undergoing synapsis, the homologous chromosomes may exchange segments, a process called *crossing over*. With this process, an exchange of chromosome segments occurs at random along the length of the chromosome, allowing gene transfer. Crossing over changes the distribution of chromatin before it divides. Together the two chromosomes of a pair have the same amount and kind of genetic material as before, but they will carry different genetic patterns when they separate.

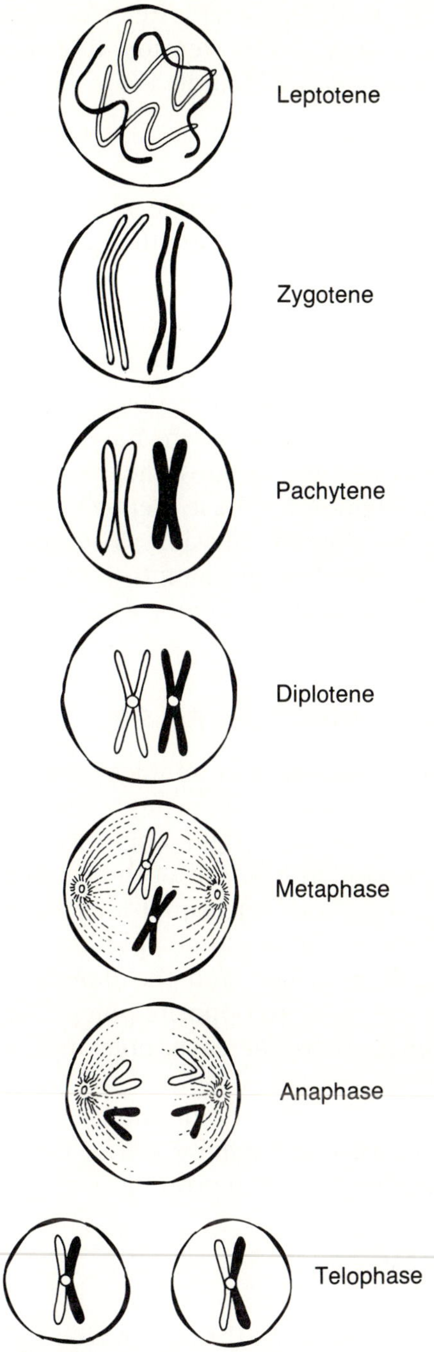

FIGURE 5-8. First meiotic division.

Metaphase

While these events are occurring, the two centrioles move to opposite poles, a spindle forms in the middle, and the nuclear membrane disappears. The tetrads line up around the equator of the spindle.

Anaphase

The daughter chromatids separate and move toward opposite poles, separating the homologous chromosomes.

Telophase

The cells become completely separated and form two daughter cells, each having 22 autosomes and one sex chromosome.

There is no clear interphase between the first and second meiotic division. The telophase on the first division blends into the prophase of the second. No synthesis of DNA occurs.

SECOND MEIOTIC DIVISION (see Fig. 5-9)

The second meiotic division resembles mitosis. The centriole divides, with a new spindle forming in each cell at a right angle to the spindle of the first division. Half of the double chromosomes line up on the equator of each spindle. No further chromosome splitting occurs. The centrioles divide and the daughter cells separate and move to opposite poles. The 23 chromosomes arrive at each pole and a membrane forms.

The two successive meiotic divisions result in the formation of four nuclei. Each of these has one of each kind of chromosome.

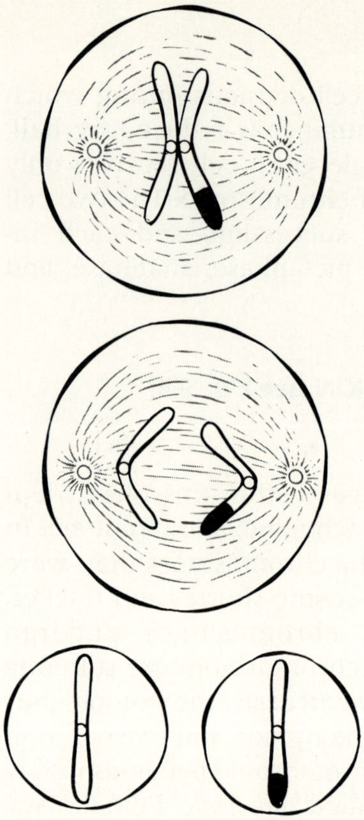

FIGURE 5-9. Second meiotic division.

GAMETOGENESIS

Gametogenesis is the process through which the primitive female and male germ cells are changed into mature gametes. This process relies on both mitosis and meiosis.

Oogenesis

Oogenesis is the formation and development of the ovum, which begins early in fetal development (see Fig. 5-10). During very early fetal development primordial germ cells migrate from the yolk sac into the developing ovaries, then differentiate into oogonia. By 12 weeks of gestation, the oogonia begin mitotic divisions to form primary oocytes. The oogonia and oocytes that develop are surrounded by a layer of follicle cells derived from the epithelium of the ovaries.

At birth the primary oocytes are in late prophase of the first meiotic division and are called *primary follicles*. There are approximately 4 million follicles present in the two ovaries at birth. These follicles remain in suspended prophase until puberty.

Division of the cytoplasm is unequal, resulting in one large cell, the *secondary oocyte*, which contains the yolk and most of the cytoplasm, and one small cell, the *first polar body*, which consists of just a nucleus. The formation of

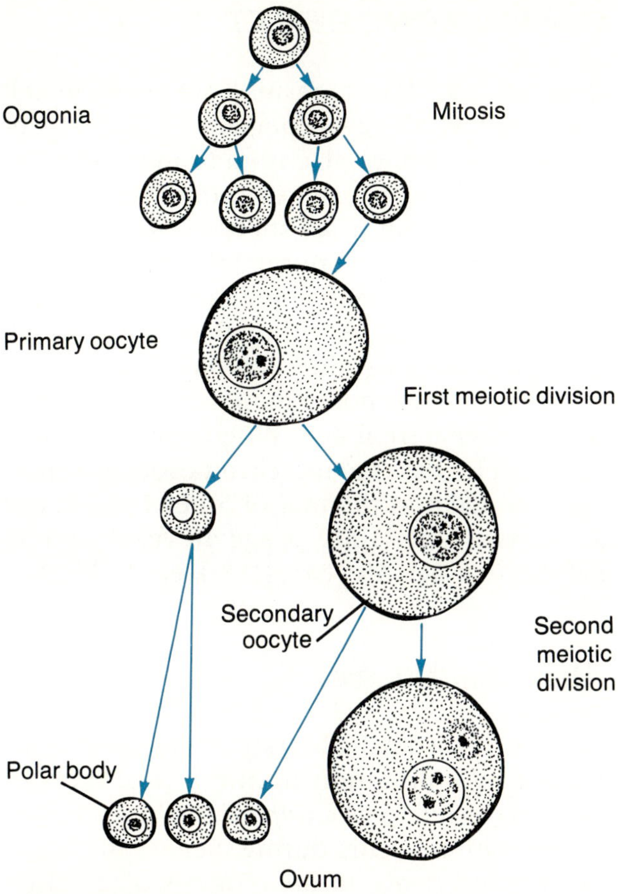

FIGURE 5-10. Oogenesis.

polar bodies enables the maturing egg to eliminate its excess chromosomes without losing yolk and cytoplasm needed for survival of the mature egg after fertilization.

The secondary meiotic division is usually not completed until after fertilization. As the ovum enters the fallopian tube, the secondary oocyte divides unequally into a large ootid and a small second polar body, each containing a haploid number of chromosomes. Each primary oocyte gives rise to one ovum (see Chapter 6).

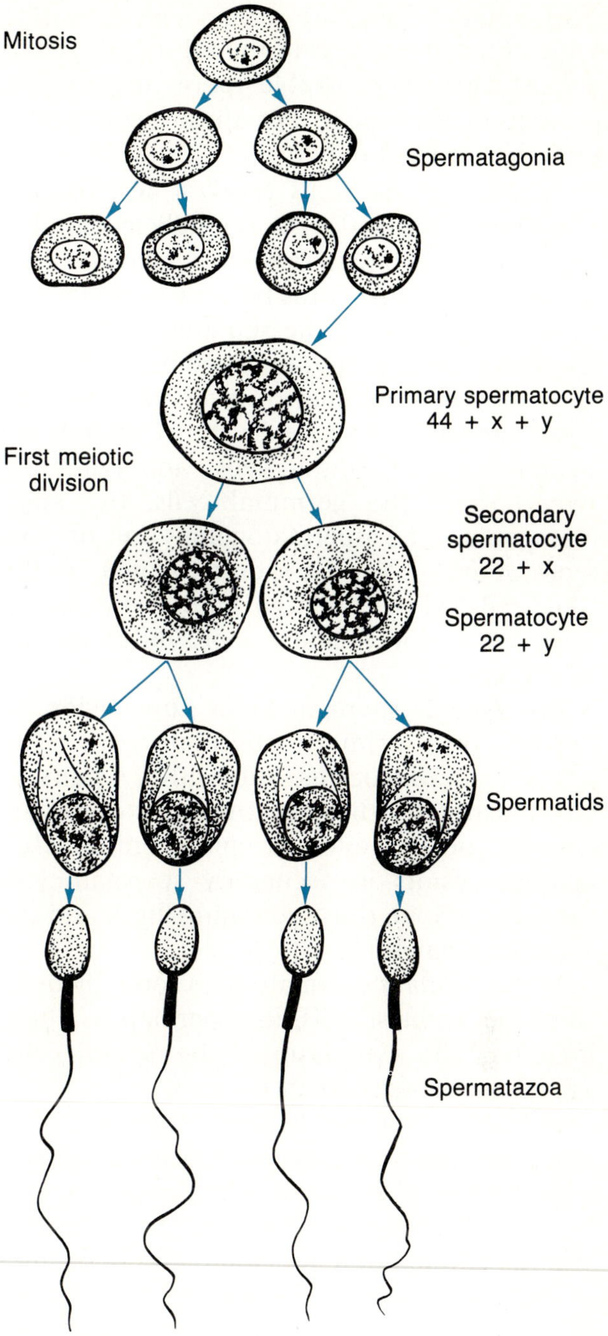

FIGURE 5-11. Spermatogenesis.

Spermatogenesis

Spermatogenesis is the sequence of events by which spermatogonia are transformed into mature spermatozoa in the male testes (see Fig. 5-11).

Primordial germ cells appear in the yolk sac at 25 days of gestation and migrate to the primary gonadal folds. By four weeks of gestation there may be more than 1000 germ cells in the area of the future gonad. At seven weeks of gestation mitosis ends and the germ cells enter a long premeiotic phase, during which the central cells of the tubules degenerate. At birth recognizable spermatogonia are present in the testes, but these lie dormant until the onset of puberty.

At puberty, about 13 years of age, the anterior pituitary gland sends out follicle-stimulating hormone (FSH), which reactivates the testes. The original cords become seminiferous tubules. The wall of the seminiferous tubules has a basement membrane lined by epithelium consisting of a number of layers of cells. The basal layer is of two types: the scattered, tall pyramid-shaped Sertoli cells, and lying between these the germinal cells, the spermatogonia. The spermatogonia are of two types, A and B. Type A spermatogonia are the stem cells which undergo mitotic division to form other type A and a more differentiated type B cell.

The type B spermatogonia now divide by mitosis into primary spermatocytes. The primary spermatocytes, still with 23 pairs of chromosomes, migrate toward the middle zone of the seminiferous epithelium. Further division results in secondary spermatocytes that are haploid, thus separating the X and the Y chromosomes.

The secondary spermatocytes soon divide to form the smallest cells, the spermatids. These imbed in the cytoplasm of the Sertoli cells. This process takes about 64 days.

To become functional sperm the spermatids must undergo a complicated process of growth and change. The nucleus shrinks in size and becomes the head of the sperm. The cytoplasm with its endoplasmic reticulum and ribosomes is shed. Golgi bodies group at the front end of the sperm to form the acrosome. The two centrioles move to a position just behind the nucleus. The mitochondria move to the junction of the tail and head, and form a spiral middle piece that provides energy.

The sperm leave the Sertoli cell and become free in the seminiferous tubules. Sperm move through the straight tubules, rete testis, and efferent ductules to the epididymis (see Chapter 6).

CHROMOSOME DEFECTS

Chromosome defects result from errors in cell division. Five to seven percent of all conceptuses have abnormal chromosomes, and the majority of these result in spontaneous abortion. Five percent of all stillborns are found to be chromosomally abnormal (March of Dimes, 1983). Chromosomal defects are found in 1 of every 200 live births, although they are not all associated with harmful defects.

One risk factor noted in many chromosomal defects is maternal age. When age is the only identifiable risk factor, chromosomal abnormalities occur at the rate of 5 per 1000 at age 35 years, 15 per 1000 at age 40 years, and 50 per 1000 at age 45 years (Hook et al., 1983).

Abnormal Number

Any chromosomal aberration that is characterized by a deviation from the total number (46) is referred to as *aneuploidy*. When a failure of separation occurs during meiosis the aneuploid gametes are formed, one with 24 chromosomes, and one with 22 chromosomes. When fertilization takes place, the resulting zygote will contain 47 and 45 chromosomes.

Numerical chromosomal anomalies can occur in multiples and nonmultiples. Multiples are those beyond the normal doubling of the haploid number. For example, in *triploidy* there are three sets of 23 chromosomes (69 total chromosomes); in *tetraploidy* four sets of 23 chromosomes are present for a total of 92 chromosomes.

Nonmultiples include monosomy and trisomy. In *monosomy* there is one less than the normal number of chromosomes (45 chromosomes). In *trisomy* an additional chromosome is present, making three chromosomes instead of the usual pair. Three of the most common trisomies are trisomy 21, trisomy 18, and trisomy 13.

Four mechanisms can lead to nonmultiple chromosomal anomalies: nondisjunction, chromosome lag, mosaicism, and translocation.

In *nondisjunction*, a chromosome pair fails to separate normally and both members of a pair move into one cell during the first or second meiotic division. One gamete then contains two of a particular chromosome while the other does not have that chromosome. When the sperm fertilizes the ovum, it contributes the third chromosome, resulting in trisomy (see Fig. 5-12). *Chromosome lag* occurs when chromosomes separate successfully during metaphase, but then one fails to migrate properly during anaphase. *Mosaicism* is present if only a portion of the body cells of an individual contain a variation in the number of chromosomes. Since the final number of chromosomes remain normal in translocation, it will be described under structural abnormalities.

Abnormal Structure

Chromosomal defects are also caused by structural abnormalities, such as deletion, translocation, ring formation, and inversion.

DELETION

In *deletion* a piece of chromosome is broken off and lost during gamete formation. One example of deletion is cri du chat syndrome, in which there is a deletion of a short arm of chromosome five. Characteristics associated with cri du chat syndrome include microcephaly, downward slanted eyes, abnormal width between the eyes (ocular hypertelorism), a rounded face, catlike cry, short metatarsals, retarded growth, and mental deficiency.

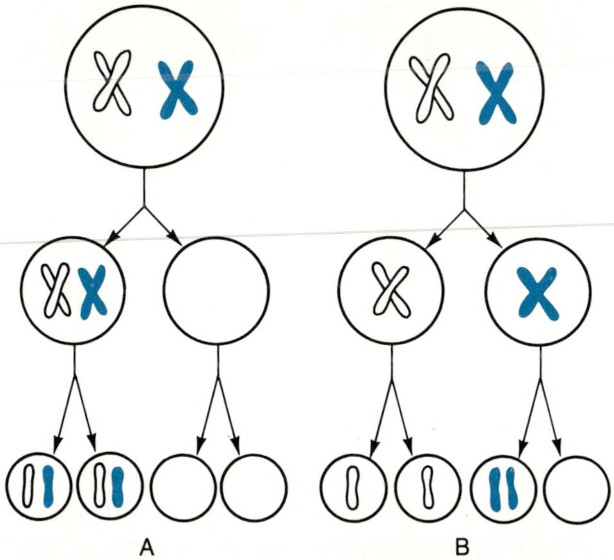

FIGURE 5-12. A. Nondisjunction. B. Normal cell division.

TRANSLOCATION

Translocation is the transfer of a segment of a chromosome to a different site on the same chromosome (reciprocal) or to a different chromosome (centric fusion).

RING FORMATION

In *ring formation* the two ends of a chromosome may reach around and touch each other, resulting in a ring-shaped structures.

INVERSION

A malfunction of crossing over can result in *inversion*, in which a section of the chromosome is taken, turned end-to-end, and reinserted in the wrong order.

Trisomies

Three of the more common trisomies are trisomy 21 (Down's syndrome), trisomy 18 (Edward's syndrome), and trisomy 13 (Patau's syndrome).

TRIMSOMY 21

Down's syndrome or *trisomy 21* is the most common trisomy, occurring in 1 of 600 births in all races. The affected individual has an extra number 21 chromosome for a total of 47. Some 94 percent of trisomy 21 cases are caused by nondisjunction, with the remaining cases caused by translocation and mosaicism.

The risk of having a child with trisomy 21 increases with maternal age (see Table 5-2)

TABLE 5-2
RISK OF DOWN'S SYNDROME

Incidence	Maternal Age
1:3000	under 30 years
1:600	30 to 34 years
1:280	35 to 39 years
1:80	40 to 44 years
1:40	over 44 years

and with the incidence of spontaneous abortions. Table 5-3 summarizes the clinical features noted in trisomy 21. A karyotype of an individual with trisomy 21 is seen in Figure 5-13.

TRISOMY 18

Edward's syndrome or *trisomy 18* occurs in 1 of every 2000 births. These individuals have an extra chromosome 18, causing certain identifiable characteristics (see Table 5-4).

TRISOMY 13

Patau's syndrome or *trisomy 13* occurs in 1 of every 4000 to 5000 births. An extra chromosome 13 causes certain clinical features to be noted (see Table 5-5).

Sex Chromosome Defects

Several syndromes are associated with defects in the sex chromosomes, including Turner's syndrome (45XO) and Klinefelter's syndrome (47XXY).

TURNER'S SYNDROME

Turner's syndrome (45XO) occurs in 1 of every 5000 females and is characterized by 45 chromosomes: 22 autosomes, plus one X and one Y chromosome with no Barr bodies seen. This syndrome occurs as a result of nondisjunction in the male gamete during meiosis. Clinical features noted in these individuals are summarized in Table 5-6.

TABLE 5-3
CLINICAL FEATURES OF TRISOMY 21

- Small rounded head
- Epicanthic folds
- Brush field spots on iris of eyes
- Strabismus
- Flat nose
- Small mouth
- Protruding tongue
- Low-set ears
- Short broad neck
- Broad, flat, square hands
- Single transverse palmar crease
- Ten ulnar loops on digits
- Short extremities
- Small loops on sole of foot
- Mental retardation
- Hypotonia
- Increased incidence of leukemia
- Increased incidence of heart defects
- Intestinal anomalies
- Susceptibility to respiratory infections
- Intolerance to atropine

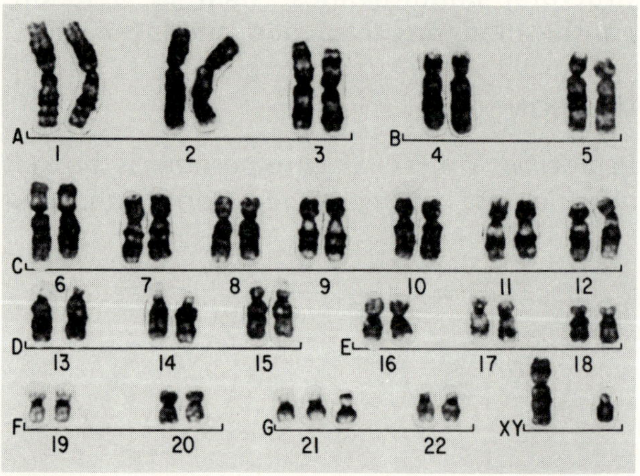

FIGURE 5-13. Karotype of an individual with Down's syndrome (trisomy 21). There are 46 chromosomes present. Note that there are three number 21 chromosomes instead of the normal two. (Photo courtesy of Alexander P. vonRothe, M.D.)

KLINEFELTER'S SYNDROME

The incidence of *Klinefelter's syndrome* is 1 in every 600 male births. This syndrome is caused by nondisjunction or mosaicism and has characteristic clinical features (see Table 5-7).

TABLE 5-4
CLINICAL FEATURES OF TRISOMY 18

Prominent occiput
Open skull sutures
High arched eyebrows
Small face
Abnormally small jaw (micrognathia)
Malformed low-set ears
Short sternum
Overlapping of fingers
Rocker bottom feet
Low birth weight
Mental retardation
Congenital heart defects
Ventricular septal defects
Patent ductus arteriosus
Horseshoe kidneys
Spasticity
Flexion contractures
Hypotonia
Failure to thrive

TABLE 5-5
CLINICAL FEATURES OF TRISOMY 13

Microcephaly
Small eyes (microophthalmia)
Scalp defects
Cleft palate
Low-set ears
Undescended testes (cryptorchidism)
Extra digits (polydactyly)
Deformed fingernails
Flexion deformities
Growth failure
Severe mental retardation
Kidney cysts
Double ureters
Deafness
Congenital heart disease
Atrial septal defect
Ventral septal defect
Patent ductus arteriosus

SINGLE GENE DEFECTS

Single gene defects are caused by the inheritance of a single abnormal gene or pair of abnormal genes. Genes occur in pairs and are located on chromosomes that are homologous. One chromosome is maternal in origin and the other is paternal. If the two genes have the same defect, the individual is homozygous for that defect.

TABLE 5-6
PHENOTYPIC FEATURES IN TURNER'S SYNDROME

Typical facies—sphinx face, carp mouth
Low-set ears
Webbed neck
Low hairline
Broad chest
No breast development
Excessive nevi
Streak ovaries
Small uterus
Hyperconvex or deep set fingernails
Hand and feet edema
Short stature
Infertility
Primary amenorrhea
Perceptual difficulties
Normal intelligence
Congenital cardiac defects
Renal anomalies

TABLE 5-7
PHENOTYPIC FEATURES IN KLINEFELTER'S SYNDROME

External genitalia male
Small testes
Sparse long hair
Abnormally large mammary glands (gynecomastia)
Unusually long legged
Tall stature
Mildly impaired IQ
Feminized habits
Often not apparent until after puberty

There are four main patterns of single gene defect inheritance: autosomal dominant, autosomal recessive, X-linked dominant, and X-linked recessive.

Autosomal Dominant

With *autosomal dominant* inheritance, an abnormal gene dominates and the normal gene of the pair is recessive. Malformations occur whether the gene comes from one or both parents. Usually the malformations are less severe than in autosomal recessive inheritance.

Paternal age does seem to be a contributing factor (Harris, 1981). This is a vertical type of inheritance, with an affected individual having a 50 percent chance of passing the gene on to each child (see Fig. 5–14).

In autosomal dominant inheritance, symptoms often do not appear until after the childbearing years. Male and female offspring are equally affected. Normal family members do not transmit the trait. Nonaffected children of an affected individual will have normal children if they mate with a normal individual. If two affected individuals should mate, 3 of 4 of their children will be affected; one of these will receive a double dose of the mutant gene and will probably not live. Examples of autosomal defects include Marfan's syndrome, achrondroplasia (a form of dwarfism), neurofibromatosis (von Recklinghausen's disease), Huntington's chorea, and osteogenesis imperfecta.

Autosomal Recessive

In *autosomal recessive* inheritance, the condition or trait is seen when mutant or defective genes have been inherited from both parents. It is a horizontal type of inheritance, with a carrier parent often being asymptomatic and having a 25 percent chance of having an affected child with each pregnancy (see Fig. 5–15).

Both parents are usually normal, but both are heterozygous carriers. Both sexes show the trait with equal frequency. The harmful recessive gene may be passed along on both sides of the family without ever being expressed. If an affected individual mates with a heterozygous carrier, half of their children will be affected and half will be carriers. When two affected individuals mate, all offspring are affected. There are more than 800 autosomal recessive disorders, including cystic fibrosis, sickle cell anemia, diabetes mellitus, muscular dystrophy, and Tay-Sachs disease.

INBORN ERRORS OF METABOLISM

These are protein disorders where defective or absent enzymes prevent metabolism of protein. This leads to eventual mental retardation or death if untreated. Some inborn errors of

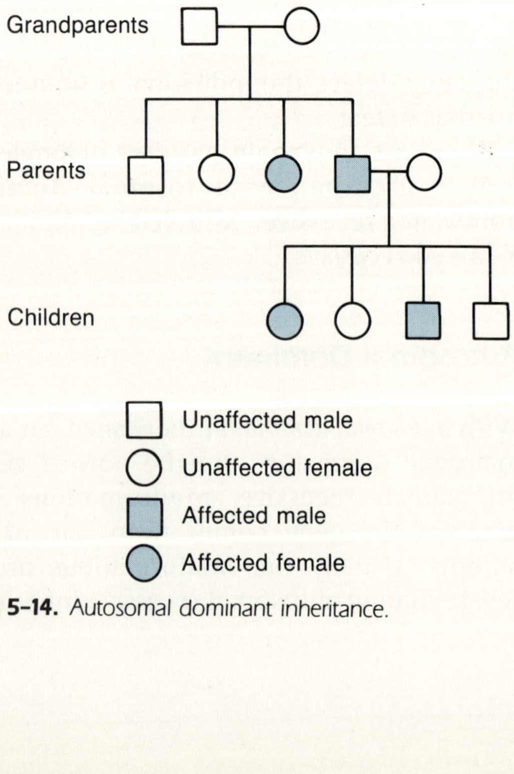

FIGURE 5–14. Autosomal dominant inheritance.

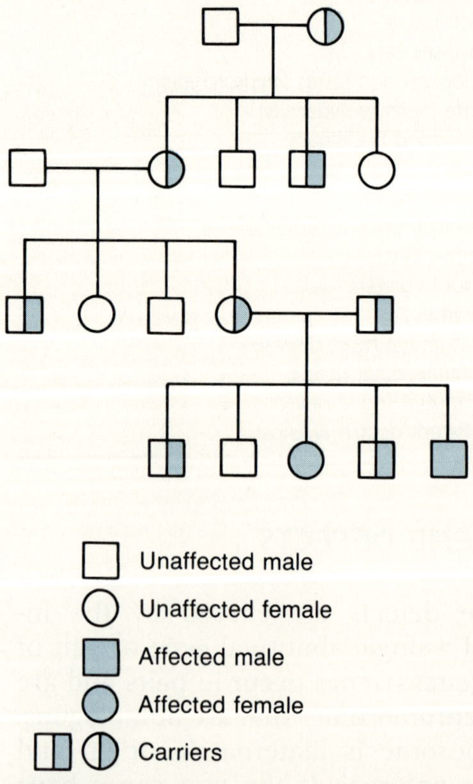

FIGURE 5–15. Autosomal recessive inheritance.

metabolism are autosomal dominant in inheritance or sex-linked, but the majority are autosomal recessive defects.

Phenylketonuria

Phenylketonuria (PKU) occurs once in every 20,000 live births. The hepatic enzyme phenylalanine hydroxylase is absent, causing an inability of phenylalanine to convert to tyrosine. Without treatment, these individuals have progressive deterioration of mental capabilities, as well as hypopigmentation, hyperactivity, convulsions, eczematoid rashes, and a characteristic musky odor.

Galactosemia

Galactosemia occurs once in every 73,000 live births. Deficient in the enzyme galactose 1-phosphate uridyl transferase, the individual is unable to convert galactose-1-phosphate to glucose-1-phosphate, a metabolically usable glucose. Soon after milk is introduced into the diet, vomiting and diarrhea occur, leading to dehydration and malnutrition. Within a few months cataracts develop and severe mental retardation occurs.

Maple Syrup Urine Disease

Maple syrup urine disease results from an accumulation of the branched chain amino acids leucine, isoleucine, and valine. This accumulation is secondary to the absence of the decarboxylase enzyme. These infants appear normal at birth, but within a week develop symptoms of vomiting, lethargy, hypertonicity, and a characteristic urine odor. Without treatment, these infants become severely retarded and die within two to four weeks. This disorder is very rare.

X-Linked Dominant

If the gene for a particular trait or abnormality is located on the X chromosome, the condition is called X-linked or sex-linked.

X-linked dominant transmission is very rare. Affected males are usually grouped in the same generation, a generation is skipped, and affected males appear in the next generation. Affected males will have normal sons; carrier daughters will transmit to the next generation. A carrier female will transmit the abnormality to half of her sons, and half of her daughters will be carriers. An example of an X-linked dominant anomaly is Vitamin D–resistant rickets.

X-Linked Recessive

Abnormal genes are carried by the X chromosomes. If the affected gene is recessive it will not express itself in heterozygous females but only in males who are homozygous.

There is no male-to-male transmission, but both sexes can be affected. A carrier female will pass the gene on to half of her sons, who will have the abnormality, and to half of her daughters, who will be carriers. An affected male will have all normal sons and all carrier daughters (see Fig. 5–16).

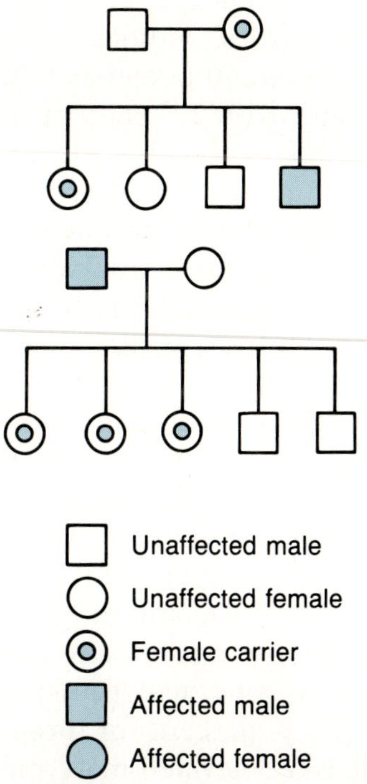

FIGURE 5–16. X-linked recessive inheritance.

Many diseases are X-linked recessive in origin. One of the best known is hemophilia, which occurs once in every 10,000 live male births. Another is glucose-6-phosphate dehydrogenase (G6PD), which occurs in 12 percent of male live births in blacks and 24 percent of female live births in blacks.

POLYGENIC DEFECTS

Several pairs of genes may interact with each other to affect a single trait. One pair of genes may inhibit or reverse the effect of another pair of genes. A given gene may produce different effects when the environment is changed. Genes are inherited as units, but they may interact in different ways to produce different traits.

Human characteristics such as height, stature, intelligence, and skin color are not inherited by a single pair of genes, but are affected by many pairs of genes. The term *polygenic inheritance* is used when two or more independent pairs of genes affect the same characteristic in the same way.

Several congenital anomalies are not inherited in one of the four main patterns, but will tend to cluster in families. Multifactorial defects contribute more than 50 percent of all congenital malformations, with 2.5 percent of all births having a defect of this origin (Simpson et al., 1984).

Examples of polygenic defects are neural tube defects, club foot, congenital dislocation of the hip, cleft lip and palate, pyloric stenosis, Hirschsprung's disease, and congenital heart defects.

Neural tube defects (NTD), including anencephaly, myelomeningocele, and spina bifida, are the most amenable to prenatal diagnosis by detection of alpha-fetoprotein (AFP) in maternal blood or amniotic fluid. AFP is a protein produced by the yolk sac and the fetal liver in up to eight times the normal amount in the presence of neural tube defects, especially open defects. Fifty percent of pregnancies with NTD will have elevated maternal plasma levels of AFP by 15 weeks of gestation, and 80 percent will have elevated AFP levels in the amniotic fluid.

GENETIC COUNSELING

Genetic counseling involves working through feelings, motivations, and defense mechanisms that families may have (Tishler, 1981). Every one of us carries recessive genes for three to eight "diseases." The vast majority of these are never transmitted to our children or grandchildren. It has been estimated that 7 of every 100 liveborn babies has a genetic defect (March of Dimes, 1983).

Genetic counseling has specific goals: (1) to provide families with information, (2) to communicate to families the risk of transmitting the defect, (3) to enable families to make informed reproductive decisions, (4) to provide psychological support in the decision-making process, and (5) to reduce the number of individuals affected by genetic diseases.

Families who should be referred for genetic counseling include:

- Women over 35 years of age
- Those with a previous child with a birth defect
- Either parent a translocation carrier
- A mother who is a carrier for a X-linked disorder
- History of two or more first trimester spontaneous abortions
- Having a previous child with a neural tube defect
- Having a known risk for metabolic disorders
- Ethnic or racial groups at increased risk for specific disorders
- Anyone who requests genetic counseling

NURSING RESPONSIBILITIES

Nurses play a unique role. They are often the first to identify families who need genetic counseling. Deviations from the normal in growth and development and other abnormalities may be noted. Information in the family history may indicate the need for referral. Specific nursing responsibilities in the genetic counseling process are summarized in Table 5–8.

Families need assistance to acquire accurate information about their problems. The nurse can help the family contact a genetic counseling center to set up appointments. After the appointment is made, families should be prepared for the counseling experience. Helping them know what to expect will help to lower parental anxiety levels and make counseling a more satisfying experience. Families can be helped to formulate their questions and collect genetic information pertaining to other family members.

During the counseling session, a careful history is taken, which includes any environmental factors that may affect pregnancy outcomes. The family history is taken in pedigree form (see Figures 5–14, 5–15, and 5–16). Chromosomal studies and appropriate laboratory evaluations may be done at the initial session. Both parents should be present in a quiet, private room for the conference.

Following the initial session, the couple is sent a summary of important points. A second conference is scheduled to identify further testing that may be needed. To date, there are well over 100 disorders that can be diagnosed or ruled out during pregnancy (March of Dimes, 1983). Tests that may be ordered include amniocentesis, x-rays, amniography, ultrasonography, fetoscopy, and chorionic villi sampling. These tests are covered in more detail in Chapter 24.

Amniocentesis is a method of obtaining amniotic fluid by inserting a needle through the abdominal and uterine wall. The procedure cannot be done until after the 13th week of gestation owing to an insufficient amount of amniotic fluid. Examination is made of the amniotic fluid, amniotic fluid cells, and cultured amniotic fluid cells. Many genetic disorders can be diagnosed by examination of amniotic fluid (see Table 5–9).

TABLE 5–8
NURSING RESPONSIBILITIES IN GENETIC COUNSELING

Identification of families who need genetic counseling
Assist families to acquire correct information about the genetic problem
Liason between the family and the genetic counselor
Help families handle the information received
Aid families in coping with this crisis
Provide information about known genetic factors
Assure continuity of nursing care to the family

TABLE 5–9
GENETIC DISORDERS THAT CAN BE DETECTED BY AMNIOCENTESIS

Adenosine deaminase efficiency
Adrenogenital syndrome
Argininosuccunicaciduria
Chronic granulomatous disease
Citrullinemia
Cri du chat syndrome
Cystic fibrosis
Cystinosis
Ellis-van Creveld syndrome
Epidermolysis bullosa
Fabry's disease
Familial hypercholesterolemia
Fancon's syndrome
Farber disease
Finnish nephrosis
Fucosidosis
Galactokinase deficiency
Galactosemia
Gaucher's disease
Glutaric aciduria, Type II
Glycogen storage disease Type II (Pompe's disease)
Hemoglobinopathies
Hemophilia A
Hunter's syndrome
Hurler's syndrome
Hypercholesterolemia
Hypophosphatasia
Hypothyroidism

TABLE 5-9 (Continued)

I-cell disease
Ichthyosis, epidermolytic hyperkeratosis
Ichthyosis, lamellar
Isocaleric acidemia
Ketotic hyperglycinemia
Klinefelter's syndrome
Krabbe's disease
Lesch-Nyman syndrome
Lysosomal acid phosphatase deficiency
Maple syrup urine disease
Maroteaux-Lamy syndrome
Meckel syndrome
Menkes syndrome
Metachromatic leukodystrophy
Kethylmalonic aciduria
Mucolipidosis I (sialidosis)
Mucolipidosis IV
Myotonic dystrophy
Neural tube defects
Neimann-Pick disease
Osteogenesis imperfecta
Philadelphia syndrome
Phosphohexoisomerase deficiency
Placental sulfatase deficiency
Porphyria, acute intermittent type
Porphyria, congenital erythropoietic type
Pyruvate, decarboxylate deficiency
Sandhoff's disease
Sanfilippo syndrome, type A
Sanfilippo syndrome, type B
Sickle cell disease
Tay-Sachs disease
α-thalassemia
β-thalassemia
Trisomy 13
Trisomy 18
Trisomy 21
Turner's syndrome
von Willebrand's disease
Wolman's disease
Xeroderma pigmentosum

X-rays may be useful when fetal skeletal problems (anencephaly, achrondroplasia, osteogenesis imperfecta) are suspected. However, the risk of radiation to the fetus is high if done before the third trimester, thus limiting the usefulness of these procedures in genetic counseling.

Amniography is used in selected mothers to diagnose fetal soft tissue defects, gastrointestinal disorders, and malformations. In this procedure an amniocentesis is done and a water-soluble contrast material is injected into the amniotic fluid, displacing the fetal soft parts to aid in diagnosing myelomeningocele or exstrophy of the bladder.

Ultrasound is used to diagnose central nervous system defects, renal agenesis, oomphalocele, and diaphragmatic hernia.

Fetoscopy is used to collect fetal tissue samples to aid in diagnosis of fetal disease. A fiberoptic scope is passed abdominally into the uterus at about 16 to 20 weeks of gestation. Fetal blood samples are taken slightly above the junction of the placenta and the umbilical cord and tissue samples are collected from the fetal body through a pair of forceps that fit through the cannula (Eleis and Esterly, 1981). Fetoscopy is usually used when both parents are disease carriers (Golbus, 1982).

Chorionic villi sampling (CVS) offers an alternative to amniocentesis for detection of fetal chromosomal and biochemical disorders. It is done in the first trimester and results are available within 6 to 24 hours and confirmed by short-term cell cultures within three to ten days. In this procedure a thin catheter is passed transcervically into the chorion frondosum under ultrasound guidance. A sample of chorionic villi is obtained for testing. CVS can detect the same chromosomal or biochemical defects as amniocentesis (see Table 5–9), with the exception of neural tube defects.

After results are obtained, the family should be allowed to make the decision that is best for them, either elective induced abortion or continuation of the pregnancy. They need to understand the meaning of the diagnosis, prognosis, and the occurrence of risk factors (see Table 5-10). Showing pictures of what a child will look like with a particular condition may assist the family in making their decision. Questions are anticipated and answered whenever possible. The nurse needs to remain as objective as possible when dealing with families. Reinforcement of data will help families to understand information. After the family has made its decision, psychological support is of prime importance.

Genetic counseling is a team effort. It requires physicians, nurses, geneticists, and social service assistants. If the team works together, the family can be assisted to make the decision that is best for them.

TABLE 5-10
RISK OF RECURRENCE OF SELECTED ANOMALIES

Anomaly	Risk (%)
Beckwith-Wiedemann syndrome	25
Calcaneovalgus	2–3
Cardiac defects	2–5
Cleft palate	2 to 5
Craniostenosis	Sporadic
Down's syndrome (chromosomal nondisjunction)	1–2
Down's syndrome (chromosomal translocation)	5–15
Equinovarus	2–3
Gastroschisis	Sporadic
Hemangioma	Sporadic
Hydrocephalus	2–5
Marfan syndrome	50
Neurofibromatosis	50
Oomphalocele	Sporadic
Potter's syndrome	Sporadic

BIBLIOGRAPHY

Adler, B. & Kushnick, T. Genetic counseling in prenatally diagnosed trisomy 18 and 21: psychological aspects. *Pediatrics*, 1982, **69**, 94-99.

Bolognese, R.J., Schwart, R.H. & Schneider, J. *Perinatal medicine management of the high risk fetus and neonate*. Baltimore: Williams & Wilkins, 1982.

Buri, C.E. & Hecht, F. Tort liability in genetic diagnosis and genetic counseling. *American Journal of Human Genetics*, 1982, **34**, 353-356.

Cadkin, A.V., et al.: Chorionic villi sampling. A new technique for detection of genetic anomalies in the first trimester. *Radiology*, 1983, **149**, 257.

Daniels, V.G. & Huang, V. L-H. *Companion to neonatal medicine*. Lancaster, England: MTP Press, 1982.

Davison, B.C. Genetic counseling and obstetrics. *Practice*, 1981, **225**, 1237.

Elias, S. & Esterly, N.B. Prenatal diagnosis of hereditary skin disorders. *Clinical Obstetrics & Gynecology*, 1981, **24**, 1069.

Epstein, M.F. & Frigoletto, F.D. Today's view in maternal and fetal medicine. *Patient Care*, 1983, **17**, 105-121.

Golbus, M.S. The current scope of antenatal diagnosis. *Hospital Practice*, 1982, **17**, 179-186.

Gray, C. Prenatal diagnosis. The demand is increasing. *Canadian Medical Association Journal*, 1982, **126**, 64.

Haddow, J.E. Screening for spinal defects. *Hospital Practice*, 1982, **17**, 128.

Hammer, R.M. & Tufts, M.A. Chorionic villi sampling for detecting fetal disorders. *MCN*, 1986, **11**, 29-31.

Harris, T.R. Genetics. In A.L. Clark, D.D. Affonso, T.R. Harris, (Eds.). *Childbearing: A nursing perspective* (2nd ed.). Philadelphia: F.A. Davis, 1981, pp. 215-232.

Hook, E.B., Cross, P.K. & Schreinemachers, D.M. Chromosomal abnormality rates at amniocentesis and in live-born infants. *Journal of the American Medical Association*, 1983, **249**, 2034.

Johnson, M. Indications and techniques for genetic amniocentesis. *Journal of Reproductive Medicine*, 1982, **27**, 557.

March of Dimes. *Birth defects. Tragedy and hope*. January, 1983.

Simpson, J.L., et al. *Genetics in obstetrics and gynecology*. New York: Grune & Stratton, 1982.

Summer, G.K. Development in genetic and metabolic screening. *Family & Community Health*, 1982, **4**, 13-30.

Tishler, C.L. The psychological aspects of genetic counseling. *American Journal of Nursing*, 1981, **81**, 732.

U.S. Department of Health and Human Services. *Amniocentesis for prenatal chromosomal diagnosis*. Atlanta, Ga.: Public Health Service Center for Disease Control, 1980.

Worthington, S. Genetic screening. *Journal of Gynecological & Neonatal Nursing*, 1984, **13**, 32s-37s.

chapter 6

PREPARING FOR REPRODUCTION

OBJECTIVES

Upon completion of this chapter, the reader will be able to:

1. Explain sexual differentiation during fetal development.
2. Discuss the effects of society on the development of sexual identity.
3. Discuss the development of sexual identity during childhood and adolescence.
4. Describe the four phases of sexual response.
5. Explain the mechanism of action of oral contraceptives.
6. Discuss the effects of oral contraceptives on bodily functions.
7. Discuss the advantages and disadvantages of oral contraceptives.
8. List the absolute contraindications for oral contraceptive use.
9. List the danger signs to be observed when using oral contraceptives.
10. Compare the methods of contraception.
11. Discuss the various methods of family planning.
12. Describe methods of permanent sterilization.
13. Discuss future methods of contraception.
14. Identify psychological causes associated with unplanned conception.
15. Describe the psychological effects of an unplanned pregnancy on the teenager.
16. Identify male and female factors associated with infertility.
17. Describe the evaluation methods and management of the infertile couple.
18. Describe in vitro fertilization.
19. Describe the AID and AIH methods of artificial insemination.
20. Discuss societal concerns related to artificial insemination.

KEY TERMS

Artificial insemination
BBT
Cervical cap
Coitus interruptus
Condom
Culdoscopy
Diaphragm
Endometriosis
Hysterosalpingogram
Impotency
Intrauterine device
In vitro fertilization
Libido
Mastodynia
Minipill
Müllerian ducts
Myomectomy
Natural family planning
Oral contraceptive
Primary infertility
RESOLVE
Rhythm
Rubin Test
Salpingitis
Secondary infertility
Sexual phases
  Excitement
  Plateau
  Orgasmic
  Resolution
Sims-Huhner Test
Spermicide
Symptothermal method
Tubal ligation
Vasectomy
Vasovasectomy
Wolffian ducts

PREPARING FOR REPRODUCTION

Reproductive maturation in both the male and female heralds the arrival of conceptual capabilities. Prior to this time, the reproductive organs have been undergoing developmental changes during embryonic and fetal periods and continuing throughout infancy and childhood. Puberty is the "alpha" of the individual as a sexual being, with the "omega" perhaps not occurring until late in the aging process or even death. Thus, at puberty, the heritage of the human race and the individual's contribution to it becomes reality.

As the reproductive organs in both male and female develop, so do the individual's sexual attitudes and values. Society provides a background filled with implications from cultural practices, family behavior, and education. The individual develops a sexual identity related to his or her background, and this identity will be subject to many changes throughout the lifespan.

The nurse can be prepared to understand the many factors which contribute to individual sexuality and at what stage of the sexual continuum a client may be. It is not within the purpose of this chapter to explore all facets of human sexuality. Yet, a basic understanding of human sexual development is necessary.

SEXUAL DEVELOPMENT

Fetal Period

From the moment of conception, biological sex determination has been potentially established. Chromosomal influences determine whether the fetus will develop male or female gonads. Hormonal influences will determine sexual differentiation. At the sixth week of gestation it is impossible to differentiate between a female and a male fetus. During the seventh week, the testes of the male begin to develop and stimulate development of the wolffian ducts (see Fig. 6–1). Before this, the wolffian ducts coexist with the müllerian ducts as the potential male and female structures. Once stimulated by the testes, the wolffian ducts become the male reproductive structures of the epididymis, vas deferens, and seminal vesicle and exert a degenerative effect on the female müllerian duct system. This degenerative effect is probably due to the antimullerian hormone and testosterone secreted by the testes. In the absence of functioning male testes, the müllerian ducts become fallopian tubes, uterus, and the upper portion of the vagina. The wolffian ducts will then degenerate.

Interestingly, it is not necessary for the female gonad (ovary) to be present for the development of the female organs. When testosterone is absent at this stage, the fetus will always develop as a female. Male sexual developmental dominance in the fetus continues until "sex typing" (Money & Ehrbardt, 1972) of the brain occurs. Weinberg (1982), describes sex typing as being crucial to the release of gonadotropin. When the fetal brain is influenced by testosterone, a noncyclic pattern of gonadotropic release is developed. Conversely, without the influence of testosterone, the female develops a cycle of gonadotropic release. It is suspected that once this crucial period of hormonal patterning is completed, susceptability to, or lack of, testosterone is limited in this effect.

Externally, the urogenital folds (see Fig. 6–2) in the female will develop into the labia and the genital tubercle will become the clitoris. The male urogenital folds, reacting to androgen stimulation, will fuse and develop into the cylindrical penile shaft containing the urethra. The male testes will remain in the abdomen until the eighth month of gestation, before descending into the scrotal sac.

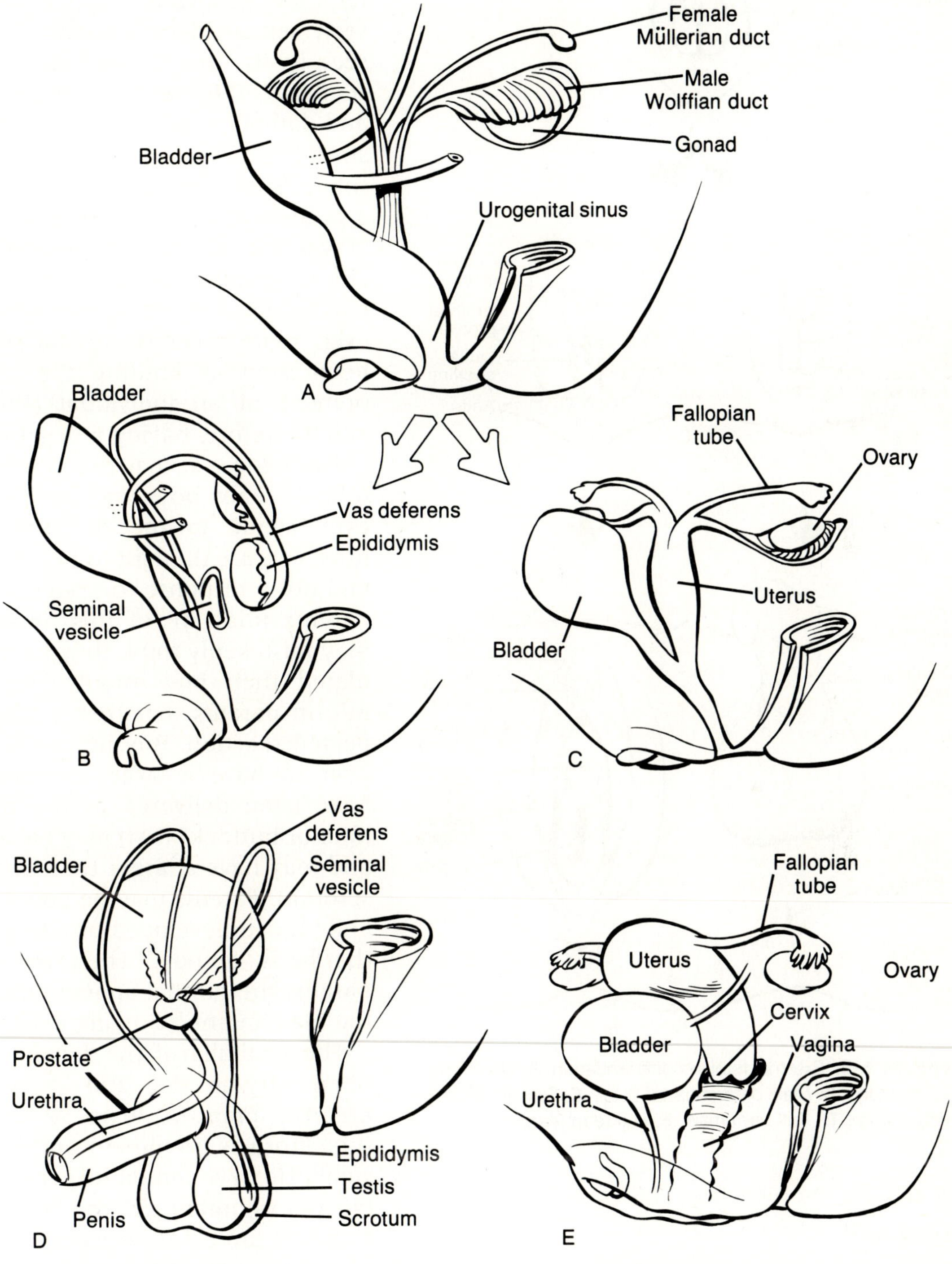

FIGURE 6–1. Internal fetal sex differentiation: A. Undifferentiated male or female. B. Male differentiated at 16 weeks gestation. C. Female differentiated at 16 weeks gestation. D. Full term male. E. Full term female.

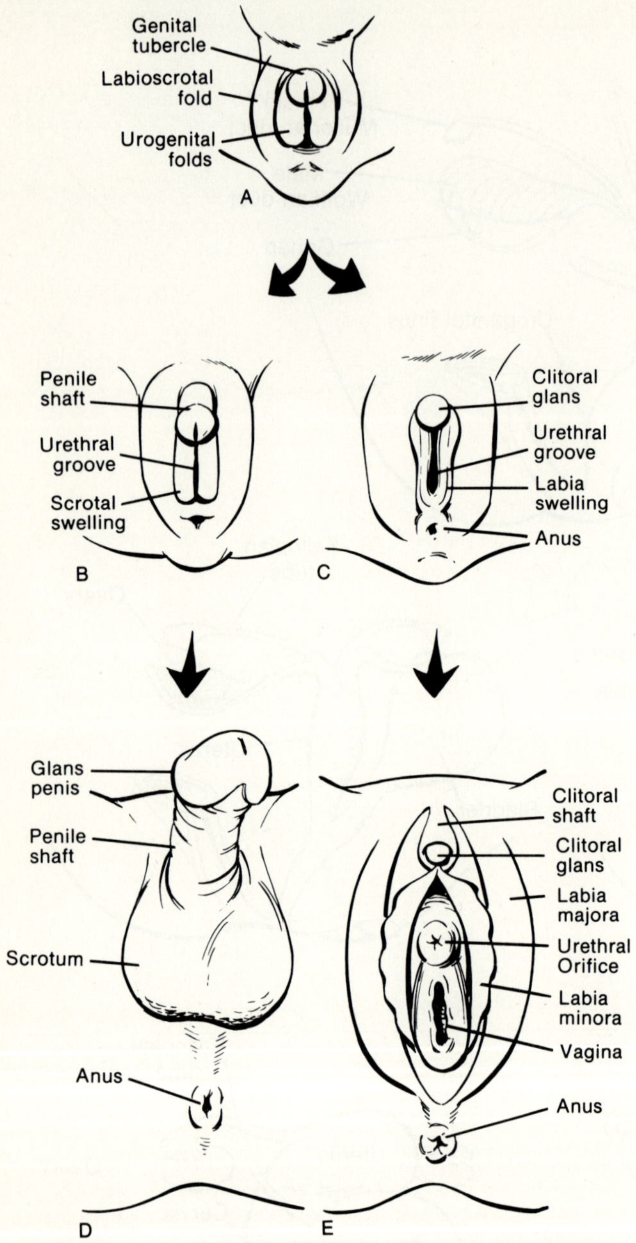

FIGURE 6-2. External fetal sex differentiation. **A.** Undifferentiated stage. **B.** Male differentiated stage. **C.** Female differentiated stage. **D.** Full term male. **E.** Full term female.

Infancy

The infant enters the world with an established sexual identification. The physical appearance of the infant genitals is termed the *sex phenotype*. Clusters of behavior center around sexual traits designated by the sex phenotype. From the first month of life society will reinforce adherence to masculine or feminine behaviors and roles. Even in the nursery, sexual identification of infants may be seen by the use of name cards in blue or pink stating "Girl Brown" or "Boy Brown." Mothers and fathers may be told they have a "big, strong boy" or a "sweet, pretty girl." This sexual stereotyping has been viewed in both a positive and a negative manner. In the past, it was felt that sexual stereotyping served to aid in gender identification and strengthen psychological components of sexuality. However, more recently, sexual stereotyping has been seen as limiting the potential development of an individual (Weinberg, 1982) and, therefore, having a negative effect.

Physiologic sexual functioning is limited in infancy. Baby boys may have penile erections even while in the delivery room. These, however, are thought to be reflexive in nature and not a response to sexual stimulation. Yet, parents unaware of this normal occurrence may mistakenly think they have sexually stimulated their boy infant. The nurse should inform parents that this is a normal and expected reaction. Boy infants at birth may appear to have a large scrotum. Infants who have been delivered in the breech position (feet or buttocks first) may have scrotal edema and may have a larger than normal appearing scrotum. Parents may be concerned that their child is overdeveloped or take pride in the fact that he is "all boy." The nurse explains to the parents the normal appearance of genitalia of the male infant following delivery.

The genitalia of the female infant at birth often vary in size and appearance. In the preterm infant of 20 to 30 weeks' gestation, the clitoris is prominent and the labia majora small. However, upon inspection of a full term (40 weeks) infant girl, the labia majora appear to cover the clitoris. Occasionally, the clitoris of a full term infant girl may be enlarged. Once again, parents who are not aware of these differences may be concerned as to the normal development of the clitoris. Parents may question if the clitoris is in fact a penis and fear their child is abnormal.

The nurse must be aware of the genetic recessive defect *adrenogenital syndrome*, which gives rise to congenital adrenal hyperplasia. In this syndrome, a lack of certain enzymes in the infant will cause a deficiency of some hormones and an excess of others (Muir, 1983, p. 235). This results in genitalia which may be difficult to distinguish between male and female at birth. Parents are told that the infant can be tested to determine the true sex and that treatment (hormonal or surgical) is possible.

The full-term infant girl may demonstrate other characteristics of a sexual concern to the parents. The *hymenal tag* is a normal piece of hymenal tissue that protrudes from the vaginal floor. The tag has no significance and will drop off within a few weeks following birth. Its presence and expected disappearance should be explained to the parents. The influence of increased levels of estrogen in the mother during pregnancy may result in a blood-tinged mucoid discharge from the vagina of the infant. Maternal estrogen can also give rise to swelling of the breast tissue in both male and female infants. Neither of these occurrences have any clinical significance.

Early Childhood

The first three years of the child's life represent the most important years in terms of sexual gender role and identity. Gender role is defined by Muir (1983) as "the behaviors of a person that indicate to others or to the self the degree to which one is male, female, or ambivalent" (p. 219). Gender identity is described by Kolodny et al. (1979, p. 50) as "the way people feel about their individuality as males or females, including ambivalence in their self-perceptions."

Obviously, many complex factors contribute to the establishment of gender role and identity in the early formative years. Chief among these factors is parental influence. In some families male children are expected to be aggressive, competitive, protective, and physical. The female child is expected to be passive, loving, delicate, and in need of protection. Boys cannot cry. Girls are expected to cry easily. A boy is taught to "look after your baby sister." A girl is taught to "pick up after your brother." These are only a few examples of early influences on gender role and identity development. They are, however, examples of sex role stereotyping, which is reinforced from day to day as the child grows. Therefore, by the time children are three years old they know which gender behaviors are expected of them. Little girls ask for dolls for Christmas and boys ask for footballs or trains. Modern society has attempted to accept the child who may differ in his or her expression of gender identity, but such acceptance is limited. Little boys who play with dolls or girls who prefer footballs are often discouraged in these activities.

During early childhood children explore their genitalia. This is a normal manifestation of the child's exploration of his or her environment. In stressful situations, boys are often seen to grasp the genitals. Parents may scold them for this, increasing the child's anxiety and imparting a negative acceptance of normal behavior. Genital manipulation by both sexes is frequent and is a part of the normal exploration and experimentation essential to the child's psychosexual development (Fromer, 1983).

Childhood

From age three years to puberty, reinforcement of sexual identity continues. Society now has an important influence on the child. Prior to this time major influences were family centered. As the children enter school, they add several new dimensions to their sexual role models. Teachers influence children by their acceptance of traditional childhood behavior. Girls are expected to be verbal and gentle. Boys are expected to be mathematical and aggressive. Textbooks illustrate the mother as the "housewife" and father as the "breadwinner." Little girls grow up to be passive mothers and boys to be fathers who are heads of the family. These are portrayed as "ideal" roles and exert a very prominent influence on children. Group activities encourage boys to engage in competitive sports and girls to be cheerleaders for the accomplishments of the boys.

Sexual activities during childhood include those of both homosexual and heterosexual natures. Interest in the genitals of the opposite and same sex is frequent and is again explorative. Sexual-type questions may be asked of parents, teachers, or nurses, and should be answered in an open, relaxed manner. Parental and societal reactions toward sexual play are important precursors of the child's future sexual attitude. Love, understanding, and guiding acceptance of the child's sexual concerns are important components for healthy psychosexual growth. Acceptable sexual behavior is conveyed to the child in the context of a loving relationship.

In nontraditional families, sexual identity and gender modeling may be difficult for the child. Role reversals in some families make it necessary for the mother to assume the role of family provider while father is engaged in the household tasks. This does not fit the traditional portrayal seen in textbooks or on television. Single parent families find the mother or father assuming both parental roles. Here again, the child may find a difference in his or her home life compared to those of his or her peers. In both situations it is necessary for contacts of the child to be aware of these differences and to give the child support in adjusting to and accepting these differences.

Adolescence

Adolescence defies all definition. It is a period beset with a series of normal crises involving the physical, emotional, and intellectual development. Characteristics used to describe this period include ambivalence, insecurity, independence, rejection of family and family values, and adherence to peer acceptance. Imbedded deep in the core of these characteristics is the reality of sexual development. Between the ages of about 12 and 20, the adolescent is confronted with not only a change in body image but also a plethora of hormonal changes and psychosexual feelings. Earlier sexual identity had been more subtle in its development. Now, at puberty, pronounced secondary sex characteristics of male or female sexuality are apparent. The male develops a deep voice, increased muscle size, increased size of the penis and scrotum, facial, arm and leg hair, increased skeletal growth, and facial acne. Girls develop increased subcutaneous adipose tissue of the breast, hips, and buttocks, menstrual periods, breast changes involving areolar and nipple changes, increased pubic hair, and ovulation. These changes make adolescents almost painfully aware of their emerging body images. Any deviations from the physical appearance of their peers become areas of great concern and anxiety.

Just as increased hormonal activity in both sexes is responsible for the development of the secondary sexual characteristics, it is also responsible for the initiation of certain sexual behaviors. Sexual activity may proceed in a number of directions but usually includes sexual experimentation, male and female masturbation, male nocturnal emissions, kissing, petting, and eventually sexual intercourse. The order and inclusiveness of these activities is influenced by many variables. Family relationships, peer pressures, religious and moral beliefs, self-image and esteem, previous sex education, and environment are prominent variables that influence sexual behavior.

Sexual permissiveness in our society is more widely accepted today than in previous generations. Although most children are taught that sexual activity should be limited to a marriage relationship, conflicting messages of sexuality are portrayed by the media and in advertisements. It is understandable that adolescents may be confused when dealing with standards and decisions concerning sexual behavior. In a study done by Kantner and Zelnik (1976), it was determined that 55 percent of unmarried women had engaged in sexual intercourse by age 19 (Kolodny et al., 1979). Akpom et al. (1976) reported in their study on teenage sexual behavior that "a significantly larger proportion of teenagers from households headed by females than from those headed by males had had their first experience of sexual intercourse at age 15 or younger." The double standard of sexual activity is not as widely accepted as in past generations. Society now accepts a more open attitude for both males and females and in so doing has created a single standard for both. Sexual situations frequently arise at a time when the adolescent is young and unprepared to make a mature decision. These decisions are often based on the need for popularity, defiance of parental authority, curiosity, affection, and simple reaction to the passions of the moment. Unfortunately, the results may not be those desired or expected. Feelings of guilt, destruction of relationships, resentment, unwanted pregnancies, and venereal disease are often the result of sexually liberated behavior and may lead to alteration of sexual identity.

Adulthood

During the adult years sexual identity broadens in its dimensions. Ideally, it encompasses the development of mature, responsible sexuality based on an intimate and sincere relationship. Sexual identity no longer is as strictly self-centered as it is during adolescence, but now reaches out to include others. Relationships involve commitments that may include marriage and a family. Often marriage is not chosen, but there is commitment to a sincere relationship. The pinnacle of sexual maturity may, for some, be reached early in adulthood. For others, it involves a continued exploration of sexual choices. These choices may include homosexuality, multiple partners, bisexuality, and varied sexual practices. Regardless of the choices made, the individual's sense of responsibility to the partners involved and adherence to personal sexual values will determine the achievement of sexual maturity.

SEXUAL RESPONSE

The pyramiding of sexual development, identity, and behavior from birth to adulthood brings the individual to the moment of sexual stimulation and expression, termed the sexual response. Research in sexuality has provided information about sexual response. Among the prominent contributors to this research is Alfred Kinsey, who collaborated with his associates to undertake the first objective studies of sexual behavior. These studies, *Sexual Behavior in the Human Male* (1948) and *Sexual Behavior in the Human Female* (1953), provided the first scientific insight into psychological characteristics of sexual behavior.

An actual description of physiological events during intercourse was described by Masters and Johnson (1966). Many critics cited this research as being too clinical, unrealistic in the population sample used, and void of the psychosocial components of sexuality. Yet, their work was the catalyst for future and more comprehensive studies.

According to Masters and Johnson (1966), there are four phases of sexual response, which are essentially the same in the male and female. One cannot discern exactly when one phase begins and the other ends. The phases are interwoven. The initial stage is the *excitement phase* of stimulation, resulting in vaginal lubrication and penile erection. If stimulation continues, there is a cresting of excitement during which the individual enters the *plateau phase*. Physiologic changes such as genital engorgement, accelerated heart and respiratory rate, increased sexual flushing, and increased lubricative secretions occur. This crescendo of physiologic sexual stimulation erupts into orgasm. The female during this *orgasmic phase* experiences pubic throbbing, uterine and fallopian tube contractions, and generalized myotonia reduction (muscle relaxation). The male climax during the orgas-

TABLE 6-1
PATHWAY OF SEXUAL STIMULI AND BODILY RESPONSES

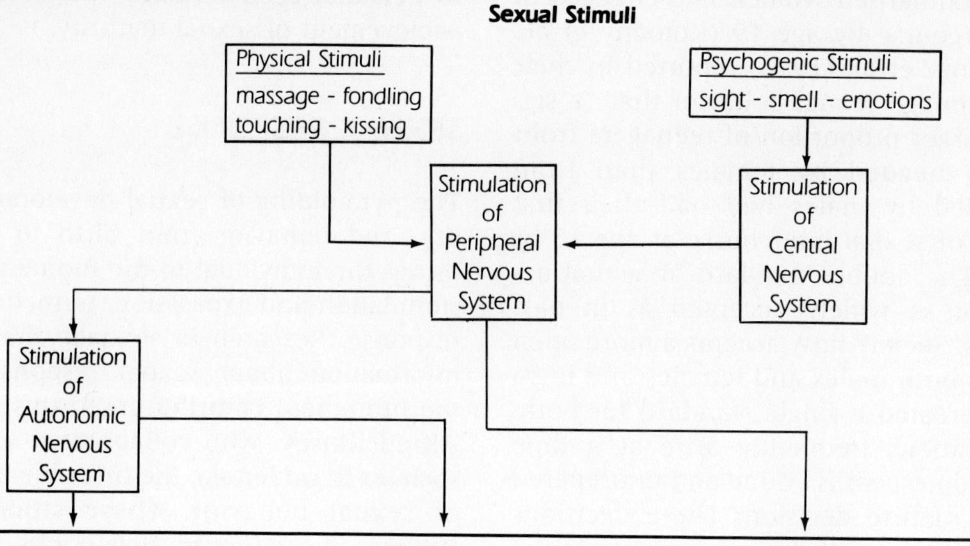

Phases of Sexual Response	Parasympathetic Effect	Sympathetic Effect	Somatic Stimulation Effect
Excitement	Dilation of arteries Increased blood supply to male penis causing erection Increased blood supply in female vulva resulting in vaginal lubrication Breast enlargement Nipple erection Skin flushing Clitoris enlargens Male bulbo urethral glands secrete mucus Lifting of scrotum Labia minora color pronounced Labia majora enlargens	Increased heart rate Increased B/P Increased respiratory rate Increased muscle strength	Contraction of voluntary muscles Generalized myotonia
Plateau	Continuation of excitement effects Increase in size of testes Labia minora turn bright red Profound flushing	Uterine elevation Hyperventilation Tachycardia Clitoris shaft withdraws into prepuce	Contraction of facial and abdominal muscles Voluntary contraction of rectal sphincter
Orgasm		Release of adrenalin causing ejaculation of sperm and spasm of vagina Rhythmic uterine contractions Strong involuntary contractions of rectum	Loss of voluntary muscular control
Resolution	Release of acetylcholine causing vasodilatation and relaxation of erection Feelings of warmth and tenderness Disappearance of flush Uterine descent and cervix emersed in seminal fluid		

mic phase results in ejaculation of seminal fluid and sperm. Each ejaculation may contain as many as 125 million sperm. The final responsive phase is the *resolution phase*. During this phase the internal and external physiologic responses return to a relaxed state. The male enters a refractory period during which he is incapable of sexual arousal or erection. This period may last as long as the initial excitement stage. There appears to be a correlation between the age and the length of the refractory period. In young males the refractory period may be relatively short, whereas in older males it is longer in duration (Table 6–1).

The female, during the resolution phase, experiences a feeling of warmth, tenderness and alertness, in contrast to the male who is sleepy and placid (Hogan, 1982). Females, unlike males, are capable of repeated sexual arousal within a short period of time.

NURSING RESPONSIBILITIES INVOLVING SEXUALITY

Sexuality is an integral part of the life of every individual. The very initiation of life is the result of a sexual relationship between two individuals. Nurses should have an understanding and respect for the sexual identity of each individual. Attitudes that foster an open acceptance of different approaches to sexuality must be cultivated. Sexual attitudes and behaviors are not formed at the time of the first sexual encounter but are ongoing from birth until death. Parents arrive in the maternity department with developed sexual values that will influence the sexual behavior of their children. The informed nurse will be able to aid parents in a nonjudgmental manner and discuss sexual functioning at all stages of development. The knowledge that the nurse conveys to the parents may serve to reinforce or change sexual attitudes that ultimately will be a part of the child's sexual identity.

FAMILY PLANNING

Contraception

When two individuals enter into a heterosexual relationship the potential for conception exists. With some, pregnancy is the desired goal, received with joy and expectation. Others view pregnancy as most undesirable and unwanted. There is little doubt that pregnancy, wanted or unwanted, has an important impact on the individual, family, and society. Family planning has become a personal reproductive choice, influenced by changes in society such as the women's liberation movement, population control, economic problems, career roles of women, family structures, and childbearing roles.

The decision to have or not have a baby is not easily made. In today's society the choice, however, does exist. If the choice is made to prevent pregnancy, then consideration is given to a method of contraception. Contraception, both in and out of a marriage relationship, has become widely accepted. Often the nurse plays an important role in assisting those who participate in sexual relationships with decisions regarding a choice of contraceptive methods.

Many effective methods of birth control are available to the sexually active person. Each of these methods has advantages and disadvantages to be considered when a decision is made. None of the contraceptive methods are 100 percent effective, safe, or convenient. It is important that individuals make informed decisions based on:

1. Thorough knowledge of the methods of contraception
2. The health risk of each method
3. Patterns of individual sexual behavior
4. Sexual preferences
5. Individual medical histories
6. Long-term effects on fertility
7. Personal and religious values
8. Ease, availability, and cost of each method
9. Acceptability by sexual partner
10. Effectiveness

Essential to the effectiveness of the chosen method is the commitment to use and a thorough knowledge of proper use.

ORAL CONTRACEPTIVES

The introduction of the birth control pill has produced dramatic effects on society. Since 1959, when oral contraceptives were approved by the Food and Drug Administration (FDA) for use in the United States, they have been considered the leading method of birth control. It is estimated that 80 million women in the world use oral contraceptives. There are two basic types of oral contraceptives, the combination pill and the minipill. The previously used sequential pills are no longer on the market.

Mechanism of Action

The intended purpose of oral combination pill contraception is to prevent pregnancy by the prevention of ovulation. The action of synthetic estrogen and progesterone in contraceptive pills mimics the hormonal state of pregnancy. Increased levels of estrogen provided by the pill diminish the hypothalmic effect on gonadotropin releasing factors, thereby inhibiting the release of follicle stimulating hormone (FSH) and luteinizing hormone (LH), both of which are necessary for ovulation to take place. If FSH is blocked, the ovarian follicle does not grow. If LH is blocked, ovulation is not triggered.

The other component of the pill, progesterone in the form of synthetic progestin, contributes to the contraceptive effect by altering sperm capacitation and reducing sperm motility. Progestin-induced alterations in the glandular epithelium of the endometrium also makes the uterine environment unreceptive to implantation.

Various combinations of estrogen and progesterone pills are available. These combinations vary in their estrogen and/or progesterone content. Intolerance to a specific pill is usually related to the estrogen content. For this reason, low dosages may range from 20 μg ethinyl estradiol to 100 μg of mestranol. The lower doses of estrogen are often associated with "breakthrough" (intermenstrual) bleeding, whereas, the higher dosages may be related to thromboembolism. It is recommended that not more than 50 μg of estrogen be prescribed for the initial regimen (Hatcher et al., 1976).

The minipill is a progesterone only type of oral contraceptive. Since there is no estrogen in these pills, there is no effect on ovulation. However, the progesterone effect of providing a hostile uterine environment and increasing the viscosity of the cervical mucus does interfere with conception. An additional effect of progesterone may be seen with minipills. There is a decrease in transporting the ovum through the fallopian tubes. Since the minipill is less effective than the oral combination pill (98 percent, compared with 99.3 percent) there does exist a remote possibility of conception. The decreased mobility of the ovum caused by the progestins may increase the risk of *ectopic* (outside the uterus) pregnancies and the implantation of a degenerated ova (Hatcher et al., 1976).

The sequential pills provided a regimen of 14 to 16 days of estrogen followed by five to seven days of estrogen and progestins. Their removal from the market in 1975 was precipitated by the increase of thrombosis and a possible relationship between the sequential pills and endometrial carcinoma. Both of these side effects were related to the high levels of estrogen, considerably over the 50 μg recommended.

Instructions for Use

The oral combination pills are taken in a very strict regimen. The user is instructed to take the pill at the same time every day. Pills are supplied in either 21-day or 28-day dispensers. When using the 21-day package, the woman counts Day 1 as the first day the menstrual flow starts, the next day as Day 2, and so on. On Day 5, she takes a pill. A pill is taken each day following for 21 days. At this time the package is empty. Menses will normally begin within three to four days following discontinuance of the pill and then the cycle is begun again. If a menstrual period does not begin following seven days after discontinuing the pill, the user is instructed to take a pill on the eighth day, and from then on until the pills are gone. Thus, she begins another 21-day pill cycle and the same instructions apply.

The 28-day pills are more convenient, in that the user takes a pill every day for 28 days. This eliminates remembering to count days between her cycle. The user must take the pill on the first day of her period and continue until 28 days of pill-taking are completed. At this time she is ready to begin another dispenser. The first five days of pills are placebos containing no hormones. The pills for days 6 to 26 contain the contraceptive hormones of estrogen and progestins. Pills for days 27 and 28 are placebos.

When taking minipills, the user is instructed to take one pill every day for as long as contraception is desired. There is no skipping of days and a pill is also taken on every day of the menstrual period.

The key factor in the success of any of the oral contraceptive methods is the commitment to responsible use. Any potential problem that would lower the effectiveness of the pill must be addressed. Simply forgetting seems to be the problem cited most often. In such cases it is important to tell the user to take the pill when she remembers it has been forgotten. This will mean that she is taking two pills in the same 24 hour period. This does not have a harmful effect. If two consecutive days are forgotten, the dosage is doubled for the following two days (Shapiro, 1977). For the remainder of the cycle, the regular regimen is continued. It is strongly suggested that another method of contraception also be employed during this cycle. Missing one of the combination pills during the cycle usually will not result in a pregnancy. However, missing a minipill during the cycle may result in pregnancy, since ovulation does take place.

Effects of Oral Contraceptives

The effects of oral contraceptives are not limited to the reproductive tract. Since the onset of usage there has been an increasing amount of research documenting the undesirable and, perhaps, harmful effects of long-term use. Frequently mentioned in the literature are the adverse effects on the blood pressure, carbohydrate metabolism, and the circulatory system. As early as 1965, a positive correlation between estrogen dosage in oral contraceptives and the occurrence of venous thrombosis was made (Inman & Vessey, 1968). The earlier contraceptive pills, with higher dosages of estrogen (over 50 μg) were also implicated as causative agents in cases of myocardial infarction and hepatic adenoma. With these considerations in mind, it is important for the nurse to be aware of the potentially adverse effects that oral contraceptives may have.

Liver Function. *Hepatic adenomas* (benign liver tumors) possibly have an increased incidence in oral contraceptive users. This problem is caused by estrogen and may be related to the type of estrogen used in the pill (mestranol). Nissen et al. (1976, p. 40) reported "the predominant lesions were focal modular hyperplasia, hepatic adenoma and hematoma." Current literature indicates that these tumors are relatively rare, although the risk increases with long-term usage (more than five years) of oral contraceptives. Since laboratory studies have indicated that oral contraceptives alter liver function (Shapiro, 1977, p. 33), it is recommended that individuals with any type of liver disease avoid oral contraceptives.

Gall Bladder Function. When oral contraceptives are used, there appears to be an increased likelihood of developing gallstones (Shapiro, 1977, p. 34). This may be the result of an increased concentration of cholesterol in the bile.

Blood Pressure. Oral contraceptive use is associated with a slight but significant increase in blood pressure (Fisch & Frank, 1977). The incidence of hypertension has been reported to be six times higher in birth control pill users than in nonusers. The mechanism for this occurrence is thought to be related to the renin-angiotensin-aldosterone system. Helmer & Judson (1967) reported an increase in renin substrate in women using oral contraceptives. Elevated levels of increased renin substrate stimulates the conversion of angiotensinogen to angiotensin. This results in arteriolar constriction and stimulates the adrenal cortex to secrete aldosterone, causing sodium retention in the kidneys. Consequently, sodium retention increases water retention, which expands the extracellular fluid volume and increases cardiac output. The combined effects of angiotensin-stimulated arteriolar constriction and aldosterone-stimulated sodium retention with increased cardiac output results in elevation of the blood pressure. Clinical variables such as age, weight, race, and family history must be considered when evaluating the influences of estrogen in oral contraceptives; therefore, it is only suggested that the estrogenic component is responsible for an increased blood pressure. It is essential that all individuals using birth control pills be monitored for blood pressure elevation. These elevations have been found to be most noticeable in the first six months of use.

Lipoproteins. It is well known that an elevated serum lipid level increases the risk of coronary heart disease. Use of lipids in the body requires combination of the lipid with proteins to form lipoproteins. Lipoproteins in turn mobilize and transport fat. Those lipoproteins containing the most protein are classified as high density lipoproteins (HDL). Lipoproteins higher in cholesterol are classified as low density lipoproteins (LDL). The very low density lipoproteins (VLDL) contain mostly triglycerides. The risk of developing coronary heart disease is inversely related to the level of HDL (Miller & Miller, 1975). The higher the HDL level, the lower the risk factor. Estrogen participates in the regulation of the synthesis of cholesterol and increases HDL concentrations, thus aiding in the prevention of risk factors associated with heart disease. This, however, is not the case with birth control pills. Concentration of HDL plasma levels is actually lowered in women taking birth control pills, thus they are at increased risk of developing coronary heart disease. Recently, attention has been focused on the progesterone content of the oral contraceptives as the causative agent for reduced HDL (Notelovitz et al., 1981). More definitive studies are needed to justify this implication of progesterone.

Thrombus Formation. Thrombus formation in contraceptive pill users can cause thrombophlebitis, cerebral thrombosis, pulmonary embolism, mesenteric thrombosis, retinal thrombi, and myocardial infarction. Causative factors enhancing thrombus formation are related to an increase in blood platelet adhesiveness and plasma proteins. When stimulated, plasma proteins activate as coagulation factors, causing clotting. Coagulation factors VI and VIII were found to be altered in contraceptive pill users (McGrath & Cataldi, 1975). An increase in factors IX and X has also been identified as a possible contributor to the hypercoagulability condition seen in oral contraceptive users (Poller, 1978). These two findings would, in themselves, indicate that oral contraceptives enhance coagulation of blood. Yet, another mechanism that alters coagulability must be considered. The mechanism that counteracts blood clotting, called the fibrinolytic system, consists mainly of plasminogen and antithrombin III. Without this mechanism the blood would not be maintained in a fluid state. Poller (1978) found a decrease in antithrombin III activity related to the estrogen content of oral contraceptives. Reduced antithrombin III alters the clot-lysis activity of the blood and contributes to thrombus formation. However, a more recent study of Notelovitz et al. (1981), showed that women using oral contraceptives with lower dosages of estrogen actually experienced stimulation of coagulation inhibitory factors and thus had a reduced incidence of thrombosis, in comparison with those receiving higher dosages of estrogen.

Warnings appearing on package inserts with all oral contraceptives emphasize the increased risk of cardiovascular side effects. Special emphasis is placed on the increased risk with age (over 35) and with heavy smoking (15 or more cigarettes a day).

Carbohydrate Metabolism. Elevations of blood glucose and plasma insulin levels have been noted in women using oral contraceptives (Spellacy, 1974). Metabolic homeostasis is dependent upon a balance of glucose and insulin in the blood. Alterations of either blood levels can have adverse effects that can ultimately lead to the development of atherosclerosis. Birth control pill users who demonstrate the most profound alterations in carbohydrate metabolism are the obese and diabetic. Discontinuing oral contraceptives is usually associated with a return of the blood glucose and plasma insulin to normal levels.

Nutritional Status. Particular emphasis has been placed on the effects of oral contraceptives on vitamin and mineral utilization. Vitamin B_6 (pyridoxine) metabolism was found to be abnormal in some women using oral contraceptives. This deficiency has been identified as having a causative relationship in the development of mental depression and fatigue (Stoehr et al., 1983). It has been suggested that all women using oral contraceptives receive a daily vitamin B_6 supplement (Shapiro, 1977).

Deficiencies in folic acid seem to be primarily associated with women having poor diets and adolescents. This effect has also been reported in women using oral contraceptives. Therefore, the possibility of folic acid deficiency must be considered when there is a pregnancy soon after discontinuing birth control pills. Folic acid deficiency occurring in the first months of pregnancy increases the risk of fetal anomalies. A decrease in zinc, riboflavin, vitamin C, and vitamin B_{12} has also been reported.

Carcinoma. Conflicting evidence has caused controversy when assessing the carcinogenic effects of oral contraceptives. Long-term use of oral contraceptives containing estrogen was thought to increase the risk of endometrial carcinoma. This risk was dependent on the dosage of estrogen and the duration of usage. The strongest supportive evidence was found in women who used the sequential oral contraceptives, which are no longer on the market. More recent data and studies have shown that the risk for endometrial cancer and ovarian cancer is actually reduced in birth control pill users (Ory et al., 1982).

Evidence of an increased incidence of cervical cancer is lacking. Precancerous cervical dysplasia is more commonly related to factors such as early marriage, frequent sex partners, and venereal type disorders rather than the use of oral contraceptives. It is essential that all birth control users have regular Papanicolaou (Pap) tests.

Hormonal sensitive neoplasias, such as breast carcinoma, have been suspected of having an increased occurrence in oral contraceptive users. Investigative studies have not found evidence to support this relationship. According to Ory et al. (1976), breast tumors are actually reduced in contraceptive pill users. It does appear, however, that once breast cancer is present, the use of birth control pills containing estrogen will stimulate growth in the cancer.

Contraceptive pills containing estrogen and/or progesterone are contraindicated during pregnancy. Conception occurring while a woman is using birth control pills is rare. When it does occur, a variety of fetal birth defects may be found. These have been collectively described by Kolodny et al. (1979) as VACTERL (vertebral, anal, cardiac, tracheoesophageal, renal, and limb) defects. Furthermore, in utero exposure of the female fetus to nonsteroidal synthetic estrogens (diethylstilbesterol, or DES) increases the risk later in life of clear cell adenocarcinoma, a rare but malignant type of vaginal and cervical cancer (Herbest et al., 1974).

There are some absolute contraindications to the use of oral contraceptives. A woman in any of the following categories should not use birth control pills.

ABSOLUTE CONTRAINDICATIONS FOR ORAL CONTRACEPTIVES

- Carcinoma of reproductive system or breast
- Coronary artery disease
- Chronic or acute liver disorders
- Pregnancy
- Thromboembolic disorders
- Thrombophlebitis

Women falling into the categories of generalized contraindications should be carefully evaluated, advised of the contraindications and counseled accordingly.

GENERALIZED CONTRAINDICATIONS FOR ORAL CONTRACEPTIVES

- Over 35 years of age
- Asthma
- Breast disease
- Cardiac problems
- Chloasma
- Depression
- Diabetic, prediabetic, or family history of diabetes
- Epilepsy
- Gallbladder disease
- Lactation
- Mononucleosis—acute phase
- Extreme obesity
- Renal disease
- Sickle cell disease
- Heavy smoking
- Surgery scheduled within four weeks
- Thyroid disease
- Vaginal bleeding—undiagnosed
- Varicose veins

Side Effects of Oral Contraception

Women using oral contraceptives may experience some side effects. Side effects are individualized and may disappear after a period of usage, or it may be necessary to consider another brand of pills. This is contingent upon the content and dosage of the progestin and or estrogen. Some of the commonly used pills, their contents and side effects are listed in Table 6–2.

Some side effects are considered dangerous when they become severe or are combined with other symptoms. They should be reported to the health professional immediately, as they may indicate cardiac or thromboembolic conditions.

DANGER SIGNS WHEN USING ORAL CONTRACEPTIVES

- Severe chest pains and shortness of breath
- Severe headaches
- Severe abdominal pains
- Severe pain in calf or thigh
- Visual disturbance associated with blurring, halo effect, flashing lights

Advantages of Oral Contraceptive Use

At this point, birth control pills appear to be the most effective method of temporary contraception. Effectiveness is based on both theoretical and actual use effectiveness of the product. Theoretical effectiveness and actual use effectiveness offer different data when measuring rates of effectiveness of contraceptive methods. Theoretical effectiveness denotes the effectiveness of a contraceptive method when used under ideal conditions with no errors. Actual use effectiveness speaks to the realistic use in field trials of women encompassing both correct and incorrect usage. Literature descriptions of theoretical effectiveness indicate there is less than one pregnancy per 100 women years in oral contraceptive users. Clinically, the actual use effectiveness may range from four to ten pregnancies per 100 women years (Hatcher et al., 1981). Overall, oral contraceptives are considered to be 99 percent effective.

Considered an advantage by many oral contraceptive users is the relationship of contraceptive hormonal action to menstrual flow

TABLE 6–2
ORAL CONTRACEPTIVE PRODUCTS AND SIDE EFFECTS

Estrogen Content	Product Name*	Progestin Content
	COMBINATION PILLS	
Ethinyl estradiol-20 mcg	ZORANE 1 + 20	Norethindrone acetate-1 mg
Ethinyl estradiol-30 mcg	LO/OVRAL	Norgestrel-0.3 mg
Ethinyl estradiol-35 mcg	MODICON	Norethindrone-0.5 mg
Ethinyl estradiol-50 mcg	DEMULEN	Ethynodiol diacetate-1 mg
Ethinyl estradiol-50 mcg	NORLESTRIN 2.5/50	Norethindrone acetate-2.5 mg
Mestranol-80 mcg	NORINYL 1 + 80	Norethindrone-1 mg
Mestranol-100 mcg	ORTHO-NOVUM 2 mg	Norethindrone-2 mg
Mestranol-100 mcg	ENOVID-E	Norethynodrel-2.5 mg
	MINIPILLS	
	OVRETTE	Norgestrel-0.075 mg
	NOR-QD	Norethindrone-0.35 mg
	MICRONOR	Norethindrone-0.35 mg
Estrogen Side Effects Excess		**Progestin Side Effects Excess**
Nausea/vomiting		Acne
Bloating		Appetite increase
Fluid retention		Weight gain—tissue
Chloasma (mask of pregnancy)		Depression
Headache		Headaches
Breast tenderness (mastodynia)		Increased Candida albicans infections
Increased cervical mucous discharge		Mastodynia
Weight gain—fluid		Decreased libido
Blood pressure increase		Fatigue
Premenstrual tension		Decreased or absent menses
		Breakthrough bleeding
		Increased facial hair
Estrogen Deficiency		**Progestin Deficiency**
Decreased libido		Hypermenorrhea
Vaginal dryness		Clotting of menstrual flow
Dyspareunia (painful intercourse)		Weight loss
Nervousness		Delayed menses
Irritability		Spotting late in cycle
Early spotting		
Amenorrhea		

*This list is not meant to be a complete list of oral contraceptives. It represents a list of a variety of types and dosages of oral contraceptives.

and duration. Individuals taking birth control pills experience decreased duration of menstrual flow and smaller amounts of blood during their periods. An indirect advantage is a reduction in the amount of iron and calcium lost through the menstrual flow. The long-term effect may be beneficial in reduction of anemia and degenerative joint disease.

Dysmenorrhea (painful menstruation) is reduced in women who use oral contraceptives, particularly the combination type pill, and occasionally this is a permanent side effect.

Ory reported a decrease in the number of cases of pelvic inflammatory disease in women using oral contraceptives (1982). He further stated that ovarian cysts and fibrocystic disease were also decreased in oral contraceptive users.

Convenience certainly must be considered when discussing the advantages of birth control pills. Simply taking a pill is more convenient and inducive to sexuality than is the use of a condom, foam, or diaphragm.

An additional benefit of birth control pills is an increase in the frequency of physical check-ups. During these examinations a Pap test, breast examination, and cervical smear are done. The supply of birth control pills or prescriptions for pills is limited to three to six months a year and can only be renewed when the client returns for her physical examination.

Nursing Responsibilities for Oral Contraceptives

The nurse is responsible for effective counseling based on sound professional knowledge. Many potential problems can be averted if the client is provided with appropriate information when needed. Complications, contraindications, side effects, and advantages of oral contraceptives must be included in all patient information. There are, however, areas of patient concern that may alter birth control usage. Often these concerns are not included in the oral or printed information given to clients. The nurse should be aware of these potential concerns and counsel the client accordingly.

A very legitimate concern of birth control pill users is the relationship between smoking and birth control pills. Evidence suggests that smoking while using birth control pills increases the risk of myocardial infarction (Jain, 1976). Another form of contraception should be considered if the client smokes. Those who are over 35 years of age are at a greater risk for developing complications.

The age of the client is an important factor when discussing oral contraceptives. Women over age 40 should be advised not to use oral contraceptives. Women under age 40 should be informed of the implied risk of thromboembolism, heart attack, and cerebrovascular accidents. It should also be noted that the frequency of these complications is greatly reduced in women under age 30 with no other risk factors. The mortality rate for women age 30 to 39 with cardiovascular problems is increased two to eight times when they use oral contraceptives (Mann et al., 1976).

The question of alterations in *libido* (sexual desire) in birth control pill users is one that remains unanswered. Women have reported both an increase and a decrease in sexual drive while taking birth control pills. Increased sexual desire may be related to a decrease in the fear of pregnancy. The shorter periods and fewer premenstrual symptoms noted may also considerably increase coital frequency. Paradoxically, a decrease in libido has been experienced by a limited number of women. It has been suggested that under these circumstances it is advisable to change to a pill containing larger amounts of estrogen. This, however, has not been reliably demonstrated in research studies.

The action of oral contraceptives has been known to be diminished by certain antibiotics (ampicillin), by anticonvulsants (phenobarbitol, primidone, phenytoin), and by antitubercular drugs (rifampin) (Stoehr et al., 1983). The list is not limited to these drugs. With many drugs, confirmative data is insufficient to warrant consideration at this time. Stoehr et al. (1983), recommend carefully monitoring the client for breakthrough bleeding, which may indicate a diminished estrogen effect. With other drugs, such as insulin and Orinase, an increase in dosage may be necessary. As mentioned previously, clotting factors may be increased by the estrogen component of oral contraceptives. Therefore, the dosages of anticoagulants such as warfarin (Coumadin) and heparin may need to be increased. Moreover, all medications taken by clients receiving oral contraceptives should be carefully monitored for signs of diminished or increased effects as well as adverse interactions. It is equally important for clients to realize they must inform physicians of any and all medications they are taking before a prescription for birth control pills is written.

The long-term effects of contraceptives on future fertility and conception is negligible. Suppression of the hypothalamus may continue for as long as three months after oral contraceptives are discontinued; however, this impairment diminishes with time. Post-pill amenorrhea is more apparent in women who have a previous history of irregular periods.

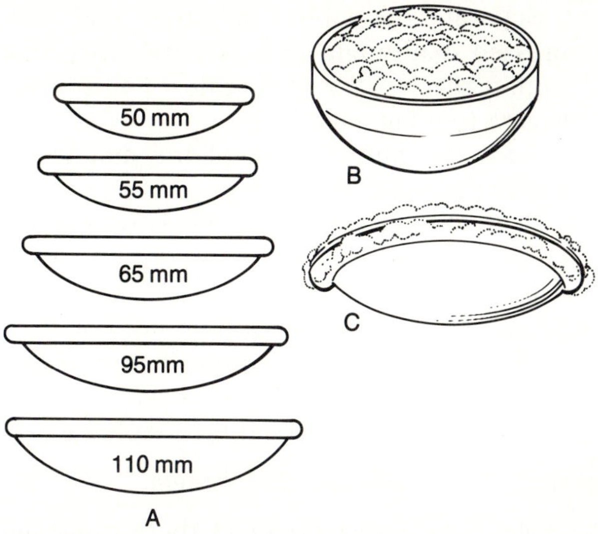

FIGURE 6-3. Sizes and types of diaphragms: **A.** Sizes ranging from 50 mm to 110 mm. **B.** Metal flat band rim diaphragm. **C.** Compressed spring band rim diaphragm.

DIAPHRAGM

The diaphragm is a mechanical method of contraception that originated in the 1800s. Initially, the method provided only a barrier for the transportation of sperm. The use of spermicidal creams with the diaphragm has enhanced their effectiveness.

Diaphragms are flexible, circular metal rings covered with a cap of latex rubber that is filled with a spermicidal cream and inserted into the vagina covering the cervix. It provides both a mechanical and chemical barrier to the entrance of sperm into the cervix.

To insure effectiveness, the diaphragm must be properly fitted by the physician or nurse practitioner. It should completely cover the cervix and be anchored in the posterior fornix of the vagina. Since diaphragms are available in many sizes and types (see Fig. 6-3), it is necessary for the examiner to determine internal measurements of the client. Measurements are taken and the proper size diaphragm is determined. The sizes range from diameters of 50 mm to 110 mm. Contraindications to the use of the diaphragm such as a cystocele, vesicovaginal fistula, rectovaginal fistula, uterine prolapse, anteversion of the uterus, and retroversion of the uterus should also be noted at the time of examination. Once the proper size has been determined, the examiner explains to the client the correct method of insertion.

Instructions for insertion would include:

Do not insert more than two hours prior to intercourse

Before insertion inspect the diaphragm to see that there are no tears or holes

Place a thin film of spermicidal cream on the rim of the diaphragm

Place a teaspoonful of spermicidal cream or jelly in the dome of the diaphragm

Assume one of the following positions:

(1) Standing with one foot elevated on the toilet seat or a stool

(2) Lying flat on the bed with the knees bent

(3) Sitting on the side of the bed with thighs separated

Compress the opposing sides of the diaphragm

Separate the labia and insert the compressed diaphragm in a posterior direction until it reaches the furthermost point of the vagina (see Fig. 6-4)

Tuck the anterior rim of the diaphragm under the pubic bone

Feel to make sure the cervix is completely covered by the cap

Do not remove the diaphragm for 6 to 8 hours after intercourse and do not douche

If intercourse is desired again insert another application of spermicide into the vagina without disturbing the diaphragm

Instructions to Remove Diaphragm

Place the index finger in the vagina and release the front rim by pulling downward and outward

Wash the diaphragm with warm soapy water, rinse well, and dry

Return to container

After the instructions for insertion and removal of the diaphragm have been given, the examiner should allow the woman to practice inserting and removing it. The examiner can then check to make sure the placement and size are correct. The woman is instructed to return for reassessment at the time of her regular yearly examination and if she has cervical surgery, a miscarriage, loses or gains 5 to 10 pounds, or experiences childbirth.

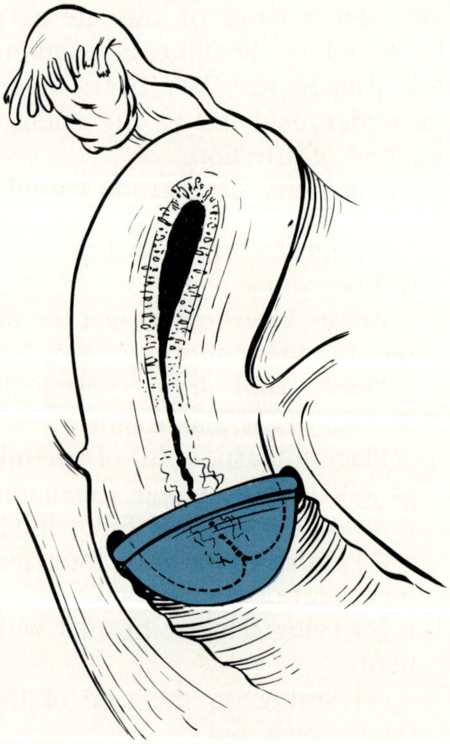

FIGURE 6-4. Proper placement of diaphragm.

Information regarding the disadvantages of the diaphragm must also be provided for the client. Dislodgement of the diaphragm is a disadvantage that can occur following frequent penile insertion. Spontaneity of lovemaking is hindered by the need to remember to insert the diaphragm and is considered by many as a distinct disadvantage. Touching of the genital area is repugnant to some women and seen as a disadvantage for insertion and checking of proper positioning. There are available plastic and metal inserters, which aid in the insertion process but are not effective for confirming proper position.

The diaphragm, when used with spermicidal cream or jelly, has a theoretical effectiveness of two to three pregnancies per 100 women years. The actual use effectiveness is 20 to 25 pregnancies per 100 women years.

When properly cared for, the diaphragm should last about a year.

INTRAUTERINE DEVICES

In ancient times everything from gold to stones was used to insert into the uterine cavities and vaginas of both animals and women to prevent pregnancy. Although, perhaps effective in their intent, these objects were also associated with a high incidence of pelvic infections and vaginal bleeding. Yet, the concept remained and with new adaptations and materials the intrauterine device (IUD) has been used as an effective means of contraception.

Recently, in the United States, the use of IUDs has produced much controversy. The safety of the IUD has become a matter of concern to the health professions as well as to the consumer. Previously utilized devices such as the Lippes loop, the Cooper Cu-7 and TCu 380A have either been withdrawn from the market or will no longer be manufactured. The increase in law suits filed by consumers against manufacturers in which IUDs have been associated with or implicated in adverse effects has promoted these actions by the manufacturers. Negative publicity associated with the Dalkon Shield IUD and a five-fold increase in the incidence of pelvic inflammatory disease associated with its use has resulted in a nationwide campaign by the manufacturers to inform women still using the device to have them removed as soon as possible. The Dalkon Shield IUD has not been manufactured since 1974.

Problems associated with IUDs include increased menstrual flow, increased uterine cramping, increased incidence of pelvic inflammatory disease, septic abortions, uterine perforations, ectopic pregnancy, and accidental expulsion of the device.

In spite of the restraints placed on the use of IUDs they still remain an effective method of contraception. IUDs have a 95 to 99 percent theoretical effectiveness. The Progestasert IUD is, at this time, still being marketed in the United States. This progesterone-treated IUD (see Fig. 6–5) slowly releases progesterone and has an irritative effect on the endometrium. In European countries, the IUD is second only to oral contraceptives in popularity.

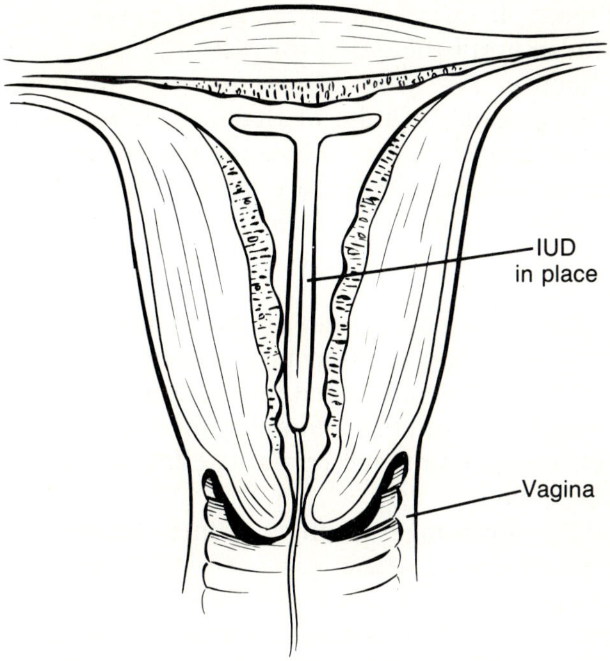

FIGURE 6–5. Progestasert intrauterine device.

CERVICAL CAP

The *cervical cap* is a 1-inch in diameter rubber cap that fits over the cervix and is secured by suction (see Fig. 6–6). Although it resembles the diaphragm in its method of contraceptive protection, it is smaller and does not rely on the spring action utilized by the diaphragm. As with the diaphragm, however, it is necessary to fill the cap with a spermicidal agent. The cap must be left in place for eight hours following intercourse. Currently, the cap has not been approved by the Food and Drug Administration (FDA) for use in the United

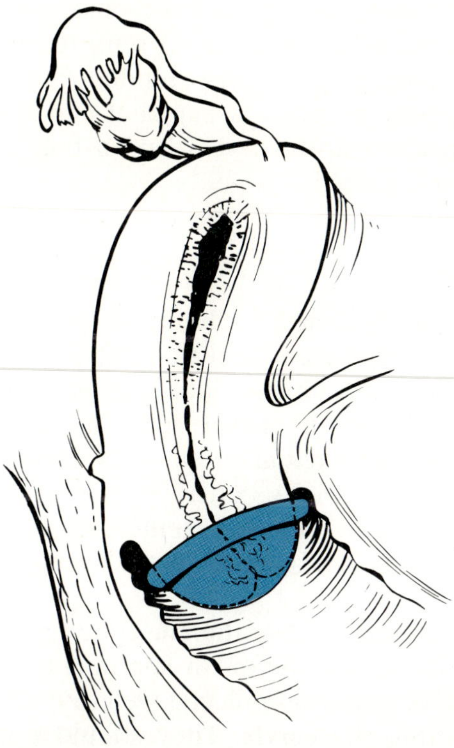

FIGURE 6–6. Placement of cervical cap.

States. It may only be used for research studies until the data proves it to be safe and effective. Two years of preliminary studies by the National Institute of Health have found it to be as effective as the diaphragm; however, further clinical studies are needed before it is approved. Data is not currently available to determine its theoretical or actual use effectiveness.

The cap may be left in place for several days, providing contraceptive protection without immediate advanced preparation. The recommended length of time that the cap may be left in place and still retain its effectiveness is three days.

The advantages of the cap include the enhancement of sexual pleasure. Although the cervical cap has advantages over the diaphragm, such as smaller size and the length of time it can be worn, it also has some distinct disadvantages. The insertion technique is more difficult, as the cap must fit directly over the cervix. Dislodgement during intercourse is also a possibility. As with the diaphragm, allergies to the latex material from which it is made may exist. Inflammatory cervical responses and foul vagina discharges have been reported in women wearing the caps for extended (more than two weeks) periods. A cap that can remain in place for up to a year and a half is now being researched.

SPERMICIDES

Spermicides are designed to be used with a diaphragm or cervical cap and as sperm-killing agents directly introduced into the vagina. They are available in cream, jelly, aerosol, foam, tablets, and vaginal suppository forms. Spermicidal preparations consist of a sperm-killing agent and an adhering creme base that holds the spermicidal agent in place over the cervix.

It is very important that the client be given complete instructions before a spermicide is used. All of the agents are placed well into the vagina covering the cervix. They should not be placed in the vagina sooner than 30 minutes before intercourse. The client is instructed to remain in a supine position and not to walk about. Before each act of intercourse a new application of spermicide must be inserted. The client is told not to douche for at least eight hours after coitus.

Special instructions accompany the different spermicidal preparations. Foams are to be shaken well before the measured amount is placed in the applicator (see Fig. 6–7). Suppositories must be stored in a cool place. When using the jellies or creams it is necessary to be sure that the applicator is completely filled with the spermicidal agent.

The chief advantage of spermicides is that they may be obtained without a prescription. Some women are embarrassed to consult a physician when in need of a contraceptive and find spermicides easily available. Teenagers will buy spermicides because they are inexpensive and there is no need for consultation with a physician, eliminating the chance that parents will be informed of their sexual activity. This may be a double-edged sword, however, as improper use of the spermicides may result in pregnancy.

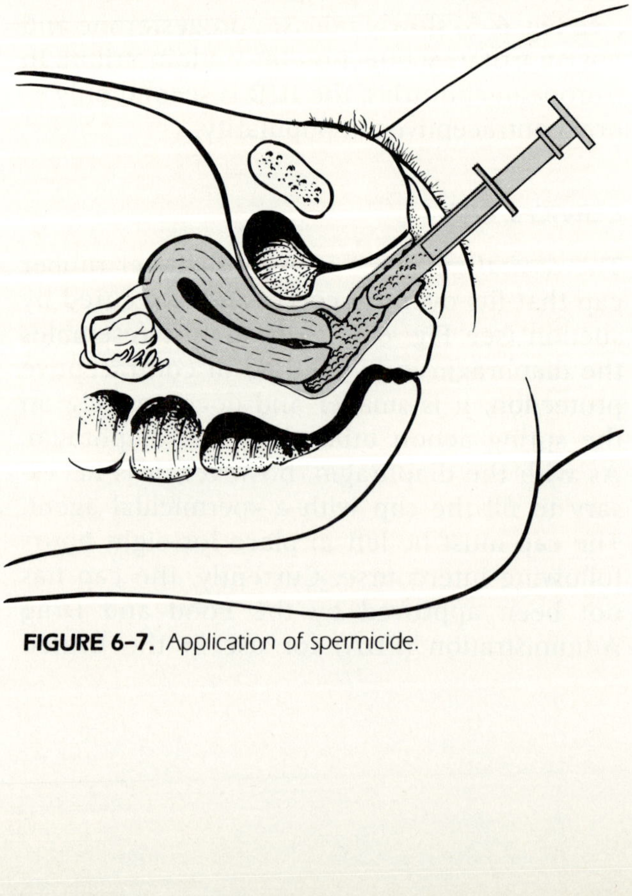

FIGURE 6–7. Application of spermicide.

Planning ahead for sexual intercourse is essential when using spermicides as the primary contraceptive. This is considered by many to be a distinct disadvantage. Other potential disadvantages are the vaginal and penile allergic reactions and irritations caused by some spermicidal preparations in susceptable individuals. Often the client complains that spermicidal residue not only burns, but is messy as well.

The greatest disadvantage of spermicides is the high rate of conception when spermicides are used alone. The theoretical effectiveness of the spermicides is 75 percent overall, but actual use effectiveness indicates the foams to be the most effective, followed by the jellies and creams, and least effective of all, the suppositories. The actual use effectiveness is less than 50 percent.

CONDOMS

The 400-year-old method of contraception, the *condom*, is still very much a part of today's scene. This mechanical method consists of a thin rubber or latex sheath placed over the erect penis to act as a depository for sperm during intercourse.

Special instructions regarding the use of condoms should be given. The condom must be in place before there is any vaginal contact. When applying the condom the tip should be compressed between the thumb and forefinger, forming an air pocket. This allows room at the tip of the condom for the ejaculated sperm. There are condoms available that have a nipplelike tip that serves to catch the ejaculate and eliminates manual formation of the pouch. Shortly after intercourse the condom-covered erect penis should be withdrawn from the vagina, eliminating any chance of sperm spillage and slippage.

Condoms should be stored in a cool dry place and discarded if old or deteriorated. Spermicidal jelly or foam may be used to lubricate the condom if necessary, but petroleum jelly such as vaseline can dissolve the rubber and should not be used. A new type of spermicidal lubricated condom was approved by the FDA in 1982. This spermicidal agent, nonoxynal-9, is very effective in reducing sperm motility when an accidental spillage of sperm does occur.

Distinct advantages are found with the use of condoms. Principal among these are low cost and ease of procurement. A unique feature of the condom is the protection it provides from the transmission of sexual diseases. It is appropriate to suggest to clients using another form of contraceptive that they also use condoms if they have a sexually transmittable disease.

Criticism of the condom is most frequently expressed by the male. Decreased sexual sensations are mentioned as the major objection by men and women. With this method of contraception coital interruption is necessary, which is viewed by some as a disadvantage.

VAGINAL SPONGES

Approved by the FDA in 1983 and on the market now, are the 2-inch diameter disposable *vaginal sponges*. The spermicidal-soaked polyurethene sponge contains the spermicide nonoxynal-9. The polyurethene sponge slowly releases the spermicide over a 24-hour period. Effectiveness of the sponge is also enhanced by its mechanical barrier effect. The sponge does not contain any hormones and is available without a prescription.

Before the sponge is inserted into the vagina it must be moistened with water. The sponge has a concave surface which fits against the cervix and is held in place by the vaginal walls. Removal is facilitated by a loop connected to the sponge.

The vaginal sponge has been implicated for its possible role in the development of toxic shock syndrome. In 1983, the Center for Disease Control reported four cases of *staphylococcus aureus*-related toxic shock syndrome in sponge users. All of the patients had worn the sponge longer than the recommended 24 hours. Studies done before the approval of the sponge, however, found it to have a bacteriostatic effect, making it hostile to these organisms.

The polyurethene material used in the sponge has been questioned as a potential cancer-causing agent. These claims have been based on the research linking polyurethene to cancerous lesions in laboratory mice. There has been no evidence to substantiate the implications relative to the sponge and cancer. Vaginal sponges have been reported as causing irritation and itching of the vulva in a limited number of cases.

The effectiveness of the sponge has not been documented.

Natural Methods of Family Planning

Natural family planning methods are chosen by those who wish to prevent conception, yet for moral, cultural, religious, or health reasons do not choose mechanical or hormonal methods of contraception. With some couples the motivation for choosing a natural method of contraception is a desire for naturalness. Other couples worry about the side effects of artificial contraceptive methods on both the woman and a possible fetus. Whatever the reason for choosing a natural family planning method, commitment to the method is absolutely essential.

The basic concept involved in most natural family planning methods is fertility awareness. The days of the cycle during which the woman is considered to be fertile (capable of conception) encompass two days before ovulation, the day of ovulation, and two days following ovulation. Therefore, the woman is instructed to abstain from sexual intercourse during this five-day period. It then remains to be determined on which day of the cycle ovulation takes place. Each of the four natural family planning methods offers a technique to make this determination. The four techniques are: the rhythm method, the basal body temperature method, the cervical mucus method, and the symptothermal method.

RHYTHM METHOD

The *rhythm method* relies on the calculation of the safe time for intercourse by mathematically determining when ovulation will take place. In order to facilitate this, the woman is instructed to keep an accurate record of the length of her menstrual periods for six to eight months. She should note the length of both the shortest and longest cycles. The first day of the menstrual bleeding is designated as day 1 of the cycle. Once cycle lengths have been determined, 18 days are subtracted from the shortest cycle and 11 days from the longest cycle. The days included between these two figures represent the fertile period. Using this method, if a client's cycles last from 26 (the shortest) to 30 days (the longest), the days of possible fertility are between days 8 and 19 of her menstrual cycle. Although this principle is sound in theory, there is no assurance that cycle variations will remain as calculated. Illness, emotional conflict, stress, and poor nutrition are but a few of the factors that can alter the client's normal menstrual cycle. Abstinence is the key word during the unsafe period. This may be inconvenient and difficult for some clients.

BASAL BODY TEMPERATURE METHOD

Observation of temperature changes is used to determine the safe period when using the *basal body temperature* (*BBT*) *method*. Temperature variations following ovulation result from the presence of progesterone produced by the corpus luteum of the follicle. Prior to ovulation the temperature will drop slightly and then elevate about 0.4°F to 1.0°F, indicating that ovulation has occurred. Thereafter, the temperature remains at the postovulation elevation until the next menstrual period. Obviously, determining ovulation by this method is after the fact. Verification of the safe period is dependent upon a continued elevation for three to four days following the initial rise. This would necessitate the client refraining from intercourse during the entire first half of the cycle.

The woman using the BBT method should be instructed to take her temperature every day before arising in the morning. This may be done orally or rectally, but always in the same manner. The temperature reading is then recorded on a graph (see Fig. 6–8). When there is a noticeable rise in temperature, notations are made on the graph, and should reflect any temperature change due to illness, emotion, lack of sleep, and other such variables. If the rise is due to ovulation, the temperature should remain elevated for the

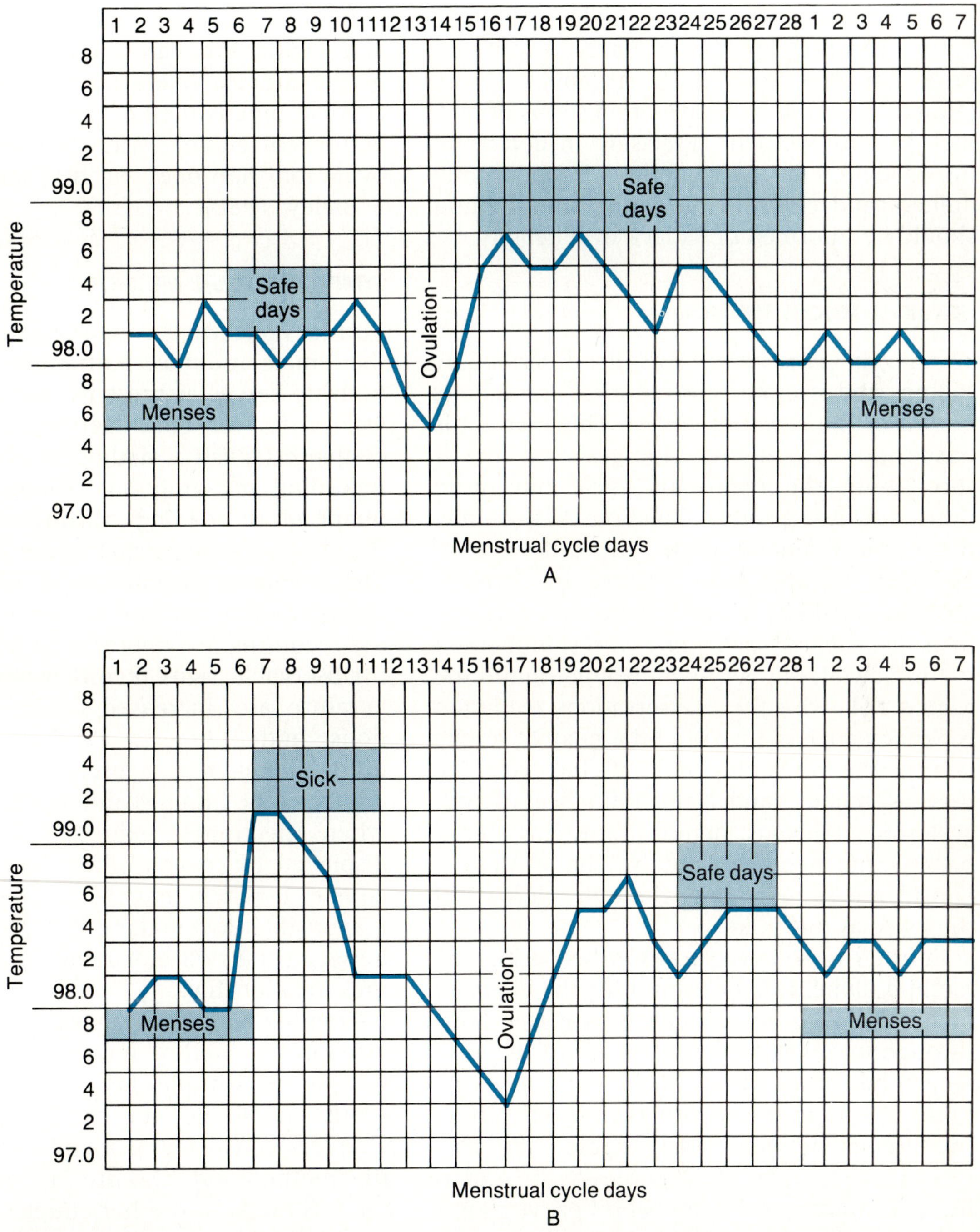

FIGURE 6–8. Basal body temperature graph: A. Ovulation—13th day. B. Ovulation—16th day.

remainder of the cycle. Accurate temperature taking and record keeping is absolutely necessary for success with this method.

The greatest drawback to the use of the BBT method is the necessity for daily temperature determinations and recordings. These essential steps can be forgotten or overlooked, completely altering the results.

According to Hilgers and Bailey (1980, p. 339), "The BBT appears to have an inherent error rate (6.8 to 9.5%) in its ability to accurately determine the ovulation status of normal, healthy women." Precision in determining ovulation by BBT method is apparently limited, and clients considering this method should be informed of its lack of reliability.

CERVICAL MUCUS METHOD

The *cervical mucus method* was first described by Billings and is often referred to as the *Billings method* or the *ovulation method*. This method is based on the mucus changes that occur throughout the menstrual cycle but more noticeably just prior to ovulation. At this time, the cervical mucus, under the influence of estrogen, becomes more profuse and stretchable. Stretchability of cervical mucus is referred to as *spinnbarkeit*. Coinciding with spinnbarkeit is a noticeable slippery-wet feeling around the vagina. Following these observations, ovulation is expected to occur within the next 24 hours. During the remaining half of the cycle the cervical mucus, under the influence of progesterone, thickens, demonstrates less spinnbarkeit and becomes cloudy. The woman is considered to be in the safe, unfertile part of the cycle at this point.

In order to achieve success when using this method alone, it is necessary for the client to be familiar with her normal cervical secretions throughout several cycles. She is instructed to record her observations of the cervical secretions. She notes the spinnbarkeit by stretching the mucus between two fingers. She also records the lubricative properties of the mucus from day to day. If she notices other symptoms during her cycle, such as mittelschmerz (ovulatory pain from rupturing follicle), heightened sexual desires, and breakthrough bleeding from increased estrogen levels, she should also record these (Britt, 1977). After several cycles, an assessment is made of the notations and determination of the fertile period is possible.

False readings of cervical mucus consistency are possible. Factors such as infection and vaginal lubricants can alter the character of the mucus. Aside from these factors, the cervical mucus method appears to have a far better correlation with the actual time of ovulation than does the BBT method (Hilgers & Bailey, 1980).

SYMPTOTHERMAL METHOD

Mutual concerned cooperative effort by both the female and male partners in a sexual relationship serves as the basis for the *symptothermal method* of contraception. Together the couple establish a method of observation and recording of symptoms. Characteristics and temperature readings throughout several of the woman's menstrual cycles are recorded. The woman is responsible for observations of the symptoms and the man is responsible for the recording of symptoms on a chart.

Observable signs recorded along with temperature are: increased libido, mucus variations, mittelschmerz, spotting, mood alterations, and increased breast size. The couple discusses the findings and together determines when affectionate expression of love is best displayed by means other than sexual intercourse. It is felt that the mutual concern for responsible lovemaking establishes a bond between the two individuals that strengthens their relationship.

Training courses designed for couples interested in this method have been offered by the Couple to Couple League (CCL). This lay group encourages the establishment of local chapters consisting of members who practice this method and who are interested in teaching this method to other couples.

COITUS INTERRUPTUS

Mention must be made of the oldest method of contraception known to man: *coitus interruptus*. This method of withdrawal of the penis from the vagina before ejaculation is considered the least reliable form of contraception.

The male assumes complete responsibility for withdrawal. He may not be able to accomplish this feat before ejaculation. Occasionally, there is a preejaculate of which the male may not be aware. This small amount of semen may contain enough sperm for fertilization.

In spite of the fact that this contraceptive method is inexpensive and natural, it is not recommended as the primary method of contraception. It can be used effectively, but not reliably. Many authorities do not consider it as a category of natural family planning methods.

Permanent Methods of Contraception

Two basic methods of permanent sterilization are used for contraceptive purposes: vasectomy in males, and tubal ligation in females. Although these methods are considered permanent, they may be reversible. In cases where successful reversal has been accomplished, the fertility rate is less than 50 percent. It is, therefore, necessary when advising couples who are seeking contraceptive advice to inform them clearly that both vasectomy and tubal ligation should not be considered unless permanent sterilization is desired. Careful consideration should be given by both partners to all the effects of permanent sterilization on the relationship and the family. If alternative methods of contraception are not acceptable and there is no future desire for children, then sterilization may be the method of choice. Before the procedure is done, informed consent followed by a waiting period is required. The choice must be voluntary, the client over 21 and mentally competent. Although consent by the other partner is desired, it is not required by law.

VASECTOMY

A *vasectomy* is a surgical procedure involving the cutting and ligation of the male vas deferens (see Fig. 6–9). In order to gain access to the vas deferens, an incision is made on either side of the scrotum, through which the procedure is performed. Following surgery, it is impossible for the sperm to pass from the testes even though they continue to be produced. When blocked, they are simply absorbed by the body. All the other manifestations of sexuality such as penile erections, orgasm, and ejaculation remain intact.

The procedure can be done in the physician's office under a local anesthetic. It does not require hospitalization. Following the procedure it is most important to explain to the client that he is not immediately sterile. He must continue to use another form of contraceptive

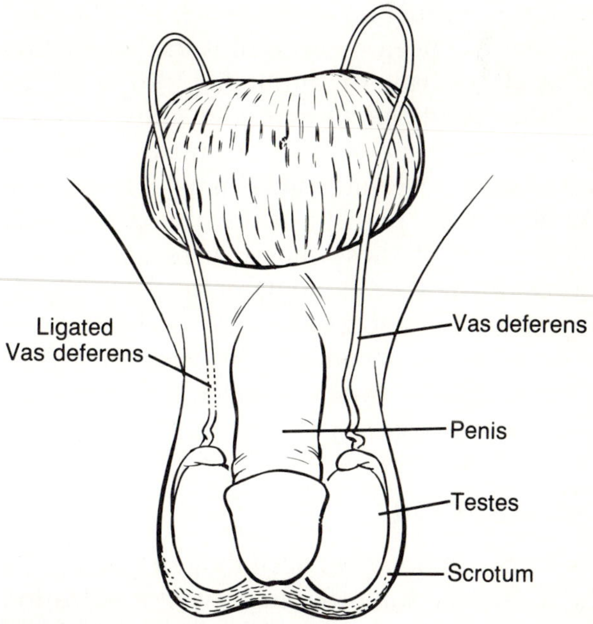

FIGURE 6–9. Vasectomy.

until he presents two ejaculate specimens that are sperm free. This may take as long as six to ten weeks and may involve as many as 15 ejaculations. The volume of seminal fluid remains essentially the same but contains no sperm.

Men are often concerned about possible diminished sexual drive following a vasectomy. Male sexual drive and characteristics are produced by the hormone testosterone, secreted by the testes. The hormone is released directly into the bloodstream and does not follow the same pathway through the vas deferens as do the sperm. There is, therefore, no effect on testosterone when a vasectomy is performed. On the contrary, some men report an increase in sexual drive owing to the relief of anxiety resulting from a diminished fear of impregnating their partner.

Vasovasectomy is the term used to describe the operation for reversal of a vasectomy. The incisionary site is in close proximity to the previous vasectomy incision. The vas deferens are then reconnected and the sperm allowed to once again pass through the vas deferens. Although anatomic restoration may be accomplished, fertility may not always be restored. In part, this may be caused by the surgical destruction of the tissue. Another factor that has been mentioned is the production of male antisperm antibodies. Royle et al. (1981) found the presence of antisperm antibodies in 79 percent of 130 males following vasectomy reversal and seminal plasma antibodies in 26 percent of the 130 males. Still, 53 percent of these males were able to impregnate their wives. Apparently, the antibody formation following vasectomy is elevated but not enough to account for an absolute reduction of fertility. Much research remains to be done in this area.

TUBAL LIGATION

Tubal ligation involves occluding or cutting the fallopian tubes in order to prevent fertilization of the egg by the sperm. There are three basic methods of tubal ligation: laparoscopy ("band-aid"), laparotomy, and vaginal tubal ligation.

Laparoscopy is performed under general anesthesia as outpatient surgery. The laparoscope is inserted into a very small incision made below the umbilicus. Carbon dioxide is then injected into the abdomen to allow visualization of the abdominal contents. The original incision site may be used or a second incision, located below the first, made to allow for the introduction of the electric cautery and the subsequent severing and coagulating of the fallopian tube. It is also possible to occlude the tubes by placing elastic bands or clips on them. These clips or bands may be removed at a later date if the client desires a reversal of the sterilization. It is important for the client to realize that the success rate is variable.

Laparotomy involves entry into the abdomen through a suprapubic incision. Here again the fallopian tubes are located and occluded by ligation, crushing, or perhaps plugging. A hospital stay is required.

The terms *colpotomy* and *culdoscopy* are used to describe the two methods of vaginal tubal ligation. Utilizing the colpotomy method, an incision is made into the vagina behind the cervix. The cul-de-sac of the peritoneal cavity is entered and the fallopian tubes brought through the incision and tied. In culdoscopy, a culdoscope is inserted into the vaginal incision while the woman assumes a knee-chest position. The area is viewed and the tubes are tied. Both of these procedures have an increased incidence of infection and are infrequently performed, since the introduction of the laparoscopy procedure.

Complications seen with tubal ligations are limited. There does, however, exist a possibility of transient cardiac arrhythmias associated with accumulation of carbon dioxide within the abdominal cavity during a laparoscopy. Some women have also reported abdominal discomfort and dysmenorrhea following tubal ligation. This may in part be due to pelvic congestion created by alterations in the vascular and lymphatic circulation. The general risks that can occur with any surgery and associated anesthesia must also be considered as risk factors during tubal ligation.

Vaginal ligations carry a greater risk of complications than do the abdominal procedures. Pelvic infections constitute the greatest risk, with bladder and bowel lacerations also occurring with some frequency. Pregnancy rates following vaginal tubal ligations are also higher than those for abdominal ligations.

Contraindications for any tubal ligation include severe cardiac and respiratory disease, obesity, intestinal obstruction, abdominal malignancy, and previous extensive abdominal surgery. Surgical procedures are also associated with cost factors and surgical risk and discomfort factors.

Less Reliable Methods of Contraception

BREAST FEEDING

Old wives' tales often refer to breast feeding as nature's contraceptive. This belief is still held by many in modern society, even though it has resulted in the conception of many children. There is unreliable contraceptive value in breast feeding and those adhering to natural child spacing should be advised to utilize another contraceptive method. Oral contraceptives should not be advised, as synthetic hormones are transmitted to the baby in the breast milk.

DOUCHING

For centuries women have unsuccessfully tried to prevent pregnancy by instilling a variety of solutions into the vagina. It did not work centuries ago, and it does not work now. Often women are misled by the labeling on the douche package, which states that the product is medicated. This is interpreted to mean that the solution kills sperm and is, therefore, effective in preventing pregnancy. Again this is in error. The medication only produces a cleansing effect and cannot kill sperm.

MORNING-AFTER PILL

Postcoital contraception can be realized with the use of diethylstilbestrol (DES) given within 72 hours following intercourse. Diethylstilbestrol is a highly potent form of a nonsteroidal synthetic estrogen. Its actions affect the endometrial implantation site and the corpus luteum of the ovary. It prevents implantation of the egg by interfering with endometrial enzymes. The corpus luteum, under the influence of DES, produces inadequate amounts of progesterone for retention of the conceptus. Both of these effects contribute to the 99 percent rate of effectiveness.

Unfortunately, reported side effects of DES are common. These side effects include nausea and vomiting, *mastodynia* (breast tenderness), vertigo (dizziness), headaches, and menstrual irregularities. All the side effects are related to the high dose of estrogen, 2.5 mg twice daily for five days.

Although DES is effective in postcoital contraception, it is viewed by many as an inadequate method of contraception. This attitude reflects the feelings that DES should be used only for emergency measures such as rape, and should not be considered as a method of family planning.

FAMILY PLANNING IN THE FUTURE

Encouraging new techniques and products have appeared on the contraceptive horizon. Efforts to produce the perfect contraceptive have resulted in innovative and promising methods. All the techniques strive for a safe, economical, convenient, comfortable, and effective means of contraception. Under consideration at this time are methods involving oral hormones for both women and men, hormonal implants, tubal plugs, injectable hormones, hormonal rings, and nasal sprays.

Hormonal components are utilized by many of the new techniques. These components offer different combinations of hormones, altered ratios of hormones, different dosages, and different methods and routes of delivery.

Research is currently being done on a five-year subdermal implant that allows the steady release of levonorgestrel, a synthetic progestin, into the blood. The steroidal hormone alters the endometrium, suppresses ovulation, and increases the viscosity of the cervical mucus, discouraging sperm motility. The capsules containing the hormone are implanted under the skin and remain effective for five years or until a pregnancy is desired, at which time they are removed. Since the implants can cause menstrual irregularities, they have not yet been approved by the FDA. The implant, called Norplant, has been shown to be safe when tested on more than 5000 women and is being manufactured in some European countries.

In addition to the hormonal implants, intravaginal rings and pessaries have been treated with the progestins, resulting in the same mode of pregnancy prevention as the implants. The rings are allowed to remain in place for three to four weeks and then removed to allow for the menstrual period. These have not been approved for use in the United States.

Preliminary studies have been done on a salve which, when applied daily to the male abdomen or chest, produces infertility. Drawbacks to this method are associated with the prolonged administration of hormones and their side effects. In China, gossyrol, a male contraceptive made from cottonseed oil, is used to suppress sperm production and mobility. It is available in pill form and appears to be highly effective. It does carry with it a number of complications associated with spermatogenesis, and therefore, is not yet available in the United States.

The hormone luteinizing hormone releasing factor (LRF) may become a new contraceptive for both men and women. LRF stimulates the surge in the production of LH just prior to ovulation. When LRF is blocked in the female, ovulation is inhibited, progesterone secretion is diminished, and the endometrial lining of the uterus is altered, interfering with implantation. In the male, blocking the release of LRF (also termed LHRH) results in the inhibition of pituitary and testicular function which alters spermatogenesis. The blocking agent for both the male and female contraceptive is a synthetic LRF analog (Sandow, cited in Jiffcoate & Sandler, 1982). These analogs have specific site receptors and are therefore more directed in action with fewer secondary effects. LRF research looks promising but still requires extensive research.

Depo-Provera (medroxyprogesterone acetate), a hormone similar to progesterone, exerts its effect on the hypothalamus, preventing ovulation. It also changes the endometrial environment, discouraging implantation and at the same time altering the cervical mucus. Depo-Provera is administered in a dosage of 150 mg, given intramuscularly every three months. The results have been very effective with successful pregnancy prevention in 99 to 100 percent of users. The drug was formerly approved by the FDA but no longer is approved in the United States. It was withdrawn from the market after researchers noted an increase in infertility following discontinuance of the drug and an increased incidence of cervical cancer. Many arguments have disputed the carcinogenic effects, but at this time the drug is used only experimentally in the United States.

ABORTION

As a means of last resort, the termination of a pregnancy by abortion is considered as a postcoital method. Although very controversial from a spiritual, moral, and ethical viewpoint, abortion remains a legal alternative. Constraints on the types of abortions available are related to the gestational period and the health of the mother (see Chapter 3). Both physical and psychological risks should be considered before the decision to have an abortion is made.

UNPLANNED PARENTHOOD

In June, 1983, the largest 12-month worldwide population increase in history was recorded. During that 1-year period, 82 million babies were born. The world population at that time was 4.7 billion. Unfortunately, not all of these babies were planned or desired.

With all the methods of contraception, one might wonder why an unplanned pregnancy occurs. Studies have shown that half of all births are not planned and two thirds of all adolescent pregnancies are unplanned. Since the probability of pregnancy is greatest for women in their teens or early twenties, it appears that this age group should provide the most information regarding unplanned pregnancies. Specific reasons do apply to the teenager, yet several commonalities relating to factors associated with unplanned pregnancy exist across all reproductive ages.

Frequent causes for unplanned pregnancies cited by women are:

Belief that they cannot become pregnant easily
Lack of knowledge about effective contraceptive methods
Inability to obtain contraceptives
Improper use of contraceptives
Moral and religious objection to contraception
Dislike for contraceptive method relative to sexual pleasure
Fear of medical effects of contraceptive
Unplanned spontaneous sexual activity
Financial inability to afford services of physician or clinic
Failure to use contraceptives even though they are available

Once it has been determined that an unplanned pregnancy exists, it may be dealt with a variety of ways. Some clients receive the news with acceptance and begin to make appropriate adjustments. Others will deny or reject the pregnancy and elect to terminate it.

The decision-making process involved in reaching these determinations is difficult and may be consuming. The individual must consider the physiologic and psychosocial changes to come. To progress on a continuum involving acceptance of these changes is arduous for even the most self-actualized. For those threatened with an unplanned event which can alter their entire lives, it may be an impossible task. The atmosphere in which an unplanned child is born may be hostile and rejecting.

Transition from a nonmothering to a mothering or additional mothering role involves resolution of a diversity of conflicts. The unplanned pregnancy may severely alter the woman's life goals and necessitate a revision of her goals or even an abandonment of previously set goals. Family lifestyles will have to accommodate a totally dependent infant who will need nuturing for many years. Personal circumstances may not accommodate the financial responsibilities involved in a pregnancy or in parenthood. Conflicts in family or personal relationships may become stressed and intensified. Coping mechanisms that have sustained psychological equilibrium at the barest of survival levels may be strained to the limit and shattered. Coupled with all of these conflicts is the reality of a changing body image and the acceptance of the pregnancy by the individual and others involved significantly in her life.

TEENAGERS AND UNPLANNED PREGNANCY

An unplanned pregnancy during the teenage years presents all of the previously mentioned problems and conflicts plus a myriad of others. Since pregnancy occurs at the rate of 1 in every 10 teenage girls, it appears that large numbers of teens are at risk for these physiologic and psychological complications.

The health consequences associated with early childbearing are many. They constitute an integral part of the total psychological well-being of the teenager and will be discussed in Chapter 28.

Unplanned Pregnancy Counseling

The individual who is confronted with an unplanned pregnancy, whether a teenager or an adult, should be made aware of community agencies which offer assistance and advice, if needed. Family planning programs offer information and consultation services to anyone interested in family planning. Before family planning methods are discussed, a thorough physical examination and pregnancy test are performed. It is often at these clinics that a woman may first confirm her pregnancy. Once the pregnancy is confirmed, decisions regarding the outcome of the pregnancy must be addressed. If the choice is to continue the pregnancy, the client is made aware of community agencies which offer help. These agencies often stress the moral and religious aspects of pregnancy continuation and emphasize the rights of the unborn child. Most of these agencies will direct the pregnant woman to economical prenatal care and nutritional assistance programs. Adoption referral, emergency shelter, and supplies are sometimes included in these services.

If the choice is made to terminate the pregnancy, then counseling should be suggested to the client before action is taken. This nonjudgmental counseling should include the psychological and physical impact and effects the abortion may have on the client, the father of the baby, and the client's family. Above all, the client should be directed to a competent physician or a reputable abortion clinic. Every effort must be made to prevent the client from attempting a self-induced abortion or securing the services of an incompetent, illegal, unsafe abortionist (a more detailed discussion of abortions may be found in Chapter 25).

INFERTILITY

In 15 to 20 percent of all married couples, the reality of childbearing is never realized.

A couple is said to be infertile if after one year of frequent, unprotected sexual intercourse they have not been able to conceive or maintain a pregnancy. If a child has never been conceived, the term *primary infertility* applies. When a pregnancy has been achieved in the past, one or more times, but present efforts are not successful, the term *secondary infertility* applies.

Alterations in fertility involve both the male and female. The responsibility seems to be evenly distributed, with 35 percent related to male infertility, 35 percent related to female infertility, and 30 percent to factors related to both male and female. These factors include male and female genital tract alterations and endocrine alterations which may result from congenital and nutritional factors, infection, chronic disease, and stress.

Female Factors Altering Fertility

When assessing factors related to female infertility, a thorough evaluation of the female reproductive and endocrine system is done. If pregnancy is to occur, an ovum must be produced, ovulation must take place, and fertilization of the ovum must occur. The fertilized ovum must be able to pass through the fallopian tube, the ovum must be implanted in the endometrium of the uterus, and the pregnancy must be maintained. Any interference with this process may render the woman infertile.

OVULATION FACTORS

Interference with ovulation results from endocrine abnormalities related to pituitary, thyroid, or ovarian dysfunction. When there is decreased pituitary function, alterations can occur in the production of luteinizing hormone (LH), prohibiting ovulation. Tumors, anemia, starvation, and Sheehan's syndrome (pituitary necrosis) are causes of hypopituitarism.

Benign pituitary adenomas are most often the cause of hyperpituitarism. These tumors stimulate the production of prolactin (an anterior pituitary hormone responsible for milk production) and are associated with the presence of a breast discharge. When significantly elevated, prolactin levels may indicate a benign pituitary adenoma. A somewhat increased prolactin level may indicate inadequacy of the luteal phase of the menstrual cycle, amenorrhea, and ovulatory alterations (Friedman, 1981).

Hyperpituitarism resulting from benign pituitary tumors is treated with medications such as bromocriptine mesylate (Parlodel), which inhibits the secretion of prolactin and prevents suppression of FSH and LH, or by surgical removal of the tumor. Hypopituitarism resulting in low levels of LH may be treated with clomiphene citrate (Clomid). This hypothalmic-reacting drug enhances the production of FSH and LH, both of which regulate ovulation. During the prescribed regimen of clomiphene, the client is told that she may experience slight bloating, mastodynia, and distention of the abdomen. She is also instructed to determine ovulation by the use of a BBT record and observation of the cervical mucus. Following ovulation, the physician examines the client for ovarian enlargement, which would necessitate discontinuing the drug. Liver disease, abnormal uterine bleeding, and pregnancy preclude clomiphene therapy. Clients should be informed that the occurrence of multiple pregnancy is increased with clomiphene.

Human postmenopausal gonadotropin (HMG) is a combination of FSH and LH obtained from the urine of postmenopausal women. It is given following an unsuccessful course of clomiphene therapy. The high cost of the drug prohibits extensive use. Its side effects are similar to those with clomiphene but may include severe symptoms related to overstimulation of the ovary. The reaction produces symptoms of electrolyte imbalance, hypovolemia, and ascites, and is most frequently seen when HMG is used in combination with HCG (human chorionic gonadotropin). HCG stimulates the release of the ovarian follicle and is given following a 7 to 14 day regimen of HMG.

Inadequate functioning of the thyroid is responsible for alterations in the menstrual cycle and the maintenance of pregnancy. Menstrual irregularities, decreased libido, and amenorrhea may be seen with hyperthyroidism. Hypothyroidism gives rise to prolonged menstrual periods, anovulation, and spontaneous abortions.

Medications given for hypothyroidism are directed toward replacement therapy using drugs such as levothyroxine. Hyperthyroidism may be treated with *thioamides* (antithyroid drugs), radioactive iodine, or surgery. These drugs may be *teratogenic* (producing birth deformities) and should be discontinued if pregnancy does occur.

Ovarian dysfunction is indicated by decreased plasma progesterone levels and is related to alterations in the corpus luteum of the ovarian follicle. It may be recalled that the corpus luteum secretes progesterone, which in turn is responsible for maintenance of the pregnancy.

Since plasma progesterone levels rise from a level of 1 mg/ml during the first half of the menstrual cycle to a level of 3 to 10 mg/ml following ovulation, it is possible to determine when these levels are insufficient. If serum progesterone levels are low, an endometrial biopsy is done on the 21st to 24th day of the menstrual cycle. This simple office procedure is performed by introducing a curette into the cervical canal and removing a small endometrial tissue sample. This tissue is examined for the absence of progesterone-influenced secretory changes. When both tests indicate a decreased progesterone level, progesterone therapy may be instituted.

Polycystic ovaries may also disturb ovulation. Symptoms that coincide with polycystic ovaries are consistent with elevated testosterone levels. The testosterone is secreted by the androgenic tissue within the polycystic ovary (Friedman, 1981). The client will demonstrate symptoms of anovulation and abnormal hairiness (*hirsutism*). A surgical ovarian wedge resection may be done to remove the androgenic tissue.

FERTILIZATION AND TRANSPORTATION FACTORS

Obviously, for fertilization to take place, there must be a union of sperm and ovum. Disruptions that alter sperm production are significant in infertility and will be discussed under male factors. However, female factors may also influence fertilization. When the fallopian tubes are obstructed, it may be impossible for the ovum to be fertilized or for the fertilized ovum to be transported to the uterus for implantation. Obstruction of the tubes is usually a result of chronic *salpingitis* (inflammation of the tubes) resulting from gonorrhea and pelvic inflammatory disease. Occasionally, a pelvic infection resulting from appendicitis will cause adhesions which will also block the fallopian tubes.

To determine tubal patency, a *hysterosalpingogram* (x-ray of the fallopian tubes) is done following cessation of the monthly menses. In this procedure, a radiopaque material is injected into the cervix. The uterus and tubes become distended and are observable under fluoroscopy. Since the material is introduced under pressure, this procedure may cause some uterine cramping and discomfort. This should always be explained to the client before the procedure is done. Interruption of the procedure for a brief interval may be necessary to allow the cramping to subside.

Hysterosalpingograms must only be done during the first phase of the menstrual cycle (days 5 to 10) to eliminate any possibility of pregnancy disruption. Beneficial results from the procedure include expansion of the tubes and a cleansing effect caused by the pressure of the injected material. Conception often occurs after a hysterosalpingogram.

In the *Rubin* test for tubal patency, carbon dioxide is injected into the cervix and through the tubes. Observations are made of the amount of pressure required for passage of the carbon dioxide through the tubes. Increasing amounts of pressure (200 mm Hg) indicate occlusion. Sharp shoulder pain present when the patient sits up, or shortly thereafter, indicates patency of the tubes. The shoulder pain is caused by pressure on the phrenic nerve resulting from the collection of the carbon dioxide in the peritoneal cavity under the diaphragm. Since this reaction is not always immediate, the client must be informed that it may occur later and that she should report it for confirmation of tubal patency. The Rubin test is infrequently performed, since other diagnostic tests, such as the hysterosalpingogram, are more reliable.

If all of the other tests prove negative, a laparoscopy or a culdoscopy can be considered. Using an endoscope, the uterus and fallopian tubes are visualized with a lighted tube inserted through a small incision in the abdomen (laparoscopy) or through the posterior fornix of the vaginal canal (culdoscopy). It is then possible to determine the presence of adhesions and ovarian and tubal abnormalities. Laparoscopy is more frequently done, since culdoscopy is an uncomfortable procedure and does not give as reliable information.

Various forms of treatment are suggested for tubal pathology. All require a surgical procedure. Patients should be informed that these procedures usually only carry a 30 to 40 percent success range. The two most frequently performed procedures are the *salpingolysis* (adhesion separation) and tubal implantations.

IMPLANTATION DIFFICULTIES

Implantation of the fertilized ovum requires a receptive site. The normal uterine implantation site may be affected by congenital, mechanical, or hormonal factors. These factors account for about 10 to 20 percent of infertility.

Congenital uterine anomalies are most often associated with disturbances of embryologic fusion of the paramesonephric ducts, causing variations in the uterus. These variations may give rise to a double uterus (*uterus septus duplex*), a uterus with one horn (*uterus unicornus*), a uterus with a split corpus (*bicornate uterus*), a uterus with a narrowing of the cervix (*uterus atresia*), or a uterus bicornate with a rudimentary horn (*uterus bicornis unilaterale rudimentarius*) (see Fig. 6–10). All of these malformations can cause an increase in the rate of spontaneous abortions.

Mechanical factors are related to the presence of uterine fibroids, which interfere with implantation. Fibroids are benign fibrous tumors located in the uterine body or in the cervical area. They are slow growing, multiple in number, and display a large range in size. Women with fibroid tumors are able to become pregnant but often experience habitual abortions. Treatment for infertility associated with these tumors may include a surgical *myomectomy* (removal of the fibroid tumor).

Uterine adhesions may also pose a mechanical difficulty for the women desiring pregnancy. Adhesions within the uterine cavity may be caused by repeated elective abortions and infections.

Uterine hormonal influences that alter fertility may be related to endometriosis. *Endometriosis* is a disorder that results in the presence of endometrial tissue at abnormal sites outside of the uterus. These endometrial sites, such as the ovaries, broad ligaments, posterior uterine surfaces, uterosacral ligaments, cul-de-sac, and bowels respond to estrogen stimulations during the menstrual cycle. They behave as uterine endometrial tissue and will bleed, causing pain and discomfort at the time of the menstrual period. It is believed that the presence of endometrial

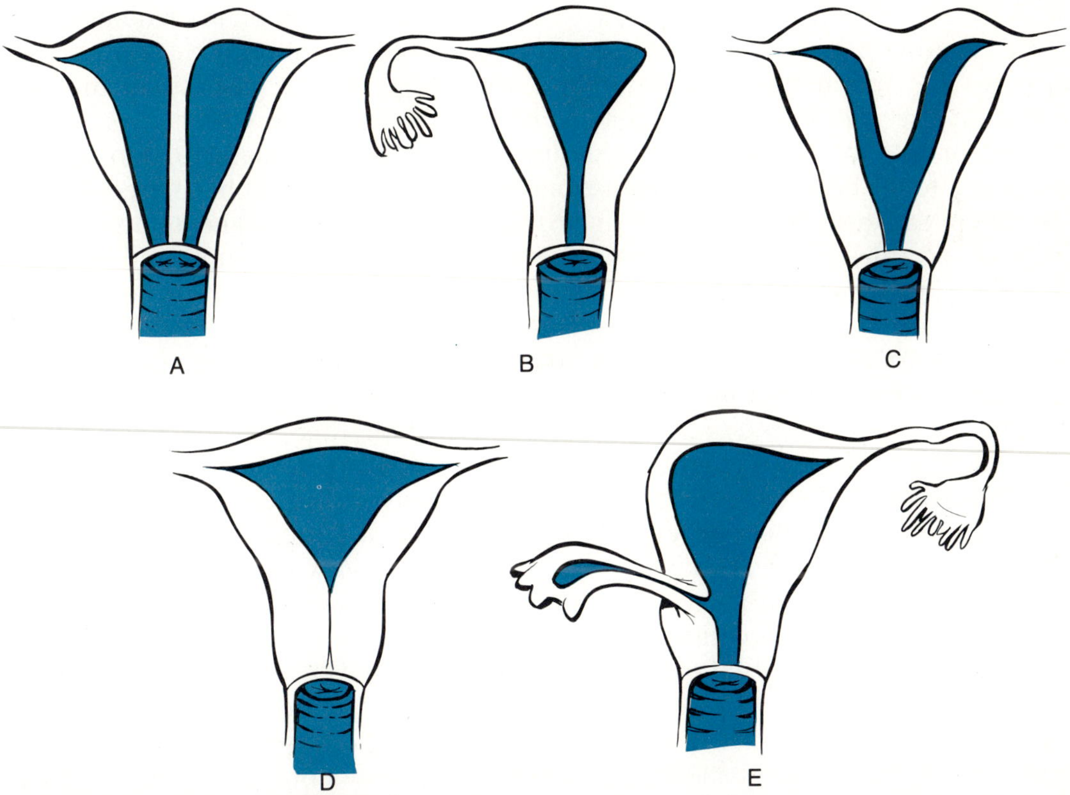

FIGURE 6–10. Uterine malformations: A. Uterus septus duplex. B. Uterus unicornus. C. Uterus bicornate. D. Uterine atresia. E. Uterus bicornis unilaterale rudimentarius.

tissue at these sites is due to a refluxive action of the tissues up through the uterus and out through the fallopian tubes, settling in the previously mentioned locations. The effects on fertility are related to interference in tubal patency when endometrial implants are located in the fallopian tubes and to endometrial fragility when endometrial implants are located at the uterine site.

Laparoscopy may confirm the presence of these implantation sites and cautery removal or surgical excision may be indicated. On occasion, hormonal therapy using oral contraceptives, which stimulate a pregnancy endometrial environment, may be useful.

The cervix of the uterus is also responsive to hormonal factors. Cervical mucus becomes more profuse, stretchable, and receptive to sperm when influenced by increasing levels of estrogen. This increases the mobility of the sperm, fostering the likelihood of fertilization. If the cervical mucus does not demonstrate the estrogenic changes, fertilization may be unlikely.

To determine the quality of the cervical mucus, the spinnbarkeit property and the Fern test are utilized. The elasticity demonstrated in the spinnbarkeit factor should be around 7 to 10 cm just before ovulation. The specimen can also be evaluated microscopically for a ferning pattern. The ferning pattern is present just before ovulation when the estrogen levels are at their peak. In the second half of the menstrual cycle the ferning pattern disappears owing to the influence of progesterone.

Medications such as Premarin may be given prior to ovulation to increase estrogen levels. Estrogen products vary in dosage and may be given for different intervals of time. If the medication does not produce the desired effect, cryosurgery may be considered. In *cryosurgery*, liquid nitrogen is used to freeze the cervical area. The superficial layers of the cervix slough off and new tissue is formed (Friedman, 1981). The cervix is allowed to heal and increased fertility is expected.

Male Factors Altering Fertility

When pursuing fertility studies, it is always advisable to begin with the male. Although males may believe the problem to be associated with the female, it is more realistic to begin with the male. Male fertility testing is less expensive and far less complicated than female infertility testing. Once it has been established that the difficulty is not related to the male, then the more extensive female testing can be initiated.

Male infertility can be caused by inadequate sperm production and motility, obstruction of the sperm passages, production of sperm antibodies, and ejaculatory problems. These conditions often result from injuries, sexual disease, mumps, substance abuse, and environmental factors such as radiation.

SPERM INADEQUACY

Sperm may be inadequate in number, motility and morphology (characteristics of normal sperm). An analysis of the seminal fluid will reveal these difficulties. A specimen is obtained by masturbation following a two-day abstinence from intercourse, and placed in a clean nonmetal container. It should be kept at room temperature and examined by a physician within a two-hour period after it is obtained.

The normal sperm count should not be less than 30 million sperm per ml. Any count less than this may decrease fertility and is significant. In such cases it may be necessary to advise the client to abstain from intercourse for a period of three to five days before the woman's expected ovulation. If the count is less than 20 million, the man is considered infertile and treatment methods should be discussed. Hormonal therapy with drugs such as Clomid may enhance sperm production. This drug causes an elevation in FSH and LH production. Testosterone has also been used, but with little success.

Sperm motility involves the examination of the specimen to determine the extent and type of movement of the sperm. The microscope examination should show a free forward progressive movement of the sperm. Fifty percent of the sperm should demonstrate this quality. When sperm motility is affected but there is an adequate sperm count, the use of HCG might be indicated to increase the motility of the sperm. Recently, the Proception fertility pack has been used to aid in maintaining the vaginal seminal pool. This polyethylene encapsulated foam vaginal tampon is introduced directly following intercourse. The tampon is introduced with its plastic cover still on and inserted as far back into the vagina as it can go. The tampon does not absorb the semen but helps in maintaining the semen close to the cervix. It may be removed by the client after six to eight hours.

Reduced sperm motility and count result from elevated scrotal temperatures. When scrotal temperature is at or above body temperature, motility of the sperm is decreased. Varioceles of spermatic veins will elevate scrotal temperature. If a variocele is noted in light of reduced sperm count and motility then a ligation of the spermatic vein may be helpful. *Cryptorchidism* (undescended testicles at birth) will also reduce sperm count if not corrected before puberty, owing to increased temperature of the testes while within the body. Increased scrotal heat may be found in men who wear extremely restrictive undergarments. Other causes include high temperature during illness, occupational exposure to heat, and work requiring a seated position during most of the working hours.

Production of sperm antibodies have been found in both males and females. Antibodies are produced in response to sperm allergies. If the female is allergic to the sperm, the male is advised to wear a condom during intercourse for a designated period of time. This reduces sensitivity to the sperm. When her sperm antibody titers are decreased, they discontinue using the condom. If the male produces sperm antibodies, little treatment is available. Some cases have been helped by the use of methylprednisolone (Medrol), a steroid that reduces the allergic response to the antibodies.

Sperm analysis following coitus (*Sims-Huhner test*) may be helpful in determining factors indicating a sperm allergy. The couple is asked to have intercourse approximately 12 hours preceding the test and at about the time of expected ovulation. Following intercourse the woman returns to the physician's office where a sample of cervical secretions is obtained. The sample is examined for cervical chemistry and the presence of viable sperm. Although this test is not exclusive for sperm allergies, it may be helpful when a normal sperm analysis is achieved during masturbation, yet infertility exists.

Ejaculatory problems are associated with anomalies, impotence, and alterations caused by sexual habits. Anomalies may be related to hypospadias or epispadias, both of which result in abnormal placement of the urethral opening, causing the sperm to be deposited away from the cervical opening.

When the male is unable to achieve or maintain an erection, he is said to be *impotent*. Impotency has many psychological implications and can be devastating to the couple faced with the situation. The male may feel he is less than a man because he cannot achieve an erection. He becomes anxious and worried, which further inhibits an erection. On the other hand, the woman feels that it is her fault because her partner no longer desires her and she is hurt and unable to help her mate. Psychological counseling is strongly recommended when an impotency problem exists over an expanded period of time. Often all that is needed is a mutual understanding that occasional impotency in the male is normal and is not reflective on his manliness or her sexual attractiveness. A brief period of relaxation away from the pressures of office and home for both of them may be all the treatment that is necessary.

Premature ejaculation is the inability of the male partner to control ejaculation in at least 50 percent of coital experiences. Problems associated with fertility arise from the inappropriate placement of the semen. In some cases ejaculation occurs before penetration. Occasionally, it may arise from urethral disorders or neurologic disease, but most cases are psychological in nature.

Sexual habits can sometimes cause male infertility problems. Too frequent intercourse may reduce fertility. Intercourse following a hot bath or shower may alter sperm motility. Some women will rise immediately following intercourse, allowing the ejaculate to be expelled. Bathing or douching following intercourse will also alter sperm capabilities. The use of alcoholic beverages and drugs to enhance sexuality may in fact reduce sexual response and inhibit erections. Excessive use of alcohol in the male is associated with decreased testosterone production and infertility.

Often a cause for the infertility cannot be determined. All tests and procedures indicate the couple to be normal and capable of conception, yet a pregnancy does not occur. In these situations well-intentioned advice such as "relax," "don't worry about it," or "let nature take its time," may be given by friends or relatives. No matter how sincere the advice, however, it often tends to make the couple feel guilty or at fault for failure to conceive. The simple truth, that there is no identifiable cause for the infertility and that other alternatives may be available, is often the most supportive and therapeutic.

Many questions are asked by the infertile couple of themselves and of each other. Feelings of failure, frustration, anger, guilt, and grief can cause stress on the relationship and within the family. The nurse is often in a position to observe the alterations in relationships and may, when appropriate, suggest the assistance of a national support group such as RESOLVE. This organization consists of infertile couples who bring understanding, sharing, and support to one another and who strive to help couples to express their feelings, recognize their loss, and regain their self-esteem.

Alternatives for Infertile Couples

When it has been determined that a fertility problem that may not be correctable exists, then alternative methods for the procurement of children may be desired. These methods include artificial insemination, in vitro fertilization, and adoption.

ARTIFICIAL INSEMINATION

Artificial insemination is the process whereby male sperm are introduced into the female vagina by artificial means. The sperm used for the insemination may be from the husband artificial insemination husband (AIH), or from a donor, artificial insemination donor (AID). AIH is the most widely accepted method, used when the sperm are present in an ejaculation but are reduced in number and/or motility. Several specimens obtained from the male may be mixed together to increase the total concentration of sperm (Fromer, 1983). On occasion, a "split ejaculate" is used. The specimen is collected by having the male ejaculate into two containers. Only the sperm from the first container are used for insemination. This provides a better concentration of sperm and increased numbers of motile sperm.

The AID method of insemination is gaining in popularity. Sperm are obtained from a donor or from a frozen-sperm bank. The identities of the donors are not known, but an effort is made to match the donor with the recipient couple. In order for a couple to be eligible for donor semen, it must be proven that the husband is incapable of producing sperm or is a carrier of a hereditary defect. Essential when considering AID insemination, is the consideration of the moral, ethical, and psychological perspectives. Both partners in the marriage must be informed of these issues and together give informed consent. A cost factor must also be considered since payment for the sperm and the insemination procedure is involved.

Some of the issues which society must address are:

Who determines the criteria for donors?
Is genetic screening essential?
Is donor semen a commercial product?
Who owns donor semen?
What are the responsibilities to the child?
Should the child be informed of the manner in which he or she was conceived?
Is the service available for both heterosexual and homosexual women?
Who has access to the records of donors and recipients?
How many times may this method be used for an individual?
Does the donor father have any parental rights?

This list is continually expanding and becoming more complex.

Definitive answers to these questions are not readily available. Society must examine these issues and make decisions based on a thorough investigation and understanding of the implications and consequences of each issue.

IN VITRO FERTILIZATION

New on the infertility scene is the use of in vitro fertilization. This term, which literally means "in glass," is synonymous with the more frequently used term "test tube baby" (Fromer, 1983). The principle facilitating this concept is the fertilization of an oocyte outside of the mother's uterus, followed by the return of the developed blastocyst to the uterus and then the successful implantation and maturation of the fetus in utero.

Although the concept sounds logical and simple in its explanation, it is a difficult and controversial procedure. The woman is superovulated using hormonal agents such as clomiphene citrate and human menopausal gonadotropin. Hormonal stimulation is begun on day 3 of the menstrual cycle and continues until follicle maturity has been determined.

Following the hormonal stimulation, the development of the ovarian follicles is monitored for size and maturity. This is accomplished by the use of daily ultrasound monitoring, noting follicular growth and maturation in a normal progression.

Cervical mucus observation is often done to denote the characteristic cervical mucus changes that preceed ovulation. The mucus becomes clear, thin, and watery with an increase in the alkalinity (pH of 7.0 to 7.5). The ferning pattern of the mucus increases, indicating impending ovulation.

Evaluation of the hormonal level of estrogen is also done after the initiation of HMG therapy. The hormone HMG contains LH and FSH hormones, which in turn cause stimulation of the ovarian follicles. The very high levels of these two hormones cause many of the primary oocytes to begin to mature. Normally, only one of the primary oocytes would reach maturity. However, when hyperstimulation occurs, many (4 to 6) oocytes mature. The theca interna cells of these maturing oocytes participate in the production of estrogen (E_2). Therefore, an increased E_2 serum level is found at the time of follicular maturity. Each maturing follicle produces a minimal level of 300 pg/ml per follicle. Combining the knowledge gained from the ultrasound observation of the number of maturing follicles with the serum levels of E_2 gives an estimation of the maturity of the oocytes. When it is determined that the oocytes are mature, the HMG injections are discontinued and HCG is given to complete the follicular maturation.

The mature ova are then harvested by performing a sterile laparoscopy. An evaluation is made of each ova according to prescribed criteria and their level of maturity. Mature eggs are inseminated within 6 to 8 hours, while immature eggs are allowed further time for maturing. Sperm, which have been collected from the husband and cultured, are placed in a petri dish containing the individual oocyte. If the desired result of fertilization occurs, the developed blastocysts are then reintroduced into the mother's womb during the proper stage of endometrial development. The mere handling of the oocyte, sperm, and blastocyst is difficult and many times the procedure is unsuccessful. Each step of the procedure must be precisely planned and carefully executed.

The nurse, as a member of the team participating in in vitro fertilization, has a very important role. She often serves as the coordinator for the activities and procedures surrounding the process. Of critical importance is the planning and coordinating of all appointments necessary for the procedure and arrangements for monitoring the effects and results of all treatments. During this time period, the nurse counsels and teaches the clients. She should always be alert for misconceptions and any client education needs that the couple may have. Her role includes coordination of the in vitro team activities to insure a smooth and cooperative team effort. It is difficult to predict and plan the performance of many of the procedures, since they are determined by the physiologic events occurring within the woman. Therefore, it is important that a degree of flexibility within the team members be maintained and that when the appropriate indications are present the team efforts be coordinated and expedited as smoothly and quickly as possible.

Ethical issues have surrounded the use of in vitro fertilization. Those issues most frequently focus on the moral responsibilities involved in alterations of the natural means of reproduction and the responsibilities involved if a defective blastocyst develops (see Chapter 3).

ADOPTION

Adoption offers another alternative to the infertile couple. This option may be suggested to the infertile couple after they have had a reasonable period of time to express and work through their feelings of loss, pain, and grief. The availability of adoptive children has become limited since the introduction of birth control pills, legalized abortion, and the more common practice of single parenting. Yet, children of mixed race, special needs, and older children are available and may well fill the desires of a loving confident couple.

NURSING RESPONSIBILITIES

In spite of the overpopulation of today's world, many remain childless not by desire but by inability to produce a child. The impact of infertility on a couple's relationship can cause feelings of inadequacy, hopelessness, and isolation. Years may be spent in efforts to achieve pregnancy, involving medical tests and treatments, vast expense, and emotional vascillations. Nurses should be aware of not only the medical management of the infertile couple, but the emotional needs as well. Nursing responsibilities and support encompass the period surrounding the realization of infertility, the period involving testing and diagnosis, the period of infertility management, and the resolution of infertility either by pregnancy or other alternatives.

BIBLIOGRAPHY

Abernathy, V. Illegitimate conception among teenagers. *Nursing Digest,* 1976, **4,** Summer, 8-9.

Akpom, C.A., Akpom, K.L. & Davis, M. Prior sexual behavior of teenagers attending rap sessions for the first time. *Family Planning Perspectives,* 1976, **8,** 203-206.

Britt, S. Fertility awareness: Four methods of natural family planning, *Journal of Obstetric, Gynecological & Neonatal Nursing,* 1977, **6,** 9-17.

Card, J. & Wise, L. Teenage mothers and teenage fathers: The impact of early childbearing on the parent's personal and professional lives, *Family Planning Perspectives*, 1978, **10**, 190.

Daniel, W. *Adolescents in health and disease*. St. Louis: C.V. Mosby, 1977.

Erickson, E.H. *Childhood and society* (2nd ed.). New York: W.W. Norton, 1963.

Fisch, I.R. & Frank, J. Oral contraceptives and blood pressure, *Journal of American Medical Association*, 1977, **237**, 2499.

Friedman, B. The infertility workup. *American Journal of Nursing*, 1981, **81**, 2040-2046.

Fromer, M.J. *Ethical issues in sexuality and reproduction*. St. Louis: C.V. Mosby, 1983.

Hatcher, R.A., Stewart, G.K., Guest, F., Finkelstein, R. & Godwin, C. *Contraceptive technology, 1976-1977* (8th ed.). New York: Irvington Publishers, 1976.

______, ______, ______, ______, ______. *Contraceptive technology, 1980-1981* (10th ed.). New York: Irvington Publishers, 1980.

Helmer, O.M. & Judson, W.E. Influence of high renin substrate levels on renin-angiotensin system in pregnancy. *American Journal of Obstetrics and Gynecology*, 1967, **99**, 9.

Herbst, A.L. Robboy, S.J., Skully, R.E., et al.: Clear-cell adenocarcinoma of the vagina and cervix in girls: Analysis of 170 registry cases. *American Journal of Obstetrics and Gynecology*, 1974, **119**, 713-728.

Hilgers, T.W. & Bailey, A.J. Natural family planning II. Basal body temperature and estimated time of ovulation. *Obstetrics and Gynecology*, 1980, **55**, 333-339.

Hogan, R.M. *Human sexuality*. New York: Appleton-Century-Crofts, 1980.

Huxal, L. Update on IUD's. *Maternal Child Health Nursing*, 1980, **5**, 186-190. 1980.

Inman, W.H.W. & Vessey, M.P. Investigation of deaths from pulmonary, coronary, and cerebral thrombosis and embolism in women of childbearing age. *British Medical Journal*, 1968, **2**, 193.

Jain, A.K. Cigarette smoking, use of oral contraceptives and myocardial infarction. *American Journal of Obstetrics and Gynecology*, 1976, **126**, 301-307.

Kantner, J.F. & Zelnik, M. Sexual and contraceptive experiences of young unmarried women in the United States, 1976 and 1971. *Family Planning Perspectives*, 1977, **9**, 55-71.

Kinsey, A.C. Pomeroy, W.B. & Martin, C.E. *Sexual behavior in the human male*. Philadelphia: Saunders, 1948.

______, ______, ______, & Gebhard, P.H. *Sexual behavior in the human female*. Philadelphia: Saunders, 1953.

Kolodny, R.C., Masters, W.H., Johnson, V.E. & Biggs, M.A. *Textbook of human sexuality for nurses*. Boston: Little, Brown, 1979.

Mann, J., Inman, W. & Thorogood, M. Oral contraceptive use in older women and fatal myocardial infarction. *British Medical Journal*, 1976, **2**, 445.

Masters, W.H. & Johnson, V.E. *Human sexual response*. Boston: Little, Brown, 1966.

McGrath, J. & Cataldi, P. Cyclical changes in coagulation factors associated with the use of progestational agents. *Haemostasis*, 1975, **4**, 73.

Miller, G.J. & Miller, N.E. Plasma high density lipoprotein concentration and development of ischaemic heart disease. *Lancet*, 1975, **1**, 16.

Money, J. & Ehrhardt, A.A. *Man and woman, boy and girl*. Baltimore: John Hopkins University Press, 1972.

Moore, K. & Waite, L. Early childbearing and educational attainment. *Family Planning Perspectives*, 1977, **9**, 220-225.

Muir, B.K. *Essentials of genetics for nurses*. New York: Wiley, 1983.

Nissen, E.D., Kent, D.R., Nissen, S.E. & McRae, D.M. Association of liver tumors with oral contraceptives. *Obstetrics and Gynecology*, 1976, **48**, 49-55.

Notelovitz, M., Guidat, J. & McKenzie, L. Contraceptives, lipids and lipoproteins: A preliminary report, Proceedings from a study published by the editors of *Drug therapy*. New York: Biomedical Information Corporation, 1981.

Notelovitz, M., Kitchens, C., Coone, L., McKenzie, L. & Carter, R. Low dosage contraceptives: usage and coagulation. Proceedings from a study published by the editors of *Drug therapy*. New York: Biomedical Information Corporation, 1981.

Ory, H., Cole, P., MacMahon, B., et al.: Oral contraceptives and reduced risk of benign breast disease. *The New England Journal of Medicine*, 1976, **294**, 419-422.

______, Layde, P.M., Webster, L.A., et al.: Oral contraceptive use and the risk of endometrial cancer. Paper presented at the 31st Annual Epidemic Intelligence Service Conference. Atlanta, Ga.: Epidemic Intelligence Service, 1982.

______, ______, ______, ______. Oral contraceptive use and the risk of ovarian cancer. Paper presented at the 31st Annual Epidemic Intelligence Service Conference. Atlanta, Ga.: Epidemic Intelligence Service, 1982.

Poller, L. Oral contraceptives, blood clotting and thrombosis. *British Medical Bulletin*, 1978, **34**, 151.

Royle, M.G. Parslow, J.M., Kingscott, M.M.B., Wallace, D.M.A. & Hendry, W.F. Reversal of vasectomy: The side effects of sperm antibodies on subsequent fertility. *British Journal Urol.*, 1981, **53**, 654-659.

Sandow, J. Inhibition of pituitary and testicular function by LHRH analogues. In S.L. Jeffcoate, & M. Sandler (Eds.). *Progress towards a male contraceptive*. New York: Wiley, 1982.

Spellacy, W.N. Metabolic effects of oral contraceptives. *Clinical Obstetrics and Gynecology*, 1974, **17**, 53-63.

Shapiro, H. *The birth control book*. New York: St. Martin's, 1977.

Stoehr, G., White, P. & White, J. Managing drug interactions with oral contraceptives, *Journal of Obstetric, Gynecological, and Neonatal Nursing*, 1983, **12**, 327-331.

Vessey, M., Yeates, D. & Flavel, R. Risk of ectopic pregnancy and duration of use of an intrauterine device. *Lancet*, 1979, **2**, 501.

Weinberg, J.S. *Sexuality—human needs and nursing practice*. Philadelphia: Saunders, 1982.

chapter 7

FETAL DEVELOPMENT

OBJECTIVES

Upon completion of this chapter, the reader will be able to:

1. List the three stages of intrauterine development.
2. Identify critical periods of tissue development.
3. Discuss environmental factors that may influence fetal development.
4. Define syngamy, fertilization, zygote, cleavage, blastomere, morula, gastrulation, embryo, and fetus.
5. State the usual site of fertilization.
6. Given a specific organ or tissue, state whether it derives from the endoderm, mesoderm, or ectoderm.
7. Define decidua vera, decidua capsularis, decidua basalis.
8. Given a specific week of gestation, identify developmental changes that occur in the embryo or fetus.
9. State the first system to become functional in the embryo.
10. Briefly describe the changes that occur during development of the following systems: cardiovascular, genitourinary, muscular, skeletal, nervous, gastrointestinal, and integumentary.
11. State the function of the placenta, umbilical arteries, umbilical vein, foramen ovale, ductus arteriosus, and ductus venosus.
12. Describe fetal circulation.
13. Briefly discuss changes that occur in fetal circulation at or shortly after birth.

KEY TERMS

Blastocele
Blastocyst
Blastomere
Capacitation
Cleavage
Decidua
Ductus arteriosus
Ductus venosus
Ectoderm
Embryo
Endoderm
Fertilization
Fetal circulation
Fetus
Foramen ovale
Gastrulation
Implantation
Mesoderm
Morphogenesis
Morula
Neural crest
Neural tube
Notochord
Syngamy
Teratogen
Umbilical arteries
Umbilical vein
Zygote

At the moment of fertilization of an ovum by a sperm, a sequence of events begins that will result, if all goes well, in a healthy neonate in 40 weeks.

DEVELOPMENTAL PHASES

Development is a series of sequential coordinated changes that move toward more complex structure and function. Cells gain a special form, shape, or structure in a process called *morphogenesis*. Several distinct mechanisms are involved in this process: cell size and shape changes, cell migration, cell recognition and adhesion, transfer of information or substances, cell proliferation or inhibition, cell death, and stabilization of new cell arrangements.

Prenatal development from fertilization of the ovum by the sperm until the completion of intrauterine life is divided into three phases: preembryonic, embryonic, and fetal.

The first three weeks of life are the *preembryonic phase*. During this phase, the fertilized ovum grows and differentiates, implantation is completed, and the primary germ layers are formed. The *embryonic phase* is from the beginning of the fourth week through the seventh week of gestation. During this phase organs and body systems are established in rudimentary form. During the *fetal phase*, from eight weeks until term, organs and systems continue to grow and develop in preparation for extrauterine life.

ENVIRONMENTAL FACTORS THAT INFLUENCE DEVELOPMENT

Embryonic and fetal development are influenced by multiple factors. The fetus is generally well protected before birth; however, agents called *teratogens* may cause congenital malformation during the development of tissues and organs. All developmental tasks are related to each other on a specific continuum. Events that occur at any given point in time will affect development of the total organism. The action of teratogens is not clearly understood. It is known that the stage of embryonic development determines the susceptibility of a teratogen.

CRITICAL PERIODS

The most critical period in the development of any tissue or organ is the time of rapid cell division (see Table 7–1).

For brain growth, the critical period extends into infancy. The skeletal system has a prolonged critical period, extending into early adulthood. Development of the embryo is most easily disturbed from day 13 to day 60, the period of organogenesis.

NUTRITION

Nutrients required for fetal growth and development are transferred to the fetus from the mother through the placenta. Maternal nutritional deficiencies have been implicated as the cause of various congenital defects.

TABLE 7–1
CRITICAL TIME PERIODS

Organ or Tissue	Time Period
Central nervous system	3 to 6 weeks
Heart	3½ to 6½ weeks
Arms	4½ to 7 weeks
Eyes	4½ to 8 weeks
Legs	4 to 7 weeks
Teeth	7 to 8 weeks
Palate	7 to 8 weeks
External genitalia	7 to 11 weeks
Ears	4 to 10 weeks

DRUGS

The teratogenesis of drugs is very complex. Some cause severe malformation, while others may only cause growth retardation. A few drugs have been positively identified as teratogens and these are to be avoided in pregnancy and prepregnancy. Other drugs are suspected of having teratogenic potential and should be taken with caution during pregnancy (see Chapter 11).

The type of malformation caused by a particular teratogen is governed by several factors: the developmental stage of the embryo or fetus, its genetic composition, the maternal physiologic state, and the intensity of the dosage administered.

ENVIRONMENTAL CHEMICALS

In recent years, there has been intensified concern about the possible teratogenicity of environmental chemicals. None has been positively identified as teratogenic in humans, although hydrocarbons, plastics, insecticides, and metals such as lead, copper, and mercury have been associated with birth defects.

INFECTIOUS AGENTS

Intrauterine infections may cause congenital malformations. Microorganisms cross the placental membrane and enter the fetal blood stream. The fetal blood-brain barrier offers little resistance to microorganisms. Infections that most commonly affect the fetus and neonate belong to the TORCH complex: T—toxoplasmosis; O—other (beta B streptococcus, etc.); R—rubella; C—cytomegalovirus; and H—herpes simplex type II (see Chapter 25).

RADIATION

Radiation of all types presents a potential hazard to the embryo and fetus. The risk is proportional to the amount of radiation and the length of exposure as well as the particular tissue involved. Although there is no conclusive proof that congenital malformations are caused by diagnostic levels of radiation, the central nervous system of the embryo or fetus is nearly always affected by radiation. The recommended limit of maternal exposure of the whole body to radiation from all sources is 500 millirads for the entire gestational period.

WEEK 1: FERTILIZATION AND IMPLANTATION

Human development begins at fertilization, when a sperm unites with an ovum to form a zygote in a process called *syngamy*.

Oocyte Transport

At the time of ovulation, a secondary oocyte is carried from the ovary into the infundibulum of the fallopian tube by movements of the fimbriae. Muscular contractions of the tubes, ciliary action of the mucosa, and fluid currents within the tube move the oocyte into the ampulla of the fallopian tube.

Sperm Transport

Approximately 125 million sperm are deposited on the cervix during intercourse. Four factors that influence sperm migration through the cervix and into the uterus are: (1) the intrinsic motility of the sperm; (2) the proteolytic activity of sperm and semen; (3) penetration of cervical mucus by the sperm; and (4) orientation of strands of cervical mucus. Passage of sperm is assisted by muscular contractions of the uterus and fallopian tubes. Prostaglandins present in seminal fluid may help to stimulate uterine motility and assist sperm movement to the site of fertilization.

Fertilization Site

The usual site of fertilization is the ampulla of the fallopian tube, the longest and widest part of the tube (see Fig. 7–1).

Viability of the Ova and Sperm

The ovum is usually fertilized within 12 hours after the secondary oocyte is expelled at ovulation. If unfertilized, the secondary oocyte usually dies within 12 to 24 hours.

The sperm usually die within 24 hours after intercourse; however, they may be capable of fertilization of an ovum for as long as 72 hours. Before a sperm is capable of fertilization, it must undergo two further changes, capacitation and acrosome reaction. During capacitation, the protective coating over the acrosomal region is removed in a conditioning process. As the sperm nears the ovum, hyaluronidase and a trypsinlike substance are released through small openings in the acrosome wall. Hyaluronidase aids in penetration of the corona radiata and the trypsinlike substance aids in penetration of the zona pellucida.

Fertilization

Fertilization is the sequence of events that begins with contact between a sperm and a secondary oocyte and ends with fusion of the nuclei of the sperm and the ovum.

Fertilization requires about 24 hours for completion. Once the sperm penetrates the corona radiata and the zona pellucida, it becomes attached to the oocyte, penetrating the oocyte membrane, and begins to move toward the cytoplasm. Both the head and the tail enter the oocyte as the secondary meiotic division of the oocyte is completed.

The sperm moves forward until it lies close to the female pronucleus. The head of the sperm, containing the paternal hereditary complement, swells as it moves through the cytoplasm. The two pronuclei move toward

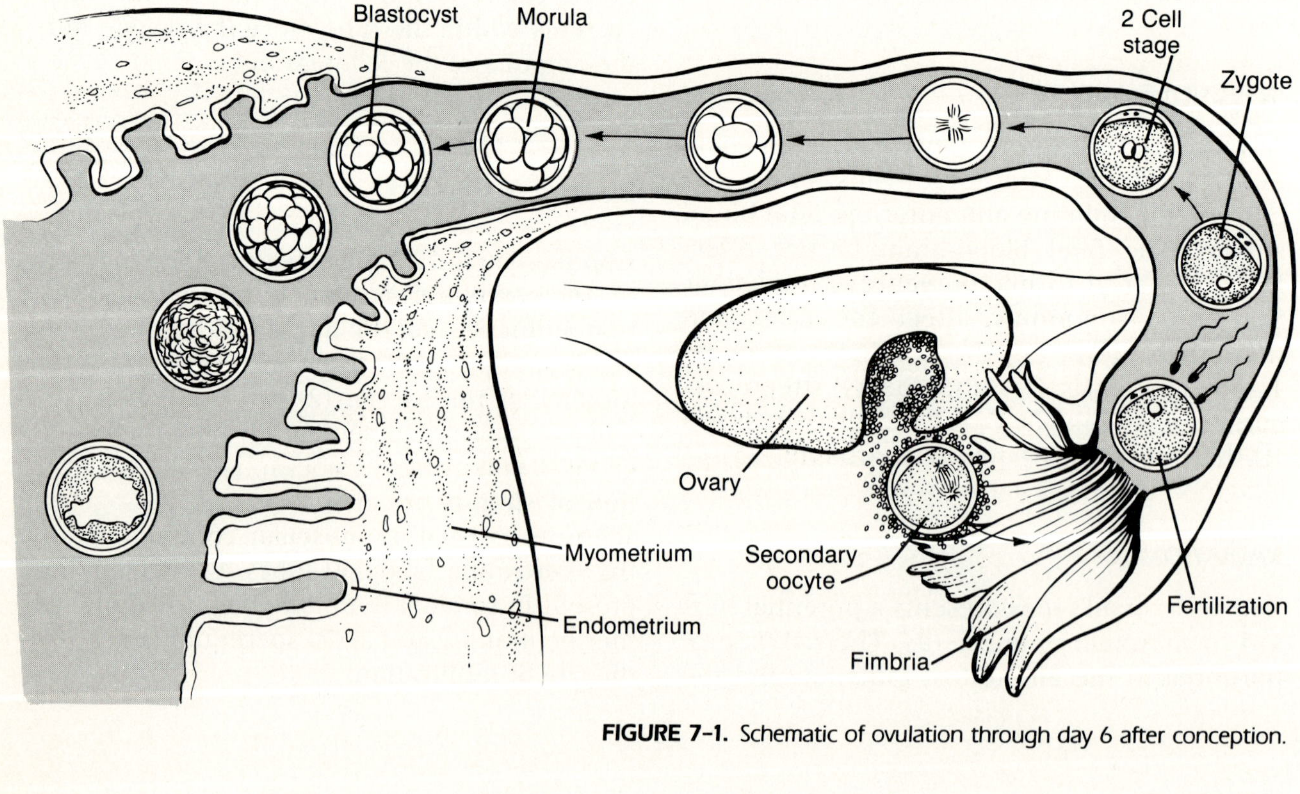

FIGURE 7–1. Schematic of ovulation through day 6 after conception.

each other and unite. When the nuclei unite, the resultant cell is called a *zygote*. It normally contains 46 chromosomes.

Fertilization results in the restoration of the diploid number of chromosomes, new combinations of chromosomes, determination of the sex of the embryo, determination of the inherited traits of the individual, and the initiation of cleavage.

The zygote immediately begins development of the embryo, the fetal portion of the placenta, the umbilical cord, and the fetal membranes (see Chapter 8).

Cleavage

Cleavage is a series of mitotic cell divisions. With each division, the cells become smaller, eventually forming the blastocyst (see Fig. 7–2).

The first cleavage occurs about 22 hours after fertilization and results in two daughter cells called blastomeres. As cleavage occurs, the embryo is slowly propelled through the fallopian tube toward the uterus (see Fig. 7–1), where it arrives about three to five days later.

When the embryo has grown to 12 to 16 blastomeres, about three days after fertilization, the *morula* stage has been attained. It is now a solid mass of blastomeres and is shaped like a mulberry.

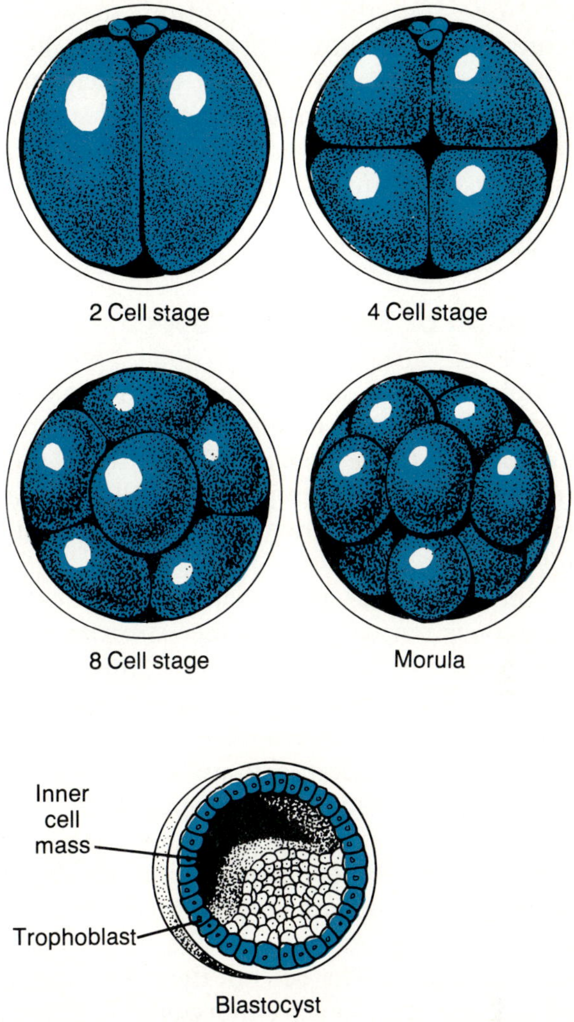

FIGURE 7–2. Schematic of cleavage, morula, and blastocyst.

Blastocyst Formation

The morula enters the uterus on about day 4 after fertilization. Fluid from the uterine cavity passes into the morula and separates it into two parts, creating a *blastocyst* (see Fig. 7–2). Some cells remain grouped together and are called the *inner cell mass*. These cells will develop into the embryo. A single layer of cells (trophoblast) compose the outer wall and will contribute to placental development. With this expansion, the zona pellucida of the ovum is stretched and eventually torn and discarded.

WEEK 2: BILAMINAR EMBRYO FORMATION

Implantation

Implantation begins at the end of the first week of gestation and ends about 12 days after fertilization. On day 6, the blastocyst attaches to the uterine epithelium in the upper portion of the uterus. The trophoblast cells invade the uterine endometrium on days 7 and 8. Proteolytic enzymes produced by the trophoblastic cells aid in erosion and penetration of endometrial tissue. As the trophoblast cells erode into the endometrium, they differentiate into an inner layer of cells, called the *cytotrophoblast*, and an outer layer with no cell boundaries, called the *synctiotrophoblast.* By day 12, the endometrium fuses above and blastocyst, enclosing the embryo in a cavity of its own.

Formation of Two Germ Layers

As implantation is taking place, small spaces appear between the inner cell mass and the trophoblasts. These spaces join to form the amniotic cavity. Some trophoblast cells form a thin membrane that encloses a cavity (primitive yolk sac).

At the same time, the cytotrophoblast cells form a loose network called the *extraembryonic mesoderm*. Large cavities develop in this tissue forming the extraembryonic coelom (cavity), which surrounds the primitive yolk sac and amniotic cavity. A connecting stalk forms between the germ disc and the trophoblast.

On the surface of the inner cell mass a single layer of flattened cells, the *endoderm*, appears. The remaining cells of the inner cell mass that are continuous with the trophoblast form the *ectoderm*. The cells of these two germ layers form a flat circular embryonic disc.

A second cavity then forms below the endoderm, called the *primary yolk sac*. The primary yolk sac becomes smaller and disappears as the secondary yolk sac develops. The prochordal plate begins to develop as a thickening of the cells at the cephalic region of the endoderm, indicating the future cranial region of the embryo.

At the end of two weeks, the future embryo is a two-layered disc that lies between two cavities, the primitive amniotic sac and the cavity of the yolk sac (see Fig. 7–3).

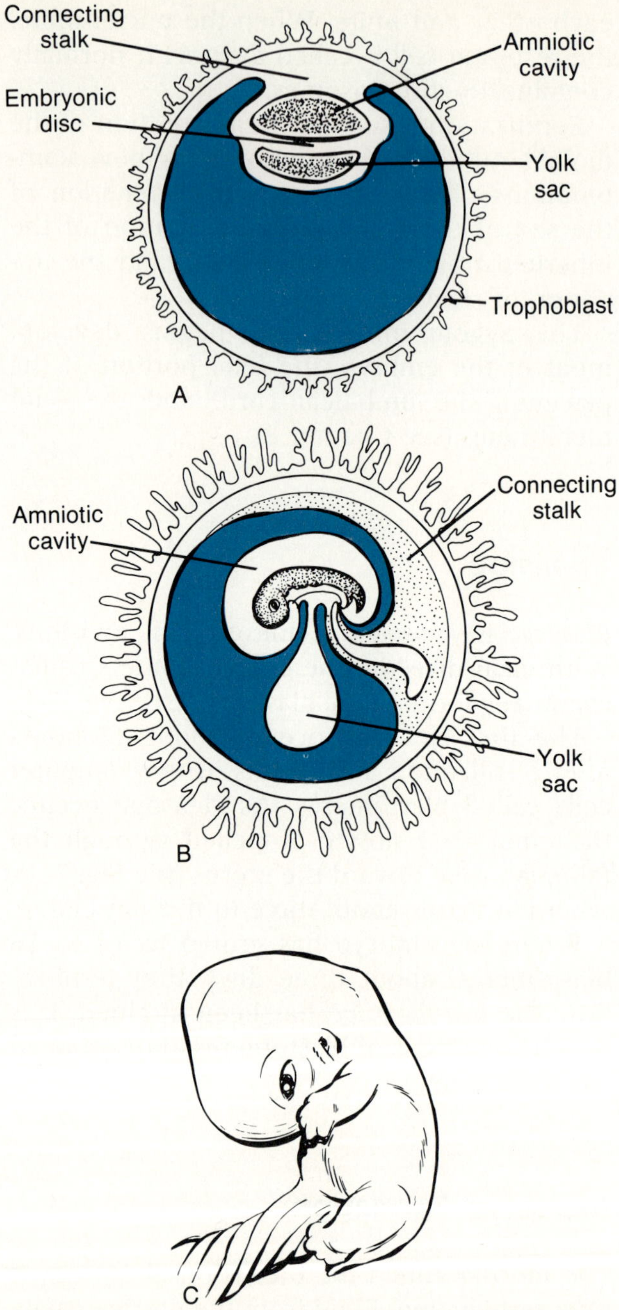

FIGURE 7–3. A. Embryo at 14 days. B. Embryo at 21 days. C. Lateral view of embryo at 56 days.

Decidua

Decidua is the endometrium of the pregnant uterus. Shortly after implantation, changes occur in the uterine endometrium near the site of implantation. The endometrium becomes edematous and vascular and contains large glands that secrete lipids and glycogen to help in nourishment of the embryo and protection of maternal tissue.

Three regions of decidual tissue have been identified: the *decidua capsularis*, which lies over the embryo; the *decidua basalis*, which is under the embryo and forms the maternal portion of the placenta; and the *decidua vera*, the remainder of the uterine lining (see Fig. 7-4). The decidua is discussed more fully in Chapter 8.

WEEK 3: TRILAMINAR EMBRYO FORMATION

During the third week of gestation, the three germ layers develop, as do the primitive streak, the notochord, and the neural tube. This period of embryonic development usually coincides with the first missed menstrual period (see Fig. 7-3).

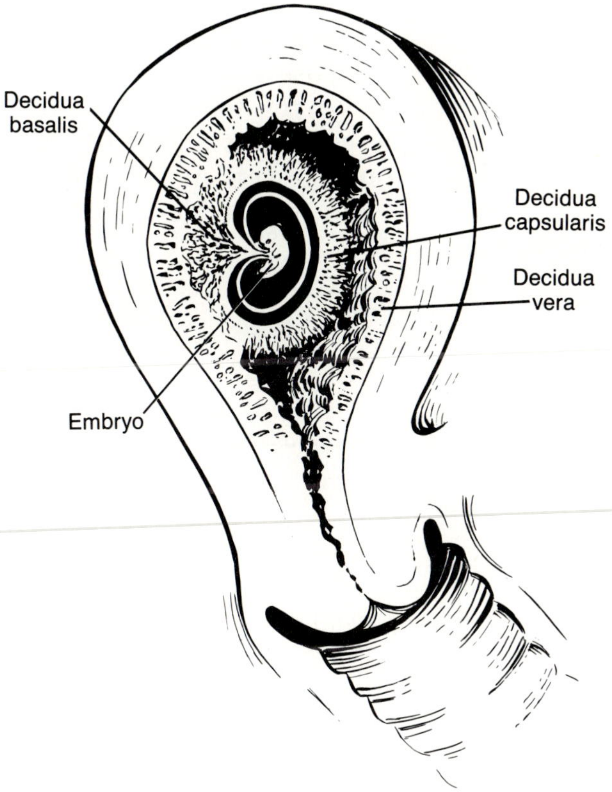

FIGURE 7-4. Diagram of the uterus shortly after implantation, showing the relation of the uterine layers to the newly implanted embryo.

Gastrulation

Gastrulation is the process by which the bilaminar embryonic disc is changed into the trilaminar embryonic disc. Gastrulation begins on day 14 and ends on day 19. During gastrulation the primitive streak and notochord are formed.

THE PRIMITIVE STREAK

The embryonic disc becomes pear-shaped. On the narrow caudal end an opaque streak, called the *primitive streak*, appears at about 15 days. A slightly elevated area appears at the cephalic end called the *primitive knot*. Cells that arise from the primitive streak migrate ventrally, laterally, and caudally between the epiblast and the hypoblast. These cells form the third germ layer, the *embryonic mesoderm*.

As the mesoderm cells extend to the side, they fuse with the extraembryonic mesoderm of the amnion and the yolk sac. At the cephalic end a small area later becomes the *buccopharyngeal membrane*. At the caudal end the ectoderm and endoderm fuse to form the *cloacal membrane*.

NOTOCHORD FORMATION

The primitive knot gives rise to cells that form the notochordal process at about 16 days. Cells from the primitive streak migrate and form mesoderm everywhere except at the oropharyngeal membrane and the cloacal membrane. A cellular rod called the notochord develops and is the basis of the axial skeleton. The vertebral column and the base of the skull will develop around the notochord.

NEURAL TUBE AND NEURAL CREST FORMATION

Following development of the primitive streak and primitive knot, a further thickening of the ectoderm, the neural plate, appears at the cephalic end. A longitudinal neural groove develops with neural folds on each side. At the edge of each neural fold is a neural crest.

These folds meet and fuse to form the neural tube, which will eventually become the central nervous system. The cephalic end will dilate to form the forebrain, midbrain, and hindbrain, while the remainder will become the spinal cord.

SOMITE FORMATION

The mesoderm on either side of the notochord thickens to form two columns. These columns begin to divide and segment into pairs of cuboidal mesoderm known as *somites*. Somites give rise to most of the skeleton of the head and trunk, associated muscles, and the dermis of the skin. Spinal nerves enter the somite portion that will form muscle.

COELOM (CAVITY) FORMATION

Isolated spaces arise in the mesoderm. These spaces eventually come together to form a horseshoe-shaped cavity, the *intraembryonic coelom*. Eventually this coelom divides into the pericardial, pleural, and peritoneal cavities.

BLOOD AND BLOOD VESSEL FORMATION

Blood vessels appear in the yolk sac, connecting stalk and chorion. At the end of the third week, the primitive heart is represented by two endocardial heart tubes that join with blood vessels in the embryo, connecting stalk, yolk sac, and chorion. A primitive cardiovascular system that circulates blood is established.

CHORIONIC VILLI

By day 15 a core of loose connective tissue has formed called the secondary *chorionic villi*. Before the end of the third week, capillaries develop in the villi. The chorionic sac becomes anchored to the endometrium and increases the surface area of the chorion for exchange between the maternal and embryonic circulations.

WEEKS 4 TO 8: THE EMBRYONIC PERIOD

During this period, all major external and internal structures begin to develop (see Table 7–2). The shape of the embryo changes as organs develop. Exposure to teratogens is especially dangerous at this time. The external appearance of the embryo is affected by the formation of various organs and structures. These weeks are the most critical weeks in development.

TABLE 7–2
SUMMARY OF DEVELOPMENT WEEK 4 THROUGH WEEK 8

Week 4	Week 5	Week 6	Week 7	Week 8
Deep neural groove Somites present Embryo curved Otic pits present Optic vesicles Upper limb buds 3 pairs branchial arches Heart prominence distinct Crown-rump length 5.0 mm	C-shaped curve to embryo Upper limbs paddle-shaped 4 pairs of branchial arches Lower limb buds present Otic vesicles Lens pits Attenuated tail Nasal pits present Optic cups present Crown-rump length 7.0 mm	Hand plates formed Lens vesicles present Prominent nasal pits Lower limbs paddle-shaped Foot plates formed Pigment in retina Finger rays Prominent cerebral vesicles Trunk begins to straighten Milk tooth buds visible Chondrification Crown-rump length 12 mm	Toe rays appear Elbow regions visible Eyelids forming Nipples visible Limbs extend ventrally Midgut herniation Tip of nose distinct Trunk elongates Crown-rump length 18 mm	Head rounded Liver can synthesize Fetal movements Thin skin Digits separate Bronchioles divide Palmprints and foot-prints Smooth muscle Eyelids Crown-rump length 31 mm

TABLE 7-3
GERM LAYER DERIVATIVES

Endoderm	Mesoderm	Ectoderm
Epithelial lining of respiratory, and gastrointestinal tracts	Muscles	Epidermis
Bronchi	Connective tissue	Hair
Lungs	Adrenal cortex	Nails
Gastrointestinal tract	Skeleton	Sebaceous glands
Liver	Dermis	Mammary glands
Pancreas	Dentine	Pituitary gland
Urinary bladder	Urogenital system	Tooth enamel
Pharynx	Serous membrane of pleura	Inner ear
Thyroid gland	Blood	Optic lens
Tympanic cavity	Lymph cells	Cranial and sensory nerves
Tonsils	Cardiovascular system	Medulla of adrenal gland
Parathyroid glands	Lymphatic system	Central nervous system
	Spleen	Retina
		Pineal body
		Sweat glands
		Peripheral nervous system

Folding of the Embryo

In order to establish general body form in the embryo, the flat trilaminar disc folds into a C-shaped cylinder because of rapid growth. Folding at the cranial and caudal ends and at the sides occurs at the same time. This results in a constriction between the embryo and the yolk sac. The dorsal part of the yolk sac gives rise to the primitive gut, which remains attached to it by a narrow yolk stalk. An epithelial covering for the umbilical cord is formed by the amnion.

Germ Layer Differentiation

Various tissues and organs develop from one of the three germ layers: the ectoderm, the mesoderm, and the endoderm (see Table 7-3).

Week 4

At the beginning of the fourth week of embryonic development, the embryo is almost straight. The neural tube is closed opposite the somites, but it is open at the caudal end. At about 24 days the first and second branchial arches, which will give rise to the mandible and maxilla, are distinct. Three pairs of branchial arches are visible by 26 days. Upper limb buds and the otic pits are visible. By 28 days the fourth pair of branchial arches and the lower limb buds are present. Lens placodes are visible on the sides of the head. A tail with somites is seen.

Week 5

Organogenesis continues, with a rapid growth and differentiation. Head growth is extensive owing to rapid development of the brain. Upper limbs begin to show differentiation as hand plates develop. The mandibular and maxillary prominences can be identified. Cardiovascular development includes septation of the heart. The midgut begins to elongate and herniate into the umbilical cord.

Week 6

The elbow and wrist regions become identifiable, and finger rays begin to form. The head appears more bent because of the bending of the brain in the cervical region. Small swellings develop that will become the auricle of the external ear. The face shows rapid development with the eyes appearing more prominent. The trunk begins to straighten.

Week 7

The yolk stalk is now the communication between the yolk sac and the primitive gut. Umbilical herniation of the intestines is present. The upper limbs are longer, with the elbows bent. Notches are present between the rays on the hand plates.

Week 8

By the end of this week the fingers are longer and toes are distinct. All evidence of the tail is gone. The head is more round and erect but is large in proportion to the body. The eyes are usually open, but the eyelids are beginning to meet. The ear auricles assume their final shape (see Fig. 7–3).

THE FETAL PERIOD

After the embryonic period, the developing human is called a fetus. The fetal period is characterized by growth and differentiation of tissues.

Weeks 9 to 12

At the beginning of the ninth week, the head constitutes almost half of the fetus. By the end of 12 weeks the crown-rump length is 87 mm, almost double the nine-week length of 50 mm. The face is broad, the ears are low set, and the eyes are widely separated with closed eyelids. The nasal septum and palate fusion are complete.

The upper limbs have almost reached their final relative lengths, but the lower limbs are still short. At about 12 weeks the external genitalia are distinguishable as male or female.

Erythropoiesis decreases in the liver and begins to occur in the spleen. Urine starts to form and is excreted into the amniotic fluid. The intestines return to the abdomen from the umbilical cord and peristalsis begins.

The fetus begins to react to stimuli during this period. Stroking of the lips will cause the fetus to make sucking movements, and stroking of the eyelids will cause a reflex response.

Weeks 13 to 16

During this period the fetal weight almost doubles to 200 gm at 16 weeks. The skin is red and transparent, blood vessels are visible, and hind limbs are well developed. Crown-rump length grows to 140 mm. Hair is present on the fetal head, and meconium is found in the intestines. Meconium consists of castoff epithelial cells, mucus and bile from the developing digestive tract, plus material entering the digestive tract from swallowing of amniotic fluid. The liver can synthesize fatty acids. Ossification of bones continues. Ovaries are differentiated and have primordial follicles that contain oogonia.

Weeks 17 to 20

At the end of 20 weeks, the fetus is 190 mm long and weighs 460 gm. The lower limbs reach their final proportions and *quickening* (maternal perception of fetal movement) is felt. Eyebrows and eyelashes are present and *lanugo* (fine downy hair) covers the body. The skin is covered with *vernix caseosa*, a greasy cheeselike material that protects the fetal skin. Enamel and dentine for teeth are present.

Brown fat, which begins to form at this time, functions as a site of heat production. Brown fat produces heat through fatty acid oxidation and is found on the floor of the anterior triangle of the neck, posterior to the sternum, and in the perirenal area.

In the female, the uterus is completely formed and vaginal formation begins. In the male, the testes have begun their descent into the scrotum.

Weeks 21 to 24

At 24 weeks gestation, the fetus appears lean with few fat pads and red wrinkled skin. The crown-rump length is 230 mm and the fetus weighs 820 gm. Fingernails are present. The alveoli of the lungs begin to form surfactant.

Weeks 25 to 29

By 29 weeks gestation the fetal lungs are capable of breathing air and providing gas exchange. Subcutaneous fat has now formed, giving the fetus a more rounded contour.

Weeks 30 to 34

The fetus is approximately 320 mm long and 2400 gm in weight by 34 weeks gestation. The pupillary light reflex is present. The skin is pink and smooth, and the arms and legs may appear chubby. Much of the lanugo is gone from the face. Fingernails reach the fingertips.

Weeks 35 to 40

At 35 weeks the fetus has a firm grasp and exhibits spontaneous orientation to light. The fetus appears plump. At term, the fetus usually has a crown-rump length of 360 mm and weighs about 3400 gm. The chest is prominent. Testes are usually in the scrotum in the male.

EMBRYONIC AND FETAL DEVELOPMENT

Head and Neck

The head and neck are formed mainly from the *branchial apparatus*, which consists of branchial arches, pharyngeal pouches, branchial grooves, and branchial membranes. Most congenital malformations of the head and neck originate during transformation of the branchial apparatus.

The tongue, face, lips, jaws, palate, pharynx, and neck originate from the branchial apparatus. The pharyngeal pouches give rise to the auditory tube, palatine tonsils, thymus, and parathyroid glands. The thyroid gland develops from a growth on the floor of the pharynx near the tongue (see Fig. 7–5).

Cardiovascular System

The first system to function in the embryo is the cardiovascular system. By the end of the third week of life, blood begins to circulate and provides the embryo with nutrients and disposes of waste products.

BLOOD

Nucleated blood cells begin to form at three weeks. By week 6 there is definite erythropoiesis in the yolk sac and liver with hemoglobin present in the erythrocytes. By week 10, the liver is the major site of hematopoiesis. During weeks 12 to 28 there is erythropoietic activity in the spleen. Bone marrow production begins during week 20. Fetal hemoglobin has two alpha and two beta chains, causing a greater

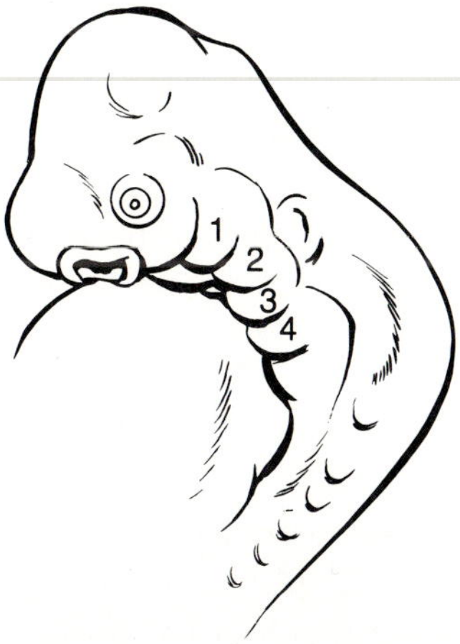

FIGURE 7–5. Head of embryo showing branchial arches.

oxygen affinity in the fetus and allowing for more efficient use of available oxygen by concentration of hemoglobin.

BLOOD VESSELS

Blood vessel formation begins in the mesoderm of the yolk sac, the connecting stalk, and the chorion during days 13 through 15 of embryonic life. About two days later, embryonic vessels begin to form. Cells called angioblasts form isolated masses (blood islands). Isolated vessels fuse to form channels that extend into adjacent areas.

The first well-defined blood vessels are the primitive aortas, which appear as extensions of the endocardial heart tube. They extend to the foregut, curve around the pharyngeal pouch and continue caudally as dorsal aortas. The vitelline arteries are initially paired vessels that supply the yolk sac. They gradually fuse and form arteries that supply the dorsal gut. Umbilical arteries course to the placenta. During week 4, each artery acquires a connection with the common iliac artery.

The three-week embryo has three pairs of veins: the vitelline, carrying blood from the yolk sac to the heart; the umbilical, carrying oxygenated blood to the embryo; and the cardinal, draining the body of the embryo.

THE HEART

During week 2 of life the heart begins to form as a straight tube (*endocardial heart tube*) through which blood flows in an undivided stream. The endocardial tube is anchored in the body at the cephalic and caudal ends. As the heart grows, it bends to the right and acquires the general external appearance of the adult heart. Between weeks 4 and 7 the heart becomes partitioned into four chambers.

LYMPHATIC SYSTEM

During week 5 the lymphatic system begins development. Six primary lymph sacs develop and later become interconnected by lymph vessels. By week 7 lymphocytes are seen in the thymus.

Genitourinary System

URINARY SYSTEM

During week 3 the mesoderm forms the nephrogenic cord while the excretory units of the nephrotome forms in the cervical region. Branches of the dorsal aorta form the glomeruli.

Three different, slightly overlapping, kidney systems are formed during embryonic life: the pronephros, the mesonephros, and the metanephros.

The *pronephros* consists of seven to ten rudimentary tubules and a collecting tube. The tubules that form first regress before the last ones are formed. At the end of four weeks the pronephros has disappeared.

During degeneration of the pronephros, the *mesonephros* begins to form, with appearance of mesonephric tubules that enter the mesonephric duct. By week 6 a large ovoid organ has formed on each side of the midline. By week 8 the majority of the mesonephric system has disappeared (see Fig. 7–6).

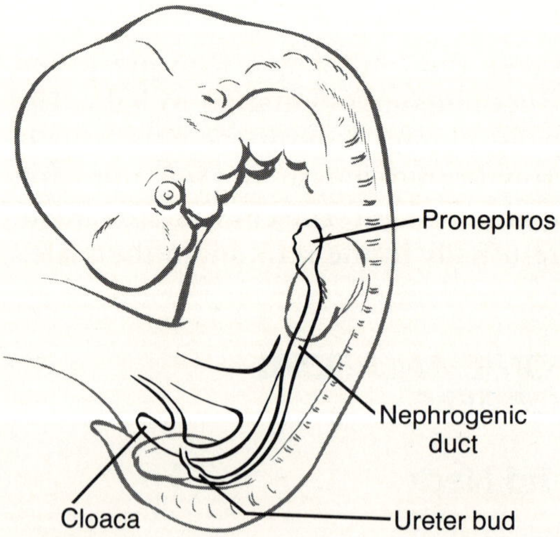

FIGURE 7–6. 32 day old embryo, showing excretory structures.

As the mesonephros disappears the *metanephros* or permanent kidney begins to appear. By week 10 the pelvis and calyces form. Urine is present and glomeruli are functional during week 12. By week 14, 20 percent of the nephrons are mature. By week 20, the kidney contains 350,000 nephrons with nephrogenesis complete by week 35. The glomerulus and loops of Henle are short. At term, fetal urine is produced in the amount of 500 ml per day.

During weeks 4 to 7 the terminal part of the cloaca divides into the urogenital sinus and the anorectal canal. The urogenital sinus gives rise to the urinary bladder, the lower portion of the vagina, and a portion of the urethra in the female. In the male it forms the urinary bladder and the urethra.

GENITAL SYSTEM

The sex of the embryo is genetically determined at fertilization. In week 7 the gonads begin to acquire male or female characteristics, although sex cannot be differentiated. By week 12 the external genitalia are distinctive in masculine or feminine characteristics.

Muscular System

The muscular system derives from the mesoderm with the exception of muscles of the iris, which develop from the ectoderm of the optic cup.

SKELETAL MUSCLE

The first indication of muscle development is the formation of myoblasts. Myoblasts fuse with one another to form elongated structures called myotubules, which then differentiate into muscle fibers. Almost all skeletal muscle fibers develop before birth.

SMOOTH MUSCLE

During early development myoblasts are differentiated from mesenchymal cells. As these myoblasts arrange themselves, they tend to be longer in the direction in which the contractile power will be exerted. By week 6 or 7, myofibrils are present.

CARDIAC MUSCLE

Cardiac muscle forms from the mesenchyme surrounding the endocardial heart tube. Muscle fibers arise by differentiation and growth of single cells.

Skeletal System

The articular and skeletal systems develop from the mesoderm. Mesodermal cells give rise to a loosely formed tissue known as *mesenchyme* or embryonic connective tissue. Mesenchymal cells differentiate into fibroblasts, chondroblasts, or osteoblasts.

CHONDROGENESIS

The first sign of cartilage formation is during week 5. The mesenchymal cells proliferate, acquire a round shape (*chondroblast*), and form a cell-rich tissue known as *precartilage*. The intercellular tissues contain collagenous fibers that are imbedded in ground substances. Three types of cartilage are formed: hyaline, fibrous, and elastic.

OSTEOGENESIS

Bone formation is of two types: membranous ossification and endochondral ossification. In *membranous ossification*, mesenchymal cells form osteoblasts that later arrange themselves in regular rows and secrete a collagen material called prebone. The prebone becomes bone matrix, which then calcifies as a result of phosphatase, an enzyme. The newly formed bone is separated from the osteoblasts by prebone. A few osteoblasts become trapped in the bone and form bone cells (*osteocytes*).

Endochondral ossification begins in week 7. The long bones of the extremities are present as hyaline cartilage covered with periosteum. A vascular band invades the center of the shaft and forms lacunae. Osteoblasts deposit bone along the cartilage and give rise to mixed spicules of calcified cartilage that later resorb and leave a narrow cavity in the center. Endochondral ossification progresses from the center of the shaft to the ends.

AXIAL SKELETON

The *axial skeleton*, which includes the vertebral column, ribs, sternum, and skull, begins to form during week 4. Sclerotome cells of the somites migrate to three main areas: around the notochord to develop into the intervertebral discs; around the neural tube to develop into the vertebral arch; and in the body wall to develop into ribs.

The skull develops from mesenchyme around the brain. It consists of a *neurocranium*, the protective case, and the *viscerocranium*, which gives rise to the facial skeleton.

APPENDICULAR SKELETON

The *appendicular skeleton* consists of the shoulder and pelvic girdles and the limb bones. It develops from endochondral ossification of the cartilage models of the bones that form in the developing limbs. The first center of ossification appears in the clavicle during week 6. In the long bones the first indication of ossification is near the center of the future long bone shaft. The secondary ossification centers of the bones at the knees are the first to appear.

Limbs

The limb buds appear as elevations on the body wall during week 4. The upper limb buds appear low on the trunk at first due to the rapid head and neck development.

Upper limb buds develop a few days before the lower limb buds. Tissues for the upper and lower limb buds derive from the mesoderm and the ectoderm. At first the limbs are directed caudally. In week 7 they extend ventrally and in week 8 they rotate on their axis in different directions and to different degrees (see Fig. 7–7).

Respiratory System

Respiratory development in the embryo and fetus is divided into four phases: (1) glandular, from 4 to 16 weeks; (2) canalicular, from 17 to 23 weeks; (3) terminal sac, from 24 weeks to birth; and (4) alveolar, from birth through eight years of age. Prior to the glandular phase, the respiratory and digestive system exists as a single tube.

GLANDULAR PHASE (WEEKS 4 THROUGH 16)

By the beginning of week 4 there is an outpouching of the fetal esophagus that results in

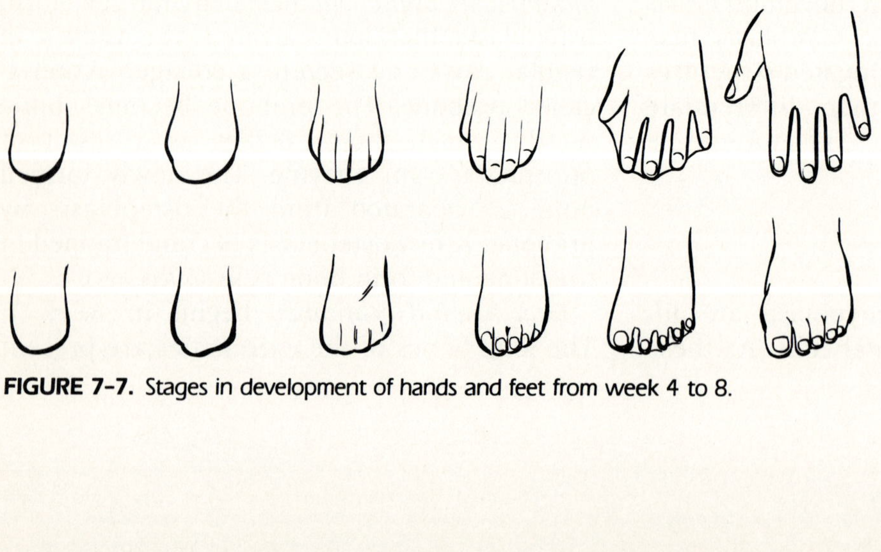

FIGURE 7–7. Stages in development of hands and feet from week 4 to 8.

formation of a ventral bud. During week 4, the right and left primary bronchi form. By week 5, the right bronchus has divided into three main branches and the left bronchus has divided into two main branches (see Fig. 7-8). The gasping reflex has been observed during week 8. During week 10 cartilage deposition begins, and during week 12 lung buds are demarcated. The main bronchi continue to divide, and at 16 weeks bronchi formation is nearly complete. The epithelial lining is pseudocuboidal and capillaries begin to grow in the alveolar sacs.

CANALICULAR PHASE (WEEKS 17 THROUGH 23)

This phase is characterized by continuing development of the respiratory bronchioles and vascular buds. This bronchial tissue becomes hollow.

TERMINAL SAC PHASE (WEEK 24 TO BIRTH)

Many more terminal sacs develop during this period. The epithelium becomes very thin, and type I alveolar epithelial cells line the terminal air sacs. Type II alveolar epithelial cells begin to produce surfactant at the beginning of this phase. Surfactant is a lipoprotein substance that lowers the surface tension at the air-alveolar exchange surface and helps to prevent alveolar collapse.

ALVEOLAR PHASE (BIRTH TO 8 YEARS)

Lung development continues after birth and alveoli increase in number up to and including age eight years. The lining of the air sacs becomes thinner and indents further, allowing an increase in the number of bronchioles and alveoli.

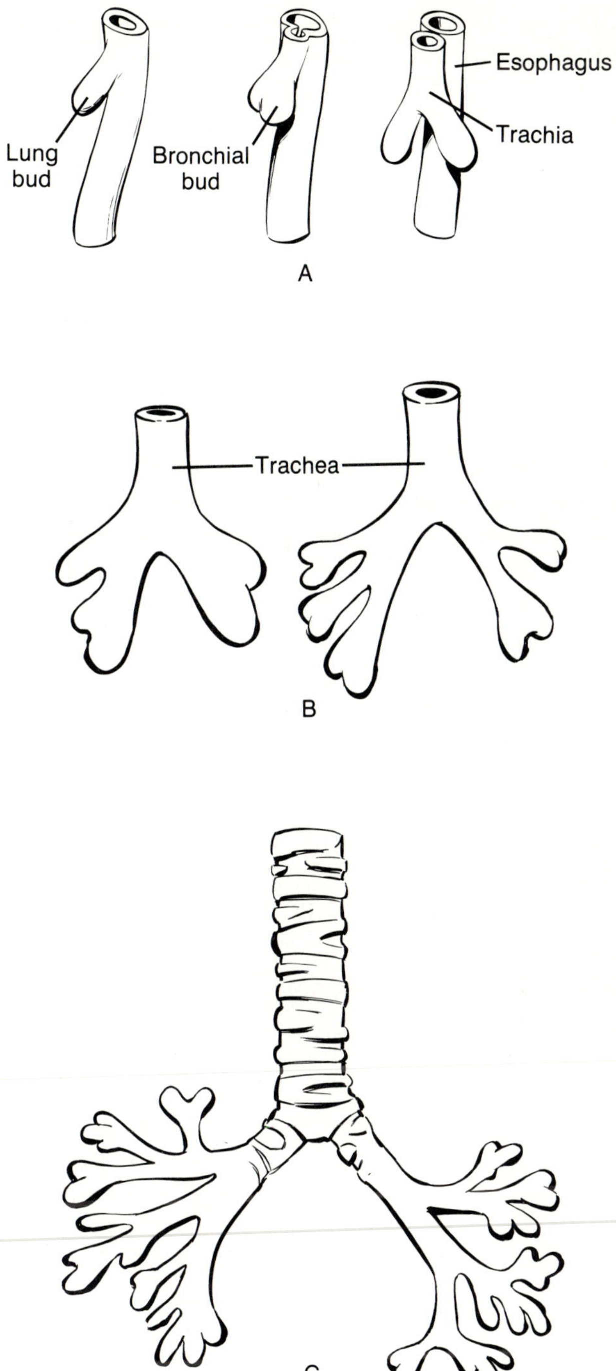

FIGURE 7-8. Stages in development of bronchi and lungs: A. 4 weeks. B. 5 weeks. C. 8 weeks.

Nervous System

The nervous system in the embryo appears at the beginning of week 3. An elongated plate of ectoderm, the neural plate, becomes visible. During the next few days the lateral edges of this plate are elevated to form the neural folds, while the depressed midline area is called the neural groove. The neural folds become fused in the midline and form the neural tube.

By the 25th day, the central nervous system is a closed tubular structure with a cylindrical caudal portion (future spinal cord) and a broader cephalic portion (future brain). The brain develops rapidly by proliferation, migration, and differentiation of neuronal cytoplasm.

Three primary brain vesicles form the prosencephalon or forebrain; the mesocephalon or midbrain; and the rhomboencephalon or hindbrain (see Fig. 7–9). The spinal cord begins formation by the middle of the fourth week from the remainder of the neural tube.

Further development transforms the brain into five regions. By week 5, the forebrain has subdivided into the telencephalon and diencephalon (thalamus and hypothalamus). The hindbrain has also divided into the metencephalon (pons and cerebellum) and the myeloencephalon (medulla oblongata). The first reflex arc becomes functional at this time.

In week 7, the telencephalon produces two bulges that become the cerebral hemispheres. In each bulge is a cavity, the lateral ventricle. The cavity in the diencephalon is known as the third ventricle. A depression in the floor of the diencephalon fuses with an upgrowth from the stomodeum and forms the pituitary gland.

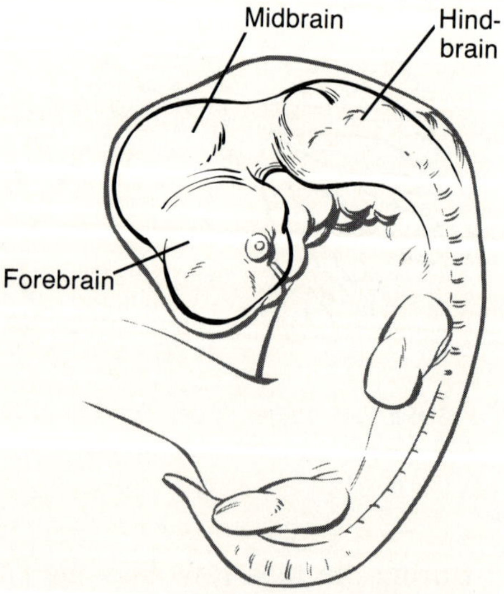

FIGURE 7–9. 28 day embryo, showing three primary brain vesicles.

During week 8, growth of the cerebellar rudiments begins. Neurons migrate toward the surface and produce the cerebellar cortex. Electrical activity is present within the brain. By week 10, the cerebral hemispheres constitute the largest portion of the brain.

Brain development is characterized by neuroblast proliferation during the second trimester. By week 16 the cerebral hemispheres have expanded to touch the smooth cerebellar hemispheres. Myelinization begins in the brain stem during week 20 and reaches the hemispheres by term. Afferent bundles are myelinated first, with motor pathways becoming myelinated after birth.

In week 26 the fetus shows the beginnings of alertness and neurovegetative behavior. Rooting and an incomplete Moro reflex are present. By week 35 the fetus has flexed limbs, a firm grasp, and a spontaneous orientation to light. The highest rate of neurologic growth is just before term.

During the third trimester the cerebral cortex proliferates and continues maturing for the first six to eight months of life. There is gradual proliferation of primary reflexes in a cephalocaudal direction with a corresponding increase in muscle tone.

Sense Organs

TONGUE

Formation of the tongue begins during week 4 of embryonic life with the development of a median tongue bud. During weeks 12 through 15 the epithelium of the tongue develops. By 24 weeks the taste buds are clearly defined.

NOSE

The first indication of nose formation is the appearance during week 4 of two thickened areas of ectoderm on the frontal aspect of the head. As development progresses, the two nasal pits and their associated processes converge toward the midline. The nasomedial processes merge with each other, forming the bridge of the nose, the upper lip, and the nasal septum. By week 9 the nose and palate are completely formed.

EYES

The developing eye first appears in the 18-day embryo as a pair of shallow grooves on each side of the forebrain. With closure of the neural tube, the optic vesicles form. By week 7, the future pupil has formed and the eyelids start to develop. The eyelids meet and fuse with each other by the end of week 9 and do not reopen until the 28th week.

EARS

In the embryo, the ear develops from three different sources: the external ear develops from the first pharyngeal cleft; the middle ear develops from the first pharyngeal pouch; and the internal ear is formed by the ectodermal otic vesicle. The first sign of the developing ear can be seen at 18 days of age as a thickening of the ectoderm on each side of the rhomboencephalon. By 12 weeks, the internal ear has formed, and the external ear has achieved its adult configuration.

Digestive System

By day 30 of embryonic life, the primitive gut has formed a blind tube with a buccopharyngeal membrane over the cephalic end (primitive mouth) and a cloacal membrane over the caudal end that develops into the urogenital sinus and rectum. This primitive gut will develop into the foregut, midgut, hindgut, liver, and pancreas (see Fig. 7-10).

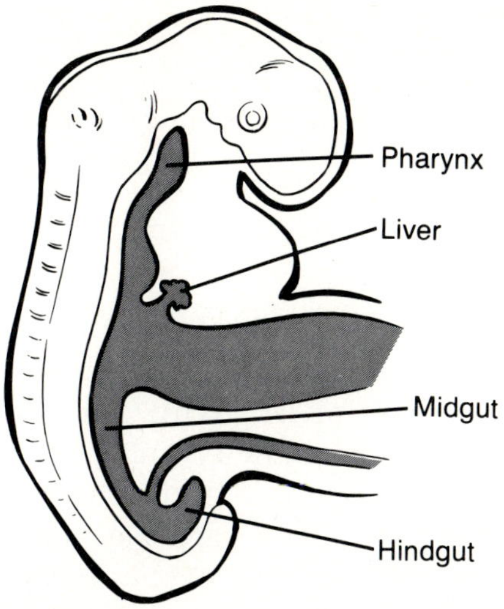

FIGURE 7-10. 4 week embryo showing early digestive system.

FOREGUT

The foregut is composed of the pharynx, lower respiratory tract, esophagus, stomach, and upper duodenum.

Cranial Part of the Foregut

At the cephalic end of the foregut the buccopharyngeal membrane forms. At the end of week 3 the membrane ruptures, creating an open connection and forming the primitive mouth. During weeks 4 and 5 the pharyngeal pouches appear, along with four pharyngeal clefts.

Pharyngeal Pouches

The human embryo has five pairs of *pharyngeal pouches* that give rise to the tympanic cavity, the eustachian tube, the palatine tonsil, the parathyroid gland, the thymus, and the thyroid gland.

Floor of the Pharynx

The tongue appears in the embryo during week 4. The mucosa covering the tongue originates from the first pharyngeal arch. On day 17 the thyroid gland is seen as an epithelial formation in the floor of the pharyngeal gut. The thyroid continues formation and reaches its final position during week 7. Thyroid function begins in week 12.

Pharyngeal Clefts

During week 5 the embryo has four *pharyngeal clefts*. Only the first continues to develop into the external auditory meatus and the eardrum.

Pharyngeal Arches

During the fourth week of development the pharyngeal clefts are separated by ridges called the *pharyngeal arches*. With further development each arch acquires a cartilaginous skeleton, a muscular component, and a characteristic artery and nerve. The cartilage component of the first arch consists of the maxillary and mandibular processes. With further development they retrogress and disappear. The mandible is formed by ossification of tissue. The cartilage component of the second pharyngeal arch forms the stapes, a portion of the temporal bone, and the hyoid bone. The cartilage of the third pharyngeal arch gives rise to another portion of the hyoid bone. The fourth, fifth, and sixth arches fuse to form the thyroid and cricoid cartilage of the larynx.

Caudal Part of the Foregut

The caudal portion of the foregut develops into the esophagus, stomach, upper duodenum, liver, gallbladder, and pancreas. The esophagus develops from the portion of the foregut that extends from the respiratory diverticulum to the fusiform dilatation. The stomach appears during week 5 and is attached to the body walls. During the next four weeks the appearance and position of the stomach change greatly owing to the different rates of growth in various regions of the walls and to a change in the position of the surrounding organs.

The duodenum is formed by a terminal portion of the foregut and the cephalic portion of the midgut. The liver appears in week 3 and by week 10 comprises 10 percent of the total body weight. Synthesis of glycogen and bilirubin begins during week 10. The pancreas begins development at 30 days and by week 20 insulin is being produced.

MIDGUT

The midgut develops into the small intestines, cecum, appendix, descending colon, and proximal transverse colon. Development of the midgut is characterized by rapid elongation, which results in the formation of a primary intestinal loop.

While the sides of the intestinal loop become fixed to the abdominal wall, the remainder continues to lengthen to such an extent that the abdominal cavity is temporarily too small. As a result, the loops enter the extraembryonic coelom in the umbilical cord during week 6. In week 10 the intestinal loops return to the abdominal cavity.

HINDGUT

The hindgut gives rise to the distal third of the transverse colon, the descending colon, the sigmoid colon, the rectum, the epithelium of the urinary bladder, and most of the urethra.

Integumentary System

The integumentary system includes the skin, teeth, nails, hair, skin glands, and mammary glands.

SKIN

The epidermis arises from the ectoderm. During the first four weeks of life the superficial ectoderm is a simple cuboidal epithelium. During week 6 the *periderm*, a thin layer of flattened cells, is formed and becomes thicker during weeks 7 and 8. The epithelium acquires its definitive structure and the cells begin to accumulate keratin by week 16. The dermis arises from the mesoderm. By week 12 pigment cells called *melanophores* are developed.

In the early stages of skin formation, the union between the epithelium and dermal tissue is smooth. During weeks 12 to 16 the epithelium thickens and its lower surface becomes irregular. By week 24 these irregularities begin to show on the palms and soles as footprints and handprints.

TEETH

Deciduous teeth begin development in week 6. Ectodermal cells migrate below the surface to form enamel organs which fit like caps over small groups of mesodermal cells that lie in the primitive jaw. The rudiments of all 20 teeth are present by week 10 and begin calcification by week 16. The permanent teeth first appear about week 18.

NAILS

The nailbeds are suggested by the molding on the tips of the digits by week 12. The nails develop from a thickened plate of epithelium known as the *primary nail field*.

HAIR

Local downgrowths into connective tissue from the epidermis mark the points at which hair starts to develop. These become recognizable on the eyebrows, eyelids, lips, chin, and scalp during weeks 12 through 16.

SKIN GLANDS

The sebaceous glands make their appearance as cell buds arising from the sides of the hair follicles. Epithelial buds that will become sudoriferous (sweat) glands appear on the palmar and plantar surfaces by week 16.

MAMMARY GLANDS

The mammary line or ridge is the first indication of mammary gland development. By the seventh week the line extends on each side of the body from the base of the forelimb to the region of the hindlimb. During the late fetal period, the epidermis at the origin of the mammary gland becomes depressed and forms the mammary pit.

FETAL CIRCULATION

The first system to function in the embryo is the cardiovascular system. The placenta functions as the organ for the exchange of wastes, provision of nutrients, and elimination of waste products. In order for the placenta to function, the fetus must have a circulatory system that allows blood to flow to and from the placenta.

Structures peculiar to the fetus that function in prenatal circulation but serve no purpose following birth include: the placenta, the organ of exchange; one umbilical vein, which carries oxygenated blood to the fetus; two umbilical arteries, which return deoxygenated blood back to the placenta; the foramen ovale, an opening between the right and left atria of the heart; the ductus arteriosus, a vessel that connects the pulmonary artery and the aorta; and the ductus venosus, a vessel that connects the umbilical vein and the inferior vena cava (see Table 7–4).

Course of Blood Through the Fetus

Arterial blood flows from the placenta to the fetus by way of the umbilical vein (see Fig. 7–11). The umbilical vein enters the fetal ab-

TABLE 7–4
CIRCULATION BEFORE AND AFTER BIRTH

Feature	Before Birth	After Birth
Placenta	Exchange	Expelled during third stage of labor
Umbilical vein	Carries oxygenated blood to fetus	Ligametum terres
Umbilical arteries	Carries deoxygenated blood away from fetus	Hypogastric ligament
Foramen ovale	Bypasses the right ventricle	Closes
Ductus arteriosus	Bypasses fetal lungs	Ligamentum arteriosum
Ductus venosus	Bypasses fetal liver	Ligamentum venosum

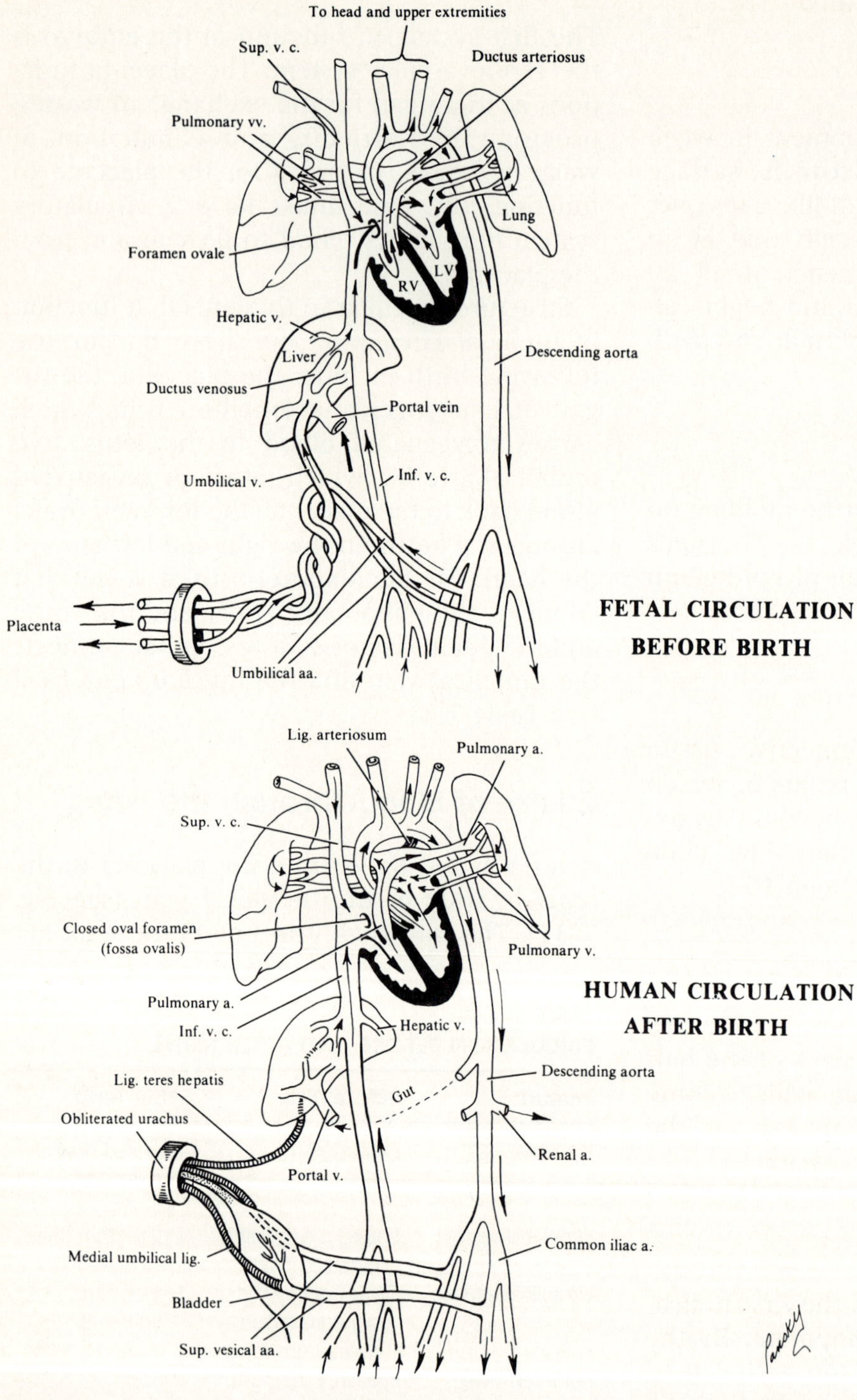

FIGURE 7-11. Fetal circulation. Reprinted with permission from Pansky, B., Review of Medical Embryology, New York: Macmillan, 1982.

domen at the umbilicus and proceeds upward to the undersurface of the liver. On approaching the liver, the main portion of the blood bypasses the liver through the ductus venosus and flows directly into the inferior vena cava. A small portion of the blood enters the liver and mixes with blood from the portal circulation.

Blood that enters the inferior vena cava from the liver bypass mixes with blood returning from the lower extremities. The blood enters the right atrium and is directed through the foramen ovale into the left atrium, thereby bypassing the right ventricle.

In the left atrium, the blood mixes with a small quantity of blood returning from the lungs through the pulmonary vein. Blood flows into the left ventricle and then into the ascending aorta. Blood is distributed to the head and upper extremities via the ascending aorta, with a small quantity continuing into the descending aorta.

BIBLIOGRAPHY

Avery, M.E., Fletcher, B.D. & Williams, R. *The Lung and its disorders in the newborn infant* (4th ed.). Philadelphia: Saunders, 1981.

Cranley, M.S. Perinatal risk. *Journal of Obstetrical, Gynecological, and Neonatal Nursing*, 1983, **12**, 13s.

Harris, T.R. Fetal development and physiology. In A.L. Clark, D.D. Affonso & T.R. Harris (Eds.). *Childbearing: A nursing perspective* (2nd ed.). Philadelphia: Davis, 1981, pp. 233-254.

Holmes, L.B. Radiation. In V.C. Vaughan, R.J. McKay & R.D. Behrman (Eds.). *Nelson's textbook of pediatrics* (11th ed.). Philadelphia: Saunders, 1979.

Loper, D.L. Gastrointestinal development: embryology, congenital anomalies and impact on feeding. *Neonatal Network*, 1983, **2**, 27-35.

Moore, K.L. *The developing human. Clinically oriented embryology* (3rd ed.). Philadelphia: Saunders, 1982.

Page, E.W., et al. *Human reproduction: Essentials of reproductive and perinatal medicine* (3rd ed.). Philadelphia: Saunders, 1981.

chapter 8

THE PLACENTA AND FETAL SUPPORT

OBJECTIVES

Upon completion of this chapter, the reader will be able to:

1. Describe the structure of the placenta.
2. Describe and state the function of the umbilical cord, amniotic sac, and membranes.
3. Discuss maternal and fetal placental circulation.
4. Describe the transfer of nutritive substances, oxygen, and waste material across the placenta and factors that affect or alter this process.
5. Identify the placental hormones and state their functions.

KEY TERMS

Amnion
Chorion
Chorionic villi
Cotyledon
Cytotrophoblastic cells
Decidua basalis
Estrogen
Human chorionic gonadotropin (HCG)
Human chorionic somatomammotropin (HCS)
Intervillous spaces
Placenta
Progesterone
Syncytiotrophoblastic cells
Umbilical cord
Wharton's jelly

PLACENTAL DEVELOPMENT

The stalk of life uniting the fetus to the maternal host is the placenta. Among the functions of this very vascular organ are the production of hormones essential to the maintenance of the pregnancy as well as the mediating of nutritive and respiratory exchange and elimination in the fetus. The placenta is essential for the promotion of life; yet, once the reproductive function is completed, the placenta is expelled from the maternal host.

The placenta, at term, is discoid in shape and weighs approximately 500 gm or about one sixth the weight of the fetus at birth (Page et al., 1976). The average placenta is 16 to 20 cm (7 to 10 inches) in diameter and 2.5 cm (1 inch) in thickness. There may, however, be many normal variations in size. The maternal surface (side attached to the uterine wall) (see Fig. 8–1*A*) is formed from the uterine endometrium and contains about 15 to 30 irregularly shaped *cotyledons* (lobes). These cotyledons impart a red, fleshy rough appearance to the placenta, when seen following delivery. In direct contrast is the smooth, shiny, bluish-white color of the fetal surface covered by the amniotic membrane. Arising from the center of the fetal surface (see Fig. 8–1*B*) of the placenta is the *umbilical cord,* which contains two umbilical arteries, one umbilical vein, and Wharton's jelly. *Wharton's jelly* is a mucoid connective tissue substance that has a jellylike consistency and separates the vessels of the cord, reducing the possibility of friction and harm to the vessels.

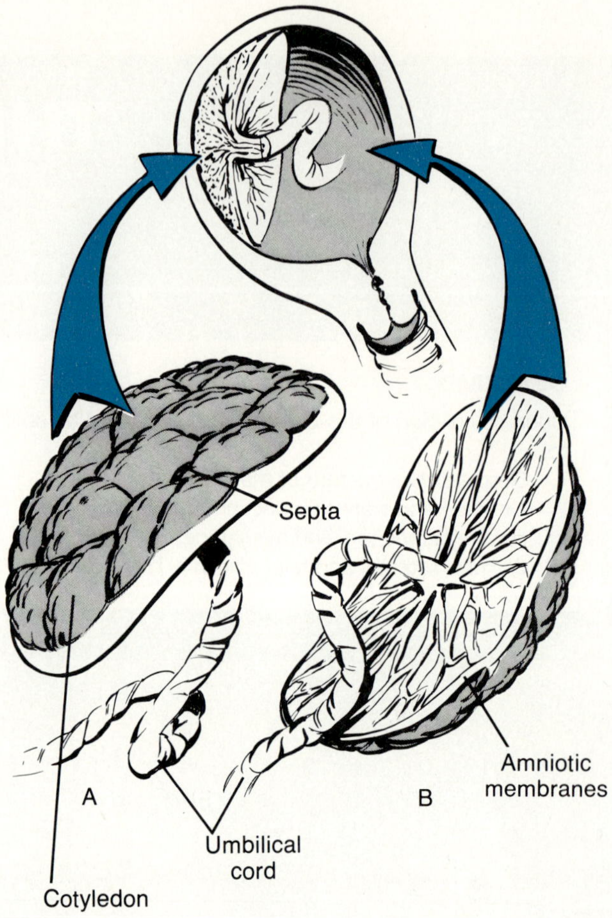

FIGURE 8–1. A. Maternal side of the placenta. B. Fetal side of the placenta.

IMPLANTATION

The *trophoblastic cells* of the blastocyst begin to invade the endometrial epithelium on about day 7 following fertilization. Although the trophoblastic cells completely surround the entire blastocyst, only those centered at the embryonic pole actually invade the endometrium. Differentiation of the trophoblast produces the inner *cytotrophoblastic* cells and an outer syncytial layer of cells called *syncytiotrophoblast* (see Fig. 8–2). These cells invade the endometrium and erode the epithelium of the maternal capillaries and uterine vessels promoting the formation of *lacunae,* spaces containing blood and glandular secretions, which will become *intervillous spaces*. The nutritive material from the maternal blood in the lacunae continue to provide nourishment for the developing embryo.

Further development of the marginless syncytiotrophoblastic cells results in the for-

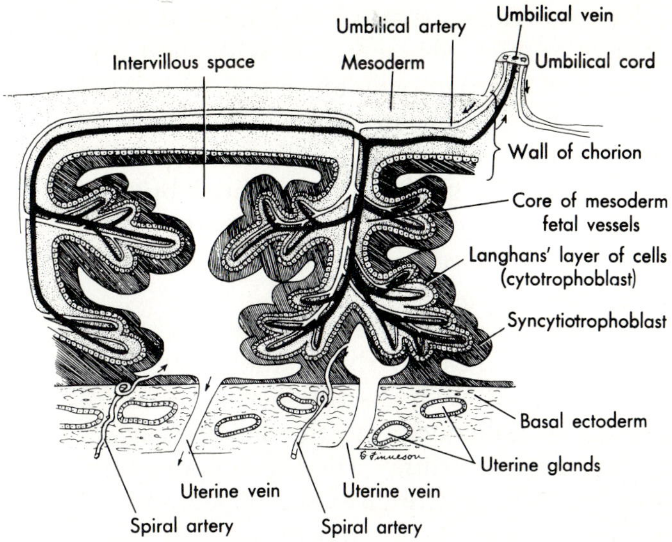

FIGURE 8-2. Differentiation of the trophoblast into the cytotrophoblastic and syncytiotrophoblastic layers of the chorionic villi. Reprinted with permission from Miller, M. et al. Kimber-Gray-Stockpole's Anatomy and Physiology, 17th ed.: Macmillan, 1977.

mation of microvilli that extend deeper into the endometrium of the uterus, continuing to penetrate until the decidual uterine tissue is reached.

DECIDUA

The stromal cells of the uterine mucous membrane, under the influence of progesterone, become decidual cells containing glycogen and lipids. These cells are shed at the time of menstruation. If pregnancy occurs, they continue to develop, becoming increasingly secretory. Upon implantation of the trophoblast, differentiation of the decidua occurs, dividing the decidua into three distinct areas. The area directly beneath the implantation site becomes the *decidua basalis* (see Fig. 7–4) and enters into the formation of the placenta. The area of the endometrium that surrounds the implanted embryo fuses and becomes the *decidua capsularis.* The remaining endometrium lining the uterus becomes the *decidua parietalis* (vera).

CHORIONIC VILLI

Columns of cytotrophoblastic cells covered with syncytiotrophoblast form and come in contact with the decidua. At this time, a fibrinoid material is produced by the decidua that prevents further penetration of the syncytiotrophoblastic microvilli into the myometrium of the uterus. With the anchoring villi now firmly attached to the decidua, the trophoblast proliferates, forming intervillous spaces containing secondary and tertiary villi. The original columns of cytotrophoblastic cells develop a mesodermal core and become main stem chorionic villi (see Fig. 8–3), containing an artery and vein which provide a linkage to the fetal circulation. The arteries and veins continue branching into the secondary and tertiary villi. The interchange of nutritive materials and fetal waste products between the mother and the fetus occurs via the capillaries of these vessels. There is no interchange of blood between mother and fetus; only nutritive, respiratory and elimination materials are exchanged.

The intervillous spaces continue to develop until two chorionic stem villi, with their secondary and tertiary villi, are engulfed in each space. The spaces are filled with maternal blood from the arterial capillaries. At about two weeks the system is functional but not complete. Each of these spaces and their contents will continue to develop into individual cotyledons.

Inspection of the placenta at the third week following fertilization shows the trophoblast to be covered with chorionic villi, some of which are embedded into the decidua basalis of the endometrium. The developed fetal chorionic villi system gives the appearance of branching roots distributed in the rich nutritive soil (blood) of the maternal intervillous spaces.

A thin membrane, the *chorionic plate* (see Fig. 8–3), which is continuous with the fetal membranes, serves as the limiting boundary on the fetal side of the placenta. The limiting boundary on the maternal side is the *basal plate.* Septa (see Fig. 8–1) protrude from the basal plate and serve as the divisions between the cotyledons. The septa do not extend to the chorionic plate.

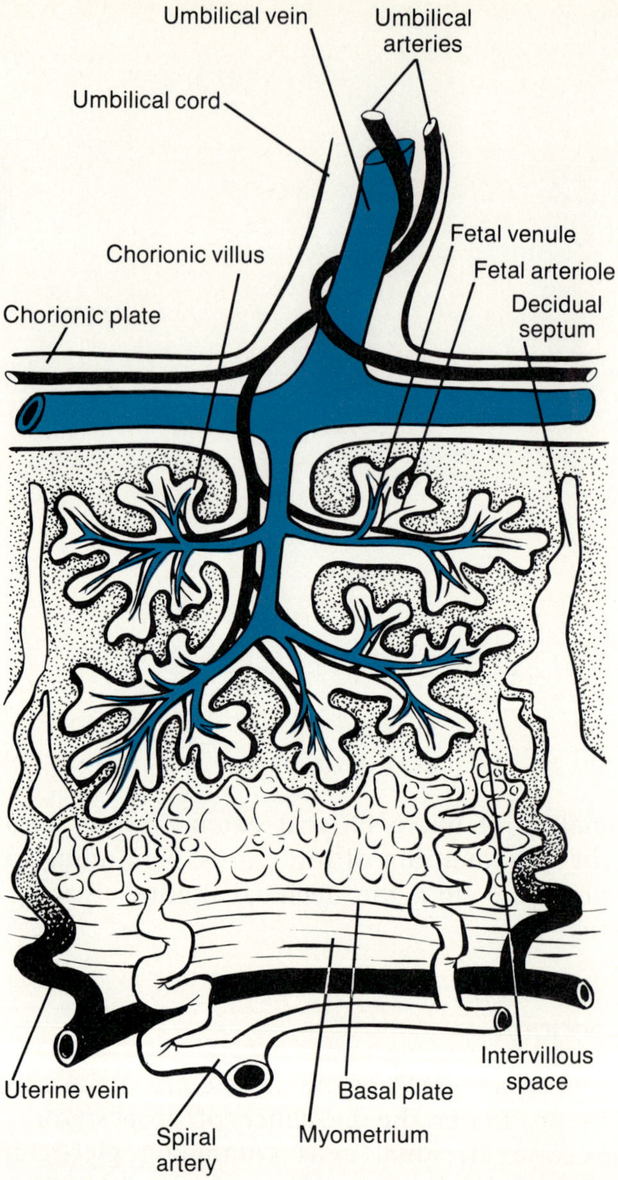

FIGURE 8–3. Chorionic structure-placement of chorionic plate at fetal surface of placenta and basal plate as limiting border of maternal surface.

COTYLEDONS

The invasion of the trophoblast into the intervillous spaces serves as the rudimentary formation of the cotyledons. Actual cotyledon formation occurs around 40 to 50 days following ovulation, at which time the 40 to 60 maternal spiral arterioles are open and placental exchange is occurring. The fetal terminal villi located in the cotyledons develop a membrane called the *syncytium,* which separates the maternal blood in the intervillous space from the fetal interstitial fluid located in the villi. The membrane is permeable, allowing the interchange of nutrients, waste, and oxygen. By this time, the original cytotrophoblastic cells have changed in nature and can no longer by distinguished as such.

Structurally, the placenta is formed at the completion of the first trimester. However, hypertrophic growth continues throughout pregnancy. There is no additional formation of stem villi during this time but continued addition of peripheral villi occurs (Martin & Gingerich, 1976). Speculation in research suggests the placenta may become a senile organ in the last month of pregnancy; however, protein synthesis by the placenta does continue until term. Adverse uterine conditions such as maternal malnutrition and vascular insufficiency may result in a decreased placental size or in abnormal placental pathology.

THE UMBILICAL CORD

Early in the development of the embryo (about 3 to 4 weeks) the rudimentary formation of the umbilical cord appears. The body stalk extends from the yolk sac of the embryo and connects with the chorionic villi of the developing placenta. Meanwhile, the heart tube and primitive blood vessels have been forming within the embryo. They begin to extend into the yolk sac and body stalk, creating a primitive circulatory link between the embryo and the chorionic villi (see Fig. 8–4).

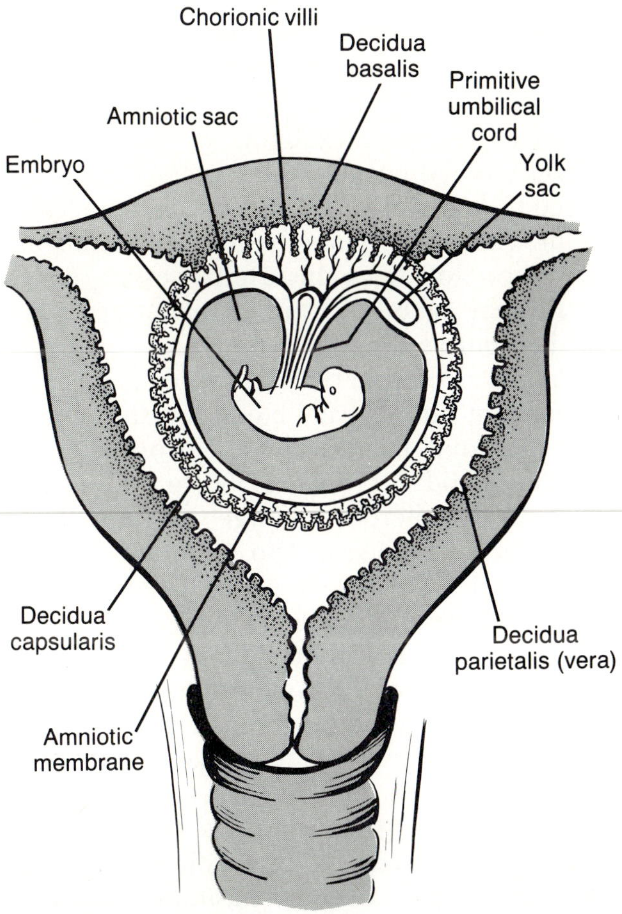

FIGURE 8–4. Primitive fetal umbilical cord and amniotic sac.

As the body stalk continues to grow, it becomes the umbilical cord, containing the two umbilical arteries, one vein, and Wharton's jelly.

At term, the cord is usually the length of the baby, ranging from 48.3 cm (19 inches) to 55.9 cm (22 inches). Observations of the cord should be made at the time of delivery. Meconium staining of the cord is an indication of previous fetal distress in utero. Fetal anomalies are often associated with absence of one of the vessels. Loops and knots in the cord are associated with a 7 percent perinatal mortality.

FETAL MEMBRANES

The placenta is covered on the fetal side by the fetal membranes. As early as the first ten days of development, the amniotic sac appears and surrounds the embryo (Fig. 8–4). It encases the embryo and continues to form the uppermost covering of the umbilical cord. The membranous sac is composed of two separate membranes called the *amnion*, which is the innermost layer, and the *chorion*, which is the outer layer. A cavity forms within the sac to accommodate the fetus and the amniotic fluid.

The origin of amniotic fluid is not certain. Transudation of the maternal serum across the placental membrane appears to be the most significant contributor to the production of amniotic fluid early in pregnancy. Thereafter, the fetus participates in amniotic fluid production. The fetus swallows the amniotic fluid in utero, it is then absorbed into its gastrointestinal tract, and excreted as hypotonic urine into the amniotic sac. The fetal kidneys thus become a participant in the regulation of the volume of amniotic fluid. Normally, the volume of amniotic fluid is 30 ml at 10 weeks, 350 ml at 20 weeks and 1000 ml at term (Page et al., 1976). Volumes of less than 400 ml (*oligohydramnios*) or more than 2000 ml (*polyhydramnios* or *hydramnios*) are abnormal.

Functions of the amniotic sac and fluid include: maintenance of thermoregulatory function of the fetal environment; prevention of injury to the fetus from external pressures; prevention of exposure of the fetus to organisms introduced vaginally; easing flexibility and movement of the fetus; promotion of fetal metabolism; and assisting in dilatation of the cervix during labor.

The constant production and exchange of the amniotic fluid within the sac allows the replacement of about 300 to 500 ml per hour, with a total exchange occurring every three hours. If abnormalities arise in the fetus and fetal amniotic exchange is impaired, accumulations or deficits of amniotic fluid may occur. Gastrointestinal obstructions such as esophageal atresia and gross malformations of the brain are frequently associated with polyhydramnios. In situations where urinary flow from the fetus is obstructed or impaired, oligohydramnios results.

The amniotic fluid consists of carbohydrates, lipids, hormones, amino acids, urea, uric acid, creatinine, enzymes, bilirubin, phospholipids, steroids, and water in varying amounts. The origin of these substances is derived from fetal structures such as the fetal kidney, ectoderm, and respiratory system, as well as the maternal contributors.

Analysis of the amniotic fluid is used to determine placental, fetal, and genetic abnormalities, fetal lung maturity, and sex. *Amniocentesis* is the procedure in which amniotic fluid is removed for analysis.

Premature rupture of the membranes may result in a slow leakage or complete loss of the fluid. In instances where just a small amount of fluid is lost through a small tear in the sac, the consequences are little or none. Usually, the amniotic sac repairs itself and the pregnancy progresses to term. However, when there is a complete rupture of the sac, labor generally ensues. The mother should be delivered within 24 hours following rupture of the amniotic sac, since prolonged rupture of the membranes increases the risk of infection and fetal demise.

MATERNAL PLACENTAL CIRCULATION

Perfusion of each lobule within the cotyledons of the placenta is facilitated by the circulating maternal blood in the intervillous spaces. The blood is propelled in spurts into the intervillous spaces from the uteroplacental arteries. Maternal blood pressure regulates the ejection and propulsion of the blood as it is forced toward the fetal surface. Some blood is channeled laterally, crossing the septa that separates the intervillous spaces. Near term, fibrin deposits between the cotyledons may interfere with this lateral circulation, creating totally separate vascular units. In instances where the arterial blood supply to these independent cotyledons is obstructed, the circulation within the cotyledon is altered or stopped. The affected unit is destroyed and replaced by an *infarct* (area of tissue necrosis). If many cotyledons become infarcted, the fetus can suffer adverse effects from placental insufficiency.

Placental venous exchange occurs when the blood circulating in the intervillous spaces is forced downward into the uteroplacental veins. This results from the force of the incoming blood flow from the arterial vessels, which causes the blood already in the spaces to be pushed outward and downward.

Filling of the intervillous spaces is not only dependent on maternal blood pressure but on other related factors as well. Normally, the uterine blood flow rate is 500 to 600 ml/min with a complete exchange of intervillous blood occurring every 3 to 4 minutes (Martin & Gingerich, 1976). In cases where the integrity of the maternal blood vessels is jeopardized, placental perfusion in the intervillous spaces may be compromised. Maternal positioning also alters blood flow to the placenta. As the uterus increases in size, pressure is exerted on the vena cava of the mother, resulting in decreased blood flow to the placenta. This is intensified when the mother assumes a supine position and is corrected by turning the mother to a left lateral position. Epidural anesthesia may also create a hypotensive reaction in the mother, resulting in less blood flow to the placenta. Blood flow to the placenta is altered during normal *Braxton Hicks contractions* (painless uterine contractions encountered throughout pregnancy) when the flow of blood is somewhat restricted through the uteroplacental arteries and veins. During Braxton Hicks contractions, the constrictive effect of the contraction is more profound on the uteroplacental veins than on the arteries. The contractions compress the veins, prohibiting drainage of the blood from the intervillous spaces. During labor, if contractions are severe or prolonged, a profound placental insufficiency may occur, resulting in fetal hypoxia.

Severe stress has been known to alter the blood flow to the placenta. Stress stimulates the sympathetic nervous system and results in constriction of the uteroplacental arteries. This same effect may be seen when vasopressor drugs are given to increase blood pressure (Martin & Gingerich, 1976).

FETAL PLACENTAL CIRCULATION

Blood flows from the fetus via the two umbilical arteries, which branch into the main chorionic villous stem and continue to the terminal chorionic villi in the intervillous spaces. Deoxygenated blood and fetal waste products pass through the fetal capillaries, connective tissue, and syncytium of the villi into the intervillous spaces. These waste products are then picked up by the mother's uterine veins and eliminated via her circulatory system.

Oxygen and nutrients, in turn, are passed from the maternal blood in the intervillous spaces through the syncytium, connective tissue, and fetal capillaries of the terminal villi to the main stem villi and into the umbilical vein. From there they are carried into the fetal circulatory system.

As the placenta matures, at about the fifth month, the cytotrophoblastic layer of the villi becomes increasingly smaller, eliminating the protective effect it provided against certain organisms such as the spirochete of syphilis. The syncytiotrophoblastic layer persists throughout pregnancy.

PLACENTAL TRANSFER OF SUBSTANCES

Assurance of an effective system for transfer of nutrients, oxygen, and waste material from the mother to the fetus is vital for the growth and development of the fetus. Placental exchange is so crucial that a number of mechanisms are needed to insure an adequate, continuous exchange. Basically, the mechanisms are operational at all times, depending on the material to be transferred.

The mechanisms of transfer are:

DIFFUSION

Simple diffusion of oxygen, carbon dioxide, water, electrolytes, certain drugs, and anesthesia occurs as these substances move from an area of higher concentration to an area of lower concentration across the semipermeable placental membrane.

FACILITATED DIFFUSION

Diffusion requiring a carrier system supplied by enzymes also occurs from an area of higher concentration to an area of lower concentration but is more rapid in its transportation. Substances such as glucose, which is in constant demand by the growing fetus, cross by facilitated diffusion.

ACTIVE TRANSPORT

Transportation of materials across the placental membrane from an area of lower concentration to an area of higher concentration occurs by active transport. Both a carrier system and metabolic energy is required in this process. Amino acids, certain water-soluble vitamins, iron, iodine, and calcium utilize active transport to cross the placental membrane.

PINOCYTOSIS

The syncytiotrophoblastic cells facilitate transfer of substances by engulfing them as they are transported across the placental membrane. This process is considerably slower than the others but accommodates larger substances such as immunoglobulins, lipoproteins, and phospholipids.

ADJUNCT MEASURES

Accidental breaks in the villi and fetal capillaries may allow some direct transfer of substances such as fetal blood cells, resulting in a slight mixing of the fetal and maternal circulations.

Factors Influencing Placental Transfer

Permeability, thickness, and size of the placenta directly affect placental exchange, as will the concentration gradient, solubility, and molecular size of materials to be transported. Occasionally, the area available for placental exchange will be lessened because the placenta is small. This may be due to the more severe diabetic conditions and hypertension. Placental infarcts also decrease the area available for exchange and are found in the placentas of diabetic mothers, mothers with pregnancy-induced hypertension, and postmature pregnancies. Premature separation of the placenta or a portion of the placenta will alter placental exchange by reducing the area available for exchange or by completely eliminating the exchange system.

The concentration gradient of a substance is altered by the amount of the substance in the maternal and fetal circulations. This normally involves a simple equalization of substances on either side of the membrane. When the difference on one side of the membrane becomes larger or smaller, diffusion takes place. However, in the case of oxygen, other factors participate with the concentration gradient to insure a constant supply of oxygen to the fetus. One such factor is the concentration of hemoglobin in the fetal blood as compared with that in the maternal blood. Fetal blood has a greater concentration of hemoglobin (15 gm per 100 ml) than maternal blood (12 gm per 100 ml). Since hemoglobin is the oxygen-carrying component of the blood, this means that the fetal circulation can carry more oxygen than the maternal circulation.

Along with the greater concentration of hemoglobin, there is a greater binding capacity for oxygen in the fetal blood. Fetal blood will more readily accept oxygen than maternal blood. This favors the transport of oxygen from maternal blood in the intervillous spaces to the fetal capillaries in the terminal villi.

Maternal and fetal blood gas levels are also affected by the pH (acidity) of the blood. The higher the pH, the more oxygen that can be carried; conversely, the lower the pH (increased acidity) the less the affinity of hemoglobin for oxygen. Fetal blood returning through the umbilical arteries to the arteries in the terminal villi has a low pH, is acidotic, and contains a larger concentration of carbon dioxide. When this blood reaches the terminal villi, the carbon dioxide diffuses across the placental membrane into the maternal circulation in the intervillous spaces. The carbon dioxide displaces the oxygen in the maternal blood of the intervillous spaces. This encourages the diffusion of the oxygen in the intervillous spaces across the placental membrane to the hemoglobin in the capillaries of the fetal villi. The blood in these tertiary veins and into the umbilical vein is now oxygenated (see Fig. 8–5).

Molecular size of the substance to be transported influences the rate of transfer. Substances with molecular weights of 700 or

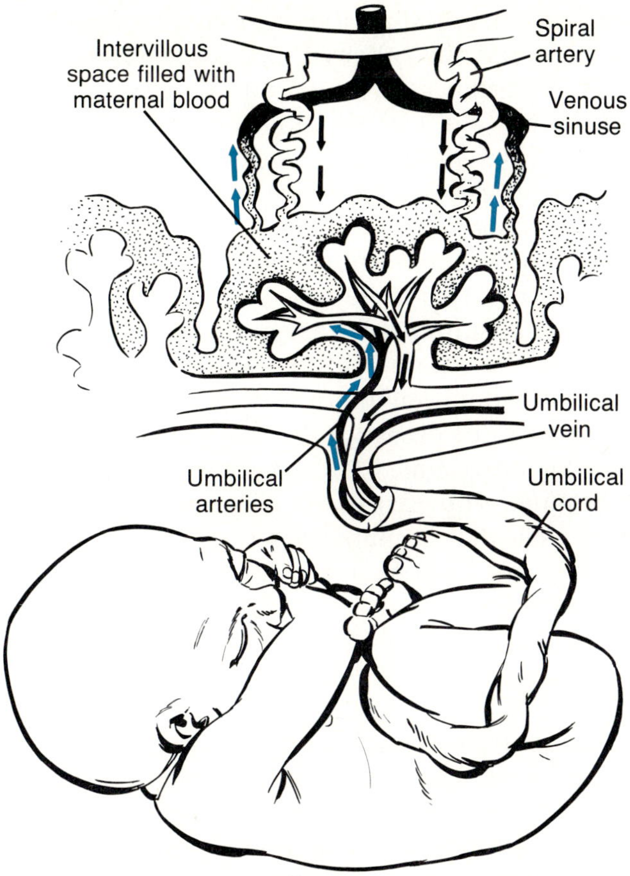

FIGURE 8-5. Direction of blood flow in umbilical vessles.

less cross the placenta by means of simple diffusion. Substances with molecular weights of 1000 or more are not candidates for exchange unless broken into smaller, more easily transported particles by enzymes.

Solubility of the substance to be transferred determines the rate of transfer. Substances that dissolve readily in lipids cross the placenta more easily owing to the high concentration of lipids in the placental membrane.

Placental Hormones

During pregnancy, the placenta becomes actively engaged in endocrine functions. Hormones secreted by the placenta play a cardinal role in the maintenance of pregnancy. These placental hormones are the protein hormones, *human chorionic gonadotropin* (HCG) and *human chorionic somatomammotropin* (HCS); and the steroid hormones, *estrogen* and *progesterone*.

HUMAN CHORIONIC GONADOTROPIN (HCG)

Syncytiotrophoblastic cells of the developing embryo participate in the secretion of HCG as early as one day following implantation and eight days after fertilization. At this time, HCG acts on the corpus luteum of the ovary, stimulating it to continue to produce progesterone, which is necessary for the maintenance of the endometrium and, therefore, the prevention of menstruation. Without the influence of HCG, the corpus luteum would degenerate, eliminating the supply of progesterone, and the pregnancy would be terminated. However, because HCG is supplied by the trophoblast, the corpus luteum continues to produce progesterone, and the uterine endometrium develops nutritive decidual characteristics.

Rapidly rising levels of HCG occur until about the 60th day of pregnancy. During this time, sexual development of the male fetus is also influenced by HCG. The HCG exerts an interstitial cell stimulating effect on the fetal testes, causing the production of a small amount of testosterone, which encourages development of the male sex organs (Guyton, 1981). It is also speculated that HCG suppresses certain cellular immunologic properties. This may protect the embryo from immunologic rejection by the maternal host.

If, during the early weeks of pregnancy, a pregnancy test is done, it is the presence of HCG in the maternal urine that indicates a positive result. The HCG can be detected in the urine as early as 26 to 49 days after the first day of the last menstrual period (Fishbach, 1984). The pregnancy test based on the presence of HCG is usually accurate but false results can occur. It must be kept in mind that a false-positive result may be related to blood and/or protein in the urine or drugs such as anticonvulsants, tranquilizers, hypnotics, and antiparkinson agents. Older women who are possibly menopausal may have false-positive results owing to the increased levels of pituitary gonadotropins. The first voided specimen in the morning contains the greatest concentrations of HCG and is usually used to perform the test. The more diluted voidings later in the day can give false-negative results. False-negative results are more common than false-positive results.

Progression of the pregnancy beyond 60 days results in decreasing levels of HCG, since at that time it is no longer needed for corpus luteum stimulation.

Human chorionic gonadotropin is also found in the urine of women who have *hydatidiform moles* (uterine cystic masses resulting from a pathologic ovum), *choriocarcinoma* (carcinomas of the chorion), and other neoplasms.

HUMAN CHORIONIC SOMATOMAMMOTROPIN (HCS)

This protein hormone produced by the trophoblastic cells is also called human placental lactogen (HPL) or human chorionic growth hormone prolactin (CGP). It is present in small amounts during the first four weeks of pregnancy with production increasing steadily at about five weeks and continuing to rise until term. There appears to be a correlation between increasing placental size and increasing levels of HCS. This is strikingly apparent in women with twin pregnancies, where placental mass is greater and HCS levels are elevated.

The physiologic roles of HCS are varied during pregnancy, when the developing fetus is in need of a constant supply of glucose. Under the influence of HCS, maternal free fatty acids are readily metabolized, providing a quick source of energy for the mother and conserving the utilization of carbohydrates. Carbohydrate metabolism is affected by the hormones' ability to decrease the peripheral effectiveness of insulin with a resultant rise in the mother's blood sugar level. At the same time, there is an increase in the level of insulin in response to the anti-insulin effect. Therefore, HCS appears to have two opposing effects, one of decreasing the peripheral effect of insulin and the other of increasing the secretion of insulin. Despite its contradictory effects, HCS does aid in the establishment of homeostasis of maternal carbohydrate metabolism while providing a constant supply of glucose to the fetus.

Protein metabolism is minimally affected by HCS. The mobilized free fatty acids readily supply a source of energy for the mother, sparing the amino acids for use by the fetus.

Included among the functions of HCS is the promotion of breast growth and development during pregnancy. The direct action of this hormone on breast tissue is controversial, but it is felt that it participates with hydrocortisone and insulin in the development of the breast alveoli.

PROGESTERONE

Continuation of the pregnancy is dependent on an adequate production of progesterone. Under the influence of HCG, the corpus luteum of the ovary continues to produce progesterone until the placenta is capable of producing sufficient quantities to sustain the pregnancy. Once this function is transferred from the corpus luteum to the placenta, increasingly larger amounts of progesterone are produced. At term, the placenta may be producing amounts as high as 1 gm per day (Guyton, 1981). Because maintenance of the pregnancy is so dependent on progesterone, any alteration or decrease in its production puts the pregnancy at risk. Such may be the case when, between six and nine weeks gestation, the corpus luteum diminishes production of progesterone. This progestoneal lag period may result in an abortion (miscarriage). It would seem that the administration of progesterone at such times might serve as a method of treatment for women with threatened abortions. However, this is not advisable as additional progesterone administration during pregnancy has not proved helpful and may cause alterations in fetal development.

Early in pregnancy, progesterone exerts its

influence by increasing the secretions of the fallopian tube, providing nutritive materials for the blastocyst. Meanwhile, the stromal cells of the endometrium become decidual under the influence of progesterone and provide nutritive materials for the implanted trophoblast. At the same time, progesterone produces a quieting effect on the myometrium of the uterus. This quieting effect also produces other maternal physiologic changes. Smooth muscles of the body are affected by progesterone, resulting in constipation, flatulence, and heartburn, as well as dilatation of the ureters. Alterations in the central nervous system produce the typically impassive, tired feelings accompanying pregnancy. The basal body temperature in the pregnant woman is also increased as much as 0.4°F to 1.0°F due to progesterone.

Pregnancy is said to be a salt-losing state because progesterone causes an increase in the excretion of sodium and chloride. This is attributed to the progesterone-antagonizing effect on the hormone aldosterone. Aldosterone is responsible for the reabsorption of sodium by the kidney tubules.

Development of breast tissue also depends on progesterone. The areolar tissue of the breast uses progesterone for development.

Respiratory function is influenced by the presence of progesterone during pregnancy. It is speculated that the respiratory threshold for carbon dioxide is lowered due to progesterone.

ESTROGEN

Although estrogen is produced by the ovaries during the menstrual cycle, this does not continue during pregnancy. Following the first few weeks of pregnancy the placenta becomes the major source of estrogen. This, however, depends on a harmonious relationship between the fetoplacental and maternal units. For estrogen to be produced by the placenta a fetal steroid precursor must be produced by the fetal adrenal cortex and the fetal liver, as well as the maternal adrenal glands (see Fig. 8–6). The fetal adrenal glands actively produce the precursors in increasing amounts throughout pregnancy. Some of the precursors from the fetal adrenal glands go directly to the placenta, where, in combination with the maternal adrenal precursor, they produce *estrone*

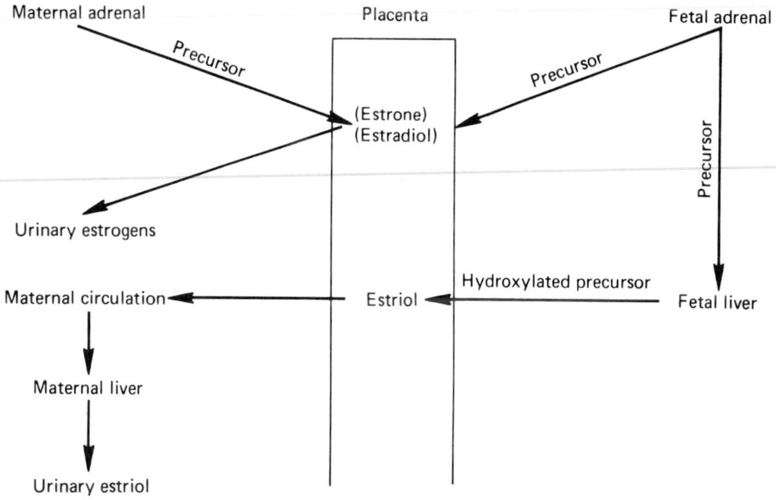

FIGURE 8–6. Simplified scheme of biosynthesis of placental estrogens in pregnancy. Reprinted with permission from Ziegel, E. and Cranley, M. Obstetric Nursing, New York: Macmillan, 1984.

and *estradiol.* Other fetal adrenal precursors are directed to the fetal liver, where they are hydroxylated. They then progress to the placenta and are transported to the mother's circulatory system as *estriol*. Estriol must be transported to the mother's liver and conjugated. Thus, it is important for both the maternal hepatic system and the fetal adrenal and hepatic systems to be functioning properly for an adequate supply of estrogen during pregnancy. Serial measurements of maternal urine estriol are used as an indicator of fetal well-being. Estriol levels will rise slightly for the first 12 weeks of pregnancy and then progress sharply upward until term. If there is a drop in estriol levels, it could indicate that the fetus is in jeopardy. Fetal distress should be based on a series of estriol level determinations, as normal fluctuations occur throughout the day. If the trend does not indicate a progressive increase, further studies of fetal well-being are indicated.

To pinpoint all of the functions of estrogen during pregnancy is difficult. Many of these functions depend on an interaction with other hormones such as progesterone. Yet, there are some actions directly related to estrogen.

The estrogens affect the growth of the uterus during pregnancy and myometrial activity, which is increased under the influence of estrogen. It is, however, kept in check by the quiescent effect of progesterone. The blood supply to the uterine vessels is also increased owing to the influence of estrogen.

Estrogen increases the sensitivity of the breast tissue to prolactin. Secreted by the anterior pituitary gland, prolactin is the hormone responsible for milk production.

Estrogens are responsible for increased vaginal secretions (normal leukorrhea) owing to hyperplasia of the epithelial cells. Increased activity of the salivary glands (*ptyalism*) may also occur, along with *gingivitis* (bleeding of the gums) and the depositing of melanin in the tissues, causing *chloasma* (mask of pregnancy). The common vascular spider nevi markings (*telangiectasias*) found on the face, neck, and arms are caused by increased estrogen production. Palmar erythema may occur in combination with the telangiectasia.

Estrogen effects on the respiratory system include increased vascularization with a tendency to nasal congestion and increased sensitivity to carbon dioxide.

ADDITIONAL PLACENTAL HORMONES

Currently, other hormones are thought to be of placental origin but their exact functions are only conjectural. One of them, *human chorionic thyrotropin*, is thought to stimulate maternal thyroid activity and may contribute to the rising levels of cortisol during pregnancy.

PLACENTAL ABNORMALITIES AND DYSFUNCTIONS

Any of the respiratory, endocrine, excretory, nutritive or regulatory functions of the placenta can be altered by abnormalities or dysfunctions of the placenta. The fetus depends on the placenta for its welfare, and impaired function may cause fetal damage or death.

Placenta circumvallata is an abnormal configuration of the placenta in which the area of the chorionic plate is reduced. The chorionic villi in the area of the deficient chorionic plate are then able to invade the decidua. The fetal membranes become deranged, forming a doubled layer of amnion and chorion with the decidua in between. When the area of disarrangement is limited, there are little or no complications. If larger areas are involved, then an abnormal adherence of the placenta to the uterine wall can occur (*placenta accreta*). This can be significant at the time of delivery, causing the placenta to adhere to the uterine wall following delivery.

Placenta succenturiata refers to the formation of an accessory lobe or lobes connected to the main placenta by the fetal arteries and veins. Although the occurrence is rare, 0.1 to 0.3

percent of mothers with this condition may develop postpartum hemorrhage if the accessory lobe is not expelled at delivery.

Five to seven percent of pregnancies will demonstrate a *Battledore placenta*, in which the umbilical cord is abnormally inserted at the margin of the placenta. Few complications arise from this abnormality, although it is postulated that fetal circulation may be compromised.

Placental infarcts produce localized areas of necrosis and subsequent alterations in placental function. Infarcts occur twice as frequently in whites as in blacks (Aladjem & Brown, 1974). On visual inspection, the infarcts may be red, white, yellow, or gray. In the early stages of infarction they appear as a deep reddish color, advancing to yellow and grayish white as time increases. They also become firm with advancing time. Infarcts are more common in mothers with toxemia, diabetes, and renal disease owing to thrombosis of the maternal decidual arteries. Localized areas of infarction seem to have little effect on the fetus. Extensively infarcted areas result in fetal distress. This is more pronounced during active labor when there is stress from the uterine contractions on the fetoplacental unit.

Degenerative changes within the placenta are the result of fibrin deposits associated with normal placental aging. These deposits extend from the decidual plate toward the fetal villi, eventually encasing the fetal vessels and causing necrosis due to ischemia of the vessels.

Placental grading has been used to determine placental changes with advancing maturation. Grades 0, I, II, and III represent the advancing ages. One would expect to find a grade 0 configuration early in pregnancy and a grade III with the mature placenta. Grannum (1982) reported the mean gestational age at which placentas are grade I, corresponding to a placenta of 31 weeks, grade II corresponds to a placenta of 36 weeks, and grade III corresponds to a placenta of 38 weeks. A grade I placenta at term suggests a delayed maturational process of the placenta, frequently seen in mothers with Rh isoimmunization and those who have Class A diabetes. Conditions of premature maturation of the placenta relate to intrauterine growth retardation, juvenile diabetes, and hypertensive disease of the mother.

The normal placenta is attached in the upper segment of the uterus. When the placenta is located in the lower uterine segment it is said to be a *placenta previa*. Categories of placenta previa are: *low lying*—placenta extending to the margin of the cervical os but not extending over the os; *partial*—placenta in the lower uterine segment with a portion extending partially over the internal cervical os; *total*—placenta located in the lower uterine segment extending completely over the cervical os.

Premature separation of the normally implanted placenta characterizes *abruptio placentae*. The etiology has not been determined, although it is associated with degenerative changes occurring with the gestational hypertensive disorders such as pregnancy induced hypertension (see Chapter 26).

BIBLIOGRAPHY

Aladjem, S. & Brown, A. *Clinical perinatology*. St. Louis: Mosby, 1974.

Fischback, F. *A manual of laboratory diagnostics tests*. Philadelphia: Lippincott, 1984.

Grannum, P. Ultrasonographic evaluation of the placenta. *Perinatology-Neonatology*, 1982, **6**, 35-45.

Guyton, A. *Textbook of medical physiology* (6th ed.). Philadelphia: Saunders, 1981.

Martin, C. & Gingerich, B. Uteroplacental physiology. *Journal of Obstetrics, Gynecological & Neonatal Nursing*, 1976, **5**, 16s–25s.

Page, E., Villee, C. & Villee, D. *Human reproduction* (2nd ed.) Philadelphia: Saunders, 1976.

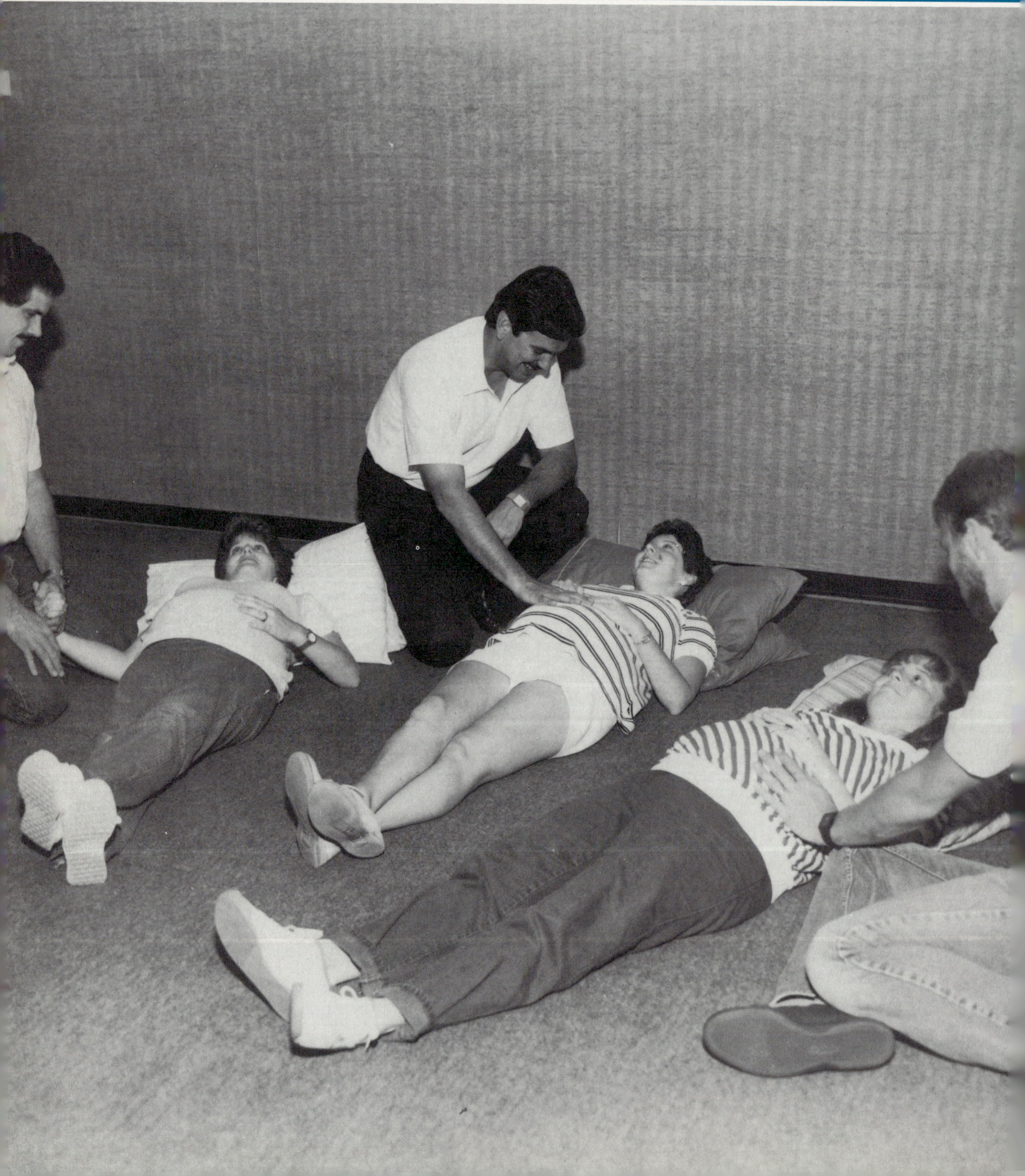

UNIT III

THE ANTEPARTAL FAMILY

UNIT III

THE ANTEPARTAL FAMILY

chapter 9

MATERNAL ADAPTATIONS TO PREGNANCY

OBJECTIVES

Upon completion of this chapter, the reader will be able to:

1. Describe the physiologic changes that occur in the reproductive system during pregnancy.
2. Describe the hormonal influences during pregnancy, and state their systemic effect and significance.
3. Discuss the hematologic and cardiovascular changes in pregnancy, and their significance and implications for nursing assessments.
4. Describe the distribution of weight gain during pregnancy.
5. Discuss the physiologic changes occurring in the renal system during pregnancy and their importance to maternal homeostasis.
6. Identify the respiratory alterations occurring during pregnancy and discuss their consequences.
7. Discuss the implications for nursing interventions related to the changes that occur in the gastrointestinal and integumentary system during pregnancy.
8. Discuss the factors influencing maternal blood glucose levels during pregnancy and state their effect.
9. Describe the psychological changes that occur during the first, second, and third trimesters of pregnancy.
10. State examples of nursing interventions that might be used when assisting the mother to adapt to the psychological changes.
11. Explain the role of the father during pregnancy and discuss factors influencing his adaptation to that role.

KEY TERMS

Chadwick's sign
Chloasma
Colostrum
Couvade
Diastasis recti
Goodell's sign
Hegar's sign
Leukorrhea
Oxytocin
Prolactin
Striae gravidarum
Supine hypotension
Tubercles of Montgomery

As a musician's instrument is finely tuned to achieve the ultimate in artistic performance, so is the body of the pregnant woman devoted and committed to the creation of a human life. The effect of pregnancy on the woman is unparalled during her life span. Adaptations and alterations of all bodily systems occur during pregnancy which are directed toward providing the ideal environment for the growing fetus. Achievement of this ideal goal may or may not be possible. However, every effort is made by the health team to assist the childbearing family to this end.

A thorough understanding of the physiologic and psychological changes that occur during pregnancy provides the cornerstone for effective maternal nursing care. Problem identification, nursing assessments, nursing diagnoses, interventions, and evaluations all depend on the nurses' understanding of the physiologic events occurring during the maternal cycle.

REPRODUCTIVE ADAPTATIONS

The most profound changes occurring in the pregnant woman are those in the reproductive system. These changes, in part, also provide the mother with the first indications of pregnancy.

Uterus

The uterine response to pregnancy begins shortly after conception. Under the influence of the hormones estrogen, chorionic somatomammotropin, and progesterone, uterine growth is stimulated in the tissues of the fundal, corpal, and cervical areas.

The most significant growth occurs in the uterine muscle. Hypertrophy of the existing muscle fibers and the formation of some new muscle fibers allows expansion of the uterus from a pear-shaped organ 6 to 8 cm long and 3 to 5 cm wide to one that measures 28 cm in length and 22 cm in width (see Fig. 9–1). Each of the three muscle layers of the uterus (see Chapter 4), responding to the effects of pregnancy, provides support during the pregnancy and hemostasis following delivery.

There is an increase in the connective tissue of the uterine walls that allows an initial thickening of the walls. However, following the approximation of the decidua capsularis with the decidua vera at about 12 weeks gestation, the walls progressively thin as the pregnancy continues. The amniotic sac now fills the cavity of the uterus and the uterine fundus begins to rise to the level of the symphysis pubis. The supporting round and broad ligaments stretch and provide additional uterine support. Displacement of the intestines occurs as the growing uterus approaches the abdominal wall.

At the fifth or sixth month there is a gradual rotation of the uterus to the right, owing to the influence of the spinal column, sigmoid colon, and rectum. Occasionally symptoms accompany these accommodations and the mother may experience "broad ligament pain," described as slight "shooting pains" in the abdomen. These are related to the stretching of the ligaments. As the uterus increases in size and weight, the supine resting position may allow the greatly enlarged uterus to rest on the aorta and inferior vena cava, altering circulation in these vessels. This can interfere with fetal circulation, and for this reason the supine position is not recommended during the later months of pregnancy. The left lateral resting position is the recommended position.

Softening of the isthmus of the uterus (*Hegar's sign*) begins in the first trimester, when the uterus becomes compressible and elongates. Elongation continues until the isthmus is about 25 mm in length (12 weeks gestation). It then shortens and interfuses with the corpus of the uterus.

The uterine cervix, influenced by an increase in the blood supply and increased hormonal levels, becomes softer (*Goodell's sign*),

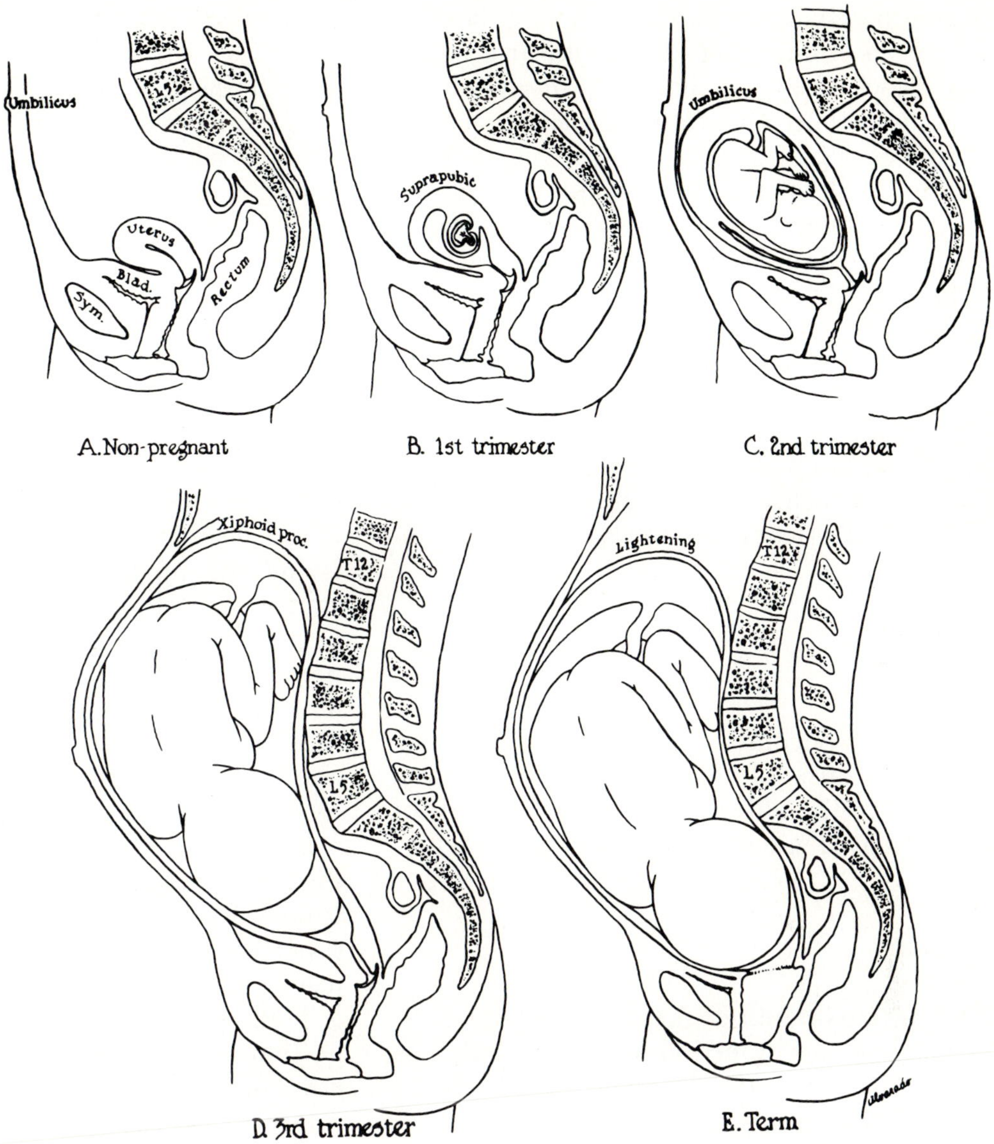

FIGURE 9-1. Relations of the body of the uterus at different gestational periods. From Iffy, L. and Charles, D. Operative Perinatology, New York: Macmillan, 1984.

edematous, and more elastic in character. The endocervical mucosa thickens, favoring an increased production of cervical mucous. Eventually the cervical canal is filled with the thick, viscid mucous and the cervical *mucous plug* is formed. This plug remains in the cervix, serving as a barrier to the external environment, protecting the fetus from ascending vaginal infections. It is expelled during labor.

Increased uterine blood supply is experienced by both the arterial and venous systems, brought about by an increase in the size and numbers of these vessels. The increased capacity is 40 to 60 times greater than in the nonpregnant state, amounting to a total uterine blood flow of 400 to 700 ml at term. Assurance of an adequate uteroplacental circulation is thus maintained.

Vagina

Hypertrophic and hyperplastic growth increases the length and capacity of the vagina during pregnancy. The elastic tissue fibers increase in number as the connective tissue undergoes changes, making it more pliable and distensible. Greatly increased vascularity produces engorged and enlarged veins, resulting in a bluish-purple discoloration of the mucous lining (*Chadwick's sign*). The vaginal epithelium also undergoes hypertrophic and hyperplastic growth, producing deep vaginal rugae.

The epithelial cells of the vagina produce an increased amount of thick, viscid mucus (*normal leukorrhea*) that is rich in glycogen. Vaginal bacilli act upon the glycogen, converting it to lactic acid, which creates an acid pH of the vagina and discourages the growth of pathogenic bacteria.

Vulva

The vulva becomes engorged during pregnancy because of the increased vascularity. Varicies of the vulva may form as a result of the increased vascular congestion and edema.

Ovaries

The corpus luteum of the ovary continues to produce progesterone following conception as a result of human chorionic gonadotropin (HCG) stimulation produced by the syncytiotrophoblastic cells of the developing placenta (see Chapter 8). Within 12 days following conception, there are sufficient amounts of HCG to halt the degenerative effects on the corpus luteum. The corpus luteum continues to grow until it has doubled in size by the eighth week. Once the placenta produces sufficient amounts of progesterone (10 to 12 weeks), HCG levels drop and the corpus luteum degenerates.

Since ovulation does not occur during pregnancy, the remaining follicles of the ovary begin to atrophy. The theca lutein cells surrounding these follicles become more extensive. These follicles are then collectively known as the interstitial glands of pregnancy.

Fallopian Tubes

Lateral displacement of the fallopian tubes occurs as the uterus grows. The upward pull on the fallopian tubes places them in the abdominal cavity perpendicular to the uterus.

Breast

The breast tissue and glands are influenced by increased hormonal production during pregnancy. Externally, the areolae of the breast broaden and darken due to the increased pigmentation (see Fig. 9–2). Sebaceous glands, called *tubercles of Montgomery*, appear and surround the nipple area. They secrete a substance that lubricates the nipples. The nipples become more erectile and early in the pregnancy there may be an appearance of the first milklike secretion called *colostrum* from the nipples (see Chapter 10). Striae (stretch marks) appear on the breast caused by the rapid growth of the breast tissue.

Increased activity of the glandular tissue of the breast necessitates a more abundant blood supply. The increased vascularity produces a superficial vein growth that is quite noticeable just below the skin. Tingling, stretching, and a feeling of heaviness are sensations experienced by pregnant women as breast growth and increased vascularity continue.

Internally, the fat and connective tissue separating each lobule of the breast increase as the alveoli differentiate into secretory cells. The alveoli are the grapelike clusters of cells which are ultimately responsible for the production of breast milk. The lobes of the breast increase in size due to the proliferation of the lobules and alveoli within each lobe (see Fig. 9–2). The milk reservoirs, known as the *ampullas* or *lactiferous sinuses*, located just adjacent to the nipple opening and continuous with the ducts of each lobe, begin to fill with colostrum at the end of the second month of pregnancy. Although some colostrum may be secreted during pregnancy, normal lactation and stimulation of the "let-down reflex" does not occur because of increased levels of pro-

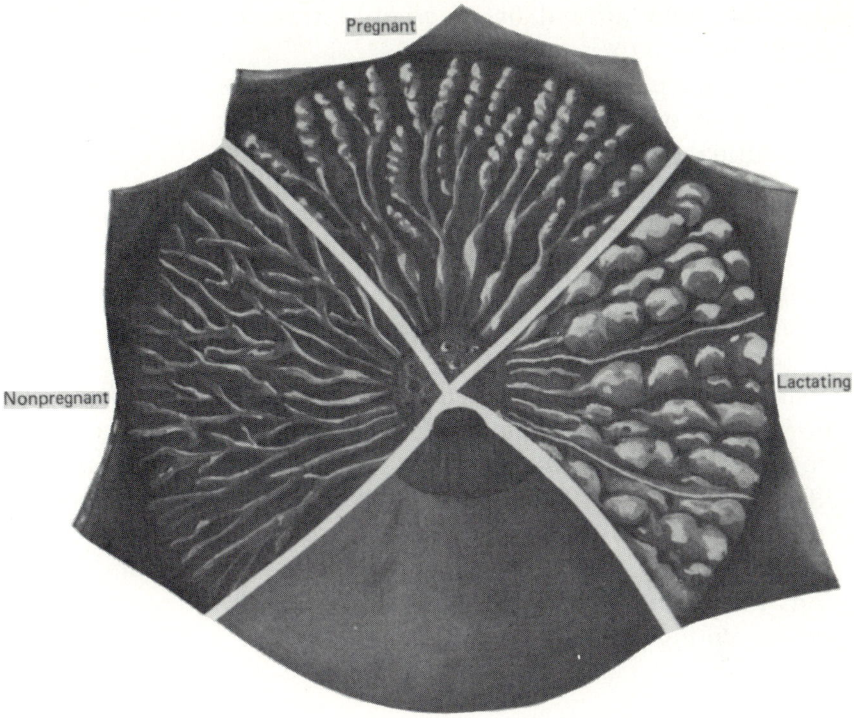

FIGURE 9-2. Changes in the breast associated with pregnancy and lactation: nonpregnant, pregnant, and lactating. Adapted from Ziegel, E. and Cranley, M. Obstetric Nursing, (8th ed.), New York: Macmillan, 1984.

gesterone and estrogen. Following delivery, however, when the levels of progesterone and estrogen drop, both the anterior and posterior pituitary glands are stimulated to produce hormones that establish lactation (see Chapter 23 for a complete discussion).

ENDOCRINE ADAPTATIONS

Conjointly linked with all of the maternal adaptations during pregnancy, the endocrine system provides the hormones which "mastermind" the pregnancy. Increased production of reproductive hormones, and even the addition of the placenta as a hormonal contributor, serve to provide the stimuli for maternal adaptations during pregnancy. Contributing to the maintenance of maternal hormonal homeostasis are the pituitary glands, ovaries, placenta, pancreas, thyroid, and parathyroid glands.

Pituitary Gland

Suppression of pituitary hormonal action is necessary during pregnancy. Although pituitary hormones are produced, the amount produced is less than usual. Follicle stimulating hormone (FSH) and luteinizing hormone (LH) normally produced during the monthly reproductive cycle are not necessary for the development of additional ovarian follicles during pregnancy. Production of these two hormones depend on the gonadotrophic releasing factors from the hypothalamus, which responds to feedback from the circulating levels of estrogen and progesterone. The higher levels of estrogen and progesterone found during pregnancy inhibit stimuli for the hypothalamic releasing factors, thus preventing the development of other ovarian follicles. The anterior pituitary growth hormone (HGH) (*somatotropin*), which effects metabolism of proteins, carbohydrates and lipids, appears to decrease during pregnancy.

Establishment of lactation is dependent on hormones secreted by the pituitary gland. During pregnancy the anterior pituitary gland secretes prolactin, which prepares the acini cells of the breast alveoli to produce milk. Increased levels of estrogen during pregnancy exert an inhibitory effect on the production of milk, however, prolonging the effects of prolactin until after delivery when estrogen levels drop.

The other pituitary hormone involved with lactation is oxytocin. Like prolactin, it is not fully utilized until after delivery. Oxytocin, produced by the posterior pituitary, supplies the stimulus for the "let-down reflex" necessary for the release of the milk from the ampulla of the breast. The infant sucking at the breast stimulates continued production of oxytocin.

Smooth muscle cell contractions of the uterine myometrium are stimulated by oxytocin. During pregnancy, progesterone inhibits this effect; however, immediately following delivery, if the infant is put to the breast to suckle, oxytocin will be secreted and uterine contractions will occur. This provides a natural method for preventing postpartum hemorrhage.

Thyroid Glands

Hyperplasia of the glandular tissue and increased vascularity cause enlargement of the thyroid gland during pregnancy. During the second month the level of thyroxine (T_4) is increased and remains elevated throughout pregnancy. High levels of thyroxine-binding proteins are also found in the maternal plasma secondary to increased estrogen production, creating a rise in the protein-bound iodine (PBI). More thyroxine is produced, but it is more readily bound and thus inactivated, resulting in essentially the same circulating levels of thyroxine as the nonpregnant state.

Elevation of the basal metabolic rate (BMR) is seen as early as the third month of pregnancy. The increased use of oxygen by the fetus and increased maternal cardiac demand are responsible for the elevation. BMR at term may be increased as much as 20 to 25 percent above the normal level. This increased metabolic activity results in increased thermogenesis in the pregnant woman.

If it is necessary to determine maternal thyroid functioning during pregnancy, it is not advisable to use radioactive iodine as a testing agent. This substance crosses the placenta quite readily and results in a high level of uptake by the fetus. Potentially harmful effects may occur if it is used after the 12th week of fetal development.

Parathyroid Gland

Metabolism of calcium and phosphorus is dependent on the secretion of parathyroid hormone. During pregnancy, especially in the last trimester, parathyroid hormone level is elevated. It is not known why hyperparathyroidism is associated with pregnancy, other than that it may be a physiologic response to the increased need for calcium by the developing fetus.

Adrenal Glands

There is a slight increase in the size of the adrenal glands during pregnancy but a significant increase in production of the adrenal hormones cortisol and aldosterone. Maternal plasma levels of both cortisol and transcortin (the cortisol-binding protein) increase throughout pregnancy. Higher cortisol levels facilitate active gluconeogenesis, which contributes to assuring an adequate supply of glucose for the fetus. Hyperacidity causing increased gastric secretions and heartburn may be related to the increased levels of cortisol, as well as the *striae* (stretch marks) found on the skin of the abdomen, buttocks, and thighs of the pregnant woman.

Aldosterone, involved in electrolyte regulation, is increased during pregnancy. High levels of progesterone produce a sodium-losing effect on the kidneys. In an effort to maintain homeostasis, the renin-angiotensin system stimulates the production of aldosterone, favoring sodium reabsorption.

Ovarian Hormones

Progesterone and estrogen are produced by the ovaries only during the first 10 to 12 weeks of pregnancy. This is necessary for the maintenance of pregnancy until the placenta matures enough to produce adequate hormonal levels. For this reason, estrogen and progesterone will be regarded as placental hormones.

Another hormone, *relaxin*, is thought to be produced by the corpus luteum of the ovary. Exact functions of this hormone are not known; however, it appears to have a relaxing and softening effect on the cartilage of the symphysis pubis and other pelvic joints. It may also promote unstriated muscle relaxation.

Placental Hormones

The placental hormones were discussed in Chapter 8. Table 9–1 summarizes hormonal influences during pregnancy and Figure 9–3 illustrates the concentration of hormones.

Pancreas

The endocrine functions of the pancreas revolve around the production of insulin. During pregnancy, insulin production is influenced by a number of factors, foremost of which is the fetal need for a continuous supply of glucose. Maternal glucose is quickly utilized by the fetus, lowering the pregnant woman's blood glucose level and decreasing her production of insulin. During the early months of pregnancy, insulin production is regulated in this simplistic manner. However, as pregnancy progresses, other influences alter the production of insulin. The increased cortisol levels encourage active gluconeogenesis, and the anti-insulin effect produced by the hormone human chorionic somatomammotropin (HCS) alters the ability of insulin to facilitate glucose use by maternal tissue cells. The higher levels of circulating glucose stimulate the pancreas to produce more insulin. Essentially two opposing effects occur, more insulin is produced, and at the same time less is able to be utilized. Insulin production continues to rise in the second and third trimesters.

Production of fetal insulin begins at 12 weeks gestation. Maternal insulin does not cross the placenta to the fetus.

Prostaglandins

Prostaglandins are a family of fatty acids for which a precise physiologic action has not been determined. They are found in many bodily tissues but in greater concentrations in reproductive tissue, amniotic fluid, semen, kidney, brain, and prostate tissue and in the corpus luteum of the ovary. Although they are classified as hormones, they are present in the tissues in a more concentrated form than in the blood stream.

Classification of prostaglandins is indicated by letters, numbers, and Greek letters. Although all the prostaglandins have an effect on pregnancy, the PGEs, which are smooth muscle relaxants and vasodilators, have the most pronounced actions. PGF_2 has been used to terminate pregnancy. Placental, endometrial, and myometrial tissue have been found to contain PGs. Prior to labor, the concentration of PGs seems to increase in these areas as well as in the amniotic fluid.

METABOLIC ADAPTATIONS

As changes occur in the maternal host throughout pregnancy, so must the metabolic responses needed to meet the demands of the growing fetus. Some of these responses may appear to be in excess of the needs of the fetus; however, they serve to insure and to enhance fetal development.

Carbohydrate Metabolism

Constant demands by the fetus for glucose alter the factors that affect the maternal blood glucose levels, creating a diabetes-like state during pregnancy. Because maternal peripheral tissue sensitivity to insulin is reduced by HCS, there is decreased tissue utilization of glucose,

TABLE 9-1
HORMONAL INFLUENCES DURING PREGNANCY

Hormone	Systemic Influence	Effect
Estrogen	**Reproductive System**	
Estriol is primarily produced by placenta in response to fetal precursor from the fetal adrenal glands and liver	Uterus	Increased uterine growth due to hyperplastic and hypertrophic growth of the myometrium
	Myometrial tissue	
	Blood vessels	Increased uterine blood flow
(Many of the effects of estrogen are a result of combined action with other hormones such as progesterone)	Endometrial tissue	Proliferation of tissue
	Breast	
	Ductal system	Proliferation of ducts
	Breast tissue	Inhibited sensitivity to prolactin
	Blood vessels	Increased blood supply
	Vagina	
	Epithelial cells	Hyperplasia and increased vaginal secretions (leukorrhea)
	Integumentary System	
	Skin	Stimulation of melantropic hormone causing chloasma of face
		Linea nigra
		Darkening of breast areolae
		Connective tissue changes striae gravidarum of breast, thighs & abdomen
	Musculoskeletal System	
	Pelvic ligaments & joints	Relaxation
	Circulatory System	Increased plasma volume
		Decreased coagulation time
		Increased fibrinogen enhancing clotting
	Hepatic System	Palmar erythema
		Spider nevi (telangiectasia)
	Renal System	
	Kidney	Increased sodium and water retention
	Endocrine System	
	Pituitary Gland	Inhibits hypothalamic releasing factor, ovarian follicles not produced
	Thyroid gland	Increased production of thyroxine and thyroxine binding proteins
	Adrenal glands	Increased transcortin levels
	Respiratory System	Increased sensitivity of respiratory system to CO_2 causing hyperventilation
	Gastrointestinal System	
	Oral cavity	Vascular swelling of gums with increased incidence of gingivitis
		Increased salivary gland secretions causing ptyalism
	Gastric secretions	Reduced
		Decreased secretory response to histamine
		Reduction in occurrence of peptic ulcers

TABLE 9–1 (continued)

Hormone	Systemic Influence	Effect
Progesterone	**Reproductive System**	
Produced by the corpus luteum of ovary until 6th to 9th week of pregnancy, then by the placenta	Uterus	Maintains endometrial stromal and decidual cells Quiescent effect on myometrium which inhibits uterine contractility
	Fallopian tubes	Increased secretions of fallopian tubes aiding in maintenance of blastocyst
	Breast	Development of breast areolar tissue and secretory ducts
	Musculoskeletal System	Relaxation of smooth muscles causing constipation, flatulence, and heartburn
	Central Nervous System	Quiescent effect causing malaise
	Gastrointestinal System	Decreased peristalsis of stomach and motility of intestines
	Gallbladder	Decreased emptying time favors formation of gallstones
	Respiratory System	Lower respiratory threshold for carbon dioxide—increasing respiratory rate
	Renal System	
	Kidney	Increasing antagonizing effect on aldosterone causing decreased sodium retention
	Ureters	Begin to dilate at 10 weeks gestation Decreased muscle tone
	Bladder	Decreased bladder tone
Human Chorionic Gonadotropin (HCG)	**Reproductive System**	
Produced by the syncytiotrophoblastic cells of the placenta	Ovary	Stimulates corpus luteum to continue to produce progesterone Interstitial cell stimulation of fetal testes
	Urinary System	HCG present in maternal urine and blood is basis for positive pregnancy test
	Digestive System	HCG implicated as a causative factor in hyperemesis gravidarum
Human Chorionic Somatomammotropin (HCS) (HPL)	**Metabolism**	
Produced by the syncytiotrophoblastic cells of the placenta	Fats	Facilitates metabolism of fats, elevating free fatty acids—increases availability of carbohydrates for fetal use
	Carbohydrates	Decreases peripheral effectiveness of insulin Diabetogenic effect increasing blood glucose level Increases insulin production
Prostaglandins	**Reproductive System**	
Produced by multiple body tissues with concentrations in reproductive tissue	Ovary	Participates in the formation of the corpus luteum

TABLE 9-1 (continued)

Hormone	Systemic Influence	Effect
	Circulatory System	Vasodilatation
	Musculoskeletal System	Smooth muscle relaxation and contractions
Relaxin	**Joints & Muscles**	
Produced by the corpus luteum of the ovary		Softening effect on cartilage and muscle relaxation
Cortisol	**Gastric System**	
Produced by the adrenal glands		Hyperacidity of gastric secretions Facilitates active gluconeogenesis

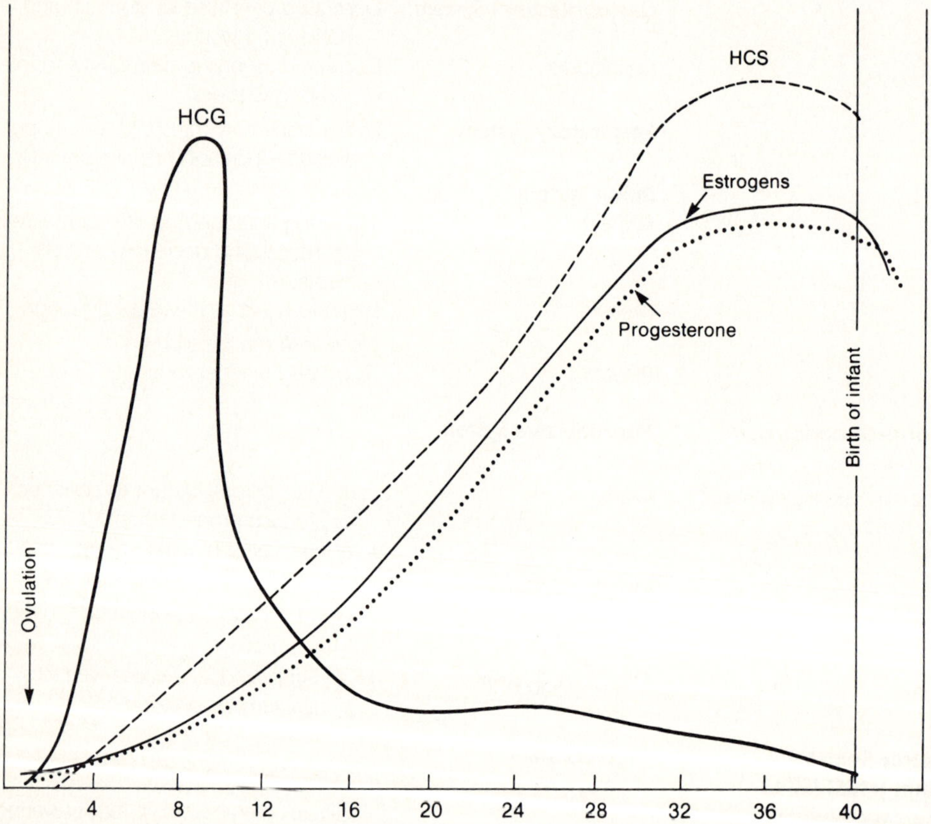

FIGURE 9-3. Concentration of hormones during pregnancy. Reprinted with permission from Ziegel, E. and Cranley, M. Obstetric Nursing, (8th ed.), New York: Macmillan, 1984.

which makes more available to the fetus. To further facilitate adequate glucose supplies for the fetus, HCS promotes maternal utilization of fatty acids and adipolysis (the breakdown of fats) as a source of energy, thereby conserving available carbohydrates for the developing fetus. If the pregnant woman does not receive an adequate amount of carbohydrates in her diet, this process is intensified and may result in excessive production of ketones from the breakdown of fats. Ketones cross the placenta and may have an adverse effect on the developing fetal brain.

A very delicate balance exists between

hypoglycemia and hyperglycemia during pregnancy. Alterations in any of the mechanisms affecting carbohydrate metabolism or insulin production can jeopardize the health of both the mother and fetus. Adequate nutrition and careful monitoring of mothers with metabolic disorders, such as diabetes mellitus, is essential to maintain homeostasis (see Chapter 25 for a complete discussion of diabetes in pregnancy). Table 9–2 summarizes factors that influence maternal blood glucose levels during pregnancy.

Protein Metabolism

Protein synthesis is increased during pregnancy in an effort to meet the increased needs for growth of maternal tissue and development of the fetus. When intake of protein is adequate, a positive nitrogen balance will be maintained. Protein needs are the greatest during the last trimester due to accelerated fetal growth.

Fat Metabolism

The increased metabolism of fats during pregnancy is associated with rising levels of HCS. Accelerated fat metabolism becomes a carbohydrate-sparing mechanism that allows increased supplies of glucose to become available to the fetus. Total cholesterol levels rise, reaching a maximum level at about 31 to 37 weeks gestation. There is a rapid drop in the cholesterol level in the first 24 hours postpartum.

TABLE 9–2
FACTORS INFLUENCING MATERNAL BLOOD GLUCOSE LEVELS DURING PREGNANCY

Factor	Maternal Adaptation	Effect
Fetal need for glucose	Early in pregnancy maternal glucose levels lowered as fetus utilizes glucose Resultant decreased insulin production by mother Less glycogen stored in maternal muscles and adipose tissue	Tendency to maternal hypoglycemia
Increased cortisol levels	Promotes maternal gluconeogenesis	Increased glucose available to fetus
Human chorionic somatomammotropin (HCS)	Increased adipolysis promoting utilization of maternal fatty acids	If this process is excessive due to poor dietary intake there may be an accumulation of maternal ketone bodies which may have an adverse effect on the fetal brain
	Produces anti-insulin effect which makes maternal peripheral tissue less sensitive to insulin, resulting in less tissue utilization of glucose as an energy source	Tendency to maternal hyperglycemia Diabetogenic state of pregnancy
	Higher levels of circulating glucose induces increased production of insulin	Promotes maternal normoglycemia
Amino acids utilized by fetus	Maternal amino acid blood levels lowered resulting in less amino acid precursors available for manufacture of glucose by the maternal liver	More protein and glucose available for fetus
Increased glomerular filtration rate	Increased filtration of glucose by maternal kidney	Maternal glucosuria

Mineral Metabolism

Metabolism of calcium and phosphorus is increased during pregnancy as a result of increased hormonal production. Maternal phosphorus concentrations are the greatest in midpregnancy, and calcium retention is the highest at term. Iron metabolism is increased to meet the demands of the increased erythropoiesis by the mother and the iron needs of the fetus. A total of 600–900 mg of iron is required during the entire pregnancy, 375 mg of which is needed to meet fetal demands.

Weight Gain

Normal weight gains in pregnancy vary with the physiologic and metabolic needs of the mother and developing fetus. The average weight gain is 22 to 30 pounds. Distribution of the weight gain may be found in Table 9-3. During the first trimester there may be a slight reduction in weight secondary to the nausea and vomiting that may occur. Overall the weight gain is as follows:

First trimester	3 pounds
Second trimester	12 pounds
Third trimester	10 pounds
Total	25 pounds

Weight restrictions should not be imposed on the pregnant woman unless a specific physiologic problem demands it. Assessment of weight gain focuses on the pattern of gain rather than on the amount. In the second and third trimesters, greater increases are expected with a gain of about one pound per week. Pregnant women who fail to demonstrate a normal pattern of weight gain or who lose weight may be at risk for alterations in fetal growth and development. Dietary restrictions imposed on the pregnant woman during the 1960s and early 1970s are no longer acceptable. Pregnant women who are restricting their weight gain should be discouraged from doing so.

TABLE 9-3
DISTRIBUTION OF WEIGHT GAIN DURING PREGNANCY

	Pounds	Grams
Fetus	7.8	3400
Placenta	1.5	595
Amniotic fluid	2.25	1000
Blood volume	3.25	1500
Extracellular fluid	3.25	1500
Uterus	2.25	1000
Breast	1	453

Water Metabolism

Alterations in fluid balance during pregnancy produce increases in both extracellular and intravascular fluid volume. Distribution of this increased fluid volume occurs in blood volume, fetal, placental, and amniotic fluid, and maternal tissue. A tendency to fluid retention is noted after the 30th week of pregnancy owing to the increase in the level of steroid hormones. Factors that contribute to retention of fluids include: increased capillary permeability, increased sodium retention after the first trimester, decreased plasma proteins, increased venous pressure in the lower extremities, and an increase in renal tubular reabsorption.

CARDIOVASCULAR ADAPTATIONS

Accommodations are made throughout the entire pregnancy in the cardiovascular system of the pregnant woman. These changes are precipitated by the hormonal influences of pregnancy and serve to facilitate the extra demands made by the fetus on maternal physiology.

Circulatory Changes

All major maternal organs experience an increase in blood flow during pregnancy; however, the uterus is the main recipient of increased blood flow, receiving 20 to 40 times the prepregnancy level. Blood flow to the breast is also increased early in the pregnancy, accounting for the feelings of tingling that many women experience. During the first trimester, renal blood flow is increased as much as 50 percent. It remains elevated during the second trimester and decreases in the third. Increased blood flow to the integumentary system stimulates growth of the hair and fingernails.

BLOOD VOLUME

Owing to a need for increased blood flow to accommodate vascular changes in the organs, total blood volume increases 30 to 40 percent over the prepregnancy level. The red cell volume increases at a slow, steady rate to 32 percent over the prepregnancy level. Plasma volume rapidly increases during the first and second trimesters, reaching a peak increase of 40 to 50 percent by 34 weeks gestation. Because of a greater expansion of plasma volume than red cell mass, there is a reduced erythrocyte count, hematocrit, and hemoglobin. These reduced levels do not jeopardize the oxygen-carrying capacity of the blood or constitute an anemia, they simply reflect a disproportionate rise in the plasma level over the red cell volume. An iron deficiency anemia does not exist until the hematocrit is less than 34 percent or the hemoglobin is lower than 11 gm/100 ml of blood.

Changes in blood volume are not only related to the increased vascular capacity of the organs but are associated with increased secretions of estrogen and progesterone. Decreased intrinsic vascular tone, as well as the increased size of the intravascular compartment, also influences blood volume during pregnancy.

WHITE BLOOD CELLS

During pregnancy there is an increase in leukocyte production. The leukocyte count will range from 5000 to 12,000 per mm^3.

PLASMA PROTEINS

A decrease in the concentration of albumin produces a reduction in total plasma proteins. The resulting reduction in colloid osmotic pressure favors fluid retention and edema.

COAGULATION FACTORS

Estrogen and progesterone influence fibrinogen levels to increase about 50 percent. The coagulation time, however, decreases but remains within a normal range of 8 to 12 minutes. Platelet production is increased and coagulation factors V, VII, VIII, IX, and X are elevated. These factors place the pregnant woman at risk for the development of venous thrombosis.

Cardiac Changes

Early in pregnancy the cardiac muscles hypertrophy, which in part accounts for the increase in the size and position change of the heart. Throughout pregnancy the position continues to change, locating the heart anteriorly, to the left, and with an upward displacement within the chest. Increased blood volume is responsible for murmurs heard at the apex of the heart and at the second intercostal space. These murmurs are not considered significant in a pregnant woman with normal prepregnancy cardiac physiology. Benign arrhythmias may produce palpitations and tachycardia.

CARDIAC OUTPUT

Cardiac output increases rapidly during the first trimester of pregnancy in response to increased circulatory changes and vascularity of the organs. Cardiac output, which is the product of stroke volume and heart rate, increases as much as 35 percent during pregnancy, peaking at the end of the second trimester. This increase is mainly caused by an increase in stroke volume.

Maternal position will influence cardiac output. In the supine position, the vena cava may become obstructed by the weight of the uterus, hindering venous return to the heart. The stroke volume is thus lowered and perfusion of the maternal organs and placenta are altered. In such instances, the pregnant woman will experience a drop in blood pressure and symptoms of dizziness and syncope. Cardiac output will rise and the symptoms will be alleviated when the woman is turned to a lateral recumbent position.

Increased demands are made on the heart, not only during pregnancy but also during labor and the postpartal period. An increase in cardiac output occurs with each uterine contraction during labor, although a return to near normal occurs in the interval between contractions. Following delivery there is a shift in the volume of blood from the uterine vessels to the systemic circulation, enhancing venous return from the lower extremities and causing a corresponding rise in cardiac output. The increased work load of the heart at this time is transient but may jeopardize a heart that is at risk for cardiac decompensation.

HEART RATE

In the early months of pregnancy (first trimester) there is a normal rise in the pulse rate that continues throughout pregnancy and peaks at a level of about 10 to 15 beats per minute above the prepregnant rate. Again, this may be attributed to the normal cardiovascular changes that influence the pregnancy.

BLOOD PRESSURE

Alterations in blood pressure during pregnancy result from reduced total peripheral resistance and the addition of the uteroplacental circulation. Overall there is a 25 percent reduction in peripheral resistance. The lowered vascular tone contributes to the drop in the blood pressure beginning in the first trimester, dropping to the lowest level in the second trimester, then rising slightly in the third trimester. The drop in the pressure is more often noted in the diastolic reading than in the systolic reading.

Monitoring blood pressure during the prenatal period is an important aspect of prenatal care. Attention is given to the maternal position when the blood pressure is taken. If the mother is in a supine position when the reading is taken, *supine hypotension* may occur, causing a decrease in the blood pressure and an inaccurate reading. Greater accuracy in blood pressure assessment is achieved by having the mother assume a left lateral recumbent position. This position will produce the lowest reading. When the blood pressure is taken with the mother seated, the highest readings are obtained.

After the 20th week of pregnancy, increases in the systolic pressure of 30 mm Hg and 15 mm Hg in the diastolic pressure, or both, are indications of pregnancy-induced hypertension. Therefore, it is of utmost importance to obtain a blood pressure assessment early in the pregnancy to serve as a baseline for future assessments.

Increased venous pressure in the lower extremities occurs as the pregnancy progresses. Again, the pressure of the expanding uterus on the vena cava and iliac veins results in marked pressure increases in the femoral veins and other veins of the lower extremities. Effects of increased venous pressure in the extremities include dependent edema of the legs, varicosities of the legs and vulva, hemorrhoids, and venous thrombosis.

When pooling of the blood occurs in the extremities, there is a corresponding increase in the capillary pressure, causing escape of fluid into the extravascular spaces. This, coupled, with a normal drop in colloid osmotic pressure during pregnancy, causes dependent edema. Standing or sitting for long periods of time will markedly increase edema in the extremities. On the other hand, periodic elevation of the feet, resting in the lateral recumbent position, and walking enhance circulation to the extremities and relieve edema.

The hematologic and cardiovascular changes occurring in pregnancy are summarized in Table 9-4.

RENAL SYSTEM ADAPTATIONS

Profound changes occur in the renal system during pregnancy owing to hormonal and mechanical effects. These changes, necessary for the normal accommodations of the mater-

TABLE 9-4
HEMATOLOGIC AND CARDIOVASCULAR CHANGES IN PREGNANCY

Physiologic Function	Maternal Alterations	Clinical Significance
Blood		
Blood volume	Increased 30-40%	Need for iron supplement in diet after 1st trimester
Plasma volume	Increased 40-50% Peaks at 34th week	
RBC	Increased 32%	Hematocrit is evaluated. It is low if less than 34%. Hemoglobin is low if less than 11gm/100ml.
WBC	May be increased from 5000/mm^3 to 12,000/mm^3 During labor increased as high as 25,000/mm^3	Elevations seen, primarily in leukocytes
Plasma Proteins	Reduced albumin	Altered colloid osmotic pressure favoring edema
Coagulation factors	Increased	
Coagulation time	Decreased	
Fibrinogen	Increased 50%	Increased possibility of thromboembolism
Platelets	Slight increase	
Heart Rate	Increased 10-15 beats per minute by 20 weeks	Benign arrhythmias may be noted
Cardiac Output	1st trimester rapid increase of 35% by the 32 week. Slight lowering thereafter	Increased workload of heart—significant in diseased heart
Stroke Volume	Increased Major contributor to elevation of cardiac output	
Blood Pressure	Slight decrease due to lowered peripheral resistance and the addition of the placental circulation Greatest decrease seen in diastolic reading	Careful monitoring of B/P After 20th week significant if there is an increase over 30mm Hg in systolic reading and/or 15mm in diastolic reading B/P should be assessed from a baseline evaluation obtained before or early in the pregnancy
Venous Pressure	Increased as pregnancy progresses	Development of dependent edema, Varicosities of the legs and vulva Hemorrhoids Supine hypotension syndrome Advise woman to assume left lateral recumbent position to increase circulation

nal-fetal unit, also place stress on the mother's urinary system.

Ureters

As early as 10 weeks gestation the ureters begin to dilate, more often noted in primigravidas (women having their first pregnancy). The dilation is thought to be primarily due to the effects of progesterone. Frequently, the right ureter is dilated more than the left. This is the result of the cushioning effect of the sigmoid colon on the left side and the compression of the right ureter by the dilated ovarian plexus and the iliac artery. Positioning of the uterus toward the right may also place pressure on the right ureter.

Muscle tone and rhythmic activities of the ureters decrease during pregnancy. This effect, combined with the dilation of the ureters, causes distention of the renal pelvis and calyces with urine. Stasis of urine and impaired drainage results, predisposing the bladder to infection. The effects of progesterone decrease bladder tone, permitting bladder distention which also increases the incidence of bacteriuria. Bladder capacity increases to about 1500 ml during pregnancy.

Increased urinary frequency begins early in pregnancy and continues until the third or fourth month, when the uterus rises from the true pelvis into the abdomen. At this time frequency decreases, only to return near the completion of pregnancy, when the uterus once again reenters the true pelvis.

Renal Functioning

Changes in renal function begin to occur during the first trimester of pregnancy (see Table 9-5). Renal plasma flow increases about 35 percent over the prepregnant level and is sustained at this level until one month from term. Glomerular filtration rate (GFR) begins to rise significantly after the first trimester and remains high until termination of the pregnancy. Increases in GFR may be as great as 50 percent over the prepregnancy level.

CREATININE, UREA, AND URIC ACID

Increases in the glomerular filtration rate of the kidney accelerate the excretion of creatinine, urea, and uric acid. This results in a lowering of blood levels of these substances during pregnancy. Decreased renal functioning may be suspected if normal prepregnant or lowered levels of creatinine, urea, and uric acid are present during pregnancy.

The most accurate test of renal function during pregnancy is the creatinine clearance test.

GLUCOSE

Two factors alter the excretion of glucose during pregnancy: increased glomeruli filtration rate, and inability of the renal tubules to effectively reabsorb the increased glucose load. Therefore, glucosuria during pregnancy is not uncommon. It is important to test the urine at each prenatal visit to determine the extent of glucosuria. If, at any time, a one plus (1+) level is found in the urine sample, it is considered significant and further assessments are needed.

SODIUM

Reabsorption of sodium keeps pace with the increased filtration rate. As pregnancy progresses, there is a slight retention of sodium to meet the increase in maternal fluid volume. The delicate balance needed involves factors that alter both the retention and the excretion of sodium.

Factors that enhance excretion of sodium are increased renal blood flow, increased glomerular filtration rate, and increased progesterone. Progesterone is postulated to have a sodium-losing effect on pregnancy, attributed to the antagonistic effect it has on aldosterone, the hormone produced by the adrenal cortex that stimulates sodium reab-

TABLE 9–5
RENAL CHANGES DURING PREGNANCY AND SIGNIFICANCE

Physiologic Change	Clinical Significance
Ureters	
Dilated & compressed	Increased tendency to urinary infections
Bladder	
Decreased tone	Bladder more easily distended
Increased capacity	
Compressed from expanding uterus	Urinary frequency Tendency for urinary infections
Renal Plasma Flow	
Increased 35% until 36th week gestation then drops to prepregnancy or lower level	Increased circulation to bladder. Small traces of protein in urine. Proteinuria is significant and needs evaluation
Glomerular Filtration Rate	
Increased 50% Lowered BUN Lowered creatinine	If elevation of BUN over 15 mg/100 ml and/or creatinine over 1 mg/100 ml may indicate kidney pathology
Increased glucose filtration	Glucosuria may be present and should be evaluated
Increased sodium filtration in early pregnancy	Tendency to sodium depletion, dietary sodium restrictions usually not advised Nocturia
Increased excretion of water	Excretion of water decreased in supine and upright positions Increased in lateral recumbent

sorption in the renal tubules. During pregnancy, increased production of progesterone reduces the level of aldosterone and decreases sodium reabsorption.

There are, however, factors that favor the retention of sodium. Chief among these is the renin-angiotensin-aldosterone system, which is stimulated during pregnancy. This system functions in opposition to the effects of progesterone, increasing the production of aldosterone and thus maintaining normal levels of sodium.

Increases in the production of estrogen, plasma cortisol, and human chorionic somatomammotropin (HCS) also have a sodium-retaining effect. These do not have as pronounced an effect as the renin-angiotensin-aldosterone system; however, their presence is significant.

In nursing, consideration is given to all factors that affect sodium regulation during pregnancy. Diets that are restrictive in salt consumption may alter the balance between sodium retention and sodium excretion. At one time these diets were popular because it was thought that they helped to prevent pregnancy-induced hypertension. Current practice requires strong supportive medical evidence for severe restrictions in dietary sodium during pregnancy. Normal dietary intake is recommended with neither a severe reduction nor an increase.

PROTEIN

Proteinuria is not a normal finding during pregnancy. When it does occur, it is significant and efforts must be made to determine the cause. Small amounts (plus 1) may be seen in individuals with orthostatic proteinuria, samples of very concentrated urine, or in the first voided morning specimen. However, proteinuria is considered abnormal and may be indicative of urinary tract infections, renal disorders, and pregnancy-induced hypertension. Contamination of specimens used for assessment of proteinuria may occur when there is maternal vaginal bleeding, in the presence of amniotic fluid, and when there is a vaginal discharge. In such circumstances a clean-catch specimen should be obtained for evaluation.

MATERNAL POSTURE AND KIDNEY FUNCTION

The most effective position to facilitate kidney function is the lateral recumbent. In both the supine and upright positions, renal circulation is decreased because of pooling of blood in the extremities and compression of the vena cava and aorta by the gravid uterus. The recumbent position, however, allows the fluid pooled in the extremities to return to the circulating blood, increasing blood volume. The lateral position reduces pressure on the vena cava and aorta, increasing cardiac output. Urinary excretion is increased during the night when the pregnant woman assumes a recumbent position. She often experiences nocturnal urinary frequency.

RESPIRATORY ADAPTATIONS

Various accommodations must be made by the respiratory system to meet the demands of increases in both maternal and fetal cells. Metabolic processes not only require increased oxygen consumption, but also an effective mechanism for the elimination of carbon dioxide.

Changing anatomic and physiologic adaptations occur throughout the respiratory system. The mucous membranes of the nasopharynx, larynx, trachea, and bronchi become hyperemic, owing to the expansion of capillary circulation, causing vocal changes, nasal congestion, and epistaxis. The diaphragm rises, the chest expands, the ribs are flared, and there is an overall relaxation of the ligamentous attachment of the ribs. After the 24th week of pregnancy, breathing changes from abdominal to thoracic.

Even with these adjustments, breathing becomes difficult during the last months of pregnancy. Dyspnea is a frequent complaint in late pregnancy, as the uterus exerts considerable pressure on the elevated diaphragm. When *lightening* (descent of the fetus into the true pelvis) occurs, about two weeks before delivery, the mother experiences relief from the dyspnea since the pressure on the diaphragm is relieved and lung expansion is increased.

Ventilation

Ventilation increases about 50 percent during pregnancy. Changes in tidal volume, minute volume, and functional residual capacity are responsible for these alterations.

TIDAL VOLUME

Tidal volume is the amount of air inhaled and exhaled during normal respiration. In the nonpregnant individual the normal tidal volume is approximately 500 ml. During pregnancy, however, there is an increase of about 40 percent, bringing tidal volume to 700 ml.

MINUTE VOLUME

Minute volume, which indicates the amount of air moved in and out of the lungs during one minute, is increased about 2 to 3 liters per minute. The nonpregnant level is about 8 liters per minute and the pregnant level is increased to 11 liters per minute. Minute volume also depends on the respiratory rate. It is determined by multiplying the respiratory rate by the tidal volume. Essentially, there is no increase in the respiratory rate during pregnancy, but the increase in the tidal volume accounts for the total increase in minute volume.

VITAL CAPACITY

One would expect, noting the changes in tidal volume and minute volume, to find an increase in vital capacity during pregnancy. This, however, is not correct. *Vital capacity,* which is the maximum amount of air exhaled following a maximum inhalation during inspiration, is not changed during pregnancy.

FUNCTIONAL RESIDUAL CAPACITY

Functional residual capacity (*FRC*), the amount of air remaining in the lungs following normal expiration, is decreased in pregnant women. Increased tidal volume and minute volume and decreased FRC result in a more efficient exchange of gases and increased alveolar ventilation. In other words, more air is brought into the lungs and less is left from the previous breath.

Changes in functional residual capacity not only enhance the exchange of oxygen and carbon dioxide in the mother and fetus, but have other effects as well. At times during labor and delivery, the mother may experience hypoventilation or hyperventilation. Because of the reduced FRC, either of these two conditions has more pronounced effects during pregnancy than in the nonpregnant woman. Stressors encountered, for instance, when the mother is holding her breath during a contraction, result in hypoventilation, increasing the risk of respiratory acidosis (increased blood levels of CO_2). On the other hand, if the mother is continuously breathing very deeply she may hyperventilate and develop *alkalosis* (increased blood levels of oxygen). Both of these situations represent an alteration in the maternal and fetal homeostasis and, if severe, may jeopardize their welfare.

During inhalation anesthesia, reduced functional residual capacity enhances the efficiency of inhaled anesthetic agents. Deep inhalations of anesthesia produce more rapid effects and at the same time, because less of these gases remain in the lungs, there is a more rapid recovery.

EFFECTS OF PROGESTERONE ON RESPIRATION

Increased concentrations of plasma progesterone during pregnancy influence the regulation of plasma pCO_2 (carbon dioxide in the blood) by the respiratory centers. When the plasma pCO_2 is elevated, there is a corresponding increase in the respiratory rate. This response is stimulated by the hypothalamus, which in pregnant women is triggered to respond at a lower level (32 mm Hg) of plasma CO_2 than in the nonpregnant woman (40 mm Hg). For this reason, there is a tendency toward hyperventilation during pregnancy.

It appears that the pregnant woman is maintained in a state of respiratory alkalosis owing to increased alveolar ventilation and decreased levels of plasma pCO_2. However, these responses are necessary to accommodate the additional CO_2 contributed by the fetus.

Renal adjustments are made to compensate for the tendency to alkalosis. Plasma bicarbonate (HCO_3) levels are lowered due to increased excretion of bicarbonate from the kidneys. Thus, the acid-base balance of the blood remains within the normal pH range of 7.35 to 7.45.

A summary of respiratory functioning may be found in Table 9–6.

GASTROINTESTINAL AND HEPATIC SYSTEMS ADAPTATIONS

Changes in the gastrointestinal system are often the first signs of pregnancy. Morning sickness combined with missed menstrual periods frequently provides the impetus for the woman to seek medical advice. As the pregnancy progresses, other changes in the gastrointes-

TABLE 9-6
RESPIRATORY ALTERATIONS DURING PREGNANCY

Physiologic Change	Clinical Significance
Oral Cavity	
Hyperemia of mucous membranes of larynx, trachea, and bronchi	Vocal changes Nasal congestion Epistaxis
Respirations	
Diaphragmatic breathing	Dyspnea common in late pregnancy
Expanding uterus exerts pressure on diaphragm	
Tidal volume increased by 40%	Plasma PCO_2 decreased Plasma PO_2 increased
Minute volume increased by 2–3 liters	Tendency to hyperventilation and alkalosis—particularly during labor
Respiratory rate remains the same as prepregnancy rate	Total oxygen consumption increased by 20%
Vital capacity remains the same as prepregnancy rate	
Functional residual capacity decreased by 20%	
Ventilation of alveoli increased by 65%	

tinal system become apparent, often causing discomfort.

Mouth and Oral Cavity

In response to the increased estrogen level, vascular swelling of the gums occurs during pregnancy, frequently beginning at about the second month gestation and continuing to the end of the eighth month. During this time the gums are more susceptible to injury and the incidence of gingivitis is increased. The salivary glands, influenced by estrogen, produce a slightly increased amount of saliva. Tooth decay does not appear to increase unless dental care during pregnancy is neglected. Good oral hygiene during pregnancy is important as are dental checkups.

Gastroesophageal and Intestinal Tract

The nausea and vomiting associated with pregnancy appears to correlate with increasing levels of human chorionic gonadotropin (HCG). Higher levels of cortisol and human chorionic somatomammotropin (HCS) also alter the metabolism of carbohydrates and can render the pregnant woman hypoglycemic. Total effects of these changes, which begin about the second month of pregnancy, may encourage a feeling of nausea and even induce vomiting.

Smooth muscle relaxation associated with the effects of progesterone contributes to decreased peristalsis of the stomach, delayed gastric emptying, and decreased motility of the small and large intestines. Constipation, heartburn, and flatulence may result.

Estrogen effects are manifested by reduced gastric secretions and acidity as well as a decreased secretory response to histamines. Because of the decreased histamine response there are also fewer peptic ulcers seen during pregnancy. Patients who have previously encountered discomfort from peptic ulcers may report relief from their symptoms.

Cholelithiasis (the formation of gallstones) is thought to increase during pregnancy as a result of a decrease in emptying time of the gallbladder and the increase in the cholesterol level. Both of these conditions are attributed to progesterone.

The development of hemorrhoids increases during pregnancy, most likely caused by constipation that occurs as the bowel is displaced by the uterine contents and pressure is placed on rectal blood vessels. Attention to bowel habits and a diet with an increased fiber content may help to alleviate the condition.

Hepatic System

There is a slight retention of bile salts during pregnancy related to an increased production of placental steroids. Suppression of bile flow encourages the accumulation of bile salts under the skin, giving rise to *pruritus gravidarum* (itching of pregnancy).

Occasionally *spider nevi* (a central arteriole with radiating small vessels found on the skin) and *palmar erythema* (redness of the palms) are present. The influence of estrogen is thought to be responsible for these changes.

A summary of gastrointestinal changes may be found in Table 9–7.

INTEGUMENTARY SYSTEM ADAPTATIONS

Hormonal changes are responsible for many alterations in the integumentary system in pregnancy. Alterations may be found in the connective tissue and in the pigmentation of the skin, complexion, and fat deposits under the skin, and in the activity of sebaceous glands, hair follicles, and fingernails.

Connective Tissue

Changes in the collagen system allow the collagen fibers in the connective tissue to relax, altering their supportive function and enabling them to separate. In areas such as the abdomen, thighs, and breast, which are overstretched, the collagen fibers separate, giving rise to streaks in the skin that may appear reddish or reddish blue in color. These streaks, called *striae gravidarum* will fade but never really disappear. Increased secretion of adrenocortical hormones are thought to be responsible for these changes. The pregnant woman usually refers to striae gravidarum as "stretch marks." Very often she uses oils and lotions to prevent or eliminate these marks; however, these alterations are caused by changes in the collagen system and the use of externally applied products will not alter them. The stretch marks do fade after birth, when they become silvery-white in color and are not as noticeable. At this time they are called *striae albicans.*

TABLE 9–7
GASTROINTESTINAL CHANGES DURING PREGNANCY

Physiologic Change	Clinical Significance
Gums	
Vascular swelling	Increased incidence of gingivitis
Salivary Glands	
More active	Increased saliva
Stomach	
Gastric acid secretion decreased	Fewer peptic ulcers
Decreased motility	Reduced emptying time of stomach causing heartburn and constipation
Increased pressure on stomach from expanding uterus	
Gall Bladder	
Reduced emptying time	Increased formation of gall stones
Liver	Accumulation of bile salts causing pruritis gravidarum

Pigmentation

The melanotropic hormone produced by the anterior pituitary gland stimulates the deposit of melanin producing hyperpigmentation in several localized areas. Often, after the eighth week of pregnancy, areas of increased pigmentation develop on the face and form a masklike appearance over the nose and cheeks. This is called the "mask of pregnancy" and is termed *chloasma* or *melasma*. Estrogen may also play a role in stimulating the melanotropic hormones, since nonpregnant women who have taken oral contraceptive medications containing higher doses of estrogen have also been known to develop chloasma. The chloasma that develops with pregnancy disappears following birth. In certain instances chloasma that develops when oral contraceptives are taken may not disappear.

Increased pigmentation is also seen extending as a line from the symphysis pubis to the umbilicus and occasionally over the height of the fundus. This line is called the *linea nigra* and is more pronounced in brunettes than in blondes or redheads.

Pigmentation changes may also be noted in the areolae and nipples of the breast. Following pregnancy the nipples and areolae generally remain darker than in the prepregnant state.

Perspiration

Increased blood flow and hormonal stimulation encourage activity of the sweat and sebaceous glands. Especially during the last trimester of pregnancy, increased feelings of warmth are experienced by the pregnant woman. Areas of erythema may be noted on the face and palms. Subcutaneous fat becomes thicker and contributes to feelings of warmth and increased perspiration.

Hair Growth

The activity of the hair follicles increases during pregnancy. Since fewer follicles are in the resting stage, less hair falls out. Following delivery, during the postpartum phase, the hair follicles return to normal activity levels. Consequently, it appears to the patient as if there is an increase in hair loss. However, it is only that an increased number of follicles have returned to the resting phase.

Complexion and Fingernails

Increased circulation to the skin, increased activity of the sebaceous glands, and elevated progesterone levels encourage the formation of facial blemishes. Most pregnant women experience only a slight increase in facial blemishes, which are usually treated with good, thorough cleansing and care. Fingernails appear to grow more rapidly during pregnancy, but they are also softer and more easily broken.

A summary of the changes in the integumentary system can be found in Table 9–8.

MUSCULOSKELETAL SYSTEM ADAPTATIONS

Postural changes occur during pregnancy in an effort to adjust to the increasing size, weight, and changing position of the uterus. An anterior shift in the woman's center of gravity necessitates a more upright posture. Increased pressure is placed on the lower spine, resulting in an abnormally increased curvature and, frequently, backache. As the pregnancy progresses the woman may develop a waddling gait.

Connective tissue changes, softening of the pelvic cartilages, increase in the elastic tissue, and relaxation of the pelvic joints facilitate increased mobility of the pelvis. This overall relaxation is attributed to increased estrogen, progesterone, and relaxin.

Separation of the recti abdomini muscles (*diastasis recti*) occurs in some women during pregnancy. Stress placed on the abdominal wall by the enlarging gravid uterus is thought to be the cause. When the separation of the

TABLE 9–8
CHANGES IN THE INTEGUMENTARY SYSTEM DURING PREGNANCY

Physiologic Change	Clinical Significance
Connective Tissue	
Separation of collagen fibers	Striae gravidarum
Pigmentation	
Increased pigmentation	Chloasma
Hair growth	
Increased activity of hair follicles	Hair appears thicker
Fingernails	
Increased growth	
Skin	
Increased blood flow	Vascular nevi
Increased activity of the sebaceous glands	Frequent facial blemishes

muscles is wide, it is possible for herniation of the uterus to occur. Complications may also be present when muscle tone is weakened during labor.

IMMUNOLOGIC ADAPTATIONS

The maternal immunologic system undergoes changes to create an immune response that is favorable to the fetus. Although many theories have been postulated for suppression of the maternal immune response to the fetus, the specific causes have not been identified. There is a decrease in the antibody IgG and in cellular immune response.

Pregnant women are more prone to bacterial and viral infections, especially in the upper respiratory tract. The incidence of complications and mortality from infections is increased. White blood cell count is increased without an increase in immunologic factors.

PSYCHOLOGICAL ADAPTATIONS

A multiplicity of factors affect the maternal psychological and emotional response to pregnancy. The physiologic influences of pregnancy produce changes that require psychological adjustments and acceptance by the pregnant woman. From the first realization of pregnancy to the birth, the complexity of the physical changes produce feelings that vary in intensity. Even as the physical cues are apparent, the psychological acknowledgment may not be realized. Acknowledgment of the pregnancy may occur without acceptance. These factors place stress on the pregnant woman, producing negative or positive responses depending on the manner in which she perceives and manages them.

Pregnancy has been described as a period of crisis during which the completion of certain developmental tasks are necessary for maternal acceptance and coping. Successful completion of these tasks is influenced by the psychosocial, cultural, family, and educational background of the pregnant woman. Identification of the stressors associated with these tasks is basic for effective management of her needs.

First Trimester

During the first trimester of pregnancy, verification of the pregnancy is one of the first concerns of the client. She may be aware of the physical signs indicating pregnancy but attribute them to other causes. As new signs continue to develop, she will consider the possibility of pregnancy. Mixed feelings may arise as she envisions herself pregnant and begins to contemplate the responsibilities involved. Although the pregnancy may have been planned, there may be moments of doubt and apprehension concerning the reality. Most women when they discover they are pregnant admit to being surprised and unsure whether they are ready for motherhood. An unplanned pregnancy may be viewed as a threat to a woman's future and evoke feelings of guilt, depression, insecurity, frustration, and anxiety.

Diagnosis of the pregnancy becomes essential. It is during this time that she will consult others who are or have been pregnant, she will become actively aware of her physical changes and possibly seek professional medical advice for confirmation of the pregnancy. Once the pregnancy is confirmed, feelings may still vacillate between those of acceptance and rejection of the pregnancy. A state of ambivalence often results, as she attempts to feel comfortable with the thought of pregnancy.

Acceptance of the pregnancy by those close to her becomes crucial. Husbands, boyfriends, parents, and other family members all influence her psychological adjustment. A shared joy and bonding occurs when she feels their acceptance of not only the pregnancy but of herself as well. She becomes secure in the knowledge that her role as a pregnant woman is supported by those she cares about. She may not have developed feelings of actualization regarding the fetus or the acceptance by her friends and family of the fetus, but she is secure in the knowledge that the pregnancy is accepted.

Preoccupation with self-concerns imparts a characteristic attitude of introversion to the pregnant woman during the first trimester. Thought is given to her changing role. Career goals are considered and the pregnancy is often seen as an interruption in the achievement of her goals. Even if the pregnancy has been planned, she must now adjust to a new role identity. Consideration is given to the value of the pregnancy versus her previous role. If this is her first pregnancy, she may see herself going from a role in which she was competent and comfortable to a role for which she feels unprepared and unsure.

An awareness of sexual identification and sexual role becomes apparent to the pregnant woman. Fulfillment of the procreative feminine function is a reality. However, if she has not been socialized to a sexual role identification, she may lack confidence in her feminine identity and, therefore, her maternal identification. Unresolved sexual conflicts may surface, threatening her relationship with her sexual partner. Stress develops when she is reluctant to share her sexual concerns.

The woman who is secure in her sexual identity also experiences alterations in her sexuality. Some women have a decrease in sexual desire that may be interpreted by the male partner as rejection. As she focuses on herself and her feminine achievement of pregnancy, she is content in her sexuality. Her partner, however, may feel a loss in their sexual relationship. At this time he is not socialized to his new role as expectant father and is only beginning to see his partner in the mothering role. The role of mother is one he had previously associated with his own childhood and it is characterized by the image of his own mother. Visualization of his sexual partner in that role may alter his sexual feelings toward her and create misunderstandings between them. Open exploration of these feelings by both partners is necessary if sexual conflicts are to be resolved.

NURSING RESPONSIBILITIES INVOLVING PSYCHOLOGICAL ADAPTATIONS DURING THE FIRST TRIMESTER

Assessment of psychological stressors during the first trimester are an important aspect of supportive nursing management of the pregnant woman. Since acknowledgment and acceptance of the pregnancy are two important tasks during this period, it is necessary for the nurse to be aware of factors that may hinder their accomplishment.

The first prenatal visit is generally directed at confirmation of the pregnancy. The nurse should be aware of this and direct her efforts toward making the client comfortable and relaxed with the techniques used to determine pregnancy. When pregnancy is confirmed, the nurse can be supportive of the reactions the client may be experiencing. Comments noting how wonderful it is to be pregnant or how lucky she is are not appropriate for every woman. If the pregnancy is rejected, the nurse must provide guiding management that will assist the client in determining her alternatives. Directional advice is not given until the client indicates a need or desire for it. Supportive, open-ended comments such as, "I see you have some concerns about the pregnancy diagnosis; would you like to share them?" are indicated. A few moments taken by the nurse to respond to the comments and reactions of the client will help to establish rapport for continued nursing management.

Quite opposite is the pregnant woman who has been eagerly anticipating confirmation of her pregnancy. She may want to immediately share her joy with the nurse and will be offended if the nurse simply walks out of the examining room following the examination. Since during the first trimester she is mainly focusing on herself and her physical changes, the client will be concerned with measures directed toward her physical care. This is not the time, however, to give her complete prenatal instructions, as her thoughts are centered on the actuality of the pregnancy and not on the details of health care. She will want to know when she should return for her next visit and the basics of prenatal health management. These measures support the reality of the pregnancy and establish confidence in her ability to see it through.

Women who have been pregnant before and have other children may initially appear ambivalent when diagnosed as being pregnant. They may have acknowledged the pregnancy before their first prenatal visit. The diagnosis of pregnancy is not a surprise to them. However, their emotions may be as confused as those of the first-time mother. Assessment of individual needs is paramount to emotional health care. Assuming that she knows everything about pregnancy since she has been through it before is not accurate. Each pregnancy presents different circumstances, attitudes, and expectations that require responsive nursing management. Listening to the client provides many clues to her physical and psychological needs. Reviewing aspects of prenatal care and management will demonstrate to her that the nurse does not expect her to remember everything about her past care and that care of the current pregnancy will be individualized. An open and communicative approach by the nurse will foster an open relationship with the client.

Second Trimester

Awareness characterizes the second trimester of pregnancy. Bodily changes have added a new dimension to the pregnant woman's appearance. Fetal movement (quickening) is felt at or around the fifth month of gestation. All of these factors actualize the existence of the baby. The pregnant woman's attention is focused on the involvement and investment in the pregnancy, as she assumes responsibility for fetal well-being.

Visible changes make the pregnant woman aware of the transformation she is undergoing. As physical changes occur there are accompanying alterations in body image. For some, these changes are traumatic; they are seen as a loss of physical attractiveness and a label of her as pregnant. For others, pregnancy signifies an achievement that evokes feelings of pride and symbolizes attainment of the epitomy of feminine sexual functioning. Still others simply accept the changes as a part of the pregnancy and accept them passively.

With the advent of quickening, a new perspective of the fetus develops. Concerns for the infant are all-consuming, and mental images of the infant begin to form. Efforts to identify fetal parts and the fetal heartbeat are shared with the father. The "baby" is a definite part of her that cannot be denied. Interpretations are given to the fetal movements such as, "He likes classical music"; "She is not active until I go to bed." She has fantasies regarding the infant as she reviews familial characteristics. She now begins to see the infant as having a separate identity formulated within the security of familiar family traits. Emphasis is placed on her desire to have the baby accepted and welcomed by those meaningful to her. Fears that the baby may not be normal arise and she worries whether she or others would be able to accept such a circumstance.

Now she places a special importance on providing a perfect environment for the developing baby. A healthy baby becomes her goal and she actively pursues activities facilitating this goal. Nutritional aspects are important and she will often eat food she dislikes but which she believes are "good for the baby." Working activities, rest periods, and recreational activities are planned with regard for what is best for the baby. Interest in prenatal education is stimulated as she explores avenues beneficial to her baby's development. She may seek out others who have experienced pregnancy or who are now pregnant, hoping to benefit from their experience.

Decision-making in areas outside of the pregnancy assume a different importance. Although she may still identify with her previous role, decisions in many areas are based on the effects they will have on the pregnancy. Concern for her welfare is important, as she views herself as the carrier of a valuable and precious treasure. It is not that she surrenders her independence; it is that she expects others to assume responsibilities supportive of her grander purpose.

During the second trimester the pregnant woman begins to form images of herself as a mother. She has recollections of her own mother's parenting and examines the negative and positive aspects of that behavior. Role modeling is used in an effort to assume a role that she may be unfamiliar with. She may mimic the mothering behaviors exemplified by her mother or by another woman she respects. When there is an opportunity to babysit with other infants she tries out her mothering behaviors. Relationships with her mother may be more intense and conflict resolution is often achieved. Viewing her own mother in the role of the baby's grandmother is not possible at this time, since she cannot project herself into the mothering role. She is still exploring, sorting, redefining, and formulating her expectations of her role as a mother. Assurance of her mother's love and support strengthens her confidence in her own mothering abilities. To think of her mother as a grandmother represents a loss to her, as she herself still is in need of mothering and nurturing. Teasing her mother about becoming a grandmother may be an attempt to "let go" of her possessiveness of her mother and to share her with the forthcoming child.

A need for reidentification of her role is also demonstrated by the mother who has other children. Thought is given by the pregnant woman to the effects the baby will have on the other children within the family. The youngest will no longer be the baby of the family but will now be a middle child. An only child will have to share his parents love and attention with another baby. The client questions how she will feel if the baby is not the sex she and the father had hoped for. Consideration is given to the practical task of caring for a new baby. She may wonder if she will have enough time and energy to give to the needs of the rest of her family. Financial concerns may make her anxious about the arrival of a new baby; however, she is more concerned with her ability to extend her nurturing to all of her children.

NURSING RESPONSIBILITIES INVOLVING PSYCHOLOGICAL ADAPTATIONS DURING THE SECOND TRIMESTER

Familiarity with the psychological and physical changes occurring the second trimester of pregnancy enables the nurse to plan nursing management tailored to the client's needs. At each of the woman's prenatal visits the nurse is aware of the client's increasing concern for her care. Explanation of the assessments that are made as well as the significance of the findings, is important. She wants to know how her pregnancy is progressing and if it is normal.

Inquiries by the nurse about fetal activity encourage the client to express concerns she may have about fetal well-being. She may wonder if it is normal to feel all the kicking on one side of her abdomen or if the baby is all right when it is quiet for a period of time. Allowing the client to listen to fetal heart tones promotes actualization of the fetus and lets her know that the baby is all right. Explanations of why the fetal heart sounds as it does and why is it more rapid than her own heartbeat helps to alleviate her concerns.

Mood swings are frequent during the second trimester and represent an area of sensitivity to the pregnant woman. Hormonal changes may be responsible for this emotional liability. Male partners are frequently confused by the mood swings and wonder what became of the woman they used to know. Indeed, the pregnant woman is herself confused when she finds herself crying one moment and laughing the next. Intervention by the nurse can be most helpful. First, an explanation of why mood swings occur and that they are normal helps the client to realize she is having a normal pregnancy reaction. The father is told that he can help by being understanding, loving, and patient but not patronizing during these episodes. It is not advisable for the father to state, "It's just your hormones, you'll get over it." In all likelihood, this will create more tears. However, just putting his arm around her and telling her he understands is often all the reassurance she needs at that moment.

As the concern for the infant increases, the need to learn more about the pregnancy and the baby also increases. Now she is interested in prenatal classes, not just for herself, but with the father. The nurse can help them choose classes that best meet their needs. Explanations of class content, scheduling of the classes, and additional sources of information are handled by the nurse.

Any indications of anxiety are noted by the nurse. When they are present, the client is encouraged to express them.

Anxieties frequently noted include: the husband's response to the pregnancy; fears about the baby's development; adjustments with the addition of a new baby; provision for the baby; mothering capabilities; feelings about the birthing of the baby; and family acceptance of the baby.

Following identification of the cause of the stress and anxiety, the nurse directs her efforts toward helping the client understand and resolve her concerns. Completion of each task of pregnancy cannot be achieved until coping or resolution of the stressors has been undertaken.

Third Trimester

The joy of pregnancy begins to fade as the third trimester is ushered in. Physical changes, altered body image, and emotional changes, which during the second trimester were accepted as a part of the pregnancy, now become a source of aggravation. She is tired of being pregnant but is not sure she is ready for birth. Her increased size makes her clumsy and vulnerable. For this reason, the pregnant woman will withdraw from situations that present any risk to herself or the baby. She tires more easily and is in need of physical and psychological renewal. When other people do things for her she is appreciative and grateful not only for their time but for their attention as well.

Plans are now activated for preparations necessary for the baby's care. The nursery or infant room is readied as choices of cribs, furniture, clothing, and a host of other items are made. As she attends to these tasks she is emotionally preparing for the physical separation of the baby from her being. She is centered on maternal tasks and finds herself departing from any roles or expectations that are not consistent with the mothering role.

Sharing plans for the baby with the father and those close to her becomes important. Discussion of names presents an opportunity for her to give the infant an identity. Acceptance of the baby by others continues to be crucial and she hopes that they will be pleased with the sex and appearance when it is born.

Her need for love and affection continues and is even more pronounced at the end of the pregnancy, when she feels awkward and unattractive because of her increased size. Her emotions are vulnerable to any feeling of rejection and she may easily misinterpret the reactions of others toward her. The most significant person from whom she usually seeks emotional support is the father. When she is assured of his love and support, she is more secure and finds the acceptance of her distorted image bearable.

As she tires of the pregnancy, the client begins to think more about the separation process. Fears and attitudes about labor and delivery are analyzed and contrasted with information she has received from childbirth education classes, friends, and other sources. She envisions what labor might be like and wonders how she will perform. Realistic or not, she develops expectations of her behavior during labor and sets goals for herself. Interest in her mother's and sister's labors develops and she may ask them to recall every detail of those events. If she and her male partner have attended childbirth classes, she practices the breathing and relaxation aids that were taught. In spite of her preparations she still may fear pain, loss of life, and death of the baby. She knows that these possibilities do exist but she is willing to face these threats in order to achieve her greater purpose of giving birth.

Both first time mothers and those who have other children are concerned with their ability to determine when they are in labor. The first-time mother reviews the signs and symptoms of labor that she has learned in classes or that others have shared with her. Those who have experienced labor before will review their past labors and contemplate if the next labor will be of the same intensity, length, and with the same onset as the others. Both types of mothers worry about being able to arrive at the hospital or delivery center on time. They begin to choose and put aside things that they will take to the hospital for themselves and the baby. They want to be ready in case the baby is early. If there are other children in the family plans are made for their care while the mother is absent. Plans are also made for notification of the father when labor begins.

The tasks have now been completed; the client has accepted the pregnancy and the baby, she has provided a safe environment for the baby for the past nine months, and she is prepared for motherhood. She is ready to give birth.

NURSING RESPONSIBILITIES INVOLVING PSYCHOLOGICAL ADAPTATIONS DURING THE THIRD TRIMESTER

At each contact with the pregnant woman during the third trimester the nurse should be aware of the woman's increasing discontentment. Comments such as

"I'm still here and getting bigger every day," "I wish the baby would come early," and "It seems like I have been pregnant forever," are frequently expressed by mothers during the third trimester.

Nursing interventions are centered on supporting the mother's self-esteem, relieving anxieties about the approaching labor and delivery, and preparing her for the transition from pregnant woman to new mother. Ideally, a supportive therapeutic environment has already been established with the client and her partner.

As the frequency of physical assessments increases during the third trimester, opportunities are provided for collaboration with the client. Feelings of vulnerability decrease when the client knows her care is carefully planned and evaluated by competent health professionals. She also derives support from the increased attention given by the nurse. She likes the special attention and concern that is exemplified by a need for closer health supervision during the last weeks of pregnancy.

Explanations by the nurse of fetal positions and the growth of the baby help the client to focus on the progression of the pregnancy rather than her distorted body image. She sees a reason for the way she looks and recognizes it as a positive image and an indication that she is achieving a successful pregnancy.

Pride in the pregnancy may sustain her emotional well-being, but the increase in physical discomforts are at times difficult to cope with. The nurse may offer suggestions for measures that might relieve these discomforts (see Chapter 11). Increased rest is one such suggestion. Time spent relaxing in a comfortable position often provides relief from many of the discomforts. The nurse should also explain the reasons for the discomforts.

Discussing the client's knowledge and concerns about labor and delivery is important during the third trimester. Although she may have attended childbirth classes, it is still necessary to assess her present understanding. The birthing process and the client's expectations should be reviewed and any misunderstanding addressed. Anesthesia options, birthing facilities, newborn facilities, and care during labor and delivery are discussed. Preferably these discussions are held when the father is present and can participate. Opportunities are given for questions, and reactions to the information are noted. Any anxiety noted in either the father or the mother is addressed. Misconceptions are corrected and additional information is presented when indicated. Cultural influences are assessed and explanations or differences that may be encountered are explained. Both the client and her partner are told that differences will be respected and accommodations made when possible. If someone other than the father of the baby is to be present during her labor and delivery, that individual is invited to participate in the discussions. The role of the father, and any other individuals she may choose to involve, is discussed and clarifications made.

The nurse's role includes assisting the pregnant woman to allow the pregnancy to terminate emotionally and to proceed on to the mothering role. Although she is not content with her distorted body image and she may be uncomfortable, the client has come to know and live with herself as a pregnant woman. Certain privileges have gone with this image and change represents another adjustment. Discussions by the nurse may be directed toward the basic needs of the newborn infant. References to the appearance of the newborn and his behavior and care help her project her thoughts into the mothering role. Assessment of factors or situations that might deter acceptance of the mothering role are made. Questions designed to make these assessments are important. The nurse often feels as if she is meddling when she directs her attention to this area. However, these assessments are just as important as physical assessments. There is no doubt that the nurse often does not have a solution to the problems that she has assessed. She can, however, explore with the client possible solutions and agencies or individuals that may be of help.

Commitment by the nurse to therapeutic nursing care is paramount throughout the pregnancy. It is during the third trimester, however, that actualizations of those nursing goals are realized.

THE EXPECTANT FATHER

Traditionally, the father's role during pregnancy has not been deemed as important as that of the mother. He is expected to provide for the family's economic welfare and to be supportive of the woman during the course of her pregnancy. As fathers become more involved during pregnancy, attention has been focused on their needs and expectations as well as the importance of their role.

A man may display a diversity of reactions when his wife or girlfriend first suspects pregnancy. These depend on his life circumstances at the time and his feelings toward impending fatherhood. In any case, acceptance of the pregnancy becomes a task that he, too, must accomplish. Unfamiliarity with the role of father creates feelings of ambivalence. One day the idea of being the proud father appeals to him while the next day he is terrified of the increased responsibilities. If he has other children and the role is not new to him, he may wonder if he can afford another child.

Acceptance of the woman in the pregnant role also creates a new dimension in their relationship. Realization that he will need to share her attention and love with another person may be viewed as a threat to their relationship. Even the additional attention that she receives from others may make him feel left out. He is concerned about their sexual relationship and considers the adjustments that may be, or are, necessary because of the pregnancy. Certainly, the mood swings that she experiences create moments of confusion for him.

When the man's expectations of the role of the father have been stereotyped by cultural influences, he may not be able to express his true feelings toward the pregnancy and fatherhood. Often he is expected to be supportive of the pregnancy and proud of his impending fatherhood while maintaining a detached attitude from the actual involvement in the pregnancy. Stressors that he may feel are not verbalized, since he is expected to take them in a "manly" way.

This pattern, fortunately, is changing in modern society. Fathers are increasingly actively involved in the pregnancy. Opportunities for sharing are presented as he accompanies the client to her prenatal visits and actively participates in prenatal classes. As he learns about the development of the fetus, hears the fetal heart tones, and feels fetal movement, he feels an emotional bonding that creates a feeling of oneness with his partner and the baby. This promotes his acknowledgment of the pregnancy and facilitates his role transition to parenthood.

Physical symptoms of nausea and vomiting, abdominal pains, heartburn, constipation, backache, and a variety of other complaints commonly seen in the pregnant woman may also appear in the father. The term *couvade* is used to denote this collection of physical ailments occurring in the father.

Although this syndrome has been documented in many cultures, the cause has not been positively identified. Earlier descriptions refer to the *ritual of couvade*, in which certain customs were observed following the birth of the infant. Practices such as confinement of the father to bed following delivery and dietary restrictions placed on the father are examples of couvade rituals. These differ from the *couvade syndrome*, in which the father experiences symptoms that may or may not be associated with ritualistic practices. Primitive societies may have seen the couvade rituals as a method of uniting the family by involving the father in the actual physical manifestations of pregnancy. Contemporary societies may see the desires of the present-day fathers to become involved in the pregnancy as analogous to the function of ritual couvade.

As the third trimester of the pregnancy begins, the father has, ideally, completed the two developmental tasks of acknowledgment and acceptance of the pregnancy. He now wants to feel fatherly and will initiate changes in his appearance to support the image of the role he hopes to achieve. Included in this changing self-concept is an increased desire to become more involved in creative activities. Generally, the activities are centered around improvements in the couple's living arrangements. These changes may be seen as movement toward the responsible father image.

A concern for responsibility is also demonstrated by his desire to know and be prepared for his role during labor and delivery. He feels it is important to practice with his partner the breathing and relaxation techniques to be used during the birthing process. Often he is the one to remind her to practice those techniques. They are achieving together and he wants to be sure that they are both prepared for their roles. He will talk with friends about labor and delivery experiences and possibly consult his own mother. Expectant parent classes become not only a source of information but an opportunity to share his feeling and reactions with other men involved in the same experience.

NURSING RESPONSIBILITIES TO THE EXPECTANT FATHER

The role of the nurse includes assessing the needs of the father as well as the needs of the mother during pregnancy. Supportive nursing functions can be instituted in each trimester. Beginning with the first contact, an assessment is made of his needs. Issues confronting the father are examined and interventions initiated.

Early in the pregnancy the nurse acquaints the father with the physical and psychological changes that will be occurring in the mother as the pregnancy progresses. Letting him know what to expect decreases anxiety when he is actually confronted with some of the changes. The pregnant woman's need for dependency and his supportive role in meeting these needs is explained and at the same time he is encouraged to express his feelings about the changes.

Alterations in sexual activity are discussed with both the mother and the father. Insight into the reason for this change is provided and a free expression of feelings is encouraged. He may fear injury to the fetus when they have sexual relations and needs to be reassured that in most instances sexual activity can be continued without any effect on the fetus.

Feelings he has toward the developing infant and even resentments he may harbor are discussed. Men frequently will express the fear that they will lose their partner's love and may be jealous of her attention to the infant. Activities that they shared previous to the pregnancy may be impossible at this time and he may feel a loss of a partner. He wonders if they will ever have any time together alone again. The nurse helps him to understand that these feelings are normal and are experienced by many people.

Education about the birthing process helps to dispel his fears of labor and delivery and even the death of his partner and the baby. The nurse invites him to share his feelings about labor and delivery. Both he and the client are encouraged to participate in tours provided by the birthing facilities. Familiarity with the surroundings they will encounter during labor and delivery helps to alleviate fears of the unknown and decreases their anxieties.

Assessment of his role perception during labor and delivery is important. He may express a desire for minimal involvement and may not wish to be present at the birth. The nurse may ask if he cares to share his reasons for these feelings, and the mother's reactions to his feelings are likewise assessed. If this attitude is harmonious for both of them, then the nurse should respect their feelings. She then provides insights into other supportive measures that he may pursue while his partner is in labor. If the father will not be present for the delivery, it is determined who, if anyone, will be present. His feelings about these arrangements should also be determined and discussed. Since the father's presence in the delivery room serves to foster his paternal role, he may have feelings of guilt related to his anticipated absence.

When the psychological needs of both the mother and father are met during the pregnancy, transitions into parenthood are facilitated.

BIBLIOGRAPHY

Curry, M.A. Variables related to adaptation to motherhood in "normal" primiparous women. *Journal of Obstetric, Gynecological, & Neonatal Nursing,* 1983, **12,** 115–121.

Grace, J. Does a mother's knowledge of fetal gender affect attachment? *MCN,* 1984, **9,** 42–45.

Hangsleben, K. Transition to fatherhood: an exploratory study. *Journal of Obstetric, Gynecological, & Neonatal Nursing,* 1983, **12,** 264–270.

Hogan, L. Pregnant again at 41. *MCN,* 1979, **4,** 174–176.

Iffy, L. & Charles, D. *Operative perinatology*. New York: Macmillan, 1984.

Kelly, M. Maternal position and blood pressure during pregnancy and delivery. *American Journal of Nursing,* 1982, **82,** 809-812.

Lee, G. Relationship of self-concept during late pregnancy to neonatal perception and parenting profile. *Journal of Obstetric, Gynecological, & Neonatal Nursing,* 1982, **11,** 186–190.

May, K. Psychologic involvement in pregnancy by expectant fathers. *Nursing Digest*. 1976, **IV,** 8-9.

Marten, L. Self-care nursing model for patients experiencing radical change in body image. *Journal of Obstetric, Gynecological & Neonatal Nursing*. 1978, **7,** 9-13.

Mercer, R., Hackley, K. & Bostrom, A. Relationships of psychosocial and perinatal variables to perceptions of childbirth. *Nursing Research*, 1983, **32,** 202-207.

O'Connell, M.L. Locus of control specific to pregnancy. 1983, *Journal of Obstetric, Gynecological & Neonatal Nursing*, **12,** 161-164.

Pridham, K. & Schutz, M. Parental goals and the birthing experience. *Journal of Obstetric, Gynecological & Neonatal Nursing*, 1983, **12,** 50-55.

Rubin, R. *Maternal identity and the maternity experience*. New York: Springer-Verlag, 1984.

Swanson, J. The marital sexual relationship during pregnancy. *Journal of Obstetric, Gynecological & Neonatal Nursing*, 1980, **9,** 267-270.

chapter 10

ASSESSMENT OF ANTEPARTAL ADAPTATIONS

OBJECTIVES

Upon completion of this chapter, the reader will be able to:

1. Describe techniques and considerations that are used by the nurse during the initial prenatal interview.
2. Identify components of the prenatal history that are the basis for antepartal assessment.
3. Describe pregnancy tests that may be used to assist in the confirmation of pregnancy.
4. Discuss the presumptive, probable, and positive signs of pregnancy.
5. Define the following terms: gravida, para, nulligravida, primigravida, multigravida, nullipara, primipara, and multipara.
6. Estimate the EDC by using Nägele's rule.
7. Describe the significance of B/P assessments during the initial prenatal examination.
8. Describe the components of the prenatal breast, abdominal, and pelvic examination.
9. Explain the significance of the laboratory tests used for prenatal evaluation of the client.

KEY TERMS

Gravida
Health history
Multigravida
Multipara
Nägele's rule
Nullipara
Para
Positive signs
Presumptive signs
Primigravida
Primipara
Probable signs
Quickening

Reproductive health care has developed into an interdisciplinary system for health delivery. The many interventions that combine in the achievement of a successful pregnancy require a solid working relationship between the physician and the nurse and the collaboration of the client and her support system. Functioning within this relationship, the nurse assesses, directs, implements, and evaluates health care and health education during pregnancy. The decision-making process related to the care of the childbearing family requires a synergistic effort by all involved. The nurse, equipped with professional training, develops skills in assessment and analysis of pertinent data, and serves as the catalyst for the successful delivery of antepartal care. The astuteness that the nurse possesses allows her to perceive the pronounced need to blend the activities of the client, the physician and the nurse. The nurse directs all her efforts toward facilitating the involvement of the client in decisions related to her health management.

ANTEPARTAL NURSING GOALS

Nursing goals during the antepartal period before the onset of labor are directed toward: (1) assisting the mother to adapt successfully to the physiologic changes occurring during pregnancy; (2) providing information and direction relevant to health education needs of the family during pregnancy; (3) assisting the client in the management of antepartal care based on the supportive and directional guidance by the nurse and other health professionals; (4) fostering the development of the client's independent goals, their adaptation to events involved in pregnancy, and the interventions needed to promote relationships within the family; and (5) assisting the client to recognize when professional health intervention and decisions become necessary for the optimal welfare of herself and the baby.

From the time the client enters the maternal health delivery system, the maternity nurse is involved in assessing health needs and planning appropriate interventions with her and the physician. A fundamental element of successful maternal care is the relationship established between the nurse and the client. Open and effective communication will enable the client to share with the nurse information and feelings pertinent to planning productive health care. When establishing this relationship, an accepting, caring attitude by the nurse will identify the client as an individual worthy of respect, capable of decision-making, and interested in receiving optimal maternal care.

Feelings of embarrassment or intimidation, or a lack of confidentiality perceived by the client will destroy effective communication and erode relationships. The client should be made as comfortable as possible by creating a supportive atmosphere. Privacy is provided, not only during physical examinations, but also during the interview. If a questionnaire is used, it may be completed by the client and then discussed with the nurse, or the nurse and client may fill it out together. Absolute confidentiality of all answers is essential.

THE HEALTH HISTORY

The health history provided by the client includes family health history, the client's past health and reproductive history, and her current reproductive profile. Each of these items is assessed at the initial visit. Ideally, this initial visit is scheduled shortly after she has missed her first menstrual period.

FAMILY HISTORY

An accurate assessment of the family health history includes information relevant to any disorders or illnesses, genetic or acquired, that might alter the outcome of pregnancy. Information is provided on the client's family, including grandparents, parents, uncles, aunts, brothers, sisters, and children. When possible, also included is information related to the father of the baby and his relatives.

Significant family history findings such as genetic problems, congenital disorders, diabetes mellitus, allergies, renal disorders, cardiovascular problems, and neurological and psychological problems are noted. When identified, continued exploration of data related to these conditions is necessary. Appropriate explanation of the need for more extensive data collection is shared with the client. Conditions known to be inherited and those which seem to occur repeatedly without known inherited patterns are investigated (Cranley, 1983). Every effort is made to elicit the concerns of the client and to explore avenues of counseling when needed.

The family health history may reveal familial disorders or conditions amenable to preventive health care. It is the responsibility of the nurse to assess the need for and to initiate health care teaching at this time. Conditions such as excessive smoking, which can cause cancer, and poor nutritional habits, which may cause obesity, are assessed. Since motivation for change in health patterns is increased during pregnancy, often just a little insight from the nurse will provide a foundation for productive changes in unsound health practices.

PAST HEALTH HISTORY

Data is obtained from the client about her own medical and surgical history. It is noted if immunizations have been given and if they are current. Live virus immunizations for German measles (rubella), mumps (parotitis), and measles (rubeola) are not given during pregnancy owing to possible teratogenic effects.

A maternal history of herpes simplex type II would alert the nurse to look for any herpes-type lesions. An assessment is made of the date of the initial occurrence, frequency, and dates of subsequent occurrences. Since an active herpes infection at the time of a vaginal delivery can cause infection in the neonate, it may be necessary to discuss the possibility of a cesarean delivery. The client is informed of the interventions that may be instituted if lesions develop and the necessity of reporting signs and symptoms. Herpes during pregnancy is further discussed in Chapter 25.

A past history of rheumatic fever indicates a need to determine functional cardiac status. During pregnancy, normal alterations in cardiac and respiratory function add stress to a heart already damaged by rheumatic fever. Once the classification of heart disease is determined, the nurse assists the client in planning her daily activities to insure minimal cardiac stress. The period of maximal cardiac stress is discussed with the client in order to plan physical activities. Cardiac problems associated with pregnancy are discussed in Chapter 25.

Tuberculosis diagnosed and treated before pregnancy necessitates followup studies. It is recommended that women be advised not to become pregnant until tuberculosis is inactive for at least two years. If the tuberculosis has been recently arrested, followup studies include sputum cultures. Even as early as the first prenatal visit, the nurse is responsible for planning nutritional interventions (increased calcium) and assessing activity stressors. Should the tuberculosis become active, the nurse must supervise medication administration (see Chapter 25).

A past history of *endometriosis* (endometrial tissue located outside of the uterine cavity) or *uterine myomas* (muscle tissue tumors) is important. Spontaneous abortion and postpartum complications are associated with these two conditions. If surgery for endometriosis or myomas has been done, a notation is made of the date and type of surgery.

Notations of previous pelvic infections are significant when assessing the status of the reproductive system. Recognizing that pelvic infection can result in the development of inflammatory masses, scar tissue, and strictures, the nurse must realize the need for continued patient evaluation. For example, pelvic infections following gonococcal and chlamydia infections may result in *salpingitis* (inflammation of the fallopian tubes). This, in turn, may be followed by the formation of scar tissue within the tubes, causing tubal narrowing and increasing the risk of ectopic pregnancy. Patient education includes the recognition of signs associated with ectopic pregnancy but should not suggest to the client that she is a possible candidate for this problem (see Chapter 25).

Notations of previous surgical procedures are made, including the postoperative recovery course, anesthesia-related problems, and postoperative complications. Diseases or conditions such as hepatitis, cholecystitis, appendicitis, cervicitis, cystitis, and hematologic disorders, which could affect the course of the pregnancy, are also noted in the history.

PAST REPRODUCTIVE HISTORY

All previous pregnancies and related information are assessed at the initial interview. The past reproductive history begins with the menstrual history of the client. Specific assessment items include the age of menarche, the frequency and duration of menses, characteristics of flow (clots; scanty or heavy amount), menstrual discomforts, emotional changes coinciding with menstrual periods, and physical changes such as fluid retention or headaches. This information will give the nurse insight into the possibility of abnormalities associated with the reproductive system or with reproductive endocrinology. For example, *menorrhagia* (heavy menstrual periods) can be associated with uterine myomas and retroposition of the uterus. A retroposed uterus caused by adhesions may become fixed, increasing the chance of abortion or urinary retention problems. A history of amenorrhea suggests disruption in hormonal production of estrogen or progesterone as well as abnormalities of anterior pituitary function, specifically follicle stimulating hormone (FSH) or luteinizing hormone (LH), or hypothalamic functioning related to the production of gonadotropic releasing factors. The intricacies of hormonal action piloting the course of pregnancy make these assessments important.

If there is a prior history of infertility, the cause and treatment should be noted. Clients treated with human menopausal gonadotropins (HMG) may be more likely to have multiple births owing to the stimulation of growth and maturation of the ovarian follicle.

Methods of contraception that have been used by the client are important factors contributing to the reproductive history. Intrauterine devices should always be removed before pregnancy. When assessing contraceptive history, inquiry is made about removal of the device.

Vaginal infections are common during the reproductive years. If the client has had previous infections, the type of infection, treatment, and date of the last occurrence should be determined. The incidence of *candidiasis* (monilia, yeast infection) is increased during pregnancy because of the increased glycogen content of the vagina. A history of prior yeast infection predisposes to repeat infection. A nursing diagnosis of knowledge deficit may be appropriate, and associated nursing interventions include informing the client to report any symptoms of a repeat infection. Neonates may develop oral infections of the mucous membranes (thrush) at the time of parturition (birth), if the mother is infected with candida albicans.

Another common vaginal infection is trichomoniasis, caused by the protozoa *Trichomonas vaginalis.* Metronidazole (Flagyl) is frequently prescribed as treatment. However, metronidazole can cross the placental membrane and enter into the fetal circulation. It is contraindicated during pregnancy, and other methods of treatment not harmful to the fetus are to be used.

The medication Nystatin (Mycolog) is often prescribed for vulvar irritation and itching (*pruritus*) caused by vaginal infections. If the client has previously used this topical antibiotic and steroid cream, she may decide to treat symptoms with the same medication but should be instructed not to do so.

When previous vaginal infections have occurred, client education includes elimination of irritants such as feminine hygiene sprays and strongly scented soaps. Undergarments should not be tight and should be made of cotton or other materials that absorb moisture. Good personal hygiene is emphasized and mention is made of the necessity to launder bath towels after each use.

Past reproductive history includes information about past pregnancies, including the number of abortions. When recording the number of previous pregnancies, certain definitions are used. *Gravida* refers to the number of times the client has been pregnant, regardless of the duration or outcome of pregnancy. The first pregnancy is recorded as gravida 1, the second as gravida 2, and so on. *Para* refers to the number of pregnancies that continued beyond 20 weeks gestation. It is important to remember that the criteria is the number of pregnancies that progressed to 20+ weeks, not the number of babies delivered. Twins born at full term are recorded as Para 1 if there have been no other pregnancies that progressed 20+ weeks. A fetus delivered before 20 weeks is not recorded as a para. Stillbirths are recorded as a para.

The obstetrical history records gravida and para together. Examples of recordings are:

Gravida 1 para 0: Denotes a woman who is pregnant with her first baby and who has had no other pregnancies that progressed 20+ weeks.

Gravida 2 para 1: Denotes a woman who is pregnant for the second time and who has had a previous pregnancy that progressed 20+ weeks. The past pregnancy may have been twins, a single birth, or a stillborn.

Gravida 4 para 2: Denotes a woman who is pregnant for the fourth time and who has had two previous pregnancies that progressed 20+ weeks and one pregnancy that terminated prior to 20 weeks of gestation.

The following terminology is commonly used in describing reproductive status:

Nulligravida: The woman who has never been pregnant.

Primigravida: A first pregnancy. The first time the uterus has been impregnated.

Multigravida: A woman who is pregnant for the second or more times.

Nullipara: The woman who has never delivered an infant of 20 weeks or more.

Primipara: A woman who has given birth to a viable infant. Common usage will describe a gravida 1 para 0 as a primipara, meaning this is her first baby. This is incorrect; the correct description for a gravida 1 para 0 is a primigravida.

Multipara: The woman who has given birth to two or more viable infants.

Another system used to describe reproductive status is the five-digit identification system, abbreviated as GTPAL.

(G)ravida: first digit—total number of pregnancies

(T)erm: second digit—total numbers of full-term deliveries including stillborns

(P)reterm: third digit—total number of preterm neonates (less than 37 weeks of gestation)

(A)bortion: fourth digit—total number of abortions

(L)iving children: fifth digit—total number of living children

The following are examples of the GTPAL system:

Mrs. Sawalha is pregnant for the fourth time.
She has had two full-term deliveries.
One of the deliveries was preterm.
She has had no abortions.
She has three living children.
4 2 1 0 3

Mrs. Hull is pregnant for the second time.
She has had no full-term deliveries.
She has had no preterm deliveries.
She has had one abortion.
She has one living adopted daughter.
2 0 0 1 1

Mrs. Kraft is pregnant for the fifth time.
She has had two previous full-term deliveries.
One neonate was born preterm.
One fetus was aborted.
She has three living children.

5 2 1 1 3

Descriptors of past pregnancies also include the birth weight of all babies previously born. Preterm, small for gestational age (neonate below 10th percentile on Colorado Intrauterine Growth Chart), and large for gestational age (neonate above the 90th percentile on the Colorado Intrauterine Growth Chart) infants should be noted. If previous infants were other than term deliveries, any knowledge the client has of the cause or related factors should be assessed.

Spontaneous abortions, stillbirths, birth defects, and neonatal problems are indicated on the prenatal record. Known contributing factors are also assessed when possible. When a genetic pattern of inherited disorders is present, the risk of recurrences is discussed (see Chapter 5) as well as the available alternatives. This discussion should involve other members of the health care team in a cooperative effort. Included in the discussion are current treatments and developments available. The decision-making process can be arduous for the client and her family. It is important that they be given reliable facts. Whatever decision the client makes, the nurse must be accepting and supportive.

Complications associated with previous pregnancies indicate a need for careful, watchful management during the present pregnancy. The assessment must include antepartal, intrapartal, and postpartal periods. If complications were present with previous pregnancies, methods of treatment and management must be noted. The nurse records information available from the client and then secures the client's past medical and reproductive records from the appropriate sources. A discussion of maternal disorders can be found in Chapters 24, 25, 26, and 27.

Data analysis at this time may identify a relationship between family or environmental factors that precipitated complications. The client is then given appropriate education, addressing the relationship of the causative factor and prevention. For example, the trend in society toward the trimline figure to enhance appearance encourages the use of severe weight reduction diets. If these diets are continued during pregnancy, there is a significant increase in maternal and neonatal complications.

Multiple pregnancies are associated with an increase in maternal and neonatal mortality. If the mother has had previous multiple births, assessment of pertinent data regarding the pregnancies and any complications is essential. Of special importance is the determination of associated preterm delivery and/or premature rupture of the membranes. Method of delivery and fetal presentations are assessed.

Information about previous labors is assessed. It should be noted whether labors were spontaneous or induced. If they were induced, ascertain the reason for the induction and the client's reaction. The length of labor and the characteristics of labor onset are noted. The relationship between the expected date of delivery and the actual delivery date is determined.

Types of previous deliveries include whether they were vaginal or cesarean deliveries. Methods of pain relief used and their success are noted. Emotional responses to past deliveries provide valuable insight into the need for an open discussion of alternative birthing methods.

CURRENT REPRODUCTIVE PROFILE

Initially, the current reproductive profile of the client begins with a determination of the expected date of delivery. The baseline data is then assessed, followed by a nutritional history and psychosocial assessment.

Expected Date of Delivery

The expected date of delivery is also known as the expected date of confinement (EDC) and is often designated as such. In the human pregnancy the EDC is considered to fall approximately 280 days from the first day of the last menstrual period. This is 10 lunar months (cycles of the moon or 29 1/2 days), 40 weeks, or 9 calendar months. Since it is difficult to know the exact day that fertilization occurred, figuring from the first day of the last menstrual period is the accepted method. A simple method known as *Nägele's rule* is used to make EDC determinations. The client is asked for the *first* day of her last normal menstrual period (LNMP). To this date add seven days and subtract three months. For example:

Date of last normal menstrual period	April 17 OR	4/17
Add 7 days	+7	4/24
Subtract 3 months (March-February-January)	January	
Expected due date	January 24	1/24

Another example would be:

Date of last normal menstrual period	June 28	6/28
Add 7 days	+7	6/35
Subtract 3 months	March 35	3/35
Extend 4 days into April	April 4	
Expected due date	April 4	4/4

Since March does not have 35 days, it is necessary to continue on into the next month. In this particular case it is April. The EDC is then April 4 of the next year.

It is explained to the gravida that this is only an estimation of her due date. Many factors can alter this date. Some women will have slight amounts of bleeding at the expected time of her normal menstrual period. This may be an implantation sign or may occur from alteration in hormonal levels, but it may be misinterpreted as her last menstrual period. This would make her EDC a month earlier than anticipated. When assessments are made, emphasis is on the date of the last normal menstrual period. The probability of error is also high when the woman does not have a regular 28-day menstrual cycle. Oral contraceptives will influence hormonal levels and, if discontinued shortly before pregnancy, the time of ovulation may be incorrect.

Other methods of determining EDC include measurement of the height of the uterine fundus, identification of quickening, and use of McDonald's Rule.

BASELINE DATA

Baseline assessments include age, height, weight, current medical condition, medications and treatments, teratogenic exposure, and symptoms associated with pregnancy.

Age Assessment

The reproductive capacity for a woman spans a period of approximately 40 years. This period extends from the onset of puberty to the menopause. Any extremes in age, either very young (16 years or younger) or old (35 years or older) increase the risk factors associated with pregnancy and fetal development. The young adolescent is at increased risk for poor nutrition, pelvic abnormalities, preterm deliveries, mental and psychosocial problems, pregnancy-induced hypertension, hypertension, and sexually transmitted diseases. Any of these factors add to the increased infant mortality rate noted among adolescents. The Task Force on Adolescent Pregnancy found that teenage mothers under 18 years are twice as likely to have low birthweight infants. Intelligence scores of children born to parents at either extreme of the reproductive years are lower than those of children born to parents in the middle reproductive years (Roberts & Engle, 1974). Youth in itself may imply an increase in risk factors; however, lower socioeconomic factors are also associated with this age group.

The risks associated with advancing maternal age increases almost two-fold when the gravida is over 35 years. Infants of these mothers are at increased risk for being small for gestational age (SGA) and having chromosome anomalies.

Weight Assessment

The normal nonpregnant weight of the client is noted. Her present weight is obtained and recorded. These two weights serve as baseline data for future determinations of adequate or inadequate weight gains. Assessment of the client's weight is made at each prenatal visit.

Low prepregnancy weights are 10+ percent under the standard weight determined for a specified height (Reeder et al., 1983). These women have a significantly higher rate of cardiac and respiratory problems and anemia, as well as an increased incidence of SGA infants, even when they have adequate weight gain during pregnancy (Edwards, 1979).

Weight loss during pregnancy is not acceptable, even when the individual is overweight. Mothers tempted to lose weight are discouraged from doing so and encouraged to concentrate on improvement of dietary habits. Severe dietary restrictions stimulate catabolism of fat stores and result in an excess of ketones in the blood. This in turn may impair fetal brain development.

A steady weight gain of 0.5 to 1.0 pound per week is recommended for the gravida. The gain over the nine months of pregnancy is approximately 4 pounds in the first trimester, 10 to 12 pounds in the second trimester, and 8 to 10 pounds in the third trimester.

Current Medical Assessment

Medical conditions associated with increased risk during pregnancy include diabetes mellitus, respiratory disorders, hypertension, sickle cell anemia, blood incompatibilities, TORCH infections, and sexually transmitted diseases.

Diabetes in the gravida is significantly altered and necessitates interventions and close supervision. Inquiries about the usual diabetic management routine and any problems maintaining this routine while pregnant will aid in planning appropriate care. Classification of diabetes according to White's classification (see Chapter 25) will aid in determining whether the mother should be referred to a tertiary facility. Blood sugar assessments are included in the laboratory evaluation. It is essential that a collaborative relationship be maintained with the client's internist.

Respiratory problems, including wheezing, coughing, and congestion, are often related to an asthmatic condition. The client is assessed for a history of asthma and allergies or both. Allergies are assessed in every client but may have special significance in the client with asthma. Client discussion focuses on the measures used to alleviate symptoms and the medications taken, both routine and for severe attacks. She is instructed to discuss her condition with her obstetrician during the physical examination and to consult him or her before continuing current medications or initiating new ones. Inclusion of her allergist in the management routine is necessary. Teamwork among those who provide care will prevent misunderstandings and mismanagement. Most commonly, asthma medications need not be abandoned during pregnancy, but they must be used judiciously and as indicated. Most xanthine bronchodilators (theophylline, aminophylline) and sympathomimetic bronchodilators (terbutaline, epinephrine) appear to be safe for use during pregnancy if monitored (Drukker, 1983). Over-the-counter medications for asthma are not to be used unless prescribed by the physician.

Sickle cell anemia during pregnancy is associated with an increased incidence of abruptio placentae, abortion, urinary tract infections, and preterm deliveries. Page et al. (1976) reported maternal mortality as high as 10 to 20 percent in mothers with sickle cell anemia. They consider it to be the medical disorder in pregnancy which carries the highest risk factor. Referral to a high-risk facility is usually advisable. Specific management can be found in Chapter 25.

Flu-like symptoms reported by the mother may be related to intrauterine viral infections (Cranley, 1983). These are often associated with TORCH complex: toxoplasmosis (TO), rubella (R), cytomegalovirus (C), and herpes simplex type II (H). Some of these infections are so subtle that the mother may not be aware she is ill. Any one of the TORCH infections can produce fetal anomalies and death.

An incompatibility may exist between the blood of the fetus and the mother when she has Rh negative blood and the infant has Rh positive blood. This can result in sensitization of the maternal blood. She produces antibodies that cause hemolysis of the red blood cells of the fetus. Maternal sensitization does not usually occur with the first pregnancy in Rh negative mothers but takes place at the time of delivery, when antibodies are formed. Thereafter, the circulating antibodies in the mother's blood will react to the presence of any Rh positive antigen produced by the fetus in a subsequent pregnancy.

A similar reaction may occur when the mother has a different blood type than that of the fetus, most commonly when the mother is type O and the fetus is type A or B. ABO incompatibilities may occur in the first pregnancy (see Chapter 25).

Venereal disease during the antepartal period presents both maternal and fetal problems. Prior to the 18th week of gestation the spirochete of syphilis does not cross the placental barrier. After 18 weeks gestation it can cross the placenta, giving rise to fetal anemia, stillbirths, or congenital syphilis. Maternal treatment before 18 weeks gestation can prevent fetal complications. If the syphilis is not diagnosed until the first prenatal visit, it must then be reported to the proper health authorities. All sexual contacts are reported and treated.

Drug Use Assessment

Screening for the use of prescribed medications and over-the-counter drugs is included in the initial client interview. This includes cigarettes, alcohol, caffeine, and illicit drugs. When interviewing the client to obtain this information, skill in addressing the issue with a nonjudgmental manner will help to obtain a true description from the client. Assessments are made of the frequency of use, amount used, period of time the drug has been used, and the indications for use. Appropriate information provided by the nurse to the client about the potential harmful effects of misused drugs may reduce the risk to the developing fetus.

Exposure to Toxic Materials Assessment

Noxious influences produced by exposure to toxic materials are suspected of causing teratogenic disorders in the developing fetus. Any exposure to chemicals, x-rays, chemical waste, industrial solvents, and nuclear materials should be documented. If the client indicates she or the father of the baby has been or is employed in occupations where these teratogens are used or produced, further fetal studies may be indicated. This should not be limited only to individuals employed in industry but also farmers, migrant workers, hospital employees, painters, and any individual exposed to teratogens.

It is thought that the fetus is most susceptible to environmental teratogens between the 13th and 60th day of development.

Pregnancy Signs and Symptoms Assessment

Data indicating signs and symptoms of pregnancy are also included in the information obtained from the client. Symptoms such as fatigue, constipation, heartburn, nausea, vomiting, spotting, breast changes, frequency of urination, quickening (feeling the fetus move), headaches, blurred vision, and edema should be noted. Any concerns by the client regarding her pregnancy are noted and explanations and suggestions offered when possible. If the nurse does not feel she can answer the client's question or offer advice, she should consult the proper authority and promptly relate that information to the client. It is not acceptable for the nurse to simply say "Why don't you check with your doctor?"

Morgan and Engel (1969) suggest the following questions to be used by the interviewer when assessing the client's symptoms:

Where is the symptom located? What is it like? How intense is it? When did it begin? What course has it followed? Under what circumstances does it take place? What alleviates it? Are there any other symptoms associated with it?

NUTRITIONAL HISTORY

Assessment of the nutritional history will aid in identifying mothers at nutritional risk. Assessment includes identification of food allergies, frequency of meals, physical conditions affecting eating habits, dental problems related to eating, dietary supplements, review of past 24-hour intake, average daily milk consumption, food likes and dislikes, use of alcohol, any special diets, and understanding of the basic four food groups. Recommendations for nutritional management during the prenatal period are found in Chapter 11.

PSYCHOSOCIAL ASSESSMENTS

Psychosocial assessment provides information which will aid the nurse when planning individualized holistic care for the childbearing family throughout the entire pregnancy. These assessments will aid in identifying factors that have potentially adverse effects on the family's adjustment to pregnancy. Factors such as behavioral development, attitude of the family toward the pregnancy, and the client's understanding of the importance of good prenatal care may be determined during the psychosocial interview.

Components of this interview include family patterns, occupation, race and culture, educational background, economic and social levels, and self-image. Certainly, not all the components of the interview may be assessed by direct questioning. The nurse invokes perceptive insight as the conversation proceeds. The nurse must be attuned to what the client is saying as well as to what she is not saying. The client's nonverbal communication can give additional insights that are meaningful in health care planning. If the father is present for the interview, it is possible to gain insights from his nonverbal communication as well. When the mother answers questions he may not respond verbally but may show negative or positive nonverbal responses. Not all the information elicited will be documentable. It is, however, important for the nurse to use her skills to interpret needs and concerns and to plan the care of the family accordingly.

Family Patterns

The role of the individual in the family and her adjustment contribute to the determination of factors affecting health care during pregnancy. It should be determined whether the family is nuclear or extended and the number of individuals included in the family household. For instance, are grandparents living with the pregnant couple? Will there be two mother figures in the household? Is there a father figure in the household? If not, will this role be assumed by a boyfriend, grandfather, uncle, or brother of the client? Are there other children in the family? What are their sexes and ages?

Equally as important in the assessment of family patterns is family management. It should be determined who is responsible for decision making within the family unit. Is this role shared by members of the family? Is it the responsibility of the father to make all the decisions in family matters? Determining the manner in which daily living responsibilities are distributed is also significant. Are certain household chores designated as his or hers? Is there a sharing of responsibility for the tasks related to family living? Are the children the full responsibility of the mother? Is the father planning on participating in the birthing process?

Insights into family relationships may not be easily assessed. A question such as "Will you have help at home with the new baby?" may encourage answers about family relationships. Listening carefully to what the client is saying and then planning the next question accordingly will provide greater insight than simply reading a list of questions. As the assessment proceeds, the nurse will find that she is also developing an understanding of how the client, partner, and others are accepting the pregnancy. If others reject the pregnancy, they are in essence rejecting her. This is difficult to live with and will hinder the emotional adjustments necessary for a positive family relationship. Knowing whether the pregnancy was planned or is wanted will markedly affect the plan of care. It may be that the mother is considering pregnancy termination and at this time only wants to know if she is pregnant. It may be that she is a single parent and she may need financial support during pregnancy. If she is an adolescent and not married, she may be anxious about her parents reactions to the pregnancy.

Family structure assessment may be as inclusive or as lengthy as the nurse or client chooses to make it. Asking meaningless questions is superfluous. At the same time, rushing through the interview imparts a feeling of insecurity and gives little on which to base assessments of family dynamics.

Occupational Assessment

Occupational assessments include the occupations of both the mother and father. This assessment provides clues to the economic status of the family, occupational environment, job satisfaction, and the placement of work priority in the family milieu. It is not uncommon in today's society to have both the mother and father working. Pregnancy may intrude on employment or preparation for employment. The level of income may be reduced if the mother is not working because of pregnancy. If she is to continue working, careful planning of her daily work schedule will need to be made to include periods of rest.

Questions pertinent to this discussion could be: Is she or he the sole support of the family? Does her job require sitting or standing for long periods of time? Will she continue to work and for how long? Is she going to work after the baby is born? What are normal working hours for the couple? Are either of their jobs seasonal? Is either parent required to be away from home for extended periods of time other than the normal work day? Are occupational hazards associated with either job? Do they find the work they do enjoyable? Do either of the parents find their jobs unusually stressful?

All of these questions may not be asked directly. The nurse can guide the discussion to obtain needed information for assessment.

Culture

Use of prenatal health facilities is markedly influenced by race, culture, and ethnic background of the individual and her family. Each culture has its own attitudes, beliefs, and customs related to health care (see Chapter 2). Knowledge of the differences and similarities of various cultures is needed by the nurse providing antepartal care. If the nurse is unaware of the values, beliefs, and attitudes inherent in the specific culture of her client, communication and the establishment of a productive relationship can be altered. The nurse should determine the cultural influences of the client and then develop a nursing care plan to accommodate these influences. Merely asking the client about her background is not enough. The nurse needs to know how significant are the cultural influences in the life of the client and her support system. The nurse should determine if the father is also from the same culture. Some cultures allow only a specific manner of expression of pain or emotion and the nurse needs to be aware of these to give appropriate and understanding care to the client. What may seem a routine question to the nurse may be perceived by the client and her family as an extreme invasion of their privacy. The adaptation of the interview to include these differences is essential.

Educational Background Assessment

The interview provides an opportunity for the nurse to assess the individual's level of understanding and the cognitive abilities needed for successful participation in health care planning. Knowing the client's educational background provides a basis for understanding, but in no way reflects the extent of the client's intelligence. When providing information to the client the nurse should not assume a superior attitude nor should she assume the client knows little or nothing about her condition. Today's health consumer is far more astute in her knowledge of health care than the woman of 20 years ago. As the nurse relays information, she continuously assesses the client's understanding by observing verbal and nonverbal responses. Individuals who are nervous will hear what is said but may not be able to internalize the information. Telephone calls, interruptions, presence of other clients, or the presence of other personnel during the interview may inhibit the client's response and reaction. Language barriers may restrict understanding and complicate comprehensibility. A keen awareness of the client's informational needs will aid in the effort to deliver this information and to ask and answer questions in the manner best suited to the client. If an interpreter is needed, one should be provided, rather than assuming the client understands.

Economic and Social Status Assessment

Reflections of the client's economic and social status are intermingled throughout the entire interview. Financial concerns can influence the care which the mother will receive throughout pregnancy. If the mother is without insurance or if her insurance does not cover pregnancy, she may not continue formal prenatal care. She may only come for the initial visit to confirm her pregnancy and then not be seen again until the time of delivery. Of course, this is not advisable and can place the client at risk for a variety of complications. Thus, if at the initial interview the nurse determines that finances are a problem, she can explore with the client alternative methods of payment for prenatal care or financial aid. Before the client leaves the office or clinic the nurse must insure that she understands the importance of continuing prenatal care.

Eliciting data applicable to assessment of the social status of the client adds another dimension when planning her prenatal care. Discussions of her membership in community organizations, participation in community programs, and the benefits derived may give insight into what the client perceives as her societal role. Families from certain income levels are often stereotyped as to social levels. When the family is stereotyped, it is difficult to achieve a true understanding of the client and her family. An understanding of how social class can affect health care is needed to plan effective nursing care.

Self-Image Assessment

Self-image may be the most difficult of all the psychological assessments for the nurse to make. Pregnancy has been described as a period of transition involving all the family members. Progression through this transitional period involves adapting to the psychological tasks of pregnancy that are interwoven with physiologic changes. Research has indicated that the self-image held by the mother and her adaptations are in a state of continuous change as she progresses through the pregnancy. Emotions ranging from anxiety to euphoria may be manifested by the mother. An awareness of the dynamics of these changes (see Chapter 9) by the nurse will allow understanding of the client's adjustments. Verbal clues may be given by the client when she says, "I'm getting so fat, nothing looks good on me anymore!" On the other hand, she may feel proud that she has conceived a child and perceives her enlarged abdomen as a sign of achievement. Teenagers who are actively involved in developing their self-images are especially vulnerable to changes in appearance.

It is essential that the nurse impart a feeling of acceptance toward the client. She should help her to resolve conflicts that weaken her self-image and support concrete efforts toward development of a positive self-image.

Table 10–1 provides an example of a prena-

TABLE 10-1
ANTEPARTAL ASSESSMENT RECORD

Client Name:	______	Father's Name:	______
Address:	______	Address:	______
Phone:	______	Phone:	______
Age:	______	Age:	______
Birthdate:	______	Birthdate:	______
Occupation:	______	Occupation:	______
Employment:	______	Education:	______
Hours worked/wk:	______	Children:	______
Insurance:	______	Ages:	______
Marital status:	______	Religion:	______
Education:	______		
Children:	______		
Ages:	______		
Religion:	______		
Date of LMP:	______		
Gravida:	______		
Para:	______		
EDC:	______		

FAMILY HEALTH HISTORY

Include history of grandparents, parents, siblings, and near relatives:

CLIENT:	FATHER:
Medical Disorders: ______	Medical Disorders: ______
Emotional Disorders: ______	Emotional Disorders: ______
Genetic Disorders: ______	Genetic Disorders: ______
Hereditary Conditions: ______	Hereditary Conditions: ______

NUTRITIONAL HISTORY

Frequency of meals: ______	Food dislikes: ______
Dietary Supplements: ______	
Special Diets: ______	Food likes: ______
	Use of Alcohol: ______
	Use of Cigarettes: ______

MEDICAL-SURGICAL HISTORY

CLIENT:	FATHER:
Immunizations: ______	Immunizations: ______
Medical Conditions: ______	Medical Conditions: ______
Surgeries: ______	Surgeries: ______
Childhood Diseases: ______	Childhood Diseases: ______
Allergies: ______	Allergies: ______

CLIENT REPRODUCTIVE HISTORY

Menstrual History:

Onset: ____________ Duration: ____________ Frequency: ____________

Characteristics: ____________

Discomforts: ____________

Contraceptive Use:

Type: ____________ Product Name: ____________

Onset of Use: ____________ Discontinued Use: ____________

Gynecological Conditions:

Disorders: ____________

Surgeries: ____________

Vaginal Infections: ____________

Sexually Transmitted Diseases: ____________

Infertility: ____________ Treatment: ____________

PAST PREGNANCIES

Date of last birth: ____________

Number of pregnancies: ____________

Characteristics:

Ectopic pregnancy: ____________

Abortion: ____________

Stillbirth: ____________

Prematures: ____________

Multiple births: ____________

Hypertension: ____________

Bleeding: ____________

Hemorrhage: ____________

Anemia: ____________

Rh incompatibility: ____________

Labors:

Preterm labors: ____________

PROM: ____________

Length of labors: ____________

Complications: ____________

Relaxation Aids: ____________

Anesthesia: ____________

Lamaze: ____________

Deliveries:

Spontaneous: ____________

Forceps: ____________

Cesarean Births: ____________

Complications: ____________

Neonatal History:

Infant Death: ____________

Anomalies: ____________

Complications: ____________

CURRENT REPRODUCTIVE HISTORY

Physical Examination:

Height: ________ Weight: ________ Usual weight: ________ EENT: ________

Heart: ____________ Abdomen: ____________

Head and Neck: ____________ Breasts: ____________

Lungs: ____________ Extremities: ____________

Vaginal examination: ____________

Pelvic Measurements:

Inlet: ____________

Midplane: ____________

Outlet: ____________

Subjective Symptoms: ____________

Laboratory Tests:

Hgb: ________ Hct: ________ Type and Rh: ____________

VDRL: ________ WBC: ________ Antibody Titer: ____________

Blood sugar: ____________

Urine: Glucose: ______________________
Albumin: ______________________
Bacteria: ______________________
Pap Smear: ______________________
Gonorrhea Smear: ______________________
Other: ______________________
Current Medications: ______________________
Summary of High-Risk Factors: ______________________
____
Examiner's Evaluation: ______________________
____
____
Signature: ______________________
Nursing Evaluation: ______________________
____
____
Signature: ______________________

tal history to be used at the initial interview. Table 10–2 provides an example of a nursing care plan developed based on information received at the initial interview.

DIAGNOSIS OF PREGNANCY

The diagnosis of pregnancy is based on data obtained during the initial interview, the signs and symptoms of pregnancy that the client experiences, and the results of the physical examination and laboratory testing. The data are evaluated in order to formulate the medical and nursing diagnoses (Table 10–2).

Signs and Symptoms of Pregnancy

The mother-to-be may have been experiencing signs and symptoms of pregnancy for several weeks before seeking confirmation of pregnancy. If she has had previous pregnancies, she may be aware of the significance of the symptoms. She may have discussed these symptoms with her husband, a friend, or her mother as a means of an anticipatory diagnosis. In some cases she may fear that she is pregnant, and in others she may fear that she is not. There does, however, come a time when she faces the reality of the situation and makes an appointment to confirm the pregnancy.

During the initial interview, she will discuss with the nurse those signs and symptoms she has experienced. They may be categorized in the following manner:

Presumptive signs: Those signs and symptoms that may be present for reasons other than pregnancy. Although frequently present during pregnancy, they are not conclusive for diagnosis of pregnancy.

Probable signs: Signs that, of themselves, are not conclusive but that are more reliable indicators of pregnancy. They are usually found on physical examination or laboratory testing.

Positive signs: Absolute confirmation of pregnancy is made when any of these signs are present.

PRESUMPTIVE SIGNS OF PREGNANCY

Amenorrhea

The first sign of pregnancy is amenorrhea or absence of menstruation. In the sexually active woman, amenorrhea most commonly means she is pregnant. There are many other causes of amenorrhea: illness, hormonal

TABLE 10–2
SAMPLE NURSING CARE PLAN: FIRST PRENATAL CLINIC VISIT

Carol S. is pregnant for the first time. On 4/12 she and her husband are entering the maternity health care system. As they embark on their first prenatal clinic visit, data is obtained by the nurse using the antepartal assessment form (see Table 10–1).

DATA BASE:

Gravida 1 para 0
Age: 25
Married
Employment: Legal secretary
Husband's age: 27
Husband's occupation: Pharmacist
LMP: 2/2 EDC: 11/9
Menstrual history: onset of menses at age 13 years
periods regular with no dysmenorrhea
Oral contraceptives used for birth control until 10/3
Weight reduction diet 1100 calories since 1/1 with no medical supervision
Family health history negative
Current health history negative

Nutritional history: eats only 2 meals a day—breakfast and supper
Smokes a pack of cigarettes daily—states "I know I should quit smoking but I can't," frequent cough when smokes too much
No alcohol intake
States "I dread being in labor."
Physical assessment: normal
Medical diagnosis of pregnancy made by the physician
Vital statistics: B/P 120/70
Temperature 98.6° F
Pulse 62
Respirations 16
Weight 110 lb on 4/12 (usual weight 120 lb)

Nursing Diagnosis	Goals	Nursing Interventions	Rationale	Evaluation
Alteration in nutrition, less than body requirements related to inadequate food intake	Client will: increase her caloric intake to satisfy the metabolic needs of her body and the fetus during pregnancy	Explain the relationship of the proper dietary intake during pregnancy and the growth and development of the fetus	Metabolic needs for the mother and growth needs of the fetus require an increase of 300 kcal over the normal nonpregnant requirements	
	Gain 25 to 30 pounds by 11/9	Weigh client at each prenatal visit and assess gain —first weight assessment to be on 4/26	All nutrient requirements are increased during pregnancy	Client weight on 4/26 112 lb
	Gain one pound per week			
	Increase daily caloric intake to 2500 calories by 4/26	Review and assess the diet of the client on last two days preceding the prenatal visit of 4/26 Graph weight at each prenatal visit	Severe restriction of calories during pregnancy results in a lowering of the blood glucose levels. Maternal fats are broken down to satisfy glucose requirements. Excessive breakdown of fats results in an increased level of maternal ketones. Ketone bodies cross the placenta and may have an adverse effect on the fetus	Review of daily intake of calories for 4/24 and 4/25 was 2500 kcal and inclusive of essential nutrients

	Describe the components of the recommended daily diet	Assess client's knowledge of basic food groups Provide chart for client with food groupings—suggest she keep it visible in kitchen as an aid in planning daily menus Discuss food likes and dislikes with the client Plan with the client a week's menu		Review of 4/24 and 4/25 diet reveals they are inclusive of all basic four food groups
	Eat 3 regular or 6 small meals per day	Discuss the importance of eating regularly	Regular meals discourage a fasting state and a lowering of the maternal blood glucose levels	Review of 4/24 and 4/25 menus shows 3 meals per day and a bedtime snack
Ineffective breathing pattern related to cigarette smoking	Client will: Discontinue use of cigarettes	Discuss the effects of smoking on the fetus	Infants born to mothers who smoke have a higher incidence of being SGA	4/26—Reduced cigarette intake to 6 per day
	Verbalize harmful effects of smoking on herself and the fetus at prenatal visit of 4/26	Discuss with the client her feelings about smoking		4/26—stated she had discussed with husband the effects of smoking on the fetus
	Note activities of daily living when engaged in smoking Develop a plan for cigarette reduction by 4/26	Discuss methods used to eliminate smoking Assist client in developing a plan for reducing cigarette usage	Low birth weight infants have an increased mortality	4/26—presented list of activities engaged in when smoking 4/26: Presented plan for elimination of cigarettes
	Experience relief from effects of smoking on respiratory system evidenced by: elimination of cough associated with smoking	Assess symptoms associated with cough Inform physician of respiratory assessment and results Teach client relaxation and breathing exercises	Cough may be related to respiratory ailment and needs to be evaluated	4/26 C/O cough—goal not met
Anxiety related to fear of labor and delivery	Client will: Verbalize confidence in her ability to meet the emotional and physical demands of labor and delivery	Discuss fears with clients, identifying areas of greatest concerns	Client will be more successful in eliminating anxiety when concerns are voiced and discussed with knowledgeable resource person	4/26 Fears discussed—stated primary fears are pain and loss of control
	Enroll in childbirth preparation class by 4/26	Inform client that husband may share in the total birth experience Inform client of childbirth preparation classes offered in the community	Knowledge that husband can share in the birth experience provides an element of comfort	4/26 Discussed childbirth preparation class with husband; decided both will attend

Table 10–2 (continued)

Nursing Diagnosis	Goals	Nursing Interventions	Rationale	Evaluation
	Prepare a list of questions regarding labor and delivery by 4/26	Review questions with client	Participation by both husband and wife offers an opportunity for explanation of labor process and answering of additional questions	4/26 Client presented list of questions which were discussed with nurse
	Discuss stages of labor and comfort and relaxation measures during these stages by 5/12	Explain and discuss labor process and comfort measures Signs and symptoms of labor Stages of labor Care during labor Delivery process Immediate care of the newborn Care in the recovery period		4/26 Discussed early signs and symptoms of labor
Knowledge deficit related to first pregnancy	The client will successfully adapt to the physical and psychological changes associated with pregnancy The client will verbalize health measures needed in pregnancy by 6/12	Assess client's knowledge of physical and psychological changes of pregnancy Instruct client in care in the following areas: Physiologic changes Daily activities Rest and exercise Danger signals Emotional changes Sexual activities Discomforts of pregnancy Infant care	Learning is enhanced when the instruction is individualized to meet the needs of the client and when the material is currently applicable	4/26 Continue teaching-learning activities, goal not met

changes, adrenal and ovarian disorders, stress, emotions, thyroid disorders, and anorexia nervosa.

Nausea and Vomiting

One of the traditional symptoms of pregnancy, "morning sickness," most commonly occurs during the second and third months of pregnancy. Some women experience this symptom as early as the first missed menstrual period. Although it is commonly called morning sickness, it occurs at all times of day. The frequency with which nausea occurs in early pregnancy varies. Some women never have morning sickness, some have it only with the first pregnancy, and others have it with every pregnancy. The cause has not been determined, but alterations in hormonal levels of human chorionic gonadotropin (HCG) have been suspected as the cause. Nausea and vomiting in a woman of childbearing age may cause suspicion but do not confirm pregnancy. Other causes include gastroenteritis, ulcers, appendicitis, and cholecystitis.

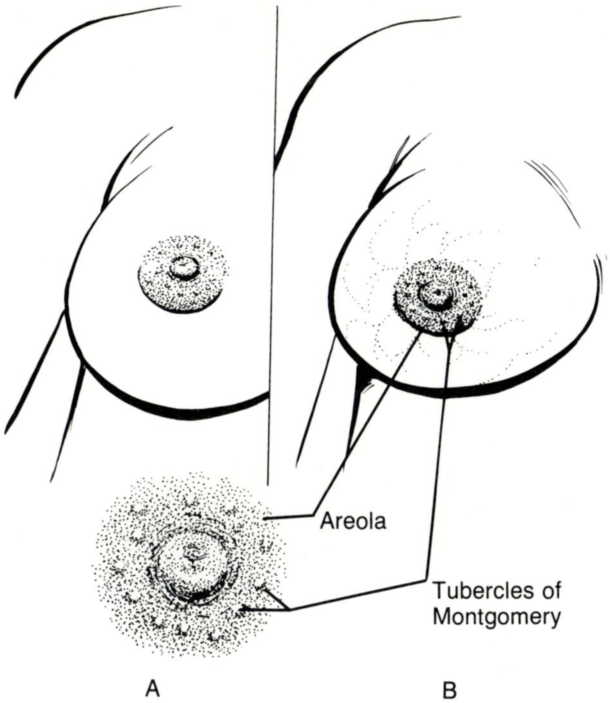

FIGURE 10–1. External appearance of the A. nonpregnant breast and B. the pregnant breast. Note the increase in the pigmentation on the areola, increased development of the tubercles of Montgomery and increased veining during pregnancy.

Quickening

Perception of fetal movements by the mother during pregnancy is considered a presumptive sign. Most commonly, the first perceptions occur at about 18 weeks gestation. Intestinal movements may also cause this sensation.

Breast Changes

There is a great deal of variability in the appearance of the breast in pregnant women. Breast changes also occur at varying times during pregnancy. Initially, there is a feeling of fullness, and a tingling accompanied by slight discomfort. As the pregnancy continues, the veins become more noticeable, the tubercles of Montgomery become more developed (see Fig. 10–1), and pigmentation of the areola of the breast darkens. In some women colostrum is secreted during the early months of pregnancy. This is the first secretion from the breast and appears yellowish in color. During the prenatal period it is secreted in small amounts, but an increased amount is noted in the early puerperium before breast milk "comes in." Some women do not secrete colostrum until after delivery, while others notice small amounts as early as three months gestation. Breast changes are related to increased levels of estrogen, which stimulates the development of the mammary ducts and is responsible for the feeling of fullness in the breast. Progesterone influences alveolar development and pigmentation changes (Benson, 1977). Breast changes may be noted in other conditions such as mastitis, fibrocystic disease, premenstruation, and hormonal changes.

Urinary Frequency

During the first trimester of pregnancy, the uterus is enlarging within the confines of the pelvic area. As enlargement occurs, pressure is exerted on the bladder, creating an increased desire to urinate. Relief from this sensation is obtained when the uterus rises out of the pelvic cavity at about 12 weeks gestation, becoming an abdominal organ. During the last six weeks of pregnancy, the presenting part of the fetus dips down into the pelvic area, once again creating an increased desire to urinate.

Fatigue

The pregnant woman will often report periods of fatigue throughout pregnancy. The increasing level of progesterone is thought to be a contributing factor. Fatigue may also be present for many reasons other than pregnancy.

Chadwick's Sign

Chadwick's sign is the bluish discoloration of the vulva and vaginal linings seen at about the sixth week of pregnancy. It is caused by increased vascularity and edema of the vaginal area. Vascularity may also be increased in conditions related to uterine and vaginal growths.

Pigmentation Changes

Throughout pregnancy many changes in pigmentation occur owing to increasing levels of estrogen and progesterone. These increased hormones stimulate the anterior pituitary to produce melanocyte-stimulating hormone. This results in production of increased melanin deposits in the skin and consequently pigmentation changes. Most noticeable are the formation of *chloasma* (mask of pregnancy) at about 16 weeks and the appearance of the *linea nigra* at about 12 weeks. Neither of these changes are caused exclusively by effects of pregnancy. Chloasma is sometimes present with oral contraceptive use. It may also occur with liver dysfunction.

PROBABLE SIGNS OF PREGNANCY

Goodell's Sign

At approximately six to eight weeks of pregnancy the increased levels of progesterone and estrogen promote vascular congestion of the cervix and stimulate growth of the cervical glands. The cervical area develops a typically soft consistency known as Goodell's sign. This consistency is described as similar to the feeling when the lips are palpated. In the nonpregnant woman the tip of the cervix feels like the tip of the nose. Goodell's sign may not be present if the woman has uterine fibroids or if she has had a previous infection that caused hypertrophic inflammatory changes. Other forms of pelvic congestion may also cause Goodell's sign.

Hegar's Sign

Softening of the lower uterine segment as early as six weeks gestation is called Hegar's sign. The physiologic basis for this sign is increased uterine edema promoted by the increase of estrogen and progesterone. Upon examination, the isthmus of the uterus may be compressed between the examiner's external hand applied on the uterus and the internal examining finger (see Fig. 10–2). Although this sign is considered one of the more reliable signs of pregnancy, it is classified only as a probable sign.

Uterine and Abdominal Enlargement

During the fourth and fifth month of pregnancy the external manifestations become apparent. The uterus increases in size and creates a larger abdominal expanse. This abdominal enlargement, called showing, is only a probable sign, since other conditions such as tumors, obesity, and ascites may be the cause.

Ballottement

As the fetus develops within the amniotic sac, it has a considerable amount of freedom of

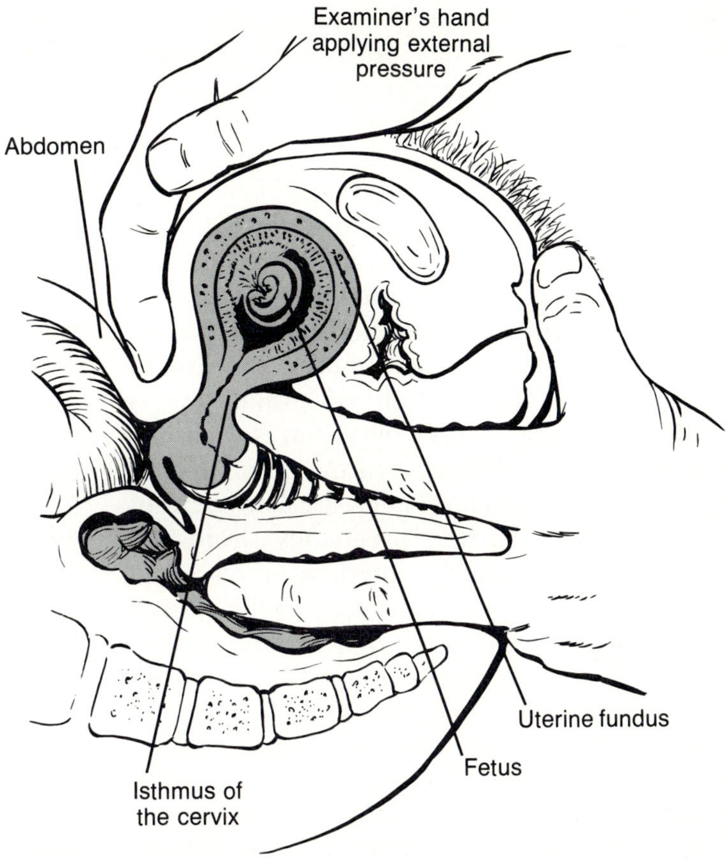

FIGURE 10-2. Examination for assessment of Hegar's sign during pregnancy.

movement, made possible by the amniotic fluid. At approximately the 16th week of gestation, if the examiner places her hand externally on the uterus and administers an abrupt rap, the fetus will move away from the examiner's hand and then rebound back. This is termed *ballottement*. Tumors may also produce the same effect; therefore ballottement is considered a probable sign of pregnancy.

Braxton Hicks' Contractions

Painless uterine contractions that begin early in pregnancy but are not usually noticed by the mother until approximately the seventh month are called Braxton Hicks' contractions. These contractions are a normal phenomena throughout pregnancy in spite of the fact that their physiologic basis is not known. Some mothers will be very aware of these contractions while others will not even notice them. The examiner will feel these as an external tightening of the abdominal wall. They are considered only a probable sign, since intestinal movements may produce similar sensations.

Palpating Fetal Contours

The examiner may be able to determine the contours of the fetus by externally feeling the configurations of the fetus through the abdominal wall as early as the fifth month of pregnancy. Asking the mother where she feels the fetus kicking will aid in determination of the position of the fetal parts. Myomas and abdominal growths may simulate the fetal outline. Palpating the contours of the supposed fetus is considered only a probable sign.

Pregnancy Tests

Improvements in pregnancy testing in the last few years have made them more reliable and less expensive. Today pregnancy testing may be done even before the first missed period. This allows early initiation of prenatal care. In cases where termination of pregnancy is desired, early pregnancy detection is desirable to allow safer termination of the pregnancy.

Various methods have been used throughout the years to diagnose pregnancy, from the "blush of pregnancy" experienced by some women, to the injection of mice, rabbits, and frogs with the urine of pregnant women (*bioassay testing*). Early pregnancy tests, used from the 1930s to the 1960s (Ascheim-Zondek and Friedman test), were based on the presence of human chorionic gonadotropin (HCG) in the pregnant woman's urine. When the urine was injected into laboratory animals, it stimulated the ovarian follicle maturation of the animal. Unfortunately, the test was not reliable until at least 14 days after the first missed menstrual period and was subject to the physiologic fluctuations of the experimental animals. The mother was required to wait as long as five days for the results of an unreliable test.

In the 1950s another type of pregnancy test, based on the presence of withdrawal bleeding following a prescribed course of estrogen and progesterone, was used. The hormones were given to stimulate the growth of the endometrial tissue of the uterus. If the woman was not pregnant, she would begin her menstrual period within 10 to 15 days after the hormones were discontinued. If she was pregnant, the withdrawal of the hormones would have no effect on the endometrial lining, since the corpus luteum, stimulated by the production of HCG, would continue to produce hormones needed for endometrial retention. Acceptable results were realized with this type of testing but acceptable effects were not. These hormones were found to produce fetal anomalies. In 1973 the Food and Drug Administration banned the use of hormones for pregnancy testing.

Current methods of pregnancy testing include home pregnancy tests, immunologic pregnancy tests (agglutination inhibitors test), radioimmunoassay, and radioreceptor assay. All these tests depend on the detection of HCG.

The *immunologic test* uses HCG antibodies produced by laboratory animals previously sensitized by HCG. The antibodies are extracted and processed for laboratory use. This test requires only one drop of maternal urine, which is then combined with HCG antiserum and latex-coated HCB. If the client is not pregnant, a clumping (agglutination) of the materials will occur. If pregnancy is present, no clumping will occur. The test may be read within two minutes. The same test may be performed by substitutions of HCG-coated red blood cells of sheep (Pagana & Pagana, 1982). This test produces the same results with more accuracy, but takes two hours to obtain results.

Radioimmunoassay and *radioreceptor assay* are both completed within one hour and are 90 to 95 percent accurate. Very small amounts of HCG can be measured in the blood as early as eight days following conception.

Home pregnancy tests are available which may be used for determination of pregnancy as early as 3 days after a missed period. These tests are also based on the presence of HCG in the woman's urine. When doing the test, the first morning urine (urine accumulated in the bladder for at least six hours) is used. Urine as directed by the manufacturer is added to the glass test tube which contains HCG on erythrocytes and HCG antiserum. A buffer solution is added to the urine in the test tube, shaken and allowed to sit for 45 minutes. Following the indicated time span the results may be read according to the directions. Home pregnancy tests have an accuracy of over 90.0%.

Despite the fact that pregnancy tests are very accurate, they are not considered positive signs of pregnancy. According to Fischbach

(1984), positive pregnancy tests also result from other conditions, including hydatidiform mole, chorioepithelioma, lung cancer, colon cancer, pancreatic cancer, stomach cancer, and choriocarcinoma. Tests that are falsely positive are seen in women taking certain medications, including some tranquilizers, antiparkinson medications, hypnotics, and anticonvulsants. They may also be positive in conditions associated with hematuria and albuminuria. Any condition that results in elevation of HCG will give a positive result.

False negative results are associated with diluted urine specimens that have a specific gravity of less than 1.005. If the test is run too early in pregnancy, before the trophoblastic activity has increased the HCG level, the test will also be negative. The incidence of false-negative results is greater than that of false-positives. Nursing responsibilities include educating the client on proper collection of the urine specimen.

POSITIVE SIGNS OF PREGNANCY

Auscultation of Fetal Heart Tones (FHT) by the Examiner

The fetal heartbeat may be heard as early as 10 weeks gestation, when a Doppler (see Chapter 16) is used. When using a fetoscope or stethoscope, the FHT are not audible until about 18 weeks. As the examiner assesses the FHT, he or she must be able to distinguish between the fetal heartbeat, the maternal heartbeat, the funic souffle, and the uterine souffle. The fetal heartbeat is a clear clicking sound produced at a rate of 120 to 160 bpm. The funic souffle is the pulsation of blood through the arteries of the umbilical cord and has the same rate and rhythm of the fetal heartbeat; it is heard as a whistling sound. The maternal heartbeat is auscultated on occasion and may be mistaken for the fetal heartbeat. If the maternal pulse rate is checked and found to be the same rate as the heart sounds being heard, only the maternal heartbeat has been heard. The uterine souffle (bruit) is the sound of the blood passing through the blood vessels of the uterus and is the same rate as the maternal pulse.

Fetal Movement Felt by the Examiner

The examiner may be able to feel fetal movements by the 18th week of pregnancy. Fetal movement is often ascertained while obtaining the FHR, owing to the stimulation of fetal movement by the slight pressure of the fetoscope.

X-ray and Ultrasound Verification

Visualization of the fetus by x-ray will give a positive diagnosis of pregnancy. This is not commonly recommended because of the potential harmful effects of radiation on the fetus. If x-ray becomes necessary, the earliest identification of fetal bone is the 16th week.

Ultrasonography (see Fig. 10–3) produces the visualization of the reflection of ultrasonic waves and will give an image of the fetus. This method has little or no effect on the fetus and is considered safer than x-ray. In 1984 the National Institutes of Health recommended that routine ultrasound not be used during pregnancy. Ultrasound usage was recommended when it was warranted for medical or obstetrical reasons. Ultrasound is used at

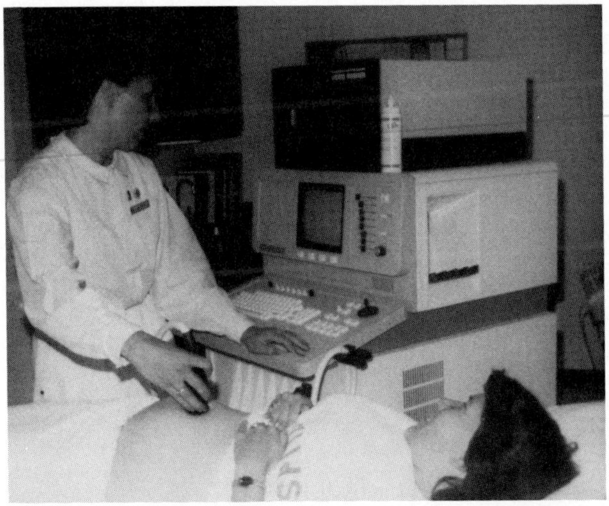

FIGURE 10–3. Ultrasound.

least once on 15 to 40 percent of all pregnant women (NAACOG, 1984). Current recommendations suggest accurate record keeping including the length, frequency, and intensity of each ultrasound exposure. The use of ultrasonography is discussed in Chapter 24.

The presumptive, probable, and positive signs of pregnancy are seen in Table 10–3. The signs and symptoms of pregnancy according to gestational occurrence are listed in Table 10–4.

PHYSICAL ASSESSMENTS OF PREGNANCY

Following the initial interview, the client history assessment, and an assessment of the signs and symptoms of the client, the physical examination is done.

The client is escorted to a private examining room, where she is instructed to remove her clothing and change into a gown. She is offered the opportunity to void and instructed to save the specimen. Sufficient time is allowed for the client to accomplish these tasks without embarrassing interruptions. It is equally important not to leave the client sitting for too long.

The nurse explains that a general examination will be done including breast assessments, along with a pelvic examination. The client is told that laboratory samples will be taken if desired by the examiner. The nurse explains that a complete physical examination will not be done at each prenatal visit once baseline parameters are obtained. Components of the physical examination are found in Table 10–1.

ASSESSMENT OF VITAL SIGNS

Maternal temperature, pulse, and respirations are recorded. Any elevation of temperature or deviation in pulse or respiratory rates are further evaluated.

Blood Pressure Assessment

Careful monitoring of maternal blood pressure is essential throughout pregnancy. Ideally, the prepregnant B/P has been obtained for a baseline; if it has not, the B/P at the first prenatal visit is used as the baseline for future comparisons.

Three factors are important when determining maternal blood pressure. First, the client should be made as comfortable as possible. Second, the B/P is taken with the client in a left lateral or sitting position. Third, the B/P cuff must be the correct size.

B/P taken when the client is hurried or anxious may cause elevations. If she is allowed a few minutes after arriving at the office to relax before taking the B/P, false elevations will be avoided. If the B/P is above the normal range, allow the client to relax for a 10-minute period, and then recheck the B/P.

The left lateral or sitting posture provides

TABLE 10–3
PRESUMPTIVE, PROBABLE, AND POSITIVE SIGNS OF PREGNANCY

Presumptive	Probable	Positive
Amenorrhea	Abdominal enlargement	Auscultation of FHT by examiner
Breast changes	Ballottement	Fetal movements felt by examiner
Chadwick's sign	Braxton-Hicks' contractions	X-ray and/or ultrasound verification
Fatigue	Goodell's sign	
Pigmentation changes	Hegar's sign	
Chloasma	Palpating fetal contours	
Linea nigra	Pregnancy test	
Quickening	Uterine enlargement	
Urinary frequency		

TABLE 10-4
MONTHLY SIGNS AND SYMPTOMS OF PREGNANCY

First Month

Amenorrhea—first missed period
Nausea and vomiting
Frequent urination
Breast tenderness
Feeling of fullness of breasts

Second Month

Frequent urination
Morning sickness
Breast vascularity
Hegar's sign
Food cravings
Slight vaginal spotting
Braxton-Hicks' contractions
Goodell's sign
Chadwick's sign
Fatigue
Positive pregnancy test
FHT heard with doppler
Ptyalism
Decreased libido

Third Month

Abdomen enlarged
Colostrum secretion
Breast pigmentation changes
Increased pigmentation
Linea nigra
Urinary frequency—gone
Uterus level with symphysis pubis
Tubercles of Montgomery
Morning sickness gone
Dizziness

Fourth Month

Chloasma
Ballottement
Showing
Fundus midway between symphysis and umbilicus
Gums bleed
Increase in "hot flashes"
Mood changes begin
Laryngeal congestion—voice changes

Fifth Month

FHT heard by examiner with stethoscope
Quickening
Varicosities
Stretch marks appear
Fundus level with umbilicus
Heartburn
Increase in libido
Increase in hair follicle activity

Sixth Month

Fundus is 1 finger above umbilicus
Fetal contours felt by examiner
Mother feels fetus kick
Ligament stretching felt by mother
Varicosities

Seventh Month

Vascular spiders
Nosebleeds
Hemorrhoids
Constipation
Flatulence
Decrease in libido
Fundus midway between the xyphoid process and umbilicus

Eighth Month

Muscle cramps
Ankle edema
Pruritis
Leukorrhea
Paresthesias
Insomnia
Increased colostrum
Fundus four fingers below the xyphoid process

Ninth Month

Shortness of breath
Backache
Fundus is one finger below the xyphoid process

Tenth Month

Lordosis
Urinary frequency
Ankle edema increased
Fundus three to four fingers below xyphoid process

more accurate measurements of B/P throughout pregnancy. Pressure measured in the brachial artery is highest when the client is in the sitting position. The left lateral position will give the lowest reading. The supine position is *not* recommended to avoid supine hypotension. A notation of the maternal position when the B/P was obtained is recorded along with the reading.

When maternal B/P readings are obtained, the same principles apply as in the nonpregnant client. The B/P cuff should be at least 20 percent wider than the diameter of the arm and is applied securely around the arm. If the cuff is too wide, a low reading will be obtained. A too-narrow cuff will give a false high reading.

Assessment of the B/P during pregnancy follows established criteria for evaluation. First, the prepregnancy or initial B/P reading is used as the basis for comparisons of subsequent readings. Second, an increase of 30 mm Hg or more over the systolic or an increase of 15 mm Hg or more over the diastolic, or both, is considered significant. Third, an absolute value of 140/90 mm Hg or greater is a significant indicator of a hypertensive disorder.

When these criteria are applied, screening of clients who are at increased risk for hypertensive disorders of pregnancy (see Chapter 25) can be identified. For instance, initial maternal B/P was 102/72. At the second prenatal visit, her B/P is 110/76. At 22 weeks gestation, her B/P is 122/90. This change from the initial B/P of 102/72 to 122/90, representing a 20 mm Hg rise in the systolic range, is considered within the normal range. The diastolic has risen 18 mm Hg, not within the normal range. Any significant rise in the maternal B/P necessitates further evaluation for hypertensive disease.

A simple screening test can identify mothers who are at increased risk for developing hypertensive disease in pregnancy. The "rollover" test (see Chapter 25) may be of value in identifying gravidas who need closer prenatal supervision and more specific education.

Clients frequently ask to be told their B/P readings. It is not acceptable to say "Ask your doctor" or "I'm not allowed to tell you." A simple direct answer followed by an open-ended question such as "Are you concerned about your B/P?" will provide a basis for communication and foster client-nurse relationships.

BREAST EXAMINATIONS

The breasts are examined at the initial prenatal visit, with emphasis placed on the contour and symmetry of the breast, vascularity, nipple condition, presence of any lumps, puckering of tissue, and pigmentation changes in the areola. If nipple discharge is noted, the cause should be determined. Colostrum secreted by the breast is considered normal. A discharge may be associated with breast cancer, ulcerations, or mastitis. The type of discharge is recorded, and is further evaluated.

The nipple is examined for the development of tubercles of Montgomery, cracks in the tissue, and nipple inversion. The areolae are somewhat darkened and enlarged during pregnancy. A warm or red breast may be an indication of infection.

The client is asked if she intends to breastfeed her newborn. She may not wish to make her decision at this time. If she is not sure, a discussion of the types of feeding available might be appropriate. Her final decision does not have to be made until the time of delivery. Instruction in the principles of good breast care is started at this time, regardless of the method of infant feeding chosen (see Chapter 11).

ABDOMINAL ASSESSMENT

Initial findings from the abdominal assessment depend on the stage of gestation at the first prenatal visit. At 12 weeks a line of dark pigmentation will appear extending from the symphysis pubis to the umbilicus. This is called the linea nigra and is considered normal during pregnancy. It is more noticeable in brunettes.

Stretch marks (*striae gravidarum*) appear on the abdomen, thighs, breasts, and buttocks of some pregnant women. Connective tissue changes that are influenced by estrogens and corticosteroids are thought to be responsible for the development of striae.

As the pregnancy progresses, abdominal configurations will change. Fundal height (height of the fundus of the uterus) is an important indication of the gestational age of the fetus. Assessment of fundal height is more accurate in determining gestational age than the menstrual history. Spotting and light menstrual periods sometimes are incorrectly interpreted and give an inaccurate estimate of the last normal menstrual period. After the 12th week of pregnancy, fundal height measurements may be made by palpating the abdomen with the palm of the hand. The symphysis pubis is identified and the top of the fundus is located. Using a centimeter measuring tape, the distance between the fundus and the symphysis is determined. Gestational age is then determined by using McDonald's rule.

McDonald's rule specifies than when determining the lunar month of gestation, the fundal height in centimeters is multiplied by 2/7. To determine the weeks of gestation, the fundal height in centimeters is multiplied by 8/7.

For a general estimate of gestational age, the following guidelines may be used: A fundal height of 12 cm is equivalent to 12 weeks of gestational age. A 16-week gestation is 16 cm; at 20 weeks the fundus is 20 cm and is even with the umbilicus.

After 26 weeks, fundal height measurement in centimeters is not accurate, and the following guidelines are used: At 28 weeks gestation the fundus is midway between the xyphoid process and the umbilicus. At 32 weeks gestation, the fundus is located four fingers below the xyphoid process. By 36 weeks, the fundus is one finger below the xyphoid process, and at term, the fundus is three to four fingers below the xyphoid process.

When fundal growth does not proceed at the expected rate, intrauterine growth retardation is suspected. Increases above the normal may indicate multiple gestation or polyhydramnios.

PELVIC EXAMINATION

Consideration for the woman's feelings is important during the pelvic examination. If the nurse has previously explained the procedure, her responsibilities now are to provide caring support for the client during the examination. For some women, this may be the first pelvic examination they have had. Other women approach the examination with reluctance for one reason or another. A gentle relaxed approach will make the examination more pleasant for the client. Explanations of what is being done during each step of the examination will alleviate anxiety and promote cooperation. Appropriate draping is important to eliminate embarrassment. The examination table should face away from the door. The client is placed in the lithotomy position, with her feet in stirrups and her buttocks at the edge of the examining table.

Inspection of the external genitalia is made, noting physical characteristics, odor, and discharge. An assessment is made of rashes, vesicles, inflammation, edema, lacerations, previous scarring, or growths. Hemorrhoids, if present, are noted. The Skene's and Bartholin's glands are palpated to determine enlargement or infection.

Before beginning the internal examination, the client is told that a vaginal speculum will be inserted. Warming the speculum by running it under warm water serves as acceptable lubrication. The proper size speculum is used and the labia gently separated by the examiner's fingers as the speculum is inserted. Proper insertion of the speculum requires the introduction of the blades closed and directed upward toward the sacrococcygeal area (see Fig. 10-4). The inserted speculum is then opened, making visualization of the vagina and cervix possible.

While the examiner has been inserting the

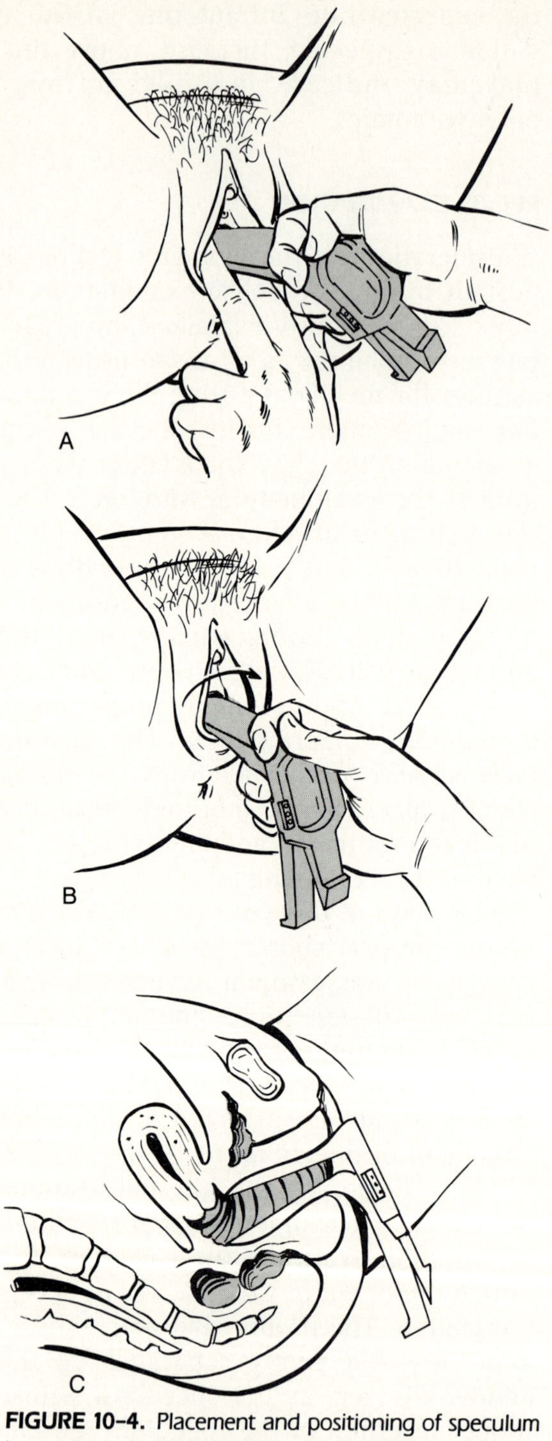

FIGURE 10-4. Placement and positioning of speculum in vagina: A. Introduction of speculum in closed, oblique position directed toward sacrococcygeal area. B. Speculum turned to horizontal position. C. Speculum in open position exposing cervix and vaginal mucosa.

speculum, the nurse assists the patient to relax. Alternately tensing and relaxing the vaginal and rectal area a few times just before insertion may make the insertion more comfortable for the client. Asking her to take slow deep breaths as she allows her body to become flaccid will assist her to relax. It may be appropriate to hold her hand as you offer support and encouragement.

Cervical inspection determines any cervical irregularities, cervical dilatation, lesions, ulcerations, infections, or growths. The vagina is observed for infections, discharge, growths, and color. Chadwick's sign is noted if present.

A Papanicolaou (Pap) smear is performed by gently scraping the endocervix and the squamocolumnar junction with a cotton applicator and a sterile tongue blade. A vaginal specimen is also taken for detection of gonorrhea. The client is informed that the tests were taken. She is told when and how she will receive the results.

After the speculum is removed, a bimanual examination is done. The gloved and lubricated index and middle fingers of the examiner are placed in the vagina, and the cervix, vaginal walls, fornix, and uterus are palpated. Any irregularities or normal variants are noted on the client's chart. With the fingers of the examining hand remaining in the vagina, the other hand is placed on the abdomen. Downward pressure is applied to bring the ovaries, fallopian tubes, and uterus into approximation with the internal fingers. Pain upon palpation is noted, as are any deviations from the normal.

The rectum is examined internally with the gloved index finger. Growths, hemorrhoids, pain, septa, fissures, herniations, and bleeding are noted.

Evaluation of the Bony Pelvis

The bony pelvis is assessed to determine adaptability of the pelvis for labor and delivery. Specific information obtained during clinical pelvimetry is discussed in Chapter 13.

On completion of the examination, the vaginal and perineal areas are wiped with a clean tissue to remove any lubricative materials. The client may then dress. An opportunity for discussion of the complete examination is provided.

LABORATORY ASSESSMENTS

Laboratory testing is a means of evaluating the health status of the pregnant woman and identifying potential risk. Determination of the tests to be performed is based on the client's history and physical examination. All tests are individualized and not done just as routine measures. To accurately interpret test results, familiarity with test results that are altered by pregnancy is needed.

Before the tests are performed, they are explained to the client. Results are presented to the client as soon as possible. Laboratory testing includes blood tests, urine tests, and cervical cultures.

BLOOD TESTS

Blood tests include hemoglobin and hematocrit determinations, differential, white blood cell counts, blood typing and Rh factor, antibody screening, rubella titer, blood sugar determination, and serology. Some alterations in normal blood values occur as a result of the physiologic changes of pregnancy.

Hemoglobin and Hematocrit

A hemoglobin below 11 gm/100 ml or a hematocrit below 34 percent, or both, indicate the possibility of anemia and the need for supplementary iron.

White Blood Cells

A white blood cell count over 15,000 mm^3 may indicate infection of blood dyscrasias. The normal value in the pregnant woman is between 5,000 and 12,000 mm^3. During pregnancy increased neutrophils elevate the white blood cell count.

Blood Typing and Rh Factor

If the mother's blood type is O or is Rh negative (or both), a potential exists for maternal-fetal blood incompatibility. If the father is known to have Rh positive blood or type A or B blood, further testing may be indicated.

Antibody Screening

The presence of antibodies indicates sensitization and formation of serum antibodies. The significance of the titer depends on the individual laboratory values. If Rh antibodies are present, repeat titers are done at intervals throughout pregnancy.

Rubella Titer

Rubella titers determine whether the mother is immune to the German measle virus. Titers of 1:10 or lower indicate a lack of effective immunity and should be repeated to verify the results. Immunization is not done during pregnancy.

Blood Sugar

Postprandial (after a meal) glucose levels over 140 mg per 100 ml indicate the possibility of diabetes and should be tested further.

Serology

A positive syphilis study indicates the presence of the spirochete Treponema pallidum. Treatment of the gravida should be initiated before the 18th week of pregnancy to prevent fetal damage. Alcohol consumed before the blood test can alter the results.

URINE TESTING

Urine is tested at each prenatal visit. Specific alterations sought include glycosuria, proteinuria, and bacteriuria. Glycosuria in the urine of 1+ or more indicates the need for blood sugar level determinations. Proteinuria of 1+ or more indicates the possibility of a urinary tract infection, kidney disease, or hypertensive disease of pregnancy. Bacteriuria indicates a urinary tract infection associated with an increased risk to the mother and fetus. Further discussion of glycosuria, proteinuria, and bacteriuria is found in Chapter 25.

Urine test results may be affected by various factors. Specimens contaminated by blood, vaginal discharge, and amniotic fluid may give positive protein readings. If the specimen is allowed to remain at room temperature for several hours after it has been obtained, false results may be obtained in some parameters. Contamination of the specimen by strong soaps or detergents may also alter the results. A clean catch midstream specimen (early morning) is preferred.

INITIAL PRENATAL ASSESSMENTS

After the collection of the information needed to establish a client data base, physical assessment is completed, and laboratory test results obtained, a diagnostic evaluation is made. Priority is given to any factors that might indicate potential or actual high-risk pregnancy. Although any pregnancy may become high-risk under adverse conditions, those known to be associated with complications have been identified (see Chapter 24) as medical, obstetrical, genetic, nutritional, and socioeconomic influences on pregnancy.

Analysis of the data and identification of problem areas serve as the basis for the diagnostic evaluation. A multiplicity of skills are needed by the nurse when applying the nursing process to formulate and actualize appropriate client goals. The nurse's theoretical knowledge base is applied to the accumulated data to identify and justify health care interventions. A blending of the physician's medical expertise and the nurse's expertise is essential. The final evaluation embodies these two professional judgments.

NURSE-CLIENT PARTICIPATORY MANAGEMENT

The health care plan formulated for the client represents a composite of the medical and nursing diagnostic evaluations and includes input made by the client. The nursing and obstetric diagnosis serves as the foundation for discussions with the client. Previously identified health management concerns are discussed. The nurse and the client determine together the desired health outcomes and the methods of achieving these goals. The need for any interventions or adjustments in health management is explained to the client. Efforts are made to determine the client's level of understanding and to guide her as she sets her own goals for good prenatal care.

Together the nurse and client discuss the need for ongoing health assessments throughout the pregnancy. Plans are made for scheduling office or clinic visits. At this time it is explained that for the first 32 weeks, monthly visits are needed. From 32 to 36 weeks, biweekly visits are planned, and weekly visits are scheduled for the last four weeks gestation.

Since the initial prenatal visit may be lengthy and comprehensive, it is important to inform the client that future visits will not be as involved, nor will they last as long. A complete physical is not done at each visit, but weight checks, B/P readings, fundal measurements, FHR assessments, urine specimen evaluations and general assessments are made at each subsequent visit. The client's partner or support person is encouraged to attend any or all visits. Special emphasis is placed on the supportive role of the nurse if she and the client are to share in continued evaluation of maternal health care. It is not enough for the client to know she will be "checked" at each visit. She needs to know that the nurse is committed to effective care, encompassing the role of consultant, teacher, care provider, and client advocate and that these services are available whenever needed.

In the teaching role, the nurse has provided information and shared her knowledge throughout the initial visit. She now encourages the client to continue her prenatal learning experience. This may be accomplished by attending prenatal or childbirth preparation classes. Times, dates, and content of these classes are described to the client and assistance is given for registration. For some, these classes are not the desired method of learning. Individual learning needs are assessed and addressed at each prenatal visit.

As the client completes the visit, she should leave with her own commitment to continued prenatal care. Feelings of trust and faith in her health care provider should be well established.

BIBLIOGRAPHY

Aladjem, S. & Brown, A. *Clinical perinatology*. St. Louis: Mosby, 1974.

Babson, S., Benson, R., Pernoll, M. & Benda, G. *Management of high-risk pregnancy and intensive care of the neonate*. St. Louis: Mosby, 1975.

Benson, R. *Handbook of obstetrics and gynecology*. Los Altos, Calif.: Lange, 1977.

Cranley, M. Perinatal risk. *Journal of Obstetric, Gynecological, & Neonatal Nursing*, 1983, **12**, 13s–18s.

Drukker, J. Antenatal assessment—part I: Maternal profile. *NAACOG Update Series*, 1983, **1**.

Edwards, L.E., et al. Pregnancy in the underweight woman: Course, outcome, and growth patterns of the infant. *American Journal of Obstetrics & Gynecology*, 1979, **135**, 297.

Fischbach, F. *A manual of laboratory diagnostic tests*. Philadelphia: Lippincott, 1984.

Gant, N.F., Chand, S., Worley, R., et al. A clinical test useful for predicting the development of acute hypertension in pregnancy. *American Journal of Obstetrics & Gynecology*, 1974, **120**, 1-7.

Gusdon, J., Anderson, S. & May, W. A clinical evaluation of the "roll-over" test: for pregnancy-induced hypertension. *American Journal of Obstetrics & Gynecology*, 1977, **127**, 1-3.

Kasser, N., et al. Roll-over test. *Obstetrics & Gynecology*, 1980, **55**, 411-413.

Marshall, G. & Neuman, R. Roll-over test. *American Journal of Obstetrics & Gynecology*, 1977, **127**, 623-625.

NAACOG Newsletter: NIH Panel suggest ultrasound limits. *National Institute of Child Health and Human Development*, 1984, **11**, 2.

Pagana, K. & Pagana, T. *Diagnostic testing and nursing implications: A case study approach*. St. Louis: Mosby, 1982.

Page, E., Villee, C. & Villee, D. *Human reproduction*. Philadelphia: Saunders, 1976.

Reeder, S., Mastroianni, L. & Martin, L. *Maternity nursing*. Philadelphia: Lippincott, 1983.

Roberts, J. & Engel, A. Family background, early development, and intelligence of children aged 6-11 years. *National Health Survey*, Series 11, No. 142, 1974.

Task Force on Adolescent Pregnancy: *Adolescent perinatal health: A guidebook for services*. Chicago: The American College of Obstetricians and Gynecologists, 1979.

chapter 11

NURSING MANAGEMENT IN THE ANTEPARTAL PERIOD

OBJECTIVES

Upon completion of this chapter, the reader will be able to:

1. Explain the relationship between maternal weight gain and fetal well-being.
2. List factors that place the client at nutritional risk during pregnancy.
3. Develop a daily diet plan containing all essential nutrients needed in the diet of the pregnant woman.
4. Cite factors that alter the absorption of iron.
5. Give examples of cultural influences that may alter the diet of a pregnant woman.
6. Discuss health management of the pregnant woman regarding rest, exercise, employment, and hygiene.
7. Describe care of the breast during the antepartal period for breastfeeding and nonbreastfeeding mothers.
8. Discuss sexuality during pregnancy and the role of the nurse when providing counseling.
9. Explain the effects of alcohol and smoking on fetal well-being.
10. Explain the important aspects of counseling the gravida in the use of caffeine during pregnancy.
11. Relate principles of health management that are used in the gravida experiencing the following minor discomforts: backache, nausea and vomiting, heartburn, constipation, varicosities, hemorrhoids, leg cramps, supine hypotension, dyspnea, and itching.
12. List the danger signals of pregnancy.
13. Discuss the role of siblings and grandparents in the childbearing event.
14. Describe the schedule used when planning continued prenatal visits for the pregnant woman.
15. Describe the nursing responsibilities involved in the care of the expectant mother at each prenatal visit.

KEY TERMS

Food allergy
Food intolerance
Nutritional risk
Overweight
Palmar erythema
Pica
Ptyalism
Pyrosis
Spider nevi
Underweight
Vegetarian

Nursing management during the antepartal period involves applying the principles of nursing care to the management of the specific client. Nursing care given without management principles is pointless and ineffective. Clients are multidimensional individuals, with varying needs and stressors. To provide nursing care that only meets basic physical needs fails to address the total person. Nursing management focuses on providing care for the client that responds to all of her needs in a mutually agreeable manner. The vehicle that directs nursing management is the nursing process. Working within the framework of the nursing process, the nurse is able to assist the client to achieve realistic goals.

The nurse cannot simply tell the client what to do; she must help her to manage her maternity care at the primary, secondary, and tertiary levels. She must also help the client understand the need for medical and nursing interventions and to make decisions that will optimize her own health management.

Ongoing assessment and individualized management of the client are continued throughout pregnancy. Continuity of care is insured when initial assessments are used as a data base to formulate the nursing diagnoses and written plan of care. At each visit, assessments are made and the nursing care plan is updated. The concept of using nursing care plans is as essential in the outpatient setting as it is in the hospital. Nursing care for any client is lacking if the nursing process is not operational.

Appropriate nursing management during the antepartal period is based on knowledge of the principles of antepartal care. This knowledge is an embodiment of physiologic, psychological, sociocultural, spiritual, and developmental concepts and their relationship to pregnancy.

NUTRITION DURING PREGNANCY

The nutritional foundation established before birth contributes to the future health of the individual. Nutritional influences interact with genetic, hormonal, and environmental factors to determine growth and development of each individual. It is known that the growth and development of a fetus can be accelerated or compromised by its nutritive environment. The task of providing this nutritive environment is assumed by the mother. Malnutrition in infancy is often caused by a lack of maternal nutritional knowledge or her failure to identify the importance of nutrition during the antepartum period.

A significant amount of research has been done in the area of fetal malnutrition. Results imply that impaired nutrition at the cellular level interferes with *hyperplasia* (increased cell division) and *hypertrophy* (increased cell growth). Subnormal organ weight caused by hyperplastic cell retardation is not reversible, regardless of future optimal nutrition. Hypertrophic cell growth involves the enlargement of existing cells. Impairment of this growth is somewhat reversible. Proper nutrition will ultimately result in normal increased growth of the cells.

Growth of the fetus proceeds in a specific pattern of 1) a period of hyperplasic growth only, 2) followed by a period of hyperplasic and hypertrophic growth, and 3) a period of hypertrophic growth only. Deficiencies at any of these three periods may result in growth alterations.

Nutritional Risk Factors

Good nutritional habits are formed almost from the moment of birth. Cultural, familial, and religious influences contribute significantly to these habits. As the individual grows, alterations in dietary habits are made according to individual food preferences, economic factors, and lifestyle. People do not always eat to sustain life but sometimes as an expression of psychological influences. Circumstances in life may also dictate alterations in nutritional habits. These factors contribute to the dietary pattern established before pregnancy. If nutritional habits and status have been good before pregnancy they are apt to remain so during the antepartal period.

Certain factors identify individuals at nutritional risk during pregnancy. These factors include: adolescent pregnancy, low prepregnancy weight related to height, increased parity, smoking, obesity, low socioeconomic level, failure to gain weight during pregnancy, pregnancy complications, special dietary restrictions, inadequate nutritional base, disorders that influence nutritional status (alcoholism, drug addiction, tuberculosis, asthma, diabetes mellitus, infection), a history of previous low birth weight neonates, and abnormal cravings.

Nutritional Management

Nutritional requirements during pregnancy differ from the requirements of the nonpregnant woman in total nutrients and quality. The pregnant woman needs to increase overall nutrition to meet the demands of the pregnancy and those of the fetus. She is not necessarily eating for two, but she is providing nutrition for two. Attention to nutritional needs must be a daily focus. Patterns of fasting, overeating, avoiding essential nutrients, or indulging in favorite foods are not consistent with good antepartal nutrition. The gravida must be made aware of the needed nutrients and their importance to her welfare and the welfare of her baby.

CALORIES

During pregnancy the metabolic needs of the pregnant woman are increased. This increase, coupled with placental development and growth needs of the fetus, requires more calories in the daily diet. To meet these demands, the woman must consume 80,000 kcal during the entire pregnancy. This results in a daily increase of 300 kcal for the gravida.

Variations in daily needs may be attributed to the activity and lifestyle of the individual woman. Those with sedentary lifestyles will not need as many calories to maintain a steady weight gain as those who are very active. The weight gain should be at the rate of 0.5 to 1 pound per week, with approximately 4 pounds in the first trimester, 10 to 12 pounds in the second trimester, and about 8 to 10 pounds in the third trimester. Failure to gain the average amount of weight during pregnancy increases the risk of both maternal and fetal complications. A positive correlation exists between maternal weight gain during pregnancy and neonatal birth weight.

PROTEINS

Since every cell of the body contains protein, the need for an adequate supply of protein throughout life is constant. These proteins must contain a sufficient amount of amino acids (complete proteins) to facilitate growth and development. The pregnant woman needs protein to maintain and replace body tissue, to accommodate placental growth, to produce amniotic fluid, and to increase circulating blood volume. At the same time, the fetus demands proteins to meet his growth and development requirements.

The Food and Nutrition Board of the National Research Council (NRC) recommends a daily intake of 44 gm protein, with an additional 30 gm for the pregnant woman, bringing the daily requirement to 74 gm per day. The adolescent, owing to her own growth demands, needs a greater amount of protein daily (6.1 gm/kg body weight/day).

Protein Sources

Protein may be found in the following food sources:

Complete proteins (should comprise at least 2/3 of the total daily requirement):
- Milk: 9 gm/8 ounce serving
- Cottage cheese: 5 gm/ounce
- Eggs: 6 gm/egg
- Meat, poultry, fish: 15 to 25 gm/3 ounce cooked serving
- American cheese: 7 gm/ounce

Incomplete proteins
- Peanut butter: 4 gm/tbsp
- Rice: 4 gm/cup
- Bread: 2 to 3 gm/slice
- Dried peas or beans: 14 gm/cup
- Pasta: 4 gm/cup

An example of daily protein intake that meets the daily requirement would be:

Four glasses of whole or skim milk	36 gm
1 egg	6 gm
1 3 oz serving of meat	15 gm
1 cup rice	4 gm
3 T peanut butter	12 gm
2 slices bread	4 gm
	77 gm protein

Vegetarian diets require substitutions of protein food, depending upon the type of vegetarian diet the client follows. The *lacto-ovovegetarian* diet omits meat, but this basic vegetarian diet is supplemented with milk, eggs, and cheese. The *lactovegetarian* diet omits meat and eggs, but milk products are included. A *vegan* diet eliminates all dairy products, eggs, meats, and animal products. Substitutions at a meal may be made by using combinations of legumes and whole grain cereals, legumes and nuts, or whole grain cereals and nuts. In the *fruitarian* diet, only dried fruits, honey, olive oil, and nuts are eaten. With this diet it is very difficult to meet the daily protein requirements.

CARBOHYDRATES

Carbohydrates are one of the fuel-producing nutrients needed for energy. They are found in sugars and starches mainly derived from plant sources. One of their main functions is to assist in the regulation of protein metabolism by their protein-sparing action. An adequate amount of carbohydrates in the diet of the pregnant woman allows protein to be utilized for the growth and development needs of the fetus, and not for the energy needs of the mother.

Carbohydrates also have an antiketogenic effect, which means that when they are present in adequate amounts less fat is broken down for energy. During pregnancy, when carbohydrates are not available, fats are readily broken down, causing an increase in ketone bodies that may have potentially adverse effects on the fetus. A constant, adequate amount of carbohydrates will deter the process.

The nervous systems of both the fetus and the mother require a constant supply of glucose. Without adequate glucose, brain and nervous tissues are incapable of functioning or developing. The need for carbohydrates is more pronounced in the last trimester, when the fetus is increasing in weight.

Carbohydrate Sources

Carbohydrates are plentiful and may be found in most food substances. Good sources of carbohydrates are:

Whole milk (8 oz)		12 gm
Vegetables:	Potato (med)	22 gm
	Corn (1/2 c)	16 gm
	Lima beans (1/2 c)	15 gm
Fruits:	Banana (medium)	34 gm
	Orange (large)	26 gm
	Raisins (1 c)	113 gm
Breads:	Whole wheat (1 sl)	12 gm
	White (1 sl)	12 gm
Whole grain:	Oatmeal (3/4 c)	20 gm

The Food and Nutrition Board of the National Research Council recommends that 48 percent of the total caloric intake be provided from the naturally occurring sugars such as sucrose, fructose, lactose in milk, and glucose in fruits. They also recommend that not more than 10 percent of the caloric intake be derived from refined sugars such as cane and beet sugars.

FATS

Fats are needed in the diet as a stored source of energy, for protective thermoregulation, synthesis of specific hormones, cell metabolism, and transportation and absorption of fat-soluble vitamins. They provide a more concentrated form of energy, supplying twice as many calories as a like amount of carbohydrates. Although it is recommended that 25 percent of the total daily caloric intake be provided by fats, the average American diet provides 40 to 45 percent. During pregnancy, the same percentage of caloric intake should be provided by fats as in the nonpregnant woman. The following foods are examples of those which may be used to obtain the daily fat requirement:

Butter (1 Tbsp)	100 cal
Egg (1 medium)	77 cal
Nuts: pecans (2 Tbsp)	104 cal
Cream (1 Tbsp)	50 cal
Avocado (1/2 small)	245 cal
Oyster (6 medium)	356 cal
Hamburger patty (1)	246 cal

CALCIUM

Calcium has a diversity of functions within the human body. It is needed for the formation and maintenance of the skeletal system, formation of the teeth, myocardial contraction and relaxation, neuromuscular stability, blood coagulation, and cell wall permeability. It is equally as important in fetal development, especially during the last two months of pregnancy when calcification of bones is occurring. The total amount needed by the fetus during in utero development is 28 gm. When calcium intake is not sufficient, demineralization of the maternal skeleton will occur in order to meet fetal needs. This is not only detrimental to the maternal skeletal system but will also adversely affect the storage of maternal calcium needed for lactation.

The recommended daily requirement of calcium is 1200 mg, an increase of 400 mg over the normal daily requirement. This requirement is not sufficient to meet the needs of the pregnant adolescent, who requires 1600 mg daily.

PHOSPHORUS

Phosphorus is needed for almost every bodily function. Some of its key roles are: participation in the acid-base buffer system, combining with fat to form phospholipids, enhancing intestinal absorption of glucose, participation in the structuring of DNA and RNA, and with calcium, mineralization of teeth and bones.

Calcium and phosphorus are so intricately linked that consideration of one necessitates consideration of the other. The recommended dietary ratio of calcium to phosphorus is 1:1. Both of these minerals are adequately supplied in milk. The daily requirement is the same as that of calcium—1200 mg daily.

Greater amounts of phosphorus are absorbed than calcium from the diet. This is significant when there is increased milk consumption. Milk contains more phosphorus proportionately than it does calcium. This results in an imbalance in the ratio of phosphorus to calcium and may precipitate leg cramps.

Milk, one of the primary sources of calcium and phosphorus, should not be eliminated from the diet either because of dislike or because of leg cramps. If leg cramps are bothersome, milk intake may be limited to two pints per day rather than the recommended one quart per day. The remainder of the calcium and phosphorus requirement would then be met by increasing the servings of meat, and eating foods rich in calcium (oysters, raisins, broccoli).

When the calcium requirement is deficient because of a dislike for milk, the same substitutes may be made, although some milk (at least 2 pints/day) should be included in the diet. In this instance, attention is focused on using milk in the preparation of soups, puddings, custards, milkshakes, and limited amounts of ice cream.

Calcium and Phosphorus Sources

Calcium and phosphorus sources can be considered together. Adequate sources of both minerals are:

Milk (8 oz whole)	291 mg calcium 228 mg phosphorus
Green beans (1 c)	63 mg calcium 46 mg phosphorus
Broccoli (1 cup)	136 mg calcium 96 mg phosphorus
American cheese (1 oz)	174 mg calcium 211 mg phosphorus
Ground beef (3 oz lean)	10 mg calcium 196 mg phosphorus
Raisins (1 cup)	90 mg calcium 146 mg phosphorus
Sunflower seeds (1 cup)	174 mg calcium 1214 mg phosphorus
Oysters (1 cup)	226 mg calcium 343 mg phosphorus

IRON

Although the amount of iron required by the body for proper functioning is very small, it is essential for the formation of hemoglobin in the red blood cells to transport oxygen to the cells.

In nonpregnant women, the daily requirement for iron is 18 mg, compared with 10 mg for men. This difference is attributed to the losses experienced during menses. During pregnancy, iron requirements are further increased owing to an increase in maternal erythropoiesis and fetal demands and storage in the fetal liver. These increased requirements cannot be met in the diet; therefore, it is recommended by the Committee on Maternal Nutrition that the diet be supplemented daily with 30 to 60 mg of iron. Iron supplements are not given during the first trimester, as they may contribute to nausea and vomiting.

To enhance the utilization and absorption of iron within the body, several factors are considered: (1) vitamin C enhances the absorption of iron; (2) calcium in the diet removes certain elements (phosphate, oxalate and phytate) that hinder iron absorption; (3) when infection is present, less iron is absorbed by the intestinal mucosa; (4) during periods of rapid growth, pregnancy, and anemia, more iron is absorbed by the intestinal mucosa; (5) the acidic environment of the stomach promotes the formation of soluble ferrous iron in preparation for intestinal absorption; (6) iron is made available to the body for use not only from dietary sources but from bodily reserves; and (7) fetal needs for iron will be met before maternal needs.

The disproportionate rise during pregnancy of blood plasma volume over red cell volume reduces the erythrocyte count, and hematocrit and hemoglobin concentrations. As a result, the hemoglobin and hematocrit levels will be lowered, causing a pseudoanemia. Normal pregnancy hematocrit levels are 32 to 42 percent as compared with the nonpregnant levels of 37 to 47 percent. Hemoglobin levels during pregnancy are 10 to 14 gm/100 ml compared with the nonpregnant level of 12 to 16 gm/100 ml. The pregnant woman who has a ready reserve of iron and who maintains an adequate dietery intake is not jeopardized by this physiologic anemia. She needs only the recommended daily supplement of iron to maintain her hematocrit and hemoglobin levels. The women who enters pregnancy with low iron reserves and has an inadequate iron intake will have difficulty meeting the increased needs for iron imposed by pregnancy. She will be at risk for developing iron deficiency anemia, with a consequent increased incidence of infection, preterm labor, abortion, and neonatal anemia.

Iron Sources

The following example illustrates the content of iron in selected plant and animal sources:

Liver (1 1/2 oz)	4.5 mg
Oysters (raw) (1/2 cup)	6.7 mg
Raisins (1 cup)	5.3 mg
Hamburger patty	2.7 mg
Turkey (3 slices)	5.0 mg
Green beans (1 cup)	2.1 mg
Watermelon (1 slice)	1.2 mg
Banana (1 large)	1.2 mg
Egg (1)	1.3 mg
Bologna (1 slice)	1.6 mg

ZINC

Zinc is one of the trace elements of the body whose significance has been long overlooked. It participates in the synthesis of DNA and RNA, is essential for enzyme action, necessary for utilization of vitamin A, and assists in the maintenance of acid-base balance. It is found in almost every tissue of the body, but concentrations are increased in eye tissue, liver, bone, hair, red blood cells, and prostate secretions. The daily requirement for the pregnant woman is 20 mg (an increase of 5 mg over the nonpregnant value).

Zinc insufficiency appears to be more common in the general population than previously known. Symptoms of growth retardation, anorexia, and an impaired sense of taste and smell are associated with zinc deficiency. A deficiency of zinc in the gravida has been implicated in the development of striae gravidarum. Pregnant women are at increased risk for developing zinc deficiency, especially teenagers, multigravidas, lactovegetarians, and vegans. Women with complications of labor (hemorrhage, prolonged labors, retained placenta, breech presentations) also exhibit zinc deficiency (LeMasters, 1981).

Zinc Sources

Zinc absorption in the diet may be prohibited by the presence of phytate in food (unleavened bread and cereal grains). Good sources of zinc are supplied by the following foods:

Oysters (100 gm)	74.7 mg
Wheat germ (100 gm)	14.3 mg
Pork (100 gm)	4.0 mg
Peas (dried)	3.2 mg
Liver (100 gm)	6.1 mg
Cashew nuts (100 gm)	4.4 mg
Beef (100 gm)	5.8 mg

IODINE

Iodine is needed for the synthesis of the hormones thyroxine (T_4) and triiodothyronine (T_3) from the thyroid gland. These hormones participate in cell oxidation affecting heat production, growth, reproduction, and other metabolic activities.

Iodine is found mainly in iodized salt and sea foods. The daily requirement is 150 mcg for the nonpregnant woman and 175 mcg for the pregnant woman. For most women, this requirement is easily met.

SODIUM

Sodium is involved with chlorine and potassium in the regulation of fluid balance, acid-base balance, muscular impulses, and permeability of the cell wall. Requirements for sodium have not been specified, since it is so readily available in the normal diet. Normal physiologic changes of pregnancy enhance the production of progesterone, which has an antagonizing effect on aldosterone and decreases sodium retention. Owing to the normal salt-losing effect of progesterone, it is important not to restrict sodium intake during pregnancy.

MAGNESIUM

All cells of the body depend on an adequate supply of magnesium. It is prevalent in bone and muscle tissue and is necessary for protein and lipid synthesis, nerve excitability, enzymatic actions, muscular activity, and synthesis of RNA and DNA. The normal daily requirement for the pregnant woman is 450 mg. The following are examples of good food sources of magnesium:

Whole wheat bread (100 gm)	78 mg
Shredded wheat (100 gm)	133 mg
Noodles (100 gm)	126 mg
Pecans (100 gm)	142 mg
Peanut butter (100 gm)	173 mg
Beet greens (100 gm)	106 mg

VITAMINS

Vitamins are necessary in the diet throughout life. They are essential to many metabolic activities such as growth and reproduction. Classification of vitamins is made according to their solubility. The water-soluble vitamins (B complex and C) are not stored by the body and, when in excess, are excreted in the urine. The fat-soluble vitamins (A, D, E) are capable of being stored in the liver when dietary intake exceeds use. They are not excreted in the urine. Fat-soluble vitamin K is not stored in the body, since it depends on bacterial flora of the intestine for synthesis.

Controversy exists over the ingestion of vitamins in larger quantities than the body can use. Many people feel that large doses of vitamins (megavitamins) are beneficial to their health. In reality, only small amounts of vitamins are needed in the daily diet. The water-soluble vitamins will simply be excreted when large doses are taken, thus providing no benefit. Over an extended period of time, large doses of these vitamins may be harmful, causing symptoms of nervous system irritability, paresthesias, renal calculi, itching, hypotension, cardiovascular disturbances, or edema.

Fat-soluble vitamins can be detrimental when taken in large doses, leading to toxicity. Symptoms of hepatosplenomegaly, jaundice, irritability, nausea, renal complications, and hypertension may develop. Megadoses of both vitamins A and D have been implicated in the development of birth defects. Reported cases of behavioral disturbances, kidney malformations, and other congenital anomalies have been identified in neonates whose mothers ingested large amounts of vitamin A; cardiovascular abnormalities, renal disorders, increased bone density, and mental retardation have been associated with vitamin D excess (Luke, 1985).

Vitamin A (retinol)

Vitamin A is found in both plant and animal sources. Plant sources exist in the form of carotene and may be found in foods such as cabbage, carrots, broccoli, apricots, spinach, sweet potatoes, cantaloupe, and peaches. Animal sources include liver, egg yolks, fortified margarine, whole milk, and butter. The daily requirement in the nonpregnant woman is 800 mg, and in the gravida 1000 mg.

Epithelial tissue growth, visual adaptations to light, protection from infection, and bone development are all functions of vitamin A. During pregnancy vitamin A is needed for growth and development of all tissues of the fetus, development of the placenta, and formation of skeletal structures and tooth buds.

Vitamin D (calciferol)

Most commercially sold milk and margarine has been fortified with vitamin D. It may only be found in the natural form in sunlight, fish liver oils, and yeast. One quart of milk (fortified) per day will meet the daily requirement of 400 IU.

Vitamin D plays an important role in the absorption, mobilization, and metabolism of calcium and phosphorus and is necessary for growth and calcification of bone.

Vitamin E (tocopherols and tocotrienols)

The main sources of vitamin E in the diet are vegetable oils, green leafy vegetables, legumes, nuts, and whole grains. Requirement for the nonpregnant woman is 8 mg daily. During pregnancy, 10 mg is recommended.

The true role of vitamin E is undefined, but its effects on cellular membrane integrity have been demonstrated. It also reportedly assumes an antioxidant role, which prevents the oxidation of substances such as vitamin A and essential fatty acids. Many other functions of vitamin E have been discussed but lack confirmation.

Vitamin K (menadione)

Synthesis of vitamin K occurs in the intestines under the influence of the normal bacterial flora. Small quantities of vitamin K may be found in green leafy vegetables and liver. No daily requirements have been established.

Vitamin K has a regulatory effect on the synthesis of prothrombin, and it is involved in blood clotting. This function is important in prevention of hemorrhage during pregnancy and the neonatal period. Until the neonate has established its own intestinal flora, vitamin K is not synthesized. For this reason, injections of vitamin K are given to the neonate shortly after birth.

WATER SOLUBLE VITAMINS

Vitamin C (ascorbic acid)

Sources of vitamin C include citrus fruits, berries, green leafy vegetables, potatoes, and tomatoes. This vitamin cannot be stored by the body. A daily intake is therefore necessary. During pregnancy, a daily allowance of 60 mg is recommended, an increase of 15 mg over the prepregnant recommendation.

Vitamin C is needed in the diet for the utilization of protein, collagen formation, absorption of iron, and as an antioxidant for polyunsaturated fats, and vitamins A and E. Studies have not confirmed its role in the prevention of colds or infection. Although it is water-soluble and excreted in the urine, untoward effects may still appear if large doses are taken over an extended period. Gastrointestinal symptoms, kidney stones, and disturbances in blood clotting have all been reported after megadoses of vitamin C (Robinson & Lawler, 1982).

Vitamin B_1 (thiamine)

Thiamine is not found in appreciable amounts in many sources. Liver, lean pork, dry beans, egg yolk and enriched flour, bread and cereals contain the greatest concentrations. An intake of 1.1 mg daily is needed in the nonpregnant diet and 1.5 mg daily in the pregnant woman.

The conversion of glucose to fat and the production of energy from glucose are two important functions of thiamine. The need for increased thiamine during pregnancy is related to the increased metabolic needs of the pregnant woman.

Vitamin B_2 (riboflavin)

Lactoflavin, found in milk, is the most abundant source of riboflavin. Other sources are liver, kidney, spinach, collard greens, and yogurt. Riboflavin requirement is increased during pregnancy from 1.3 mg to 1.6 mg. Like many other vitamins in the B complex, riboflavin is involved as a coenzyme in both protein and carbohydrate metabolism.

Niacin (nicotinic acid)

When protein intake is adequate, the dietary intake of niacin is usually also adequate. Foods such as meats, fish, poultry, peanut butter, potatoes, and legumes are good sources of niacin. The recommended daily intake during pregnancy is 16 mg, a 2 mg increase over the nonpregnant requirement.

Niacin is needed as a coenzyme in the synthesis of fats, and, in partnership with riboflavin, is necessary for glycolysis and oxidation of glucose.

Vitamin B_6 (pyridoxine)

Vitamin B_6 can be found in foods such as yeast, wheat germ, sunflower seeds, liver, and eggs. The daily adult requirement is 2 mg, with an increase of about 0.6 mg during pregnancy.

The metabolism of amino acids is affected by the coenzymatic action of pyridoxine. It is also necessary for carbohydrate and fat metabolism but these effects are not pronounced. The large demands of the fetus on the mother during pregnancy account for the needed increase in requirements.

Pantothenic Acid

Many foods contain pantothenic acid, but the best sources are skimmed milk, egg yolk, liver, kidney, salmon, yeast, tomatoes, and potatoes. Because of its availability, there is no established adult daily requirement. The average intake is about 5 to 10 mg per day, which is adequate during pregnancy. It is needed for its coenzymatic action on protein, carbohydrates, and fats, and also for the production of antibodies.

Vitamin B_9 (folic acid)

Folic acid is found in green leafy vegetables, liver, kidney, yeast, eggs, and whole grain cereals. The daily requirement for the adult woman is 0.4 mg, and 0.8 mg during pregnancy. The requirement for folic acid is doubled because of increased fetal growth demands, especially during the last trimester of pregnancy. When there is a deficiency of folic acid, megaloblastic anemia may occur owing to alterations in the formation of red blood cells. These red blood cells are immature and contain little, if any, hemoglobin. Symptoms of anemia appear, characterized by headache, irritability, weight loss, fatigue, apathy, and depression. The incidence of maternal and fetal complications is increased.

To prevent the occurrence of megaloblastic anemia, most women will receive supplements of folic acid during pregnancy, in dosages of 0.2 to 0.4 mg.

Vitamin B_{12} (cobalamin)

Animal sources provide the best supply of vitamin B_{12}. It is found in milk, eggs, meat, and cheese. Requirements for the nonpregnant woman are 3 μg daily and 4 μg for the pregnant woman.

Vitamin B_{12} must be acted upon by gastric secretions before it can be absorbed. It is necessary for the formation of red blood cells, and in that capacity it is invaluable for the treatment of pernicious anemia.

A list of the dietary needs of the pregnant woman prepregnancy and during pregnancy is seen in Table 11–1.

TABLE 11–1
RECOMMENDED DIETARY ALLOWANCES BEFORE AND DURING PREGNANCY AND LACTATION*

Nutrient	11–14 Years	15–18 Years	19–22 Years	23–50 Years	Pregnancy	Lactation
Energy, kcal	2,200	2,100	2,100	2,000	+300	+500
Protein, gm	46	46	44	44	+30	+20
Vitamin A, RE	800	800	800	800	+200	+400
IU						
Vitamin D, μg	10	10	7.5	5	+5	+5
Vitamin E, mg αTE	8	8	8	8	+2	+3
Ascorbic acid, mg	50	60	60	60	+20	+40
Thiamin, mg	1.1	1.1	1.1	1.0	+0.4	+0.5
Riboflavin, mg	1.3	1.3	1.3	1.2	+0.3	+0.5
Niacin, mg equiv.	15	14	14	13	+2	+5
Vitamin B-6, mg	1.8	2.0	2.0	2.0	+0.6	+0.5
Folacin, μg	400	400	400	400	+400	+100
Vitamin B-12, μg	3.0	3.0	3.0	3.0	+1.0	+1.0
Calcium, mg	1,200	1,200	800	800	+400	+400
Phosphorus, mg	1,200	1,200	800	800	+400	+400
Magnesium, mg	300	300	300	300	+150	+150
Iron, mg	18	18	18	18	†	†
Zinc, mg	15	15	15	15	+5	+10
Iodine, μg	150	150	150	150	+25	+50

*Recommended Dietary Allowances (9th ed.). Food and Nutrition Board, National Academy of Sciences, National Research Council, Washington, D.C., 1980.

†Supplemental iron, 30–60 mg daily, is recommended.

From Robinson, C., et al. **Normal and Therapeutic Nutrition** (17th ed.). New York: Macmillan, 1986.

NURSING RESPONSIBILITIES CONCERNING ANTEPARTAL NUTRITION

As a member of the antepartal health team, the nurse is responsible for nutritional counseling of the gravida. Following an assessment of dietary patterns, the nurse analyzes the information that has been supplied and then plans the appropriate interventions. This counseling is individualized to meet the needs of each client. It is useless to tell a woman whose family has financial difficulties that she would meet her protein requirement by eating meat twice a day. It is equally useless to tell the mother who does not like milk to drink a quart of milk every day.

Dietary assessments are included in the initial history taken at the first prenatal visit. Following the assessment, both the client and nurse plan realistic objectives that will help the woman to meet dietary needs. At each prenatal visit thereafter, an evaluation of success in meeting objectives should include any difficulties or concerns the client has about her diet. A brief review of the foods that should be included in the daily diet of the pregnant woman may be given (Table 11–2). A summary of the client's diet on the day previous to her visit may alert the nurse to dietary inadequacies. These deficiencies are discussed with the client in a nonthreatening way without insinuating failure when objectives are not met. Together different approaches to the situation are explored, developing a workable solution. Table 11–3 provides a sample diet for the pregnant woman.

On occasion, the nurse may find that there are special dietary concerns which alter or have the potential to alter nutritional status. These concerns may not be noted as problematic by the client, but should be evaluated.

TABLE 11–2
FOOD ALLOWANCES IN THE DAILY DIET OF THE PREGNANT WOMAN

	Pregnant Woman	Pregnant Teenage Girl	Lactating Woman
Milk, whole or low-fat	3–4 cups	4–5 cups	4–5 cups
Meat, fish, poultry (liver once a week), cooked weight	4 ounces	4 ounces	4 ounces
Eggs	3 to 4 per week	3 to 4 per week	3 to 4 per week
Vegetables, including			
Dark green leafy or deep yellow	½ cup	½ cup	½ cup
Potato	1 medium	1 medium	1 medium
Other vegetables	½–1 cup	½–1cup	½–1 cup
One vegetable to be raw each day			
Fruits, including			
Citrus	1 serving	1 serving	1 serving
Other fruit	1 serving	1 serving	1 serving
Cereal, whole grain or enriched	1 serving	1 serving	1 serving
Bread, whole grain or enriched	4 slices	4 slices	4 slices
Butter or fortified margarine Desserts, cooking fats, sugar, sweets	to meet caloric needs	to meet caloric needs	to meet caloric needs
An iron supplement is usually prescribed.			
Iodized salt			

From Robinson, C., et al. **Normal and Therapeutic Nutrition** (17th ed.), New York: Macmillan, 1986.

TABLE 11-3
SAMPLE DAILY DIET FOR THE PREGNANT WOMAN

Breakfast	Lunch	Dinner
Orange juice, 5 oz	Sandwich	Roast beef, 6 oz.
Oatmeal, ½ c	Whole wheat bread	Broccoli, ¾ c
Toast, 1 slice	2 slices	Baked potato
Butter or margarine	Tuna fish, ½ c	butter or margarine
Milk, 8 oz	Diced celery	Green salad
Decaffeinated Coffee	Mayonnaise	with tomatoes
or tea, 1 c	Lettuce	Milk, 8 oz.
	Banana	Decaffeinated coffee
	Milk, 8 oz	or tea
	Oatmeal cookies	
Midafternoon snack: apple, 1; milk, 4 oz		Evening snack: milk, 4 oz

Pica

Pica is the craving for, and ingestion of, substances not normally considered as food, such as coal, clay, cornstarch, or dirt. The list is not confined to these foods and may include any substance the client finds appealing. During pregnancy, many women will have cravings for specific food substances that are edible; this is not considered pica. Women with pica would not normally consider eating the substances they seem to crave during pregnancy. They cannot explain the reasons for their choices and often will not reveal their cravings. The substances most commonly craved are not, as a rule, harmful to either the mother or the fetus. They may, however, interfere with the absorption of certain nutrients (iron) and affect maternal nutritional status.

Underweight

The underweight woman who enters pregnancy 10 percent or more below the standard weight determined for her height and age is at risk for maternal and neonatal complications. These women often have protein deficiencies and anemia; they may deliver low birth weight infants.

Correction of the weight deficiency during pregnancy is a tedious task. The nutritional needs of the pregnancy are superimposed on the nutritional requirements needed for restoration and gain of weight. The weight deficit exhibited ideally is gained back during the remainder of pregnancy along with the weight gain needed to support the fetus. Leonard (1984) suggests the following formula for calculation of weight correction.

$$\text{Kg to be gained per week} = \frac{\text{Kg underweight}}{\text{Weeks until EDC}}$$

This would then be added to her normal expected weight gain of 0.5 to 1.0 pounds per week.

An important factor to be considered when assessing the underweight woman is the reason for the low weight. Counseling will not help if the underlying cause is not corrected. Nutritional habits, body image, economic status, culture, occupation, nausea, medical problems, emotional concerns and lifestyle are factors that are considered as possible contributors to weight deficiency.

The underweight woman needs motivation to gain weight during pregnancy. Motivation can be curtailed when there is pregnancy denial by the woman or her significant others. If the pregnancy is unwanted, rejection may be manifested by refusal to nourish this conceptus. Mothers who feel there is body image distortion by pregnancy often go to great lengths to avoid weight gain. Even though figure-conscious, some women realize they must provide good nutrition for the fetus. In this case, they may endeavor to eat nutritious foods while at the same time avoiding foods generous in needed calories. The importance of nutrition for a healthy fetus is emphasized.

Financial difficulties may cause some women to be underweight. Exploring the foods that are nutritious and within the budget is important for these women. Food supplement programs are available within most communities; the nurse is responsible for awareness of such programs. Two frequently used programs are the federally funded Food Stamp Program and the WIC Program (Supplemental Food Program for Women, Infants, and Children). The Food Stamp Program was established in 1964 and is available within a specified income range. Food stamps are issued for food purchase. The WIC Program is a supplemental food program available to pregnant and lactating women as well as infants and children up to age five. Women receiving benefits from this program are evaluated for nutritional risk due to income.

Food Allergies

Clients will avoid certain foods because of food allergies or intolerance. Allergic reactions to food substances are the result of immunologic responses, while intolerance denotes an enzyme deficiency. In either case, clients will avoid the food because of the discomfort or symptoms noted when the food is consumed.

Food allergies are often related to the protein content of the food and are manifested by gastrointestinal symptoms, although allergic reactions of a respiratory, neurologic, or cutaneous nature may occur. Even minute quantities of the offending food may make the client symptomatic. Common allergies include milk, chocolate, oranges, legumes, shellfish, and eggs. Food allergies are taken seriously, and dietary alterations are made. In addition to noting the allergy on the dietary history, the nursing care plan should address the allergy and the planned interventions.

Food intolerances produce many of the same gastrointestinal symptoms as food allergies. An intolerance to milk is fairly common and may be related to any enzyme necessary for sugar digestion. Most commonly, it is related to a lack of the enzyme lactase, which is needed to hydrolyze the disaccharide lactose. Certain population groups have a higher incidence of lactose intolerance. Orientals, Native Americans, American blacks, Mexican-Americans, and Jews most commonly exhibit this trait. Milk substitutions or calcium supplements may be ordered. Food processing used in the making of some cheeses will alter the lactose and make it tolerable for some individuals with lactose intolerance.

Cultural Influences

Relationships between food and culture have existed throughout the centuries. Food has been thought of as a means of socialization, an expression of religious belief, and an integral part of tradition. Variations may exist, not only in food preparation but in foods eaten. When food is intertwined with religious beliefs, elimination of certain foods from the diet is common. Any of these factors will affect the pregnant woman.

Biblical influences may determine the dietary habits of certain cultures. Jewish dietary beliefs do not allow the consumption of milk and meat at the same meal and allow only four—footed cloven-hoofed cud-chewing animals (beef, sheep) to be eaten. Koshering of the meat by soaking it in salted water is needed to remove the blood of the animal. Food preparation is not allowed on Saturday (the Sabbath). Religious holidays require the preparation of special foods to commemorate the day and may include fasting.

Fasting is also an important part of the Roman Catholic religion. Although pregnant women are exempt from fasting, meal preparation by the pregnant woman must include these restrictions. Days of abstinence from meat include Ash Wednesday and all Fridays during Lent.

Muslim religious practices require fasting during one month of the year from dawn to sunset. Food may be eaten twice during the period from dusk to dawn. This fasting does not include the pregnant woman, but she is required to make allowances for those fast days by adding them to the number of days she will fast following pregnancy. A special religious ceremony is followed in slaughtering meat to insure its purity. Only meats prepared in this fashion may be used, with the exception of koshered meats. Pork is not included in the diet.

Seventh Day Adventists abstain from meat, fish, and poultry, but do eat dairy products and plant foods. Zen macrobiotic diets are derived from the Zen Buddhist religion and require a balance between the use of "yin" and "yang." "Yin" foods are thought of as hot and masculine, while "yang" foods are cold and feminine. These foods are eaten on one of ten levels including various combinations. Lower level foods include vegetables, animal products, fruits, and salad. The highest level includes only cereals and brown rice with limited amounts of fluid. Pregnant women who follow the higher level requirements face nutrition deficits.

Puerto Ricans may also classify foods as "hot," "cold," or "cool." This classification is not according to food temperature but to the benefits derived from the food. In order for a person to be healthy, there must be a balance of "hot" and "cold" foods in the diet (see Chapter 2). The diet is very high in starchy carbohydrates and is limited in protein, milk, fruits, and vegetables. Dietary patterns often favor obesity and encourage the development of iron deficiency anemia.

Vietnamese natives adhere to the "cold" and "hot" use of food during pregnancy. "Hot" foods are eaten during the first trimester and "cold" foods during the second and third trimesters (see Chapter 2). Rice is an important food substance and may be combined with seafood and vegetables. Since meat is considered a "hot" food, it is not eaten during the second and third trimesters. Peanuts and soybeans are readily used and may provide the needed protein. Lactose intolerance is also common among this group.

The diets of the Japanese and Chinese include the extensive use of vegetables. Meat is used in combination with vegetables. Protein is provided from plant sources. Rice is considered a staple and is served at almost every meal. Milk intolerance is common. Eggs are widely used.

Within the United States, various regions will have differing dietary patterns. Midwesterners are traditionally "beef eaters" and consumers of dairy products. Fresh fruits and vegetables are not always available and may be lacking in the diet. The South is noted for the use of vegetable greens such as collards and turnips. Pork, chicken, and nuts are widely used and serve as good sources of protein. "Soul food" (chitterlings, blackeyed peas, collards, ham hocks, hoecakes, barbequed ribs) is native to the black population of the South but is widely included in the diets of both southern and northern populations.

In areas on the eastern seacoast, large amounts of seafood are eaten. Fish provides high-quality protein as well as a good supply of vitamin A, vitamin D, iodine, and calcium. In the Southwest, the Mexican-American influence is seen in the use of pinto beans, corn flatcakes, and hot peppers. This type of diet is usually blended with the use of beef products and vegetables and provides adequate amounts of protein and vitamins.

Dietary habits within the United States may be influenced by the cultural patterns of various areas. Within these various patterns, nutritious foods are available. Dietary counseling is centered on acquainting the client with what is available and how it will enhance her diet. Cultural influences must be included in dietary planning while still targeting optimal nutrition.

HEALTH MANAGEMENT DURING PREGNANCY

EMPLOYMENT

Employment outside the home is common for women in the childbearing age group, for financial and career reasons. One of the first concerns expressed by pregnant women is whether they will be able to continue their employment. The answer depends upon the woman and her health during pregnancy. If there is a desire to work, there is no reason most women cannot continue to be employed, providing their working conditions do not adversly affect their health or the health of the fetus. Employment in areas where pregnant women are in contact with toxic substances or experience physical stress is not recommended. If employment requires extended periods of standing, manipulation of heavy objects, or abnormal posturing, it is advisable for the woman to discuss other arrangements or options with the employer. Employers who employ 15 or more employees must adhere to federal laws that insure the pregnant woman the right to be employed or continue employment during pregnancy, maternity leaves, and benefits, and reinstatement of employment following maternity leaves. If there are no high-risk factors, employment may be continued until the time of delivery.

EXERCISE

Activity and exercise are recommended during pregnancy for most women. Exercise helps to improve and maintain good circulation and muscle tone needed for physiologic adaptations. Physical activity also imparts a sense of well-being to the individual and promotes relaxation. Planned exercises are beneficial to the woman as she prepares for delivery (see Chapter 12). Strenuous activities that place stress on the muscles or alter body alignment are not recommended. Women who have been actively engaged in a sport before pregnancy can usually continue the activity if it does not interfere with comfort or present a health risk. Swimming and walking are two recommended exercises. Exercising should be a daily activity and not just engaged in sporadically.

REST

Although the need for sleep and rest normally increases during pregnancy, the amount of sleep needed varies. Some women complain that they want to sleep all day, while others have difficulty sleeping. Physiologic changes during pregnancy place greater demands on the body. In order to meet these demands without fatigue, the pregnant woman needs periods of rest throughout the day and uninterrupted sleep at night. When helping the client to plan her rest periods, consideration must be given to responsibilities and activities that are a part of the normal daily routine. A home with several small children is not conducive to frequent rest periods for the mother. Rest periods may be planned to coincide with nap times or quiet times.

As the pregnancy progresses, it becomes difficult to find a comfortable position for rest and sleep. Suggestions that may promote comfort include side lying, with the abdomen supported by the bed or pillows, the top leg flexed toward the abdomen and the bottom leg slightly flexed at the knee (Fig. 11–1).

Extended periods of sitting or standing will cause fatigue and discomfort. Maintaining good posture while sitting or standing will

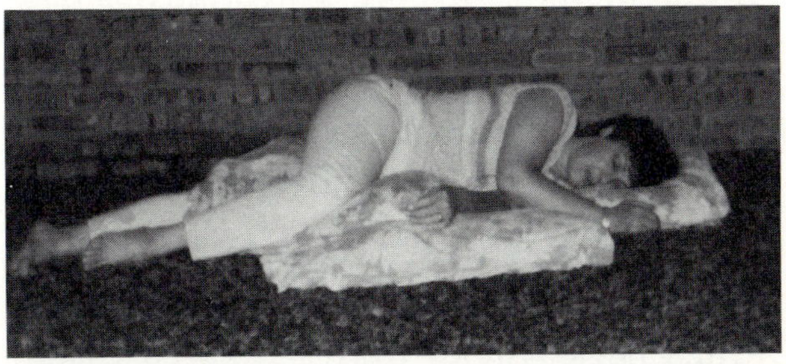

FIGURE 11–1. Resting position during pregnancy.

help to lessen strain. Women who sit at a desk most of the day will find it beneficial to change positions frequently or walk about when possible. If the job requires extended periods of standing, it may be helpful to elevate the feet during break periods and to use a chair or stool when possible.

Rest and relaxation are important during pregnancy. They are as important as other aspects of pregnancy care and should not be left to chance. These two elements are stressed by the nurse in planning care.

CLOTHING

Garments that are loose and nonconstrictive are the most comfortable during pregnancy. These garments may be in the form of maternity wear, which is most commonly put on during the third month of gestation. Specially designed girdles may be worn to relieve backache and muscle fatigue by providing support for the enlarging uterus, lifting it upward and toward the back. Tight girdles worn during pregnancy are not recommended, since they do not provide the proper support and may be constrictive.

Support hose may be worn if the woman finds them comfortable or if she has varicosities. Garters, knee socks, and knee high hose should not be worn, as they impede circulation, causing discomfort and contributing to the development of varicosities.

Brassieres, properly fitted and supportive, will prevent sagging and discomfort from the increasing weight and size of the breasts. Bras that have wide backs and wide straps will provide the best support. Wired bras or half-bras are not recommended, as they interfere with good circulation and do not support the entire breast. If colostrum is secreted before delivery, absorbent breast pads are placed inside the bra cups. Plastic-lined pads are not used, since they can be irritating to the nipple and encourage the development of infections.

High heeled shoes worn during pregnancy interfere with good balance and accentuate the spinal curvature. Shoes that are low-heeled will provide a better base of support.

GENERAL HYGIENE

Good health requires good hygiene during pregnancy and throughout life. General hygiene principles are included in antepartal assessments and teaching.

Bathing may be continued in the manner preferred. Showering or tub bathing is acceptable, as long as safety precautions are taken. In the last months of pregnancy, uneven weight distribution can cause the mother to easily lose her balance and it increases the possibility of falling. Bath mats and railings should be used. Long periods of soaking in the tub are not recommended, as hypotension may occur and cause syncope. If the membranes are leaking or ruptured, tub bathing is not advised. Sauna bathing for long periods is not recommended, since elevated body temperatures over 102°F may interfere with brain development of the fetus.

Feminine hygiene is continued throughout pregnancy, but douching is not recommended, since it may contribute to the incidence of spontaneous abortions. The normal leukorrhea of pregnancy causes an increase in clear mucus vaginal discharge. The normalcy of the discharge is stressed. Cleanliness measures are recommended but the use of strong vaginal sprays are not.

Breast Care

Breast care during pregnancy is important for all mothers, regardless of the method of infant feeding chosen later. Care begins with the use of a properly fitted brassiere that can be adjusted to allow for increase in breast size. Cleanliness is important, although strong irritating soaps are not used on the nipples. Breast secretions (colostrum) may be cleansed from the nipple by using a washcloth and warm water. If secretions are allowed to dry on the breast they may cause irritation and promote nipple cracking. Some women find it helpful to apply a mild ointment such as Mammol ointment, lanolin, or even Vaseline to the nipple when secretions have become crusted.

If the client is planning to breastfeed, preparation of the breast begins during the antepartal period. The nipples must be "toughened" before breast feeding is undertaken. This can be accomplished by oral stimulation provided by her sexual partner or by nipple rolling. Nipple rolling involves gently rolling the nipple between the thumb and forefinger for about 15 seconds twice a day (Fig. 11-2). Massage of the nipple can be done after bathing by gently rubbing the nipple with a rough towel.

During nursing breast assessment, inspection may reveal nipple retraction or inversion (see Fig. 11-3). The pinch test, performed in the following manner, is used to determine nipple protrusion: with the thumb and forefinger placed at the outer edge of the areola, the nipple is gently pinched. The normal nipple will protrude, while the introverted nipple will retract. If the nipple appears flat with no protrusion, it is retracted. When the nipple appears inverted within the areola, it is introverted. Massage of the nipple will usually cause it to extend. The infant presented with retracted or introverted nipples during breastfeeding may experience difficulty grasping the nipple. It is important to assist the mother to institute measures to correct the problem during the prenatal period. Nipple rolling and massage are helpful. Hoffman's exercise (Fig. 11-4) has been suggested by Riordan (1983) to aid in stretching nipple tissue. When performing this exercise, the mother places her

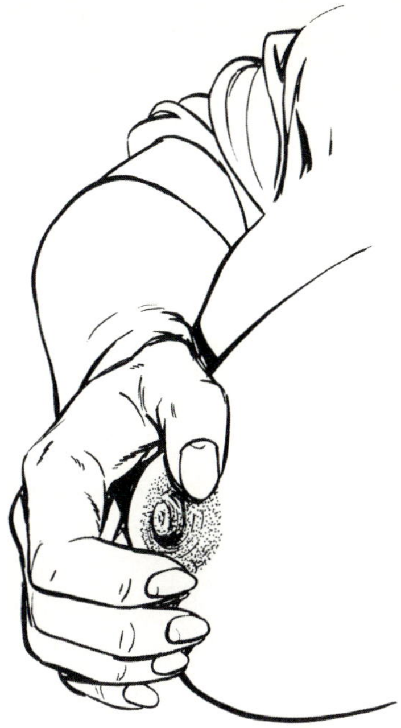

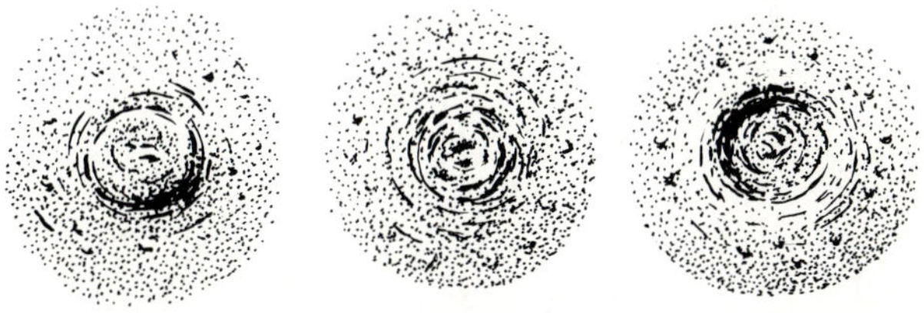

A B C

FIGURE 11-3. Assessment of nipples during pregnancy using pinch test to determine: A. Normal nipple protrusion. B. Flatness of nipple indicating moderate retraction. C. Inward retraction indicating inverted nipple.

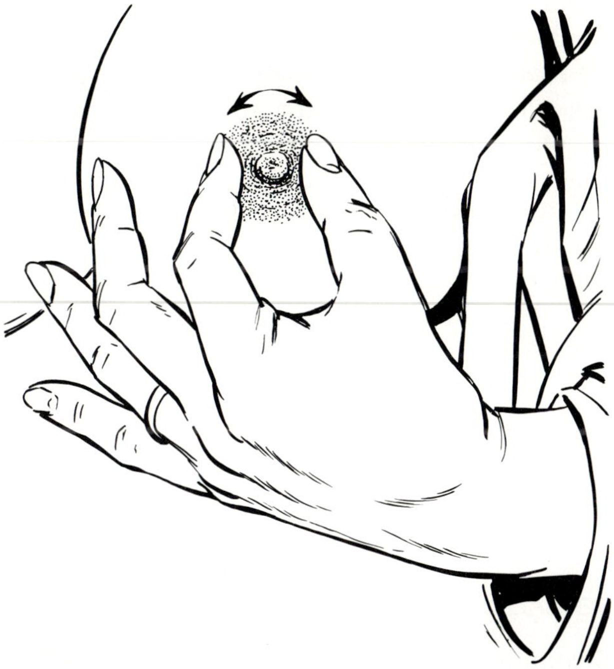

FIGURE 11-2. Nipple rolling.

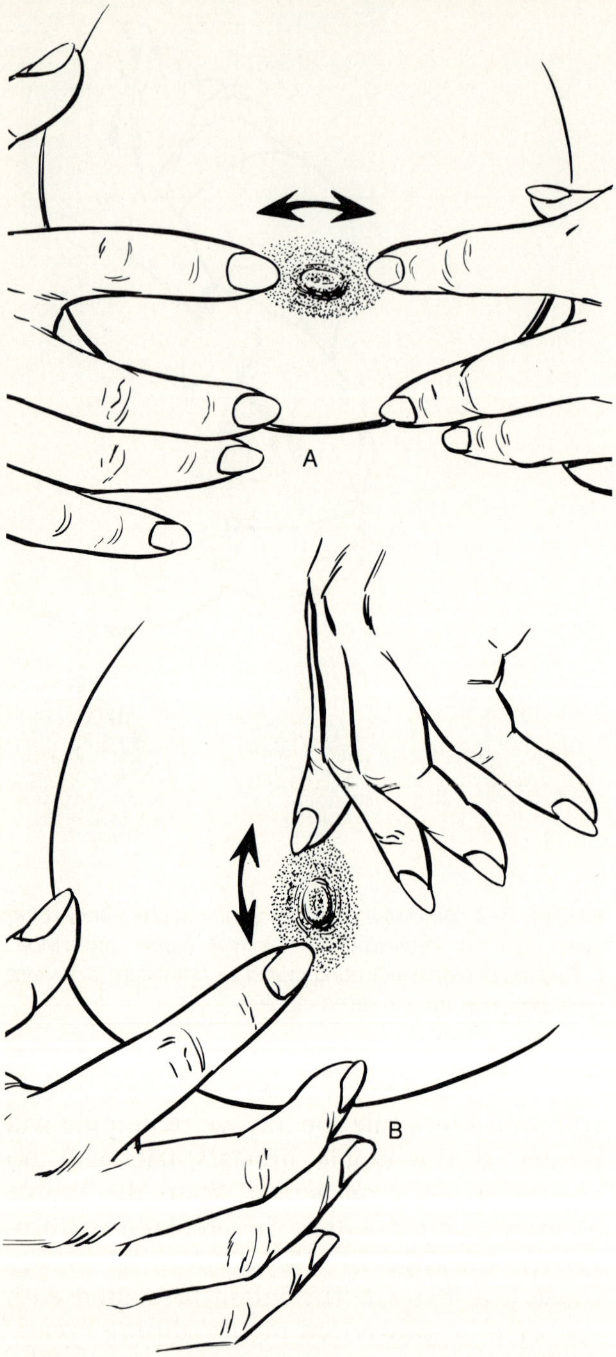

FIGURE 11-4. Hoffman's exercise for nipple stretching. A. Stretching the nipple sideways. B. Stretching the nipple upward and downward.

forefingers on either side of the nipple and gently stretches the nipple to each side; she then places her fingers below and above the nipple and stretches the nipple tissue in that direction. Massaging the nipple may promote uterine contractions and should be stopped if these uterine contractions begin.

Another device recommended to correct inverted nipples is the breast cup. This cup, shaped like a doughnut, is worn over the nipples and inside the bra during the second and third trimesters of pregnancy. The pregnant woman is instructed to begin wearing the cup for one hour and then gradually to increase the time to several hours throughout the day. The cup places suction on the areola, causing the nipple to protrude through an inner opening in the shield. Use of this device is discontinued when breastfeeding is started, as constant suction on the lactating breast encourages plugged milk ducts. The milk expressed within the cup is considered contaminated and is not to be fed to the infant.

Oral Hygiene

Continued good oral hygiene is encouraged during pregnancy. Dental examinations and care are promoted, although dental x-rays are not recommended during the first trimester. Irritation, bleeding, and hypertrophy of the gums are common during pregnancy owing to increased estrogen production. Vigorous brushing with a hard bristled tooth brush is not recommended, but brushing should not be neglected. *Ptyalism* (excessive salivation) caused by increased estrogen levels may accompany pregnancy. This is generally irritating to the mother but does not cause tooth decay or gum irritation.

Fetal calcium needs will not cause decalcification of the pregnant woman's teeth. Cavities occur when good oral hygiene or dental care is not practiced during pregnancy. Most dental work can be undertaken, although extensive procedures are not.

SEXUALITY DURING PREGNANCY

Sexuality is as much a need during pregnancy as it is throughout the life cycle. Many factors enter into the sexual expression of love during pregnancy. Sexual needs are present for both the gravida and her partner. Although it may not be mentioned by the pregnant couple, it is a genuine concern. Nursing assessment of this facet of the client's life is important in preventing misconceptions and anxiety. Discussion of the sexual aspects of pregnancy should begin early in the first trimester.

Frequently assessed concerns of couples include fear of harming the baby during intercourse, altered sexual desires, attractiveness of the pregnant woman, and stimulation of labor through lovemaking. Each of these factors has the potential to alter the couple's sexual relationship.

Sexual abstinence was previously the byword but is no longer considered necessary during a normal pregnancy. In the absence of complications, the mother may engage in intercourse throughout pregnancy. If symptoms such as uterine activity or bleeding appear at any time, intercourse is not recommended. Abstinence is also recommended if the mother has habitual abortions or has an incompetent cervix. Diagnosis of placenta previa, premature rupture of the membranes, or threatened preterm labor will preclude coitus.

Coitus and orgasmic response during intercourse have been implicated in contributing to the onset of preterm labor, premature rupture of the membranes, and amniotic fluid infections. Research data are conflicting and confusing, neither supporting these contentions nor denying them. Lack of sufficient data seems to compound the problem but does highlight the need for continued research in this area.

When counseling the pregnant couple, the nurse may find it helpful to consider the following. Sexual activity during pregnancy may be maintained if there are no complications. Orgasms, either by coital activity or masturbation, may produce uterine contractions, although these have not been demonstrated to have a precise effect on the stimulation of labor or PROM. Penile penetration has not been found to have an irritating effect on the cervix or uterine contents. When the membranes are intact, there is no increased incidence in amniotic fluid infections or chorioamnionitis associated with coitus. Sexuality may be expressed in a number of ways during pregnancy, including oral genital sex; however, air embolisms and subsequent death have occurred when air is blown into the vagina. Many pregnant women have one sustained contraction during an orgasm instead of the normal rhythmic contractions experienced during sex before pregnancy.

Sexual desire may range from decreased levels to increased interest at various times during pregnancy. It is generally agreed that the majority of women will have lessened desire during the first trimester. It is difficult to determine if this decrease is the result of physiologic changes or is influenced by the woman's concerns over the pregnancy. Nausea, breast tenderness, and fatigue are frequently cited as causes of decreased interest.

As the woman becomes accustomed to both the physiologic and psychological aspects of pregnancy during the second trimester, her level of sexual interest appears to increase. Accompanying her increased comfort is an awareness that the pregnancy is well underway and presumably safe. Sexuality is heightened by increased circulation to the pelvic area, creating pelvic congestion that intensifies sexual stimulation. Some women will experience orgasm for the first time during pregnancy. The onset of uterine contractions with orgasm during the second trimester may frighten some women. This response should be explained to the couple early in pregnancy. Gentle massage of the small of the back or the lower abdomen may relieve the discomfort.

Disenchantment characterizes most aspects of the woman's psychological response during the third trimester, including her sexual desires. As her size increases, sexual positioning becomes awkward and for some even uncomfortable. The male-superior position is probably the least recommended, since it creates pressure on the female abdomen and causes discomfort. In this position, the pregnant woman may develop supine hypotension from the pressure of the fetus and the added weight on the inferior vena cava. A rear entry or x-position may be suggested as more comfortable during coitus. When there has been a previous history of incompetent cervix, preterm labor, or PROM, it is recommended that the woman refrain from intercourse during the last three to four weeks of pregnancy.

If limitations on sexual activity are recommended for obstetrical reasons, the nurse may suggest alternatives that will satisfy the sexual needs of both partners. An assessment is made of the nature of the limitation, indicating if only orgasm is contraindicated, if penile penetration with orgasm is not recommended, or if only masturbation, which produces stronger orgasm, is prohibited.

The expression of love is not centered just in the coital act but is a response to the feelings of loving and being loved. Sexual feelings may be experienced through tactile stimulation and positions of closeness. Bodily massage, caressing, kissing, and oral genital stimulation are noncoital alternatives. Some couples may be uncomfortable with sexual activity that they feel is nontraditional. In these instances, the nurse may suggest that they discuss and explore their feelings with each other, reaching decisions that are mutually agreeable. Before the nurse enters any discussion with the client concerning alternative sexual expression, she must first explore her own feelings toward sexuality. Above all, she must be sincere with the couple and show respect and acceptance of their feelings.

The father's response to the pregnancy and the bodily changes occurring in the woman are often of concern to both of them. If either he or she perceives her body as distorted and unattractive, sexual relationships may be altered. A sense of sharing in the creation of life and joy in watching the baby grow inside the womb may counteract the negative feelings. Frank discussions of these feelings are often necessary to help alleviate the tension created by misunderstandings. Although the gravida may see her body as unattractive when compared with the standard of beauty in today's world, the father may look upon her enlarging abdomen with pride and see her as even more beautiful than before.

Cultural and social factors are also responsible for alterations in sexual expression during pregnancy. When procreation is seen as the woman's main role, the sexual feelings may be denied during pregnancy. In some cultures abstinence from sexual activity is expected for both male and female. Other societies practice coitus interruptus; still others look upon pregnancy as a visible sign of shameful sexual activity. Assessments of these beliefs and practices are necessary before any interventions are undertaken. Prenatal education classes should discuss sexuality during pregnancy. These classes will often provide the appropriate atmosphere for exploration of values pertinent to sexual matters. The nurse must remember not to force her values or opinions on the couple. If they are satisfied with their sexual roles, intrusion by the nurse into their sexuality is unnecessary and may be resented.

TRAVEL

There are no restrictions on travel during pregnancy, providing the woman is comfortable and there are no obstetrical or medical complications. Periods of prolonged sitting will favor pooling of blood in the lower extremities and will contribute to edema of the legs and feet. For this reason, it is suggested that when long automobile trips are taken, rest stops be provided every two hours. This allows the woman to walk about for several minutes before resuming her trip. Travel by air provides the shortest travel time and is the preferred method of transportation.

Automobile seat belts are worn to provide safety from sudden stops or in the event of an accident. The belt is positioned under the abdomen and over the shoulder. It is fastened securely but should not apply pressure on the abdomen.

DRUGS AND PREGNANCY

In most cases, the mother shares quite generously with the fetus all substances that are taken into her system by ingestion, absorption, injection, or inhalation. To determine which of these substances will affect the fetus is a difficult task that involves many factors. Since any chemical agent that has an effect on a living organism can be classified as a drug, the list of possibilities becomes endless. The desirability or consequences of the drug at various times throughout the pregnancy must also be considered. Not every drug will have the same effect on the fetus.

The placenta, as the organ of transport, holds the key to determining drug influences on the fetus. Substances must cross the placenta in order to affect the fetus. The chemical characteristics of a drug will determine its ability for transplacental carriage. Drugs with a molecular weight of more than 1000 (e.g., heparin) are not readily transported. Most drugs have a molecular weight of 200 to 300 and will easily cross through the semipermeable membrane of the placenta. Protein binding characteristics of the drug will also alter its diffusion. The fetus has less ability (a lower protein level) to bind certain drugs than does the mother, leaving a larger amount of the drug remaining within the fetal tissues. Drugs such as the sulfonamides will displace bound bilirubin and result in neonatal jaundice. Lipid solubility is another chemical characteristic that will alter transfer. If a substance is fat-soluble and un-ionized (salicylates, for example), it will diffuse more rapidly.

In addition to the drug's ability to cross the placenta, the gestational age will affect the teratogenicity. During the first 17 days gestation, drugs that cross the placenta will either cause death of the conceptus from effects on cell division or will have no effects at all. If the drug is toxic, death of the zygote will result. Organogenesis continues during the period from 18 to 55 days. When developing cells are exposed to toxic agents, structural malformations may result. During this period the brain, central nervous system, and cardiovascular system are particularly susceptible. Growth retardation is the principle manifestation of adverse effects from drugs taken from the 56th day of gestation until birth. Even years after birth, the effects of drugs with extended latency periods, such as the carcinogens, may be realized. Vaginal adenocarcinoma in young women has been reportedly caused by in utero exposure to diethylstilbesterol (DES).

Directly related to the effects of drugs during pregnancy is the dosage and duration of administration of the drug. Exposure to even small doses of a drug for an extended period of time may have adverse effects on the fetus. A large dose of a medication taken only a few times may be teratogenic if taken during a vulnerable gestational period.

Determination of the safety of drugs during pregnancy is complicated and unpredictable. Retrospective studies, although inconclusive in many cases, have provided valuable information on the effects of drugs. Humans may demonstrate different reactions to drugs than animal models, making controlled animal studies inapplicable. In these instances, animal research cannot be used as an indicator of drug safety for pregnant women. A case-in-point is the tragic result from the use of thalidomide. Thalidomide was proven safe in laboratory animals, yet produced *phocomelia* (absence of the proximal portion of a limb) in the infants of mothers who took the drug during pregnancy.

Judicious and prudent use of drugs appears to be the most acceptable approach during pregnancy. Instances where the risk of using a drug must be weighed against the potential complications are encountered with complications of pregnancy, either medical or obstetrical. A thorough knowledge of the drug, its beneficial and adverse effects, contraindications, acceptable and safe dosages for both the mother and the fetus, and interaction with other drugs is needed before any drug can be recommended during pregnancy.

Nursing Responsibilities

The nurse should make a careful assessment of drug use by the gravida. This assessment should be made during the first prenatal visit, enabling the mother to avoid certain drugs that are not recommended during pregnancy. Important considerations when counseling the mother include: (1) all medications taken during pregnancy should be approved by the obstetrician; (2) the first three months gestation is the period when the fetus is the most susceptible to toxic agents; (3) of the 3 percent of newborns born with abnormalities, 10 percent or less are caused by teratogens; (4) toxic agents may be ingested as drugs, chemical and air pollutants, radiation, environmental contamination, and megadoses of nutritional supplements; (5) the dosage and duration of drug administration affects the teratogenicity of a drug; (6) over-the-counter drugs are not always safe during pregnancy and should not be taken indiscriminately.

Critical developmental periods of teratogenic sensitivity are indicated in Table 11-4, and fetal and neonatal effects from certain drugs are listed in Table 11-5.

TABLE 11-4
CRITICAL DEVELOPMENTAL PERIODS OF TERATOGENIC SENSITIVITY

Critical Area	Weeks of Gestation
Central Nervous System	3rd to 6th week
Heart	3rd to 7th week
Eyes	4th to 9th week
Ear	4th to 12th week
Arms	4th to 7th week
Legs	4th to 7th week
Palate	6th to 12th week
Teeth	6th to 8th week
External genitalia	7th to 12th week

ALCOHOL

Alcohol is a drug that has the potential to affect the fetus severely. There appears to be no minimal level of alcohol intake compatible with fetal development. Even small amounts of alcohol are considered unsafe for the fetus. During pregnancy, the mother is advised to abstain from alcohol for the entire gestational period.

The fetus of a pregnant woman with an alcohol problem is at risk for development of *fetal alcohol syndrome*. This syndrome is characterized by undergrowth, facial anomalies, mental retardation, joint anomalies, cardiac murmurs and microcephaly. About 45 percent of the fetuses whose mothers are alcohol-dependent will develop this syndrome.

Careful assessment of drinking habits is needed during the prenatal interview. Chronic alcohol abusers will attempt to conceal their drinking habits and may put off seeking prenatal care to avoid divulging this problem. If the pregnant woman admits to a drinking problem, the nurse helps her to understand the necessity of abstinence during pregnancy without adding guilt feelings. Further assessment may reveal that alcohol is used as a coping mechanism. The thought of eliminating alcohol may be threatening. Professional alcoholic counseling is advised in these situations, and continued support by the health care team is imperative.

SUBSTANCE ABUSE

Substance abuse includes the use of illicit drugs as well as commonly used substances such as tobacco and coffee.

TABLE 11-5
FETAL AND NEONATAL EFFECTS FROM CERTAIN DRUGS

Drug	Effects on Fetus/Neonate	Known Teratogen	Contraindicated in Pregnancy	Caution in Use During Pregnancy
Anticoagulant				
Warfarin derivatives (Coumadin)	Decreased synthesis of clotting factors II, VII, IX and X; fetal hemorrhage, microcephaly; stillbirth, neonatal hemorrhage, nasal hypoplasia	x	x	
Anticonvulsant				
Diphenylhydantoin (Dilantin)	Congenital heart disorders; cleft palate, digital hypoplasia; microcephaly, folic acid deficiency, IUGR, eyelid ptosis, congenital hernia, mental deficiencies	x	x	
Paramethadione (Paradione)	Abortion, congenital heart disorders, mental retardation; facial abnormalities			x
Trimethadione (Tridione)	Abortion, congenital heart disorders, neural & skeletal malformations, facial anomalies—cleft lip and palate	x	x	
Antidiabetic				
Chlorpropamide (Diabinese)	Neonatal respiratory distress, prolonged hypoglycemia		x	
Tolbutamide (Orinase)	Multiple congenital defects, fetal death (X 3) thrombocytopenia, neonatal hypoglycemia		x	
Antihypertensive				
Reserpine	Bradycardia, respiratory distress, nasal stuffiness, hypothermia, hypotonia, anorexia			x
Antimalarial				
Chloroquine hydrochloride	? abortion			x
Quinacrine hydrochloride	? congenital anomalies		x	
Quinine	Abortion, anomalies of eye & ear thrombocytopenia, CNS abnormalities		x x	
Pyrimethamine	Fetal risk		x	
Antineoplastic				
Antimetabolites				
Folic acid antagonist (aminopterin) (methotrexate)	Abortion, ocular defects, multiple skeletal defects	x	x	
Busulfan	Decreased WBC, IUGR, renal malformations, malformations of extremities, ovarian agenesis, hydrocephalus	x	x	

TABLE 11-5 (continued)

Drug	Effects on Fetus/Neonate	Known Teratogen	Contraindicated in Pregnancy	Caution in Use During Pregnancy
Antiemetic				
Meclizine hydrochloride (Antivert) (Bonine) (Bonamine)	? Cleft palate			x
Bendectin (not currently used)	? Limb defects		x	
Diuretics				
Ammonium chloride	Thrombocytopenia, hyperbilirubinemia, hypokalemia, respiratory distress, low platelet counts, hyponatremia, hemolysis, death			x x
Thiazides	Low platelets			
Infection Preventitives				
Aminoglycosides (Streptomycin) (Gentamicin) (Neomycin)	Eighth nerve damage, skeletal anomalies, renal abnormalities, ototoxic damage		x	
Tetracyclines (Vibramycin) (Chlortetracycline) (Terramycin)	Delayed bone growth, enamel hypoplasia, stained teeth, hemolytic anemia, icterus, thrombocytopenia		x	
Chloramphenicol	? fetal death ? gray baby syndrome ? bone marrow suppression		x	
(Erythromycin)	None known			x
Antiamebics				
(Metronidazole) Flagyl	Mutagenic 1st trimester malformations		x	
Sulfonamides	Hemolytic anemia, icterus, thrombocytopenia, growth retardation			x
Hormones				
Androgens	Congenital limb reduction, increased production of androgen by adrenal glands, masculinization of females	x	x	
Corticosteroids	Immunologic disorders in first few weeks of neonatal life SGA, cleft palate, adrenal insufficiency			x
Estrogens (Diethylstilbesterol)	Cardiovascular anomalies, vaginal adenocarcinoma in young women exposed during fetal gestation, hypertrophic testes in males epididymal cyst, cleft lip & palate	x	x	

TABLE 11-5 (continued)

Drug	Effects on Fetus/Neonate	Known Teratogen	Contraindicated in Pregnancy	Caution in Use During Pregnancy
Gonadotropins				
(Clomiphene citrate) Clomid	? Trisomy 21, abortion, neural tube defect			
Oxytocin	Abortion, neonatal hyperbilirubinemia		x	
Inorganic iodine	Excessive amniotic fluid,		x	
(Mucolytic agents)	thyroid enlargement, cretinism,		x	
Radioactive iodine	Destruction of fetal thyroid tissue		x	
Progesterones	Transposition of great vessels, limb anomalies		x	
Narcotics	Large amounts cause hypothermia, apnea, respiratory depression, lethargy, low apgar scores, death			x
Psychotropics				
Antidepressants				
Tricyclics (Adapin) (Elavil) (Luidomil) (Tofranil)	Limb anomalies, CNS anomalies, irritability, withdrawal symptoms, respiratory distress, colic, urinary retention		x	
Diazepam				
(Valium)	Hypotonia, poor suck reflex, low apgar scores, hypothermia, ? cleft lip, thrombocytopenia			x
Lithium	Altered cardiac rhythm and thyroid function, jaundice, cyanosis ?anomalies		x	
Phenothiazine	Delayed respirations, ocular abnormalities, hypotonia			x
Salicylates				
(Aspirin)	Skeletal defects, decreased protein binding, decreased platelet aggregation, decreased clotting factor XII			x
Sedatives Barbiturates	Premature closure of the ductus arteriosus (large doses) ? anomalies, apnea, poor sucking reflex lethargy, weight gain decreased			x
Bromides				
(Chloral hydrate)	Large doses cause fetal death, neonatal skin irruptions, IUGR			x
Magnesium sulfate	Respiratory depression, hypotonia, apnea, (convulsions?)			x
Thalidomide	Phocomelia, ocular defects, congenital heart disorders, intestinal disorders	x	x	

TABLE 11-5 (continued)

Drug	Effects on Fetus/Neonate	Known Teratogen	Contraindicated in Pregnancy	Caution in Use During Pregnancy
Tocolytics				
Alcohol	Fetal alcohol syndrome, hypotonia, depression, intoxication			x
Sympathetic amines (beta receptors)				
Ritodrine hydrochloride	Tachycardia, hypothermia, hypoglycemia, hypocalcemia			x
Vitamins				
Vitamin A (megadoses)	Renal anomalies, behavioral disorders, congenital anomalies			x
Vitamin D (megadoses)	Mental retardation, renal disorders, ? aortic stenosis, increased bone density			x

"Street drugs" may be used by the pregnant woman, just as they are by other segments of the population. The use of mind-altering drugs is increasing and the fetus of a pregnant woman may be victimized from the moment of conception. Although the data are unclear on many drugs (marijuana, cocaine), there has been no evidence that can proclaim them safe during pregnancy. Lysergic acid diethylamide (LSD) has been implicated in the increased incidence of limb bud abnormalities and chromosomal damage. Narcotic addiction appears to be responsible for intrauterine growth retardation (IUGR), preterm and breech deliveries, and neonatal death during withdrawal. Pregnant women using drugs often suffer from malnutrition, compounding the effects on the fetus.

Smoking during pregnancy has been documented as a definitive developmental and health risk to the fetus. If the pregnant woman smokes during pregnancy, her unborn child also smokes. A wide range of adverse fetal and neonatal effects are associated with maternal smoking. Those reported include spontaneous abortion, impaired brain development, impaired physical growth apparent in length and head and chest circumference, preterm deliveries, hyperkinesis, abnormal placental attachments, SGA neonates, sudden infant death syndrome, and an increase in perinatal and neonatal deaths. The data concerning pregnant women who smoke indicate a clear relationship between the number and frequency of cigarettes smoked and the weight of the neonate at birth. Several theories have been offered to explain this relationship; (1) vasoconstrictive properties of nicotine can alter placental perfusion, (2) elevated carbon monoxide levels in the maternal circulation cause fetal hypoxia, and (3) suppression of maternal appetite causes problems associated with poor nutrition.

During the initial interview, the nurse assesses the smoking pattern of the client. Health teaching begins at this time, with an explanation of the adverse effects of smoking on the fetus. It is not realistic to expect the mother to throw away her cigarettes at that moment, but the nurse can help her to formulate a plan for cutting down and eventually quitting. The client is not only told of the harmful effects of each cigarette but she is also told of the harmful effects to the fetus.

Although quitting is best, cutting back on the number of cigarettes she smokes per day will benefit the fetus.

The Food and Drug Administration (1981) recommended caution in the use of caffeine during pregnancy. This warning was based on data obtained from animal studies that showed fetal death, low birth weight, limb anomalies, and retarded bone development resulting from maternal caffeine ingestion. Retrospective human studies have suggested relationships between caffeine intake and preterm labor, stillbirths, and fetal anomalies. Pregnant women are advised of the possible adverse effects on the fetus from high levels of caffeine consumption.

Caffeine is widely used in many households and may be found in coffee, tea, chocolate, soft drinks, cocoa, appetite suppressants, diuretics, over-the-counter pain relief medications for headaches and menstrual cramps, medications to keep awake, and cold and allergy remedies. The most concentrated amounts are found in coffee and tea. Five ounces of brewed coffee contains between 100 and 145 mg of caffeine, depending upon the method of preparation. Instant coffee contains about half the amount of caffeine found in brewed coffee. Tea will yield between 10 and 50 mg per cup, depending on brewing time (the longer the brewing the more caffeine) and the type of tea (black tea has the most caffeine and green tea the least). Many consumers do not realize the caffeine content of soft drinks, which contributes to overall consumption of caffeine. Colas contain between 30 and 50 mg caffeine per can.

Assessment of caffeine intake should be made for all gravidas, even if they do not drink coffee or tea. The pregnant woman who consumes five or six cans of cola per day may consume more caffeine than the woman who has two cups of coffee. Limitation of caffeine intake is recommended by using decaffeinated coffee and tea, and caffeine-free soft drinks, as well as reading the labels on over-the-counter medications that may contain caffeine. A safe level of caffeine has not been established for the gravida, but no more than two to four cups of coffee (or its equivalent) or about 400 mg daily is suggested.

SUPERSTITIONS OF PREGNANCY

To the health practitioner, superstitions are unfounded and of no value during pregnancy. To the pregnant woman, superstitions may have a profound effect on her perceptions and practices. Familiarity with these superstitions will enable the nurse to realize when superstitions are exerting a negative influence on the pregnancy. Following are examples of superstitions believed to be true in the past and some that are currently believed.

Sex of the Child

If the mother's face had a greenish cast, the baby is a boy. If the baby is carried on the right side, it is a boy. A male fetus will bring a good mood to the mother. Placing the marriage bed in a north-south direction will favor the conception of a boy. Fetal heart tones that are slow indicate a boy. Boys are carried higher than girls.

Birth Marks and Anomalies

Markings on the baby are caused by the sins of the parents. Climb a ladder during pregnancy and the baby will be born with a bald spot. If the mother has a lot of heartburn during pregnancy the baby will have a lot of hair. If the woman gives birth and the right arm of the child is short, the land will become rich. If a woman gives birth and the child has no hands, the enemy will gain possession of the city in which the birth occurred. If a pregnant woman sits on one or both of her feet habitually, the baby will have club feet. If a woman raises her arms above her head during pregnancy, the cord will become tied around the baby's neck. Cravings cause birthmarks. Craving for gingerbread will cause a brown spot in the eye of the baby. An unsatisfied craving will cause a strawberry mark on the baby. Tying an amulet and stones of jade, jasper, and agate around the neck or to the upper arm will protect the baby from blood incompatibilities and prevent hard labor and postpartum hemorrhage.

Delivery

The baby comes at the same time it is conceived. Babies born during the seventh month of gestation have a better chance of survival than those born at eight months. Drinking a cola will bring on the baby if it is time, or ease off the pain if it is not. A knife, razor, or scissors placed under the bed until delivery is over will cut the labor pains.

None of these superstitions have an actual factual basis or are true, yet many women subscribe to them. The nurse should tactfully explain to the client the inaccuracy of the superstitions and provide accurate information.

MINOR DISCOMFORTS OF PREGNANCY

BACKACHE

Alteration in weight distribution during pregnancy, coupled with the stretching of muscles and ligaments, softening of the pelvic cartilage and connective tissue, and the relaxation of the pelvic joints, all place pressure on the lower spine. As the pregnancy advances, the pressure on the lower spine is further increased and backache becomes a frequent complaint. Proper body alignment and good body mechanics are the most therapeutic measures that can be suggested. To help align the back properly, the client is told to stand and sit with the back straight and the tilt of the pelvis accommodated by the lower back and abdominal muscles.

To further relieve the discomfort of backache, the mother may be taught the use of pelvic rocking (see Chapter 12). It is also suggested that she wear low-heeled shoes and support her back during rest and sleep periods by using a firm mattress. Back rubs may be given by her partner, not only for pain relief but as a means of closeness during periods of sexuality. Heat applications may also provide a measure of relief from backache.

In addition to suggestions given for relief of backache is the differential diagnosis needed to rule out medical causes of backache. The incidence of urinary infections is increased during pregnancy, and backache may indicate their development. A herniated disk also causes back pain and may produce intense discomfort. The character and onset of the back pain are assessed, since labor contractions are often felt as low back pain.

NAUSEA AND VOMITING

"Morning sickness" is the term frequently used in association with the nausea and vomiting of pregnancy. The feelings of nausea may be experienced all through the day and night. The hormonal influences of pregnancy (HCG and estrogen) have been suggested as causative factors, as have psychological factors. Neither claim has been substantiated by research, and both may be viewed as indirect or direct contributors to nausea and vomiting.

Although the exact mechanism responsible is not known, the feeling experienced by the pregnant woman is indeed real and uncomfortable. The intensity of the nausea will vary from woman to woman, with some merely feeling queasy and others experiencing vomiting. Symptoms will usually subside by the end of the first trimester.

Nausea and vomiting may influence nutritional intake and psychological adjustments to pregnancy. It is difficult to look upon pregnancy with joy if there is a constant feeling of nausea. The father may feel he is in part responsible for the discomfort his partner is feeling and have doubts about the pregnancy. Since the odor of food often adds to the nausea, meal preparation may be difficult, leading to nutritional alterations for the family.

Assessment of the frequency, severity, and pattern of the nausea and vomiting is done by the nurse. When nausea occurs upon awakening, the suggestion of eating a few crackers immediately upon awakening, remaining in bed for a short time, then rising, may offer some relief. If this is difficult to do because of work or school obligations, the father may be of some help by fixing breakfast for the children before the mother arises.

When the nausea occurs at intervals throughout the day, suggestions include eating several (6) small meals during the day rather than the normal three meals. This provides a constant supply of carbohydrates and avoids fluctuations in the blood glucose level. Starchy carbohydrates are more easily tolerated than other foods when nausea is present. Consumption of rich or greasy foods may contribute to the nausea and should be avoided. Overeating is not usually a problem, but it is to be avoided since it may add to the feelings of nausea. Limiting intake of liquids at meal times may also help to alleviate the nausea.

Ideally, the nausea and vomiting are controlled without the use of medications. Medications formerly used to treat nausea and vomiting are no longer routinely used owing to teratogenic effects. If nausea and vomiting remain uncontrolled, continuing past the third month of pregnancy, alterations may occur in maternal electrolyte balance which affect fetal growth and development. Hospitalization is then recommended to prevent further dehydration and restore fluid and electrolyte balance.

As with other discomforts of pregnancy, nausea and vomiting may be caused by disorders other than pregnancy. Gastroenteritis, appendicitis, cholecystitis, and inner ear problems are but a few of the conditions that should be considered.

HEARTBURN

Heartburn (*pyrosis*) is the burning sensation felt in the throat and esophagus caused by eructations of gastric contents. Acid indigestion, as heartburn is frequently called, is influenced by the increased production of progesterone during pregnancy. The muscle relaxing actions of progesterone cause a decrease in peristalsis, a relaxed cardiac sphincter, and decreased stomach emptying time. These factors combine with the altered position of the stomach from the enlarging uterus to produce symptomatic heartburn in 35 to 50 percent of pregnant women, especially during the third trimester.

To relieve the discomfort of heartburn several suggestions may be offered. Small frequent meals are advised to avoid placing added pressure on the stomach. A small glass of milk before and between meals will often relieve the discomfort. Avoiding spicy, rich, greasy foods and avoiding heavy meals before bed may be of some benefit. Antacids, if taken in large amounts, may disturb fetal electrolyte balance and should be avoided unless specifically recommended by the health care provider. Chewing gum or sucking on hard candy will benefit some clients, while in others the stimulation of digestive secretions intensifies heartburn. Remedies such as baking soda or some antacids are not recommended because of the high sodium content.

GINGIVITIS

Increased estrogen production produces increased vascularity of the gums. This, together with the progesterone-induced changes in connective tissue, encourages the development of gingivitis. Good oral hygiene and consumption of fresh fruits containing vitamin C will decrease symptoms. The expectant mother is told to avoid harsh toothbrushes.

PTYALISM

Elevated levels of estrogen contribute to increased production of saliva during pregnancy. This condition is more often noticed at night when the mother is in a supine position. Sucking on hard candy and using an astringent mouthwash are methods employed to reduce saliva.

CONSTIPATION

Progesterone exerts its effect on the gastrointestinal tract by slowing peristalsis. This effect, added to the pressure on the bowel by the enlarging uterus, causes constipation. Although the expectant mother may have had good bowel habits prior to pregnancy, there still remains an increased tendency for constipation to occur. Exercise, adequate fiber in the diet, and increased fluid intake are measures instituted early in pregnancy.

If constipation does occur, she may be advised to further increase her dietary intake of fiber by including foods such as bran cereals, apples, broccoli, peanuts, pears (with skin), and whole meal breads. Bowel habits should include the establishment of regular elimination times when the client is relaxed and unhurried. Laxatives and enemas are not advised unless specifically prescribed by the physician. The use of mineral oil is discouraged, since it interferes with the absorption of fat-soluble vitamins A, D, and E. Foods such as rice, chocolate, and cheese are sometimes found to be constipating.

HEMORRHOIDS

Hemorrhoids are large, distended varices of the rectum. Constipation and pressure on the perineal veins from the enlarging uterus predispose a patient to hemorrhoids. The discomfort of hemorrhoids may be somewhat relieved by avoiding constipation, increasing fluid intake, sitz baths, topical anesthetic sprays, and application of ice to the perineal area.

VARICOSITIES

Varicose veins usually appear in the second or third trimester of pregnancy, caused by the reduced tone of the unstriated muscles of the vein walls, the increased vascularity of the pelvic organs, and the predisposition to pooling of blood in the lower extremities. Varicosities may be found in the vulva and perineal area as well as in the legs. To prevent obstruction of venous return to the heart, the client is instructed to avoid any tight or constricting garments, to avoid sitting or standing for prolonged periods of time, to elevate the legs when sitting, to exercise in moderation, and to use elastic hose to promote muscle tone. Attention is directed toward assessments for thrombophlebitis when the client complains of pain, redness, or warmth in an extremity.

EDEMA

Physiologic changes (see Chapter 9) occurring during pregnancy contribute to the development of edema in the extremities. Assessments of the extent and physiologic characteristics associated with the edema are necessary to distinguish between normal physiologic edema and the edema associated with pregnancy-induced hypertension (PIH).

Dependent edema is most often noted at the ankles, and occurs after periods of standing or in the evenings following daily activities. Edema of the extremities may be relieved by resting with the feet elevated several times a day. It is reasonable to advise the expectant mother to elevate her feet every time she sits down and to avoid standing for long periods of time. To increase venous return to the heart and relieve edema, she is instructed to assume a left lateral position when sleeping. Avoiding constrictive garments and using support hosiery may also be recommended.

SUPINE HYPOTENSION

Feelings of faintness are often experienced by the client when she is in a supine position. Hypotension from a reduction in blood volume returning to the heart caused by pressure on the inferior vena cava results in a feeling of lightheadedness and vertigo. Relief is obtained by rolling to the left side and remaining in that position for a few minutes.

Dizziness experienced by the client is related to postural hypotension from pooling of the blood in the extremities and to periods of hypoglycemia resulting from hormonal changes of pregnancy. The client is advised to avoid quick movements and standing in the upright position for extended periods. Small frequent meals provide relief from the hypoglycemia by providing a ready supply of glucose.

LEG CRAMPS

Leg cramps result from an imbalance in the ratio of calcium to phosphorus. Pressure of the gravid uterus on the nerves of the extremities also increases the discomfort. Adjustment in calcium and phosphorus intake may be needed to restore the proper ratio. This may be done by assessing the amount of milk the client is drinking and the high phosphorus foods she is eating.

Leg cramps most commonly occur at night when the client stretches in her sleep. She awakens with pain in her calf. The first reaction is to massage the area. This is not recommended and should be advised against, owing to the increased possibility of thromboembolic conditions. She may place pressure on the knee while dorsiflexing the foot of the cramping leg. Standing up and applying pressure on the affected foot is also sometimes successful in relieving the cramp. Moderate exercise such as walking will increase muscle tone and is a preventive measure.

ITCHING

In about 20 percent of pregnancies woman complain about itching of the skin that intensifies as pregnancy progresses. Any skin area may be involved, although complaints of itching usually involve the abdomen or perineal area. Inspection of the skin will not reveal skin eruptions, even though evidence of scratching of the area may be noted. Explanations for this type of pruritis are not known, but it is suggested that stretching of the skin over the abdomen may cause itching as will the increased exudative properties of the skin.

Lotions, salves, or creams that contain cortisone or phenol are not recommended, owing to the possible teratogenic effects on the fetus. Baking soda added to the bath water and followed by application of a lotion containing menthol will help to relieve itching.

Another form of itching specific to pregnancy is *pruritis gravidarum*. During the last trimester the gravida complains of itching which may or may not be associated with jaundice. The exact mechanism of this condition is not known but is thought to be related to the increased production of placental steroids, which favors the accumulation of bile salts under the skin. The condition subsides following pregnancy.

Perineal itching may be the result of normal leukorrhea or vaginal infections such as *Trichomonas vaginalis* or *Candida albicans.* Pregnant women are instructed to report episodes of vaginal itching, foul odor, eruptions, or tenderness to identify the causative factor and institute treatment (see Chapter 25). Normal leukorrhea cannot be eliminated. Good perineal hygiene is advocated. Douching during pregnancy is not recommended.

SPIDER NEVI AND PALMAR ERYTHEMA

The two conditions often appear together in the last two trimesters of pregnancy. Spider nevi appear on the skin of the legs, arms, face, and cheeks as central arterioles with radiating smaller vessels. They are red or bluish red and create a spiderlike look under the skin. Palmar erythema imparts a red appearance to the palms and fingertips. Increased levels of estrogen are thought to be responsible for these conditions, and the client is reassured that these changes are normal. Palmar erythema disappears, but spider nevi only fade after delivery.

DYSPNEA

Shortness of breath during the later months of pregnancy is caused by pressure of the enlarged uterus on the maternal diaphragm. Energetic activities should be limited to lessen the stress on the respiratory system. Reclining with two pillows under the head and shoulders or deep abdominal breathing will provide some relief. When lightening occurs in the last few weeks of pregnancy, breathing will become less difficult.

ROUND LIGAMENT DISCOMFORT

Stretching of the ligaments that support the uterus during pregnancy occurs as the pregnancy advances. Discomfort may be experienced as gripping pains in the lower abdomen and groin that occur at irregular intervals. When a complaint of this nature is offered by the client, it should not be assumed that it is round ligament pain. Careful assessment is needed to rule out ectopic pregnancy, labor contractions, appendicitis, ovarian cysts, pelvic inflammatory disease, endometriosis, and abruptio placentae. Proper body mechanics and avoidance of positions that stretch the ligaments may help to reduce this discomfort.

DANGER SIGNALS DURING PREGNANCY

All expectant mothers are told to report any of the following signs to the physician immediately:

- Vaginal bleeding
- Visual disturbances, blurring of vision, spots before the eyes, double vision, dimness of vision
- Severe continuous headache
- Chest pain
- Persistent vomiting
- Swelling of the face and fingers
- Chills and fever
- Severe abdominal pain
- Sudden escape of fluid from the vagina prior to term
- Lack of fetal movement
- Epigastric pain
- Burning on urination

FAMILY-CENTERED CARE

The needs of each member of the family, their involvement, and roles in the childbearing period are important in the promotion of family-oriented care. The extended family of past years automatically included aunts, uncles, siblings, and grandparents in the childbirth experience. Today's nuclear family limits the involvement of those not within the immediate family circle. Grandparents, aunts and uncles, friends, and even other children may feel left out of this special event.

Identification of the psychological needs of both the mother and father have been identified in Chapter 9. The needs of others whose lives are touched by the pregnancy deserves consideration.

A crisis occurs when a new brother or sister enters the life of a child. The former love, adoration, and attention centrally focused on the child is now threatened by an intruder who demands equal rights to those amenities. He or she is still dependent on parents and, if very young, is unable to express the frustration in an acceptable manner.

When there are several siblings, the adjustment may still be difficult. Parental attention now must be divided further. Each child must assume a new role in the family whether he desires it or not. Even the physical environment may be altered as he is changed from a crib to a bed like big brother or sister. Previously accepted behavior becomes "babyish" and he is no longer looked upon as the baby in the family.

Family routines are altered to accommodate the new arrival that the unprepared child may view as a threat. From his perspective, the new baby is someone who cries a lot and either sleeps or eats most of the time and is no fun to play with.

The task of adjusting to the new arrival may seem overwhelming and monumental for the other siblings. Children are resilient and with parental help and guidance can make a successful adjustment. Preparation of children before the new arrival appears is very important. The nurse may suggest several ways in which parents can prepare other children for the anticipated event.

When children are young (under 4 years), preparation for the new baby is begun during the last months of pregnancy. Earlier preparation makes the waiting too long, and it becomes unbelievable for the child. Parents may begin the preparation by telling the child about the new baby in mommy's "tummy" and allowing them to feel the baby. Story books that portray the arrival of the new baby may be read and even visits with other families who have new babies are helpful. Detailed explanation of the origin of the baby are not necessary but simple truthful answers to questions as they arise are appropriate.

Older children are told of the new arrival as soon as expectations are visible or when the arrival is being talked about between family members. Trying to conceal the pregnancy may create feelings of insecurity, as the child wonders why the mother is tired, perhaps nauseated, and changing in appearance. Early explanations will prevent or relieve anxiety the child may be experiencing. Including these children in preparations for the new arrival allows them to feel a part of the event.

Children are made to feel that something special is happening to them as well as to mommy and daddy. It will be *their* new brother or sister and should not be presented as a new playmate since this creates unrealistic expectations. Alterations in the environment are not explained as needed for the arrival of the baby but are presented as changes that benefit them. For instance, changing older children from the crib to a new bed is explained as a special new bed for them, not just because they are older but because they are special and loved by mommy and daddy.

Whether children are toddlers, preschoolers, or school age, they are told about the absence that will occur when their mother has the baby. They need to know that there will be someone to care for them, get them ready for school, say their prayers with them, and do all of the other functions that are important to their developmental level. They need to know that daddy will be there and who the other person will be if there is to be additional help in the home. If they are going to stay with their grandparents or someone else, they will want to know the details about where they will sleep and eat. It is important that they have some understanding of how long two or three days will be, if that is the number of days mother will probably be gone. Most hospitals provide sibling visitation programs as well as a visit to the hospital before the baby comes. These programs are very helpful and reassuring to the child. If sibling visitations are available, the child is told about visiting his mother and the new baby.

Jealousy is to be expected when the new baby arrives. It is normal and is dealt with in a loving manner. Acting out and behavioral changes may occur with some children. Reassurance of parental love is always important to children but especially as they prepare to share that love with another.

GRANDPARENTS

Grandparents are often among the first to hear the news of the expected arrival. When harmonious relationships exist between the parents and grandparents there is great joy and pride shared in both telling and receiving the news. The grandparenting role is usually not acknowledged at first, when there are mixed emotions about their child becoming a mother or a father. As time progresses, they accept their role and will even joke and tease about it.

Many factors affect the attitudes of the grandparents as they identify with their new role. If they have young children still living at home, they may find themselves facing a dual role. Grandparents are traditionally looked upon as old, gray-haired, doting on their grandchildren, and financially comfortable and secure. In truth, this picture is not applicable to many of today's grandparents. The man and woman of 40 have difficulty in viewing themselves as old and sedate. The family who is still involved in the parenting of young children will find their lives anything but sedate. As they begin to work through their change in role, they begin to develop an individualized role, viewing themselves as fulfilling an important place in the lives of the parents-to-be and the expected baby (see Fig. 11–5).

If a trusting relationship exists, the expectant mother feels comfortable and secure in seeking the advice of her mother. Advice concerning the choice of a physician, midwife, clinic, or hospital for maternity care is often sought from the mother or grandmother. Suggestions may be given, but it is important for parents to realize that the final decision is ultimately that made by the expectant couple. Relationships can become strained if the mother assumes a controlling role, giving advice when not consulted and monitoring every aspect of her "little girl's" pregnancy. Even though the expectant mother still needs to be nurtured by her mother, her own developmental tasks require that she make independent decisions. When she is not allowed to make decisions or when her decisions are looked upon as inadequate, the pregnant woman is prevented from conceptualizing herself in the mothering role.

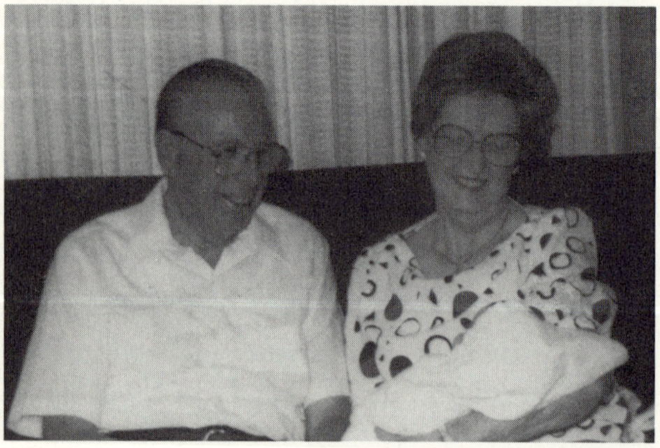

FIGURE 11–5. Grandparents are a special source of interaction and support.

Grandfathers may find it difficult to envision their son or son-in-law capable of assuming the responsibilities necessary for providing for a family and assuming fatherhood. The role of their daughter as mother is unfamiliar to them and they are often uncomfortable with the realization of the sexuality of their daughter and the image of her fulfilling a role previously identified with their wife. They will ponder what their own responsibility to this newcomer will be.

Prenatal classes for grandparents provide an opportunity for grandparents to become acquainted with their anticipated role. Discussions in these classes include topics such as current health management during pregnancy, the family and the birthing process, management of the newborn, role expectations, and the positive contributions of grandparents on childbearing and rearing. Involvement of the grandparents in preparations for the new baby seems to be a healing panacea for the doubts and concerns they may feel. When the family unit is healthy, the months of expectation provide time for adjustments to their new role. As they work together in preparation, the strengths of both the parents and grandparents provide a firm foundation for the parenting of the new baby.

CONTINUED HEALTH MANAGEMENT

Regardless of the type of health care facility the client chooses for her prenatal care, the nurse assumes the role of health care manager. Functioning within this role, she is responsible for the organization of care for each client. As the needs of the client and her family change throughout pregnancy, the nurse is responsible for evaluation and revision of the plan of care. Visits to the health care facility are planned in collaboration with the client and continued assessments of all dimensions are needed. The recommended scheduling for visits is once a month for the first 32 weeks, every two weeks until 36 weeks, then once a week until delivery. Nursing responsibilities at each subsequent visit after the initial visit are found in Table 11-6. A sample nursing care plan for the third trimester is provided in Table 11-7.

TABLE 11-6
NURSING RESPONSIBILITIES AT SUBSEQUENT VISITS

Assessments	Significance & Responsibilities
REVIEW	
All previous assessments	
Nursing diagnosis	
Nursing care plans	
ASSESSMENTS	
Maternal Parameters	
Temperature-Pulse-Respiration	See Tables 9-4 and 9-6
B/P	
Assess for	See Table 9-4
Pressure over 140/90	
Systolic + 30 over baseline	
Diastolic +15 over baseline	
Weight	See Table 9-3
Assess total gain and pattern of gain	
RBC	See Table 9-4
If Hematocrit below 30% repeat weekly; repeat on all gravidas at 24 & 34 weeks; blood sugar levels at 28 & 36 weeks	
Repeat Rh antibody screening of Rh^{-} gravidas	Repeat at 24, 28, 32, and 34 weeks
Urine	See Table 9-5
Assess for proteinuria, glucose, bacteria, and ketones	
Edema	
Assess for edematous areas and extent of edema	Dependent edema of ankles & feet in last trimester normal. Edema progressing to hands & face may be indicative of pregnancy induced hypertension. Consult physician. Determine correlation with elevated B/P, proteinuria, blurred vision & headache
Vagina Assess for vaginal discharge and bleeding Assess for amniotic fluid	Leukorrhea of pregnancy normal. If accompanied by itching, inflammation, or eruptions may indicate pathology. Consult physician. Presence of bloody discharge abnormal unless at term. Amniotic fluid leakage may indicate premature rupture of the membranes unless at term. Consult physician
Cervix Assess for softening, dilation and effacement in last weeks of pregnancy only	Do not assess if placenta previa, abruptio placenta, or premature labor suspected

TABLE 11-6 (continued)

Assessments	Significance & Responsibilities
ASSESSMENTS	
Breast Assess for lumps, secretion, inflammation and tenderness	Mastitis abnormal finding, colostrum may be present in last weeks of pregnancy
Uterus Assess for fundal height Correlate with gestation age	Decreased height for gestational age may indicate IUGR or fetal demise. Increased height may indicate polyhydramnios or multiple gestation
Assess for uterine contractions	Braxton-Hicks' contractions normal—Do Leopold's maneuver after 28th wk.
Assess for monthly physiologic adaptations	See Table 10-4, Monthly signs & symptoms of pregnancy
Fetal Parameters	
Fetal Heart Tones Assess rate, rhythm, quality, and location	Report absence of FHT or rate below 120 or above 160
Fetal Movement Assess for fetal movement during examination	If fetus is sleeping active fetal movement is not felt by examiner
Inquire about frequency of fetal movement within past 24 hours	Report if mother has not felt movement, may indicate fetal demise
Fetal Age Correlate with fundal height and gestational date	Report if discrepancies with EDC, ultrasound examination may be indicated Record when engagement of presenting part occurs
Nutritional Parameters	
Assess and discuss diet with client	Note any dietary deficiency and review nutrition with client
Assess for use of drugs and medications (including alcohol, tobacco & caffeine)	Note any medications taken, reason, and frequency of usage
Psychosocial-spiritual Parameters	
Assess and discuss aspects which may cause anxiety or alter pregnancy outcome Familiarize client with agencies providing economic or social aid when indicated	Refer when appropriate
Educational Parameters Assess for knowledge deficit in all area of antepartal care Correlate teaching with appropriate gestational period, learning level and readiness to learn	Familiarize all clients with availability of prenatal education but continue to assess learning needs throughout pregnancy
EVALUATION	
Evaluate assessment data Evaluate client goals and nursing interventions from previous care plan Discuss evaluations with client	Data evaluation and planning includes input from all members of the health team
PLANNING	
Formulate Nursing Diagnosis Revise Nursing Care Plan Discuss plan of care with client and plan for next visit	Office or clinic visits: once a month for the first 32 weeks, every two weeks until week 36 and then once a week until delivery

TABLE 11-7
SAMPLE NURSING CARE PLAN: PRENATAL CLINIC VISIT—THIRD TRIMESTER

Carol S., a gravida 1, para 0, has been receiving antepartal care since 4/12 when she made her first visit to the prenatal clinic. Her due date is 11/9. She has returned approximately every four weeks for her clinic visits. At her visit on 10/11 the prenatal history, clinic assessments, and nursing care plans are reviewed. Nursing diagnoses have been indicated on each of her care plans and goals, intervention and evaluations stated. A review of the nursing diagnoses reveals:

Nursing Diagnoses	Date Formulated	Dates Evaluated
Alteration in nutrition, less than body requirements related to inadequate food intake	4/12	4/26–5/23–6/23–7/25–8/23–9/23 Steady weight gain but goal of 25–30 pounds not met
Ineffective breathing patterns related to cigarette smoking	4/12	4/26–5/23 Goal met—client is not smoking
Anxiety related to fear of labor and delivery	4/12	4/26–5/23–6/23–7/25–8/23–9/23 Remains anxious about delivery—goal not met
Knowledge deficit related to first pregnancy	4/12	4/26–5/23–6/23–7/25 Goal met—attending childbirth preparation class starting 7/25
Self-concept, disturbances related to body-image	6/23	7/25–8/23–9/23 Improved self-image—stated she feels proud of her developing pregnancy. Goal met
Oral mucous membrane, alteration related to gingivitis	7/25	8/23–9/23 Gingivitis improved. Goal met

Assessments 10/11

Vital statistics:	B/P 128/72 Pulse 64 Respirations 16 Temperature 98.6°F Weight 138 lb
Laboratory values:	Urine: Neg for protein and acetone Neg for Glucose Neg for Bacteria Blood: Hemoglobin 12 gm Hematocrit 36%
Fetal assessment:	FHT 128 LLQ Fundal height 2 fingers below xyphoid process Weeks gestation 34 weeks
Physical assessment:	Vaginal: No bleeding or discharge Breast: No lumps, no secretions, nipples erect Cervix: Softening, no dilatation Edema: None apparent or described

TABLE 11-7 (continued)

Assessments 10/11

Extremities: No varicosities, no leg cramping
Respiratory: Dyspnea upon exertion, no cough, lung sounds clear
Elimination: Constipated, no hemorrhoids

Nutritional assessment: Eating well, balanced diet three times a day
Understands principles of good nutrition
No alcohol or tobacco, 2 cups of coffee per day

Psychosocial-spiritual: Anxiety over impending labor. Family support system intact. Father with mother at clinic visit.
Discussed preparations for newborn, sustaining spiritual values

Nursing Diagnosis	Goals	Nursing Interventions	Rationale	Evaluation
Alteration in nutrition, less than body requirements related to inadequate food intake	Client will: Gain 25 to 30 pounds by 11/9	Weigh client	To determine total weight gain	10/11 Weight 138 Gain of 28 pounds since 4/12. Goal met
		Continue to stress importance of adequate diet	To maintain weight & nutritional status	
Anxiety related to fear of labor and delivery	Verbalize confidence in her ability to meet the emotional & physical demands of labor and delivery	Assess knowledge of labor & delivery gained in prenatal class	Knowledge decreases anxiety from fear of the unknown	Client understands labor & delivery process Fear related to reality of approaching delivery
		Reinforce learning with review of labor and delivery by both husband and wife	Confidence gained with realization of own knowledge base Realization of team approach to labor & delivery	Able to discuss comfort and relaxation measures with accuracy
		Encourage practice of relaxation and breathing techniques daily	Develops attitude of preparedness	States they will set aside a time every evening for practice of techniques
Ineffective breathing pattern related to pressure of uterus on diaphragm	Client will: Institute measures to relieve pressure of uterus on diaphragm Experience relief from shortness of breath during daily activities and resting	Assess respiratory and cardiac status Explain measures client may utilize to relieve pressure Deep abdominal breathing	To assess for medical cause of dyspnea Relieves abdominal wall tension allowing thoracic expansion & greater intake of air	Respiratory and cardiac functions within normal range. Refer to assessment data Practiced abdominal breathing, performed well

		Practice stretching exercise with hands extended over head while doing abdominal breathing	Allows complete expansion of the thoracic cavity.	Practiced exercise, performed well
		Use two pillows under head when resting	Relieves pressure on the diaphragm	
		Rest in sitting position when experiencing discomfort	Decreases pressure on diaphragm	
		Limit strenuous activities such as climbing stairs	Avoid unnecessary stress on respiratory functioning	
		Secure help when lifting heavy articles.		
		Reassure client that pressure will be relieved when baby drops in pelvis (lightening)	Descent of fetus removes pressure off diaphragm	Stated she would welcome the occurrence
Bowel elimination, alteration in, related to constipation secondary to decreased smooth muscle tone	Client will: Experience relief from altered bowel function	Explain the causes of constipation during pregnancy	To relieve anxiety about constipation	Client understands relationship of pregnancy and constipation
	Understand dietary approach to control of bowel functioning	Stress importance of adequate fluid intake, 6 glasses daily	Decreased motility of bowel causes reabsorption of fluid, creating hard stools	Understands need for increased fluid intake and fiber containing foods
	Increase fluid and fiber intake in diet	Explain need for increase fiber content of diet	Fiber-containing foods stimulate peristalsis	
		Review with client foods that contain increased amounts of fiber (whole grain cereals, & bread, fresh fruit, & vegetables)	Increases client's awareness of foods in her own diet which provide fiber	States she likes fresh fruits with skins such as pears. Will include them as snacks and also eat more raw vegetables
	Establish regular bowel habits	Explain need for defecation when urge is first present	Delaying urge promotes stasis of bowel contents creating constipation	States she often ignores urge to defecate
	Avoid use of laxatives or enemas	Explain labor-stimulating effects of enemas and possible effects of strong laxatives on fetus	Continued use of laxatives increases constipation	
		Explain why use of mineral oil is not recommended	Interferes with absorption of vitamin A, D, & E	
		Bulk-producing laxatives may be used if recommended by physician		

BIBLIOGRAPHY

Allen, E. & Mantz, M.L. Are normal patients at risk during pregnancy? *Journal of Obstetric, Gynecological & Neonatal Nursing,* 1981, **10,** 348-353.

Alter, B. Prenatal diagnosis of hemoglobinopathies and other hematologic disease. *Journal of Pediatrics,* 1979, **95,** 501-503.

Brucker, M. & MacMullen, N. What's new in pregnancy tests. *Journal of Obstetric, Gynecological & Neonatal Nursing,* 1985, **14,** 353-359.

Ellis, D. Sexual needs and concerns of expectant parents. *Journal of Obstetric, Gynecological & Neonatal Nursing,* 1980, **9,** 306-308.

Goodlin, R., Schmidt, W. & Creevy, D. Uterine tensions during maternal orgasm. *Obstetrics & Gynecology,* 1972, **39,** 125-127.

Griffith, S. Childbearing and the concept of culture. *Journal of Obstetric, Gynecological & Neonatal Nursing,* 1982, **11,** 181-184.

Hawley, C. The older primipara: implications for nursing. *Journal of Obstetric, Gynecological & Neonatal Nursing,* 1981, **10,** 182-185.

Jameson, S. Variations in maternal serum zinc during pregnancy. Correlations, congenital malformations, dysmaturity, and abnormal parturition. *Acta Medica Scandinavia,* 1975, **Suppl,** 79.

LeMasters, G. Zinc insufficiency during pregnancy. A review. *Journal of Obstetric, Gynecological & Neonatal Nursing,* 1981, **10,** 124-125.

Leonard, L. Pregnancy and the underweight woman. *MCN,* 1984, **9,** 331-335.

——— Twin pregnancy. Maternal-fetal nutrition. *Journal of Obstetric, Gynecological & Neonatal Nursing,* 1982, **11,** 139-145.

Luke, B. Megavitamins and pregnancy. A dangerous combination. *MCN,* 1985, **10,** 18-23.

Mills, J.L., Graubard, B.I., Harley, E.E., et al. Maternal alcohol consumption and birth weight. How much drinking during pregnancy is safe? *Journal of the American Medical Association,* 1984, **252,** 1875-1879.

———, Harlap, S. & Harley, E. Should coitus late in pregnancy be discouraged? *Lancet,* 1981, **2,** 136-138.

Mueller, L. Pregnancy and sexuality. *Journal of Obstetric, Gynecological & Neonatal Nursing,* 1985, **14,** 289-294.

Naeye, R. Factors that predispose to premature rupture of the fetal membranes. *Obstetrics & Gynecology,* 1982, **60,** 93-97.

——— Influence of maternal cigarette smoking during pregnancy on fetal and childhood growth. *Obstetrics & Gynecology,* 1981, **57,** 18-21.

——— Weight gain and the outcome of pregnancy. *American Journal of Obstetrics & Gynecology,* 1979, **135,** 3-9.

Rankin, S. & Duffy, K. 15 problems in patient education and their solutions. *Nursing 84,* 1984, **14,** 67, 71-72, 74.

Rayburn, W. & Wilson, E. Coital activity and premature delivery. *American Journal of Obstetrics & Gynecology,* 1980, **137,** 972–974.

Reamy, K., White, S., Daniell, W. & Levine, E. Sexuality and pregnancy. *Journal of Reproductive Medicine,* 1982, **6,** 321–327.

Riordan, J. *A practical guide to breastfeeding.* St. Louis: Mosby, 1983.

Robinson, C., et al. *Normal and therapeutic nutrition* (17th ed.). New York: Macmillan, 1986.

Rosso, P. Nutrition and maternal-fetal exchange. *American Journal of Clinical Nutrition,* 1981, **34 S.** 744-755.

Rudman, D. & Williams, P. Megadose vitamins: use and misuse. *New England Journal of Medicine,* 1983, **309,** 488-490.

Winick, M. *Nutrition and fetal development.* New York: Wiley, 1974.

Worthington, B.R., Weigle, A. Caffeine and pregnancy outcome. *Journal of Obstetric, Gynecological & Neonatal Nursing,* 1983, **12,** 21-24.

chapter 12

PRENATAL EDUCATION

OBJECTIVES

Upon completion of this chapter, the reader will be able to:

1. Identify areas of assessment when planning a prenatal education program for the childbearing family.
2. Discuss the formulation of objectives appropriate for a prenatal education program.
3. Identify factors in the environment that enhance or distract from the learning environment.
4. Discuss group dynamics as a factor influencing learning in the class sessions.
5. Discuss factors influencing the structuring of course content in the prenatal education program.
6. Identify topics appropriate for a general prenatal education program. Discuss why these topics were chosen and their value.
7. Explain the basis for the psychoprophylactic method of prepared childbirth.
8. Identify the concepts and techniques that are the foundation for "prepared childbirth."
9. Demonstrate exercises used to enhance body alignment, relaxation, and breathing techniques.
10. Discuss the role of the labor coach during childbirth.
11. Explain product and process evaluation of a prenatal program.

KEY TERMS

Abdominal breathing
Accelerated/decelerated breathing
Conditioning
Effleurage
Labor coach
Lamaze technique of prepared childbirth
Open glottis breathing
Pant/blow breathing
Psychoprophylactic technique of prepared childbirth
Rhythmic chest breathing
Support person

Prenatal education is as much of a commitment to responsible nursing as is the delivery of maternity nursing care. It is the catalyst necessary for synthesis of the client's knowledge, gained throughout pregnancy. Nurses, in response to the ever-emerging changes in the delivery of family-centered maternity care, serve as a vanguard for the provision and implementation of instruction and programs dedicated to the dissemination of information concerning the childbearing experience.

From the moment of the first birth, childbirth education began. Women shared experience, whether good or bad, with daughters and other women. Cultural aspects and customs became an ingrained part of the childbearing experience; some were beneficial and others ladened the experience with fear and pain. Rituals served as the knowledge base upon which women entered and embraced the birthing experience. Control of the rituals was in the hands of the tribal leader, or medicine man, who performed the sacred and magical rites necessary for a successful birth. Pain was to be expected and the cry of the woman in childbirth a symbol of childbearing.

Throughout history, this legacy has persisted with variations and refinement in its adaptations. Decisions surrounding childbirth traditionally have been delegated to and assumed by the medical profession with limited input from pregnant women. These decisions were dutifully carried out and monitored by nurses. Fathers were interested bystanders who watched the enigma unfold. Although these roles were passively accepted by most individuals, slowly an awareness emerged for exploration and examinations of the foundations upon which these premises were based. New approaches to childbearing were offered by Grantly Dick-Read (1933), Lamaze (1951), and advocates of psychoprophylactic pain control (1958) and gate-control theory of pain control. Interested women became informed, and the impetus for necessary changes ensued.

However arduous the change, progress has been made toward the involvement of women in the decisions related to childbirth. Preparation for childbirth has become a team process involving physician, nurse, and parents working in a concentrated, coordinated effort to produce a satisfying and rewarding experience for the family.

APPROACHES TO PRENATAL EDUCATION

Many approaches to childbirth education have been proposed and aptly executed. All have goals directed toward assisting the parents to achieve a successful birth. Each program, however, is directed toward addressing the individual needs of the clients. When considering these needs, the nurse must assess the following:

- Client's readiness to learn
- Client's knowledge base
- Client's learning needs
- Client's learning level
- Past experiences related to childbirth
- Client's attitudes and fears about pregnancy
- Knowledge resources and support systems available to the client

Motivation for learning principles of health care is increased during pregnancy. This concept can be used when planning care for the childbearing family. Prenatal education that emphasizes a healthy pregnancy and a healthy baby provides incentive and goal direction for both the mother and father.

In view of these motivational aspects, the nurse who is planning a prenatal education program takes into consideration the factors influencing motivation. Acceptance or rejection of the pregnancy, trust and confidence in health providers, recognition of learning needs and conflicts that inhibit learning, and incentives all may influence the learner's motivation. Behavioral motivation is important as a learning force that directly influences the assimilation of knowledge and, ultimately, the welfare of the expectant family.

Each person brings a unique perspective to the process. Although goals may be similar for two participants in a prenatal education program, each has needs that reflect her individual characteristics and background. Previous education, experiences, and activities play an important role when assessing learning needs. The gravida with three children has different learning needs than the teenage mother with her first pregnancy. Yet, each can still learn something that will help her through the prenatal period and childbirth.

An initial assessment of the background of each individual in a prenatal class supplies information regarding her knowledge base. This assessment is informal, as individuals and instructors become acquainted. Free exchange of information between the participants and the instructor is encouraged during each class, and many times the expertise of a participant may be used to enhance the class. The multigravida may share her feelings or experiences with the class, providing an element of reality.

The learning needs of various clients reflect their concerns, goals, and objectives related to the childbearing experience. They may state that they desire to gain information or insight into the birthing process or that they know nothing about the care of the newborn. They have expressed a desire to learn and a need to internalize information perceived as meaningful. Respect for these learning priorities should be considered when planning course content. Active participation by clients in planning course content enables them to assume responsibility for their education and fosters participation in the learning process.

Sequencing of content may also be suggested by the participants. This may or may not concur with the opinion of the instructor and, in some instances, may make her a bit uncomfortable with the course organization. Discussion usually reveals, however, that the learners are addressing those topics about which they have anxieties and which may adversely effect future learning if not dealt with early in the class. With these factors in mind, it is then appropriate for the instructors to make suggestions for the ordering of the topics that provides continuity.

Learning levels of the participants are as individualized as the client's themselves. Ongoing assessments of the effectiveness of the instructor's teaching method are essential to class management. Efforts should continually be made to draw each participant into discussions, with questions framed at the appropriate learning level. Verbal and nonverbal cues are valuable indicators of teacher effectiveness. Fidgeting, sleeping, or distractive behaviors indicate a need to employ another teaching technique. Lecturing is the least effective method of teaching. It does present the information but does little to encourage involvement of listeners. A skillful blending of lecture, questions, discussion, and audio visual aids may stimulate the group, enhancing the experience for all participants and the instructor as well.

Past childbearing experiences will have a pronounced effect on learning health care concepts related to pregnancy. These experiences may be personal or a potpourri of experiences shared by others. Negative experiences with the health care system, misconceptions, old wives' tales, and distorted perceptions are obstacles to effective learning. Unless these obstacles are made known and explored, the client will not become an active participant in the learning process. Each person must believe the information presented by the instructor is reliable, accurate and applicable to her own situation. If the instructor presents herself as the authority whose information can not be questioned, an atmosphere of mistrust and doubtfulness is sometimes created. On the other hand, when the instructor is challenged or conflicting opinions are expressed, if she truthfully and openly explores and acknowledges questions, trust in the instructor's credibility develops. Correction of misinformation often requires a measure of sensitivity by the instructor. Attentively and patiently allowing the client to relate her experiences, attitudes, and conclusions gives insight into the reasons for false assumptions and the emotional response associated with these feelings. It should be remembered that each person believes what she is saying is true and worthy of expression. Response by the instructor such as "I'm glad that you called that to our attention, as it is a point which many others may be concerned about," sets the stage for productive interaction between the learner and the instructor. Moreover, if answers to questions or explanations of the client's past experiences can not be given, an honest, "I don't know but I'll see what I can find out for you," insures the client that the instructor is sincerely interested and committed to extracting the truth from the situation.

There is no doubt that most pregnant women have some fears and concerns about the delivery process and their capabilities when confronted with the situation. These fears may or may not be realistic but do place added stress on the mother. Fathers may also have feelings about their capabilities during labor and delivery and may even worry about the welfare of their partner and child. As the instructor explores these feelings with clients, she fortifies them with a sense of control over the events of labor, built on understanding and preparedness. Negative, self-limiting fears are replaced with positive feelings of anticipation for the challenges presented during labor and delivery. Pain during labor is not denied but methods of control that can be employed by both mother and father are emphasized.

Cultural differences may alter the client's perception of the events involved in childbearing. An understanding of these differences and respect for these beliefs must be expressed by the instructor. When in conflict with the instructor's view, these beliefs are examined with the clients in a nonjudgmental manner. Change is not forced on the client, but information that demonstrates sound reasons for change is provided.

Throughout class sessions the instructor shares resources that may be helpful and will add to clients' knowledge about pregnancy, labor, and delivery and care of the newborn. These resources may be reading material, other classes, audiovisual aids, or other knowledgeable individuals. It is important that referrals be appropriate to each client's level of understanding. Watching a movie of a Lamaze delivery is generally more appropriate than viewing a movie depicting the intricacies of a Cesarean delivery. Research articles may be enlightening for the instructor but cumbersome and boring for the teenage mother. On the other hand, individuals more knowledgeable about health care might find the same article valuable.

The instructor also determines whether other individuals might serve as sources of information and support. If, for instance, Aunt Mary is a nurse she may answer many questions and be a very reliable resource. Other clients may turn to friends who, in themselves, have limited maternity experience and rely on memories of their own deliveries. Some clients are interested in reading every bit of material they can secure regarding pregnancy and will be very informed. Each of these resources may have value for the individual and can contribute significantly to learning. The instructor who is aware of each client's resources will help them all to examine the information, extracting that which is beneficial and disregarding that which is not.

LEARNING ENVIRONMENT

The classroom environment has a profound effect on learning. Within this environment are psychological, physical, and social influences. All are interrelated and, when in harmony, create positive learning situations. Feelings of discomfort, annoyance, intimidation, or dissatisfaction all tend to exert a negative influence, producing less-than-desired results.

When considering the physical environment, comfort is a top priority. Luxury accommodations are not necessary, but attention to relaxation and comfort is important. Individuals seated on a small circle of blankets placed on the floor in a cheerful room are far more amiable than participants seated in a row of straightbacked chairs in a stark, cold room. A flexible seating arrangement encourages movement within the group and promotes eye contact with each other. Sitting in a circle draws individuals into the core with no space barriers, whereas a military seating arrangement places an invisible barrier between the learner and the instructor. This seating arrangement encourages the learner to listen with eyes straight forward unaware of the actions and reactions of others in the class. All eyes are focused on the instructor who utters great words of wisdom. Obviously, this method is not in keeping with today's view of learning as a reciprocal process. Other measures include good lighting, comfortable room temperature, and adequate ventilation. Attention to these details before the beginning of each session will improve the learning atmosphere.

Enhancement of the learning environment is increased by the use of appropriate audiovisual aids. Movies, slides, videotapes, and filmstrips can be used to increase the understanding of the subject material. Their use must be carefully planned to meet the desired objectives and not just to cover the material quickly. Effectively used, these aids can strengthen discussion or present visual descriptions of anticipated situations such as labor and delivery. Appropriate timing is essential when using audiovisual material, and a movie or video tape should not be shown just because it is available. All audiovisuals should be previewed and evaluated before use in the classroom. The level of information presented should be consistent with the learning level of the client or group. Before the material is presented, an explanation of the material and the objectives of the presentation should be mentioned. Upon completion of the presentation, questions and discussion should be encouraged.

The psychological status of the client is paramount to her learning. The manner in which the learning environment is perceived by the learner influences her behavioral response. If the learning environment is perceived as nonthreatening and supportive, personal involvement is increased and learning enriched. The instructor who views her role as that of a facilitator guiding the learner with her knowledge and expertise creates a climate that optimizes the learning potential of each student. The nurse need not be thought of as the client's best friend; however, a sincere interest in each student is important. When the client feels unable to ask questions because the instructor will think of them as "dumb," learning is blocked. Conversely, the student who views the instructor as a resource person with whom communication and interaction are easy, responds with eagerness and enthusiasm. Mutual collaboration between learner and instructor provides an atmosphere conducive to the achievement of learning goals.

Interaction takes place not only between student and teacher, but also between the student and the other individuals involved in the learning situation. Within the first few sessions of a class, patterns of socialization can be seen. Pregnancy provides a common base for those in the class; however, alliances develop based on other needs and values. For effective learning to occur the student must feel somewhat comfortable with her role in the group. As interaction between the group members takes place, other group dynamics become apparent. Members begin to share experiences, concerns, and fears. Feelings of understanding and empathy evolve as the group becomes united in its efforts to reach learning goals. Plans are frequently made for class members to notify each other when the babies begin to arrive and for a postpartum meeting of all the members and their new babies.

Fundamental to the success of the group is the inclusion of the teacher as a part of the group. Observation of the group process and its dynamics will enable her to assume a leadership role. Efforts to solidify the group are not made at the first class meeting, but subtle indications of group involvement are noted and used as a foundation for the growth. Indications of impeded group growth may also be identified by nonverbal clues and behaviors of individual members. Attempts can then be made by the instructor to determine and correct the deterrents.

In her leadership role, the instructor serves to facilitate the learning process. The quality of the instruction is a direct result of the planning and organization done by the instructor. Her knowledge of the subject is essential to effective instruction but does not insure successful teaching. A blend of teaching skills, knowledge, planning, and organizing are fundamental to the teaching-learning process.

Diversity of teaching methods is recommended when planning teaching strategies for the adult learner. Consideration is given to the effectiveness of each method as it relates to the material to be presented. Although an instructor may be more comfortable with one teaching method over another, it is not advisable to use only one method consistently. Following the determination of objectives and course content, the instructor decides which teaching method will be most successful for the group involved. With some, group discussion may be the predominant method. Other groups may benefit from a more structural approach to the material, such as lecture. No matter how many times the course is taught by the instructor, consideration must be given to the method of teaching best suited for the current class.

STRUCTURING THE CLASSES

When designing the program of instruction for expectant parent classes, the needs of the group determine the type of program to be offered. In some instances the class will focus on prenatal care and preparation for delivery. Other classes emphasize methods of relaxation and coping behaviors helpful during labor and delivery. Ideally, a variety of courses may be offered, providing clients an opportunity to choose the program most applicable to their needs.

Much controversy exists concerning the best time during pregnancy for prenatal education. Many believe clients should receive instruction in the first trimester so they can benefit from it throughout pregnancy. Others believe that instruction in the last trimester of pregnancy focuses on the actual concerns of the clients and prepares them better for the upcoming labor and delivery.

Early first trimester instruction offers a foundation of information as physiologic and psychological changes begin to occur. Insight into the needs of the developing fetus and the mother provides the basis for the maternal understanding and health care planning. Information offered during this time may assist clients to make decisions regarding labor and delivery which are consistent with their needs.

Courses offered in the mid or last trimester generally focus on preparation for labor and delivery. Mechanisms and techniques that may be employed to promote comfort and reduce anxiety during childbirth are stressed. Classes demonstrate physical exercises and breathing techniques that are practiced at each session with the aid of their support person (labor coach). Group support is an integral part of the class, with practice sessions creating a shared atmosphere. Care of the infant and preparations for its arrival are frequently client priority items during the last trimester.

The length of the course is influenced by the purpose and objectives of the program. Time constraints are needed to provide a framework for course organization, but flexibility within these time constraints is desired. Organization of each class session should include a preview of the material to be presented at the beginning of each class and a summary at the completion of the class period. These techniques provide continuity to the presentation and allow the learner to realize a sense of achievement as highlights are summarized at the end of the class.

CONTENT OF CHILDBIRTH EDUCATION CLASSES

While developing the objectives for a prenatal or childbirth preparation class, the needs of the clients are considered. Similarities and common needs may be identified, allowing the instructor to delineate topics as she designs the program. These topics provide the components of the course outline, which is presented for discussion at the first class session. Data derived from the assessment of the learners' needs will then allow the instructor to modify and restructure the course outline. Topics that may be suggested to the group for consideration are:

Basic anatomy and physiology of the reproductive system
Conception and fetal growth
Physical and emotional aspects of pregnancy
Nutrition and care during pregnancy
Signs of labor
The laboring process
Comfort measures during labor and delivery
Physical fitness as preparation for labor and delivery
Analgesia and anesthesia used during labor and delivery
The birthing process—vaginal and cesarean deliveries
Characteristics of the newborn infant
Newborn and maternal care following delivery
Parenting and the family

The group may be interested in all of these topics or they may wish to concentrate on certain topics or even offer suggestions for other topics. Topics such as the anatomy and physiology of the reproductive system may generate little interest; however, it is then the responsibility of the instructor to integrate this material into the course content in an interesting, comprehensible manner.

Preparing the body for the physical and psychological stressors encountered during labor and delivery is often a topic of interest to all the class participants. These concepts and techniques may be introduced as early as the first class session and reviewed and practiced at the following classes. This preparation includes the employment of relaxation aids, breathing techniques, and physical exercises.

Two of the foremost leaders in prepared childbirth were Grantly Dick-Read (1933) and Ferdinand Lamaze (1951). Dr. Dick-Read, an English obstetrician of the 1920s and 1930s, identified childbirth as an experience innundated with distortions and fear, that creates an unnatural anxiety in women. He believed that childbearing was a natural process that could be enhanced by childbirth education. This would enable the mother to break the fear-tension-pain cycle that bound her to the pain and unpleasantries of the birthing process. Once this ingrained cycle was broken, he believed, the mother would be able to participate in childbirth with a measure of control over the events of labor and delivery. He felt that, without the burden of fear and anxiety, the woman would experience childbirth as a natural process without the need of medication for pain.

Dr. Dick-Read's concepts were largely ignored by his fellow colleagues until 1951, when Dr. Ferdinand Lamaze, a French physician, introduced painless childbirth based on the psychoprophylactic method of prepared childbirth (PPM). Although previously introduced in Russia, its use did not become widespread until Dr. Lamaze modified the technique and applied it to his practice.

The psychoprophylactic and Lamaze methods of prepared childbirth differ from the Dick-Read method in their structural approach of "conditioning." The mother is taught to respond to a verbal clue in order to elicit the behavioral response of relaxation. She is not told to just relax with each contraction, but, through practice, she automatically relaxes when the verbal clue is given by her labor coach. The term contraction is used to replace the term pain, and when she hears the word contraction she associates it with relaxation.

The couple learns that relaxation and comfort during labor and delivery is their responsibility, giving them control over the experience. However, this control can only be gained by practice, discipline, and dedication to the method. Both the woman and her labor coach see the experience in a positive manner, enabling them to cope and adapt as labor progresses.

The role of the labor coach is vital as he or she provides clues of a verbal and tactile nature. When interruptions in coping occur, the labor coach reenforces the techniques with words of encouragement and direction. These interruptions are to be expected and not viewed as an indication of the client's failure. Through practice, the couple is able to make the necessary adjustments when the situation occurs.

The original methods used by both Dick-Read and Lamaze did not incorporate the role of a support person such as the father. However, as the methods became more widely accepted, the concept of the "labor coach" chosen by the mother was adopted, enabling the support person to become actively involved in the birthing process. The support person is not limited to just the father but may be the client's friend, sister, mother, or any individual chosen by the pregnant woman.

Concepts involving relaxation repeatedly appear as components of the methods of prepared childbirth. First found significant by Dick-Read and Lamaze, they have become some of the most important elements of childbirth education. These concepts are based on preparedness of the childbearing couple through techniques involving:

Physical fitness
Breathing techniques
Relaxation techniques

Physical Fitness

During the entire life span, physical fitness enhances all the dimensions of man. It is an integral part of successful adaptation to many of life's experiences. The childbearing experience is no exception. Physical fitness during pregnancy is a decided asset when meeting the physiologic and psychological needs of labor and delivery.

Success in achieving physical fitness during pregnancy may, for some, be a continuation of previously established health practices. In the modern sedentary lifestyle of many individuals, however, physical fitness is more of an ideal than a reality. A large percentage of pregnant women engage in some sort of physical activity that is neither planned nor regular. These activities may be beneficial to the overall fitness of the mother, but because of their unstructured nature will not provide conditioning of all the muscle groups. In these circumstances, a program of exercises that prepares the body for the physical stress of those muscles involved in childbirth is initiated.

Vigorous exercising programs are not recommended during any stage of pregnancy. Exercises that speak to conditioning, body alignment, and positioning are the most helpful. The best physical fitness program for the pregnant woman is one that addresses her individual physical fitness needs. However, this may be difficult to determine or to actualize in a class with many participants. The following exercises are offered as examples of some of the many exercises which may be employed during pregnancy.

BODY ALIGNMENT

Good posture during pregnancy enables the pregnant body to accommodate to the physical changes and stress placed on the muscles, pelvis, and spine. Principles of good body alignment include posture when walking, standing, and lifting. When walking, emphasis is placed on standing erect with shoulders back, allowing free expansion of the thoracic cavity and enhancing deep breathing.

EXAMPLE

Stand erect with the shoulders and the back of the head against the wall and arms at the side. Inhale deeply and slowly raise the arms to a horizontal position against the wall (see Fig. 12-1,*A*). Continue raising the arms over the head in an arclike fashion until they touch (Fig. 12-1,*B*). Slowly exhale as the arms are returned to their original position. Repeat three times.

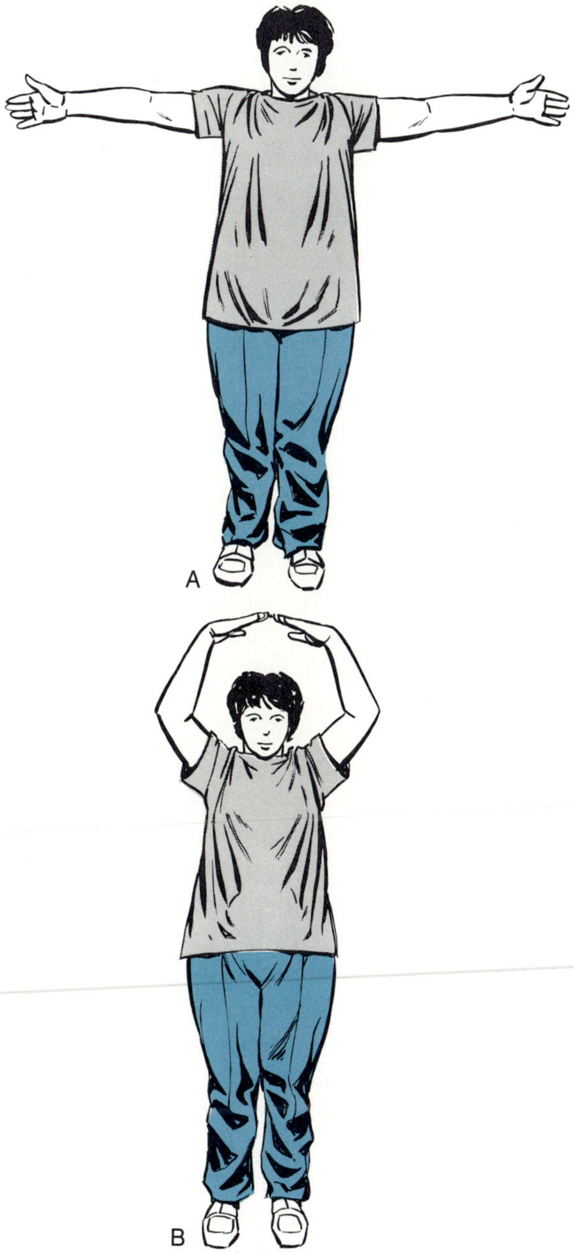

FIGURE 12-1. Body alignment arc: A. Inhale as arms are raised to a horizontal position. B. Raise arms in an arclike fashion.

EXAMPLE

Pelvic tilt alterations during pregnancy are related to the softening of the pelvic joints. This, coupled with the weight of the enlarging uterus, causes an increase in the curvature of the spine, resulting in backache. The discomfort created by this anatomic change may be relieved by pelvic rocking, which decreases the lumbosacral curvature of the spine.

Assume a position on the hands and knees. Inhale deeply as the chin is tucked down on the chest, the abdominal muscles and buttocks are contracted, and the back is arched upward. Exhale as the head is raised and the abdomen allowed to drop toward the floor (see Fig. 12-2). Repeat three times.

During labor, pelvic rocking may be done to relieve backache while in the supine position. The back is arched, the knees are flexed and the abdominal muscles and buttocks are contracted, creating a space between the floor and the back. Inhale as the back is arched and exhale as the spine is allowed to return to the resting position.

IMPROVED MUSCLE TONE

Good muscle tone allows the muscles needed during labor and delivery to function at their full potential. Muscle tone may be improved by participation in planned exercise sessions such as swimming, walking, and aerobics designed for the pregnant woman. The following exercises will improve muscle tone in the muscles used during the birth process.

EXAMPLE

Stand erect with the feet about 1 foot apart and the arms relaxed at the sides. Inhale deeply as the right arm is extended over the top of the head, stretching from the waist to the opposite side. Allow the left arm to slide down the left side as the degree of extension is increased (see Fig. 12-3). Exhale while returning to the upright position. Repeat, bringing the left arm over the head and sliding the right arm down the side. Repeat the entire sequence three times. This exercise increases the intercostal dimension of the chest, facilitating deep breathing.

EXAMPLE

While sitting on the floor in an upright position, flex the legs, placing the soles of the feet together. Place the

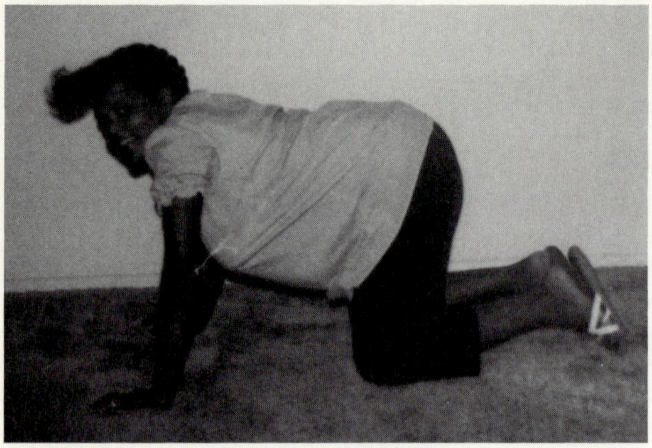

FIGURE 12-2. Body alignment—pelvic tilt.

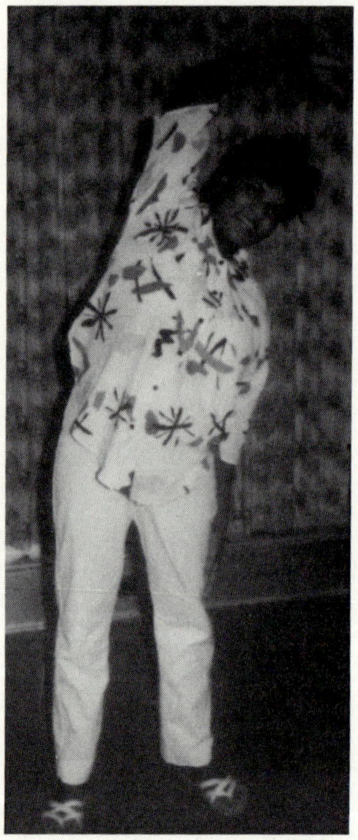

FIGURE 12-3. Muscle tone erect waist stretch.

hands under the knees of each leg. Using the thigh muscles, push the knees toward the floor while the arms are pulling upward on the knees (see Fig. 12-4). Resistance should be felt as the two forces work in opposition. The inner thighs and the muscles of the hips are strengthened when performing this exercise.

EXAMPLE

This exercise aims to improve the muscle tone of the perineal area. The area contains the pubococcygeal

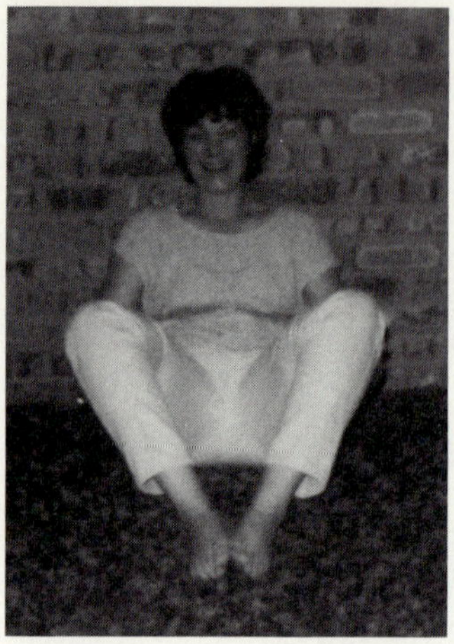

FIGURE 12-4. Muscle tone tailor press.

muscles, which are responsible for contraction of the urethral, vaginal, and rectal openings. Control may be acquired in each of the separate areas by individually contracting and relaxing each muscle.

While urinating, purposely stop the flow of urine by contracting the muscles surrounding the urethra. Relax them and allow the flow to resume.

During intercourse, contract and relax the muscles of the vagina. Contracting and relaxing the vagina may also be utilized to provide relaxation during a pelvic examination.

Contract the area surrounding the rectum, drawing the muscles upward and inward. Allow the muscles to relax, and repeat the procedure 5 times.

Relaxation Techniques

The overlying basis for the techniques used in labor and delivery is the concept of controlled relaxation. Relaxation physiologically spares the body from the effects of pain, eliminating untoward effects from poor circulation, tension, and altered oxygenation of the tissues and muscles. Without relaxation, even a body that is physically fit, is unable to function at peak performance.

Relaxation is not achieved during labor and delivery without conscious awareness and directed concentration. Simply telling oneself to relax will not accomplish the task. There must be motivation and awareness based on learned principles of conditioning, concentration, and controlled relaxation techniques.

These principles are employed in a team effort involving the laboring woman and her labor coach.

Conditioning begins with an awareness of relaxation. Tension is not always perceived by the individual, even when muscles are constricted; therefore, learning to relax is essential. The combined efforts of the pregnant woman and her coach are employed to learn controlled relaxation. As the mother learns the techniques of relaxation, the coach is taught to recognize signs of increasing tension that the mother is experiencing. A sequence of progressive muscular relaxation techniques may be taught to the couple in the following manner.

1. The mother is asked to assume a supine position, with pillows supporting her head, shoulders, and knees. She then directs her attention to an object within her view. Taking several deep breaths in and out, she progressively relaxes her body beginning with the head. The head may be rotated in a circular fashion several times in both directions. The muscles of the face, mouth, and neck are then relaxed followed by the shoulders and arms. Each arm should lie limply at the side. Progressive relaxation continues down the body until the entire body has been consciously relaxed.
2. The labor coach then instructs the mother to tense several areas of her body. Either verbal or tactile cues may then be given by the coach to assist the mother to relax specific areas of her body while deliberately maintaining contractions in other areas. The verbal cues are in the form of commands such as, "Breathe deeply, exhale, and relax your right arm." Tactile cues are given by stroking the part which is to be relaxed in a proximal to distal manner. After each area of the body has been tensed and relaxed, the mother is asked again to relax completely. The coach then checks all parts of her body to determine if relaxation is complete. The coach gently raises her hand, feeling for limpness at the wrist, and continues in this manner with the other parts of the body. There should be no resistance as each part is manipulated.
3. At each session this routine is followed as the mother learns to trust the cues given by her coach. The practice sessions consist of isolating areas to be tensed, followed by relaxation cues directed toward other areas of the body. This method of neuromuscular disassociation enables the mother to maintain a voluntary state of relaxation during labor while the uterus involuntarily contracts. Her attention is focused on a response when the cue word "contraction" is given and away from the discomfort of the contraction.

Through concentration and practice, the conditioned response of relaxation is realized. Ideally, the practice session is held frequently, if not daily, during the later months of pregnancy. In this manner, when labor does begin, the mother feels confident, well prepared, and assured of the support and capabilities of her coach. She feels in control and able to make decisions in the birthing process. In turn, the coach feels responsible and prepared for the role he or she will assume during the labor. The coach realizes that he or she is a significant contributor to the comfort and safety of both the mother and the baby.

Breathing Techniques

A variety of breathing techniques designed to assist in relaxation may be used during labor and delivery. Although some instructors may be proponents of specific breathing techniques, strict adherence to a certain method is seldom seen. Clients generally become acquainted with the various techniques but are free to choose the technique most appropriate for them. In the past years, breathing and relaxation techniques were used to replace pain medications or anesthesia. Although this concept is currently accepted, the client should be told that she and her coach have a choice and may combine breathing and relaxation techniques with medication and anesthesia if desired. Mothers should not be burdened with the thought of failure if they choose to receive assistance in relaxation. At the same time, medications and anesthesia must not be forced on the mother who chooses to experience birth without them.

Breathing techniques are started at the beginning of each contraction. As the deep breath is taken, the cue for focusing the attention is given and the conditioned response of relaxation is begun. Throughout the contraction breathing techniques are employed. At the conclusion of the contraction another deep cleansing breath is taken.

1. Abdominal Breathing. This breathing technique is initiated when contractions begin to produce discomfort. The mother is instructed to take a deep breath at the onset of the contraction. During the practice sessions she is instructed to place one hand on her abdomen and the other on her chest. As the breath is taken she should feel the hand on the abdomen rising more than the hand on the chest (see Fig. 12–5). The breath is held as long as the contraction lasts. This type of breathing allows the uterus to expand without resistance from the abdominal wall. As the contractions increase in intensity and duration, it may no longer be possible for the mother to sustain a breath during the entire contraction. In this case she may find it necessary to take several chest breaths while she maintains the abdominal wall expansion. The focus of attention is on the sustained abdominal breathing while the remainder of the body is relaxed. Abdominal breathing is difficult to sustain during the transition phase of labor, necessitating the mother to change to a shallow chest breathing.
2. Lamaze Rhythmic Chest Breathing. Different levels of breathing are used with the Lamaze techniques. At the onset of true labor, during the latent phase, slow, rhythmic chest breathing is begun with each contraction. The mother is told to take a deep cleansing breath, inhaling through the nose and exhaling through the mouth. Following the cleansing breath, the mother should invoke a breathing pattern of 6 to 9 breaths per minute, inhaled through the nose and exhaled through the mouth.
3. Accelerated/Decelerated Breathing. When contractions increase in intensity, frequency, and duration, slow, rhythmic breathing may no longer reduce discomfort. As she advances to the second level of breathing, the contractions last from 45 seconds to more than 60 seconds, with cervical dilation increasing (about 4 to 7 cm). During this active phase of labor, she begins an accelerated/decelerated type of breathing. After taking a cleansing breath, a shallow rapid breathing pattern is begun. The rate begins slowly and increases with the intensity of the contraction, reaching a peak at the height of the contraction (acme), and slowly decelerating as the contraction subsides (see Fig. 12–6). This pattern depends on the mother's perception of the intensity of the contraction and may vary from one contraction to the next.
4. Effleurage. Effleurage is used to enhance breathing techniques during the more active phases of labor. The mother begins this technique by using her fingertips to lightly massage the uterus. As she inhales she places her fingertips on the abdomen at the level of the symphysis pubis and massages upwards toward the navel. During exhalation the fingertips are moved downward on the lateral aspects of the abdomen (see Fig.

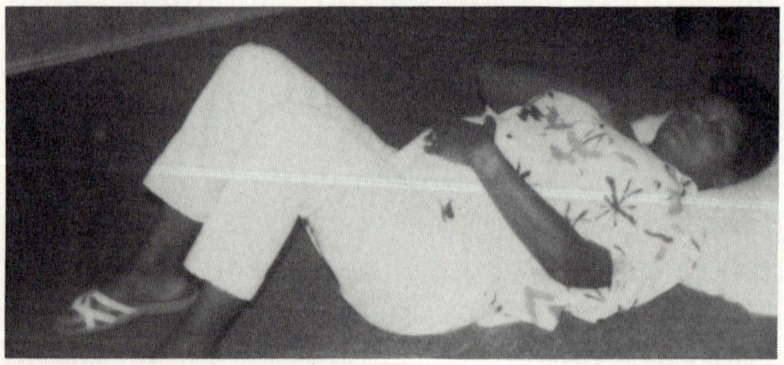

FIGURE 12–5. Relaxation abdominal breathing.

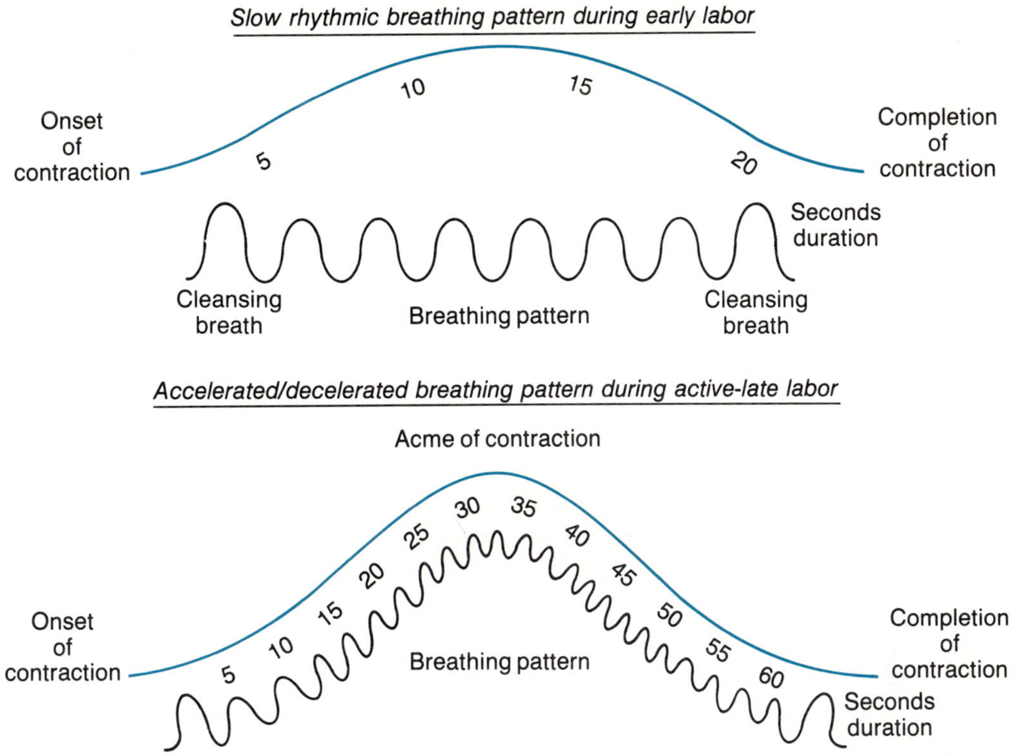

FIGURE 12-6. Relaxation accelerated/decelerated breathing.

12–7). The technique may be done in the reverse manner, depending on the preference of the mother.

5. Pant/Blow Breathing. The transition phase of labor produces the most intense contractions of the laboring process. During this phase the mother is often threatened with the loss of control. Contractions now occur one after the other with only short intervals between contractions. Following the cleansing breath, she inhales and exhales through the mouth creating a sound resembling "hee-hee." Three of these breaths are taken. The next breath is exhaled through pursed lips with a slight blow. The pattern thus consists of 3 pants followed by 1 blow repeated throughout the entire contraction. At the completion of the contraction a cleansing breath is taken.
6. Second Stage Breathing. With the onset of the second stage of labor the mother experiences the urge to push. At the beginning of each contraction she takes a cleansing breath and then pushes for four to five seconds while maintaining an open glottis and exhaling slightly with an audible grunt. The glottis remains open during the push to avoid the effects of the Valsalva maneuver, encountered while pushing with a closed glottis. During the entire contraction there may be 5 or 6 episodes of pushing.

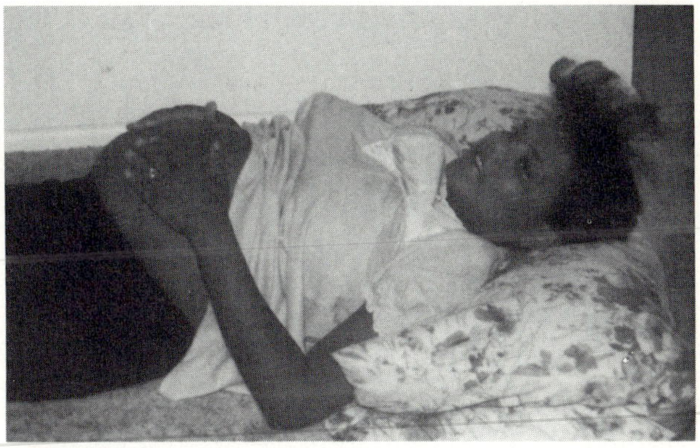

FIGURE 12-7. Effleurage.

Following the contraction she relaxes and breathes, using chest breathing techniques. This manner of breathing differs from the Lamaze technique and from the formerly accepted breathing technique of pushing and holding the breath during the entire contraction. Caldeyro-Barcia (1979) found open glottis breathing effective in preventing maternal cardiovascular stress effects and fetal effects from decreased placental blood flow associated with breath holding and pushing (Carr, 1983). When practicing the technique, the mother is asked to assume a squatting position, which will facilitate a bearing down effort at the time of delivery. Since not all hospitals or birthing centers can accommodate delivery in the squatting position, the gravida may also practice the exercise while assuming a position on the floor with the knees flexed. The shoulders and head are placed on pillows and elevated about 35 degrees. She places her hands behind her knees and pulls her knees outward. After her verbal cue, "contraction begins," is given, she begins the following pattern of breathing:

A cleansing breath is taken.

Pushing is begun with an open glottis and no thoracic pressure. A grunt may be heard.

Pushing continues for not more than five seconds.

The short spurts of pushing are repeated with an open glottis throughout the entire contraction.

Between contractions she rests and uses chest breathing.

When instructing couples in the use of breathing techniques, several considerations must be kept in mind. The techniques are demonstrated by the instructor before each class practice session. During these sessions the instructor monitors each couple as they perform the breathing techniques. Observations are made for too rapid a rate, shallow ineffective breaths, sustained expirations, tenseness during the breathing patterns, and disharmony between the mother and coach when practicing. Characteristics and symptoms of hyperventilation are discussed. Couples are made aware that hyperventilation results in a decrease of CO_2 with a concomitant rise in the pH of the blood. This respiratory alkalosis produces symptoms that include ringing in the ears, tingling in the fingers and toes, and vertigo. Each couple is shown how to correct this condition by breathing slowly into a paper bag or cupped hands.

Responsibilities of the Coach

The labor coach makes a direct, positive contribution to the success of the childbearing experience. From the onset of the first class, the coach's role is defined as that of the support person for the laboring mother. Dedication of both the mother and the father or other support person to a positive childbearing experience is the key to a successful delivery. The coach's involvement in and knowledge of the process must be as zealous as that of the mother. Both become aware of the process of delivery and the stressors involved. Before the onset of labor they should be able to conceptualize the entire experience, including the physical and psychological aspects. The techniques they can employ cooperatively are emphasized, and each knows that the other is there to share the experience.

During the practice sessions, the coach must not only be aware of the techniques involved but of the stimuli and cues that provoke a positive response from the mother. Some women will respond to the verbal cues and resent the use of tactile cues, while others will benefit more from the stroking. The coach will also learn the manner in which she is best able to focus her attention and concentrate on conscious relaxation. Together they can discuss the most useful approaches for the stressful periods.

Using knowledge of the childbearing events, the coach is able to encourage the mother by reminding her of the progress she is making during labor. Since the coach is aware of the characteristics of the transition phase, he or she does not become alarmed when the mother vascilates between control and moments of inadequate coping. The coach is prepared for her reactions during these moments and provides positive support in the ways most helpful to her.

During the entire labor process the coach watches for signs that indicate physiologic reactions to stress. If controlled breathing gives way to hyperventilation, awareness of the symptoms and measures that can be taken to alleviate the problem is needed. Careful assessment of muscular relaxation of each part of the mother's body provides clues to signs of increasing muscular tension, which, if allowed to continue, could contribute to muscular spasms and lower pain tolerance. Overt responses such as withdrawal, crying out, lip biting, and fist clenching are viewed by the coach as negative responses and indicators for coaching interventions. Reassuring words, a take-charge attitude, and reminders of control measures are often actions which, if instituted by the coach at the appropriate time, may help the mother to regain control.

The coach is not only responsible for filling the coaching role but also for controlling his or her behavioral responses during labor and delivery. This is particularly important when the father assumes the coaching role. In years past, when a passive role was assumed by the father, his needs or responses were seldom considered. Today, however, exploration of the father's psychologic responses to labor are examined before the onset of labor. The father is taught to be aware of the feelings he may experience seeing the mother of his child in pain and realizing the limitations of his ability to help her. He also learns that the events of labor may be lengthy, with both mother and father becoming weary, yet neither being able to step out of the process and rest.

In the same vein, his instruction during prenatal education teaches him the roles of the nursing personnel and ways in which the team of nurse, physician, mother, and father may work together. He comes to realize that when difficulties in the laboring process occur he may depend on the professionals for support and direction. It may be necessary for him to express his feeling of helplessness and ask for assistance to help him relax, refocus, and once again assume his supportive role.

The support person if other than the father may also feel uncomfortable as labor progresses. Feelings of inadequacy are intermingled with an overwhelming sense of responsibility. The support person who was relaxed at the onset of labor may now show signs of tension, becoming quiet while watching the physical manifestations of the transitional stage. Once again, the nurse must be supportive of this individual as well as the client.

EVALUATION PROCESS

Evaluation of instruction enables the instructor to modify the program and to make needed content additions or alter teaching techniques. Effective evaluation provides assessment of the outcome in relation to the desired goals and objectives of the program. Instructional programs may provide enlightenment and entertainment, but if the objectives have not been met, the program has been less than effective in attaining its goals.

The evaluation process should provide an assessment of the structure, content, and method of instruction. These items have been collectively defined as product and process evaluation. The product component refers to the attainment of objectives and the achievement of desired behavioral outcomes. The process refers to the design and structure of the course, including instructional approaches.

Since decisions regarding future programs and instruction are based on the decisions made following the evaluation, careful identification of the purposes and areas of evaluation must be identified and incorporated into evaluation. The who, what, where, when, and how of the evaluation process should be addressed. Repetitious or redundant items can be excluded, as careful attention is given to the evaluation tool. Variations of check list, written narratives, discussion, and audiovisual recording may be included in the evaluation. Questions should be objective rather than subjective as well as pertinent and to the point.

The evaluation process is no better than the purpose for which it was intended. If the instructor merely wants a pat on the back for her efforts, a simple "Did you enjoy the class as much as I enjoyed teaching you" directed to the entire class will probably result in the desired accolade. However, if the instructor is truly interested in the effectiveness of the product and process, she will critically plan and analyze all aspects of the evaluation process.

Administration of the evaluation should be planned to allow adequate time and anonymity. Open-ended questions will invite truthful and frank answers if names are not on the questionnaires. If the evaluation is considered a last minute item, to be completed in the last two minutes of class, serious consideration of the questions may not be given.

Upon completion of the evaluation process, the data must be analyzed, summarized, and utilized for decision making. The data may reveal information that is critical as well as supportive. In either case, the information must be included in the overall analysis. Ignoring information that is ego-deflating allows an inaccurate assessment and an invalid basis for decision making.

Evaluation provides the keys to the success of any future programs. The evaluation process cannot be overstated, as it provides the insight for improvements which are prerequisites for effective teaching and learning.

BIBLIOGRAPHY

Beck, N. & Hall, D. Natural childbirth: A review and analysis. *Obstetrics and Gynecology*, 1978, **52**, 371-379.

Caldeyro-Barcia, R. The influence of maternal bearing-down efforts during second stage on fetal well-being. *Birth Family Journal*, 1979, **6**, 17-21.

Carey, J. First trimester prenatal counseling in private practice. *Journal of Obstetric, Gynecological and Neonatal Nursing*, 1981, **10**, 336-339.

Carr K. Management of the second stage of labor. *NAACOG Update Series* (CPEC), 1983, **1** (9).

Dick-Read, G. *Childbirth without fear*. New York: Harper & Row, 1957.

Genest, M. Preparation for childbirth-evidence for efficacy. *Journal of Obstetric, Gynecological & Neonatal Nursing*, 1981, **10**, 82-85.

Humenick, S. Pregnant adult learners. *NAACOG Update Series* (CPEC), 1984, **1**, 1-8.

Jimenez, S. Application of the body's natural pain relief mechanism to reduce discomfort in labor and delivery. *NAACOG Update Series* (CPEC), 1983, **1**, 1-7.

———. My way: the new Lamaze. *Childbirth Educator*, 1982, **1**, 37-42.

Sasmor, J. & Grossman, E. Childbirth education in 1980, *Journal of Obstetric, Gynecological & Neonatal Nursing*, 1981, **10**, 155-160.

———. *Childbirth education—A nursing perspective*, New York: Wiley, 1979.

Simkin, D. *The complete pregnancy exercise program*, St. Louis: Mosby, 1980.

Walls, J. An instruction guide for educating expectant mothers, *MCN*, 1983, **8**, 274-276.

UNIT IV

THE INTRAPARTAL FAMILY

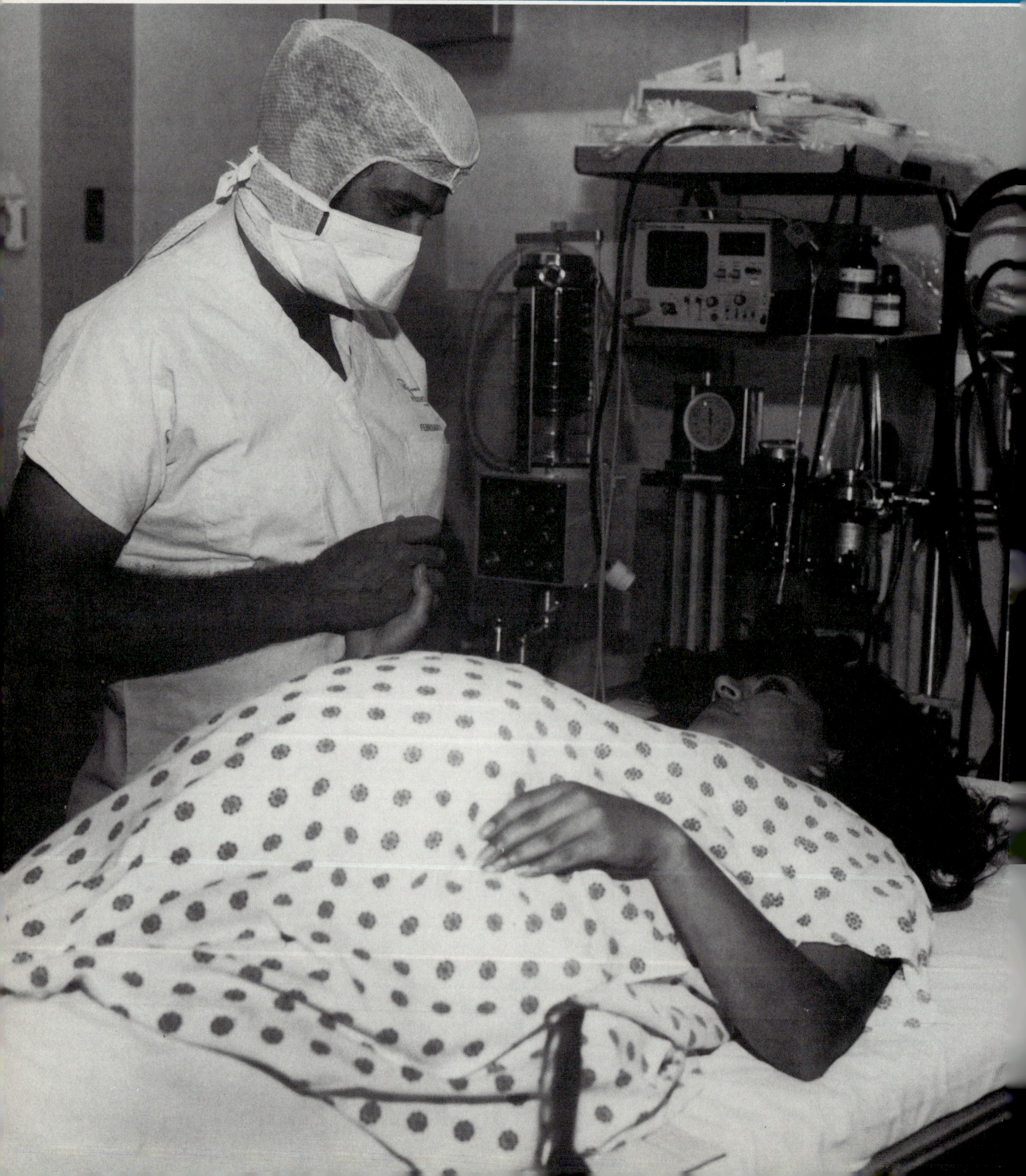

UNIT IV

THE INTRAPARTAL FAMILY

UNIT IV

THE INTRAPARTAL FAMILY

chapter 13

MATERNAL-FETAL RELATIONSHIPS

OBJECTIVES

Upon completion of this chapter, the reader will be able to:

1. List the five "p's."
2. Describe the bony structure of the pelvis.
3. Differentiate between the false pelvis and the true pelvis.
4. Given a diameter of the pelvic inlet, cavity, or outlet, state the normal measurement.
5. Briefly describe the four types of pelvis.
6. State the diameters of the pelvis that may be measured with clinical pelvimetry.
7. State the importance of x-ray pelvimetry.
8. Define attitude, lie, and presenting part.
9. Describe the process of molding of the fetal head during labor.
10. Define engagement and station.
11. Briefly describe Leopold's manuevers and the information that is obtained with assessment.

KEY TERMS

Android pelvis
Anthropoid pelvis
Breech presentation
Bregma
Cephalic presentation
Engagement
False pelvis
Fetal attitude
Fetal lie
Fontanel
Gynecoid pelvis
Labor
Lambda
Leopold's manuevers
Molding
Occiput
Passage
Passenger
Pelvic cavity
Pelvic inlet
Pelvic outlet
Pelvimetry
Platypelloid pelvis
Position
Presentation
Sinciput
Station
Sutures
Transverse lie
True pelvis
Vertex

Labor can be defined as the series of processes by which the products of conception are expelled from the mother. Five factors known as the five P's affect the process of labor: passage, passenger, powers, placenta, and psyche. The *passenger* is the fetus who travels the *passage,* the maternal pelvis. The *powers* are uterine muscle contractions that aid in moving the fetus through the maternal pelvis. The site of placental implantation in the uterus may affect the labor process. Psyche can be a powerful factor in labor. The childbearing couple who is "prepared" both physically and emotionally for labor often have a more satisfying labor experience. The passage and passenger are discussed below. Powers, placenta, and psyche are discussed in Chapters 14 and 15.

THE PASSAGE

The passage is composed of the rigid bony pelvis and the soft tissues of the cervix, vagina, and introitus. The size and shape of the pelvis are important in the progress of labor. Slight disproportions between the fetal head and the maternal pelvis may make vaginal delivery extremely difficult or even impossible.

Pelvis

The *pelvis* is a bony ring between the moveable vertebrae of the vertebral column and the lower limbs on which the vertebral column rests (see Fig. 13–1).

STRUCTURE

The pelvis consists of two innominate bones that make up the front and sides and the sacrum, and the coccyx, which makes up the back portion of the pelvis. These bones articulate through four joints: the symphysis pubis, the sacrococcygeal joint, and the two sacroiliac joints.

Each innominate bone is formed by the fusion of three bones around the acetabulum: the ilium, the ischium, and the pubis. The symphysis pubis is located between the two pubic bones in front.

The *ilium* is the fan-shaped upper part of the hipbone. The anterior superior iliac spine is felt as the front angle of the hipbone. The iliac crest extends backward from the anterior superior iliac spine to the posterior superior iliac spine.

The *ischium* consists of a body that forms part of the acetabulum. An important landmark, the ischial spine, separates the greater sciatic from the lesser sciatic notch. The distance between the ischial spines is important obstetrically because it is the shortest diameter of the pelvic cavity. The ischial spines are palpated during vaginal or rectal examination to determine the descent of the presenting part of the fetus into the true pelvis (station). The lower part of the ischium is the ischial tuberosity, the bone on which humans sit.

The *pubis* consists of the body and two rami, and forms the front of the pelvis.

The *sacrum* is a triangular bone with the base above and the apex below. It consists of five vertebrae fused together and lies between the innominate bones. The *sacroiliac joints* attach the sacrum to the innominate bones. At the upper edge of the first sacral vertebrae is a slight protrusion called the *sacral promontory*. The protrusion reduces the anteroposterior diameter of the pelvic inlet.

The *coccyx,* or tail bone, is composed of four vertebrae. The coccyx and the sacrum are attached to each other by the *sacrococcygeal joint,* which allows flexion and extension during labor. Extension increases the anteroposterior diameter of the pelvic outlet during labor.

Only slight movement of the pelvis at the site of the four joints is possible. During pregnancy the hormones progesterone and relaxin

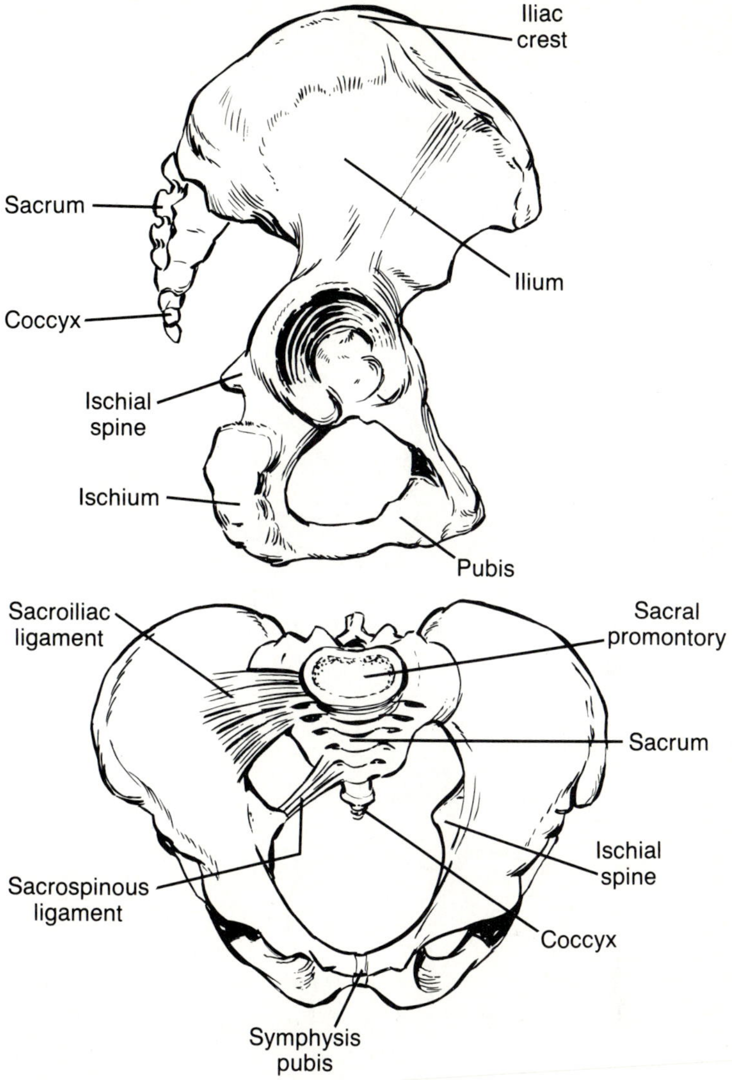

FIGURE 13-1. Two views of the female pelvis showing bones and joints.

cause increased flexibility of the symphysis pubis and the sacroiliac joints.

DIVISIONS

The four pelvic bones are united so they form two cavities, the false pelvis and the true pelvis. Dividing the false pelvis from the true pelvis is the linea terminalis, a slight constriction also called the pelvic brim (see Fig. 13–2).

False Pelvis

The false pelvis lies above the linea terminalis. Its boundaries are the lumbar vertebrae posteriorly, the iliac fossae laterally, and the anterior abdominal wall anteriorly. Functions include support of the enlarged uterus during pregnancy and directing the fetus into the true pelvis.

True Pelvis

The true pelvis lies below the linea terminalis. It is through this canal that the fetus must pass for vaginal delivery. Boundaries are the sacrum posteriorly, the inner surface of the ischial bones laterally, and the pubic bones anteriorly. It is divided into three parts: the inlet, the pelvic cavity, and the outlet.

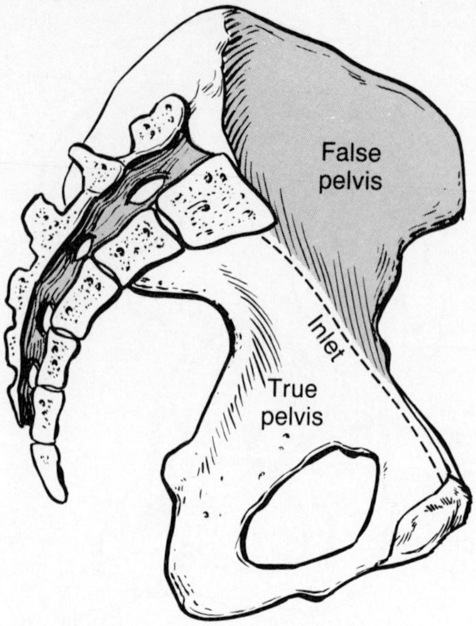

FIGURE 13-2. Divisions of the pelvis, showing the false pelvis and the true pelvis.

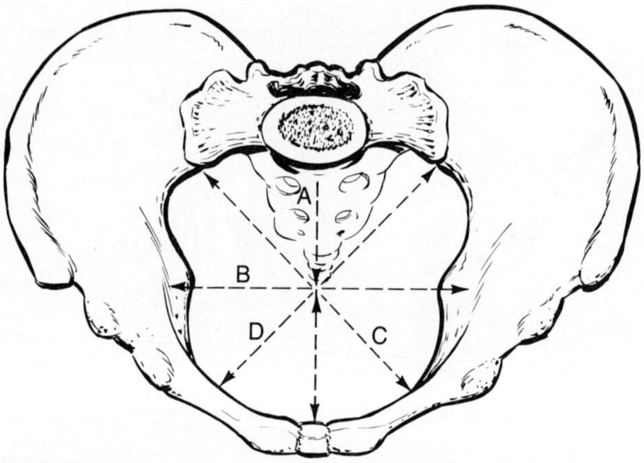

FIGURE 13-3. Pelvic inlet showing the following diameters: A. Anteroposterior. B. Transverse. C. Right oblique. D. Left oblique.

Pelvic Inlet

The inlet, or pelvic brim, is bounded by the pubic crest and spine anteriorly, the iliopectineal lines laterally, and the sacral promontory posteriorly. The inlet is usually nearly round in shape in the gynecoid pelvis (see Fig. 13-3).

Diameters of the pelvic inlet include anteroposterior, transverse, right and left oblique, and posterior sagittal. The *anteroposterior diameter* extends from the middle of the promontory of the sacrum to the upper margin of the symphysis pubis. This is the most important inlet diameter, since it is through here that the fetus must pass. Three different anteroposterior diameters can be measured: the anatomic (true) conjugate, the obstetric conjugate, and the diagonal conjugate. The *anatomic conjugate,* extending from the middle of the sacral promontory to the superior surface of the pubis, measures 11.5 cm. The *obstetric conjugate* extends from the middle of the sacral promontory to the posterior superior margin of the symphysis pubis. This diameter measures 11.0 cm and is the most important anteroposterior diameter. The *diagonal conjugate* extends from the subpubic angle to the middle of the sacral promontory and measures 12.5 cm. This diameter can be measured by clinical pelvimetry with a pelvimeter.

The *transverse diameter*, the greatest distance between the linea terminalis on either side, measures 13.5 cm. The *left and right oblique diameters* extend from one sacroiliac joint to the opposite ileopectineal eminence; they measure 12.5 cm each. The *posterior sagittal diameter,* extending from the intersection of the anteroposterior and transverse diameters to the middle of the sacral promontory, measures about 4.5 cm.

Pelvic Cavity

The pelvic cavity is a curved canal that extends from the pelvic inlet to the pelvic outlet. It is divided into the plane of greatest dimensions and the plane of least dimensions. The plane of greatest dimensions is the roomiest part of the bony pelvis. Its boundaries are the midposterior pubis anteriorly, the upper portion of the obturator foramina laterally, and the second and third sacral vertebrae posteriorly. The plane of greatest dimensions is of little importance obstetrically.

The most important plane of the pelvis is the plane of least dimensions (see Fig. 13-4). It is the smallest pelvic plane, extending from

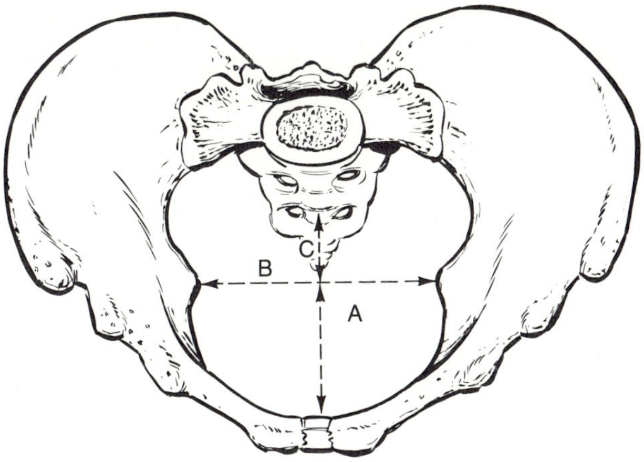

FIGURE 13-4. Pelvic cavity: Plane of least dimensions. A. Anteroposterior diameter. B. Transverse diameter. C. Posterior sagittal diameter.

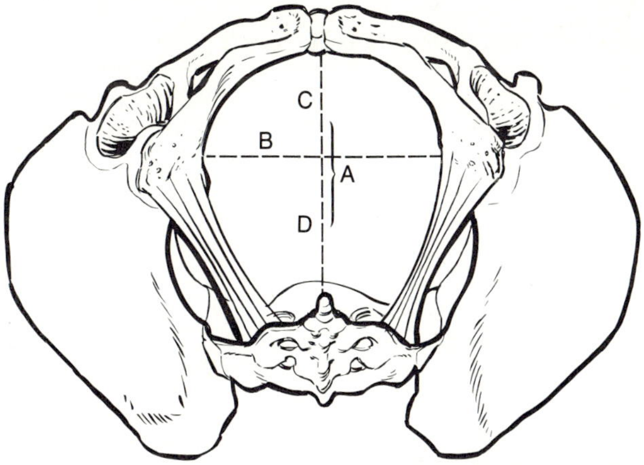

FIGURE 13-5. Pelvic outlet: A. Anteroposterior diameter. B. Transverse diameter. C. Posterior sagittal diameter. D. Anterior sagittal diameter.

the apex of the subpubic arch through the ischial spines to the sacrum at or near the junction of the fourth and fifth sacral vertebrae. There are three important diameters: the anteroposterior, the transverse, and the posterior sagittal. The *anteroposterior diameter* extends from the lower symphysis pubis to the junction of the fourth or fifth sacral vertebrae and measures 12.0 cm. The *transverse diameter* is the distance between the ischial spines and measures 10.5 cm. The *posterior sagittal diameter* extends from the bispinous diameter to the junction of the fourth and fifth sacral vertebrae and measures 4.5 to 5.0 cm.

Pelvic Outlet

The pelvic outlet, or inferior strait, consists of two triangular planes with a common base of transverse diameters between the ischial tuberosities (see Fig. 13-5). The anterior triangle has the following boundaries: the base is the bituberous diameter, the apex is the subpubic angle, and the sides are the pubic rami and the ischial tuberosities. The posterior triangle has as boundaries the bituberous diameter at the base, the sacrococcygeal joint at the apex, and the sacrotuberous ligaments.

The four diameters of the pelvic outlet are anteroposterior, transverse, posterior sagittal, and anterior sagittal. The *anteroposterior diameter* extends from the inferior symphysis pubis to the tip of the coccyx and measures about 9.5 to 11.5 cm. The *transverse diameter* between the ischial tuberosities measures about 11.0 cm. The *posterior sagittal diameter,* extending from the middle of the transverse diameter to the junction of the sacrum and coccyx, measures 9.0 cm. The *anterior sagittal diameter* extends from the middle of the transverse diameter to the subpubic angle; it normally measures 6.0 cm.

Table 13-1 summarizes the diameters of the maternal pelvis. In assessing the pelvis, the most important parameters are:

Obstetric conjugate of the pelvic inlet
Distance between the ischial spines
Subpubic angle
Transverse diameter
Posterior sagittal diameters of the inlet, cavity, and outlet
Curve and length of the sacrum

Pelvic Variations

The pelvis presents many different variations—no two pelves are exactly alike. Differences may be due to heredity, accidents, disease, or development.

There are four major pelvic types: gynecoid, anthropoid, android, and platypelloid. The

TABLE 13-1
DIAMETERS OF THE FEMALE PELVIS

Diameter	Measurement in CM
Inlet	
Anteroposterior	
Anatomic conjugate	11.5
Obstetric conjugate	11.0
Diagonal conjugate	12.5
Transverse	13.5
Left and right oblique	12.5
Posterior sagittal	4.5
Pelvic cavity	
Plane of least dimensions	
Anteroposterior	12.0
Transverse	10.5
Posterior sagittal	4.5 to 5.0
Outlet	
Anteroposterior	9.5 to 11.5
Transverse	11.0
Posterior sagittal	9.0
Anterior sagittal	6.0

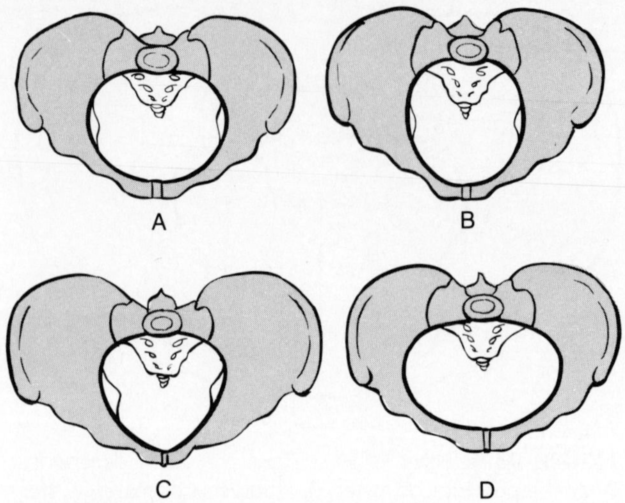

FIGURE 13-6. Pelvic types: A. Gynecoid pelvis. B. Anthropoid pelvis. C. Android pelvis. D. Platypelloid pelvis.

type of pelvis is determined by the shape and measurements, and influences the course of labor and delivery. The closer the pelvis is to the gynecoid classification, the more likely the labor and delivery will be normal.

GYNECOID PELVIS

The *gynecoid or female pelvis* is present in 50 percent of all women. The inlet is almost round or is a transverse oval with an anteroposterior measurement a little shorter than the transverse measurement (see Fig. 13-6). The posterior segment is roomy and the sacrosciatic notch is wide. The pubic rami form a pelvic angle of about 90 degrees. The fetal head usually engages in a transverse diameter with good flexion (see Chapter 14). Occiput anterior positions at delivery are common. Good uterine function is present and spontaneous delivery usually occurs. There is less perineal tearing because of the wide pubic arch.

ANTHROPOID PELVIS

The *anthropoid or apelike pelvis* is the next most common type. The inlet is oval with a longer anteroposterior diameter than transverse diameter (see Fig. 13-6). The pelvis is deep and the sacrosciatic notch is broad and shallow. The fetal head usually enters the pelvis in a posterior position. Labor and delivery are not difficult and posterior positions are common at delivery.

ANDROID PELVIS

The *android or male pelvis* has a heart-shaped inlet and a shallow posterior segment (see Fig. 13-6). The side walls of the pelvis are usually convergent and the subpubic notch is narrow. The fetal head often enters the pelvis in an occiput posterior position and may exhibit extreme molding at delivery. During labor the occiput posterior position may persist, with midforceps rotation needed for delivery.

PLATYPELLOID PELVIS

The *platypelloid or flat pelvis* is disproportionately wide from side to side (see Fig. 13-6). The true pelvic cavity is shallow with a short diagonal conjugate measurement. During labor disporportion often exists and cesarean section may be needed owing to cephalopelvic disproportion.

PELVIMETRY

During pregnancy, measurements of the pelvis are important maternal assessments in determining if the passage is adequate for the passenger. Pelvic measurements can be made clinically or by x-ray pelvimetry.

Clinical Pelvimetry

Measurement of the maternal pelvis with a pair of calipers called a pelvimeter is called *clinical pelvimetry*. All pelvic measurements cannot be determined clinically. Internal measurements that may be obtained clinically are:

Diagonal conjugate diameter of the inlet
True conjugate diameter of the inlet
Transverse diameter of the outlet
Posterior sagittal diameter of the outlet

Clinical measurements are usually made in the office early in pregnancy and may be repeated later if necessary.

DIAGONAL CONJUGATE

The distance between the subpubic angle and the middle of the sacral promontory is called the *diagonal conjugate*. The patient is placed in the lithotomy position. Two fingers are introduced into the vagina and pressed inward and upward as far as possible until the sacral promontory is touched with the middle finger (see Fig. 13-7). The point on the back of the hand just under the symphysis pubis is marked, and the fingers are withdrawn and measured. The distance from the tip of the middle finger to the marked point is the diagonal conjugate, which normally measures 12.5 cm.

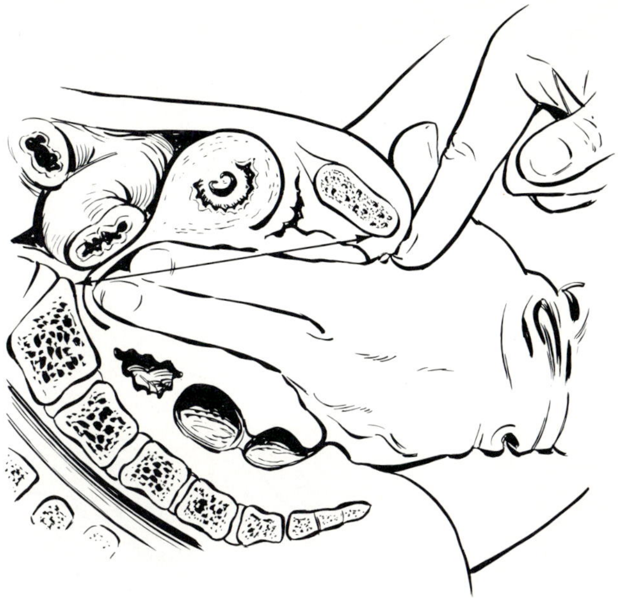

FIGURE 13-7. Method of measuring the diagonal conjugate by clinical pelvimetry.

During measurement of the diagonal conjugate the examiner also assesses the contour of the pelvis by evaluating the height of the symphysis pubis, the shape of the pubic arch, the mobility of the coccyx, the inclination of the pelvic walls, and the prominence of the ischial spines.

TRUE CONJUGATE

The important anteroposterior diameter is the *true conjugate*, which lies between the posterior symphysis pubis and the sacral promontory. Measurement of this diameter is determined by subtracting 1.5 cm from the diagonal conjugate measurement.

INTERTUBEROUS DIAMETER

The most important diameter of the pelvic outlet, the *intertuberous or transverse diameter*, lies between the inner surfaces of the ischial tuberosities and normally measures 11.0 cm. A pelvimeter (see Fig. 13-8) or the examiner's hand may be used to obtain this measurement.

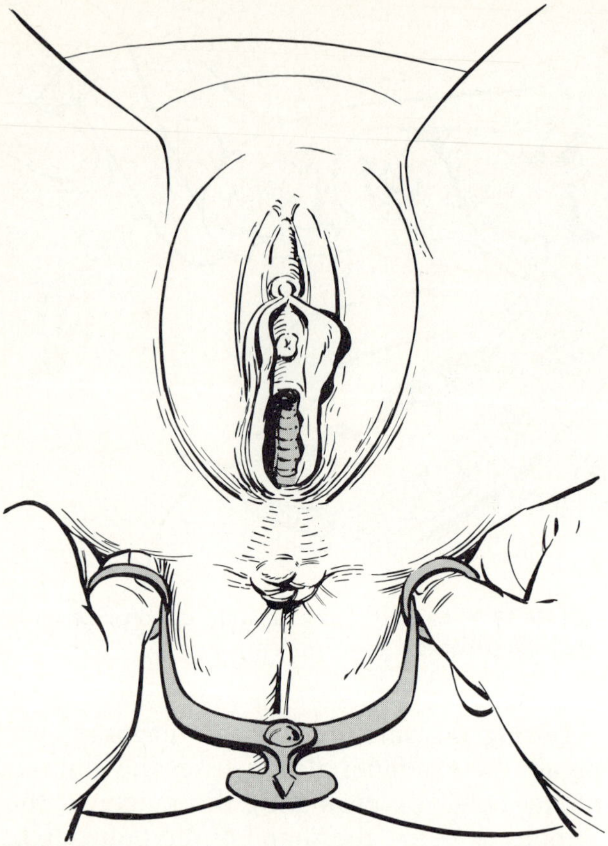

FIGURE 13-8. Method of measuring the intertuberous diameter of the outlet with a pelvimeter.

When a pelvimeter is used, the patient is placed in a lithotomy position. The measurement is taken externally from the inner lower edge of the ischial tuberosities at the level of the anus. When the examiner's hand is used, a closed fist is placed between the tuberosities and the distance across the portion of the hand that fits into this space is measured.

In addition to obtaining the intertuberous diameter, the examiner assesses the coccyx for mobility, the general contour of the pelvic outlet, and the width of the pubic arch.

POSTERIOR SAGITTAL DIAMETER

The *posterior sagittal diameter* is the distance from the middle of the transverse diameter to the junction of the sacrum and coccyx and measures 9.0 cm. This distance is of importance when the intertuberous diameter is short.

> **NURSING RESPONSIBILITIES**
>
> When clinical pelvimetry is calculated in the office setting, it is important for the examiner and the nurse to thoroughly explain all procedures that will be done. A relaxed patient will be much more comfortable during the measurements. The nurse should stay in the examination room while the measurements are being taken.

X-ray Pelvimetry

X-ray pelvimetry (see Fig. 13-9) is used to measure the shape and the inclination of the maternal pelvis, the length of the pelvic diameters, and the relationship and fit of the fetal presenting part into the maternal pelvis. This information, along with clinical examination and judgment, will help to determine labor outcome.

There is minimal exposure to irradiation with this procedure. Pelvic x-rays involve not only the mother but also the fetus. The decision to do a pelvimetry examination must be made with this fact in mind. Pelvimetries are not usually done until the third trimester, and often not until after the start of labor. Gravidas who have had previous difficult deliveries or a damaged fetus at a previous delivery may have pelvimetry ordered to determine whether a safe vaginal delivery is possible. When an abnormal or grossly contracted pelvis is suspected from history or confirmed by physical examination during pregnancy, a pelvimetry may be indicated. Breech presentations in a primigravida or in multiparas who have previously had small neonates may also require pelvimetry. Pelvimetry may be ordered when there is suspected malpresentation or malposition, or a very difficult slow progress-

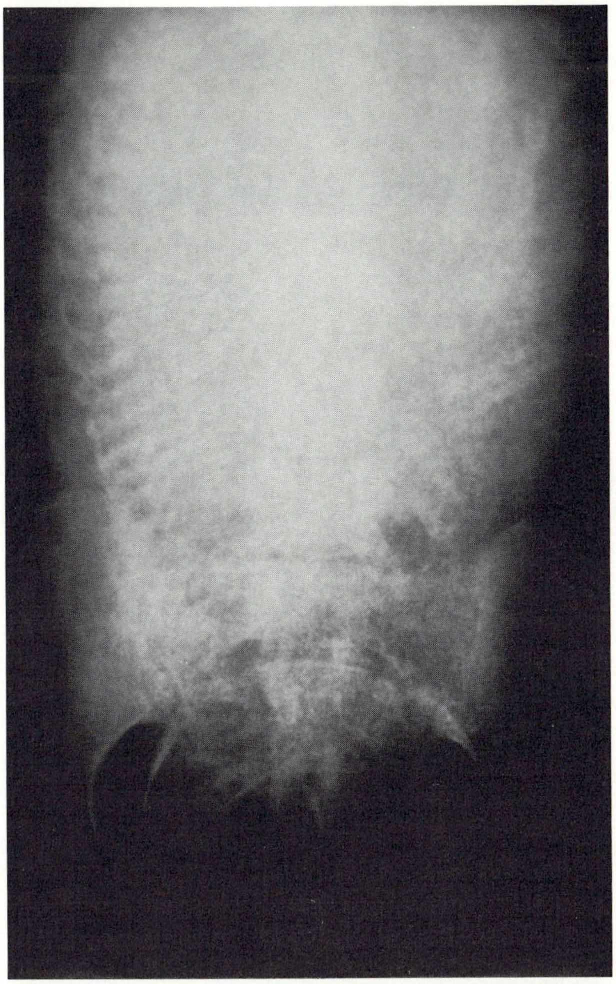

FIGURE 13-9. X-ray pelvimetry. View of the pelvis shows a single floating term fetus in cephalic presentation with the fetal spine on the maternal right. Measurements are: Inlet—anteroposterior 12.2 cm; transverse 13.0 cm. Midplane—anteroposterior 9.8 cm; transverse 10.0 cm.

ing labor with extreme molding of the fetal skull and lack of descent.

NURSING RESPONSIBILITIES

Regardless of the indication for x-ray pelvimetry, the risks and procedure technique must be explained and understood by the gravida. A nurse should accompany the patient to the radiology department to offer support, help position the patient, observe the pattern of uterine contractions, auscultate fetal heart tones, and initiate interventions in an emergency situation such as imminent delivery.

TECHNIQUES

Usually three films are taken: the first an abdominal view, the second a lateral view, and the third an anteroposterior view. The abdominal view gives information about fetal attitude, fetal lie, presentation, and position, as well as a rough estimate of the size of the fetus, the presence of multiple fetuses, and some fetal abnormalities. With a lateral view, information is obtained on the length and curve of the sacrum, pelvic depth, narrowness or wideness of the sacrosciatic notch, and the anteroposterior diameters of the inlet. The posterior sagittal diameter of the midpelvis and outlet can also be measured, as well as the size and shape of the ischial spines, the station of the fetal presenting part, the presence of synclitism or asynclitism, fetal attitude, and relationship of the presenting part to the maternal pelvis. The anteroposterior view helps to identify the shape of the pelvic inlet, the widest transverse diameter of the inlet, the distance between the ischial spines, the slope of the pelvic sidewalls, and the classification of the maternal pelvis (gynecoid, anthropoid, android, or platypelloid).

THE PASSENGER

The passenger is the fetus, who will travel through the birth passage during labor.

Fetal Head

The head is the most important part of the fetus during passage through the maternal pelvis (see Fig. 13–10). It is the largest part of the fetus and is the part that most commonly

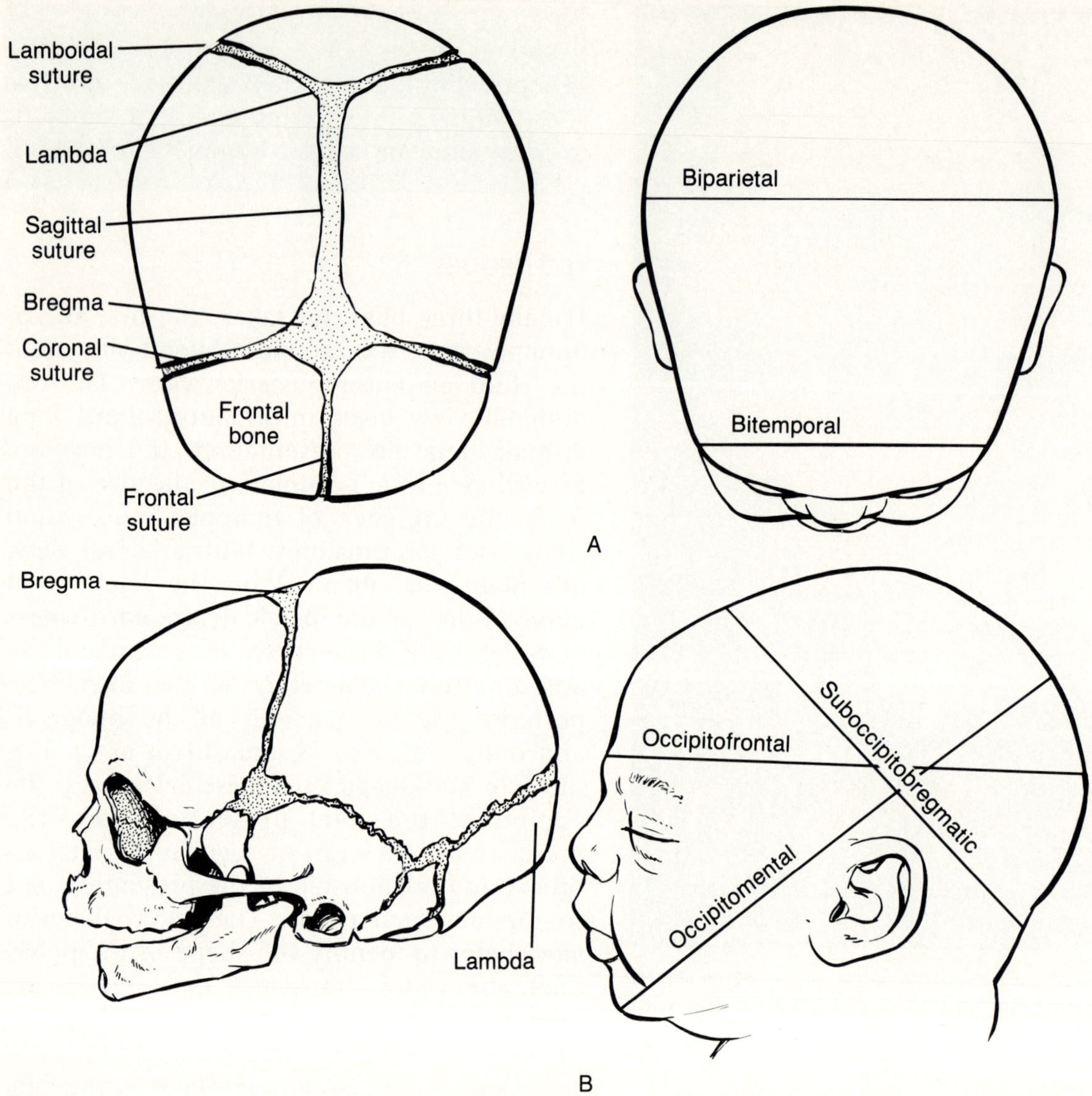

FIGURE 13-10. Fetal skull: A. Top of skull. B. Lateral view.

presents first during labor. During labor the fetal head should adapt to the maternal pelvis for delivery. If the head cannot adapt owing to excessive size or limited moldability, vaginal delivery may be extremely difficult or impossible.

SKULL BONES

The cranium of the fetus forms the top, sides, and back of the head. Eight bones form the fetal cranium. The frontal bone, two parietal bones, and the occipital bone are the important ones obstetrically. The other four bones (sphenod, ethmoid, and two temporal bones) also compose the fetal skull but are of little significance obstetrically, since they are near the base of the cranium.

SUTURES

Sutures are the spaces between the skull bones that aid in molding of the fetal skull. During vaginal or rectal examinations sutures may be felt and outlined to aid in identification of the position of the fetal head during labor.

There are four sutures. The *sagittal suture* lies between the parietal bones. The *lamboidal suture* lies between the occipital bone and the two parietal bones. The *coronal suture* extends transversely from the anterior fontanel and lies between the parietal and frontal bones. The *frontal suture* lies between the two frontal bones and is an anterior continuation of the sagittal suture.

FONTANELS

The membrane spaces where the sutures intersect are called *fontanels*. There are two fontanels of obstetrical importance: the anterior and the posterior (see Fig. 13–10).

The *anterior fontanel* or *bregma* is located at the junction of the sagittal, frontal, and coronal sutures. It measures approximately 3 × 2 cm and is diamond-shaped. Normally this fontanel closes by 18 months of age.

The *posterior fontanel* or *lambda* is smaller, triangular-shaped, and located at the junction of the sagittal and lamboidal sutures. It normally closes at six to eight weeks of age.

AREAS OF THE FETAL SKULL

The skull is divided into four areas. The *occiput* is the area behind the posterior fontanel. The *vertex* lies between the two fontanels and extends to the parietal bones. The *bregma* is the area of the anterior fontanel and the *sinciput* is located in front of the anterior fontanel.

DIAMETERS OF THE FETAL SKULL

The diameters of the fetal skull are important in determining the relationship between the size of the maternal pelvis and the fetal head. Six diameters are usually described (see Fig. 13–10):

1. The *biparietal diameter* is the largest transverse diameter. It is measured between the parietal bones, and normally is 9.25 to 9.5 cm.
2. The *bitemporal diameter* is the greatest distance between the temporal bones. It measures 8 cm, and is the shortest transverse diameter of the fetal skull.
3. The *suboccipitobregmatic diameter* is measured from the undersurface of the occipital bone, where it meets the neck to the center of the bregma. Measuring 9.5 cm, this diameter presents when the head is well flexed.
4. The *occipitofrontal diameter* presents in the military attitude. It extends from the external protuberance of the occiput to the glabella or forehead and measures 11.0 cm.
5. The *verticomental diameter* runs from vertex to chin and is important in brow presentations. It is the largest anteroposterior diameter, at 13.5 cm.
6. The *submentobregmatic diameter* measures 9.5 cm and extends from the junction of the neck and lower jaw to the center of the bregma. It is important in face presentations.

MOLDING

The ability of the fetal head to change its shape to adapt to the maternal pelvis is called *molding*. The fetal bones are joined loosely by membranes so that actual spaces exist between the edges of the bones, allowing the bones to alter their relationships as pressure is exerted on the head during labor. Molding is accomplished without a reduction in the actual volume of the skull.

Fetal Attitude

During the third trimester, the fetus becomes curved on itself to occupy the smallest possible space in the uterus. The relationship of the parts of the fetal body to one another is called the *fetal attitude* (see Fig. 13–11). Characteristically, this attitude is one of flexion. The back is convex, the head is sharply flexed with the chin almost on the chest, the thighs are flexed over the abdomen with the legs bent at

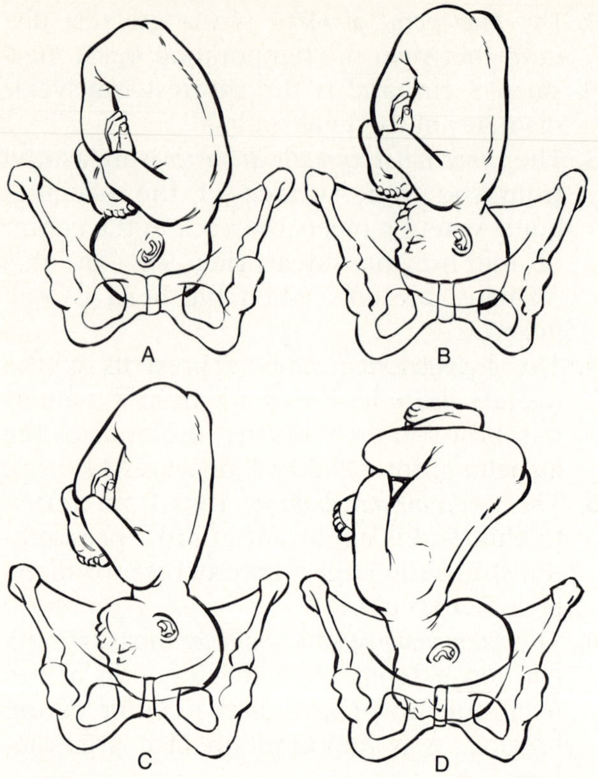

FIGURE 13-11. Fetal attitude: A. Flexion. B. Neither flexion nor extension. C. Partial head extension. D. Complete head extension.

the knees. The arms are usually crossed over the chest, or may lie parallel to the sides. The umbilical cord lies in the space between the arms and the lower extremities (see Fig. 13-11,*A*).

Fetal Lie

Fetal lie refers to the relationship of the long axis of the fetus to the long axis of the mother. There are two lies: (1) *longitudinal*, when the long axis of the fetus and mother are parallel; and (2) *transverse*, when the long axis of the fetus is perpendicular or oblique to the long axis of the mother. In 99 percent of all pregnancies at term the fetus is in a longitudinal lie.

In the following descriptions of fetal presentations, all directions refer to the mother in a standing position. Upper means toward the mother's head. Anterior, posterior, right, and left refer to the maternal front, back, right and left. Denominator refers to a chosen point on the presenting part of the fetus and is used to describe fetal position.

LONGITUDINAL LIES

Longitudinal lies are grouped into: (1) *cephalic*, when the head comes first; and (2) *breech*, when the buttocks or lower limbs come first.

Cephalic Presentations

Cephalic, or head presentations account for 96 to 97 percent of all presentations. They are classified into four main groups:

1. *Occiput presentation* is present when fetal attitude is one of flexion and the fetal chin is near or on the chest (see Fig. 13-11,*A*). The presenting part is the posterior vertex and the denominator is the occiput.
2. *Military presentation* occurs when there is no flexion and no extension of the fetal head (see Fig. 13-11,*B*). The occipitofrontal diameter presents and the occiput is the denominator.
3. *Brow presentation* is one of halfway extension (see Fig. 13-11,*C*). The forehead presents and is the denominator.
4. *Face presentation* occurs when there is complete extension of the fetal head. The neck is sharply extended so that the occiput and the fetal back may be in contact with each other. The presenting part is the face and the chin (mentum) is the denominator (see Fig. 13-11,*D*).

Breech Presentations

Breech presentations account for 3 to 4 percent of all deliveries. They are classified according to the attitude of the hips and knees into four main groups:

1. *Complete breech*, in which there is flexion at the hips and at the knees, has the buttocks

as the presenting part, and the sacrum as the denominator (see Fig. 13–12,*A*).

2. *Frank breech* is the most frequent breech presentation. There is flexion at the hips and extension at the knees, with the lower limbs anterior to the fetal abdomen (see Fig. 13–12, *B*). The buttocks are the presenting part and the sacrum is the denominator.
3. *Footling breech,* in which there is extension at the hips and the knees (see Fig. 13–12, *C*), can be either single footling (one foot presenting) or double footling (both feet presenting).
4. *Kneeling breech,* with extension at the hips and flexion at the knees (see Fig. 13–12, *D*), has one or both knees as the presenting part and the sacrum as the denominator.

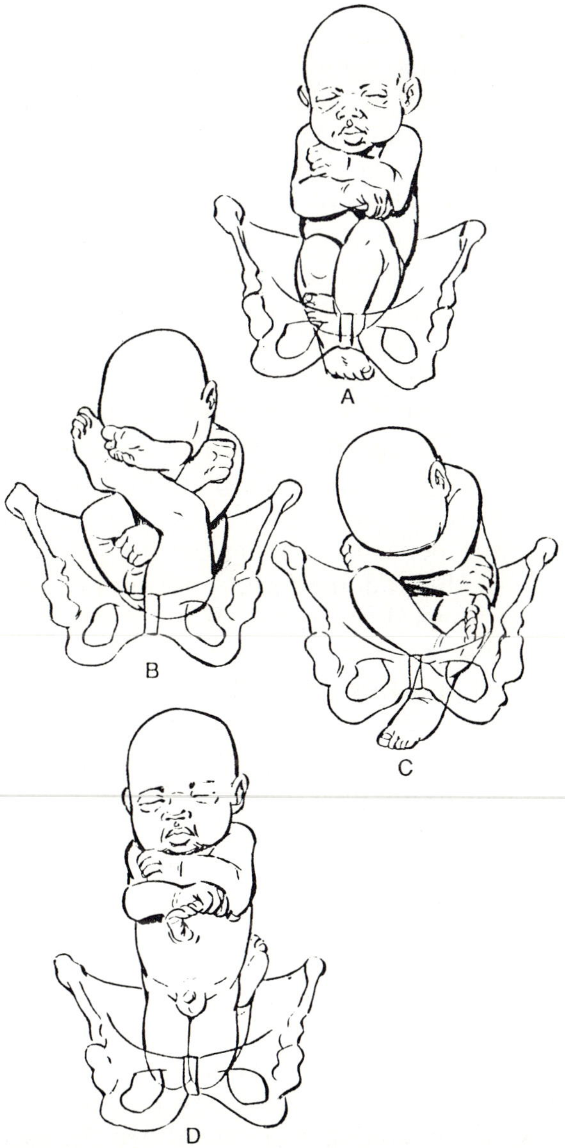

FIGURE 13-12. Breech presentations: A. Complete breech. B. Frank breech. C. Footling breech. D. Kneeling breech.

TRANSVERSE OR OBLIQUE LIE

A transverse or oblique lie is present when the long axis of the fetus is perpendicular or oblique to the long axis of the mother (see Fig. 13–13). Usually the shoulder is the presenting part, although the arm may present. The scapula is the denominator.

Presentation is not fully established until the presenting part enters the maternal pelvic inlet. The fetus may change position throughout pregnancy. After 32 weeks, the fetus will usually assume a cephalic presentation because the more movable part of the fetus finds greater freedom in the roomier part of the uterus, the fundus.

Position

The relationship of the fetal denominator to the mother's pelvis is called the *position*. The maternal pelvic girdle has a 360 degree cir-

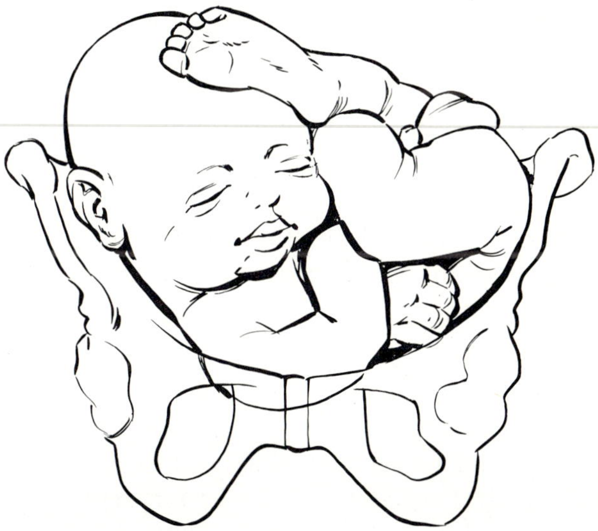

FIGURE 13-13. Transverse lie.

cumference. The maternal symphysis pubis is anterior and the sacrum posterior. Eight points that are 45 degrees apart are marked, and the position of the fetus is described as the relationship of the denominator to one of these marks.

Positions are usually described in abbreviations determined by the first letter of each word: the left occiput anterior position is stated as LOA; left occiput transverse is stated as LOT and so forth. There are eight positions for each denominator.

In a vertex presentation the occiput is the presenting part. Possible positions are (see Fig. 13-14):

OA:	occiput anterior	OP:	occiput posterior
LOA:	left occiput anterior	ROP:	right occiput posterior
LOT:	left occiput transverse	ROT:	right occiput transverse
LOP:	left occiput posterior	ROA:	right occiput anterior

In a face presentation, the chin or mentum is the denominator. Positions are:

MA:	mentum anterior	MP:	mentum posterior
LMA:	left mentum anterior	RMP:	right mentum posterior
LMT:	left mentum transverse	RMT:	right mentum transverse
LMP:	left mentum posterior	RMA:	right mentum anterior

In a breech presentation the sacrum is the denominator. Positions are (see Figure 13-15):

SA:	sacrum anterior	SP:	sacrum posterior
LSA:	left sacrum anterior	RSP:	right sacrum posterior
LST:	left sacrum transverse	RST:	right sacrum transverse
LSP:	left sacrum posterior	RSA:	right sacrum anterior

With a shoulder presentation in a transverse lie, there are only four positions. The shoulder is either anterior or posterior on the left or right side of the mother's pelvis. Positions are:

LScA:	left scapula anterior	RScP:	right scapula posterior
LScP:	left scapula posterior	RScA:	right scapula anterior

Engagement

Engagement means that the widest diameter of the fetal presenting part has passed through the maternal pelvic inlet. In a cephalic presentation the biparietal diameter is the widest (see Fig. 13-16), and in a breech presentation, the intratrochanteric diameter is the widest.

Engagement may occur several weeks before the onset of contractions in the primigravida. In multigravidas, engagement may not occur until the onset of labor or during labor owing to the relaxed abdominal muscles.

Engagement can be determined by abdominal, vaginal, or rectal examinations. With abdominal examination, the nurse can palpate the presenting part for the degree of descent into the pelvis by placing her hands on each side of the abdomen and pushing her fingers down toward the pelvis. If the lower part of the head cannot be felt with the fingers, the head is probably engaged.

During a vaginal or rectal examination the nurse feels for the relationship of the presenting part to the maternal ischial spines.

Station

Station is the relationship of the presenting part to an imaginary line drawn between the maternal ischial spines. It is expressed in centimeters above or below this line. When the presenting part is at the level of the ischial spines, the station is zero. Above the ischial spines the station is minus one, minus two, etc. Below the spines the station is referred to as plus one, plus two, plus three, etc. At a plus

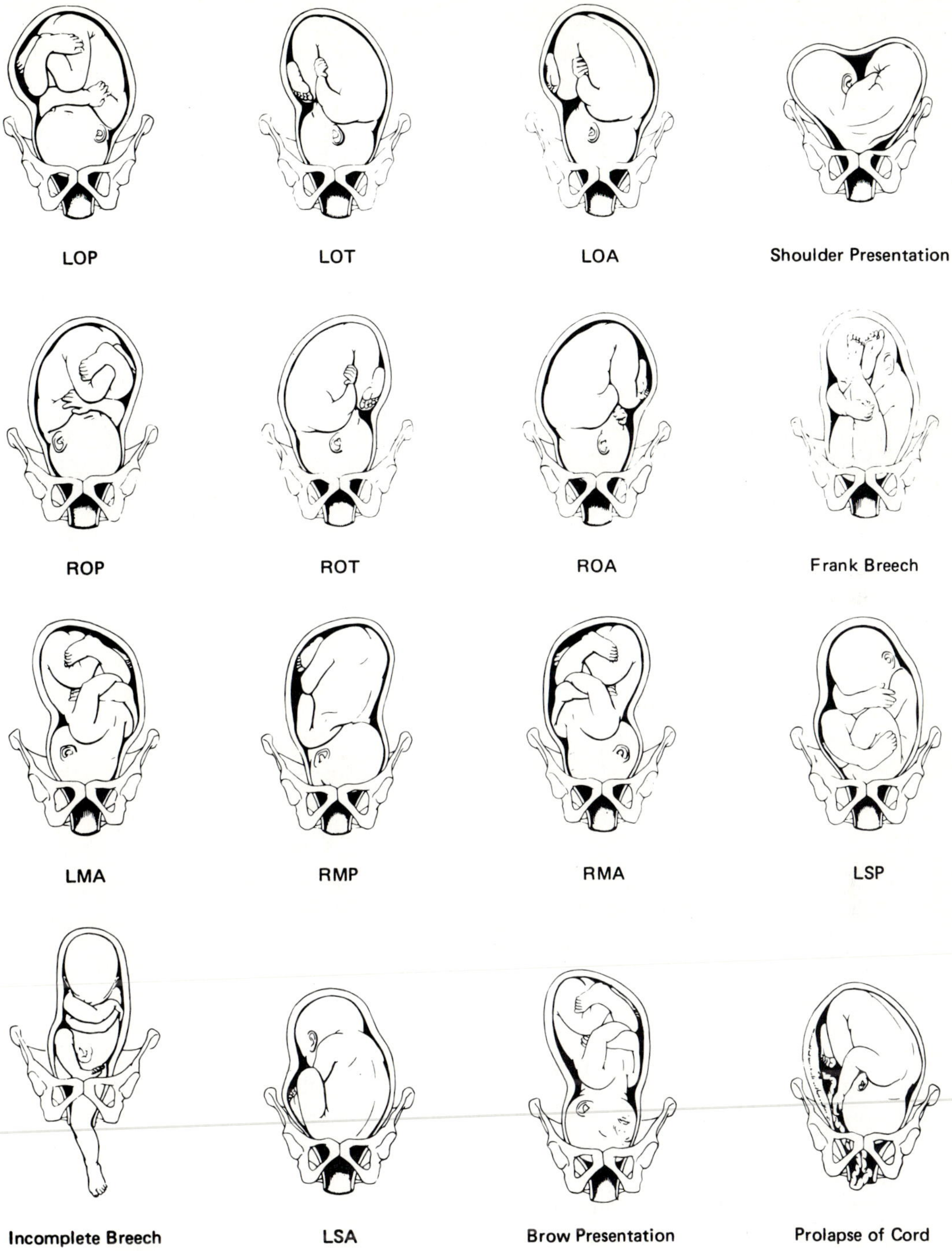

FIGURE 13-14. Fetal positions. (Reprinted with permission from Obstetrical Presentation and Position, Ross Laboratories, Columbus, OH).

four station there is bulging of the perineum (see Fig. 13-17).

General terms are sometimes used to describe station. A *high* presenting part is one that is not engaged, as is a *floating* presenting part. When the presenting part is entering the pelvis, but is not yet engaged, the presenting part may be described as *dipping*.

It is important to determine the station when labor begins and to keep accurate

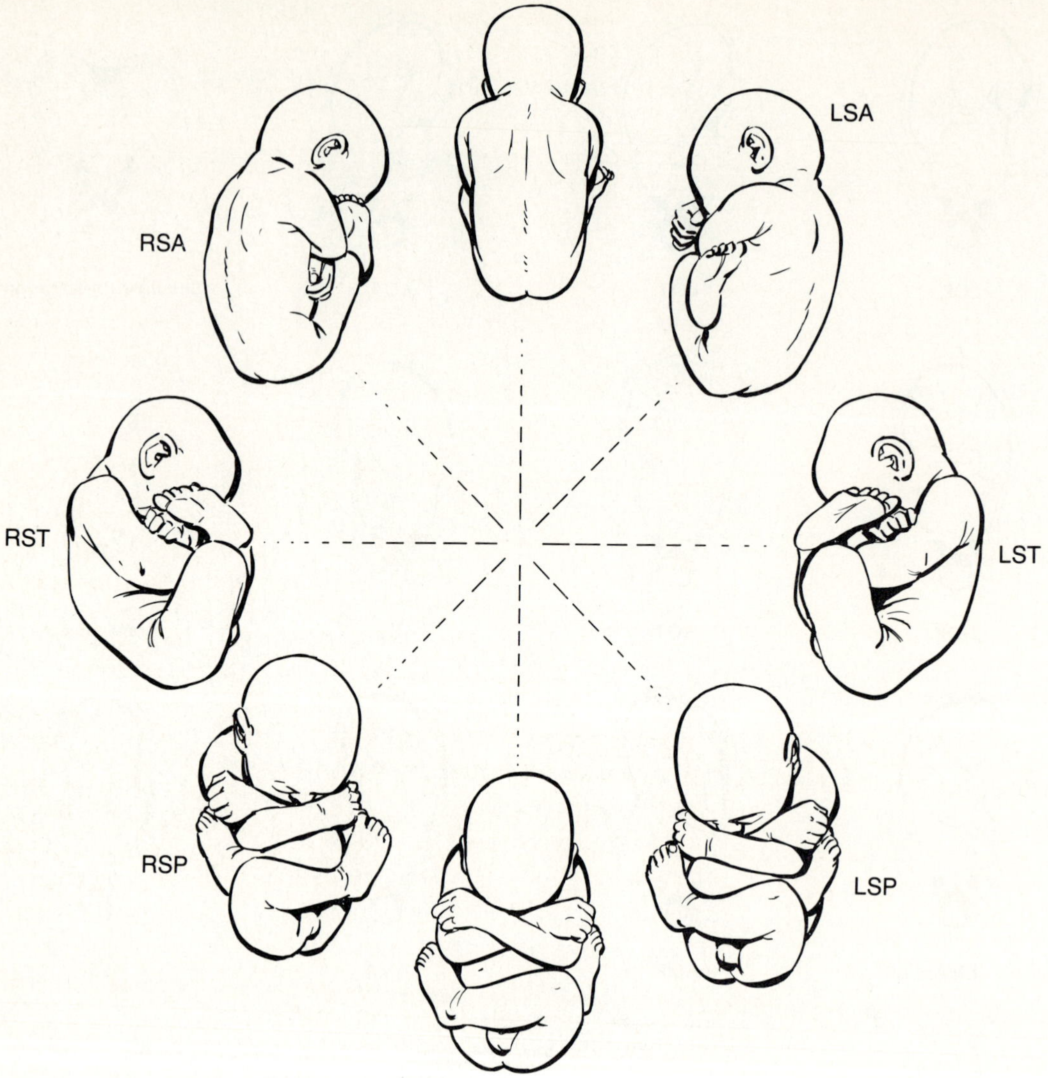

FIGURE 13-15. Breech positions.

documentation of the rate of descent of the presenting part during labor. A nulliparous woman in labor with an unengaged presenting part may have cephalopelvic disproportion. When the presenting part remains high during labor, especially in the primigravida, cephalopelvic disproportion or dysfunctional labor may be suspected.

Examination of the Patient

In order to predict the course of labor, fetal presentation and position should be determined. There are four methods of doing this: (1) abdominal inspection and palpation, (2) auscultation, (3) vaginal or rectal examination, and (4) x-ray or ultrasound.

ABDOMINAL INSPECTION AND PALPATION

Explain the procedure to the patient. Have her empty her bladder and lie down on her back with her knees flexed and her abdomen exposed. Warm your hands by washing them in warm water before touching her abdomen. Cold hands may stimulate muscle contraction, not only making the patient uncomfortable, but also making accurate palpation difficult.

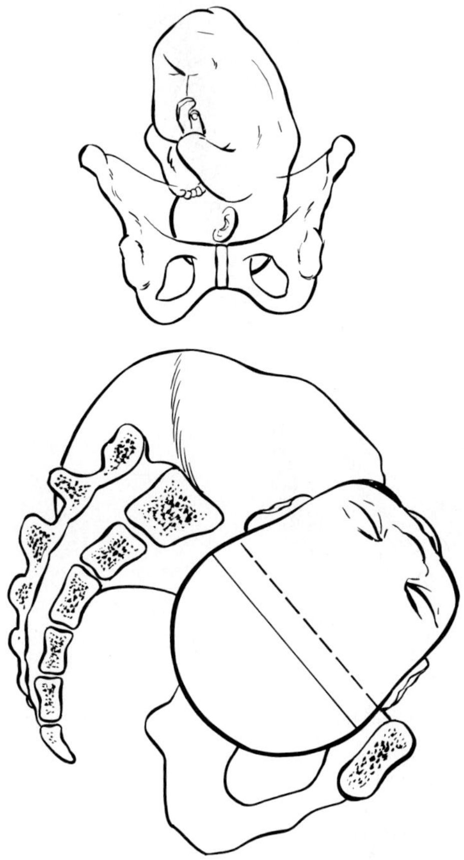

FIGURE 13-16. Engagement of the fetal skull.

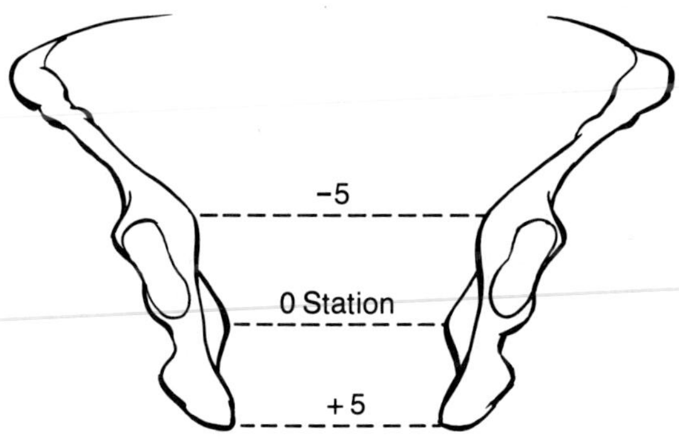

FIGURE 13-17. Station.

First inspect the abdomen visually. Ask yourself the following:

Which diameter of the abdomen appears to be the longest?

Is the long diameter horizontal or vertical?

If there is fetal movement, where is it noted?

Where is the fetal back?

How big does the fetus appear?

Abdominal palpation should be done in a systematic manner. One system that may be used in Leopold's manuevers, a four-step method of abdominal evaluation (see Fig. 13-18).

First Manuever

Stand facing the patient and place the fingers of both hands on the upper part of the abdomen in the area of the uterine fundus. Outline the pole of the fetus that occupies the fundus. A head will feel hard, round, and movable, while a breech will be softer, irregularly shaped, and less movable.

Second Manuever

Next locate the back and small parts of the fetus in relation to the mother's right and left sides. Slide your hands down the sides of the abdomen while exerting a firm even pressure. On one side a smooth, hard resistant surface (the back) can be felt. On the opposite side you will feel a number of angular nodulations (the knees and the elbows). While palpating the fetal back, note whether it is in an anterior or lateral portion of the maternal abdomen.

Third Manuever

Gently grasp the lower portion of the abdomen just above the symphysis pubis between thumb and index finger and try to press thumb and fingers together. If the presenting part moves upward to allow you to press your thumb and fingers together, the presenting part is not engaged. The head or breech can be identified as the lower pole with this manuever.

Fourth Manuever

Turn toward the patient's feet and place the tips of the fingers of each hand on either side

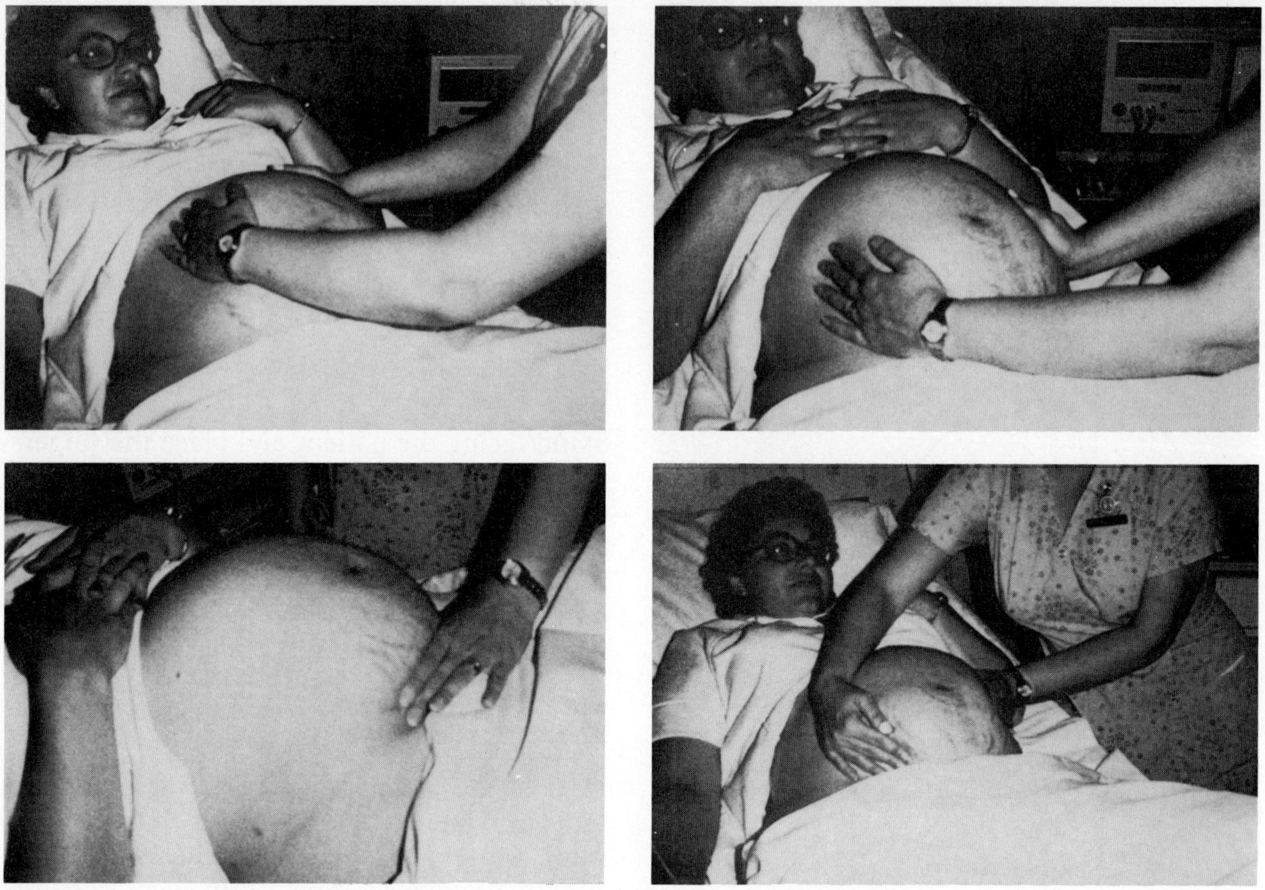

FIGURE 13-18. Leopold's maneuvers: First maneuver (top left). Second maneuver (top right). Third maneuver (bottom left). Fourth maneuver (bottom right).

of the midline in the lower abdomen. Make deep (but gentle) pressure in a downward and inward direction. If the head is presenting, the fingers of one hand will feel the cephalic prominence while the other hand will descend farther. If the cephalic prominence is on the same side as the small parts, it is the brow and indicates flexion of the fetal head. If you feel the cephalic prominence on the same side as the back, the face is presenting. Once the head is well down into the maternal pelvis, it is difficult to feel the cephalic prominence.

AUSCULTATION

The fetal heart rate is auscultated. Fetal heart sounds are transmitted through the convex portion of the fetus. If the presentation is vertex or breech, the fetal heart is heard through the fetal back. If the presentation is face, the back is concave and the fetal heart is heard through the fetal thorax.

If the fetal heart is heard at or above the umbilicus, the fetus may be in a breech presentation. With a cephalic presentation, the fetal heart is usually heard in the lower abdomen. If the position of the fetal head is LOA, the heart is best heard in the maternal right lower quadrant.

VAGINAL OR RECTAL EXAMINATIONS

When a vaginal or rectal examination is done during pregnancy, the station of the presenting part, the softness and length of the cervix, and the basic pelvic configuration can be determined.

When a vaginal or rectal examination is done during labor, information about the presentation, position, and station of the fetus, and about cervical dilation, effacement, and landmarks can be obtained.

X-RAY OR ULTRASOUND

In women who are very obese or who have rigid abdomens, abdominal palpation may be difficult or even impossible. If fetal malposition is suspected, an ultrasound or x-ray may be ordered to determine the presentation, presenting part, station, and flexion of the fetus.

chapter 14

PHYSIOLOGY OF LABOR

OBJECTIVES

Upon completion of this chapter, the reader will be able to:

1. Identify factors that may affect the progress of labor.
2. Describe the signs of labor and explain the related physiology.
3. Differentiate between false labor and true labor.
4. Discuss theories for the onset of labor.
5. Describe the physiology of uterine contractions.
6. State the four stages of labor; identify changes that take place during each stage.
7. Identify the functional divisions of labor.
8. Describe the mechanisms of labor.

KEY TERMS

Active phase
Amplitude
Cervical effacement
Constriction ring
Contraction
Descent
Dilatation
Duration
Expulsion
Extension
External rotation
Flexion
Frequency
Intensity
Internal rotation
Latent phase
Lightening
Mechanism of labor cervical
Pathologic retraction ring
Physiologic retraction ring
Retraction
Show
Tonus
Transition

FACTORS AFFECTING LABOR

Many factors enter into the progress and outcome of labor. Factors of importance may be maternal, uterine, or fetal in origin.

Maternal Factors

AGE

The gravida under 18 years of age is at increased risk for deviations in labor progress and outcome owing to pelvic, physiologic, and psychological immaturity (see Chapter 28). Also at risk is the gravida over 35 years of age.

PARITY

Primigravidas usually have longer labors than do multigravidas. Mortality is lowest with the second child and increases after the sixth.

INTERVALS BETWEEN PREGNANCIES

The intervals between pregnancies will affect labor and neonatal outcome. Infants born less than one year apart tend to be lower in birth weight.

PSYCHOLOGICAL FACTORS

Progress in labor can be related to psychological factors. Three variables have the most influence on the progress of labor: pregnancy acceptance, identification of the role of motherhood, and a history of psychological counseling (Lederman et al., 1979).

OTHER FACTORS

The size and shape of the maternal pelvis in relation to the size, presentation, position, and attitude of the fetus will influence labor progress, as well as maternal physical characteristics.

Uterine Factors

UTERINE CONTRACTIONS

Effectiveness of uterine contractions can shorten or prolong labor. Uterine contraction efficiency is influenced by maternal positioning during labor. The supine position increases the frequency of uterine contractions but decreases the intensity. Lateral positioning decreases uterine contraction frequency but may increase the intensity. Semiupright and upright positions in labor favor cervical dilatation and contraction regularity with complete uterine relaxation between contractions.

CERVIX

The consistency, effacement, and dilation of the cervix will affect the progress of labor.

STATUS OF MEMBRANES

Premature rupture of the membranes can result in poor labor progress. Membranes that rupture after 2 cm cervical dilation are associated with an increase in the progress of dilation.

PLACENTAL LOCATION

A placenta that is located over or next to the cervical os (placenta previa) will hinder or make vaginal delivery impossible. A placenta that is located high in the uterine fundus is associated with a slow or prolonged labor in some women.

Fetal Factors

GESTATIONAL AGE

Smaller babies usually deliver after shorter labors. Neonates who are delivered before 38 or after 42 weeks are at increased risk for labor difficulties than are neonates delivered at term.

FETAL HEAD

The position of the fetal head will affect labor progress. Increased uterine efficiency is associated with occiput anterior positions. The size of the fetal head will affect labor progress.

PRESENTATIONS OTHER THAN CEPHALIC

Noncephalic fetal presentations will affect the length and progress of labor.

PREMONITORY SIGNS OF LABOR

In the majority of parous women a prodromal stage precedes true labor. The premonitory signs may be very noticeable, or so slight that they go unnoticed. These premonitory signs include lightening, false labor, show, cervical effacement, increased vaginal secretions, increased backache, increased sacroiliac pressure, frequency of urination, weight loss, an energy spurt, gastrointestinal symptoms, and sleep disturbances.

LIGHTENING

The settling of the fetal presenting part into the lower uterine segment is referred to as *lightening*. It may occur two to three weeks before labor in the primigravida, but may not occur until active labor in the multipara. The abdomen undergoes a change in shape, the fundal height decreases, and the gravida may say that the baby has "dropped." Lightening occurs as a result of myometrial contractions, a well-formed lower uterine segment, and descent of the presenting part to or through the maternal pelvic inlet.

As a result of lightening, respirations become easier. Lordosis is increased, and the increased pelvic pressure causes frequency of urination, leg cramps, dependent edema, or a sensation of pelvic fullness.

FALSE LABOR

Braxton-Hicks' contractions occur throughout pregnancy but are usually not felt by the patient until the latter part. The uterine contractions of false labor are irregular in frequency, duration, and intensity. They occur especially at night, and tend to subside toward morning. Although usually painless, they may cause lower abdominal discomfort.

SHOW

Discharge of possibly blood-tinged mucus from the vagina is called *show*. Show represents the expulsion of the mucus plug from the cervical canal. The bloody tinge to the mucus is caused by rupture of superficial blood vessels by the increasing pelvic pressure when the mucus plug separates from the cervical mucus.

CERVICAL EFFACEMENT

In preparation for labor the cervix may become softer and thinner. In primigravidas the external os of the cervix may be sufficiently dilated to permit one finger to be inserted in the cervical canal. In multiparas, this dilation may be 2 to 3 cm. Thinning of the cervix occurs as a result of uterine myometrial contractions that pull the cervix upward and thin the dense fibrous connective tissue.

INCREASE IN VAGINAL SECRETIONS

Vaginal secretions increase owing to the congestion of the vaginal mucous membranes.

INCREASED BACKACHE AND SACROILIAC PRESSURE

During the latter part of pregnancy the hormone relaxin will cause relaxation of the pelvic joints and increase the incidence of backache and sacroiliac pressure.

FREQUENCY OF URINATION

The increased pressure of the fetal presenting part limits the capacity of the urinary bladder and increases the sensation of bladder fullness. This leads to an increase in the frequency of urination.

WEIGHT LOSS

A weight loss of one to three pounds may occur owing to fluid loss. A change in estrogen and progesterone levels will result in an electrolyte shift, leading to fluid loss.

ENERGY SPURT

An energetic need to accomplish various household tasks (sometimes referred to as a "nesting urge") frequently occurs within 24 to 48 hours before the onset of labor.

GASTROINTESTINAL SYMPTOMS

Diarrhea, indigestion, nausea, and vomiting may occur shortly before the onset of labor. The cause of these disturbances is unknown, but diarrhea may stimulate uterine contractions.

SLEEP DISTURBANCES

Many women report increasing difficulty in sleeping or changes in their sleep patterns shortly before the onset of labor.

False Labor vs. True Labor

Distinguishing between false labor (Braxton-Hicks' contractions) and true labor can be difficult. Often false labor is diagnosed only after uterine contractions have completely stopped. When a patient arrives in the labor and delivery area with uterine contractions, it becomes a nursing responsibility to aid in differentiation of false labor and true labor (see Table 14-1).

FALSE LABOR

False labor contractions are inefficient uterine contractions, usually of irregular frequency and variable duration. Discomfort is felt mainly in the lower abdomen or groin. The uterine contractions are mild in intensity. These contractions result in no cervical changes and do not push the presenting part into the maternal pelvis.

TRUE LABOR

With the onset of true labor, uterine contractions occur at regular intervals and become more frequent, of longer duration, and increasing intensity. Discomfort is felt during the contractions, and often starts in the lower back and radiates to the abdomen. Cervical dilation occurs and the presenting part descends into the maternal pelvis.

TABLE 14-1
TRUE LABOR VS. FALSE LABOR

True Labor	False Labor
Contractions regular	Contractions irregular
Contractions become more frequent	Contraction frequency unchanged
Contraction duration increases	Contraction duration remains same
Contraction intensity increases	Contraction intensity unchanged
Discomfort starts in back and radiates to front	Discomfort mainly in abdomen and groin
Intensity is increased by walking	Walking does not change intensity
Show usually present	Show seldom present
Cervix dilates and effaces	No cervical changes
Presenting part descends	No change in station of presenting part
Sedation does not stop contractions	Effective sedation stops contractions

ONSET OF TRUE LABOR

Many theories have been proposed to explain why true labor begins. None of these theories has been universally accepted as the actual cause of the onset of true labor. In all likelihood, a combination of maternal and fetal factors are responsible for labor initiation.

UTERINE STRETCH THEORY

Distention of the uterus has been implicated in triggering the onset of labor. Any organ that is hollow will contract and empty itself when stretched. With the progression of pregnancy the uterus stretches to many times its nonpregnant size. Distention is a direct stimulus to the mechanical activity of the uterus and causes an increase in the electrical activity. When the uterus distends far beyond its volume, labor begins. This theory explains the preterm labor common in polyhydramnios and multiple gestations.

MENSTRUAL CYCLE THEORY

It has been postulated that an association exists between the menstrual cycle and the onset of labor. Labor normally begins 40 weeks or 10 menstrual cycles after the last normal menstrual period.

POSITIVE FEEDBACK THEORY

According to this theory, the fetal head pushes against the cervix with enough pressure that a reflex increase in uterine contractility occurs. This increased contractility pushes the fetus downward against the cervix, stretching the cervix further and initiating a new cycle.

DESCENT OF THE PRESENTING PART

As the fetal presenting part descends into the maternal pelvis, there is an increase in afferent nerve impulses. These impulses in turn increase oxytocin release.

ROLE OF THE DECIDUA

As the pregnancy nears term, there is degeneration of the uterine mucosa, causing a release of lysosomal enzymes that initiates prostaglandin synthesis. Smooth muscle contraction will then follow.

OXYTOCIN STIMULATION THEORY

Uterine muscle is increasingly responsive to oxytocin as pregnancy progresses to term. Oxytocin is produced by the hypothalamus and stored in the posterior pituitary gland. Just before the onset of labor, the amount of oxytocin is believed to increase, possibly due to the influence of the fetal posterior pituitary gland.

Braxton-Hicks' contractions may cause stretching of the cervix, sending impulses to the hypothalamic-neurohypophyseal axis. Oxytocin is released and causes uterine contractions.

PROGESTERONE WITHDRAWAL THEORY

Estrogen production reaches a maximum before labor begins. Estrogens have many myometrial effects:

- Estrogens are essential for the coordinated activity and reactivity of the uterus
- Estrogens restrict the growth response of the uterus to distention
- The energy sources for uterine contractions are affected by estrogens
- The resting membrane potential of the myometrial cells of the uterus is elevated by estrogen
- Estrogens appear to cause the synthesis of prostaglandin A_2 from the uterus
- Under the influence of estrogens, the contraction wave of the uterine muscle is propagated in an orderly manner from one part of the uterus to another

At the same time that estrogen production is increasing, progesterone production is diminishing, allowing estrogen to dominate. A decrease in placental production of progesterone also occurs as a result of placental aging. The primary myometrial effect of progesterone is interference with the propagation of the contraction wave. When the proper concentrations of estrogen and progesterone are reached, uterine contractions begin.

FETAL ENDOCRINE THEORY

Peak placental function is from 38 to 40 weeks of gestation. After that time, placental trophoblasts degenerate and alter the placental vasculature. The fetal adrenal glands secrete corticosteroids that may trigger the onset of labor by activating myometrial-stimulating agents. Shortly before labor begins, the sensitivity of the fetal adrenal glands to adrenocorticotropic hormone (ACTH) is increased. This sensitivity increases cortisol production, stimulating the release of prostaglandin precursors. Prostaglandin precursors, in turn, stimulate uterine contractions.

UTERINE CONTRACTION PHYSIOLOGY

In order to understand the essentials of uterine contraction physiology, several terms must be defined:

Contraction: The shortening of a muscle in response to a stimulus, with return to its original length following the contraction.

Retraction: The muscle shortens in response to a stimulus but does not return to its original length when the contraction has passed. The muscle becomes fixed at a shorter length, but maintains tension. Retraction is responsible for descent of the fetus during labor.

Physiologic retraction ring: As labor proceeds, the upper part of the uterus becomes shorter and thicker and the lower portion becomes longer and thinner. The boundary between these two segments is the physiologic retraction ring (see Fig. 14–1).

Pathologic retraction ring: When labor is obstructed, the physiologic retraction ring becomes pathologic.

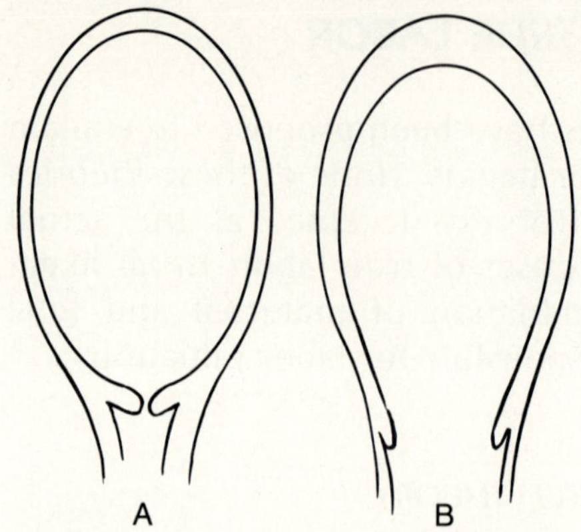

FIGURE 14–1. Schematic of physiological retraction ring: A. Latent phase of first stage of labor. B. Second stage of labor.

Constriction ring: A local spasm of myometrial muscle that grips the fetus and prevents descent.

Tonus: The lowest intrauterine pressure between uterine contractions expressed in mm Hg. The normal resting tone of the uterus is 8 to 12 mm Hg.

Intensity: The rise in intrauterine pressure during uterine contractions. The normal increase is 30 to 50 mm Hg.

Amplitude: The difference between the peak pressure during a contraction and the tonus.

Frequency: The number of uterine contractions per unit of time.

Duration: The length of time measures from when intrauterine pressure begins to rise until the pressure returns to tonus.

Properties of Uterine Muscle

Uterine muscle has the same properties as other smooth muscle: contraction, relaxation, coordination, and elasticity.

CONTRACTION AND RELAXATION

The contractile properties of uterine muscle are functions of actinomycin and calcium ions in the cells. Uterine muscle contractility is influenced by estrogens that increase the binding of the calcium ion in the muscle cells. The sarcoplasmic reticulum that surrounds the uterine myofibril is a storage system from which calcium can be released to the myofibril, causing a muscle contraction.

Uterine muscle relaxation occurs when calcium is bound by the sarcoplasmic reticulum. Autonomous, spontaneous contraction and relaxation are inherent properties of smooth muscle.

COORDINATION

The uterus remains relatively quiet during the first half of pregnancy, although some myometrial activity occurs. There may be frequent, localized contractions of uterine muscle that increase the intrauterine pressure only 1 to 5 mm Hg above tonus. The resting pressure between uterine contractions remains constant throughout normal pregnancy.

Near the end of the second trimester, the regional activity continues, with occasional interruptions by isolated contractions that are similar to those of true labor. These Braxton-Hicks' contractions are triggered from various portions of the uterus and spread for variable distances along the uterine muscle.

During late pregnancy, Braxton-Hicks' contractions become more frequent and are accompanied by increasing discomfort. When these contractions come in bursts, the woman may feel she is in labor. As true labor approaches, they become more regular in frequency, duration, and intensity, and spread over larger areas of the myometrium.

The uterus contains two pacemakers: the primary pacemaker in the left cornus, and the secondary pacemaker in the right cornual area near the broad ligament. In normal uterine contractions, the contraction wave begins at the primary pacemaker and spreads downward in the next 15 seconds. The duration of the contraction diminishes progressively as the wave moves away from the pacemaker area. The contraction phase begins later in the lower portion of the uterus, but the peak of the contraction occurs simultaneously in all portions of the uterus. The intensity of the contractions decreases from above downward. For normal uterine action there must be good coordination between the upper and lower halves of the uterus and between the upper and lower uterine segments.

ELASTICITY

Elasticity, or adjustment in length without adjustment in tension, allows expansion of the uterus during pregnancy. Under the influence of estrogen, the uterine muscle cells undergo hypertrophy and hyperplasia to accommodate the growing fetus. Elasticity permits the following to occur:

Increase in uterine volume
Descent of the presenting part
Uterine tonus
Rapid descent of the uterine fundus after delivery

Hemodynamic Stressors

During labor, there are four major areas of hemodynamic stress: uterine circulation, intervillous circulation, umbilical circulation, and fetal circulation.

UTERINE CIRCULATION

Uterine blood flow depends upon the anatomic arrangements of blood vessels, their tone, contractility, arterial perfusion pressure, and venous outflow. During labor the total decrease in uterine blood flow depends on uterine tonus and the frequency, duration, and intensity of contractions.

INTERVILLOUS CIRCULATION

The intervillous space is divided into smaller spaces, filled with maternal blood. The fetal villi dip in to absorb oxygen and nutrients into the fetal capillaries. During labor the inflow and drainage of maternal blood is increased. The outflow is nearly shut off, resulting in pooling of blood to provide the fetus with a reserve from which to draw nutrients during uterine contractions.

UMBILICOFETAL CIRCULATION

The umbilical cord normally consists of two arteries, one vein, Wharton's jelly, the allantoic duct, and a cord covering. If the cord is compressed by a true knot, cord around the fetal neck or body, or cord prolapse, the blood supply to the fetus is compromised. The fetus will attempt to compensate for this decrease in oxygen (see Chapter 16: Fetal Monitoring).

THE LABOR PROCESS

Stages of Labor

Labor is divided into four stages: the stage of dilation, the stage of expulsion, the placental stage, and the stage of recovery.

FIRST STAGE

The first stage of labor is called the stage of dilation. It begins with the onset of true labor and ends with complete cervical dilation (10 cm). In the primigravida this stage averages 13.3 hours and in multipara 7.5 hours.

SECOND STAGE

The second stage of labor is the stage of expulsion, beginning with complete cervical dilation and ending with delivery of the fetus. The primigravida averages 57 minutes for this stage and the multipara 18 minutes.

THIRD STAGE

The third stage is the placental stage, beginning after delivery of the newborn and ending with placental expulsion. This stage averages 5 minutes in both the primigravida and the multipara.

FOURTH STAGE

Stage four, or the stage of recovery, begins with placental expulsion and ends when the mother's physiologic status is stable. It lasts a *minimum* of one hour, regardless of parity.

Phases of Labor

The first stage of labor is divided into two phases: latent and active (see Fig. 14–2).

LATENT PHASE

The latent phase begins with the onset of labor and lasts until the beginning of the active phase of cervical dilation (3 to 4 cm). This is the longest phase of the first stage of labor. The cervix dilates at a rate of approximately 0.3 cm per hour. In the primigravida the latent phase lasts 8.6 hours, with an upper normal limit of 20 hours. For the multipara the latent phase averages 5.3 hours, with an upper limit of 14 hours.

ACTIVE PHASE

The active phase of the first stage begins with the upswing of the contraction curve (5 cm) and ends with the beginning of the second stage of labor at 10 cm cervical dilation. In the primigravida the active phase averages 5.8 hours, with an upper limit of 12 hours, and in the multipara the average duration is 2.5 hours, with an upper limit of 6 hours. The cervix dilates at a *minimum* rate of 1.5 cm per hour in the multipara and 1.2 cm per hour in the primigravida.

The active phase can be further divided into the acceleration phase, the initial portion of the active phase; phase of maximum slope, from 5 cm to 9 cm cervical dilation; and deceleration phase, from 9 to 10 cm dilation. The phase of cervical dilation from 8 to 10 cm is often referred to as the transition phase of labor.

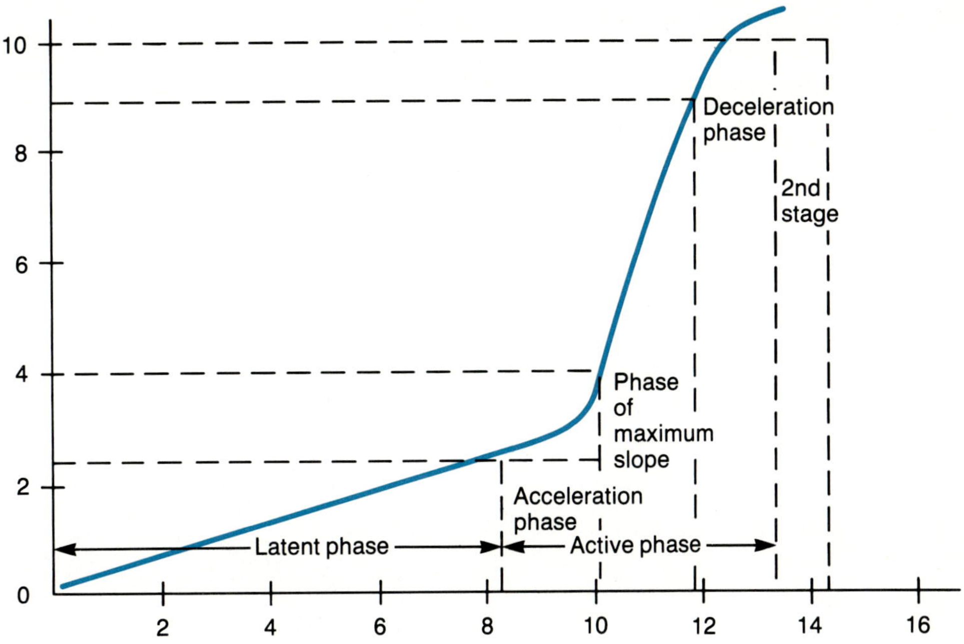

FIGURE 14-2. Schematic of average labor pattern.

Functional Divisions of Labor

Labor can be divided into three functional units that are based on cervical dilation and descent of the present part (see Fig. 14-3).

PREPARATORY DIVISION

Changes during this functional division are subtle, and include coordination of uterine myometrial activity and cervical softening and effacement. The preparatory division is basically equivalent to the latent phase of labor. During this division, the uterus is particularly sensitive to sedation. Medication given to the mother during the preparatory division can disrupt the coordinating efforts of the myometrium and prolong labor.

DILATIONAL DIVISION

The majority of cervical dilation occurs during this division. The inclination of the maximum slope is considered a measure of the efficiency of the uterine contraction pattern. The slope averages 3 cm per hour in nulliparas and 5.7 cm per hour in multiparas.

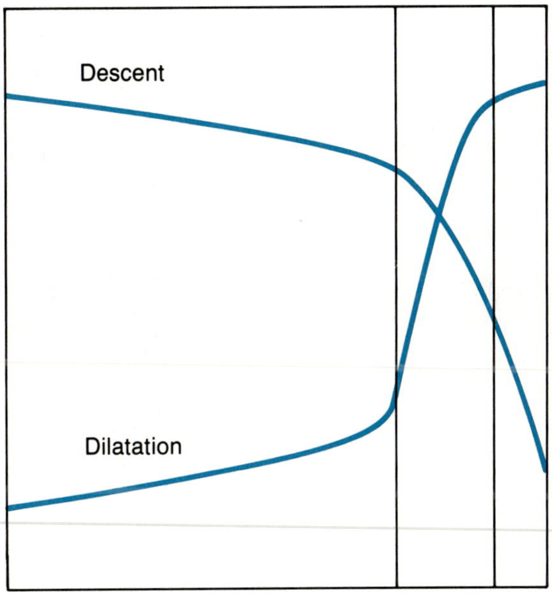

FIGURE 14-3. Functional divisions of labor showing interrelationship of cervical dilatation and descent of the presenting part.

PELVIC DIVISION

The end of the dilational division marks the onset of the pelvic division of labor. The descent pattern during this division measures the overall efficiency of the labor process. The slope of fetal descent averages 1.6 cm per hour in nulliparas, and 5.4 cm per hour in multiparas.

Mechanism of Labor

The mechanism of labor involves the progressive rotational movements of the fetus that enable the diameters of the presenting part (and entire fetus) to pass through the maternal pelvis. There are seven movements which overlap each other:

Engagement
Descent
Flexion
Internal rotation
Extension
External rotation
Expulsion

The following descriptions of these seven movements assumes a fetus presenting in a left occiput anterior (LOA) position, the most common position for labor.

ENGAGEMENT

Engagement of the presenting part is passage of the biparietal diameter of the fetal head through the maternal ischial spines (see Fig. 14–4).

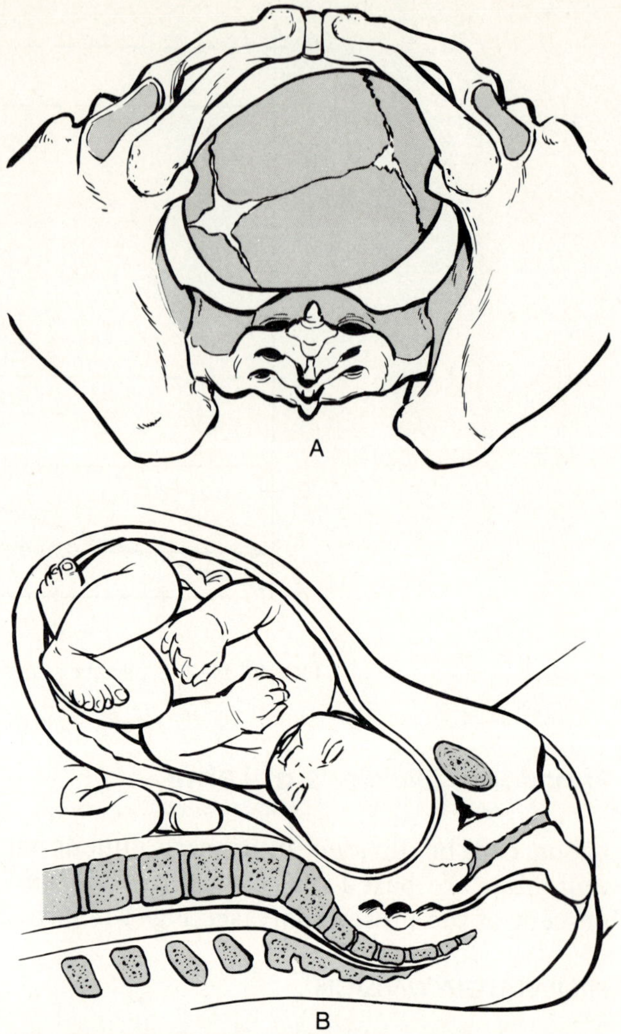

FIGURE 14–4. Engagement of the presenting part at the onset of labor: A. Vaginal view. B. Lateral view.

DESCENT

The process of descent begins with engagement and continues throughout labor. Other fetal movements are superimposed upon descent through the maternal pelvis. In primigravidas considerable descent may occur before labor begins. In multiparas descent may not take place until well into active labor.

Most frequently, the fetal head engages in the transverse diameter of the maternal pelvic inlet. If the fetal head enters the pelvis squarely, the plane of the fetal head will parallel the planes of the maternal pelvis, and the head is said to be in *synclitism* (see Fig. 14–5). If the fetal head is tilted laterally toward one of the fetal shoulders, the sagittal suture will be closer to either the maternal sacral promontory or symphysis pubis. The fetal cephalic planes will be oblique to the maternal pelvic planes and the head is said to be *asynclitic* (see Fig. 14–6).

Descent occurs as a result of the downward pressure of the uterine contractions, bearing down efforts by the mother during the second stage of labor, and by gravity (see Fig. 14–7).

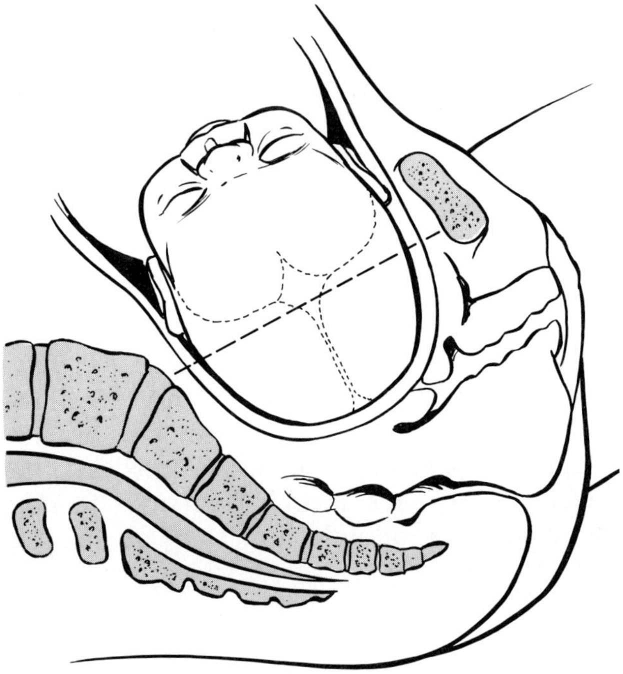

FIGURE 14-5. Synclitism of the fetal head during labor.

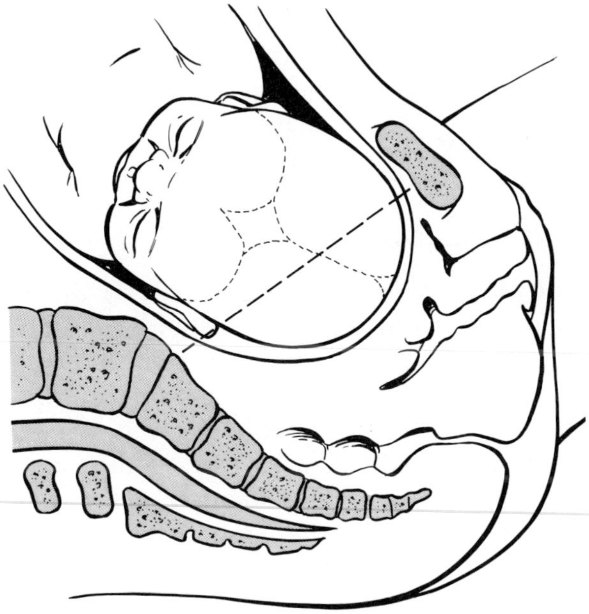

FIGURE 14-6. Asynclitism of the fetal head during labor.

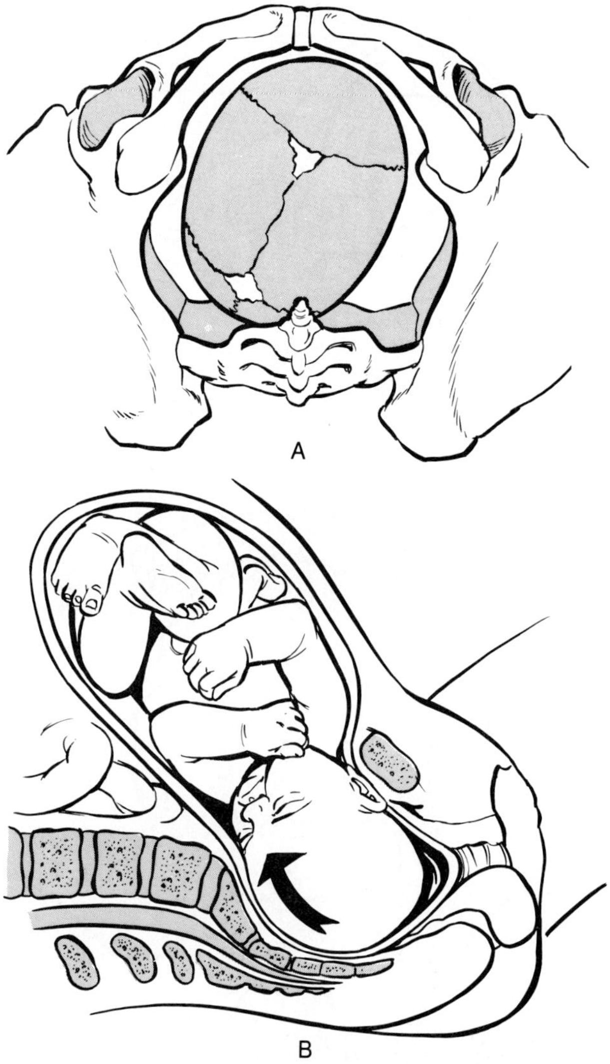

FIGURE 14-7. Descent and flexion of the fetal head in a LOA position. A. Vaginal view. B. Lateral view.

FLEXION

Flexion is the forward tipping of the fetal head so that the chin lies close to the chest. When the fetal head is completely flexed, the presenting diameter changes from the occipitofrontal diameter (11 cm) to the smallest diameter of the fetal head, the suboccipitobregmatic (9.5 cm). Flexion (see Fig. 14-7) is the result of pressure from the pelvic floor and the force transmitted along the fetal spine to the junction of the head and the first cervical vertebrae.

INTERNAL ROTATION

For labor to progress, the long axis of the fetal head must fit into the long axis of the maternal pelvis. The head turns from the transverse or oblique diameter to an anteroposterior diameter (see Fig. 14-8).

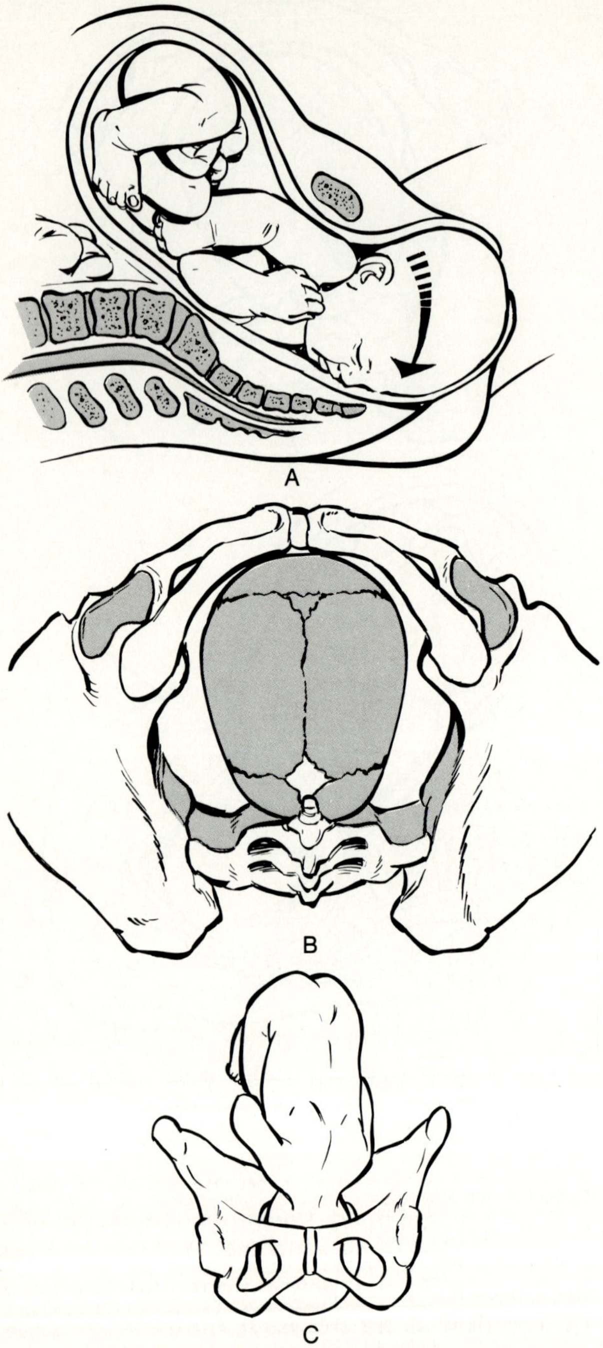

FIGURE 14-8. Internal rotation of the fetal head in LOA position. The fetal head rotates from LOA to OA to fit the long axis of the maternal pelvis. A. Lateral view. B. Vaginal view. C. Anteroposterior view.

The occiput of the fetal head makes contact with the maternal levator ani muscles and fascia, and rotates 45 degrees to the right. The sagittal suture turns to a OA position. As a result of the rotation, the occiput lies near the symphysis pubis and the sinciput lies near the sacrum.

While the head rotates, the shoulders remain in the left oblique diameter of the maternal pelvis and the neck twists 45 degrees. Internal rotation takes place mainly during the second stage of labor, just before or as the fetal head reaches the pelvic floor.

EXTENSION

As the flexed head continues its descent, there is bulging of the maternal perineum. The occiput passes through the outlet slowly and the back of the neck pivots. Then the sinciput, bregma, nose, mouth, and chin are born in succession over the maternal perineum (see Fig. 14-9). Extension is essential for the head to pass through the vulvar outlet, which inclines upward and forward with distention. Extension results from two forces: uterine contractions that exert downward pressure, and the pelvic floor resistance. Once the head is born and is free of the maternal pelvis, *restitution* occurs. The neck untwists and the occiput rotates 45 degrees back to its original position (see Fig. 14-10).

EXTERNAL ROTATION

The process of external rotation of the fetal head is the outward manifestation of internal shoulder rotation. The shoulder that is anterior encounters resistance and rotates 45 degrees toward the symphysis pubis, while the posterior shoulder turns toward the sacrum. In this way the long diameter of the fetal shoulders can fit the long diameter of the maternal pelvic outlet. Externally, the fetal head rotates another 45 degrees to maintain a normal relationship with the shoulders (see Fig. 14-11).

EXPULSION

The anterior shoulder is born under the symphysis pubis and pivots there. Then the posterior shoulder delivers over the perineum (see Fig. 14-12). The rest of the body delivers with no special mechanism.

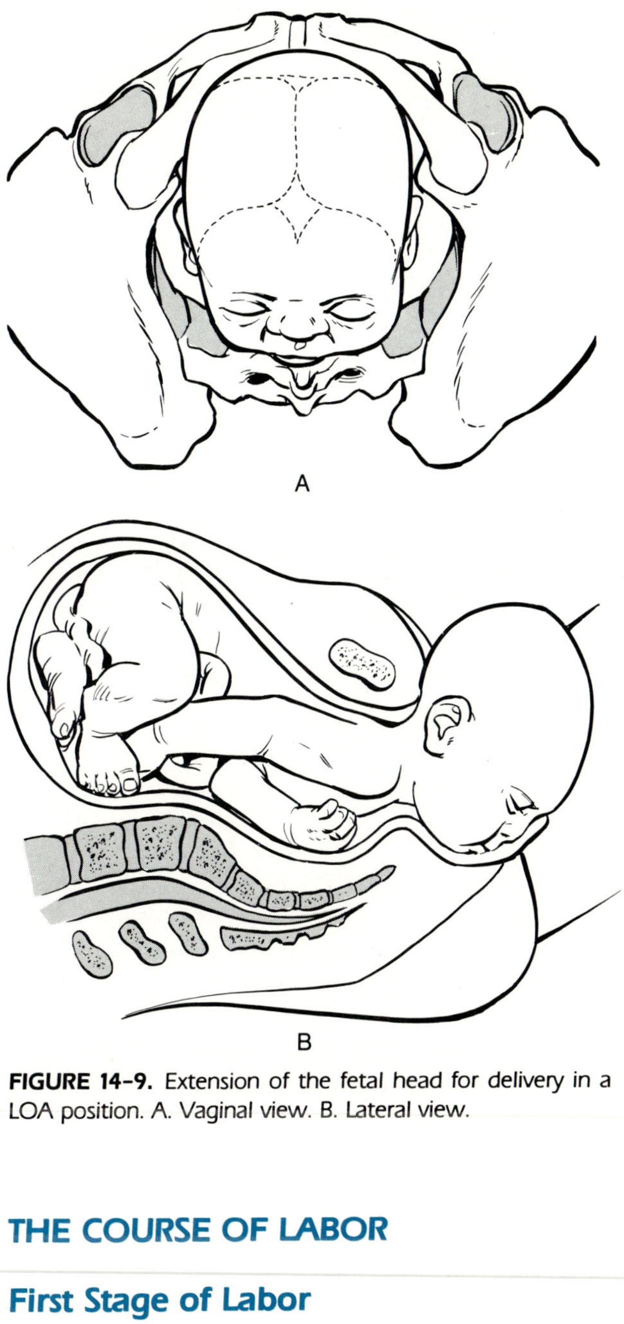

FIGURE 14-9. Extension of the fetal head for delivery in a LOA position. A. Vaginal view. B. Lateral view.

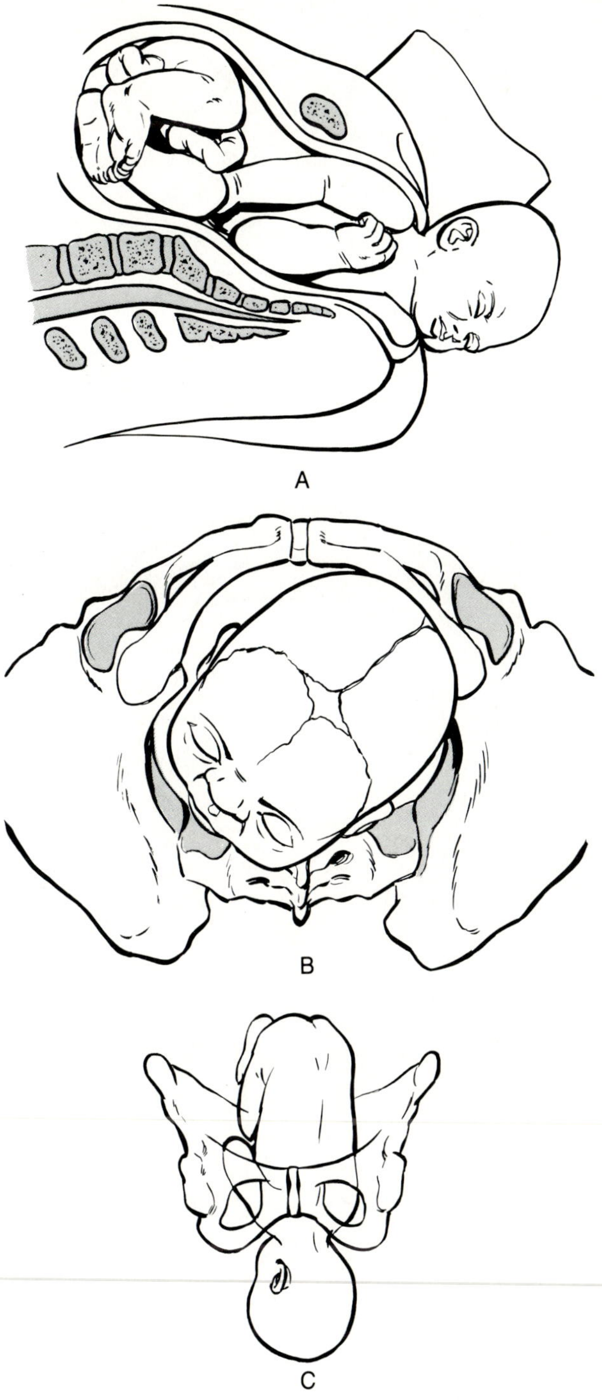

FIGURE 14-10. Restitution from OA to LOA at delivery. A. Lateral view. B. Vaginal view. C. Anteroposterior view.

THE COURSE OF LABOR

First Stage of Labor

UTERINE CONTRACTIONS

Uterine contractions are involuntary and generally independent of extrauterine control. Efficient uterine contractions exhibit *fundal dominance,* in which contractions are initiated in the uterine fundus and radiate over the body of the uterus toward the cervix. Contractions begin in the fundus owing to the greater concentration of myometrial cells in that portion of the uterus.

The interval between uterine contractions diminishes gradually from about 10 minutes to as little as 1 or 2 minutes. Periods of relaxation between uterine contractions are essential to fetal well-being. The duration of con-

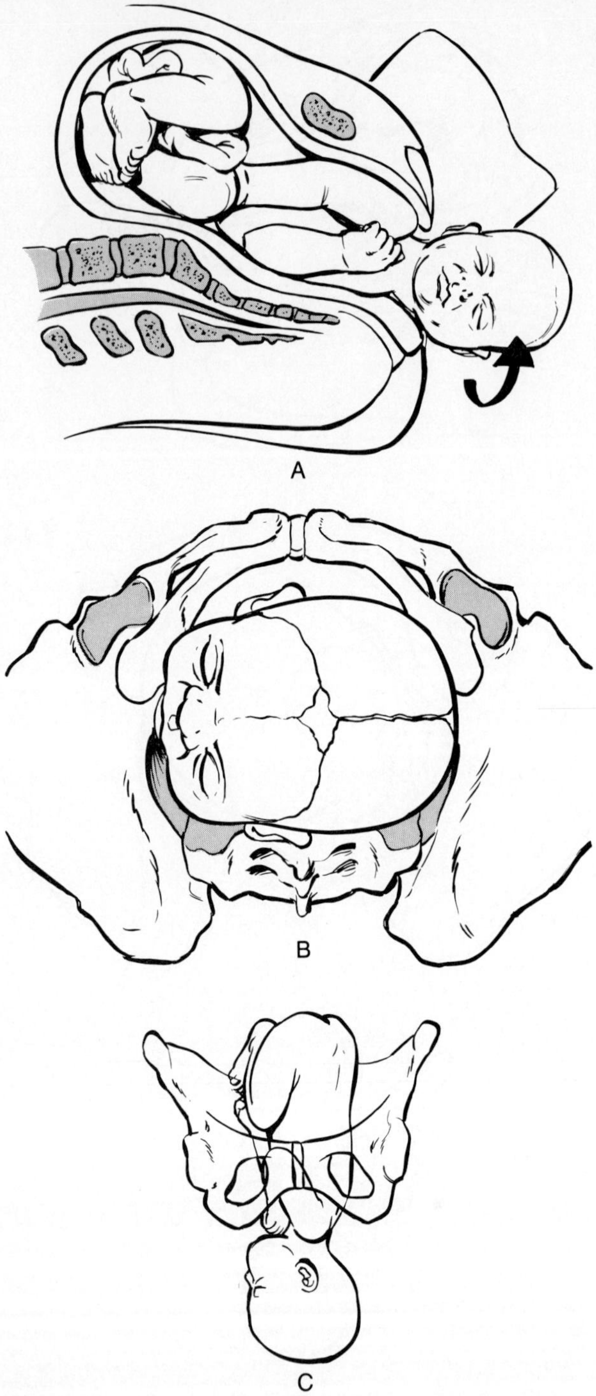

FIGURE 14-11. External rotation from LOA to LOT for shoulder delivery. A. Lateral view. B. Vaginal view. C. Anteroposterior view.

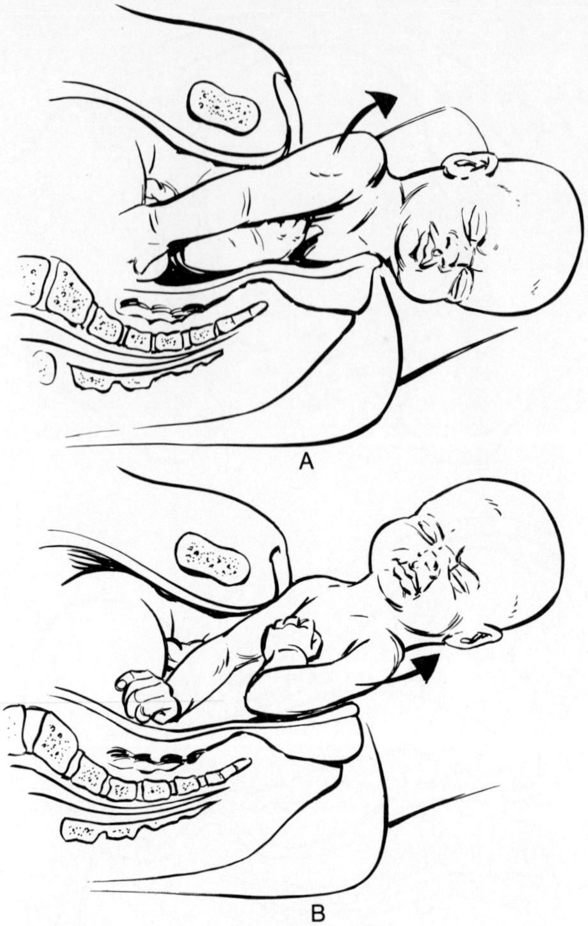

FIGURE 14-12. A. Delivery of the anterior shoulder. B. Delivery of the posterior shoulder.

tractions ranges from 30 to 90 seconds and averages 1 minute. The intensity of contractions varies considerably during labor, and may range from 30 to 50 mm Hg.

Upper and Lower Uterine Segments

With the onset of labor, the uterus differentiates into two distinct segments. The upper segment becomes thicker as labor advances, while the lower segment is less active and becomes thinner.

The lower uterine segment develops gradually as pregnancy progresses and then thins during labor. The two uterine segments can be differentiated during a contraction by abdominal palpation. The upper segment is firm and the lower segment feels much less firm.

During labor the upper segment contracts, retracts, and finally expels the fetus. In response to upper segment contractions, the lower uterine segment and cervix dilate, forming a greatly expanded, thinned-out tube that is pulled upward around the presenting part.

The physiologic retraction ring marks the junction of the upper and lower segments.

The upper segment myometrium does not relax to its original length after contracting. It becomes fixed at a shorter length while maintaining the same tension (*brachystasis*). With each successive contraction the upper uterine cavity becomes slightly smaller and thicker and gradually propels the fetus downward.

At the same time, the lower uterine segment lengthens without changing tension (*mecystasis*) to accommodate the fetus. The progressive lengthening is accompanied by thinning of the segment.

Changes in Uterine Shape

Uterine contractions produce an elongation of the ovoid uterus, with a decrease in the horizontal diameters. The decreased horizontal diameters produce a straightening of the vertebral column of the fetus, which presses the upper fetal pole into the fundus and the lower fetal pole down into the maternal pelvis. As the uterus lengthens, longitudinal fibers are pulled taut, causing the lower segment and cervix to pull upward over the lower fetal pole and enabling the cervix to dilate.

Ligaments

The round ligaments contract at the same time as the upper uterine segment, resulting in a pulling of the uterine corpus (body) in the same direction. This pulling contributes to fetal descent. The contractions of the uterosacral ligaments help to pull the cervix backward.

CERVICAL CHANGES

Two cervical changes occur during the first stage of labor: effacement and dilation.

Effacement

Prior to labor, the cervix usually softens and is described as "ripe." The position of the cervix changes within the vagina so that the external os is aligned with the vaginal canal rather than lying toward the posterior vaginal wall. *Cervical effacement* is the shortening of the cervical canal from approximately 1 to 2 cm in length to a circular opening with almost paper-thin edges (see Fig. 14–13). To accomplish this thinning, the cervical muscular fibers in the vicinity of the internal os are pulled up and into the lower uterine segment during contractions. The initiation of effacement before true labor begins is facilitated by the expulsion of the mucus plug from the cervical canal.

Dilation

In order for the fetus to pass through the cervix, the cervix must dilate to a diameter of

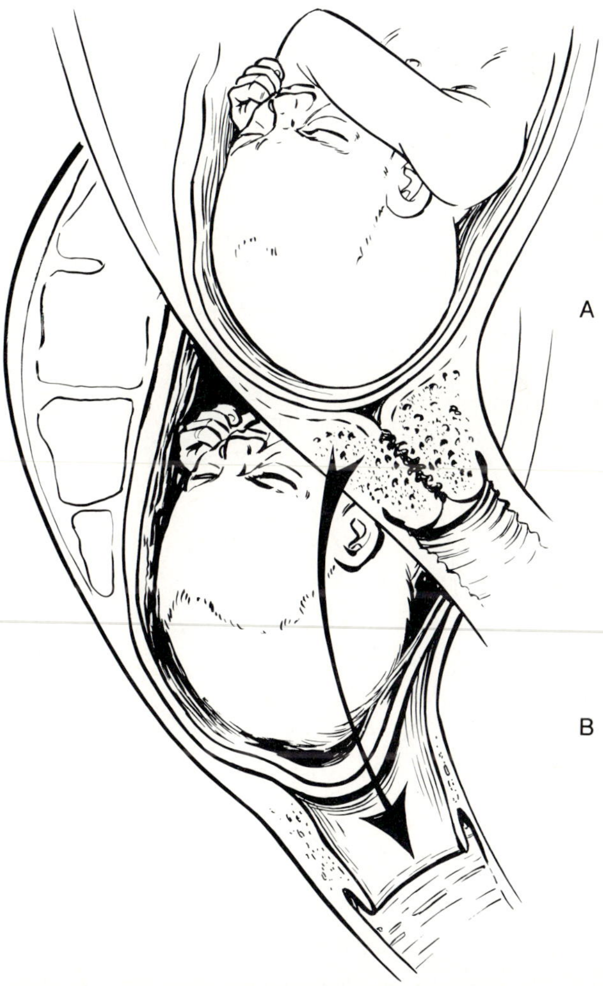

FIGURE 14–13. Cervical effacement. A. Cervix thick and closed. B. Cervical effacement.

10 cm (see Fig. 14–14). Dilation of the cervix is caused by two mechanisms: the pressure on the cervix by the bag of waters or the presenting part, and the longitudinal retraction on the cervix by the upper uterine segment as it contracts and retracts (see Fig. 14–15).

CHANGES IN MEMBRANES

The fetus lies in a sac covered with an inner layer (*amnion*) and an outer layer (*chorion*) that is filled with amniotic fluid. As labor progresses and the cervix dilates, the membranes separate from the lower uterine segment. The lower pole of the membranes bulges a little with each uterine contraction and may adopt several shapes (see Fig. 14–16). A bag of waters that hangs in the vagina is of little help in dilating the cervix and may hinder labor by preventing descent of the presenting part. In normal labor, the rupture of the membranes causes uterine contractions to be more efficient and labor to progress faster.

UMBILICAL CORD CHANGES

The umbilical cord is also subjected to the increased intrauterine pressures exerted by uterine contractions. This pressure may be sufficient to impede blood flow in the cord vessels.

PLACENTAL CHANGES

Uterine contractions also affect the placenta. During contractions the uterine blood vessels are compressed and may be occluded. Since exchange of blood, gases, and nutrients at the placental site depends on maternal circulation, contractions represent a potential threat to oxygenation and nutrition of the fetus.

MATERNAL PHYSIOLOGY

During labor, there are normal alterations in maternal physiology. These changes will affect all the body systems, but especially the car-

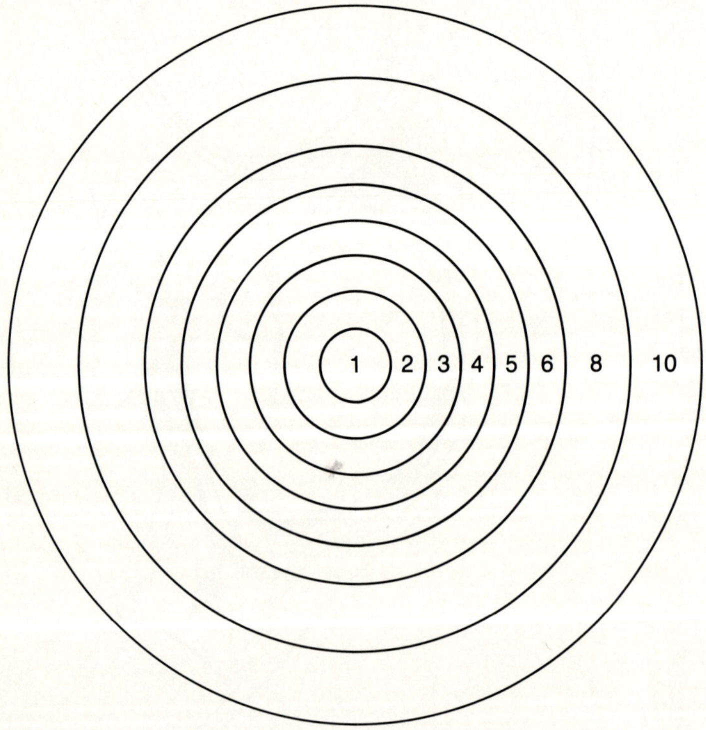

FIGURE 14–14. Cervical dilatation with circles to scale.

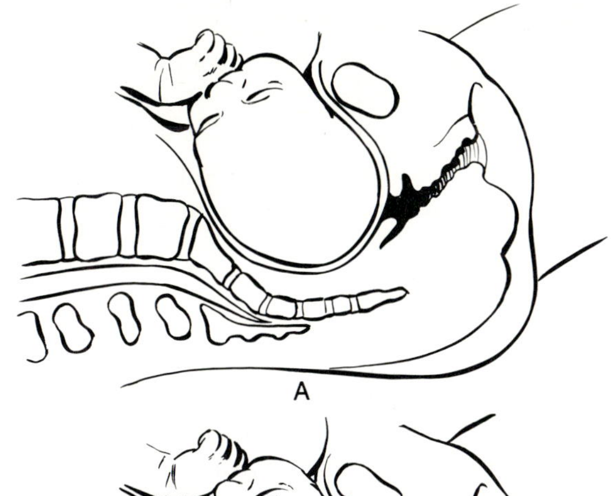

FIGURE 14-15. A. Cervix dilated 2 to 3 cm and thinning. B. Cervix 5 cm dliated. C. Complete effacement and dilatation.

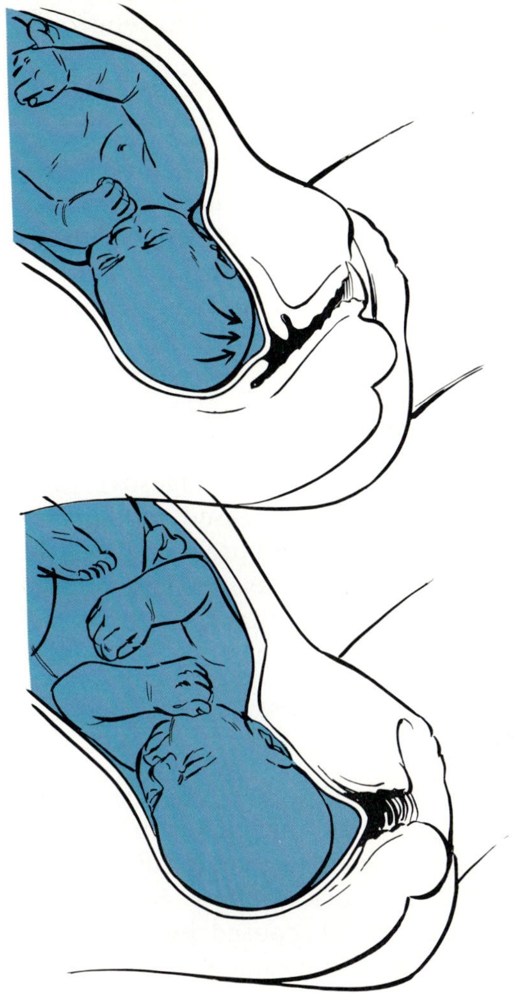

FIGURE 14-16. Bulging of the membranes.

diovascular, respiratory, gastrointestinal, and renal systems.

Cardiovascular System

Uterine contractions are associated with hemodynamic changes. With each contraction, the cardiac output increases 15 to 20 percent, owing to return of blood from the placental circulation, increased physical activity, and catecholamine release. This increase begins before the contraction and returns to normal as the contraction ends.

At the same time, arterial blood pressure rises and a reflex bradycardia occurs. The distal aorta and the common iliac arteries are compressed during a uterine contraction, causing a redistribution of the cardiac output to the upper portion of the maternal vascular system.

The pulse rate increases because of increased metabolic activity, anxiety, and increased muscular activity.

Usually blood pressure remains normal between uterine contractions but may increase during a contraction. Blood pressure decreases may be seen in supine hypotension syndrome (see Chapter 16).

Respiratory System

The respiratory rate between uterine contractions remains within the normal range. During contractions the rate will increase, owing to the increased metabolism and oxygen consumption that is normal during labor.

Gastrointestinal System

When active labor begins, the digestive processes cease. There is decreased motility of the gastrointestinal tract and prolonged gastric emptying time. This decrease in gastrointestinal activity is the reason that solid foods are not given during active labor.

Renal System

Polyuria is common during labor as a result of the increased cardiac output, with a corresponding increase in the glomerular filtration rate and renal plasma flow. Slight proteinuria may be noted, caused by increased metabolic activity. Ketonuria is seen in dehydration and maternal exhaustion, as well as in nutritional deficiencies and electrolyte imbalances.

Acid-Base Balance

The maternal blood pH usually remains within the normal range of 7.35 to 7.45, with a slight trend toward acidosis. The body does not fully compensate for this acidosis during active labor for several reasons:

Muscular activity produces acid metabolites and elevated blood lactate and pyruvate levels

Starvation causes ketosis associated with acidosis

Respiratory rate is commonly increased during uterine contractions and hyperventilation may occur

Parity; in the primigravida the plasma bicarbonate is decreased and the plasma lactate is increased

Length of labor; a prolonged labor will increase lactate and pyruvate levels owing to the additional increase in muscular activity

Laboratory Values

Hemoconcentration is common during labor because of increased muscular activity and dehydration. The white blood count may be markedly elevated due to increased muscular activity during labor. The differential count remains within normal limits.

Second Stage of Labor

As the second stage of labor is reached, the uterine contractions occur every 1.5 to 2 minutes and last from 60 to 90 seconds. The intensity of the contractions is about the same as in the active phase of the first stage of labor until voluntary bearing-down efforts take place.

UTERINE SHAPE

The uterus changes shape and continues to become longer vertically while the transverse and anteroposterior diameters shorten.

SHOW

If no bloody show has been present prior to the second stage, it will now appear. If it has been present, the amount will increase and the color will be brighter owing to capillary rupture and separation of the fetal membranes from the decidua in the lower uterine segment.

UTERINE SUPPORTS

After complete cervical dilation, the uterine supports (cardinal ligaments, pubocervical fascia, and uterosacral ligaments) begin their role. The supports act as stout ropes against which the uterus works. If the supports were elastic in nature, a second stage uterine contraction, instead of advancing the fetus down the birth canal, would merely pull the cervix higher. When the second stage of labor is prolonged, injury and ecchymoses may occur within these ligaments.

BEARING-DOWN EFFORTS

Maternal voluntary bearing-down efforts are superimposed on the uterine contractions as the powers during stage two. Bearing-down efforts are the result of strong contractions of the diaphragm and the rectus, oblique, and transverse abdominal muscles. Each bearing-down effort causes a rise to 50 mm Hg intra-abdominal pressure that is added to the intrauterine pressure, raising the intrauterine pressure to 110 to 130 mm Hg.

Expulsive efforts are also reflexly elicited by vaginal and perineal dilation, as the presenting part descends during a uterine contraction.

Pelvic Molding

During the second stage, there is a 20 to 30 percent increase in the pelvic outlet area by a gradual increase in the maternal sagittal and transverse diameters. This increase occurs as a result of an increase in the bispinous diameter, an increase in the intersacroiliac distance, and posterior movement of the sacrum.

POSITIONING FOR DELIVERY

Left Lateral or Sims' Position

The left lateral position may be used when the gravida is delivering at home in bed. Advantages include:

- Patient comfort
- Avoidance of supine hypotension syndrome
- Avoidance of aspiration if vomiting occurs
- Bearing-down efforts are controlled
- Lowered incidence of perineal lacerations

Disadvantages of this position include:

- Difficult to handle emergencies that may arise
- Third stage of labor is awkward
- Perineal repair is very difficult

Dorsal Position

In the dorsal position the patient lies on her back on the bed or table with her knees flexed. Advantages of this position include:

- Patient comfort
- Accessibility to the perineum
- Bearing down is more effective

Disadvantages include:

- Supine hypotension is a possibility
- An uncooperative patient will make a controlled delivery difficult
- Decreases the normal intensity of uterine contractions

Lithotomy Position

In this position the patient lies on her back with her legs in stirrups and her buttocks close to the lower edge of the birthing bed or delivery table. Advantages of this position include:

- Easy access to the perineum
- The attendant can easily deal with any complications that may occur
- Easier perineal repair

Disadvantages include:

- May have adverse effect on maternal blood pressure, cardiac return, and pulmonary ventilation
- Decreases normal intensity of uterine contractions
- Inhibits the voluntary efforts to delivery spontaneously

May increase the need for forceps deliveries

Inhibits spontaneous expulsion of the placenta, which in turn increases the need for cord traction or manual removal of the placenta

Increases the need for episiotomy due to increased tension on the pelvic floor and stretching of the perineal tissue

Maternal discomfort

BIRTH OF THE NEWBORN

With each uterine contraction the presenting part descends farther, receding slightly as the uterus relaxes. The vaginal introitus becomes an anteroposterior slit, then an oval, and finally a circular opening. The pressure of the fetal head stretches the fibers of the levator ani muscles and thins out a central portion of the perineum from a wedge-shaped mass of tissue 5 cm in thickness to a thin, almost transparent membranous structure less than 1 cm in thickness. Feces may be forced out of the rectum at this time.

As the anus opens, the anterior wall of the rectum bulges through. With continued fetal descent, the occiput of the fetus comes to lie under the symphysis pubis. The head continues its advancement with each contraction, forcing the largest diameter of the head through the vulva (*crowning*). Once this has occurred, the head is born as the bregma, forehead, nose, mouth, and chin appear over the perineum.

The fetal head then falls back toward the anus, and restitutes as the neck untwists. After a few moments, external rotation takes place as the shoulders move from the oblique to the anteroposterior diameter of the pelvis.

Controlled Birth of the Head

A slow, gradual birth of the fetal head reduces the incidence of perineal lacerations. A sudden thrusting out of the fetal head should be avoided to prevent large and jagged lacerations. During the actual delivery of the head, a too-rapid emergence can be prevented by having the gravida pant through an open mouth during the uterine contractions. When the patient is panting, the diaphragm moves, making it impossible for effective intra-abdominal pressure to build and bearing down to occur.

Gentle manual pressure against the emerging fetal head may be employed to prevent too rapid expulsion. The head should never be held back forcibly.

Another method of slowing expulsion of the fetal head is use of the *Ritgen manuever*. Ideally performed between uterine contractions, it will encourage extension of the fetal head to expedite birth. The attendant's hand is covered with a towel and placed so that the fingers are behind the maternal anus. Extension of the head is aided by pressing against the face, preferably the chin, through the maternal rectum. The other hand is placed against the fetal head to control the speed of delivery.

Episiotomy

When perineal lacerations cannot be avoided, an episiotomy (incision into the perineum) may be done before delivery of the head. (See Chapter 16 for discussion of episiotomies.)

Following Delivery of Head

The fetal head is supported as it restitutes and rotates externally. The face is wiped and mucus aspirated from the mouth. The attendant feels around the neck to determine if loops of umbilical cord are present. If loops are present resting loosely around the neck, they can be slipped over the head. If the loops are coiled tightly around the neck, the cord must be double clamped, cut between the clamps, and then unwound.

Birth of the Body

By the time the shoulders are ready for delivery, restitution and external rotation of the head have taken place. The mother is asked to bear down during a uterine contraction. The head is grasped with the hands on the parietal bones and depressed toward the rectum. This enables the anterior shoulder to emerge under the symphysis pubis. The head is then raised so that the posterior shoulder can be delivered over the perineum. The lowering and raising of the head is achieved by merely lifting and lowering the head without exerting traction. Once the head and shoulders have been delivered, the rest of the body slips out easily, usually with a gush of amniotic fluid. (Care of the newborn immediately after birth is discussed in Chapter 16.)

MATERNAL PHYSIOLOGY

During the second stage of labor, the overall cardiac output increases approximately 40 percent. The pulse rate will remain within normal limits or may increase 20 BPM. The respiratory rate will remain within normal limits between contractions or it may increase less than 8 per minute. The temperature may be slightly elevated (1 to 2° F) owing to the increased metabolic rate at this time.

Immediately following delivery there is a sudden release of inferior vena cava obstruction. The uterine vascular channels decrease and the venous return to the heart increases.

Third Stage of Labor

After delivery, the intrauterine pressure increases dramatically, up to levels of 250 mm Hg. Uterine content is reduced by 7/8 with delivery.

Expulsion of the placenta occurs in two stages: (1) separation of the placenta from the wall of the uterus into the lower uterine segment or vagina; and (2) expulsion of the placenta through the vagina.

SEPARATION OF THE PLACENTA

Within a few minutes of delivery of the newborn, uterine contractions begin again. The extent of the retraction of the upper uterine segment is larger than during the first or second stages of labor. In order to accommodate itself to this reduced area, the placenta increases in thickness and folds on itself. This tension causes the weakest layer of the decidua to give way and separate from the uterine wall.

The membranes usually remain in place until the separation of the placenta is complete. They are then peeled off the uterine wall by myometrial contraction and traction exerted by the separated placenta. The body of the uterus at this time forms an almost solid mass of muscle, with the anterior and posterior walls lying close to each other. During the process of separation, blood accumulates between the placenta and the uterus. When the detachment is complete, the blood is released and gushes from the vagina (see Fig. 14–17).

EXPULSION OF THE PLACENTA

After placental separation, the placenta is expelled into the vagina by uterine contractions. It is then delivered by bearing-down efforts of the mother or by *gentle* traction on the umbilical cord, which is protruding from the vagina.

Mechanisms of Expulsion

Two mechanisms of placental expulsion have been identified. In the *Duncan mechanism*, the

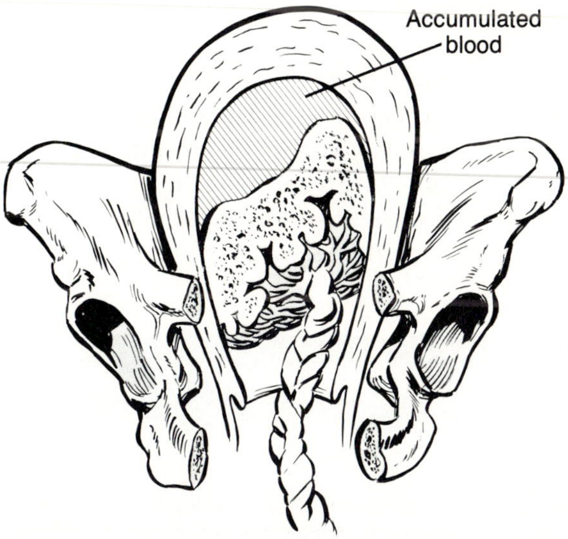

FIGURE 14–17. Placental separation.

lower edge of the placenta comes out first with the maternal and fetal surfaces appearing together at the introitus. The rough looking maternal edge comes first ("dirty Duncan"). In the *Schultze mechanism* the placenta expels like an inverted umbrella, with the shiny fetal side appearing first (shiny "Schultze"). The method of expulsion is of little practical importance.

The membranes are mechanically drawn off the uterine wall by the descending placenta. After placental expulsion, the membranes are expelled still adhering to each other.

EXAMINATION OF THE PLACENTA

The expelled placenta is examined to ascertain that no parts are missing. If torn blood vessels are seen along the placental edge, an accessory lobe may have been retained in the uterus.

Under normal circumstances, the uterus contracts firmly and remains well contracted after placental expulsion. The vessels and sinusoids of the uterus are closed, and bleeding from the placental site is controlled. Oxytocics are usually administered to maintain uterine contraction and control uterine bleeding (see Chapter 16).

Fourth Stage of Labor

UTERUS

During the fourth stage of labor, the uterus continues to relax and contract. The placental implantation site becomes an irregular, nodular, somewhat elevated region approximately the size of the palm of the hand with thrombosed vascular sinuses.

The uterus may be felt as a solid, firm mass that lies approximately 12 cm above the symphysis pubis at approximately the level of the umbilicus. Weight of the uterus during the fourth stage is approximately 1000 gm.

CERVIX, VAGINA, AND UTERINE LIGAMENTS

The cervix is soft and collapsed, and the cervical os slowly retracts with an opening of approximately 2 cm. The walls of the vagina are smooth. The broad and round ligaments that support the uterus intra-abdominally are relaxed, owing to the release of tension after evacuation of the uterine contents.

URINARY SYSTEM

The bladder is characterized by edema, hyperemia, sometimes extravasation of blood, and increased capacity. Diuresis begins during the fourth stage of labor.

MATERNAL PHYSIOLOGY

During the fourth stage of labor, physiologic stability is achieved. The pulse rate is decreased (puerperal bradycardia) owing to vagal nerve counterregulation in response to an increase in sympathetic activity. The circulating blood volume begins to increase. Leukocytes may increase and the erythrocyte sedimentation rate may rise to 50 mm during the first hour after delivery. The fibrinogen level remains elevated. Thrombocytes are increased.

By the end of the second hour after delivery, there is a cessation of pressure on the heart from the enlarged uterus and maternal vital signs are normal.

BIBLIOGRAPHY

Friedman, E. *Labor. Clinical evaluation and management* (2nd ed.). New York: Appleton-Century-Crofts, 1978.

Liggins, G.C. Initiation of spontaneous labor. *Clinical Obstetrics & Gynecology*, 1983, **26**, 51.

Roberts, J., Malasanos, L. & Mendez-Bauer, C. Maternal position in labor. Analysis in relation to comfort and efficiency. *Birth Defects, Original Article Series*, 1981, **17**, 97-128.

chapter 15

PSYCHOLOGICAL ASPECTS OF LABOR AND DELIVERY

OBJECTIVES

Upon completion of this chapter, the reader will be able to:

1. Discuss the role expectations of parents in relation to the labor process.
2. Identify emotional stresses of labor.
3. Differentiate between maturational and situational crises.
4. Discuss models of coping during labor.
5. Given a patient in labor, identify appropriate nursing interventions that can be used to facilitate labor.
6. Describe benefits to the patient when a support person is included in the labor process.
7. Discuss appropriate and nonappropriate coping behaviors and techniques used during labor.

KEY TERMS

Anxiety
Coping
Crisis
Maturational crisis
Sensory alteration
Sensory deprivation
Sensory overload
Situational crisis

Reactions of parents-to-be to the labor process vary greatly and are influenced by many factors. To provide effective care during labor, a basic understanding of the psychological aspects of the labor process is needed.

Nurses have a responsibility to help others give support to the patient during labor and delivery. Angry behaviors and hostile remarks from patients and support persons during labor may be an expression of fear and anxiety or a plea for help. Support persons may verbalize a desire to escape or may express anger and helplessness during labor. It is an important part of the nurse's role to help the patient and the support person cope effectively with labor.

STRESSES OF LABOR

Labor and delivery are experiences unlike any other. During the third trimester of pregnancy, the pregnant woman has ambivalent feelings about labor and delivery, since these pose a threat to her welfare and to the welfare of her baby. She also becomes aware of the possibility that the baby she carries may be defective in some way.

She is uncomfortable and awkward. During the first trimester she asks "Am I really pregnant?" In the second trimester she states, "I am pregnant." By the third trimester, physical and emotional changes give rise to the response "I am pregnant, and I'm tired of being pregnant. I don't think I want to be pregnant any more."

Maternal tasks include dealing with concerns about self and the baby. "Will my baby and I survive labor and delivery?" is a common thought as labor approaches.

Anxiety

All women experience fears and anxieties during labor and delivery. These two words—fear and anxiety—are sometimes referred to synonymously. In fact, these are different concepts.

In fear, the individual is afraid of some actual thing or event. Common fears include helplessness, the mystery of labor itself, death, old wives' tales, gossip of others, and lack of knowledge.

Fears predispose to various degrees of anxiety. In anxiety, the person is unaware of the source of apprehension. She knows she is afraid and this fear may be attached to something. She really doesn't know why she feels so apprehensive. As the level of anxiety increases, there is a corresponding decreased ability to understand what is happening and what is expected of her.

The degree of anxiety exhibited by a woman in labor depends upon many variables:

- Basic personality of the woman
- Attitude towards the pregnancy
- Perception of her mother's labors
- Childbirth preparation
- Amount of trust in the clinic, midwife, and doctor
- Effect of and response to medication
- Progress of labor

SELF-IMAGE IN LABOR

Labor may have a positive or a negative impact on the self-image of the patient. While childbirth is a meaningful event during the life cycle, culture and society may emphasize birth as a significant activity, or birth may be viewed as a negative stressful event. Maternal attitudes may be positive, with childbirth a logical step towards self-fulfillment, or negative with motherhood an undesirable goal.

Goals and expectations of the labor process also influence self-image. When there is an understanding of labor and goals are realistic, a positive self-image is maintained. Unrealistic perceptions and goals may lead to a negative self-image.

Feedback may be positive or negative. Maternal efforts to cope with labor and appreciation of support persons contribute to a positive self-image. When the nurse gives negative feedback, i.e., telling a patient that her behavior is inappropriate, or neglecting to offer full explanations at a level understood by the patient, a negative self-image is perpetuated.

SOURCES OF ANXIETY

Anxiety is not necessarily detrimental. When anxiety is mild or moderate, it makes a person more alert and responsive to stimuli. Anxiety enhances learning at mild or very moderate levels because hearing, seeing, and retaining of information is increased. Anxiety at severe or panic levels will immobilize the ability for problem solving.

To assess anxiety levels during labor, the nurse identifies potential or actual sources of anxiety. Upon arrival in the labor room, strange faces, sounds, and smells greet the patient. For many primigravidas, labor is their first exposure to hospitals with their overwhelming and intimidating rules and physical structures.

Labor beds and delivery tables are uncomfortable and the patient may not be able to find a comfortable position. Glaring lights, hospital routines such as perineal preps and enemas, and equipment such as fetal monitors may all increase levels of anxiety.

Loneliness and uncertainty, a perceived lack of support from nurses and significant others, conflicting advice from nursing staff, and upsetting environmental factors ("noisy" labor patients, hospital noises) also increase anxiety.

Labor may begin before the expected due date, adding to other anxieties the uncertainty of fetal outcome. Frustration and discouragement may be evident when the labor begins well after the due date.

Unexpected events can occur during labor. A primigravida may anticipate that regular uterine contractions will be present before the membranes rupture. When the membranes rupture prior to the onset of uterine contractions, she may become anxious. A multipara who expects the progress of labor to be like previous labors may become anxious if labor is longer than expected.

Other anxiety-producing stimuli during labor include vaginal examinations, discomfort from uterine contractions, and disruption of the individual's activities. Removal of clothing and personal belongings, enforced activity limitations, using the bedpan for urination and defecation, lack of privacy, and frequent interruptions for vital signs and other assessments all contribute to disruptions.

FEARS

There are three classic fears identified during labor: fear for self, fear for the baby, and fear of the unknown.

Fear for Self

Both women and their partners report fears of injury, mutilation, complications, unmet expectations, and death during labor.

Fear for the Baby

Fear for the unborn child is expressed in terms of abnormality, injury, complications, or death. Frequently, questions about fetal welfare are asked repeatedly during the process of labor.

Fear of the Unknown

The unfamiliar hospital environment, strange faces, sensory overload, isolation, and unpredictable behavioral responses all contribute to a fear of the unknown.

Sensory Alteration

Sensory alteration occurs in any situation in which there is an increase or decrease in sensory stimulation, and may be described in terms of sensory overload or sensory deprivation.

SENSORY OVERLOAD

Sensory overload occurs when there is an increase in the amount or intensity of sensory stimulation. Physiologic events during labor and delivery may increase sensory input. During the first stage of labor, uterine contractions, increased mucous or blood tinged vaginal discharge, rupture of the membranes, cervical dilation and effacement, and trauma of soft tissue can increase stimuli. In the second stage of labor, stimuli are increased by the urge to bear down, descent of the fetus, and uterine contraction intensity.

Preparations for delivery are often associated with increased sensory input. Vaginal examinations are more frequent, and transfer to the delivery or birthing room exposes the patient and her partner to another new environment.

Strange equipment and procedures may increase sensory input. Extra stimuli also occur from inappropriate staff conversations or rapidly progressing labor, and may interfere with the ability to assimilate and deal with stimuli.

SENSORY DEPRIVATION

Sensory deprivation is a decrease in the amount or intensity of sensory input. Restrictions imposed during labor on visitors, activities, food, intravenous fluid administration, and altered sleep patterns contribute to sensory deprivation.

Pain

Pain interpretation during labor and delivery is influenced by culture, past experiences with hospitalization and injuries, previous childbirth experiences, and educational preparation for labor.

The increased emphasis during labor on the feminine parts of the body in terms of exposure and manipulation will influence pain perception. Negative attitudes toward femininity and motherhood will also increase the perception of pain.

As labor progresses, perceived or actual threats to self and the fetus will intensify pain. A support person in addition to nursing staff can aid in modifying pain perception.

THE CRISIS OF LABOR

Crisis is characterized by increased anxiety and increased depression. Coping mechanisms previously employed are no longer adequate. As anxiety and depression increase, the patient becomes less and less able to solve problems.

Many situations hold a potential for crisis. Maturational crisis occurs as a normal accompaniment of growth and development and lasts for a length of time. A situational crisis occurs with a specific event that creates increased stress.

Labor and delivery can be both a maturational and a situational crisis. If the mother-to-be is a teenager, a combination of crises is present.

The crisis of labor and delivery is not necessarily detrimental. It may provide a turning point that has the potential to weaken or strengthen the family unit. Structural and psychological assets and liabilities all enter into resolution of this crisis.

Loss

Loss during labor is usually seen in one of three ways:

Loss of a valued object or person
Loss of expectations
Loss of a portion of self

Loss of the valued object or person most commonly refers to the threatened loss of the baby.

Loss of expectations occurs when the developed set of concepts and expectations about childbirth and the baby are not fulfilled. Most commonly, the intensity of the loss is associated with the length of time that the expectation has been held. Expectations about the sequence of events during labor and delivery may be unmet when labor progresses faster or slower than expected, or when the father is not allowed in the delivery room because of complications or his unavailability.

Loss of a portion of self usually refers to self-esteem, roles, ability to perform activities of daily living, and body image. Self-esteem loss during labor is most commonly noted with loss of control, negative feedback, and loss of expectations. Loss of role occurs with confinement during labor and lack of recognition of career and accomplishments other than pregnancy.

Body image loss is associated with the loss of the pregnant figure after delivery. For nine months, the figure has been gradually expanding. In the course of several hours, the expanded figure is gone, creating a change in body image.

Models of Coping During Labor

People provide themselves with mechanisms for coping with problems as they progress towards certain goals. Many methods of coping are possible.

In one model people take total responsibility for creating and solving their own problems. Home births with only the assistance of family and friends are examples of this model. If the home delivery is unsuccessful or requires assistance from health professionals, the parents may feel inadequate or incapable of solving their problems.

In another model, people are not blamed for their problems but are responsible for solutions. To solve problems, these individuals must be assertive and accept appropriate help from others. The assistance of childbirth education groups directs energy into creating a more positive environment for delivery.

A third model assumes that people neither create nor solve problems. People who are ill get well by seeking professional help. In labor, this model says, health professionals make decisions and dictate the progress and outcome of labor.

FATHER'S PARTICIPATION

The father fills a unique role during pregnancy, labor, delivery, and early puerperium. His presence aids in accomplishing maternal goals when he is actively involved in this developmental phase of the family.

Male roles are traditionally instrumental, whereas female roles are traditionally expressive. He is responsible for economic security and she is responsible for family nurturing and domestic activities. In our everchanging society, these traditional roles are gradually changing to a sharing or blending of both roles.

During labor, the father's role is ideally one of sharing the work. His involvement helps the mother to cope successfully with labor. Fathers are encouraged to attend childbirth preparation classes and become effective labor coaches. His involvement provides comfort and support during labor.

Benefits of his participation in labor and delivery accrue not only to the mother, but to himself. Bonding to the baby begins during pregnancy and continues throughout labor and delivery. Participation in labor and delivery can be ego-building and emotionally nourishing, helping him to take on the fatherhood role.

NURSING ROLE

Supportive nursing care during labor and delivery requires an understanding of both physiologic and psychological aspects of the labor and delivery process. Support is anything that will strengthen the ability of an individual to function capably and to his or her satisfaction. The supportive nurse displays not only the technical skills needed for labor and delivery, but also warmth, compassion, and empathy.

Assessment Data

To support the childbearing family effectively, accurate and specific nursing observations and assessments are needed.

INITIAL PATIENT ASSESSMENT

On admission, an initial patient assessment is undertaken by the nurse (see Table 16-1). In addition to the many physiologic parameters to be assessed, interviewing techniques are needed to obtain accurate data. The ideal time for interviewing is during the latent phase of labor. At this time, stresses are at a minimum and the patient is alert and responsive. Nonverbal communication signals, such as autonomic reactions to pain, stress, and muscle tension are also important areas for assessment.

LABOR EXPECTATIONS

Data about the couple's expectations of labor are obtained. Information about the amount and type of childbirth education will give clues to expectations. Specific requests should be identified; for example, the type of analgesia or anesthesia desired. Identification of patient expectations of staff is also helpful in planning care.

MEANING OF LABOR

Attitudes and values attributed to the labor process are also identified. Cultural views of labor are assessed. Conflicts between the couple's perceptions and the protocol of the hospital or birthing center need to be resolved or, at a minimum, identified at the onset of labor.

STRESS-INCREASING FACTORS

Factors that will increase stress are identified and assessed. Concerns, fears, and understanding of hospital policies are assessed, as are basic attitudes toward pregnancy and labor. An increase in psychological stress will increase the physical discomforts of labor.

DESIRED SUPPORT

The patient's support person during labor is identified. The level of support desired by both the patient and her coach is assessed to better formulate nursing diagnoses based on the patient's goals and desired or expected outcomes.

Creation of a Therapeutic Environment

A therapeutic environment that communicates a sense of trust and security is important to the labor patient. The patient and her coach should be addressed by name and the nurse should introduce herself by name and state that she is the patient's nurse.

Priorities must be identified through interviewing, observation, and listening. Eye contact while listening will help to pick up clues.

ANXIETIES AND FEARS

Anxieties and fears are identified and assessed. An expressed fear of labor may be vocalized by the patient as a specific need for the baby or an identified fear for herself. Statements such as "Is my baby all right?" "Do you think this will be another long labor?" or "My girlfriend hemorrhaged when she had her baby," all give clues to emotional tension and anxiety.

Behavioral signs of tension and anxiety may also be noted. The voice may be tremulous. The pupils may be dilated. The patient may seem on the verge of tears or may be crying. Inability to concentrate or comprehend what is said may be noted. Extreme shyness or fearfulness may exist. The presence of one or more of these signs indicates a degree of anxiety and tension.

Vital sign assessments also provide clues to anxiety. An elevation of blood pressure or pulse rate over the baseline prenatal parameters can indicate anxiety.

After identification of the cause of anxiety or stress, the nurse can help to decrease or eliminate stressors. If the anxiety is from lack of knowledge, teaching at an appropriate level is instituted. A brief but thorough orientation to the unit, that includes the physical layout and operation of nurse call lights, will often decrease anxiety. Policies and procedures that will be implemented or used during labor are explained.

Anxiety related to the patient's ability to maintain control during labor should be identified and appropriate interventions planned and implemented. When childbirth education classes have been completed, reinforcement of information already learned may be all that is needed. If no childbirth classes were taken, simple coping techniques can be introduced and reinforced as labor progresses.

Conscious relaxation techniques will aid in coping. Relaxation helps to promote normal labor progress. Touch and verbal instructions can help the client to relax, as can involvement of the labor coach. Signs of increased tension such as clenched fists can be pointed out so the support person can identify them and aid in promotion of conscious relaxation.

Use of a focal point to maintain relaxation is often helpful. The focus can be a picture or object, or it can be internal, e.g., heartbeat. As labor progresses, the client can focus on the nurse or support person to follow breathing patterns.

Deep chest breathing helps the client during labor. The breath is taken slowly and deeply as in normal breathing. Slow deep breathing can help to maintain relaxation and it can be used as a focal point throughout a uterine contraction.

A controlled, slow panting type of mouth breathing pattern will help when deep chest breathing is no longer effective. The patient is instructed to take light quiet breaths through the mouth at a rate of approximately 30 per minute. The main problem with this shallow chest breathing is the increased possibility of hyperventilation. The nurse and labor coach need to be aware of the depth, rate, and pattern of breathing.

A therapeutic environment is maintained when the same nurse cares for the patient throughout labor and delivery. As labor progresses, the nurse can aid the client simply by "being there." The nurse should position herself so that her presence can be felt and some eye contact can be maintained.

Assess and Meet Informational Needs

On admission to the labor or birthing room, the knowledge of the client and her partner about the normal physiologic progress of labor and the expected sequence of events is assessed. Misconceptions can be corrected and teaching of needed information can be initiated.

Teaching is difficult during labor. As labor progresses, the client's attention span narrows and less information can be integrated for effective learning. Repetition and reinforcement of previous teaching is needed as labor progresses.

LATENT PHASE

The latent phase of labor is a good time to assess informational needs and to teach. Anxiety is usually mild and the patient is receptive to learning. Physiology of labor, expected body sensations, and self-help measures can all be taught during this phase.

ACTIVE PHASE

The active phase of labor is accompanied by increases in stress and anxiety. Teaching new information is very difficult. Previous teaching can be reinforced by the use of short sentences or phrases to increase retention.

TRANSITION PHASE

Transition narrows the perceptual field and further decreases learning capabilities. Short phrases are used and the focus of teaching is on the present—information needed to complete this phase.

Promotion of Relaxation

The cycle of fear–tension–pain can be interrupted or broken by education, purposeful activity, and supportive care. As this cycle is broken, the components are replaced and instead a cycle of confidence–controlled relaxation–decreased perception of pain is created.

Relaxation during labor can be increased through use of conscious relaxation techniques, hygiene, a decrease in the effects of immobility, a decrease in environmental stimuli, and positive reinforcement.

Conscious relaxation methods enable the client to obtain maximum benefits from intervals between uterine contractions. A discussion of methods of relaxation taught in childbirth preparation classes is in Chapter 12.

Nursing actions designed to promote hygiene during labor will aid in promoting relaxation. Keeping linens dry will decrease irritation and friction on the skin. Perineal cleansing will decrease discomfort and the incidence of ascending infection. Sponge baths and oral hygiene will help to increase patient comfort and relaxation.

Decreasing the effects of immobility include correct anatomic positioning and changing maternal positions at frequent intervals. Ambulation for short periods (if allowed) will help to maintain circulation. Back rubs will stimulate circulation and decrease muscle fatigue from decreased levels of activity.

There are many ways to decrease environmental stimuli, including control of glaring lights and decreasing extraneous noises and traffic. Organization of nursing care will avoid unnecessary interruptions. As much privacy as possible should be provided. Avoidance of unnecessary conversation will aid in decreasing stimuli.

Positive reinforcement can be used by the nurse and support person to minimize discouragement and frustration as labor progresses.

Provision of Comfort

Support during labor and delivery serves as a way of providing help and assistance in a situation that is difficult to handle alone. To be most effective, support is provided by the nurse in conjunction with a partner or labor coach. The partner or labor coach may be the husband, another relative, or a friend. A support system during labor will reduce pain perception and the amount of analgesia or anesthesia received.

SUPPORT BY THE NURSE

The nurse provides support by developing a helping relationship. This relationship has two major components: understanding and caring.

Understanding Relationship

An understanding relationship during labor can be achieved and maintained in many ways. The use of therapeutic touch through hand holding, back rubs, and stroking the brow communicates understanding of the dependency needs of the client. It also serves to establish rapport and enhances communication between the nurse and the client. A few of the appropriate indications for therapeutic touch are anxiety, fear, pain, and joy.

Recognizing clues indicative of stress and anxiety also contribute to the understanding relationship. Clues may be verbal or nonverbal, obvious or subtle. Stressful stimuli should be decreased to keep anxiety and stress at acceptable levels. If he is not present, ask the client for the name of her support person, who should be included in care of the client and kept informed of the progress of labor.

Verbal encouragement as labor progresses is also part of the relationship between nurse and client. Positive reinforcement, encouragement that coping behaviors are appropriate, and alteration of inappropriate behaviors are all methods used to develop and maintain an understanding relationship.

Caring Relationship

A caring relationship is established by addressing the client by name and orienting her to the unit and policies and procedures necessary to her care during the labor process.

Physical needs should be met upon request and without specific request. A cool cloth to the forehead and a change of linen for comfort are only two ways this can be done.

The patient and her partner must be kept informed of labor progress. This will help to decrease anxiety, discouragement, and frustration, and at the same time reinforce appropriate relaxation techniques and breathing patterns.

The client should be allowed and encouraged to participate in decisions that affect her care whenever possible. Follow-through with commitments is important. When you tell the patient that you will return in 15 minutes, return in 15 minutes.

SUPPORT OF THE PARTNER

The role of the nurse doesn't end with her support of the client in labor. A responsibility also exists to help other persons give support to the client.

The level of participation desired by the support person is assessed on admission. These wishes are respected as much as possible. Breathing and relaxation techniques are reinforced as needed when prior childbirth education has taken place. If the patient and support person have no educational preparation for labor, appropriate measures are taught and demonstrated.

The nurse provides encouragement for the support person while respecting privacy and monitoring the client's progress. If the support person is properly encouraged when appropriate, self-esteem will rise and efficiency as a labor coach will result.

Clues to increasing anxiety and stress level of the support person are assessed as labor progresses. An increasing anxiety level may be noted by hostile comments to nursing staff or unrealistic demands or commands to the patient. Reinforcement of previous teaching and positive reinforcement of appropriate actions may be all that is required.

Promotion of Initial Infant Bonding

The neonate begins bonding with parents immediately after birth when in the alert state. The nurse can facilitate parent-infant bonding in the delivery room or in the birthing room. The parents are encouraged and allowed to see, touch, and listen to the neonate. A non-judgmental approach by the nurse is essential. Comments by the nurse such as "Here is your cute little boy," may inhibit spontaneous initial impressions of the neonate by the parents.

Immediately after the initial neonatal assessment is completed, the newborn is given to the mother to hold. She is encouraged to explore her newborn by touch and sight as she desires. When the father has been an active participant during labor and delivery, neonatal interactions are perceived as more positive by the mother. Initial maternal-infant interactions and paternal-infant interactions usually follow an orderly progression that includes touch and eye contact.

The parents are allowed to progress with bonding at the pace they desire. The neonate is not pushed on the parents; the parents indicate the amount of interaction desired.

Integration of the Labor Experience

For individual growth to proceed, resolutions of situations and crisis must take place. Pregnancy is a crisis that culminates in the birth of the neonate. It needs to be resolved before the next stage, parenthood, can be entered.

Feelings about labor and delivery need to be verbalized. A woman will define her performance during labor in terms of her own experiences and the responses of others to her.

Accurate knowledge about the process of labor and delivery prior to the onset of labor is usually associated with positive feelings about labor. The ability to maintain control during the labor process is associated with positive feelings, as is a positive relationship with a support person, most commonly, the husband.

The patient is encouraged to verbalize feelings and perceptions about the labor experience and to ask questions. Feedback from the nurse will emphasize positive behavior, progress, and so on. A nonjudgmental attitude is needed by the nurse to aid in the process of integration.

Accurate recognition and assessment of coping behaviors and coping mechanisms during the four stages of labor will aid the nurse to plan and provide appropriate interventions during each of the stages. A summary of usual behaviors during labor with suggested nursing responsibilities is given in Table 15–1.

TABLE 15-1
SUMMARY OF LABOR BEHAVIORS

Behaviors	Suggested Nursing Interventions
FIRST STAGE OF LABOR: LATENT PHASE	
Exhibits high energy and activity level	Listen
Happy with admission	Good time for assessment of expectations, attitudes, past experiences with hospitalizations
Relief that pregnancy will soon be over	Assess what she has been told or heard
Smiling, talking, laughing	Create a positive atmosphere
Comfortable	Eye contact important
Spontaneous expression of feelings	Excellent time for teaching
Focus on others besides self	Involve patient in care
Asks questions	Involve her in decision making
Mild anxiety	Do not ask her questions during contraction
Alert: sees, hears, retains information well	Assess relaxation and breathing techniques
Anxiety enhances learning	
Pain tolerance high	
Exerts efforts to gain approval	
FIRST STAGE OF LABOR: ACTIVE PHASE	
Serious, determined	Take measures to promote relaxation
May be weary	Organize care to minimize disturbance to patient
Upset when routines involve restrictions	Assess and meet dependency needs
Less talking	Facial sponges, dry linen, back rubs, straighten sheets
Dependency needs noted	Use short sentences, phrases
Breathing labored	Increase contact time with patient
Preoccupied with self	Provide pain relief measures
Increased discomfort	Meet requests and demands courteously
Increased diaphoresis	Do not make demands on patient
Restless	Allow behaviors
Anxiety moderate to severe	Positive reinforcement
Perceptual field reduced	
Decreased attention span	
Increased focus on "now"	
Difficulty in retaining new information	
Isolation	
Less pain tolerance	
Increased attention to pain	
Less concentration on coping	
Makes frequent demands for praise from others	
Tremors during contractions	
FIRST STAGE OF LABOR: TRANSITION PHASE	
Focus on self only	Do less talking and explaining to patient
Exhausted, wants to give up	Do not expect patient to respond to you as before
Increased sensations in perineum	Stay with patient as much as possible
Shaking, chills, nausea	Make no demands
Restless	Positive reinforcement
Details may be blown out of proportion	Support
Difficult to get attention	Encouragement
Decreased ability to make decisions	Keep informed of labor progress
Increased stimuli for sensory overload	
May have amnesia between contractions	

TABLE 15-1 (continued)

Behaviors	Suggested Nursing Interventions
SECOND STAGE OF LABOR	
Fatigue Desire to defecate Exhausted Cannot guard self against injury Amnesic episodes Decreased ability to cooperate with labor process May lose coping abilities Aggressive behaviors	Praise efforts in breathing or pushing Keep informed of progress Encourage rest between uterine contractions Accept behaviors Safety measures to decrease chance of injury Remain with patient Decrease anxiety levels
THIRD AND FOURTH STAGES OF LABOR	
Focus on others Sense of relief Excitement Dozing, sleeping, talking Anxiety decreased Alert Frequent questions Apologizes for behaviors Focus on neonate Focus on family	Encourage and allow contact with infant—sight, touch Breast feed if desired Answer questions Encourage verbalization Give feedback about labor as desired or requested

BIBLIOGRAPHY

Anderson, S.V. Siblings at birth, A survey and a study. *Birth and Family Journal*, 1979, **6**, 80-88.

Arakelian, M. An assessment and nursing application of the concept of locus of control. *Advances in Nursing Science*, 1980, **3**, 25-42.

Bloom, K.C. Assisting the unprepared woman during labor. *Journal of Obstetric, Gynecological, & Neonatal Nursing*, 1984, **13**, 303-307.

Butani, P. & Hodnett, E. Mother's perceptions of their labor experiences. *MCN*, 1980, **9**, 73-82.

Campbell, A. & Worthington, E.L., Jr. Teaching expectant fathers how to be better childbirth coaches. *MCN*, 1982, **7**, 28-32.

Cogan, R. Effects of childbirth preparation. *Clinical Obstetrics and Gynecology*, 1980, **23**, 1-4.

Cronewett, L. & Brickman, P. Models of helping and coping in childbirth. *Nursing Research*, 1983, **32**, 84-88.

Fishbein, E.G. Expectant father's stress—due to the mother's expectations? *Journal of Obstetric, Gynecological, & Neonatal Nursing*, 1984, **13**, 325-331.

Gabel, H. Childbirth experiences of unprepared fathers. *Journal of Nurse Midwifery*, 1982, **27**, 5-8.

Grossman, F., Eichler, L. & Winickoff, S. *Pregnancy, birth and parenthood*. San Francisco: Josset-Bass, 1980.

Heggenhougen, H.K. Father and childbirth: An anthropological perspective. *Journal of Nurse Midwifery*, 1980, **6**, 21-26.

Klaus, M. & Kennell, J. *Parent-infant bonding* (2nd ed.). St. Louis: Mosby, 1982.

MacLaughlin, S. & Taubenheim, A.: A comparison of prepared and unprepared first-time fathers' needs during the childbirth experience. *Journal of Nurse Midwifery*, 1983, **28**, 9-16.

Mercer, R.T., Hackley, K.C. & Bostrom, A.G. Relationship of psychosocial and perinatal variables to perception of childbirth. *Nursing Research*, 1983, **32**, 202-207.

O'Connell, M.L. Locus of control specific to pregnancy. *Journal of Obstetric, Gynecological & Neonatal Nursing*, 1983, **12**, 334.

Philips, C.R. & Anzalone, J.T. *Fathering: Participation in birth* (2nd ed.). St. Louis: Mosby, 1982.

Roberts, F.B. Infant behavior and the transition to parenthood. *Nursing Research*, 1983, **32**, 213.

Stephany, T. Supporting the mother of a patient in labor. *Journal of Obstetric, Gynecological & Neonatal Nursing*, 1983, **12**, 345-356.

Weaver, R.H. & Cranley, M.C. An exploration of paternal-fetal attachment behavior. *Nursing Research*, 1983, **32**, 68-72.

chapter 16

NURSING MANAGEMENT DURING THE LABOR PROCESS

OBJECTIVES

Upon completion of the chapter, the reader will be able to:

1. State the factors involved in the initial assessment of the patient.
2. List information that can be obtained from the prenatal record.
3. State specific information that can be derived from physical assessment of the gravida.
4. Discuss behaviors, anxiety, and pain levels and appropriate nursing interventions during the phases of the first stage of labor.
5. Identify ways in which the nurse can support labor coaches.
6. For each stage of labor, discuss appropriate nursing assessments and interventions.
7. Given a specific oxytoxic drug, state the action, route of administration, usual dosage, side effects, contraindications, and nursing actions.
8. Describe indirect and direct methods of fetal heart rate and uterine contraction monitoring: state advantages and disadvantages of each.
9. Define the following: baseline fetal heart rate, variability, tachycardia, bradycardia, early deceleration, late deceleration, variable deceleration, sinusoidal fetal heart rate pattern; identify the significance of each; indicate appropriate nursing interventions.
10. Identify relationships between medications given to the mother and fetal heart rate patterns.
11. Describe fetal blood sampling.
12. Identify appropriate nursing interventions when fetal monitoring is used during labor.
13. State fetal monitoring information that should be documented on the fetal monitoring strip and on the patient's chart.
14. Discuss patient reactions to fetal monitoring
15. State three forces that must be overcome to initiate breathing in the neonate.
16. Describe Apgar scoring.
17. Identify nursing responsibilities if the Apgar score is 7–10; 4–6; 1–3.
18. Discuss neonatal resuscitation.
19. Identify priorities of neonatal care immediately after delivery; discuss appropriate nursing interventions.
20. Discuss initial infant bonding.
21. State four signs that placental separation has occurred.

KEY TERMS

Accelerations
Acme
Apgar score
Baseline changes
Baseline FHR
Decelerations
Decrement
Direct FHR monitoring
Duration
Early deceleration
Episiotomy
External uterine activity
Fern test
Fetal blood sampling
Fetal bradycardia
Fetal tachycardia
Frequency
Increment
Indirect FHR monitoring
Intensity
Internal uterine contraction monitoring
Late deceleration
Metabolic thermogenesis
Nitrazine paper
Perineal lacerations
Periodic changes
Sinusoidal FHR pattern
Supine hypotension
Variability
Variable deceleration

When a gravida arrives in the labor and delivery suite in active labor, the nurse is in a unique position. The nursing care given during the labor and delivery process requires skill and knowledge. With individualized nursing interventions, the culmination of nine months of waiting for the miracle of birth can be a positive and satisfying experience for the parents. By setting nursing goals and objectives and then using the nursing process to meet these goals, the nurse can aid in the experience of labor. Knowledge of the normal labor and delivery process and of deviations from the normal is necessary to plan effective interventions. Cultural and psychological understanding is essential to nursing interventions during labor. An environment that communicates warmth, security, and trust must be established and maintained. The education and informational needs of the parents are evaluated and perceptions of danger of the unknown are minimized. Therapeutic listening is a vital component of care.

INITIAL ASSESSMENT

The initial assessment of the gravida is completed on admission. The initial assessment should include greeting the patient, review of the prenatal record, patient assessment information, obtaining baseline physiologic parameters, assessing labor expectations, and assessing psychological, social, and cultural factors.

Initial Greeting of the Patient

The initial greeting that the patient receives upon arrival to the labor area is very important. She may arrive accompanied by the father of the baby or other support persons. All persons should be made to feel welcome. Visiting regulations in hospitals will vary; in some hospitals only the father may visit during labor and delivery while other hospitals allow several support persons. The gravida and the support person are shown to the labor room. An unhurried and unrushed approach when greeting them avoids intensifying normal anxiety.

Review of the Prenatal Record

Prenatal records are sent from the physician's office or prenatal clinic prior to the patient's due date (see Chapter 9). The format will vary but certain information will be noted on the record. These data should be reviewed before the initial assessment is completed.

Patient Assessment Information

The initial patient assessment is completed by the nurse (see Table 16–1). Information must be obtained quickly yet in an unhurried manner. The patient whose labor is well advanced will have only a short time in which to provide

TABLE 16-1
LABOR AND DELIVERY INITIAL PATIENT ASSESSMENT

Date: ________ Time: ________
Husband's Name: ________________
Maiden Name: ________________
Mode of Admission: Ambulatory: ______ Wheelchair: ______ Cart: ______
Type & Rh: ______ Age: ______ Religion: ______
Gravida: ______ Para: ______ Abo: ______ LMP: ______ EDC: ______
Height: ______ Weight: ______
Rubella titer: ______ Needed: ______
Allergies: ________________________________
____
Allergy Band: ______ Identaband: ______
Reason for Admission: Labor: ______ Induction: ______ Bleeding: ______
Other: ________________________
Pertinent Medical Conditions: ________________________
____
____
Medications Currently Taking: ________________________
Brought In: ______ Sent Home With: ____________
Emotional State: Calm: _____ Anxious: _____ Fearful: _____ Angry: _____
Depressed: _____
Physical Assessment Results: ________________________
____
____
____
Prosthesis: ____________
Valuables: ______ Sent Home With: ______ To Vault: ______
Retained: ______
Childbirth Preparation Classes: ________________________
Support Person In Delivery: ____________ Birthing Room: ____________
Visitor: ____________
Anesthesia Desired: ____________
Pediatrician: ____________ Breast: ______ Bottle: ______
Informant: ____________
Prep: Abdominal: ___ Perineal: ___ Partial: ___ None: ___
Done by: ____________
Urine Specimen: Voided: ___ Catheterized: ___
To Lab: ___ Discarded: ___ Not Obtained: ___
pH: ___ Protein: ___ Sugar: ___ Ketone: ___
Other: ________________________
Enema: SS: ___ Fleets: ___ Hold: ___
Membrane Status: Intact: ___
Ruptured: ___ Date: ___ Time: ___ Color: ___
Ate or Drank Last: ____________
Temp: ___ Pulse: ___ Resp.: ___ B/P: ___ FHT: ___
Fetal Monitoring: ____________
RE/VE @ : ______ By: ______
Dilatation: ___ Station: ___ PP: ___ Effacement: ___
Doctor/Attendant: ______ Notified At: ______
Lab Work Ordered: ________________
R.N. Signature: ________________

pertinent data with which to plan effective nursing interventions. The majority of patients arrive at the hospital in time for a thorough assessment.

NAME AND AGE

Ask the gravida to spell her name and state her age. Ask who her support person or persons are.

EXPECTED DATE OF CONFINEMENT

Ask her the date of her last normal menstrual period (LNMP) and her expected date of confinement (EDC) or due date. Has she had any testing to verify the EDC? This information will help alert staff to the possibility of a preterm or postterm birth.

PRENATAL CARE

If no prenatal record exists or if it is not available, ask her about prenatal care. When did she first go to the doctor or clinic? How often did she go? When was her last prenatal visit? At times patients will arrive at the hospital for delivery without any prior prenatal care. If she has been seen at the office or clinic more frequently than the average patient, she may have a medical or obstetrical problem relevant to her labor care. Were any special tests done during pregnancy?

PAST PREGNANCIES

Review the prenatal record. Information about past pregnancies and their outcome can be validated or supplemented as needed.

RELIGION

Ask her religion or religious affiliation.

HEIGHT AND WEIGHT

Ask her how tall she is and assess her weight. How much weight did she gain during this pregnancy? Was her weight gain within the normal range? Did she notice any swelling of the hands and feet during this pregnancy?

ALLERGIES

Does she have any allergies? What reactions does she have to the specific allergens? Is she currently taking any allergy medication? Has she been taking it throughout this pregnancy?

PAST MEDICAL AND SURGICAL HISTORY

Ask her about any previous surgeries or current medical problems. Medical problems of special significance during labor include diabetes mellitus, heart disease, anemia, tuberculosis, hypertension, kidney disease, and venereal disease (see Chapters 25 and 26 for specific discussions of pertinent medical problems).

Family history needs investigation owing to the congenital nature of many diseases.

If she has any past or present medical problems, is she taking any medication? What is the name of the medication and what dosage does she take? For what length of time has she been taking this medication? Did she bring the medication with her?

EMOTIONAL STATUS

Is she calm, apprehensive, fearful, or angry? What is the emotional status of her support person? If she is not emotionally calm, determine the reason for the deviation. Is she fearful because of a knowledge deficit? Is she fearful because of problems with previous pregnancies? Information obtained will need to be incorporated into her plan of care.

Determine the attitudes, values, and feelings toward this pregnancy. Was this pregnancy planned? Is this pregnancy emotionally acceptable to her?

PROSTHESES

Determine if she wears glasses or contact lenses, has dentures, capped teeth or loose teeth. Does she wear a wig or a hairpiece? Does she have a glass eye or other artificial prosthesis?

VALUABLES

Did she bring anything of value to the hospital? If she did, be sure to note and record the disposition of such valuables. Were they sent home? With whom? Were they locked up in the hospital vault? Did she retain them?

CURRENT LABOR STATUS

Contractions

When did her contractions start? About how far apart were the contractions at that time? What quality did the contractions have? Ask her to describe the contractions. What is the current status of uterine contractions? Are they getting progressively closer and harder or are they remaining the same frequency, duration, and intensity?

Show

Does she have a bloody show? When did it start? What amount of bloody show is present? If she says it is a large amount, ask her to describe the amount to you. If she cannot do that, ask her the number of perineal pads she has worn in a specific time frame and the amount of bleeding on each pad.

Rupture of the Membranes

Did her "bag of waters" break? If so, when? What was the amount? What color was the fluid? Was there a foul odor to the fluid? If the fluid has a foul odor, intrauterine infection may be present. If the fluid is yellow-stained, a blood incompatibility between the mother and the fetus may be present owing to fetal red blood cell breakdown by bilirubin. The fluid may be green-stained owing to passage of meconium by a stressed fetus. Heavy meconium passage in early labor is associated with intrapartum and neonatal hypoxia. Passage of meconium in the amniotic fluid occurs normally in breech presentations.

If there is a question of whether the membranes have ruptured, two simple tests can determine the presence of amniotic fluid: Nitrazine paper and the fern test.

Nitrazine Paper. To test for the presence of amniotic fluid with Nitrazine paper, insert a sterile, cotton-tipped applicator into the vagina and then touch it to a strip of Nitrazine paper. The strip of wet paper is then compared with a chart that accompanies the paper. If amniotic fluid is present, the chart will show an alkaline reaction of 6.5 pH or higher and will turn the paper a dark blue color. A bloody show may also give a false-positive reading, since blood is alkaline in nature.

Fern Test. The fern test can assess the presence of amniotic fluid. A drop of vaginal fluid is obtained using a vaginal speculum and a sterile, cotton-tipped applicator. The fluid obtained is spread on a clean slide and allowed to dry. If there is no blood in the specimen and no gross infection, the dried slide will show a frondlike (fernlike) pattern when viewed under a microscope.

OTHER

Ask when she ate or drank last to determine the risk factors for aspiration in the event an anesthetic is needed during labor or delivery.

If the hospital allows fathers in the delivery room or birthing rooms, determine the patient's preference and eligibility for such a program.

Ask her if she is breast or bottlefeeding her newborn, and the name of the newborn's pediatrician.

Determine whether she and her partner have attended childbirth education classes and, if so, which ones. These classes have somewhat different philosophies and give the patients slightly different expectations of the labor and delivery process.

What type of analgesia or anesthesia have

the client and her doctor discussed for this labor and delivery?

PHYSIOLOGIC PARAMETERS

Various physiologic parameters must be obtained during the initial patient assessment.

Vital Signs

Temperature, pulse, respirations, and blood pressure are measured, and the fetal heart rate (FHR) is auscultated to obtain baseline parameters. These are compared with the prenatal vital signs. Temperature may be elevated owing to maternal dehydration, maternal infection, or environmental factors (extremely hot day outside, very warm room temperature). The pulse, respirations, and blood pressure may be elevated owing to anxiety, excitement, fear, or the presence of uterine contractions. She may be hypertensive or have pregnancy-induced hypertension. Vital signs are assessed in the intervals between uterine contractions.

Physical Examination

A brief but thorough head-to-toe assessment is undertaken by the nurse during the initial assessment. Physical assessment begins with observation of the patient's overall appearance. Is she pale? Flushed? Does she appear ill? Does she appear frightened? Is dehydration or edema present? Are there any obvious open lesions?

Look at the conjunctiva of the eyes. Are they pale? Paleness may indicate anemia. Assess the mucous membranes of the mouth. If anemia is present, they are pale. What is the general condition of the teeth? Are they loose or in need of repair? Does she wear dentures or retainers? Does she wear braces? Are there symptoms of upper respiratory infection? Are the lips cracked? Are there lesions present on the lips?

Are the lungs clear to auscultation? Are heart sounds and rhythm normal? Check the color of the nailbeds and assess capillary refill.

Leopold's manuevers are used at this time to determine fetal size and presentation (see Chapter 13). Palpate the bladder area to detect a full bladder.

Inspect the lower extremities for varicose veins and edema. If varicosities are present, the gravida is more prone to develop a phlebitis during the postpartum period. If edema is present, note its location and the degree of edema present.

Vaginal or Rectal Examination

Vaginal or rectal examinations can help to determine the progress of labor. They may be contraindicated in certain circumstances, such as unexplained bright vaginal bleeding and extreme fetal immaturity.

It was previously felt that only rectal examinations should be done by the nurse during labor to avoid possible introduction of bacteria into the lower reproductive tract. Over the years, this view has changed. Many studies have shown little difference in infection rates when comparing patients having vaginal or rectal examinations.

To perform a rectal examination, a clean examining glove and lubricant is needed. Explain the procedure and provide privacy. Use your index finger and tuck your thumb under your remaining fingers. The index finger should be well-lubricated with a water-soluble jelly and then introduced gently into the rectum while the patient takes a deep breath. By sliding your finger along the rectal wall, the cervix can be felt as a circular ridge with a depression in the center. Determine the cervical dilation, effacement, fetal presenting part, and station. After the examination, discard the glove. Wipe the client from front to back and cover her with the top sheet.

Rectal examinations have several distinct disadvantages. They are less accurate than vaginal examinations. The condition and dilatation of the cervix is often difficult to determine, especially if the bag of waters has not ruptured. The station may be difficult to determine owing to inability to palpate the ischial spines. During a rectal examination, the posterior vaginal wall is pushed against the cervical opening, increasing the chance of vaginal bacteria entering the cervical canal. The rectal examination is painful to the patient and aggravates existing hemorrhoids.

Vaginal examinations are considered preferable. They are more accurate and cause less discomfort to the client. Deviations from the normal are more easily identified. There is no documented increase in infection rates.

To perform a vaginal examination, the client should be positioned on her back with her knees flexed. The procedure is explained and privacy is provided. After washing the hands, a sterile examination glove is put on. A lubricating solution is used on the fingertips. Place the ungloved hand on the outer vulva and spread the labia majora so the external genitalia can be inspected for lesions. The index and middle fingers are introduced gently into the vagina, directing the fingers backwards and upwards. The cervix is touched with the fingers. Cervical dilation is determined by comparing the cervical opening with a centimeter scale. On the average, an index finger measures 1 cm, and the middle finger measures 1.5 cm in diameter. If both fingers can fit into the cervical opening, the cervix is dilated 2 to 3 cm. Other dilations are determined by estimating the width of the cervical opening. If no cervix can be palpated, the dilation is 10 cm, or complete.

Determine the consistency of the cervix. Is it hard or soft? Estimate the degree of cervical effacement. Before effacement occurs, the cervix is approximately 2 cm thick. It is easier to estimate the percentage of effacement if you know what points on your examining finger are 1 and 2 cm. When the cervix is very thin, it is difficult to accurately assess dilatation, because it is difficult to tell if fetal scalp is felt or a very thin cervix is palpated.

What is the fetal presenting part? Is it cephalic, breech, or a shoulder? Is there caput succedaneum present and is it small or extensive? What is the relationship of the presenting part to an imaginary line between the ischial spines? Is the presenting part above or below the ischial spines? How many centimeters above or below the ischial spines is the presenting part?

If the presenting part is breech, where is the sacrum? Are the legs flexed or extended? If the presenting part is cephalic, identify the sagittal suture. What is its direction? Is it in the anteroposterior, oblique, or transverse diameter of the maternal pelvis? Is the bregma right or left? Is it anterior or posterior? Where is the posterior fontanel? Is the head in flexion or extension?

Are the membranes ruptured? If not, are they bulging through the cervix? If the membranes are ruptured, what color is the fluid? How much fluid is there? Does it have a foul odor?

Is a bloody show present? If so, note the color and amount.

How does the presenting part fit into the pelvis? Is there engagement or does the presenting part rebound when touched with the finger? Does the presenting part ride over the symphysis pubis?

Following a vaginal examination, withdraw the examining fingers. Wipe the perineum from front to back and replace the top sheet. Tell the client and support person the progress of dilation. They are usually anxious to have positive progress reported.

Laboratory Tests

On admission a urine specimen is obtained and blood is drawn for admission laboratory tests. A clean catch urine specimen is tested for the presence of protein, blood, glucose, and ketones, as well as for specific gravity. Admission blood tests vary from hospital to hospital. The usual tests ordered include a hemoglobin and hematocrit determination. Any prenatal blood work that has not been done or needs to be repeated is drawn with the admission laboratory tests.

Perineal Preparation

The area to be prepped varies from no shaving at all to completely shaving the vulvar and perineal area. The physician's orders are checked for the amount of shaving ordered. Gather the equipment and explain the procedure to the client. A protective pad is placed under the client's buttocks and she is draped for privacy. The area to be shaved is lathered. The skin is held taut while shaving to prevent pulling and a long, smooth stroke is used with the razor. Be sure to direct razor strokes downward toward the rectum. When shaving is completed, the perineum is thoroughly washed.

Enema Administration

An admission enema may or may not be given. The reasons for administering an enema in early labor include preventing feces from impeding descent of the presenting part, stimulating uterine contractions, and preventing contamination of the sterile field during delivery.

During initial assessment of the patient, the nurse will ascertain the patient's bowel status. If she is constipated, an enema can be helpful. If she has diarrhea, an enema is not needed and may increase the chances of infection. An enema is not to be given if labor is well advanced, there is active unexplained bleeding, or a preterm birth is suspected. A presenting part that is not engaged is also a relative contraindication to enema administration.

If an enema is ordered for the labor patient, several points are relevant in administration. It may be more difficult to insert the tip of the enema tube into the rectum because of pressure on the rectum from the presenting part. The enema solution is to be given slowly, between uterine contractions. The presence of hemorrhoids may make the procedure more uncomfortable for the patient. Results are noted by the nurse and documented on the chart.

NURSING INTERVENTIONS: FIRST STAGE OF LABOR

Ongoing Physiologic Assessments

After the initial patient assessment is completed, specific physiologic parameters are assessed on an ongoing basis during the first stage of labor (see Table 16–2). These include maternal vital signs, uterine contractions, progress of cervical dilatation and effacement,

TABLE 16–2
NURSING INTERVENTIONS: FIRST STAGE OF LABOR

Intervention	Admission	Latent Phase	Active Phase
ASSESS AND DOCUMENT:			
Temperature	Yes	q 4 hours (q 2 hours if membranes ruptured or temperature elevated)	q 4 hours (q 2 hours if membranes ruptured or temperature elevated)
Pulse	Yes	q hour	q hour
Respirations	Yes	q hour	q hour
B/P	Yes	q hour (unless abnormal)	q hour (unless abnormal)
Urination	Yes	q 3–4 hours	q 3–4 hours
FHT	Yes	continuously with fetal monitor or q 30 minutes	continuously with fetal monitor or q 15 minutes
VE/RE	Yes unless contraindicated	q 1–2 hours or PRN	q hour or PRN
Contractions	Yes	continuously with fetal monitor or q 30 minutes	continuously with fetal monitor or q 15–30 minutes

descent of the fetus through the maternal pelvis, and fetal heart rate and patterns. A sample nursing care plan for the first stage of labor is found in Table 16–3.

Cultural, Social and Psychological Assessment

The nurse needs an awareness of cultural norms and expectations to plan pertinent nursing interventions during labor (see Chapter 2).

Social relationships play an important role in labor. Different members of the hospital and medical staff will come in contact with the prospective parents during labor. The variance and diversity of personnel can be frightening and overwhelming to the client and her partner. The nurse needs to assess and possibly limit the number of hospital personnel to which the woman is exposed. Family members and other support persons play an important role in maternal perceptions and anticipations of labor. Labor is fatiguing and extra people providing sensory input may interfere with coping ability. Usually it is recommended that the number of family members and others be limited during labor. The gravida can then devote her attention, concentration, and energy to the process at hand, that of labor. The nurse can assess the family situation to aid in determining the number of persons that should be allowed into the labor area.

Assessment of the psychological status of the parents is important. Most parents-to-be arrive at the hospital excited, and quite possibly anxious. A few minutes taken to explain policies and procedures will aid in decreasing this natural anxiety.

The expectations of the labor process are assessed. Have the parents attended any type of childbirth preparation classes? If so, what kind? What expectations do they have for labor? What relaxation techniques are they prepared to use? Nursing interventions will vary according to the type of preparatory class the parents have attended. Some parents have had no preparation for labor and delivery and have no idea of what to expect or what is expected of them. A careful assessment of the education and expectations of the parents will aid in appropriate planning.

Maternal Vital Signs

Vital signs are assessed frequently during labor to ensure that maternal physiologic status remains stable.

TEMPERATURE

Temperature is taken on admission and every four hours during labor. A temperature over 99° F (37.2° C) is reported to the physician and is taken more frequently. An elevated temperature may indicate dehydration or an infection.

PULSE AND RESPIRATORY RATE

Maternal pulse and respirations are taken every hour during active labor. The pulse rate in labor will usually remain within normal range. An elevated pulse may indicate anxiety, nervousness, or dehydration, or it may be sign of developing complications. Respirations counted between contractions should remain within normal limits.

BLOOD PRESSURE

The blood pressure is assessed and recorded every hour during active labor. Readings are obtained between uterine contractions since during a uterine contraction, the systolic blood pressure may rise as much as 20 mm Hg. Elevated blood pressure may be caused by anxiety, chronic hypertension, or pregnancy-induced hypertension (PIH). Hypotension may be due to supine hypotension syndrome or hemorrhage. Supine hypotension is characterized by dizziness, faintness, pallor, tachycardia, diaphoresis, and nausea. The B/P will

TABLE 16–3
SAMPLE NURSING CARE PLAN: FIRST STAGE OF LABOR

Sylvia B., a 27-year-old white married gravida 4 para 2 abo 1, is admitted to labor room 3 at 1:35 a.m. on 12/28. The prenatal record was reviewed and the Labor and Delivery Initial Patient Assessment was completed (see Table 16–1). Spontaneous rupture of membranes at 10 p.m., moderate amount clear fluid.

Data Base:

EDC 1/5
Usual childhood diseases
Blood type O positive
2 previous vaginal deliveries at term, no intrapartal, postpartal, or neonatal complications
Baptist
Height 5′5″ Weight 159 lb (weight gain 24 lb during this pregnancy)
Rubella titer 1:80
Other prenatal blood work within normal limits
No known allergies
No pertinent medical conditions, on no medications except prenatal vitamins
Physical assessment within normal limits
Wears glasses
Vital signs: Temperature 97.9°F
Pulse 76
Respirations: 20
B/P: 112/76
FHT: 144 BPM

Vaginal examination at 1:35 a.m. reveals: Cervix 3 cm dilation, 90% effaced, presenting part cephalic at 0 station
Contractions: Onset at 11:15 p.m. 12/27 15–20 minutes apart
Now 10 minutes apart, lasting 35–40 seconds, moderate intensity
Support person: husband, Paul
Admission urine obtained: pH 7.0, blood-neg, protein-neg, glucose-neg, ketone-neg
Admission laboratory work done: CBC, PTT, Prothrombin time, Type & Screen—all within normal limits
Requesting standby anesthesia only with local for episiotomy (if needed)
Partial perineal prep completed per standing orders Dr. P
Soda phosphate enema given with good results per standing orders Dr. P.
Dr. P. notified of admission and status

Nursing Diagnosis	Goals	Nursing Interventions	Rationale	Evaluation
Knowledge deficit related to labor and delivery process	The patient and her support person will be prepared for labor and delivery	Assess knowledge level of patient and support person Allow opportunity for questions Identify learning needs and use this time for teaching and/or reviewing	Explanations of and/or reinforcement of labor and delivery process are individualized	Sylvia and Paul attended childbirth preparation classes with all 3 pregnancies Policies, procedures, breathing techniques reviewed with them

Potential ineffective breathing patterns related to a lack of knowledge and anxiety Potential alteration in tissue perfusion related to hyperventilation	The patient will remain as physically and psychologically comfortable as possible throughout labor	Assess preferred breathing techniques on admission Avoid hyperventilation Assess use of techniques frequently during labor process	Knowledge of preferred breathing techniques will aid the nurse in reinforcing these during labor	Sylvia and Paul knowledgeable in appropriate breathing techniques Able to maintain techniques throughout labor with minimal reinforcement No hyperventilation noted
		If fetal monitor is used, can aid in coordinating breathing techniques		
		Be physically present at bedside as much as possible	Fear can inhibit labor progress	
		Accept coping behaviors Reassure of progress—keep informed of labor progress	As labor progresses and more discomfort is present, it becomes more difficult to maintain control. The nurse and/or support person will provide support and encouragement	Kept informed of labor progress
Alteration in comfort related to uterine contractions and cervical dilatation	The patient will remain as comfortable as possible during labor	Decrease sensory overload Keep perineum clean and dry Wipe perineum from front to back Keep linens clean and dry		Room lights dimmed Sylvia kept clean and dry
		Offer backrubs and other comfort measures		Paul utilized lumbosacral support for backache
		As transition approaches, offer more encouragement to maintain breathing patterns until complete cervical dilatation Encourage to rest between contractions	Transition is the most difficult to maintain breathing	

TABLE 16-3 (continued)

Nursing Diagnosis	Goals	Nursing Interventions	Rationale	Evaluation
Potential for injury to related to analgesic medication administration Potential alteration in tissue perfusion of fetus related to analgesic medication administration		Analgesic medications: Assess patient wishes in regard to possible administration during initial assessment Determine physician preference and orders for medication, dosage, route, and time of administration Be knowledgeable about fetal and maternal effects of specific medication	Analgesia given at inappropriate times can prolong labor or cause respiratory depression in the neonate	No analgesic medication requested or needed during labor
		Administer at the proper time Do VE, take vital signs, FHT prior to and 30 minutes after administration Decrease environmental stimuli to allow for rest Side rails up	When analgesics are given at appropriate time (4–5 cm), may enhance labor progress	
Potential activity intolerance related to decreased activity during labor	The client will understand and adjust to activity limitations	Encourage ambulation early in labor Encourage to change position frequently Assist client to comfortable position if restricted to bed Avoid backlying position Provide pillows for comfort	Avoidance of flat backlying position will decrease the incidence of supine hypotension Upright positions will allow gravity to aid in fetal descent. Sidelying position allows for improved fetal oxygenation	Sylvia preferred sidelying position during labor
Potential alteration in tissue perfusion of mother and fetus related to abnormal maternal vital signs	A stable maternal/fetal physiologic unit will be maintained throughout labor	Monitor vital signs throughout labor: Temperature q4 hr Pulse q hr Respirations q hr B/P q hr Assess more frequently if needed Assess between uterine contractions	Alterations in maternal vital signs indicate potential complications	Temperature 97.6° to 98°F Pulse ranged from 68 to 84 BPM Respirations ranged from 16 to 24/min B/P ranged from 110/74 to 124/80

Potential for maternal or fetal injury related to abnormal presentations, abnormal positions, or alterations in normal process of cervical dilation or fetal descent		Vaginal/rectal examinations done on admission and as needed to determine labor progress Do before and after analgesic medication After ROM Maintain aseptic technique	Abnormal fetal presentations or positions can hinder labor progress Abnormalities in labor progress are identified	VE on admission: 3 cm cervical dilatation, 90% effaced, PP 4:38 am: VE 4–5 cm at 0 station 6:17 am: VE 5–6 cm at 0 station 7:20 am: VE 7–8 cm at +1 station 7:30 am: VE 9–10 cm at +2 station 7:55 am: VE complete at +2 station
Ineffective coping related to discomfort of labor		Inform patient/support person of labor progress	Keeping patient/support person informed helps to decrease anxiety and aids in maintaining or changing breathing techniques	Kept informed of progress No problems coping with discomfort
Potential alterations in tissue perfusion of mother and fetus related to hypertonic UC patterns		Monitor uterine contractions for: Frequency Duration Intensity UC that deviate from normal are reported to physician: Evaluation interval: q 30 minutes in active labor q 5–15 minutes in transition	Hypertonic uterine contraction patterns increase incidence of fetal distress Hypotonic uterine contraction patterns prolong labor and exhaust mother Normal UC are fundal dominant. Become more frequent, of longer duration, and more intense as labor progresses	On admission, UC were q 10 minutes, lasting 35–40 seconds, of moderate intensity. 4:30 am: UC q 8 min, moderate intensity 6:30 am: UC q 3–4 minutes, 50 seconds, stronger 7:00 am: UC q 2–3 minutes, 60 seconds, intense 7:45 am: UC q 2 min, 60–70 seconds, intense
		Evaluate show: Amount Type	Excessive show may indicate marginal placenta previa. Sudden increase in show may indicate rapid labor progress	Small amount bloody show on admission—amount and color remain unchanged throughout labor
Potential alteration in fetal tissue perfusion related to uteroplacental insufficiency, cord compression, or maternal hypotension		Assess fetal heart rate Intermittent auscultation: Take for one full minute before, during, and after UC	Normal FHR 120–160 BPM Alterations in rate and rhythm are signs of changes in fetal oxygenation	FHR 144 on admission Evaluated at 30 min intervals. No alterations in rate or rhythm noted

TABLE 16–3 (continued)

Nursing Diagnosis	Goals	Nursing Interventions	Rationale	Evaluation
		Note deviations from normal Assess and document q 15–30 minutes in active labor Following ROM Following interventions With change in UC pattern Fetal monitoring: If used, see Table 16–15		
		Assess amniotic fluid: Time of rupture Amount Color Odor Consistency	Normally amniotic fluid is essentially clear. Any discoloration should be documented and reported to the physician	Amniotic fluid clear on admission—no change during labor
Potential electrolyte imbalance related to inadequate fluid intake Potential alteration in nutrition related to limited intake during active labor		Assess need for food and fluids: Amount of oral intake determined by MD orders If oral intake allowed, clear liquids If NPO, IV fluids usually ordered Strict intake and output	Fluid and electrolyte balance needs to be maintained during labor Digestion stops when labor begins	Ice chips given in small amounts until 4:30 am IV of 1000 ml D5LR started at 4:30 am 8 hr intake: 100 ml oral 1000 ml IV
Alteration in pattern of urinary elimination related to labor progress		Encourage to void at least q 3 hours Assess bladder for distention May need to catheterize	A full bladder will increase patient discomfort and may hinder labor progress	Up to bathroom X2 550 ml clear yellow urine Catheterization not needed
Coping, family: Potential for growth	The support person will participate in the labor process according to his expectations	Determine the level of participation in the labor process desired by the patient and support person Answer any questions	The support person is important in the care of the labor patient	Paul had attended Childbirth Preparation Class and planned on being in the delivery room
		Keep informed of labor progress Explain procedures Support the coach's role Offer coffee, tea, etc Relieve at intervals to allow a break if desired	Keeping the support person informed of labor progress will aid in maintaining breathing and relaxation techniques	He coached Sylvia well; offered appropriate support; praised her breathing techniques

TABLE 16-4
NURSING INTERVENTIONS: SUPINE HYPOTENSION SYNDROME

Turn the gravida to her side (preferably the left side)
If no relief of symptoms is obtained after the position is changed, then:
  Elevate her legs
  Increase her intravenous rate (if present)
  Start oxygen at 6-8 L/min per face mask
Document all vital signs and patient response

drop rapidly and the gravida appears shocky. Appropriate nursing interventions are summarized in Table 16-4. Maternal B/P is taken before and after administration of any analgesic or anesthetic agent and after oxytocin administration.

Uterine Contractions

The word "pain" is often used as a synonym for uterine contractions. When "pain" is used to denote contractions, a negative connotation is given to a positive labor process. The word pain is associated with hurting and feelings of an uncomfortable nature. With the increase in childbirth education and childbirth preparation classes, an effort has been made to instill a more positive view of uterine contractions.

Uterine contractions often become uncomfortable as labor progresses. The nurse has a responsibility to help the client distinguish between the anticipation of discomfort and actual discomfort. If this distinction is made, she can cope with labor more effectively. The management of pain during labor is discussed in Chapter 17.

Uterine contractions create a stress situation for both the mother and the fetus. The cycle of fear-tension-pain must be broken to minimize client discomfort. If this cycle cannot be broken, the perception of discomfort is greatly increased. The client will react to even minimal stimulation with exaggerated discomfort. Vaginal examinations will cause severe discomfort. The nurses fingers or hand on the maternal abdomen will "hurt."

CHARACTERISTICS OF UTERINE CONTRACTIONS

Uterine contractions are assessed for frequency, duration, and intensity (see Fig. 16-1). During uterine contractions the maternal arterial pressure will rise, owing to the increase in peripheral resistance. Oxygenation of maternal, placental, and fetal cells is impaired during uterine contractions.

The *frequency* of uterine contractions is timed from the beginning of one contraction to the beginning of the next contraction.

The *duration* of the contraction is from the onset of uterine tightening until the uterus is completely relaxed.

The *intensity* of the contraction may be described as weak, moderate, or strong when assessed by manual palpation. During a weak contraction, the nurse's fingers will easily indent into the maternal abdomen and uterus. With a moderate contraction, the fingers will only slightly indent the abdomen or the uterus. The fingers will not indent the abdomen or the uterus during a strong contraction. Intensity is impossible to interpret without being at bedside.

To accurately assess uterine contractions manually, the fingers of one hand are lightly placed on the fundus of the maternal uterus. Points to be remembered when assessing uterine contractions include:

- Contractions begin in the uterine fundus.
- The fingertips are placed gently on the uterine fundus.
- The contraction will be felt as a tightening that will increase (increment), peak (acme), and decrease (decrement).
- Contractions that are abnormal in pattern are reported to the physician to prevent deleterious effects for the mother and the fetus (see Chapter 26).

During uterine contractions the client will need encouragement and support from her coach or the nurse in using and maintaining her breathing and relaxation techniques.

Uterine contractions are evaluated every 30 minutes from the onset of active labor until

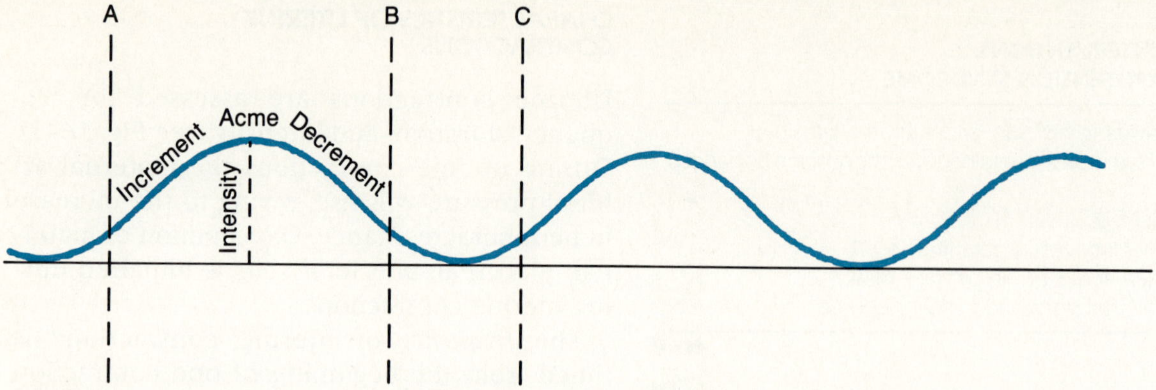

FIGURE 16-1. Characteristics of uterine contractions. A to C = frequency. A to B = duration.

the cervix had dilated to approximately 5 cm, then every 15 to 30 minutes from 6 cm to until complete dilatation of the cervix.

Show

As labor progresses and the cervix dilates and effaces, a blood-tinged secretion called show, caused by superficial capillary rupture in the cervix, may be noted. If the amount of show increases, it may indicate rapid labor progression. A perineal pad should not be worn to evaluate the amount of show during labor because of the increased risk of infection. A protective pad under the buttocks will absorb the vaginal discharge and is easily changed to keep the mother clean and dry. The amount and type of show present is noted and documented.

Fetal Heart Rate

Assessment and on-going evaluation of the fetal heart rate (FHR) during labor is a prime nursing responsibility. Intermittent auscultation of the FHR may be done with a DeLee-Hillis fetoscope, a Leff stethoscope, or a doppler unit (see Fig. 16-2). The fetal heart tones are best transmitted through the fetal back or chest, as explained in Chapter 13. They are usually located in the lower quadrants of the maternal abdomen, but they are sometimes located in the upper quadrants if the fetal presenting part is not engaged or if the presentation is breech or a shoulder.

The FHR is to be auscultated and counted for 1 full minute. The maternal pulse is checked to differentiate between her pulse and the FHR. Maternal pulse and the FHR are to be checked before, during, and after a uterine contraction to note any alterations in rate or rhythm. Deviations from the normal rate of 120 to 160 BPM are noted and reported.

Intermittent auscultation of the FHR is documented every 15 to 30 minutes during the first stage of labor and every 5 minutes during the second stage. The FHR is checked immediately in the following instances:

- Following rupture of the membranes, whether spontaneously or by amniotomy
- After any interventions such as enemas or medication administration
- Following any change in the uterine contraction pattern
- With any indication of labor complications

There are advantages and disadvantages to intermittent auscultation of the FHR. Errors in counting are easily made, especially during a uterine contraction when the uterine muscle is tense. A large portion of the continuous FHR is not heard as the uterus contracts, and early signs of fetal distress may not be iden-

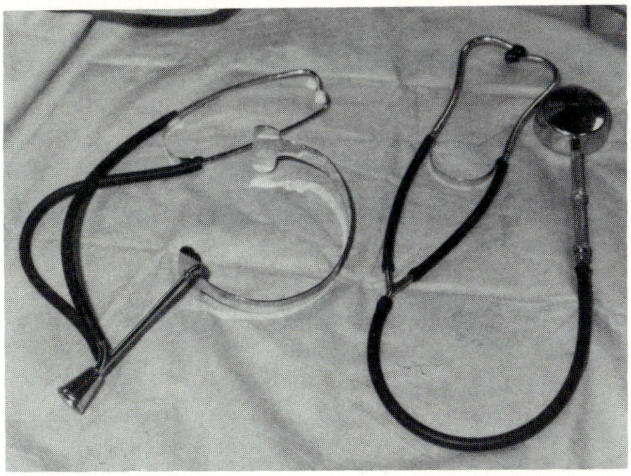

FIGURE 16-2. DeLee-Hillis fetoscope (left) and Leff stethoscope (right).

tified. No permanent record of the FHR (continuous) is obtained for legal documentation.

Electronic fetal monitors using external or internal methods, or both, to record the FHR continuously are often employed during labor and are discussed later in this chapter.

Vaginal or Rectal Examinations

Vaginal or rectal examinations are performed to determine the progress of labor as necessary. An examination should be performed before and approximately 30 minutes after the administration of analgesic medication and when the membranes rupture, in addition to every one to two hours.

Amniotic Fluid Evaluation

The "bag of waters" may rupture before labor begins or at any time during labor. Artificial rupture of the membranes (amniotomy) may be performed by the physician to initiate or stimulate uterine contractions. If an amniotomy is to be performed, prepare the client by explaining the procedure and expected results (see Chapter 26).

Normally, amniotic fluid is clear in color. A foul odor to the amniotic fluid may indicate infection. Amniotic fluid that is green or greenish-brown indicates that meconium has been passed by the fetus in utero. A hypoxic episode in utero will cause the fetus to increase peristalsis, relax the anal sphincter, and pass meconium. A yellowish staining of the amniotic fluid can indicate a hypoxic episode to the fetus that occurred 36 or more hours prior to the rupture of the membranes or an Rh incompatibility. A port wine stain to the fluid indicates the presence of abruptio placentae, uterine rupture, or cervical bleeding. If the fluid is thick in consistency, intrauterine infection may be present.

Nursing interventions appropriate to amniotic fluid evaluation include the following:

Note the time of rupture, whether spontaneous or by amniotomy

Observe the amount, color, odor, and consistency of the fluid

Assess the FHR

Maintain bedrest until the presenting part is well engaged

Do a vaginal examination to rule out prolapsed cord

Record the time of the observations

Assess uterine contractions for an increase in frequency, duration, and intensity

Keep the patient as clean and dry as possible

Prevention of Infection

Nursing interventions to help protect the mother and fetus from infection during labor include:

Maintain aseptic technique when doing vaginal examinations

Keep the perineal area clean and dry—remember to wipe the perineal area from front to back

Screen visitors for infections

Enforce hospital policies with regard to dress codes and hand washing

Enforce infection control policies specific to the hospital relating to good handwashing techniques, clothing, care of instruments, and cleaning of labor and delivery rooms

Positioning During Labor

A gravida may be ambulatory or sitting in a chair during the early portion of labor if the fetal presenting part is engaged, no active bleeding is present, and there are no maternal complications. Various studies (Caldeyro-Barcia, 1979; Carr, 1980) have concluded that women who were ambulatory during early labor had shorter labors than those who were recumbent throughout labor. The use of electronic fetal monitoring equipment does not necessarily confine the mother to bed. She must stay close to the monitor but may ambulate or sit.

If the patient prefers or is required to be in bed early in labor, she is encouraged to lie on her side (see Fig. 16–3), thereby causing the uterus to fall away from the vena cava and allowing free blood return from the lower extremities. She is often more comfortable overall when lying on her side and the respiratory, urinary, and cardiovascular systems benefit. There is less danger of aspiration of gastric contents. Bedrest is maintained following administration of a barbiturate, analgesic medication, or anesthetic agent.

The upright position is prefered by some women during labor. This position may facilitate the descent of the presenting part through the maternal pelvis. It has been documented that labors are shorter with the mother in an upright position (Caldeyro-Barcia, 1979).

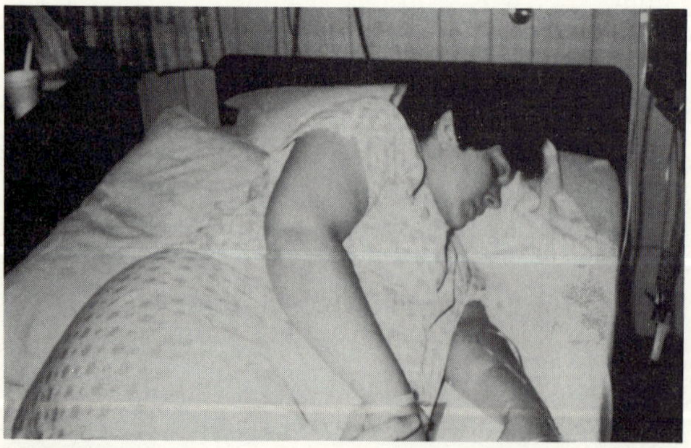

FIGURE 16–3. Side lying position during labor.

Protect From Aspiration

During labor, almost all gastrointestinal functions stop. Food that is in the stomach will not continue to digest. The incidence of vomiting during labor is relatively high. A side-lying position helps to facilitate drainage if the gravida should vomit. Oral intake is normally limited or restricted during active labor.

Food and Fluids

The amount of food and fluids allowed during labor varies greatly according to physician preference. The patient is usually restricted to clear liquids in early labor with no solid foods allowed because of cessation of digestion. Other physicians prefer nothing by mouth (NPO) for their patients in labor. If the patient is NPO, intravenous fluids may be started to maintain adequate fluid and caloric intake, and to prevent dehydration and exhaustion.

Elimination

During active labor the patient may feel either a decreased or increased need to urinate. Voiding should be encouraged at least every three to four hours. A full bladder during labor intensifies the discomfort associated with uterine contractions, impedes labor by hindering the descent of the fetus, and predisposes to maternal urinary stasis and urinary tract infections during the postpartum period.

If the bladder can be palpated above the symphysis pubis and the mother is unable to void, she may need to be catheterized. Several points are important when catheterizing the patient in active labor:

Strict asepsis is necessary
Explain the procedure
Provide privacy
Uterine contractions will make it more difficult for the patient to cooperate
Vaginal discharge may make it more difficult to maintain strict aseptic technique
The catheter is inserted between uterine contractions
The catheter is inserted farther into the urethra (it must go around the fetal presenting part) before urine will flow

Breathing Techniques

During the initial patient assessment, information is obtained about the type of childbirth preparation classes the parents have attended. All of these classes teach useful breathing techniques that are employed during labor (see Chapter 12). An awareness of the various breathing techniques will help in supporting the parents during labor.

One aspect of breathing techniques will be of particular concern to the nurse is that of possible hyperventilation. Hyperventilation increases the rate and depth of respirations and causes an excess of carbon dioxide. If the pattern is not corrected, respiratory alkalosis may develop and the gravida will complain of feeling dizzy, faint, or have tingling of the extremities, especially the fingers. The nurse can intervene by having the patient hold her breath or breathe into a paper bag. Observe the pattern of breathing with the next few contractions. If necessary, recoach the patient in the proper breathing techniques.

Analgesia

In order not to impede labor progress, analgesic medication is not routinely administered to the client until cervical dilatation has reached 3 or 4 cm. If analgesic medication is given at the appropriate time, it may actually serve to increase the intensity of uterine contractions and shorten labor. When analgesics are given too early, they may decrease the intensity, duration, and frequency of uterine contractions and prolong the labor process (see Chapter 17).

The nurse must know the medications that are ordered by the physician. She needs to be aware of the drug actions, maternal and fetal effects, side effects, and contraindications. The bladder should be emptied prior to administration, so rest will not be interrupted. Vital signs, including FHR, must be documented before the medication is administered and 30 minutes after administration. A vaginal examination to determine labor progress is done before and 30 minutes after administration. Bedrest is maintained, and environmental stimuli are decreased to allow maximum medication effect. Side rails should be raised, even though her coach is at the bedside. Explain the rationale for this to the patient and her coach. If labor has progressed rapidly, so that delivery is imminent or expected within the next two hours, the analgesic medication should be withheld to prevent possible respiratory depression in the neonate.

Other Discomforts

In addition to the discomfort of uterine contractions and cervical dilatation, many gravidas experience discomfort from leg cramps, back pain, and rectal pressure.

LEG CRAMPS

Leg cramps during labor may be caused by poor anatomic positioning and poor relaxation. The legs are never rubbed to relieve the cramps. Relief may be obtained by elevating and extending the leg, keeping the leg straight (pressure may be needed on the knee to keep the leg straight), and forcibly pushing the upper half of the foot toward the knee if the client is in bed. If the client is able to get up, stepping on the foot and walking about may help to relieve the cramp.

BACKACHE

Low backache, especially over the lumbosacral region, is common during labor. It may occur with each contraction or be present constantly. In some women, backache is a greater source of discomfort than the actual uterine contractions. Nursing interventions include massage of the lower back with the palm of the hand, application of pressure to the lumbosacral area with the hand, application of pressure to the lumbosacral area with a pillow, avoid backlying positions, and heat application to the lower back.

RECTAL PRESSURE

Rectal pressure from a well-engaged presenting part is a source of discomfort. Nursing interventions include explanation of the cause and assessing for labor progress.

Safety Measures

It is important to provide safety measures for the mother and the fetus. When the mother is in bed, the siderails should be raised. If she is allowed out of bed, a footstool and a supporting hand are needed when getting up. Indirect lighting will allow the mother to rest and still allow accurate assessments and observations by the nurse. Labor rooms and hallways should be uncluttered to avoid the possibility of falls.

Maternal Reactions to Phases of Labor

Maternal reactions to the phases of the first stage of labor are influenced by many factors, including the nursing staff providing care. Beginning at the time of admission to the labor unit, an atmosphere of trust must be created. Informational needs of the client and her partner are assessed and met.

The client brings to the labor experience her attitudes, values, and feelings toward this pregnancy, her cultural and social makeup, and her previous experiences with hospitalization. These all contribute to her behavioral responses to labor.

Time spent at the bedside should be unhurried. When you leave the bedside, tell the parents when you will return (and return promptly as promised) and how to use the nurse call system to reach you. A genuine interest will do much to promote trust and alleviate anxiety.

Certain behaviors are evidenced by women in the various phases of labor. Assessment of these behaviors not only as clues to appropriate interventions during the various phases, but also as clues to labor progress is important.

EARLY LATENT PHASE

The latent phase of the first stage of labor begins with the onset of true labor and ends at 4 cm cervical dilation. The client is excited and relieved that she is finally in labor. She smiles, is talkative, and may play cards or watch television (see Fig. 16–4). She is interested in her environment and will often inquire about other patients who may be in labor. She easily expresses attitudes and feelings about pregnancy, the fetus, her partner,

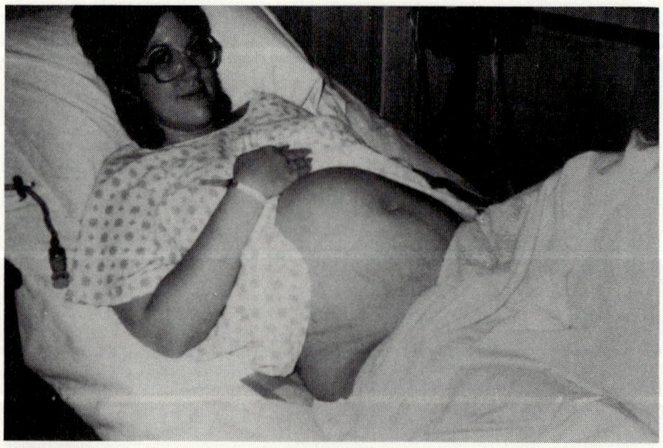

FIGURE 16–4. Patient behavior during the latent phase of labor.

and her family. The discomforts of uterine contractions and cervical dilation are tolerated, and distraction with measures such as a soft voice, touch, and light conversation are useful.

Nursing Responsibilities

The latent phase of labor is normally an excellent time for teaching. The patient can retain information. Anxiety factors need to be carefully assessed and dealt with in an appropriate manner. Breathing techniques can be taught to the patient if no childbirth preparation classes were attended. If the patient has gone to classes, breathing techniques can be reviewed.

LATE LATENT PHASE

Toward the end of the latent phase the patient needs more energy to cope with work of labor. She may appear flushed, and respirations are deeper. Nausea and vomiting are common. She may complain of a dry mouth and diaphoresis can be present. The force of uterine contractions is greater and she may verbalize feelings of helplessness during contractions. The need for support may be expressed, and support with breathing techniques is important.

Nursing Responsibilities

Teaching is still appropriate, but must be accomplished within the patient's narrowed attention span. The purpose of the more intense uterine contractions is emphasized and the client is reassured about labor progress. Analgesic medication may be administered if ordered. Support and reassurance needs to be given to the labor coach.

ACTIVE PHASE

The client becomes serious and determined, as she focuses her energy on coping with uterine contractions. She may appear tired and talk less, only verbalizing about necessities for her comfort and labor. She may be restless and verbal with her expressions of discomfort. Respirations become labored and hyperventilation is common. Routines that involve restrictions such as using the bedpan instead of getting up to use the bathroom, and limitations of oral fluids may upset her. Difficulty in concentration on breathing techniques is common. She has difficulty in retaining new information and in concentrating. Perception of discomfort is increased owing to uterine contractions, descent of the presenting part, cervical dilation, pressure, fatigue, increased anxiety, and verbalized or nonverbalized fears.

Nursing Responsibilities

Physical presence and touch are important. Explanations are brief and dependency needs are anticipated. Positive reinforcement is given frequently.

TRANSITION PHASE

The transition phase of labor is the most difficult for the client and for her labor coach. Pelvic and rectal pressure is increased and leg cramps may be present. Behavior will change with drowsiness noted between uterine contractions, along with increasing irritability. Diaphoresis, shaking, chills, nausea, and vomiting may become apparent or will become more marked. It may be difficult to get her attention owing to the short attention span at this time.

Nursing Responsibilities

A calm organized approach and avoidance of unnecessary chatter will help to decrease sensory overload. Positive reinforcement after each contraction and acceptance of individual coping behaviors is important. The client should not be left alone.

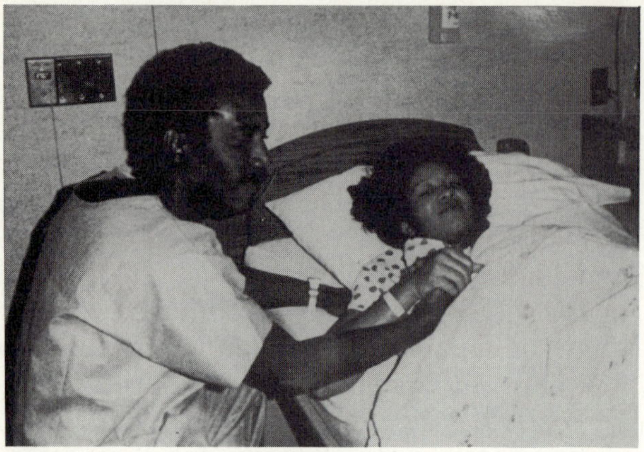

FIGURE 16-5. Gravida and husband during the active phase of labor.

SUMMARY OF SUPPORT PERSON ROLE

With much of the nursing focus on the client during the different phases of labor, the father or support person should not be forgotten. Coaching is encouraged (see Fig. 16-5). The nurse can act as a resource about labor progression, so correct breathing techniques can be instituted. Putting a comfortable chair by the bedside, offering coffee or other fluids, or offering a warm blanket will aid in keeping him comfortable.

FETAL MONITORING

Mortality from 20 weeks gestation through the first four weeks of life (the neonatal period) is roughly equivalent to the number of deaths in the next four decades of life. A large percentage of this mortality is concentrated in the last week of gestation and the first week after birth.

Labor is a fetal stress test, in which the fetus may be handicapped by maternal medical problems, analgesia, anesthesia, or maternal hypotension or hypertension. Each contraction is a repetitive stress to the fetus. The mechanical forces associated with uterine contractions may compress the fetal head or the umbilical cord. They will interfere with intervillous blood flow.

The fetus who has used its reserves during pregnancy because of maternal, fetal, or combined problems has little compensatory capacity left when the stress of uterine contractions begin with the onset of labor.

Fetal Heart Rate Instrumentation

For continuous tracings of the FHR and uterine contractions, a fetal monitor is needed that meets certain guidelines. Once the monitor is in place, an understanding of the clinical significance of the various fetal heart rates and fetal heart rate patterns is needed. If continuous fetal monitoring is used as an adjunct to nursing care during labor, the medical and nursing staff must be aware of the idiosyncrasies of the particular monitor they are using.

With an electronic fetal monitor, the instantaneous fetal heart rate is displayed on a meter or on a digital display (see Fig. 16-6).

The fetal heart rate and uterine contraction tracings will record simultaneously on printed graph paper. Heavy vertical lines are printed at 1-minute intervals and lighter vertical lines are printed at 10-second intervals. The fetal heart rate tracing is recorded on the upper part of the chart paper and uterine contractions are recorded on the lower scale.

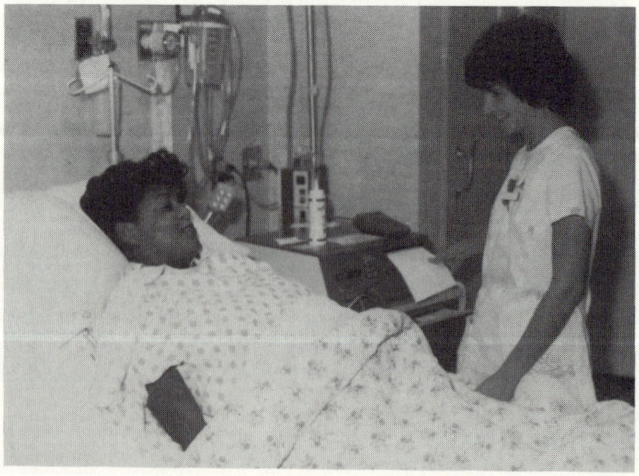

FIGURE 16-6. External fetal monitoring in place during labor.

Monitoring Methods

Electronic monitoring of fetal heart rate and uterine activity can be done using indirect or direct methods.

INDIRECT FETAL HEART RATE MONITORING

Phonocardiography

A transducer similar to a microphone is tightly fixed to the abdominal wall and the mechanical energy associated with the fetal heart rate is detected. The series of signals received demonstrate the first and second heart sounds. This method can be used during the antepartum and intrapartum periods with no hazards to the fetus or to the mother.

Ultrasonography

Ultrasonography is based on an echo technique for object location. A Doppler signal is created by a difference in frequencies of waves. Continuous sound signals are sent out from transmitting crystals that bounce off the object and reflect back to the receiving crystals. If the object that reflects back is in motion, the frequency of the reflected signal will change. The ultrasonic signal is directed toward the fetal heart. As the fetal heart pumps blood, the movement of the walls of the heart can be detected, since the reflected signal is altered with each heartbeat. The receiving crystals recognize this change in frequency and acknowledge it as a heartbeat. Each time a beat is recognized, an audible signal is heard called the Doppler signal.

Electrocardiography

Indirect or external fetal electrocardiography is based on the detection of the electrical energy of the fetal heart as recorded from the abdominal wall of the mother. Certain interferences may be encountered with this technique: the maternal electrocardiogram may be superimposed on the fetal electrocardiogram, the electrical activity of the abdominal wall muscles may be detected, and electrical interference may give an artifact appearance to the tracing.

Advantages

External fetal monitoring is simple and convenient. The patient may readily accept the procedure—it is noninvasive, no cervical dilatation is needed, and the membranes need not be ruptured. There is no infection hazard. The indirect methods can be used at any point of gestation. The monitor may be applied by the nurse, and the sound heard is similar to that heard with a fetoscope.

Disadvantages

External monitoring is difficult to use with an obese patient, a patient who is very restless or active, or a patient with polyhydramnios. The fetal heart record contains more artifacts, and variability cannot be determined. Some maternal restrictions in positioning may be required in order to obtain an accurate tracing. The belt may cause discomfort and it may require frequent repositioning to give reliable data. For some, the cost may be prohibitive. More attention may be paid to the monitor than to the patient.

DIRECT FETAL HEART RATE MONITORING

The fetal heart rate may be continuously recorded by attaching a small electrode to the fetal presenting part and recording the fetal electrocardiogram. A cardiotachometer within the fetal monitor converts the fetal electrocardiogram into a continuous and instantaneous fetal heart rate tracing.

Advantages

The main advantage of the direct method of fetal heart rate monitoring is a clear and precise fetal heart rate tracing. There are no restrictions in maternal positioning in bed, although bedrest is usually necessary.

Disadvantages

The cervix must be dilated at least 2 cm, with ruptured membranes. The nurse or physician must be able to identify accurately the presenting part and the position. The electrode cannot be placed on a face, the genitalia, or the fontanel. There is a possibility of maternal or fetal trauma, as well as an increased risk of infection. The patient is confined to bed and may occasionally complain of discomfort from the wire protruding from the vagina.

EXTERNAL UTERINE ACTIVITY MONITORING

During a uterine contraction, the uterus becomes more convex and also rotates anteriorly. These changes in uterine shape and position are reflected, to some extent, by changes in the maternal abdominal wall and can be detected with a gauge containing a form of counterpressure that is applied to the maternal abdomen with a belt. By displaying these changes, the frequency and duration of uterine contractions can be recorded.

Advantages

The technique is noninvasive and does not increase the infection potential to the fetus or to the mother. It can be used even in very early labor and can be applied by the nurse. A continuous recording of uterine contraction frequency and duration can be seen on the tracing.

Disadvantages

The external method of monitoring uterine contractions does not provide a reliable measurement of intrauterine pressure during contractions because of the uterine muscle and abdominal wall tension of the mother. The belt that is used to hold the gauge may loosen and alter the tension, thus giving an incorrect reading of contraction frequency and duration. Changes in maternal position will affect the recording. Difficulties in obtaining useable tracings are encountered when the patient is obese, very restless, or the fetus is preterm. It is important to remember that the intensity or quality of uterine contractions cannot be assessed with the indirect method.

DIRECT OR INTERNAL UTERINE CONTRACTION MONITORING

To monitor uterine contractions directly, a transcervical catheter and a pressure transducer or strain gauge are needed. The pressure transducer converts the amniotic fluid pressure to an electrical signal that is amplified and displayed on the monitor chart paper as uterine contractions.

Advantages

The recording of uterine contractions is clear, precise, and accurately reflects the frequency, duration, and intensity of contractions.

Disadvantages

To use direct uterine contraction monitoring, the cervix must be dilated to at least 2 cm and the membranes must be ruptured. Because it is an invasive procedure, strict aseptic techniques must be employed when inserting the catheter. There is also a risk factor of maternal or fetal trauma during catheter insertion and an increased incidence of infections.

APPLICATION OF FETAL MONITORING

The procedure for applying and adjusting fetal monitors varies with the equipment used, the method of monitoring, and the policies of the hospital.

COMPLICATIONS OF FETAL MONITORING

There have been no documented complications of external fetal heart rate or uterine contraction monitoring. A survey of studies revealed a wide variance in reported complications of fetal scalp electrodes and intrauterine catheter placements. The use of internal scalp electrodes was related to an increase in the overall Cesarean section rate (Neutra et al., 1980). The rate of scalp abscesses in the neonate ranged from infrequent to 0.4 percent to 4.5 percent. One case of neonatal herpes related to electrode placement has been reported (Parvey and Chien, 1980).

Complications in using the intrauterine catheter have also been documented in the literature. The incidence of intrauterine infections varies from no increase to a doubling. Increases in febrile mortality have also been reported. Uterine perforations have been reported in the literature, but the incidence is infrequent.

Risk Factors

Electronic fetal heart rate and uterine contraction monitoring is used in more than 80 percent of all labors today. Previously, fetal monitoring was reserved for women at increased risk or for the high-risk fetus. Some physicians and nurses feel that all patients in labor should be monitored. Others feel that only gravidas and fetuses identified as high risk should be monitored, since they are the most likely to develop problems that may require medical or nursing interventions. Identified risk factors are summarized in Table 16–5. Continuous monitoring is recommended for the gravida and fetus in the high risk categories.

Fetal Heart Rate

Maintenance of fetal welfare during labor depends upon several factors: (1) the placental blood flow must be adequate and unimpaired; (2) placental oxygen transfer must proceed unimpaired; and (3) the fetus must have normal blood properties that favor oxygen uptake. Anything that affects placental function will affect fetal oxygenation and the fetal heart rate. There is one spiral artery for every intervillous space or unit in the placenta. If that unit is obliterated or otherwise compromised, then it is no longer available for fetal oxygenation (see Chapter 8).

FACTORS THAT DECREASE UTERINE BLOOD FLOW

Certain factors will decrease uterine blood flow and thereby decrease fetal oxygenation. These include maternal hypotension, uterine contractions, maternal hypertension, and vasoconstriction due to sympathetic discharge.

TABLE 16–5
RISK FACTORS

Maternal Factors	Fetal Factors	Uterine Factors	Complications of Pregnancy
Chronic hypertension	Heart rate variations	Failure to progress	PIH
Diabetes mellitus	Stained amniotic fluid	Possible cephalopelvic disproportion	Premature rupture of the membranes
Heart disease	Breech presentation	Medical induction of labor	Abruptio placentae
Anemia	Postmaturity	Uterine inertia	Placenta previa
Rh negative	Preterm	Surgical induction of labor	Prolapsed umbilical cord
Age: $<$ 18 years $>$ 35 years	Failure to descend during labor	Oxytocin augmentation	Amnionitis
Previous cesarean section	Other	Multiple gestation	
Poor obstetrical history			
Physical anomalies			

FACTORS THAT INCREASE UTERINE BLOOD FLOW

Certain factors will increase uterine blood flow and thereby increase the amount of oxygen available to the fetus. These include bedrest, estrogen administration, nitroglycerin administration, and the transient effect of acetylcholine.

UMBILICAL BLOOD FLOW

Blood flow in the umbilical vessels comprises approximately 50 percent of the fetal cardiac output at any one time. At term, there is a turnover of 300 ml per minute. Mild hypoxia will increase umbilical blood flow. Severe hypoxia, maternal hypertension, and cord occlusion will decrease the blood flow through the umbilical vessels.

Normal Fetal Heart Rate

The normal fetal heart rate or the heart rate pattern in which the fetus remains well oxygenated throughout labor (see Fig. 16–7) is characterized by a basal rate of 120 to 160 BPM, no significant basal changes throughout labor, and no slowing of the FHR during or following uterine contractions.

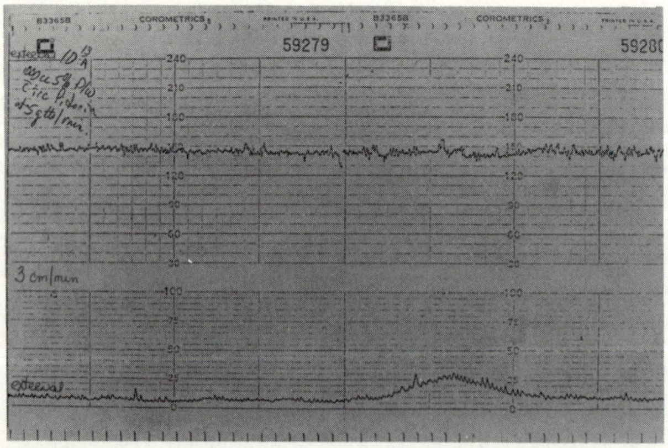

FIGURE 16–7. Normal fetal heart rate. FHR baseline 140 to 150 BPM. Average variability. No periodic changes noted. One uterine contraction noted on strip of 60 seconds duration, mild intensity on palpation.

REGULATION OF FETAL HEART RATE

The fetal heart rate is intrinsic: the rate is set by the sinoatrial node and influenced by both the parasympathetic and sympathetic nervous systems. The parasympathetic nervous system is responsible for vagal stimulation which decreases the fetal heart rate. The parasympathetic nervous system also controls heart rate variability. The sympathetic nervous system functions as a mechanism to increase the fetal heart rate.

The parasympathetic and sympathetic nervous systems are influenced by the baroreceptors and the chemoreceptors. The baroreceptors are located in the aortic arch and the carotid sinus of the fetus. They function as stretch receptors and provide a rapid response. They provide a stabilizing, protective function in the fetus. Chemoreceptors are located in the periphery and the central nervous system. They mainly affect respirations, and respond to changes in oxygen and carbon dioxide tensions to help maintain pH.

FACTORS AFFECTING THE FETAL HEART RATE

Many different and varied factors affect the fetal heart rate by either increasing or decreasing the rate. Medications administered to the mother, such as oxytocin, may decrease the FHR by increasing uterine activity, which will in turn decrease placental blood flow. A decrease in the variability of the FHR is seen with maternal administration of medications that affect the central nervous system: (1) narcotic analgesics, such as meperidine hydrochloride (Demerol) and morphine sulfate; (2) barbiturates, such as secobarbital and phenobarbital; (3) tranquilizers, such as diazepam (Valium); and (4) phenothiazines such as promethazine hydrochloride (Phenergan). Parasympatholytics, such as atropine sulfate and scopolamine hydrochloride, may also decrease the variability of the FHR.

General anesthetics decrease FHR variability, although regional anesthetics usually have

TABLE 16–6
FACTORS THAT INCREASE OR DECREASE THE FETAL HEART RATE

Analgesia
Anesthesia
Fetal rest periods
Vena cava syndrome
Maternal fever
Fetal malformations
Fetal immaturity
Cord compression
Cord constriction
Inadequate uteroplacental exchange
Head compression

little effect on the FHR unless there is associated maternal hypotension. If maternal hypotension occurs, it can be correcting by turning the mother to a left lateral position, increasing the intravenous fluid rate, administration of oxygen, and administration of ephedrine. Paracervical blocks are associated with fetal bradycardia that may last up to 10 minutes (see Chapter 17).

The fetal heart rate is also affected by fetal rest periods (decreased variability), vena cava syndrome (bradycardia), maternal fever (tachycardia), fetal malformation (bradycardia or tachycardia), and fetal immaturity (tachycardia and decreased variability) (see Table 16–6).

FETAL HEART RATE PATTERNS

The fetal heart pattern represents the output of physiologic control systems. If an imbalance exists in the cardioaccelerator and the cardiodecelerator mechanisms, it is reflected in a corresponding fetal heart rate acceleration or deceleration.

Two segments are present in any fetal heart rate pattern: baseline changes and periodic changes. *Baseline changes* are alterations in the fetal heart rate with no periodic changes in or between periodic changes. *Periodic changes* are associated with uterine contractions.

Baseline Changes

DETERMINATION OF THE BASELINE FETAL HEART RATE

Determination of the baseline fetal heart rate is accomplished by:

Evaluating the FHR at 10-minute intervals throughout labor

Describing the FHR by identifying the range in which the rate is located during the major portion of that 10-minute interval

If the change in FHR lasts more than 10 minutes, a new baseline is present

FETAL TACHYCARDIA

Fetal tachycardia is sustained elevation of the FHR over 160 BPM. It is often the first sign of fetal hypoxia and develops gradually as the oxygen-deficient atmosphere of the fetus causes the heart rate to increase in order to improve tissue oxygenation. When the fetus lacks adequate amounts of oxygen, glucose is not completely metabolized and lactic acid is produced instead of carbon dioxide and water, leading to an accumulation of lactic acid and a lowering of the blood pH, as well as an increase in the heart rate. An increased heart rate allows greater flow of blood through the placenta.

Causes

There are many causes of fetal tachycardia (see Table 16–7). Fetal hypoxia causes the fetus to attempt to compensate for the decrease in uterine blood flow by increasing sympathetic stimulation. In maternal infection the fetus may have tachycardia up to 24 hours before the maternal temperature is elevated, most probably caused by accelerated metabolism in the fetus.

Types

Fetal tachycardia is divided into two types according to the number of beats per minute.

TABLE 16–7
CAUSES OF FETAL TACHYCARDIA

Prematurity
Immaturity
Maternal fever
Fetal hypoxia
Fetal infection
Fetal stimulation
Fetal activity
Maternal anxiety
Fetal arrhythmias
Maternal hyperthyroidism
Parasympatholytic medications
Fetal hypovolemia
Idiopathic

Mild fetal tachycardia is defined as 161 to 180 BPM and *marked tachycardia* is 180+ BPM (see Fig. 16–8).

Significance

Prolonged tachycardia may be an early sign of fetal distress and has been associated with respiratory depression of the neonate at birth. Tachycardia in the presence of late or prolonged variable decelerations indicates acute fetal distress.

Nursing Responsibilities

When periods of fetal tachycardia are identified on the fetal monitor strip, appropriate nursing interventions include the following:

- Take and record maternal temperature
- Administration of oxygen
- Increase intravenous fluid rate
- Discontinue oxytocin infusion
- Change maternal position (preferably to left lateral)
- Continued observation of the FHR
- Documentation

FETAL BRADYCARDIA

Fetal bradycardia is defined as a sustained fetal heart rate under 120 BPM.

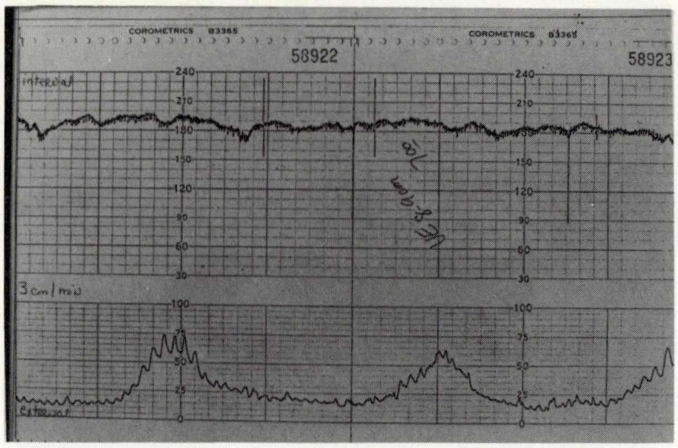

FIGURE 16–8. Fetal tachycardia. FHR baseline 180s. Variability present. Occasional decreases in FHR to 170 and 176 BPM of undetermined origin. Uterine contractions q 3 minutes, lasting 60 seconds of moderate intensity on palpation.

Causes

Fetal bradycardia can be caused by fetal or maternal factors (see Table 16–8). It may be a reflex response to a persistent increase in fetal vagal tone or a late occurrence following direct depression of the myocardial metabolism in fetal hypoxia. Maternal hypothermia may cause fetal bradycardia, as will medications that are beta-adrenergic agents such as propranalol hydrochloride.

Types

Fetal bradycardia is classified as moderate or marked. *Moderate bradycardia* is defined as 100 to 119 BPM, *marked bradycardia* is a fetal heart rate less than 100 BPM (see Fig. 16–9).

Significance

Fetal bradycardia alone is usually not associated with depressed neonates at birth. The significance normally depends upon the degree of bradycardia present. Moderate bradycardia is not associated with fetal acidosis. Bradycardia present with normal variability has been associated with congenital heart lesions in the neonate. If there is little or no variability and marked bradycardia is present, it is considered a sign of fetal distress.

TABLE 16–8
CAUSES OF FETAL BRADYCARDIA

Fetal hypoxia
Persistent increase in vagal tone
Fetal arrhythmias
Maternal hypothermia
Maternal drug administration
Idiopathic

Nursing Responsibilities

Appropriate nursing interventions when fetal bradycardia is noted include:

Close observation of the FHR
Administration of oxygen via face mask
Increase intravenous infusion rate
Discontinue oxytocin infusion
Change maternal position
Documentation

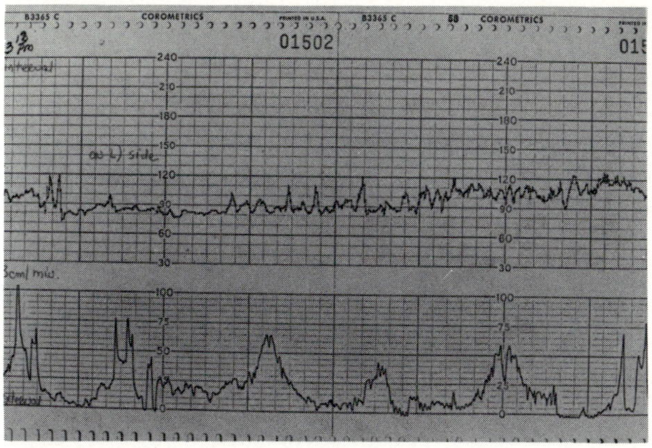

FIGURE 16–9. Fetal bradycardia. FHR baseline 80 to 90 BPM. Variability moderate to marked. No periodic changes noted. Uterine contractions q 1 1/2 to 2 minutes, of short duration, hypertonic in nature.

Periodic Changes

Periodic changes are classified according to the shape of the change in the FHR pattern and the time relationship between the beginning of a uterine contraction and the onset of the FHR change. These changes may be accelerations or decelerations.

ACCELERATIONS

Accelerations are transitory increases in the FHR caused by bursts of sympathetic nervous system activity. They are primarily of two basic shapes: uniform and variable. *Uniform accelerations* have an onset shortly after the beginning of the uterine contraction. The shape is usually similar to that of the contraction. *Variable accelerations* have an angular shape and a variable time relationship to the uterine contraction. They are usually associated with fetal movement. Accelerations can occur at any time (see Fig. 16–10) or they may be associated with uterine contractions (see Fig. 16–11). When accelerations are noted with fetal movement, contractions, or external stimulation, they are usually considered indicators of fetal well-being. During periods of stimulation and activity, the accelerations may merge to produce a fetal tachycardia.

Nursing Responsibilities

Nursing interventions appropriate when accelerations are noted include:

Observation of the FHR
Documentation

VARIABILITY

Variability is defined as a FHR fluctuation around a given FHR level and represents a continuous interaction between the fetal sympathetic and parasympathetic nervous systems.

Short term variability is the interval difference in baseline FHR with each successive fetal ECG. *Long term variability* is rhythmic fluctuations that occur with the fetal heart beat described in terms of frequency (2 to 6 cycles per minute) and amplitude of the change in the beats per minute (6 to 10 is normal). These rhythmic fluctuations are one parameter of fetal well being.

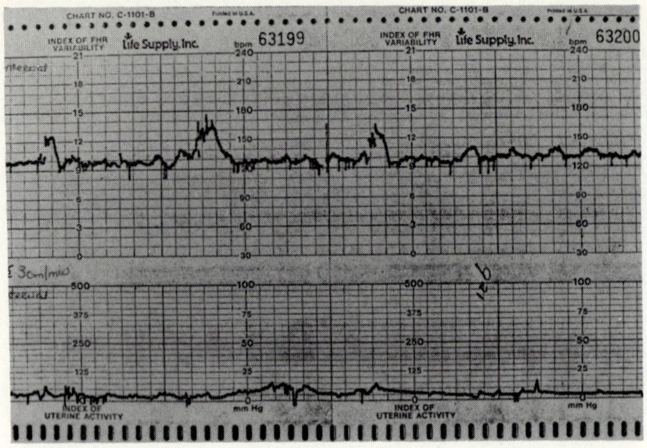

FIGURE 16-10. Accelerations. FHR baseline 124 to 130 BPM. Average variability. Accelerations of 15 to 30 BPM noted without other periodic changes. No uterine contractions noted.

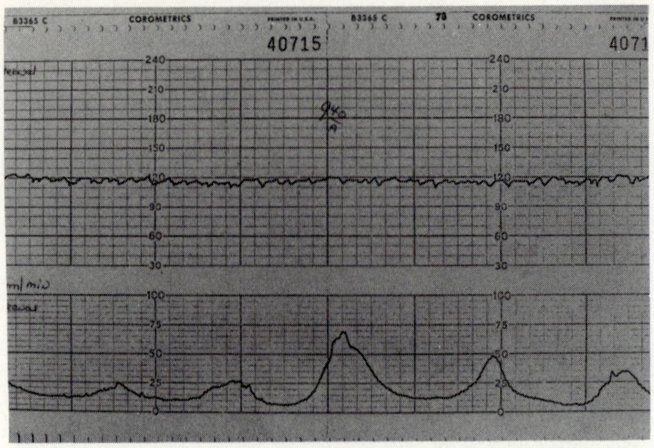

FIGURE 16-12. Normal variability. FHR baseline 110 to 120, mild bradycardia noted. Average variability present. Long-term and short-term variability on strip. No periodic changes noted. Uterine contractions q 1 to 2 minutes, moderate intensity.

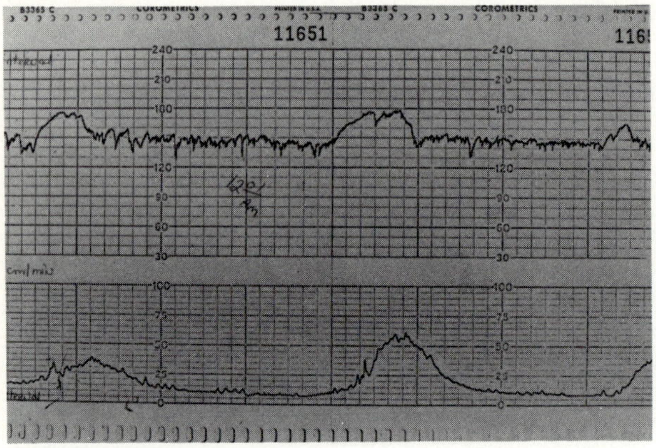

FIGURE 16-11. Accelerations associated with uterine contractions. FHR baseline 140 to 150 BPM. Normal variability with 2 episodes of marked variability noted. Accelerations of 30 to 40 BPM lasting 40 to 60 seconds noted with uterine contractions. No other periodic changes noted. Uterine contractions q 3 to 4 minutes, lasting 60 seconds, of moderate intensity.

TABLE 16-9
CAUSES OF DECREASED BASELINE VARIABILITY

Prematurity
Maternal drug administration
Fetal arrhythmias
Quiet fetal sleep
Fetal asphyxia
Fetal tachycardia
Fetal cardiac anomalies
Fetal central nervous system anomalies

Ranges

Long term variability is divided into five ranges:

Marked	over 25 BPM
Moderate	11 to 25 BPM
Normal	6 to 10 BPM
Minimal	3 to 5 BPM
None	0 to 2 BPM

Short term variability is recorded as present, absent, or decreased. Marked variability may follow fetal activity or fetal stimulation and usually indicates a well-developed mechanism for heart rate control in the fetus. Normal variability is seen in Figure 16-12. Decreased variability may have both fetal and maternal causes (see Table 16-9). Prematurity is a common cause owing to incomplete maturation of the cardiac control systems. Decreased variability is commonly seen during periods of quiet physiologic sleep in the fetus. Maternal drug intake is also a frequent cause of decreased variability (see Figures 16-13 and 16-14).

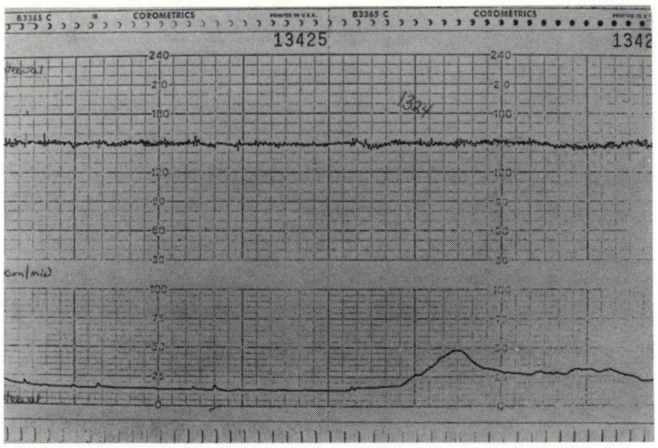

FIGURE 16-13. Minimal variability. FHR baseline 150s. Minimal variability of 3 to 5 BPM present. No periodic changes. One uterine contraction noted lasting 60 seconds with delayed return to uterine resting tone.

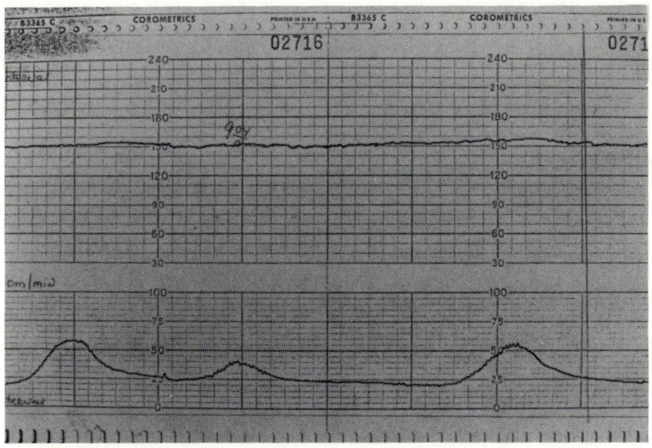

FIGURE 16-14. No variability. FHR baseline 150s. No variability noted, either long-term or short-term. No periodic changes noted. Uterine contractions q 2 to 3 minutes, lasting 40 to 60 seconds, mild intensity on palpation.

Significance

Variability cannot be assessed accurately using external methods of monitoring. Decreased variability is associated with placental insufficiency. When decreased variability becomes associated with decelerations in the fetal heart rate, low Apgar scores are often seen at birth.

Nursing Responsibilities

When decreased variability is noted, appropriate nursing interventions include:

Observation
Documentation

DECELERATIONS

When the periodic changes are decelerations in the FHR, four assessment steps are needed to identify the deceleration pattern.

1. Note the beginning of the uterine contraction, since that denotes the onset of the fetal stress. Compare the shape of the uterine contraction with the shape of the FHR deceleration.
2. Identify the time relationship between the onset of the uterine contraction and the onset of the FHR deceleration.
3. Look at the relationship of the peak of the uterine contraction and the lowest level of the FHR deceleration.
4. Identify the range of the FHR deceleration.

Early Deceleration

One type of deceleration pattern is early deceleration (see Fig. 16–15). The onset of the FHR deceleration is early in the uterine contraction. The heart rate normally does not fall below 100 BPM and the deceleration is normally over before or as the uterine contraction is completed (see Table 16–10).

The cause of early decelerations is probably fetal head compression during uterine contractions. When there is a change in cerebral blood flow, the vagus nerve is stimulated, vagal tone increases, and the fetal heart rate slows. Early decelerations are usually considered innocuous.

Nursing Responsibilities

Appropriate nursing interventions include:

Close observation of FHR
Careful differentiation from late decelerations
Documentation

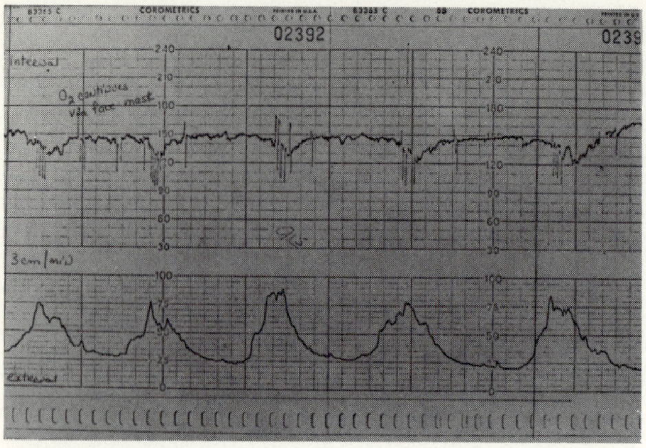

FIGURE 16–15. Early deceleration. FHR baseline 146 to 150 BPM. Variability decreased. FHR decelerations to 120 to 130 BPM lasting 30 seconds with uterine contractions. Uterine contractions q 1 1/2 to 2 minutes, lasting 50 to 60 seconds, of moderate intensity.

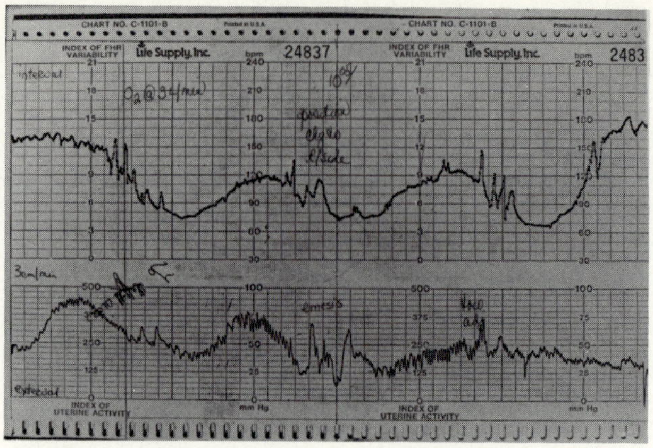

FIGURE 16–16. Late decelerations. FHR baseline 160 BPM. Average variability present with some loss of variability during deceleration pattern. Late decelerations noted to 70 to 80 BPM lasting approximately 1 1/2 minutes without return to baseline FHR. Uterine contractions lasting 60 to 80 seconds, of moderate intensity.

TABLE 16–10
EARLY DECELERATION CHARACTERISTICS

Early onset in the uterine contraction
Uniform shape that mirrors uterine contraction curve
Usually does not fall below 100 BPM
Usually lasts <90 seconds
Usually associated with a baseline FHR in normal range
Due to fetal head compression
Is not affected by high concentrations of maternal oxygen
Is not usually associated with acidotic neonates at birth

TABLE 16–11
LATE DECELERATION CHARACTERISTICS

Onset late in the uterine contraction
Consistent, specific FHR pattern, uniform in shape
Usually does not fall below 120 BPM, but may fall to 60 BPM
Usually less than 90 seconds duration
Usually associated with normal baseline range
Denotes uteroplacental insufficiency
Can usually be altered by maternal oxygen administration

Late Deceleration

Late decelerations are hypoxic FHR deceleration patterns associated with a decrease in maternal-fetal oxygen exchange. Their onset comes *after* onset of the uterine contraction and they have a specific, uniform shape (see Fig. 16–16). They may stay within the normal FHR range of 120 to 160 BPM (see Table 16–11) and often occur with every uterine contraction.

Late decelerations are frequently associated with uterine hyperactivity, maternal hypotension, and placental insufficiency. Each of these decreases intervillous space blood flow and leads to decreased maternal-fetal oxygen transfer. Other associated conditions include PIH, Rh isoimmunization, diabetes mellitus, and intrauterine growth retardation (IUGR).

Nursing Responsibilities

Late decelerations are ominous, indicative of fetal hypoxia. Appropriate nursing interventions include the following:

Identification of the deceleration pattern

Change maternal position to lateral or Trendelenberg to redistribute the mechanical forces and decrease uterine contraction frequency

Relieve maternal hypoxia by giving oxygen at 7 L per minute by face mask to raise the maternal-fetal oxygen gradient

Relieve maternal hypotension by changing position, elevating the legs, and increasing intravenous fluid administration

Decrease uterine activity by discontinuing oxytocin infusion to increase the perfusion of intervillous spaces and decrease the frequency of contraction stress

Notify physician

Documentation

Medical Interventions

Fetal blood sampling is used when there is a periodic pattern of repetitive late decelerations or repetitive moderate to severe variable decelerations that cannot be improved by appropriate nursing interventions.

Fetal blood sampling provides information about fetal pH, oxygen pressure, and carbon dioxide pressure. There are certain prerequisites: the cervix must be dilated 2 to 3 cm, the membranes must be ruptured, and the presenting part must be reasonably immobile.

A small specimen of blood is collected by the physician in a heparinized glass tube after a superficial puncture of a prepared area of fetal skin. Two or more successive specimens are taken to rule out inaccurate readings. Interpretation is as follows:

scalp pH	7.25 to 7.35	normal
	7.20 to 7.24	prepathologic
	< 7.20	acidosis

Delivery

Vaginal delivery may be indicated if an ominous FHR deceleration pattern is present, but delivery is imminent (will take place within 30 minutes). If the pattern cannot be corrected and acidosis increases, a cesarean section is performed.

Variable Deceleration

Variable decelerations have a variable onset and tend to drop and then rise suddenly. The shape of the FHR pattern will vary from a V-shape (see Fig. 16–17) to a wide U-shape (see Fig. 16–18). The FHR may drop to 50 or 60 BPM. Characteristics of variable decelerations are summarized in Table 16–12. They are described as mild, moderate, or severe and are almost always caused by umbilical cord compression. They tend to occur frequently in occiput posterior positions. If the deceleration is profound enough, fetal cardiac arrest may occur.

Nursing Responsibilities

Appropriate nursing interventions include the following:

Identification of the FHR deceleration pattern

Vaginal examination to determine if a prolapsed umbilical cord is present

Change maternal position to remove pressure from the umbilical cord and de-

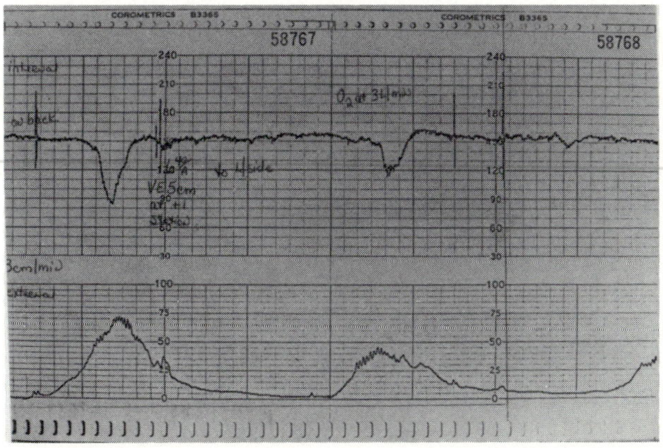

FIGURE 16–17. Mild variable decelerations. FHR baseline 150 to 160 BPM. Decreased variability. Mild variable decelerations of 20 to 30 seconds occurring with uterine contractions decreasing to 86 BPM and 120 BPM with rapid return to baseline. Uterine contractions q 3 1/2 minutes, lasting 90 seconds, of irregular quality.

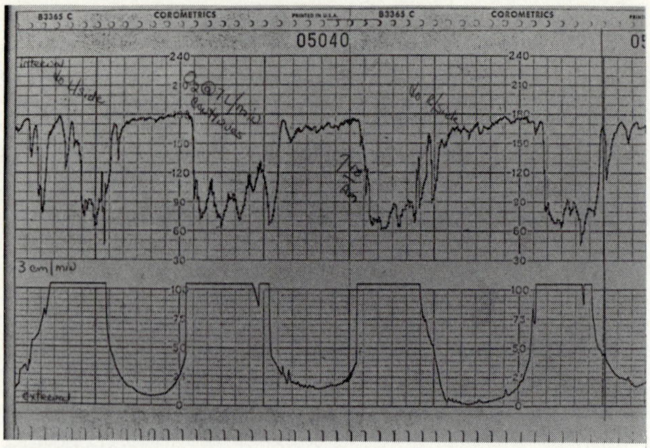

FIGURE 16-18. Variable decelerations. FHR baseline of tachycardia, 170 to 180 BPM. Short-term and long-term variability present. Variable decelerations lasting 30 to 60 seconds occurring with uterine contractions. Uterine contractions q 2 minutes, lasting 50 to 60 seconds, severe intensity. Patient is pushing with contractions.

TABLE 16-12
VARIABLE DECELERATION CHARACTERISTICS

Variable onset—tend to drop and rise suddenly
May occur before, during, or after a uterine contraction
Varied FHR pattern shape—V shape to wide U shape
May fall as low as 50 BPM
Duration of slowing varies from a few seconds to minutes
Due to umbilical cord compression
Markedly altered by maternal position changes
Baseline is usually within the normal range

crease uterine activity. Several position changes may be needed

Increase intravenous fluid infusion rate

Administer oxygen at 7 L per minute via face mask

Discontinue oxytocin infusion

Notify physician

Documentation

Mixed Decelerations

Mixed deceleration patterns may occur (see Fig. 16-19), as a combination of early, late, or variable deceleration patterns.

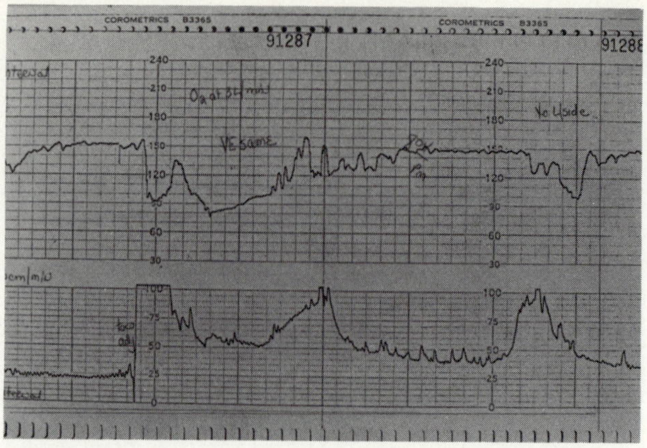

FIGURE 16-19. Mixed decelerations. FHR baseline 140 to 150 BPM. Minimal variability noted. Variable decelerations combined with late decelerations or a slow return to the baseline, giving a late component to deceleration pattern. Uterine contractions q 2 to 3 minutes, moderate intensity.

Nursing Responsibilities

Appropriate nursing interventions include:

Identification of the FHR patterns

Change maternal position to lateral or Trendelenberg to redistribute mechanical forces and decrease uterine activity

Relieve maternal hypotension by changing position, raising the legs, and increasing intravenous infusion rate

Relieve maternal hypoxia by administration of oxygen per face mask at 7 L per minute

Decrease uterine activity by discontinuing oxytocin infusion to increase perfusion of intervillous spaces

Notify physician

Documentation

Sinusoidal Pattern

A sinusoidal fetal heart rate pattern is characterized by a fixed, regular, amplitude of 2 to 5 BPM (see Figure 16-20). The wavelength averages 15 to 30 seconds and has a flutter type of rhythmicity.

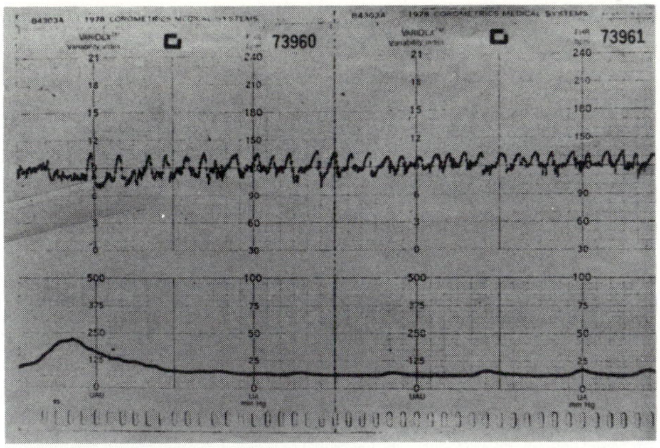

FIGURE 16-20. Sinusoidal pattern. Note the characteristic jagged configuration to the FHR pattern.

The etiology seems to be a virtual absence of central nervous system control of the heart rhythm. This could be caused by derangement of autonomic centers from hypoxia, acidosis, or impaired cardiac response to autonomic stimulation.

Incidence of this pattern is very low. It is most commonly associated with Rh isoimmunization with anemia and fetal-maternal hemorrhage. In the non–Rh immunized pregnancy, the sinusoidal pattern is seen in women who have received alphaprodine as an analgesic during labor.

The significance of this pattern is unclear. It is associated with a high neonatal mortality. When it is documented during labor, fetal blood sampling is performed to determine fetal status.

Nursing Responsibilities

Nursing interventions include the following:

Recognition of the pattern
Administer oxygen to alleviate fetal hypoxia
Notify the physician
Prepare the patient for fetal blood sampling
Documentation

Fetal Heart Rate Patterns

INNOCUOUS PATTERNS

Innocuous FHR patterns are associated with a normal fetal acid-base balance and with a good 5-minute Apgar score. These patterns include no periodic changes, accelerations, early decelerations, mild variable decelerations, and normal to marked variability.

OMINOUS PATTERNS

These patterns require prompt intervention to correct them and include: late decelerations; variable decelerations with a rising baseline, decreasing variability, drop to 70 BPM or less for longer than 30 seconds, or a slow return to baseline; prolonged decelerations; sinusoidal pattern; or tachycardia or bradycardia combined with decreased variability.

Acute Fetal Distress

Acute fetal distress is a situation in which the fetus is compromised in direct association with uterine contractions. The potential for acute fetal distress exists when any of the following occur: a progressive rise in the FHR baseline, tachycardia, mild variable decelerations, or a progressive decrease in variability. When prolonged variable decelerations lasting longer than 1 minute and dropping to 60 BPM, a smooth baseline with minimal or no variability, or late decelerations are noted, acute fetal distress can be identified.

NURSING RESPONSIBILITIES

When acute fetal distress is noted, seven major nursing interventions are appropriate (see Table 16–13):

1. Maternal position change. A change in the mother's position will help to correct one of the several causes of

TABLE 16–13
NURSING INTERVENTIONS IN ACUTE FETAL DISTRESS

Maternal position change
Correct maternal hypotension
Decrease uterine contractions
Oxygen administration
Maternal glucose administration
Notify physician, nursery, pediatrician
Prepare for delivery of the fetus

fetal distress. If the cause is umbilical cord compression, a change in maternal position will redistribute the mechanical forces and alleviate pressure on the umbilical cord. If the cause is supine hypotension, changing the gravida to a side lying position will lift the heavy uterus away from the vena cava and allow free return of venous blood to the heart. If the cause is pressure of the uterus on the aorta or common iliac arteries, the arterial pressure in the pelvis and lower extremities will drop (Poseiro effect). Having the gravida lie on her side will relieve the pressure.

2. Correct maternal hypotension. When maternal hypotension exists, there is poor perfusion of blood through the placenta. Corrective measures include elevation of the legs, rapid administration of intravenous fluids, and maternal position changes.
3. Decrease uterine contractions. Strong uterine contractions will cause a decrease in intervillous blood flow. If the contractions are also frequent, oxygen-carbon dioxide transfer across the placenta is impaired, and the fetus may not be able to recover adequately between the stresses of uterine contractions. Oxytocin infusions need to be carefully regulated and the uterine contractions closely monitored. If the contraction pattern becomes abnormal, the oxytocin infusion must be decreased or discontinued.
4. Oxygen administration. The administration of oxygen to the mother at 7 L per minute via face mask will increase the blood oxygen tension in the mother, increase the transfer of oxygen to the fetus, and help to maintain the oxygen tension of the fetal blood.
5. Maternal glucose administration. When the fetus suffers a hypoxic insult, glucose is rapidly mobilized. If the fetus is not receiving adequate glucose from the mother, his own glycogen stores become depleted. Glucose readily crosses the placenta from the mother to the fetus and is administered via intravenous infusion to the mother.
6. Notify physician, nursery, pediatrician. When fetal distress is noted, appropriate nursing interventions are instituted and the obstetrician, nursery, and pediatrician are notified of fetal status.
7. Prepare for delivery of the fetus. Vaginal delivery is feasible even with acute fetal distress if delivery can be accomplished within a short time, no more than 30 minutes. If vaginal delivery is not imminent and the distress patterns do not improve with appropriate interventions, a cesarean section is indicated.

A comprehensive nursing care plan for fetal distress is found in Table 16–14.

Nursing Role in Fetal Monitoring

The nursing care of a monitored patient is basically the same as nursing care given to any labor patient, with a few special nursing interventions that directly relate to the fetal monitor (see Table 16–15).

The procedure is explained to the patient and her coach. Many people associate monitors with critical illnesses and the parents may be concerned that something is wrong with the fetus. The purpose of fetal monitoring and how the monitor functions should be included in the explanation.

Maternal positioning is usually not restricted unless the fetal heart tracing cannot be maintained. The gravida can be in a comfortable position and should be encouraged to change positions to maintain a more effective labor pattern. If fetal heart rate and uterine activity are normal, the belts can be removed for short periods of time.

When external fetal monitoring is used, the presence of the two abdominal straps may cause irritation and discomfort. A small amount of powder can be applied to the skin under the belts if care is taken not to get powder on the ultrasound transducer or the tocotransducer. The belts and transducer can be removed every one or two hours and repositioned, with fresh gel applied to the ultrasound transducer.

The monitor tracing can be a useful adjunct to maintaining breathing patterns and techniques during labor. The uterine contraction may be displayed on the monitor paper several seconds before the patient feels the contraction.

Nurses must be careful to avoid giving nursing care to the monitor instead of to the patient. Fetal monitoring will actually free the nurse from counting the fetal heart rate at specified intervals and will make her more available to provide bedside nursing care to the patient.

LEGAL CONCERNS

The nurse is legally responsible for making a nursing diagnosis, which includes observation of symptoms and institution of appropriate nursing interventions. She must know the proper use and operation of the equipment and be able to interpret FHR patterns. She needs to take appropriate actions when the monitor tracing is abnormal.

The nurse's role is to apply external monitoring and assume responsibility for the quality of the tracing. The application of the internal monitoring modes is reserved for the specially trained obstetrical nurse or the physician.

Application of a fetal monitor when the patient refuses is considered battery. If attempts at education of the patient regarding the fetal monitor are futile and she still refuses the application of the monitor, a release of responsibility will need to be signed by the patient. Proper documentation of educational attempts must be made. If continuous fetal monitoring is not used, intermittent fetal heart rate assessment is then done at specified time intervals and as needed.

DOCUMENTATION

Fetal Heart Rate Patterns and Uterine Activity

Interpretation of the fetal monitor tracing is to be done systematically in four specific steps (see Table 16-16). Documentation of the interpretation is done at least every two hours or when changes occur.

Ominous Patterns

When an ominous pattern is identified, the nurse must initiate appropriate nursing interventions, notify the physician, and document the interventions, along with orders received, and FHR response.

Fetal Heart Tracing

In addition to identifying information pertinent to the patient (identification number, date, name—on tracing) and pertinent obstetrical history, the fetal monitor record strip should include documentation of paper speed (1 cm per minute or 3 cm per minute), calibrations, and type of monitoring used. Any maternal position changes, medication administra-

TABLE 16-14
COMPREHENSIVE NURSING CARE PLAN: CARE OF THE GRAVIDA WITH FETAL DISTRESS

Nursing Diagnosis	Goals	Nursing Interventions	Rationale	Evaluation
Knowledge deficit related to fetal distress	The client and support person will verbalize an understanding of fetal distress	Assess client/support person's knowledge of fetal distress Assess ability to understand explanations Explain fetal distress: Causes Clear up misconceptions	Explanations are to be given at a level easily understood	Fetal monitoring explained to patient and support person Understanding of explanation verbalized Fetal distress explained and understanding verbalized
	The client and support person will understand nursing interventions for fetal distress	Explain interventions: Purpose Expected outcomes Reinforce and/or repeat explanations as needed	Understanding of interventions will aid in compliance and prevent further insult to the fetus	Understanding verbalized
Potential for injury to the fetus related to uteroplacental insufficiency, cord compression, or maternal hypotension	Injury to the fetus is minimized by early nursing assessments	Assess and document continuous FHR tracing every 15 minutes: Baseline FHR Variability Periodic changes Assess FHR tracing for: Bradycardia Tachycardia Decreased variability Late decelerations Variable decelerations	Frequent assessments will detect subtle changes in FHR that are indicative of fetal distress	Documentation of FHR tracing assessment on chart every 1-2 hours or prn

		If alterations in FHR noted: Change maternal position Administer oxygen per face mask Increase non-oxytoxic IV infusion rate Discontinue oxytocin infusion (if present) Vaginal examination Notify physician Document Prepare for delivery if pattern not corrected by interventions	These interventions will increase intervillous space blood flow and increase oxygen to fetus	Documentation of any and all intervention on chart, as well as result of interventions
		Assess and document UC pattern for: Increased frequency Increased duration Increased intensity	Hyperstimulation pattern of UC will decrease blood flow to the fetus and increase fetal distress	Document assessment of UC pattern and any interventions
Anxiety related to uncertain fetal outcome	The patient and support person will verbalize fears/concerns regarding fetal outcome	Assess anxiety related signs: Trembling Tears Restlessness Depression Anger Hostility Expressed fears Verbalized concerns	Explanations will help to allay some fears and anxieties Do not give false hope	Document explanation given and client/support person's reaction

TABLE 16–15
SAMPLE NURSING CARE PLAN: FETAL MONITORING

Mary P., age 19 years, is a gravida 2 para 1 who is 40 weeks of gestation. She has been in active labor for 3 hours.

Data Base:

Normal prenatal history
Maternal blood type AB+
Maternal vital signs within normal limits
Cervical dilatation 3 to 4 cm, 75% effaced
Presenting part cephalic at +1 station
Contraction frequency 3 minutes, 40 seconds duration, of moderate intensity
FHR 142 BPM
Membranes ruptured spontaneously—moderate amount green-tinged amniotic fluid

Nursing Diagnosis	Goals	Nursing Interventions	Rationale	Evaluation
Knowledge deficit related to fetal monitoring	The patient and support person will verbalize understanding of the fetal monitor and its purposes	Assess knowledge level about fetal monitoring Provide information about fetal monitor, procedure and purpose Allow opportunity for questions	Assessment of knowledge level will aid in identifying level of teaching needed	Understanding of the fetal monitor verbalized by Mary and John
Potential for injury to fetus related to uteroplacental insufficiency or cord compression	The fetus will remain oxygenated during labor	Institute internal FHR monitoring according to hospital policy and procedure Institute external UC monitoring according to hospital policy and procedure Assess and record continuous FHR tracing q 15 to 30 minutes for: Baseline FHR	Amniotic fluid is green-tinged Internal FHR monitoring will aid in minimizing fetal insult by early identification of fetal distress	FHR baseline 130–140 BPM. Average variability of 6–10 BPM noted Occasional acceleration of 10–20 BPM noted with no other periodic changes at this time Contractions q 3 minutes, lasting 40 seconds, moderate intensity

		Baseline variability Presence and type of periodic changes Assess UC pattern for: High amplitude Increased frequency Long duration If abnormalities are noted: VE for possible cord prolapse Change maternal position Administer oxygen per face mask Increase nonoxytoxic IV infusion rate Discontinue oxytocin infusion (if running) Notify physician of status and/or further changes in FHR or UC pattern Document Observe for further changes	Nursing interventions can often alleviate the cause of the decreased fetal oxygenation and improve fetal outcome	FHR pattern normal Uterine contraction pattern normal Continue to evaluate for changes in UC pattern No interventions needed at this time
Anxiety related to possible fetal distress	Patient and support person have opportunity to verbalize fears and concerns	Explain all actions taken Reinforce explanations as needed	Many concerns can be readily alleviated with explanations	No signs of fear now Continue to evaluate and assess

TABLE 16-16
FOUR STEPS IN INTERPRETATION OF FHR AND UC TRACINGS

1. Identify the Baseline Fetal Heart Rate

This should be described as being within the normal range, bradycardia, or tachycardia. The number of BPM is specified.
Example: Fetal heart rate baseline of moderate tachycardia, 170 to 176 BPM

2. Assess the Degree of Baseline Variability

The variability present in the baseline FHR is to be assessed, along with the presence or absence of long-term and short-term variability.
Example: Average variability of 6 to 10 BPM on internal tracing

3. Identify Periodic Changes

Periodic changes are noted as accelerations, early decelerations, late decelerations, variable decelerations, sinusoidal patterns, or mixed patterns. The range of increase or decrease is documented.
Example: Accelerations of 15 to 20 BPM for 25 seconds noted with each contraction. No other periodic changes noted at this time.

4. Assess Uterine Activity

The frequency, duration, and intensity of uterine contractions is assessed. If the uterine contraction tracing is external, the intensity can be assessed as mild, moderate, or severe.
If an intrauterine catheter is in place, the resting tone and intensity of uterine contractions is measured in mm of Hg and documented.
Example: Contractions every 3 minutes, lasting 40 to 50 seconds, of moderate intensity.
Example: Uterine resting tone 10mm Hg, contractions every 3 minutes, lasting 40 to 50 seconds, intensity of 40 mm Hg.

tion, administration of oxygen, increase or decrease of the intravenous infusion rate, or oxytocin rate, as well as other patient care information is noted on the fetal monitor tracing. The fetal monitor record is retained by the hospital.

Patient Response to Fetal Monitoring

Routine fetal monitoring is done in the majority of labors in the traditional hospital setting. In alternative birth environments use is somewhat less.

Monitoring is used in both low- and high-risk patients. The value of monitoring in the low-risk patient has been extensively studied. Results vary from no improved fetal outcome to a decreased incidence of stillbirths, perinatal mortality, and low Apgar scores.

In the high-risk patient there is little disagreement that fetal outcome improves with fetal monitoring. Fetal deaths after admission and total perinatal mortality are reduced in these patients. When fetal monitoring is routinely used in labor, parents may feel that the monitor is an important part of labor care or they may feel that the monitor is an intrusion into a natural process.

NURSING INTERVENTIONS: SECOND STAGE OF LABOR

Transfer of the Patient

If delivery is to be in a traditional delivery room and the patient is a primigravida, transfer is usually made at the beginning of the second stage of labor. A multigravida would usually be transferred to the delivery room at approximately 7 to 8 cm cervical dilation.

Patient Behaviors

During the second stage of labor, the patient will have bearing down sensations on the perineum and she may verbalize feelings of tearing or ripping, pressure, and a need to defecate.

NURSING INTERVENTIONS

Do not leave the patient alone. Support and positive reinforcement are needed during this stage. No new information should be introduced. Aggressive behaviors are accepted. Physical care is directed at providing patient safety, conserving energy, and relieving incidental discomforts. The perineum is kept clean. Cold cloths to the forehead and small pillows under the lower back or sacrum are helpful. A sample nursing care plan for a patient in the second stage of labor is found in Table 16–17.

Bearing Down

When the cervix is completely dilated, the patient may begin to bear down or push. Bearing down before complete cervical dilation may cause the cervix to become edematous, dilate slowly, and lacerate.

POSITIONING

The gravida may push in a variety of positions: high Fowler's, low Fowler's, squatting, knee chest, or side lying.

High Fowler's Position

A high Fowler's position for bearing down is associated with increased efficiency of expulsion of the fetus. The pelvic inlet tilts forward and the pelvic outlet downward while the anteroposterior diameter of the pelvic outlet is increased. The duration of the second stage of labor is decreased by half when the mother is upright. The well-being of the fetus may be improved with a decreased incidence of deceleration patterns.

Low Fowler's Position

Traditionally, the patient pushes in a low Fowler's position. When a traditional delivery room is used, several pillows can be placed under the patient's shoulders and head to prevent her from being supine (see Fig. 16–21). When the patient is completely supine, her pushing efforts will work against gravity (McKay, 1981), and supine hypotension may result.

Whether the mother is in high or low Fowler's positions, pushing will be more effective when she assumes a C shape. Her chin is tucked into her chest and her back is curved. Her legs should be flexed and apart. She needs to grasp her knees, the backs of her thighs, side rails, or handlebars for counterbalance. Elbows should be bent.

PUSHING EFFORTS

For effective pushing, the diaphragm needs to be fixed to increase intra-abdominal pressure. Pushing efforts may be of a vigorous expulsive type, spontaneous bearing down, or exhale breathing type.

Vigorous Expulsive Efforts

Vigorous expulsive efforts are made by taking several deep breaths, then holding the breath while pushing as long as possible. The handlebars are grasped and the elbows are bent out when pulling on the handlebars. While pushing the chin is pulled forward onto the chest. When needed, another breath is taken and pushing repeated until the contraction is over. Following the contraction, the patient takes a cleansing breath and relaxes until the next contraction.

With this method of pushing the patient

TABLE 16-17
SAMPLE NURSING CARE PLAN: SECOND STAGE OF LABOR

Data Base:

See Table 16-3
First stage of labor progression normal
Maternal vital signs remained within normal limits during first stage
Uterine contraction pattern normal
FHT remained within normal limits; no fetal distress noted
Cervical dilation progressed without difficulty

Nursing Diagnosis	Goals	Nursing Interventions	Rationale	Evaluation
Alteration in comfort related to the second stage of labor	Maternal physiologic status will remain within normal limits Fetal status will remain within physiologic limits	Instruct the patient in correct pushing techniques Assist her to find a comfortable, correct position for pushing	The second stage of labor begins with complete cervical dilatation and ends with delivery of the neonate	Sylvia was completely dilated at 7:55 a.m. and was instructed to begin pushing with each contraction and rest between them following transfer to the delivery room
	The support person will provide effective support for the client	Encourage support person as coach	When the cervix is completely dilated, she can begin pushing	Paul was seated at Sylvia's right side after completing his scrub
		Keep client and support person informed of progress of fetal descent	Ineffective pushing will prolong 2nd stage Pushing is more effective if a "C" position is assumed	Paul and Sylvia are kept informed of fetal descent
		Set up for the delivery according to policy Provide comfort measures (cold, wet cloths, etc.) Do not leave patient alone Offer support and positive encouragement	There is an air of excitement during the second stage of labor due to imminence of delivery	Delivery room set up according to protocol Wet washcloth used by Sylvia to keep lips moist After each pushing effort, praise was given by nurse and by Paul

Potential alterations in tissue perfusion of mother and fetus related to abnormal maternal vital signs and/or abnormal uterine contraction patterns		Monitor maternal vital signs q 15 minutes Monitor the FHR continuously by monitor or q 5 minutes by intermittent auscultation UC monitored for frequency, duration, and intensity	Continuous assessments are needed to maintain maternal and fetal well-being	B/P ranged from 110/70 to 116/74 P ranged from 84 to 92 R ranged from 16 to 24 FHR remained 132 to 136 BPM by fetal monitor. No periodic changes noted with or following push efforts UC remained normal
Potential for anxiety related to disorganized preparation of delivery room		Dress codes are to be followed Have all equipment prepared for delivery	Hasty, disorganized preparation will increase anxiety levels and decrease coping abilities of mother	All persons in delivery room wore scrub outfits & caps, and shoe coverings Delivery room set up without haste
		Place mother's legs in stirrups or leg support when needed Raise legs together Check for proper alignment		Legs placed in stirrups when Dr. P. scrubbed and gowned for delivery
		Do perineal scrub Drape patient with sterile drapes Make sure patient can reach handlegrips Offer constant support and encouragement		Perineal scrub done Draping done
		Adjust mirror so patient and support person can see delivery		Mirror adjusted
				Sylvia delivered a live boy at 8:06 am over an intact perineum in a LOA position

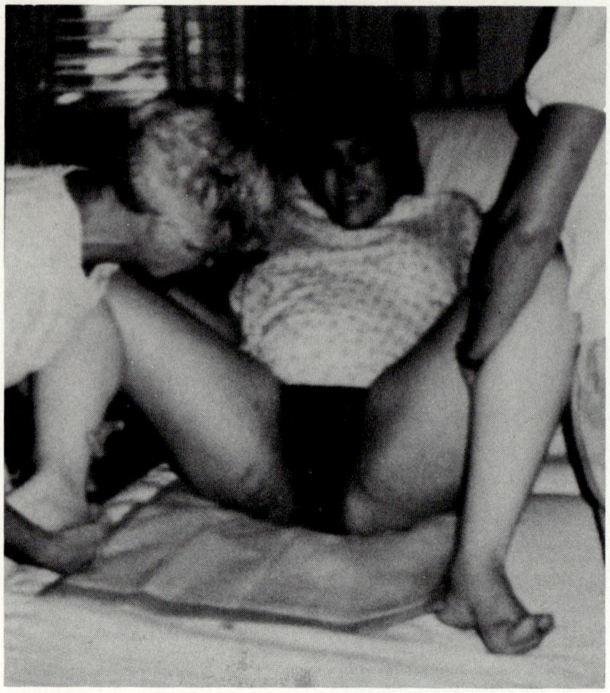

FIGURE 16–21. Pushing efforts with gravida in Low-Fowler's position.

may have petechiae on the face and ruptured small blood vessels in the eyes. Vigorous pushing efforts initiate a sequence of events called the Valsalva maneuver. Phase 1 initiates the process by increasing maternal intrathoracic and arterial pressures. Phase 2 is the period of straining, in which intrathoracic pressure is greater than pressure in the great system veins. The resultant decrease in venous return will cause decreased cardiac output and decreased blood pressure. The neck veins become engorged and the eustachian tubes are inflated. Phase 3, or reflex vasoconstriction, is accompanied by fetal hypoxic effects, increasing the incidence of FHR deceleration patterns. When the patient quickly takes one or two breaths between pushing efforts, the abdominal muscles vigorously retract. When pushing efforts stop, there is a sudden surge of blood to the heart, causing maternal tachycardia and late deceleration patterns in the fetus. With Phase 4, there is a period of rest. The maternal cardiac output and blood pressure increase and aortic pressure rises.

Vigorous pushing efforts are traditionally taught to patients for use in the second stage of labor. An alternative method of bearing down is spontaneous bearing down.

Spontaneous Bearing Down

With spontaneous bearing down efforts, the patient follows the dictates of her body in pushing. She pushes when she feels the need to push and in the method she feels like using. This spontaneous bearing down may make the second stage of labor somewhat longer but has several advantages to the fetus and to the mother. The fetus will suffer less hypoxia during contractions. The mother will suffer less cardiac stress, the perineal muscles will distend more slowly, thus decreasing the need for episiotomy, and the cardinal ligaments will have less strain, thereby decreasing the incidence of cystocele or uterine prolapse.

Exhale Breathing

A third type of pushing taught in some childbirth preparation classes is a modified Valsalva maneuver. With this method, the client takes several deep breaths, holds her breath for five or six seconds to fix the thoracic and abdominal muscles, then begins slow exhalation with the lips parted. As she feels the urge to push, abdominal muscles are employed, with the pelvic floor muscles relaxed. With the next breath, the patient will slowly inhale and repeat as before. When the contraction ends, a deep breath is taken to relax muscle tension.

Delivery Phase

The actual delivery phase traditionally takes place in the delivery room, as does all of the third stage of labor. The traditional delivery room is similar to an operating room (see Fig. 16–22). The same principles are used to prevent infection in both, and adequate equipment is readily available. If a birthing room is

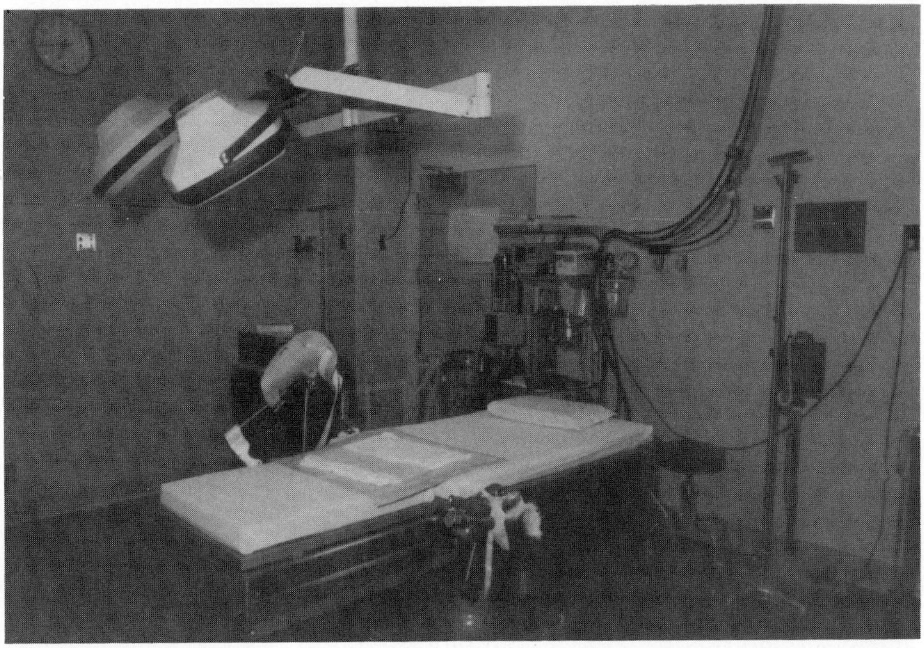

FIGURE 16-22. Traditional delivery room.

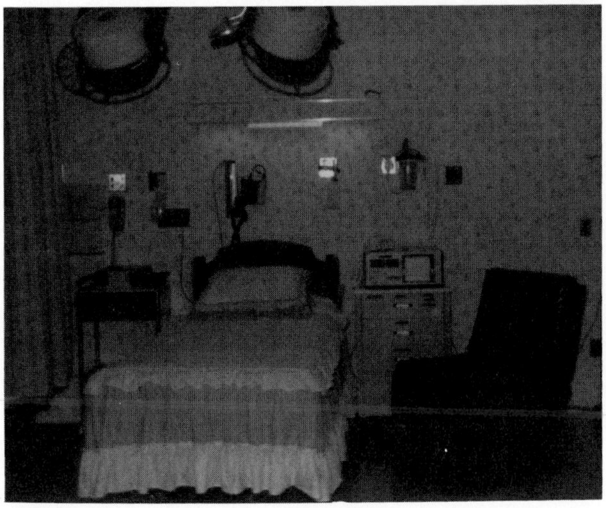

FIGURE 16-23. Birthing room, one view.

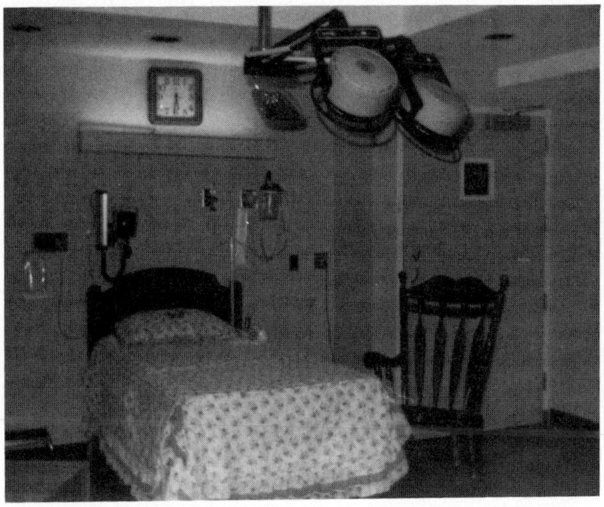

FIGURE 16-24. Birthing room, one view.

used, the client remains in the birthing room for stages two, three, and four of labor (see Figs. 16-23 and 16-24).

PREVENTION OF INFECTION

Important to the welfare of both the client and the fetus is prevention of infection. Delivery room personnel are dressed in cotton uniforms that are not worn outside the labor and delivery area. The hair is covered, and a mask is worn covering the nose and mouth. Personnel with upper respiratory infections are not permitted.

A long scrub is done by personnel at the beginning of the work shift. Frequent hand washing with a bacteriostatic agent is important. All equipment used for the delivery itself is sterile, and this sterility must be maintained to prevent infection in the gravida or fetus.

If the father or other support person is to be in the delivery or birthing room, he must wear proper attire, shoe coverings, a hat and mask, and scrub before entering the delivery or birthing room.

EQUIPMENT

Sterile gowns, gloves, and drapes used in the delivery room are similar to those used in an operating room. Instruments used for the actual delivery are sterile (see Fig. 16–25). The delivery table is made of two sections, an upper section, which is stable, and a lower section that can be rolled in or removed for the actual delivery. The birthing bed or delivery table is adjustable: it can be raised or lowered as a whole and put into various positions. A fetal monitor should be available in the birthing or delivery room. Anesthesia equipment is available and is similar to that found in the operating room.

Newborn care equipment is available (see Fig. 16–26). A radiant warmer or heated unit is needed to maintain thermal stability of the neonate and suction, oxygen, and resuscitation equipment is available as are cord clamps, identification materials, caps to cover the newborn head to conserve heat, and eye prophylaxis, if eye prophylaxis is to be performed in the delivery or birthing room.

Suction and oxygen equipment are available for the patient, as are intravenous equipment and medications. Some type of emergency call device must be operational. Adequate lighting is important.

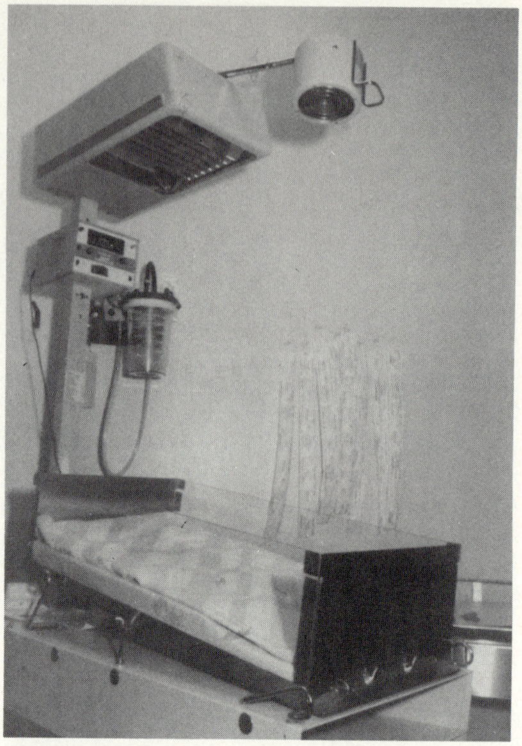

FIGURE 16–26. Infant radiant warmer unit in the delivery room.

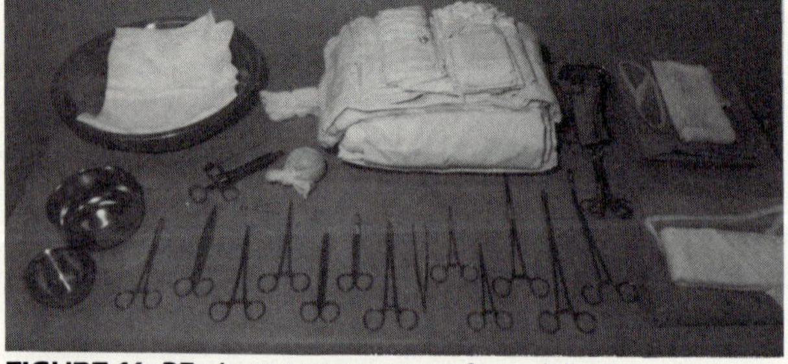

FIGURE 16–25. Instruments set up for a delivery.

The majority of these items will not be used for delivery, but must be readily available if an emergency arises that requires more sophisticated care for the gravida or for the neonate.

Maternal, Paternal, and Fetal Observations

During the second stage, both mother and fetus need to be continuously monitored. The client should never be left alone during this stage.

MATERNAL OBSERVATIONS

Uterine contractions are assessed carefully by either palpation or monitor tracing. The client is coached in her pushing efforts by the nurse or partner (see Fig. 16-27).

Vital signs are monitored for deviations from normal. The temperature is checked every two hours. Blood pressure, pulse, and respirations are assessed every 15 minutes and as necessary.

Anxiety and coping levels and behaviors must be assessed continuously. Constant and consistent support, encouragement, and positive reinforcement are offered.

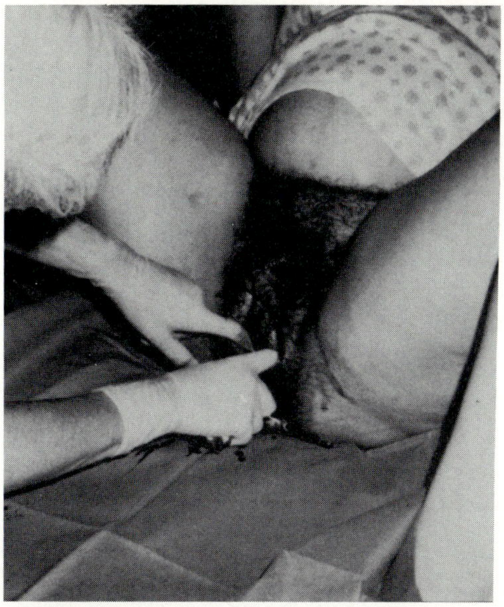

FIGURE 16-27. Pushing efforts—note the fetal head crowning.

STIRRUPS OR LEG SUPPORTS

In the delivery or birthing room, the mother's legs may be placed in stirrups or leg supports for the actual delivery, or foot supports may be used. Important points to remember when stirrups are used include elevation of the legs simultaneously to prevent ligament strain, spreading the legs wide enough to visualize the perineum, raising the legs to the same height to prevent pressure on the nerves, and checking under the knees to make sure no undue pressure is exerted on the popliteal space. When removing the legs from the stirrups, they must be brought down together slowly to prevent sudden hemodynamic changes.

The stirrups or leg supports help to maintain a lithotomy position for delivery. This position gives better visualization of the perineum, allows easier access to the perineal area, and reduces the time needed for preparation if operative intervention becomes necessary. Disadvantages of the lithotomy position include an increase in maternal back strain and an increased need for episiotomy, caused by the tightening and narrowing of the vaginal opening as the perineum is pulled forward (McKay, 1981).

PERINEAL PREPARATION IMMEDIATELY BEFORE DELIVERY

Immediately prior to delivery, the perineal area, inner thighs and lower abdomen are scrubbed with an antiseptic solution (see Fig. 16-28). Precautions are taken to prevent bacteria from being brought to the mother and to avoid carrying maternal bacteria into the reproductive tract. All equipment used is sterile.

When the perineal scrub is complete, sterile drapes are applied. During the draping procedure, the attendant scrubs as if for surgery and puts on a sterile gown and gloves. The lower half of the table is then removed.

PATERNAL OBSERVATIONS

If the father has attended childbirth preparation classes, he is directed to change into proper attire (if not already done) and scrub his arms and hands well with a bacteriostatic solution while the mother is being prepared for delivery. When he has completed this preparation, he can enter the room with the mother. Usually he is seated at the mother's side near her head. From this position his physical presence can be felt by the mother and he can coach and offer encouragement. He may help to elevate her shoulders while she is pushing, wipe her face with a cold cloth, and offer any other appropriate comfort measures.

FETAL OBSERVATIONS

The fetal heart rate is monitored during the second stage of labor. If intermittent auscultation is done with a fetoscope or Leffscope, the fetal heart rate is documented every 5 minutes. If an electronic fetal monitor is used, continuous observation and assessment of the FHR and associated FHR pattern must be documented.

TABLE 16-18
NURSING RESPONSIBILITIES IN THE DELIVERY ROOM

Keep the mother comfortable
Support the father in his role
Monitor fetal heart tones
Monitor uterine contractions
Assess maternal vital signs
Obtain sterile supplies
Notify the physician of the imminence of delivery
Notify the anesthesia department of the imminence of delivery
Assist the anesthesiologist or anesthetist in regional anesthesia
Monitor intravenous infusions
Scrub perineal area
Catheterize if the bladder is distended
Prepare newborn identification
Obtain and ready all equipment needed for the newborn
Assist the physician or attendant
Reassure the mother
Assist with coaching (if father present)
Coach the patient (if father absent)
Explain procedures as needed

SUMMARY OF NURSING RESPONSIBILITIES IN THE DELIVERY OR BIRTHING ROOM

Before the actual delivery, the nurse must set priorities for providing care for the mother and fetus. Some of the important nursing responsibilities in the delivery room are summarized in Table 16-18.

Perineal Lacerations and Episiotomy

PERINEAL LACERATIONS

Perineal lacerations may occur during the delivery of the fetus. They are classified into four types, by degree:

First degree: involves only the skin and mucous membranes

Second degree: involves skin, mucous membrane, and perineal muscles

Third degree: involves skin, mucous membranes, perineal muscles, and anal sphincter

Fourth degree: involves skin, mucous membranes, perineal muscles, anal sphincter, and anterior rectal wall

EPISIOTOMY

An episiotomy is an incision of the perineum at the time of delivery to facilitate expulsion of the newborn. There are two types (see Fig. 16-29):

Median. The incision is made in the midline down to the rectal sphincter.

Mediolateral. The incision is begun at the lower introitus and is directed laterally and downward away from the rectum to either the right or left side.

The median episiotomy is easily repaired, heals well, and causes minimal discomfort to the mother in the puerperium. The mediolateral episiotomy allows more room for delivery and is often performed if operative assistance such as forceps are to be used or if the newborn is large.

Indications

An episiotomy is sometimes performed as a prophylactic measure to preserve the integrity of the perineal floor and to prevent uncontrolled tears when a large newborn is anticipated. Maternal indications include a resistant perineum with thick and heavy muscles

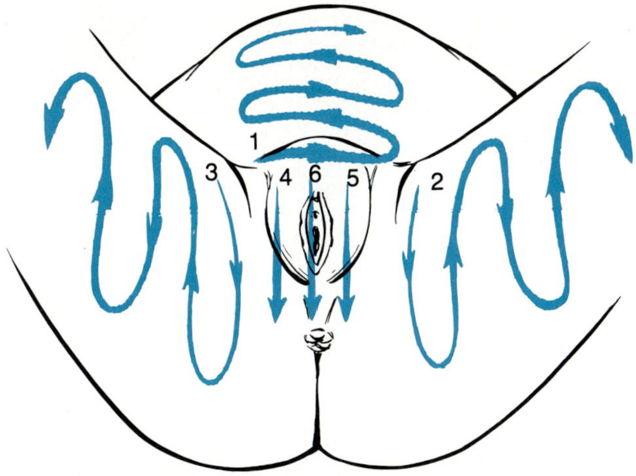

FIGURE 16-28. Perineal scrub before delivery.

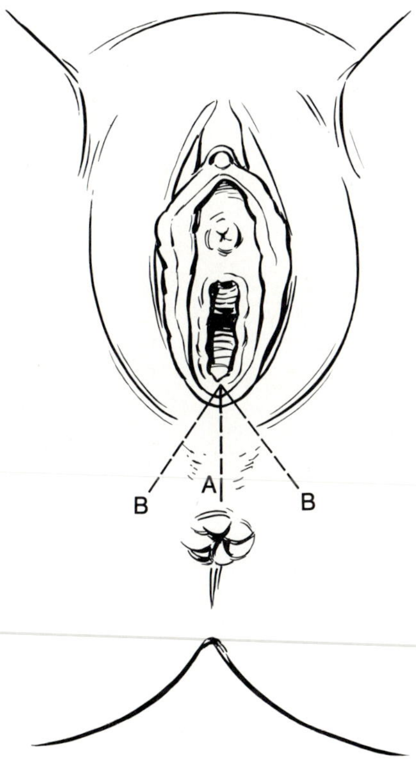

FIGURE 16-29. Episiotomy: A. Midline. B. Mediolateral.

or old scarring that may impede fetal descent. Fetal indications include preterm delivery, fetal distress, large size, and abnormal position of the presenting part.

Advantages

Routine episiotomies do have several distinct advantages. A straight incision is easier to repair and heals better than a jagged tear. The perineal floor is preserved to prevent cystocele and rectocele formation and uterine prolapse. Episiotomy avoids tears into the rectum and decreases pressure on the fetal head by the maternal perineum. It will also serve to shorten the second stage of labor.

Disadvantages

Disadvantages of routine episiotomy include possible extension of the incision, especially the midline incision, increased maternal blood loss, unsatisfactory repair, maternal discomfort, and an increased risk of infection. In addition, the incision may detract from initial bonding. There is an increased risk of infection. An episiotomy may not have been needed in all cases.

BIRTH OF THE NEWBORN

At birth the newborn begins an extrauterine existence and continues the process that began with fertilization. The metabolic support of the placenta is lost at delivery and the baby must now begin the transition to extrauterine life. Nursing interventions to support the newborn during this adjustment are important. A sample nursing care plan for a newborn at birth is found in Table 16-19. Care of the newborn includes both primary and secondary priorities (see Table 16-20).

Establishment of Respirations

Delivery of the fetal head is controlled to prevent forceful and rapid expulsion. If an episiotomy is needed, it is usually done when the head distends the perineum. Immediately after the head is delivered, palpation around the neck is done to determine if loops of the

TABLE 16–19
SAMPLE NURSING CARE PLAN: CARE OF THE NEWBORN IMMEDIATELY FOLLOWING DELIVERY

Newborn male G. was delivered at 3:33 p.m. over a midline episiotomy from a gravida 5 para 4 at 40 weeks gestation.

Data Base:

Maternal prenatal history normal
Maternal blood type A+
Labor and delivery progress within normal limits
Fetal heart rate tracings remained within normal limits during labor and delivery
Delivery was spontaneous, ROA
Infant G's mouth and nose were suctioned by Dr. T., with a small amount of mucus obtained
He was dried off and placed in a radiant warmer

Nursing Diagnosis	Goals	Nursing Interventions	Rationale	Evaluation
Potential for ineffective breathing pattern related to stress of labor and delivery	The newborn will begin to establish extrauterine physiologic stability	Determine and record Apgar scores at 1 and 5 minutes after birth	Apgar scores determine the degree of resuscitation needed during the first minutes of life	1-minute Apgar score: Heart rate 2 Respiratory effort 2 Muscle tone 2 Reflex irritability 2 Color 1 9 5-minute Apgar score: Heart rate 2 Respiratory effort 2 Muscle tone 2 Reflex irritability 2 Color 1 9 Apgar scores of 9 at 1 minute and 9 at 5 minutes indicate newborn G. is in good condition and requires no resuscitative measures
Potential impaired gas exchange related to copious airway secretions	Spontaneous respirations of 30 to 60 per minute will be established and maintained	Place newborn on side in slight Trendelenberg position	Assist mucus drainage by gravity	No mucus drainage noted
		Gently suction mouth and nose with bulb syringe	Suction is gentle to prevent irritation of the throat and to prevent vagal stimulation	Small amount white mucus obtained with bulb syringe
		Stimulate crying by gently flicking feet		Newborn cry lusty

Inability to control body temperature related to unstable temperature regulating mechanism	Skin temperature will remain within normal range	Skin temperature probe applied to maintain skin temperature at 98 to 99° F	If skin temperature is not maintained in neutral thermal range, newborn will suffer cold stress	Skin temperature 98.7°F
		Leave newborn uncovered on a dry surface under a radiant warmer	Radiant heat warms the skin surface of the newborn	Radiant warmer used to maintain skin temperature
		Keep newborn head covered with an infant stocking cap	Covering the head prevents heat loss	Head kept covered with infant stocking cap
Potential alteration in cardiac output related to improper cord clamping	Umbilical cord will remain clamped	Make sure cord clamp is applied properly with no excess bleeding	Clamping the umbilical cord prevents neonatal hemorrhage	Cord clamp in place
	Normal number of vessels are present in the umbilical cord	Check umbilical cord for presence of 3 vessels—2 arteries and 1 vein	An abnormal number of vessels is associated with congenital anomalies	2 arteries, 1 vein
Potential for infection related to contamination of the umbilical cord	Cord infection will be prevented	Maintain aseptic technique	The incidence of infection is reduced when aseptic technique is maintained	Aseptic technique maintained
Parental fear related to improper newborn identification	The newborn will be properly identified	Apply identification bands to newborn's ankles and identification band with matching number to mother's wrist	Identification is to be done before mother and newborn are separated	Identification bands #7047 applied
		Obtain newborn's footprints and mother's fingerprints	Footprints and fingerprints are permanent methods of identification	Maternal right index finger and newborn footprints obtained
Potential congenital anomalies related to abnormal genetic development	Initial physical assessment within normal limits	Complete initial physical assessment before giving mother newborn to hold	Physical assessment will identify anomalies and potential neonatal complications	Initial physical assessment within normal limits
Potential alteration in parenting related to delay in bonding process	Initial parent–infant bonding is instituted	Give newborn to parents to hold as soon as possible	Altered parent–infant bonding is more common when the process of bonding is delayed	Both parents held newborn
		Unwrap newborn so parents can see and touch		Newborn unwrapped
		Assist mother with breast feeding if desired		Breastfeeding deferred per mother's request
		Observe for eye contact		Eye contact established with both parents

TABLE 16-20
PRIORITIES OF NEWBORN CARE

Primary Priorities
Establish respirations
Monitor the cardiovascular system
Provide temperature regulation and support
Secondary Priorities
Cord care
Eye care
Identification
Initial physical assessment
Provide for initial bonding

umbilical cord are present. If they are present but loose, the loop may be slipped over the baby's head. If the loop is wound tightly around the neck, the umbilical cord is double clamped and cut immediately.

CLEARING THE AIRWAY

As soon as the head is delivered, the mouth is aspirated to prevent reflex gasping and aspiration of oral secretions (see Fig. 16-30). A rubber bulb syringe may be used for suction of the mouth. The bulb is compressed before insertion to prevent secretions in the oropharynx or nasopharynx from being forced into the bronchi. After the mouth is suctioned, the nares are suctioned to remove secretions. A plastic catheter with a mucus trap may be used to clear the airway. The catheter is placed in the newborn's mouth, reaching to the oropharynx with the opposite tube in the attendant's mouth. Suction is created by sucking as the catheter is withdrawn and rotated. Suctioning should be brief and gentle to avoid trauma to the delicate mucosa.

The physician or attendant may wait until the newborn is completely delivered to suction the mouth and nose (see Fig. 16-31). If the newborn is delivered before suctioning, positioning is head down to facilitate drainage from the oropharynx by gravity. The neonate should not be suspended by the feet, as this position will increase cerebral venous pressure and the possibility of intracranial hemorrhage.

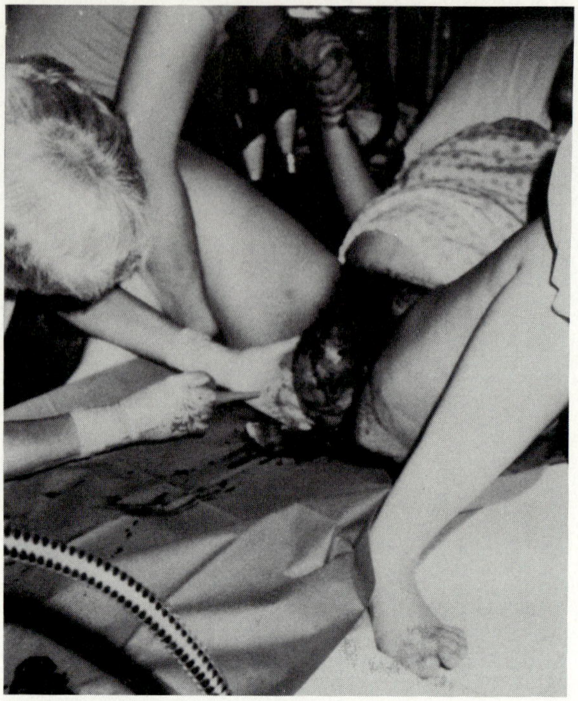

FIGURE 16-30. Suctioning the newborn's mouth as the head is delivered.

The narrow nasal passage of the neonate makes him more subject to obstruction of air flow. Newborn infants have very narrow nasal passages. Clearing the airway may be enough of a stimulation to initiate respirations in the newborn.

FIRST BREATH

For a newborn to take the first breath, three major forces must be overcome: (1) viscosity of the fluid in the airway, (2) surface tension, and (3) tissue resistive factors.

Biochemical Changes

When the umbilical cord stops pulsating, anoxia results from interruption of the blood flow and maternal oxygen. Carbon dioxide accumulates in the blood and lowers the pH to the point where the respiratory centers in the medulla are stimulated to initiate breathing. At birth, the average arterial pO_2 is 20 to 30 mm Hg, denoting a mild hypoxia.

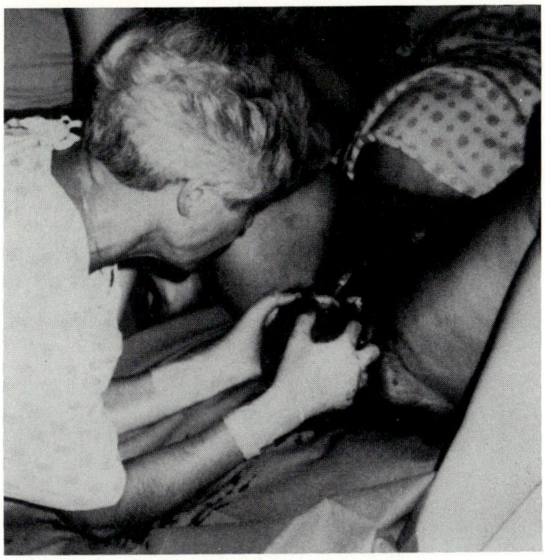

FIGURE 16-31. Delivery of the anterior shoulder.

Physical and Sensory Changes

The onset of respirations is facilitated by four physical and sensory changes. First, there must be rapid expansion of the chest following compression during passage through the birth canal. Second, stimulation of the tactile receptors is accomplished through handling during and immediately following delivery. Third, the infant undergoes an abrupt change from a fluid to an air environment. Finally, there is a change from a higher in utero temperature to a lower environmental temperature.

Most newborns begin to breathe within the first minute of life and many will take the first breath within seconds. The nurse notes and documents the time of birth and the Apgar scores.

Apgar Scores

Most hospitals and alternate birth centers use the scoring system for evaluating the newborn condition at 1 and 5 minutes after birth that was developed by Dr. Virginia Apgar. With this screening method, five signs are observed at exactly 1 minute and at exactly 5 minutes after birth: heart rate, respiratory effort, muscle tone, reflex irritability, and color. Each of these five signs is evaluated and given a score of 0, 1, or 2. The individual scores of these items are totaled for an Apgar score (see Table 16-21).

Scoring is done by a designated person in the delivery or birthing room. If two persons are doing Apgar scores, the scores may be slightly different, but should not differ to any great degree.

SIGNS

Heart Rate

The most important sign is the heart rate. It can be assessed with a pediatric stethoscope or by visually observing the junction of the umbilical cord and the skin. The heart rate is between 120 and 160 beats per minute.

Respiratory Effort

The respiratory effort of the newborn is second in importance. A healthy newborn will establish respirations at a rate of 30–60/minute within 1 minute following birth. Apnea requires immediate attention.

Muscle Tone

Muscle tone refers to good flexion of the extremities. The arms and legs are actively flexed and resist efforts to extend them.

Reflex Irritability

The response to a stimulation is called reflex irritability. Often flicking the soles of the feet is used to determine response and to stimulate the newborn. A catheter tip placed just inside the nose can also be used to test this sign.

Color

Color is the least important sign. Most newborns have a blue tinge to the body extremities immediately after birth. Acrocyanosis (blue hands and feet) is still common at 1 minute after birth and for several hours after.

TABLE 16–21
APGAR SCORING SYSTEM

	0	1	2
Heart rate	None	<100 BPM	>100 BPM
Respiratory effort	None	Irregular Slow	Regular Newborn is crying
Muscle tone	Absent Flaccid	Extremities are slightly flexed	Active movement of extremities
Reflex irritability	None	Grimace	Active crying
Color	Blue Pale	Blue extremities Body pink	Body pink

SIGNIFICANCE

The Apgar score at 1 minute will denote the neonate's condition at birth, while the 5 minute Apgar score will give a better prognostic indicator of survival.

USE IN NEONATE MANAGEMENT

Apgar scores at 1 minute will indicate the care needed by the neonate during extrauterine transition.

Apgar Scores of 7 to 10

Neonates with Apgar scores of 7 to 10 at 1 minute usually do not need additional treatment other than the routines to ensure a patent airway, temperature regulation, and assessment.

Apgar scores of 4, 5, and 6

Neonates who have an Apgar score at 1 minute of 4, 5, or 6 may have problems initiating respirations. They may need support with ventilation. Visualization of the larynx may be needed with tracheal suction for clots, meconium, mucus, or vernix caseosa. An airway can be inserted and oxygen given at 3 L per minute. With these interventions, the neonate will usually begin to breathe spontaneously.

Apgar scores of 1, 2, and 3

Time is important in neonates with Apgar scores of 1, 2, or 3 at 1 minute of life. If the heart rate is under 100 BPM with no response to stimulation, resuscitation must be started. The neonate may need endotracheal intubation, inflation of the lungs with oxygen, external cardiac massage, cardiac stimulants, and correction of metabolic acidosis and hypoglycemia.

Resuscitation

When a newborn does not breathe at birth, it will have a rapid decrease in blood pO_2, a rise in blood pCO_2, and a fall in blood and tissue pH, resulting in acidosis. Resuscitative efforts must be started at once.

The delivery or birthing room is equipped with newborn resuscitation equipment (see Table 16–22). An individual should be present at the delivery (usually the anesthesiologist) who is experienced in newborn resuscitation.

The ABC's for resuscitation of the newborn are:

A: establish airway
B: institute breathing
C: maintain cardiac support
D: administer medications as necessary
E: evacuate to high risk nursery

TABLE 16–22
NEWBORN RESUSCITATION APPARATUS

Source of oxygen, suction, and compressed air
Self-inflating breathing apparatus
Face masks
Laryngoscope handle
Laryngoscope blades—size 0 and 1
Extra batteries and bulbs
Endotracheal tubes—size 2.5, 3.0, 3.5, 4.0
Stylet
Suction catheters
Bulb syringe
Syringes and needles
Intravenous supplies
Umbilical catheters
Tape
Doppler blood pressure apparatus
Medications

A: ESTABLISH AIRWAY

Oral suctioning is used first to establish a patent airway. The newborn is positioned with the head lower than the body. The head should be turned to one side so secretions will collect in the cheeks. If the airway is not established with oral and nasal suctioning, the newborn is placed in a supine position with the neck *slightly* extended. A laryngoscope is inserted by trained personnel and the larynx is visualized and suctioned. An airway is inserted to keep the base of the tongue from blocking the glottis.

B: INSTITUTE BREATHING

A mask is placed over the nose and mouth to create a seal. The proper mask size is important: if the mask is too small, a seal cannot be obtained; if the mask is too large, it may extend over the eyes and cause injury. Warmed humidified 100 percent oxygen is administered. Insufflation with an anesthesia bag is begun at 40 mm H_2O at a rate of 40 to 50 times per minute. As soon as the chest wall rises, this pressure is decreased to 15 to 20 mm H_2O to prevent overexpansion of the alveoli. If this is effective, the newborn will begin spontaneous respirations within 1 minute. If no improvement is noted, or if the neonate's condition deteriorates, endotracheal intubation is done.

C: MAINTAIN CARDIAC SUPPORT

If heart activity is absent after endotracheal intubation and three or four bag insufflations, external cardiac massage must be initiated by a second person. The heart is compressed with the fingertips at a rate of 75 to 100 times per minute in conjunction with 40 to 50 ventilations per minute.

D: ADMINISTER MEDICATIONS AS NEEDED

Drugs that may be indicated for a severely depressed newborn include sodium bicarbonate to reduce metabolic acidosis, epinephrine to increase the heart rate and myocardial contractility, 25 to 50 percent dextrose to correct hypoglycemia, atropine sulfate to increase the heart rate, naloxone to counteract maternal narcotic administration, dopamine to increase the cardiac output, isoproterenol to correct hypotension and bradycardia, and calcium gluconate to increase cardiac output.

E: EVACUATE

As soon as possible, the newborn is transferred to the high-risk nursery or to a tertiary neonatal center for intensive medical and nursing care.

GENERAL NURSING RESPONSIBILITIES

Assessment and observations of the newborn and documentation of any resuscitative efforts are completed. Asepsis is maintained as much as possible because the depressed newborn is at an increased risk of infection. To help maintain body temperature and avoid further stress, the newborn is placed in a warmed blanket or in a warm environment (preferably a radiant warmer).

Explanations are made to the parents in terms that they can understand. They also need support and reassurance during this time.

Monitoring the Cardiovascular System

The second priority of newborn care in the delivery room is monitoring the cardiovascular system. Clamping the umbilical cord at birth eliminates the supply of oxygenated blood from the placenta (see Fig. 16-32). Thereafter the newborn must obtain oxygen from its own lungs. The ideal time to clamp the umbilical cord and cut it has been studied (Yao, 1977). Early clamping of the cord is defined as less than 10 seconds after birth. Late clamping is defined as 3 minutes or longer. Early clamping of the umbilical cord is thought to lengthen the third stage of labor and increase the likelihood of maternal hemorrhage and retained placenta. Conversely, late clamping is associated with transient cyanosis and pulmonary rales in the newborn. It would appear from the studies done that the optimal time to clamp and cut the umbilical cord is between 10 seconds and 3 minutes after birth.

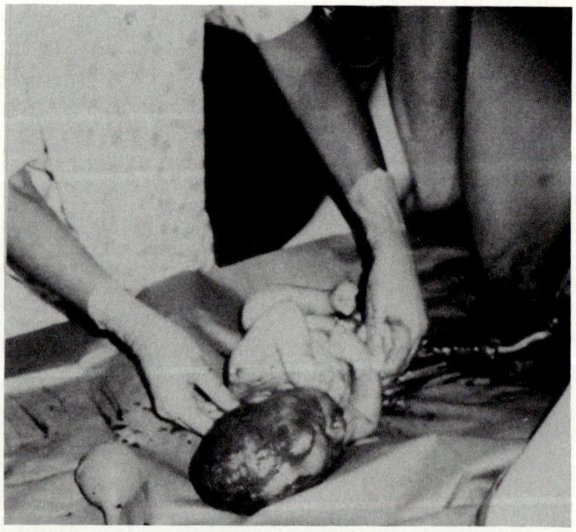

FIGURE 16-32. Newborn before the umbilical cord is clamped.

Newborns who are hypoxic at birth will have inadequate organ perfusion and become hypotensive. The neonate will appear pale, with cold extremities and weak peripheral pulses. When the skin is blanched with a firm pressure, the color may return slowly. When shock symptoms are present, treatment includes albumin for initial volume expansion, plasma, and whole blood. Vital signs must be monitored frequently.

Temperature Regulation and Support

The third priority of newborn care is the provision of temperature regulation and support. The newborn's chances for survival increase when the temperature is regulated properly.

Even the normal full-term newborn has difficulty adapting to temperature variations. Infants have relatively poor resources to resist the effects of heat and cold because of decreased function of the sweat and sebaceous glands for the first four weeks of life, a large surface area in relation to body mass, small amounts of subcutaneous fat, and the closeness of blood vessels to the skin.

The newborn who is exposed to cold environmental temperatures will draw on brown fat (see Chapter 21) reserves to aid in body temperature control. An increase in the respiratory rate to increase oxygen intake when exposed to cold is a process called *metabolic thermogenesis*. As the body temperature decreases, metabolism increases, thus elevating the newborn's oxygen need above normal, predisposing to inadequate oxygenation.

In order to maintain ideal body temperature in the newborn, the environmental tempera-

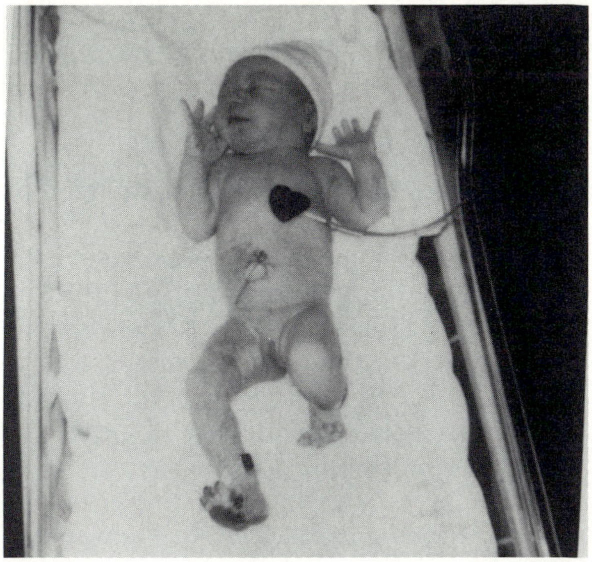

FIGURE 16–33. Skin temperature probe applied to regulate temperature. Note the cap on the head to conserve heat.

ture is carefully controlled after birth. Immediately after birth, the newborn is dried off quickly, including the face and head, to reduce heat loss by evaporation and radiation. Prewarmed blankets will help to reduce heat loss by conduction. Ideally, the newborn is placed in a preheated radiant warmer. A skin temperature probe is placed midway between the sternum and umbilicus (see Fig. 16–33) to maintain the skin temperature between 97.6° F and 98.6° F (36.3° C to 37.0° C). A cap is placed on the head of the newborn to reduce heat loss.

Cord Care

After birth the umbilical cord is clamped with a sterile cord clamp and cut with sterile scissors. The optimum place to clamp the cord is about 1 inch from the skin. The nurse will examine the cord for the presence of three vessels—two arteries and one vein. There should be no bleeding from the stump, which is left uncovered to promote drying. Cord clamps are usually left on for 12 to 24 hours after birth to prevent bleeding and are removed when the umbilical vessels are crushed and thrombosed.

Care of the Eyes

A mandatory regulation is the instillation of a prophylactic agent into the eyes to protect from ophthalmia neonatorum, a gonococcal infection that may cause blindness. Care of the eyes may be done in the delivery or birthing room or it may be postponed until admission to the nursery.

Within one hour after birth, the eyes are treated with either silver nitrate or an ophthalmic antibiotic ointment (erythromycin or tetracycline). Silver nitrate is effective against gonorrheal ophthalmia neonatorum but is not effective against chlamydial ophthalmia neonatorum, whereas erythromycin and tetracycline are effective against both.

When silver nitrate is used for prophylaxis, the eyelids and surrounding skin are cleansed with sterile cotton moistened with sterile water. The eyelid is gently opened and two drops of 1 percent silver nitrate are instilled on the conjunctival sac and allowed to run across the sac. With a new ampule of silver nitrate, instill two drops into the other eye. In 1 minute, the excess silver nitrate can be wiped from the eyelids with sterile water to prevent staining of the skin. The eyes should not be irrigated.

With administration of an antibiotic ointment, the eyelids and surrounding skin are cleansed with moist sterile cotton. The newborn's eyelids are gently opened and a ribbon of ointment 0.5 to 1 cm long is instilled into each conjunctival sac, being careful not to touch the tip of the tube to the eyeball or eyelid. The excess ointment is wiped from the eyelids after 1 minute. Do not flush the ointment from the eye. As with any antibiotic, hypersensitivity reactions may occur.

Parents express concern that eye prophylaxis may interfere with initial bonding. It may be advisable to postpone eye prophylaxis until the newborn is admitted to the nursery to take advantage of the quiet and alert eye contact with the parents.

Identification

Proper identification must be completed before the mother and newborn are transferred from the delivery or birthing room. Identification consists of bands with identical numbers, maternal fingerprints, and newborn footprints.

Identification bands are usually three-part bands with identical numbers on each band. Inserts with the mother's name, the date, time of birth, sex of the infant, and delivering physician are placed in the bands before applying. One band is placed on the mother's wrist and the other two are applied to the newborn's wrists or ankles (see Fig. 16–34). A second person should check the band numbers and band information and document this check.

The mother and newborn wear these bands throughout the hospital stay. Numbers are checked each time the newborn is brought to the mother. Upon discharge from the hospital, one band is removed from the newborn after verification and retained by the hospital as a permanent part of the newborn chart.

Another method of identification is the footprint or fingerprint. Newborn footprints and maternal fingerprints are taken before transfer from the delivery or birthing room. The form used for fingerprints and footprints usually contains other important information such as the mother's name, identification band number, the name(s) of the personnel who applied the bands, the name(s) of the personnel who obtained the footprints and fingerprints, date and time of birth, and sex of the newborn. The form is then signed by the physician, the delivery room nurse, and the nursery nurse who receives the newborn on admission to the nursery (see Fig. 16–35).

Footprints and fingerprints must be taken accurately. Ridges in the fingers, toes, and soles of the feet are specific to each individual and provide a means of permanent identification.

Initial Physical Assessment

An initial physical assessment of the newborn is performed at this time. This initial brief

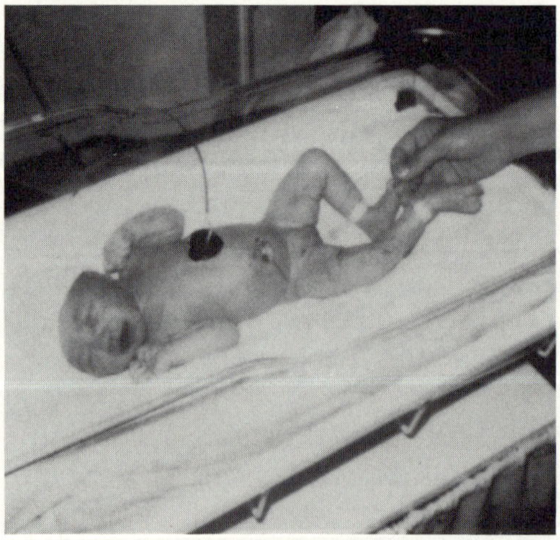

FIGURE 16–34. Identification bands in place on the newborn's ankles.

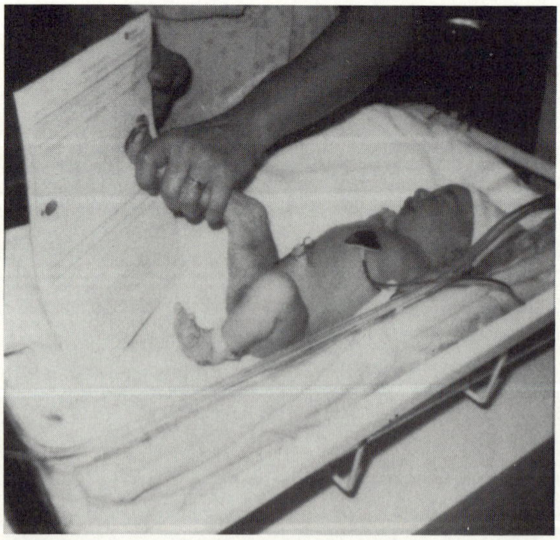

FIGURE 16–35. Footprints being taken for identification.

assessment does not preclude a complete physical assessment and examination in the nursery, but serves as a rapid assessment tool for the delivery room nurse. The only equipment needed is a pediatric stethoscope. The entire assessment takes only a few minutes to complete and consists of five steps:

1. Observe the newborn for obvious anomalies. For example, look at the head size, count the number of fingers and toes.
2. Note if there was polyhydramnios (excessive amount of amniotic fluid). Polyhydramnios is commonly associated with an increased incidence of gastrointestinal, central nervous system, and genitourinary anomalies.
3. Observe the shape of the abdomen. A convex abdomen may indicate intestinal obstruction or an abdominal mass. A concave abdomen is present with diaphragmatic hernia.
4. Assess respirations. Note if the newborn can breathe with its mouth closed to rule out choanal atresia.
5. Count the number of umbilical vessels (2 arteries and 1 vein are normal). Abnormalities in the number of vessels are associated with trisomies and genitourinary anomalies.

Initial Bonding

Newborn behavior at birth is divided into three periods: the first period of reactivity, sleep, and the second period of reactivity (see Chapter 21). In the first 15 to 30 minutes of life, the newborn is in the first period of reactivity and exhibits alert, exploratory behavior. It is at this time that initial bonding ideally occurs. The newborn is given to the mother or father to hold (see Fig. 16–36). Concerns about the newborn chilling while being held are largely unfounded (Gardner, 1979). Hearing the newborn cry, seeing and touching, holding him or her close to the body, and breastfeeding encourage the attachment process. See Chapter 19 for a further discussion of bonding. The nurse may remain with the newborn and parents during this initial period to assess both positive and negative signs of attachment or she may leave the parents alone if desired.

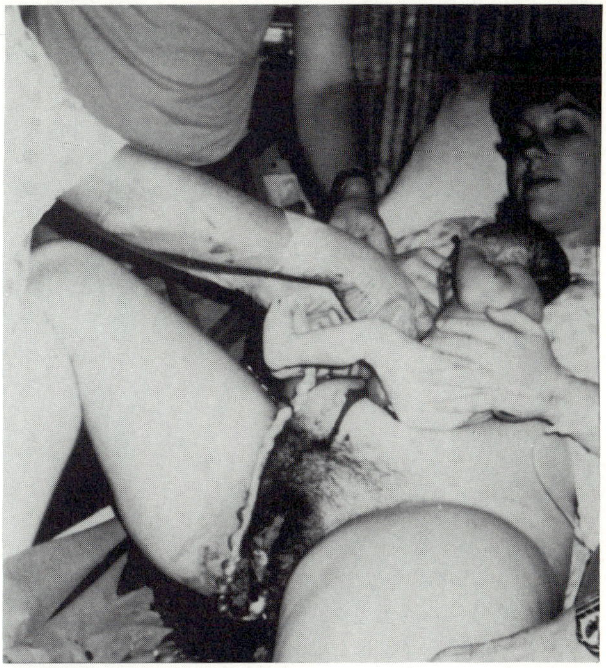

FIGURE 16–36. Initial bonding taking place. Note the umbilical cord is not yet clamped or cut.

Positive signs of attachment include realistic comments about the newborn, the use of affectionate terms, acceptance of the sex of the newborn, and behaviors such as touching, hugging, and smiling. Negative signs of attachment may also be noted and include refusal to look at or hold the newborn and hostility over the sex of the newborn. All attachment assessments are evaluated within the total context of the situation. A particularly long and exhausting labor will influence parental reactions.

NURSING INTERVENTIONS: THIRD STAGE OF LABOR

During the third stage of labor, care includes the mother and the newborn. Both need to be assessed frequently (see Table 16–23).

TABLE 16–23
SAMPLE NURSING CARE PLAN: THIRD STAGE OF LABOR

Data Base:

See Table 16–17
First stage of labor normal
Second stage of labor normal, within accepted time limitations

Sylvia delivered a live baby boy at 8:06 am over an intact perineum in an LOA position

Nursing Diagnosis	Goals	Nursing Interventions	Rationale	Evaluation
Alteration in cardiac output related to placental separation	The mother will remain physiologically stable during the third stage of labor	Observe for signs of placental separation: Uterus rises upward in abdomen Uterus becomes globular in shape and firm Umbilical cord protrudes from vagina Sudden gush of blood from vagina Instruct mother to push to expel the placenta	The third stage of labor begins with delivery of the newborn and ends with placental expulsion	Placenta separated at 8:09 am
		After placenta expelled, massage the uterine fundus to contract the uterus	Inadequate contraction of uterus will lead to excessive blood loss	Spontaneous Duncan placental expulsion at 8:10 am

		Monitor maternal vital signs Administer oxytoxics as ordered		P 84, R 16, B/P 120/74 Oxytocin 10U IM methylergonovine maleate 1 cc IV
		Check the placenta for the presence of all cotyledons and membranes		Placenta intact
Potential alteration in parenting related to impaired parent-infant attachment immediately after delivery	Initial infant bonding is initiated with parent(s) as evidenced by visual tactile, and auditory contact	Allow mother and father to hold newborn as soon as possible after delivery: Do initial newborn assessment Assist parents to hold newborn Encourage to visually examine newborn from head to toe Encourage to touch newborn Encourage to talk to newborn Allow and assist with breastfeeding if desired	Initial newborn bonding immediately following delivery is important to development of parent-infant bond. Many factors can alter bonding	Initial newborn assessment done by nurse Mother and father both held newborn Breast feeding deferred per mother's request Continue to assess

TABLE 16–24
OXYTOCIC DRUGS

Name	Dosage	Route	Onset of Action	Duration of Action	Contraindications	Side Effects	Nursing Interventions
Oxytocin injection (Pitocin)	5–10 U	IM	3–7 min	30–60 min	Hypersensitivity	Hypertension, water intoxication	Inject deep into muscle Massage injection site for quick absorption Check vital signs
	Induction or stimulation: 1–2 mU/min titrate to good labor (10 U in 1000 ml IV fluid)	IV	1 min	Continuous while infusion running	Hypersensitivity	Fetal: bradycardia, hypoxia, intracranial hemorrhage, trauma, neonatal hyper-bilirubinemia Maternal: uterine hypertonus, tetanic contractions, anaphylaxis, water intoxication, hypo-natremia, hypotension, ECG changes	Monitor maternal vitals q 15 minutes Intake and output Monitor FHR Monitor UC Accurate flow with infu-sion pump Physician must be immediately available Monitor for water intoxi-cation Always infuse via piggyback
	Control of postpartum bleeding: 10–40 U to 1000 ml IV fluid: titrate	IV	1 min	Continuous while infusion running	See above	See above	Monitor maternal vitals q 15 minutes Intake and output Monitor uterine firmness Monitor vaginal bleeding

Ergonovine maleate (Ergotrate)	0.2–0.4 mg 0.2 mg 0.2 mg	OS IM IV	5–15 min 2–5 min immediate	3 hours 3 hours 45 min	Hypersensitivity, induction of labor, uterine sepsis, hypertension, PIH	Nausea, vomiting, hypertension, bradycardia, shock, ergotism	Monitor maternal vitals Monitor uterine firmness Monitor lochia Check for severe cramping, may need to reduce dosage Check for symptoms of ergotism: Nausea Vomiting Cramping Diarrhea Drowsiness Dizziness Headache Confusion
Methylergonovine maleate (Methergine)	0.2 mg 0.2 mg 0.2 mg	OS IM IV	5–10 min 2–5 min immediate	1–3 hours 1–3 hours 1–3 hours	Hypersensitivity, hypertension, PIH, induction of labor, uterine sepsis	Allergy, nausea, vomiting, hypotension, hypertension, bradycardia, headache, dizziness, tinnitus	Monitor maternal vital signs Monitor for uterine relaxation Monitor lochia If IV, GIVE SLOWLY

Placental Separation and Expulsion

Placental separation usually occurs 1 to 5 minutes following delivery of the newborn. Signs that signify placental separation include: (1) the uterus rises upward in the abdomen because the placenta has moved down into the lower uterine segment; (2) the umbilical cord protrudes from the vagina owing to descent of the placenta; (3) the uterus assumes a globular shape and becomes firmer; and (4) a sudden gush of blood from the vagina may occur owing to placental separation.

Once the placenta has separated, the patient is coached to push as she did for delivery to expel the placenta. If the patient cannot push and the placenta is separated, the nurse can assist by palpating the uterus for firmness. If the uterus is firm, gentle fundal pressure is applied with one hand to push the placenta out of the vagina.

As the placenta is expelled, the fundus is massaged to contract the uterus and to decrease blood loss. The time of placental expulsion, method of expulsion (Duncan or Schultze), spontaneous expulsion or manual removal, and an estimate of maternal blood loss are documented as are any other pertinent data.

The mother's vital signs are taken and recorded. The placenta is inspected to determine if all cotyledons and membranes are present. If they are not, the missing cotyledon or membranes are removed from the uterus by the attendant to prevent postpartum hemorrhage.

Oxytoxics

An oxytoxic drug is one that promotes uterine contraction. These are sometimes given prior to or at the completion of the third stage of labor. The time and route of administration of any of the oxytoxics depends upon physician preference. Oxytoxics are given intramuscularly (IM) or intravenously (IV) either with delivery of the newborn or following placental expulsion.

The nurse who prepares and administers oxytoxics needs to be aware of the physician's order for the proper timing and route of administration (see Table 16–24).

NURSING INTERVENTIONS: FOURTH STAGE OF LABOR

The fourth stage of labor follows placental expulsion and lasts until maternal vital signs and condition are stable, a minimum of one hour. Stable maternal condition indicates: fundus firm, lochia dark and small or moderate in amount, no bladder distention, alert and responsive, stable vital signs, and no signs of hematoma formation. Ideally the mother, father, and newborn remain together (see Fig. 16–37) to facilitate further attachment. This section will deal exclusively with maternal assessments and appropriate nursing interventions (see Table 16–25). Neonatal assessments and nursing interventions on admission to the nursery are discussed in Chapter 22.

Repair of the Perineum

If a perineal laceration is present or if an episiotomy was done, it will be sutured at this

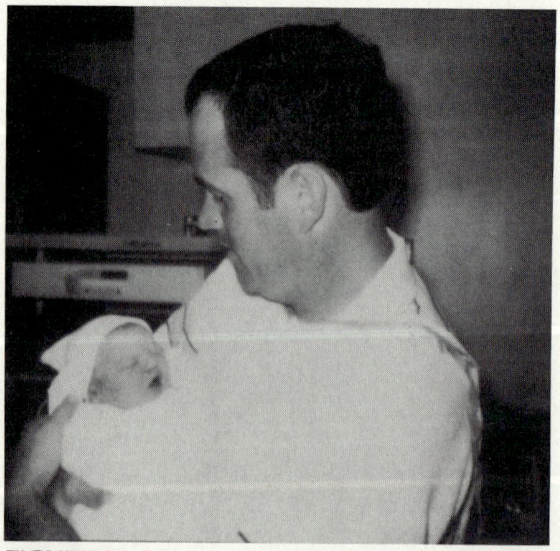

FIGURE 16–37. New father bonding immediately after delivery.

TABLE 16–25

SAMPLE NURSING CARE PLAN: FOURTH STAGE OF LABOR

Marian P. is a 24 year old gravida 4 para 4 who is admitted to the recovery room at 3:30 pm on February 8.

Data Base:

A live girl was delivered over a midline episiotomy at 3:01 pm
Infant Apgar scores 9 and 9
Upon transfer from delivery, her fundus was firm and at the umbilicus
lochia was moderate and red
EBL for delivery: 200 ml
Local anesthesia for episiotomy repair
No analgesia given during labor
Blood type B+
Physician orders: Discontinue present IV when vital signs stable
Ice to perineum for 12 hours

Last voiding: 250 ml at 2:10 pm
No intrapartal complications
No medical problems
Wishes newborn returned to recovery room when newborn assessment completed in nursery
400 ml D5/LR infusing at 28 gtt/min
Vital signs: Temperature 98.9° F
Pulse 100
Respirations 16
B/P 128/74

Nursing Diagnosis	Goals	Nursing Interventions	Rationale	Evaluation
Knowledge deficit related to policies and procedures	Client verbalizes understanding of the physical facilities, policies, and procedures related to the fourth stage of labor	Assess client knowledge of the physical facilities, policies, and procedures of the recovery room	Anxiety is heightened by a lack of knowledge	Marian oriented to the recovery room policies and procedures
		Orient client to the recovery room Answer questions		Verbalized understanding of recovery room policies and procedures
Alterations in comfort related to uterine involution and episiotomy	Client verbalizes that discomfort is manageable, and the normalcy of some discomfort	Assess client perception of discomfort: Location Intensity Quality		No c/o discomfort on admission
		Identify other factors that may contribute to discomfort: Fatigue Bladder distention Hunger	Bladder distention will inhibit uterine involution and increase discomfort level	No other factors identified

TABLE 16–25 (continued)

Nursing Diagnosis	Goals	Nursing Interventions	Rationale	Evaluation
		Assess perineum q 15 min for 1 hour, q 30 min for 1 hour for: Swelling Presence of hematoma Approximation of episiotomy	Perineum may be swollen or discolored	Perineum not discolored or swollen
		Apply ice to perineum	Ice will aid in decreasing swelling and pain	Ice to perineum
		Palpate bladder for distention q 15 min for 1 hour, then q 30 minutes for 1 hour	Urinary stasis predisposes to urinary tract infections	No bladder distension noted on admission
		Encourage to void Catheterize when distended with physician's order		Voided 450 ml urine at 4:45 pm
		Administer pain medication as ordered Keep clean and dry		Darvon compound 65 mg given at 4:30 pm for episiotomy discomfort
Potential for fluid volume deficit related to excess blood loss	Maternal physiologic parameters remain within normal limits	Assess uterine status q 15 min for 1 hour, q 30 min for 1 hour Tone Fundal height Position	Uterine should remain firm and even, in midline	3:30 pm—uterus firm, even in midline 3:45 pm—uterus firm, even in midline 4:00 pm—uterus firm, up one, to right 4:15 pm—uterus firm, up two, to right 4:30 pm—(after voiding) uterus firm, down one, in midline

		Assess amount and color of lochia and presence of clots Monitor number of perineal pads used Turn to side to assess blood loss	Deviations from the normal in amounts, color, or odor are indicative of complications	3:30 pm—lochia moderate red, no clots 4:30 pm—lochia small, dark, no clots 3 peri pads used
		Monitor and record B/P, P, and R q 15 min for 1 hour, then q 30 min for 1 hour	Vital signs normally remain in normal limits	3:30 pm—B/P 124/75, P84, R16 3:45 pm—B/P 120/74, P80, R20 4:00 pm—B/P 112/74, P84, R20 4:15 pm—B/P 110/70, P88, R16 4:30 pm—B/P 108/64, P80, R20 5:00 pm—B/P 114/70, P80, R20 5:30 pm—B/P 116/76, P84, R16
		Take and record temperature Assess LOC		Temperature 98° F Alert and oriented
Alterations in self concept related to birthing experience	Patient verbalizes concerns and perceptions of birth	Assess mother and father's feelings about labor and delivery Encourage to talk about feelings Explain normalcy of concerns if any		No concerns at this time Both parents happy, "glad it's all over"

time. During the perineal repair, the nurse is responsible for checking the uterus. The uterus should be firm and at about the level of the umbilicus. Maternal vital signs are monitored.

Transfer to the Recovery Room

When perineal repair is completed, the vulva is cleansed with warm sterile water. The vulva, thighs, and buttocks are dried, and a sterile perineal pad is applied. The legs are removed from the stirrups or leg support together and lowered slowly to prevent sudden hemodynamic changes. The uterine fundus is assessed for firmness and position, the lochia is assessed for color and amount, and vital signs are taken. The mother is moved into a clean bed. If she is chilled, a warm blanket may be used to promote comfort. The newborn is wrapped in a warm blanket and given back to the mother to hold.

Neonate Arrival in the Nursery

When the newborn is transferred to the nursery for assessment, a report is given, so the nursery nurse can institute appropriate interventions. Pertinent information includes:

Newborn condition at birth
Apgar scores at 1 and 5 minutes
Amount and type of maternal analgesia or anesthesia and time given
Type of newborn resuscitation (if any)
Sex of newborn and condition at birth
Any intrapartal complications, such as premature rupture of the membranes, stained amniotic fluid, FHR deceleration patterns
Responses of the parents to the newborn
Present maternal physiologic status
Newborn feeding method chosen by mother
Type and amount of medication given to the newborn
Identification band numbers
Pediatrician name
Any abnormal findings from the initial assessment in the delivery room

When initial newborn assessments are completed, the newborn is usually returned to the parents to continue the attachment process.

Maternal Assessments

REPORT OF MATERNAL STATUS

The nurse who will be responsible for maternal assessments during the fourth stage of labor is given a report that includes the following information:

Gravida and para
Last assessment of the fundus and lochia
Estimated blood loss during delivery
Amount and type of medication received that might affect her recovery room care, i.e., analgesics, anesthetic agents, etc.
Type of perineal laceration or episiotomy
Specific physician's orders
Time of last voiding or catheterization
Predisposing factors for postpartum hemorrhage
Parental response to newborn
Parental desires regarding seeing and holding newborn
Intravenous solutions or transfusions currently infusing
Last vital signs
Sex and condition of newborn
Pertinent medical conditions

TIME INTERVALS

Assessment is made at least every 15 minutes for the first hour after delivery, every 30 minutes for the next hour, and every hour until stable (see Table 16–26).

UTERINE FUNDUS

Before assessing the uterine fundus, explain to the client what you are going to do and provide privacy. Tell her she will be uncom-

TABLE 16-26
ASSESSMENT PARAMETERS FOR THE FOURTH STAGE OF LABOR

Uterine fundus
Bladder
Perineum
Lochia
Vital signs
Pain
Level of consciousness
Need for food and fluids
Comfort and safety needs
Emotional status

fortable during this assessment; explain the importance of keeping the uterus firm to prevent excessive bleeding. The uterine tone immediately postpartum depends on many factors: oxytocin administration, polyhydramnios, size of the newborn, parity, multiple births, uterine inertia, length of labor, and amount of urine in the bladder. Have the mother flex and spread her legs. Unhook the perineal pad and palpate the uterine fundus by cupping one hand over the fundal area and placing the other hand just above the symphysis pubis to support the lower uterine segment. The fundus is normally in the midline at the level of the umbilicus.

If the uterus is soft and not contracted, gently massage until it contracts and stays firm. Do not overmassage the uterus; the muscle may become overstimulated, fatigue, and relax, increasing blood loss.

A firm uterus that is enlarged above the umbilicus may indicate clots and whole blood retained in the uterine cavity. Clots and blood are expressed by applying pressure to the firm uterus for approximately 5 seconds, resting, and reapplying pressure as necessary.

The height of the fundus is measured after expressing all clots and blood by measuring the number of fingerbreadths above or below the umbilicus.

BLADDER

Observe the bladder area for distention. If the bladder is full, a bulge is evident above the symphysis pubis. The uterus may be several fingers above the umbilicus and displaced to the right of the midline. A full bladder will inhibit normal postpartum uterine contraction. Anesthesia received during labor or delivery may interfere with the patient's recognition of the need to void.

PERINEUM

The perineal area is inspected for discoloration and swelling that indicates hematoma formation (a collection of blood in tissue). With hematoma formation the client will complain of intense perineal pain and rectal pressure and will become increasingly restless. Hypovolemic shock may result. If the client received a regional anesthetic for delivery, she will have minimal or no perineal feeling and will not be uncomfortable. If a hematoma is detected, the physician should be notified; evacuation of the hematoma is usually necessary.

Normal perineal discomforts during the early puerperium result from trauma to the area from perineal lacerations or an episiotomy after the local anesthetic used for repair wears off. Burning and a dull, aching, or pulling sensation are common complaints. An ice bag may be ordered during the first 12 hours postpartum to decrease edema and discomfort. A small double walled ice bag wrapped in sterile gauze is filled with ice and applied to the episiotomy or laceration area.

Check for the presence of hemorrhoids and perineal varicosities. They may be irritated and engorged from pushing efforts and can be a source of discomfort.

LOCHIA

The lochia is assessed for amount, color, consistency, and odor. Normal lochia has a fleshy odor and is composed of blood from the placental site, shreds of membranes, vernix caseosa, lanugo, decidua, and possibly meconium. Saturation of two perineal pads in 15 minutes or three perineal pads in 30 minutes is considered excessive. A *saturated* perineal pad contains approximately 100 ml of fluid. Roll the patient to her side to check for lochia that has collected under the buttocks. Perineal pads should be changed as necessary to keep her clean and dry.

VITAL SIGNS

Temperature is taken and should remain within normal limits. An elevated temperature may be due to dehydration or infection. Blood pressure and respirations should be within normal limits for the patient, based on prenatal and intrapartal assessments. The pulse rate may be slower during the early puerperium, but it may be elevated if excessive bleeding is or was present. The blood pressure may be elevated owing to excitement, medication administration (i.e., methylergonovine maleate or ergonovine maleate), or pregnancy-induced hypertension, or it may be lowered owing to excessive bleeding or certain types of anesthesia.

PAIN

Pain during the fourth stage of labor is most commonly due to episiotomy discomfort and uterine contractions. Multiparas will have more uterine cramping than will primiparas. Cramping is also increased with a distended bladder, breastfeeding, and blood or clot retention within the uterus. Nursing interventions include an explanation of the source of pain, and analgesic medications when ordered.

LEVEL OF CONSCIOUSNESS

The maternal level of consciousness is assessed.

NEED FOR FOOD AND FLUIDS

Many clients begin the fourth stage of labor with intravenous fluid infusions. The intravenous infusion can usually be discontinued with a physician's order when the mother is stable. When fluids or food are allowed, encourage small amounts at first.

COMFORT AND SAFETY NEEDS

Both the mother and father need reassurance and rest at this time. A clean dry bed, frequent perineal pad changes, and a warm blanket will help to make the mother more comfortable so she can rest. The father can be made comfortable in a chair by the bed or by an opportunity to change from delivery room clothing or get something to eat.

EMOTIONAL STATUS

A wide range of emotions is displayed by the new parents. They may laugh, cry, shout, embrace, and talk. The same questions are often asked repeatedly.

BIBLIOGRAPHY

Berman, L.S. & Saunders, B.S. Newborn resuscitation. *Perinatology/Neonatology,* 1980, **4,** 22.

Blank, J.J. Electronic fetal monitoring. Nursing management defined. *Journal of Obstetric, Gynecological & Neonatal Nursing,* 1985, **14,** 463ff.

Butterfield, P.M., et al. Effects of silver nitrate on initial visual behavior. *American Journal of Diseases of Children,* 1978, **132,** 426.

Caldeyro-Barcia, R. The influence of maternal bearing-down efforts during second state on fetal well-being. *Birth and Family Journal,* 1979, **6,** 17.

———. The influence of maternal position on time of spontaneous rupture of the membranes, progress of labor, and fetal head compression. *Birth and Family Journal,* 1979, **6,** 7-15.

Carr, K.C. Obstetric practices which protect against neonatal morbidity: Focus on maternal position in labor and birth. *Birth and Family Journal,* 1980, **7,** 249.

Gardner, S. The mother as incubator—after delivery. *Journal of Obstetric, Gynecological & Neonatal Nursing,* 1979, **8,** 174-176.

Ingemarsson, E., et al. Influence of occiput posterior position on the fetal heart rate pattern. *Obstetrics & Gynecology,* 1980, **55,** 301.

Johnson, T.R.B., et al. Significance of the sinusoidal fetal heart rate pattern. *American Journal of Obstetrics & Gynecology*, 1981, **139,** 446.

Krebs, H.B., et al. Intrapartum fetal heart rate monitoring: III. Association of meconium with abnormal fetal heart rate patterns. *American Journal of Obstetrics & Gynecology*, 1980, **137,** 936.

Langerdorfer, S., et al. Pediatric follow-up of a randomized controlled trial of intrapartum fetal monitoring techniques. *Journal of Pediatrics*, 1980, **97,** 103.

Mandanes, A.E., David, D. & Cetrulo, C. Major complications associated with intrauterine pressure monitoring. *Obstetrics & Gynecology*, 1982, **59,** 389.

Martin, C.B. & Gingerich, C. Uteroplacental physiology. *Journal of Obstetric, Gynecological & Neonatal Nursing*, 1976, **5,** 16s-25s.

McDonough, M., Sheriff, D. & Zimmel, P. Parent's response to fetal monitoring. *MCN*, 1981, **6,** 32.

McKay, S.R. Second stage labor—has tradition replaced safety? *American Journal of Nursing*, 1981, **81,** 1016.

McManus, T.J. & Calder, A.A. Upright posture and the efficiency of labour. *Lancet*, 1980, **1,** 72.

Neutra, R.R., et al. Effect of fetal monitoring in neonatal death rates. *New England Journal of Medicine*, 1978, 299, 324.

______ ______. Effect of fetal monitoring on cesarean section rates. *Obstetrics & Gynecology*, 1980, **55,** 175-180.

Okada, D. M., et al. Neonatal scalp abscesses following intrapartum fetal monitoring: Prospective comparison of two spiral electrodes. *American Journal of Obstetrics & Gynecology*, 1977, **8,** 875-878.

Parvey, L.S. & Ch'ien, L.T. Neonatal herpes simplex virus infection introduced by fetal monitor scalp electrode. *Pediatrics*, 1980, **65,** 1150.

Perloe, M. & Curet L.B. The effect of internal fetal monitoring on cesarean section morbidity. *Obstetrics & Gynecology*, 1979, **53,** 3,354-357.

Petrie, M., et al. The effect of drugs on fetal heart rate variability. *American Journal of Obstetrics & Gynecology*, 1978, **130,** 294.

Powell, O.H., et al. Fetal heart rate acceleration in labor: Excellent prognostic indicator. *American Journal of Obstetrics & Gynecology*, 1979, **124,** 36.

Sampson, M.B., Mudalier, M.S. & Leie, A.S. Fetal heart rate variability. *Postgraduate Medicine*, 1980, **67,** 207.

Wagner, P.G. Continuous fetal tissue pH monitoring: A preliminary experience. *Journal of Obstetric, Gynecologic & Neonatal Nursing*, 1981, **10,** 164.

Whitley, N. & Mack, E. Are enemas justified for women in labor? *American Journal of Nursing*, 1980, **80,** 1339.

Yao, A.C. & Lind, J. Cord clamping time—influence on the newborn. *Birth and Family Journal*, 1977, **4,** 91-98.

Young, B.K., Katz, M. & Wilson, S.J. Sinusoidal fetal heart rate. I. Clinical significance. *American Journal of Obstetrics & Gynecology*, 1980, **136,** 587.

chapter 17

PAIN RELIEF DURING LABOR AND DELIVERY

OBJECTIVES

Upon completion of this chapter, the reader will be able to:

1. Describe causes of pain in labor.
2. Discuss factors that influence pain perception.
3. State how nonpharmacologic methods can relieve the discomfort of uterine contractions.
4. Given a specific analgesic, state its action and maternal and fetal effects.
5. List two advantages and two disadvantages of peripheral nerve blocks.
6. Given a patient receiving nerve root block anesthesia, discuss appropriate nursing interventions.

KEY TERMS

Analgesia
Anesthetic
Biofeedback
Caudal anesthesia
General anesthesia
Inhalation anesthesia
Lumbar epidural block
Nerve root block
Pain
Paracervical block
Peripheral nerve block
Pudendal block
Regional anesthesia
Subarachnoid block

Pain may be defined as a feeling of distress or suffering caused by stimulation of specialized nerve endings. Most women in labor experience some degree of pain. The amount of pain expressed by the client during labor varies greatly.

One difficulty nurses may have in caring for clients in labor is management of pain. Failure to recognize and accept pain as an integral part of the labor process will interfere with the ability to give appropriate nursing care. The inequality of the client's perception of pain and the nurses' recognition and acceptance of it will lead to ineffective nursing interventions and a less than optimal outcome for the client.

CAUSES OF PAIN

Physiologic Events

UTERINE ISCHEMIA

During the first stage of labor, uterine contractions occur at progressively closer intervals, last longer, and become more intense. When the uterine muscle contracts, there is a resultant lack of oxygen and a buildup of waste products in the myometrial cells. As the uterine contractions become more frequent, there is insufficient time to allow adequate reoxygenation of cells, with resultant pain.

CERVICAL DILATION

As the cervix effaces and dilates during labor, impulses from the cervix are transmitted via afferent nerve pathways to the spinal cord at the level of the tenth, eleventh, and twelfth thoracic vertebrae. These spinal cord segments supply the skin area of the lower abdomen, lower lumbar, and upper sacral spine.

OTHER CAUSES

Pain during labor is also caused by traction on and stretching of the uterine ligaments, ovaries, fallopian tubes, and peritoneum. Pressure on nerve ganglia near to the cervix and vagina, soft tissue distention, and distention of the perineal and pelvic floor muscles also contribute to discomfort during labor.

Psychological Factors

Response to pain is very personal and is modified or intensified by many factors. Few reliable predictors accurately identify clients who will experience more pain in labor. Age, social status, parity, and race have no direct relationship to expressed pain during labor.

Anxiety or fear about labor and delivery is common. Anxiety and pain do have a cyclical relationship in which anxiety generates tension leading to increased pain perception. Women who are highly anxious during labor show more intense discomfort. High levels of anxiety require support by the nurse and a support person to attempt to diminish them.

Pain interpretation during labor is also influenced by previous experiences. Past experiences with pain and hospitalization or previous labors affect current pain perception.

A woman's acceptance of pregnancy and the role of motherhood will affect the amount of pain experienced during labor, as will her relationship with her sexual partner (Lederman et al., 1979). Most commonly the amount of pain perceived increases as labor progresses, peaks during transition, and declines during delivery.

Apparent tolerance to pain by the patient can be misleading. Pain-associated behaviors do not necessarily include increased intensity of pain. Fatigue as labor progresses interferes with the ability to relax, as will emotional stress. Anemia intensifies anoxia of compressed myometrial cells during a contraction. Cultural norms often dictate expected pain-associated behaviors.

Feelings of helplessness and lack of control also intensify pain perception during labor (Butani and Hodnett, 1980).

NURSING APPROACHES TO PAIN RELIEF

Nurses are in a unique position to assist with pain relief during labor owing to their personal and prolonged contact with the client. To accomplish this, the nursing process is implemented.

Nursing Assessment

Ongoing assessment of pain during labor must include both objective (nursing observations) and subjective (client description) components.

Pain is a personal experience, with physiologic and psychological factors interacting to produce discomfort. These factors need to be identified as part of the assessment. Each person will experience and express pain in a unique way; therefore, it is imperative that each person be considered individually.

Emotional and behavioral responses to pain are assessed before interventions are planned. A systematic assessment of the pain includes the client's statements about the pain.

PAIN INDICATORS

Indications of pain include both sympathetic and parasympathetic responses and behavioral responses. Sympathetic responses usually occur with moderate pain and include pallor, elevated blood pressure, dilated pupils, skeletal muscle tension, tachypnea, and tachycardia.

More intense pain responses are usually of a parasympathetic type and include pallor, decreased blood pressure, bradycardia, nausea, vomiting, weakness, a feeling of faintness, and possibly loss of consciousness.

BEHAVIORAL RESPONSE TO PAIN

Behavioral responses to pain are varied, but may include protective positioning, moaning, grimacing, clenched fists or jaws, crying, fright, restlessness, withdrawal, muscle twitching, diaphoresis, holding the painful area, and refusing to change positions.

Nursing Interventions

During labor, the nurse can: (1) assess the need for assistance in coping with and reducing stress; (2) acknowledge the discomfort; (3) help with distraction and relaxation techniques; (4) eliminate distressing environmental factors; and (5) encourage participation of the support person. These have been discussed in Chapter 16.

The nurse works with the client, seeking ways to reduce or relieve pain, evaluate effectiveness of pain relief measures, and readjust interventions as necessary.

RELIEF OF ANXIETY

The greater the anxiety, the more discomfort is felt by the client. Measures employed by the nurse to relieve anxiety include staying at the client's side, allowing her to have more input into her care, and a willingness to listen.

Therapeutic touch, backrubs, and cool cloths will help to promote relaxation. If you need to leave the bedside, make sure the patient knows when you will return and that the nurse call button is readily available.

USE OF DISTRACTION AND DIVERSION

Perception of pain will be reduced if the awareness of pain is decreased. Small talk, idle chatter, and excessive noise are tiring rather than helpful. Some people find a barely audible noise such as a radio playing very softly relaxing, while others find it irritating.

On admission, determine the type of childbirth preparation classes attended (if any). This will aid in planning appropriate nursing interventions.

COMBAT ANTICIPATORY FEARS

Anticipatory fears are common in pregnant women. Old wives tales and friendly advice from relatives and friends combine with the reality that is felt during labor.

Childbirth education will decrease or alleviate anticipatory fears. The kind of pain or discomfort that will be experienced is discussed in class as are ways to relieve the distress. When relaxation is increased, muscle resistance is reduced and less pain is perceived. Proper positioning and body alignment will also aid in relaxation.

PHYSICAL CARE

In addition to psychological aspects of labor care, general principles of physical care are used to minimize irritations that lower pain tolerance. The client is protected from pain-producing stimuli, i.e., muscle spasms, interference with local blood supply and venous drainage with frequent position changes, and distention of the bladder or bowel.

Painful procedures should be performed at a time when the client is more comfortable, i.e., between uterine contractions or after analgesic medications have been administered. Excessive fatigue decreases pain tolerance, so measures to avoid fatigue are important.

ADMINISTRATION OF ANALGESICS

The administration of medications to reduce or relieve pain during labor, another important nursing intervention, is discussed later in the chapter.

Nursing Evaluation

Pain-relieving measures have a reduced value if they are not evaluated for their effectiveness. Changes in pain perception can be assessed by asking the client to rate her pain on a scale of 1 to 10, both before and after interventions.

Changes in the client's behavior are also assessed. As pain is reduced, removed, or becomes more tolerable, the behavioral responses associated with pain are altered.

NONPHARMACEUTICAL PAIN RELIEF IN LABOR

Pain and discomfort during labor and delivery may be relieved by many methods, including the use of analgesic medications. Today the trend is toward less and less use of analgesics, with relief or lessening of pain by alternate methods. Prenatal childbirth education classes help clients prepare for labor and delivery. Classes are usually structured according to one of three methods: Dick-Read, Lamaze, or Bradley.

Common Premises

All three of the methods for management of stress and pain during labor have certain principles in common. The partners wish to share in the birth of their child as part of the concept of family unity and togetherness. The woman uses the support of a partner, who is trained to provide this support. There is an opportunity to develop mechanisms for coping with pain or discomfort during labor and delivery by relaxation, diversion, or disassociation to maintain self-control and control of the immediate environment. Also included are discussion and practice in parenting activities to be used after delivery. With all three methods, anxiety is decreased, and personal satisfaction is increased.

One problem common to all three teaching methods is that the body's physiologic response to pain is not blocked. This leads to increases in serum epinephrine levels and may in turn lead to decreased uteroplacental blood flow (Schnider, 1985). Hyperventilation may occur to the point of maternal respiratory alkalosis, which causes decreased oxygen transport across the placenta.

Methods of Coping with Pain

All three methods are discussed fully in Chapter 12. A brief summary of the central premise and characteristics of each method follows.

GRANTLEY DICK-READ

The Dick-Read method of childbirth education is commonly referred to as "natural childbirth" and is based on the premise that labor and delivery are natural processes. According to this method, pain results from tension plus fear. If fear is removed and tension is decreased, pain will be minimized. Breathing techniques aid uterine contraction patterns and relax the perineum. The importance of a support person throughout labor is stressed. Women who use this method may feel they are improperly prepared or remiss in their duties as mothers if they request or require medication to aid in relief of discomfort.

LAMAZE (PSYCHOPROPHYLACTIC) METHOD

With the Lamaze method of childbirth preparation, knowledge is employed to remove fear of the unknown. Pain perception is dulled by use of a conditioned response to monopolize the nerve pathways. Concentration on a focal point aids in relaxation through diversion. Breathing control assists uterine contractions and prevents or increases effective bearing down when appropriate. Adequate ventilation is maintained by the use of cleansing breaths prior to and after each contraction.

BRADLEY METHOD

The Bradley method is commonly referred to as partner-coached or husband-coached natural childbirth, and is based on the premise that, in the presence of a loved one, the woman can work with each contraction to facilitate childbirth. Knowledge removes fear of the unknown. Kegal exercises permit proper control and relaxation during birth and return to normal function postpartum. Relaxation and abdominal breathing are used during the first stage of labor to facilitate working with uterine contractions.

General Nursing Interventions

When a labor patient and her partner elect to use one of the three methods summarized here, the nurse provides supplies for comfort measures, such as cool wet washcloths or ice chips (if allowed). The coach may need to be reminded of proper breathing techniques to use during the various stages of labor. Moral support, encouragement, and appropriate praise are important aspects of nursing care. The client and coach are kept updated regarding labor progress and any procedures. The coach needs to be relieved for breaks at intervals. If hyperventilation occurs, one of the following may be suggested to decrease symptoms of faintness and dizziness: (1) breathing into a paper bag; (2) breathing into cupped hands; or (3) holding the breath for short intervals. Demonstrating the appropriate breathing for a few uterine contractions may help reestablish the rate and rhythm desired.

During transition and delivery, only one person should give the client directions. Her attention span is narrowed and too many people giving instructions will only serve to confuse her. Extraneous chatter should be kept to a minimum at this time.

The decision to receive or not to receive pain medication should be supported by the nurse during labor and delivery. Childbirth is not an endurance test. The patient in labor should not feel that she has "failed" if she needs or requests medication to relieve uterine contraction discomfort, nor should she feel "forced" into taking pain medication.

All breathing patterns and interventions must be individualized during labor and delivery. No two labors are exactly alike, nor do people react the same way to the stress and pain associated with labor.

Biofeedback

Biofeedback is a relaxation-based form of pain relief that employs distraction devices and autonomic nervous system control (*vasodilatation*) to decrease pain perception. The ability to relax during labor aids in increasing maternal comfort and maintaining physiologic and psychological control.

The biofeedback method usually used during labor is electromyography or EMG biofeedback. The desired biological signal, muscle tension, is detected through the use of skin electrodes. As muscle tension is detected by the electrodes, the degree of tension is displayed on a visual monitor and an audible click or tone is heard. Pain perception is reduced in two ways: through reduction of abdominal muscle tension, and concentration and focus on relaxation of the abdominal muscle that provides distraction from pain.

The use of biofeedback equipment during labor has several advantages: the low cost of biofeedback equipment ($200.00–$400.00), the ease of instruction and training in the use of the unit, and the ability to use biofeedback without a support person. There are no reported physiological hazards to the mother or fetus.

Transcutaneous Electrical Nerve Stimulation

Transcutaneous electrical nerve stimulation (TENS) is used for pain relief during labor and delivery, as well as episiotomy discomfort during the postpartum period. The only possible side effect is skin irritation from the electrodes; on occasion, the current interferes with external fetal monitor tracings. The TENS unit delivers a pulsed alternating current to the body that stimulates beta neurons, in turn decreasing the nervous system's capability to recognize pain. The use of TENS poses no risk for the mother or fetus, and is associated with a decreased need for analgesia and anesthesia, as well as an increased sense of control during labor.

ANALGESICS DURING LABOR

An *analgesic* is a substance that reduces or abolishes suffering from pain without producing unconsciousness. In analgesia the sensation of pain and the associated psychic reactions are abolished and the perception of pain is altered. By changing the patient's attitude and mood toward pain, analgesics induce apathy to the pain and promote feelings of well-being and freedom from anxiety.

Analgesics given during labor are used to manipulate pain perception. Factors that affect the pain threshold are important in determining which, if any, analgesics should be given. These factors include maternal fatigue, lack of sleep, decreased nutritional intake, frequency, duration and intensity of uterine contractions, anxiety, fears, labor status, and maternal cellular changes that may occur with complications.

All systemic drugs given to the mother will affect the fetus, owing to placental passage of the medication. The result may be indirect, affected by changes in maternal physiologic status, or direct, affecting primarily the fetal heart rate and central nervous system. Some medications given to the mother during labor have an effect on the neonate for the first 48 to 72 hours after birth. The action of medication in the body depends, to a great extent, on the rate at which the drug is metabolized by the liver and excreted by the kidneys. The fetus has immature liver enzymes and renal system and will have difficulty eliminating drugs given to the mother.

The fetal brain will usually receive a greater amount of the medication, owing to the increased blood supply to the brain in utero.

During labor, medications are administered by the intramuscular or intravenous route. Oral medications are not used, because of the prolonged gastric emptying time and decreased absorption of medication that occurs when labor begins.

The optimal time for medication administration varies from patient to patient, according to the purpose for which the medication is being given. In a labor with normal progression, the optimal time to administer a narcotic analgesic is usually considered to be at 4 to 5 cm cervical dilation.

With intramuscular injections, the onset of pain relief is usually 30 to 45 minutes, although intramuscular medication is not released at a predictable rate. Intravenous medication is given slowly in small doses at the beginning of each of three to five consecutive uterine contractions. During a uterine contraction, blood flow is decreased through the intervillous spaces, thus increasing maternal pain relief and decreasing placental transfer of the medication to the fetus. Pain relief is accomplished with smaller doses of the medication.

General Nursing Interventions

On admission, history of allergies and renal or liver disease is noted. Unusual reactions to medications are assessed. Hydration status is assessed by determining the amount and type of intake and output in the eight hours preceding admission, character of the mucous membranes, and skin turgor. The expectations for analgesia or anesthesia during labor are determined. Throughout labor, the need for pain relief is assessed at frequent intervals.

Before administering medication, the nurse should provide an explanation of the medication and its expected action and effect to the client and support person. The client is asked to void. Baseline parameters of maternal vital signs, fetal heart rate, and status of labor are obtained.

After administration, side rails are raised, and the call light is placed within easy reach of the client. Tell her when you will reassess labor status and vital signs. Close observations are needed to assess pain relief and labor status. The medication administered is documented on the client's chart and on the fetal monitor tracing, noting the amount and type of medication administered, the time, reason for administration, and effects.

Several classifications of systemic medications are used during labor. These include sedative/barbiturates, ataractics/tranquilizers, phenothiazine derivatives, narcotic analgesics, anticholinergics, amnesics, and narcotic antagonists. Examples of each of these classifications are given in Table 17–1.

ANESTHESIA DURING LABOR

Anesthesia generally refers to loss of feeling or a loss of sensation, particularly the loss of the sensation of pain. Labor pain is associated with increased maternal catecholamine secretion and hyperventilation. Both of these result in decreased uteroplacental perfusion and resultant fetal hypoxia. Well-performed anesthesia may produce positive effects not only in the mother but also in the fetus.

The goal of obstetrical anesthesia is *safe* relief of pain and discomfort for mothers who request or require it, and safety for the fetus. Safe obstetrical anesthesia depends upon the knowledge, skill, and expertise of the anesthetist or anesthesiologist.

Choice of Anesthesia

When selecting anesthesia for an obstetrical patient, many factors are considered. No one method is used for all obstetrical patients. Preexisting medical problems in the obstetrical patient such as cardiac disease, diabetes mellitus, and anemia will influence the choice

TABLE 17–1
ANALGESIA DURING LABOR

Classification	Maternal Effects	Fetal Effects	Nursing Interventions
			General: Explain expected action Determine need for medication Institute safety measures Proper recording Monitor FHT Monitor UC Assess labor status Utilize comfort measures
Sedative/Barbiturate			
Secobarbital sodium (Seconal) Pentobarbital sodium (Nembutal) Amobarbital (Amytal)	Relief of anxiety and promotes sleep	Neonatal depression Crosses placenta freely Decreased sucking reflex for 4 to 5 days after birth Decreased muscle tone	Best effect if given early in latent phase of first stage of labor Give with extreme caution if maternal liver or renal involvement Review chart for allergies Assess B/P, P, R, level of consciousness, FHR, uterine contractions
Ataractics/Tranquilizers			
Diazepam (Valium) Hydroxyzine pamoate (Vistaril)	Acts on limbic system, thalamus, and hypothalamus and induces calming effects Potentiates effects of narcotics (can reduce dose of narcotics by 1/3 to 1/2)	Decreased muscle tone High doses of diazepam may produce lethargy, hypothermia, respiratory depression Crosses the placenta rapidly	If diazepam given IV, inject slowly, taking at least 1 minute for each 5 mg given. Inject into a large vein. Do not mix with or dilute with other solutions or drugs Monitor maternal vital signs, FHT, labor status
Phenothiazine Derivatives			
Promethazine hydrochloride (Phenergan)	Potentiates the action of narcotic analgesics due to sedative and antihistamine effect	Decreased muscle tone FHR monitoring effects are loss of short-term variability	Maximum total dose in 24 hours should not exceed 100 mg
Narcotic Analgesics			
Meperidine (Demerol) Morphine sulfate Fentanyl (Sublimaze) Alphaprodine (Nisentil) Nalbuphine (Nubain)	May accelerate labor as patient relaxes Analgesia Sedation If given in latent phase can depress contractile patterns and prolong labor	Neonatal respiratory depression Fetal/neonatal blood level is 70% maternal Bradycardia Hypothermia Readily crosses through placenta	Administer in active phase of first stage of labor Do not give if delivery is expected within 2 hours Check maternal vital signs, FHR, cervical dilation before and 30 minutes after administration Assess for pain relief

TABLE 17-1 (continued)

Classification	Maternal Effects	Fetal Effects	Nursing Interventions
Amnesics			
Scopolomine hydrochloride	Dulls memory May cause extreme restless and agitation Does not affect pain Depresses parasympathetic nervous system	Respiratory depression Crosses the placenta Fetal tachycardia or bradycardia	Give with narcotic to decrease incidence of excitement and hallucinations Stay with patient Monitor maternal vital signs, FHT, UC, labor status
Narcotic Antagonists			
Levallorphan tartrate (Lorfan Injectable) Naloxone hydrochloride (Narcan)	Reverses narcotic depression Narcan prevents or reverses pain relief intensity	Reverses narcotic depression	Note medications given to mother, time, amount, route Ineffective against respiratory depression due to barbiturates Do not give Narcan to addicted mother, it will cause immediate withdrawal symptoms

of anesthesia, as will the presence of complications peculiar to pregnancy, such as antepartum bleeding, pregnancy-induced hypertension, and labor complications. Other factors important in choosing anesthesia include assessment of the time and amount of food ingested before the onset of labor, fetal maturity, anesthesia availability, and the client's wishes.

Inhalation Anesthesia

NITROUS OXIDE AND OXYGEN

A mixture of nitrous oxide and oxygen is one of the safer inhalation agents used for pain relief during labor and delivery. It affords excellent analgesia without accumulation in the body. Used intermittently with each uterine contraction, the patient is able to cooperate in bearing down. The depth of anesthesia obtained can be altered quickly if necessary. Unless maternal anoxia occurs, there is no untoward effect on the circulatory, respiratory, or nervous system.

When a nitrous oxide and oxygen mixture is administered to the client, fetal concentrations approach maternal concentrations within 15 to 19 minutes, increasing the danger of neonatal depression with continued use. The client may become confused or apprehensive with continued administration.

Nursing Responsibilities

Before nitrous oxide and oxygen mixtures are administered, assessment of maternal intake of food is important. Check for the presence of dentures, chewing gum, or anything else that the patient may choke on or aspirate. Oxygen and suction must be available. Maternal vital signs and the fetal heart rate are monitored. Only one person should give the patient instructions on breathing, pushing, and relaxing.

During second stage uterine contractions the patient is instructed to take two or three deep breaths of the mixture, hold her breath, and bear down. If necessary, she should take another breath of the mixture and bear down again. As the contraction begins to decrease in intensity, pure oxygen is given to increase fetal oxygenation.

TRILENE

Trichloroethylene (Trilene) is a volatile liquid inhalation anesthetic that has a pleasant odor, is nonirritating, and does not cause an increase in salivary or tracheobronchial secretions. It can be self-administered with an inhaler under supervision by regulating the setting on the inhaler that is held by the patient.

Trilene remains in the body for 12 hours or more. With prolonged administration, the neonate may be depressed at birth. Other potential effects include maternal narcotic depression, tachycardia, and cardiac arrhythmias. Nausea and vomiting may also occur.

Easily decomposed by light and heat, Trilene can cause cranial nerve damage. It becomes toxic when mixed with alkalis. Anesthesia machines that have soda lime absorbers must not be used during delivery if Trilene has been administered during labor.

Nursing Responsibilities

Assessment of maternal food intake is done before Trilene is administered. Check for the presence of anything that may predispose to choking. Oxygen and suction should be available. Maternal vital signs and fetal heart tones are monitored.

With self-administration, continuous inhalation is not allowed, to prevent drowsiness and disorientation. If the client becomes drowsy or if narcotics are given, the concentration setting should be lowered. Discontinue Trilene if maternal tachypnea, irregular pulse rate, or nausea occur. The anesthetist or anesthesiologist must be advised that the patient has used Trilene during labor.

Teaching of proper administration to the client should be accomplished between uterine contractions. She is instructed to hold the mask lightly over her mouth and nose during uterine contractions and to breathe in room air along with the anesthetic. Hyperventilation and shallow respirations should be avoided.

PENTHRANE

Methoxyflurane (Penthrane) can also be self-administered by the client during labor. This potent nonflammable analgesic has a pleasant odor. It usually has no adverse effects on uterine contractions or on neonatal Apgar scores at birth.

The effects of Penthrane are cumulative. Once an analgesic level has been reached, it is easily renewed when the client inhales at the onset of a uterine contraction. Prolonged administration throughout labor and delivery is not recommended because maternal restlessness and lack of cooperation may result. Overdosage leads to serious maternal depression, cardiac arrhythmias, and renal and hepatic toxicity, as well as to accumulation in the fetus.

Nursing Responsibilities

As with any inhalation anesthetic, assessment of maternal food intake is important. Check for the presence of anything that may lead to choking. Maternal vital signs and fetal heart rate are monitored, particularly noting decreases in the blood pressure and respiratory rate. She may experience transient dizziness, and tingling and numbness of the extremities.

Teaching proper self-administration is accomplished in the same way as with Trilene. It is important that no one hold the mask for the client. The mask must not be propped, as this would prevent the mask from falling away from the face if she loses consciousness.

General Anesthesia

General anesthesia is rarely indicated in uncomplicated vaginal deliveries but may be necessary in obstetrical emergencies. These anesthetics reach the fetus through placental transfer, and may cause neurologic and respiratory depression in the newborn.

During general anesthesia administration, an adequate airway is maintained at all times to prevent the sequelae of improper ventilation hypoxia, and hypercarbia that may lead to ventricular fibrillation or cardiac arrest.

The greatest incidence of maternal mortality occurs with aspiration pneumonitis. Digestive action of the gastrointestinal tract is inhibited during labor, and any food in the stomach when labor begins remains undigested. When general anesthesia is given to the obstetrical patient, about 1 in 10 have an emesis. If the vomitus is aspirated, hypoxemia from the airway obstruction occurs, followed by an intense bronchospasm. The patient becomes restless and may be quite agitated. The respiratory rate increases as air hunger, cyanosis, and tachycardia occur. Rales, rhonchi, and wheezing occur, and frothy pink pulmonary secretions are noted. If the sequence of events is not altered, heart failure and shock may occur, with fatal results.

The maternity nurse should never be involved with administration of general anesthesia. These agents are only to be administered by a person trained in anesthesia administration, i.e. a certified registered nurse anesthetist (CRNA) or an anesthesiologist.

Peripheral Nerve Blocks

Peripheral nerve blocks anesthetize a specified anatomic area. They block neural pathways and result in a temporary interruption in the pain pathway. Anesthetic agents commonly used in a 0.5 to 2 percent solution include lidocaine hydrochloride, procaine hydrochloride, bupivacaine hydrochloride, tetracaine hydrochloride, and mepivacaine hydrochloride. Drugs used for nerve blocks are vasodilators. It is possible to potentiate the action of these anesthetic agents by supplementing them with epinephrine, a vasoconstrictor. Adding a vasoconstrictor makes it possible to prolong the effects of the anesthetic agent by causing local vasoconstriction, which allows the agent to stay in contact with the tissue for a longer time. It also reduces the possibility of the anesthetic agent reaching a toxic blood level.

LOCAL INFILTRATION

Local infiltration of the perineum is useful for perineal repairs. Administration is done by the physician.

Nursing Responsibilities

On admission, assessment of allergy history is done. After administration, maternal response is monitored for pain relief, adverse reactions, and hypotension.

PUDENDAL BLOCK

A pudendal block is a form of anesthesia in which a local anesthetic is injected near the pudendal nerve next to the ischial spines. The pudendal nerve derives from sacral 2, 3, and 4 and supplies the perineal area, vulva, and vagina.

Administration is through the vagina, with a 5- to 6-inch needle guided by an Iowa trumpet (see Fig. 17–1). Impulses from the pudendal, posterior femoral cutaneous, ileoinguinal, and

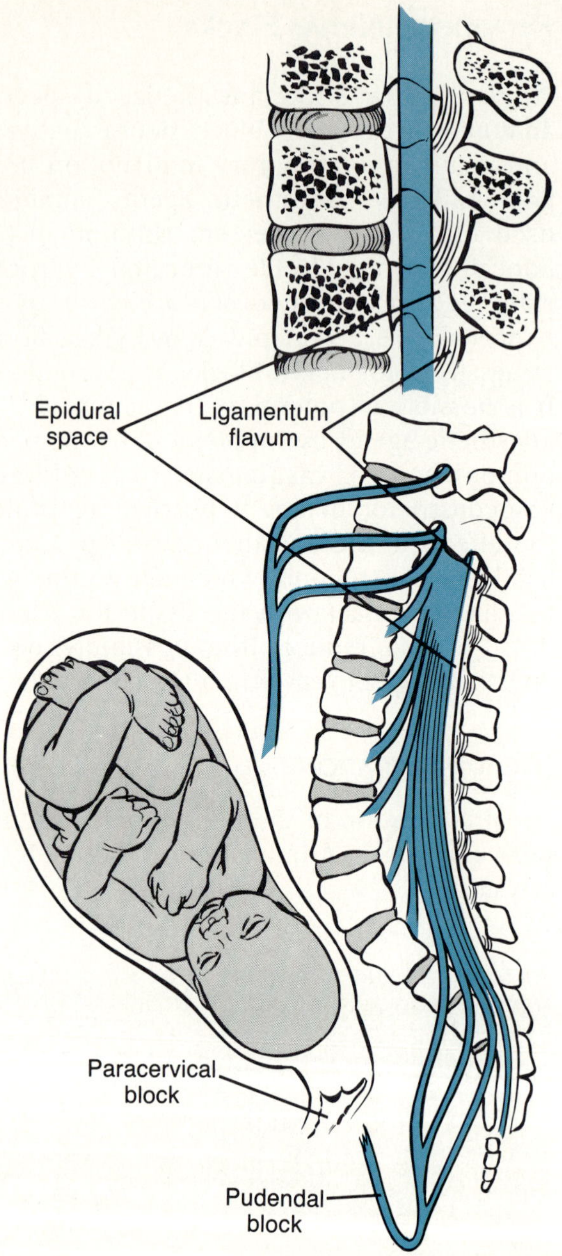

FIGURE 17-1. Schematic of full term gravida illustrating sites for injection of pudendal block, paracervical block, caudal anesthesia, lumbar epidural, and spinal anesthesia.

hemorrhoidal nerves are blocked, and the lower two thirds of the vagina and the perineum are anesthetized, without relief of uterine contraction discomfort.

Pudendal block is of short duration, lasting approximately 30 minutes to 1 hour. The patient is conscious and can take an active part in birth. No fetal depression occurs.

Nursing Responsibilities

Thorough explanation to the client is essential to obtain her cooperation. History of allergies is assessed before administration. The bearing-down reflex may be inhibited, and additional instruction and encouragement during pushing is needed. Maternal vital signs, fetal heart rate, and uterine contractions are monitored.

PARACERVICAL BLOCK

Paracervical block is transvaginal injection of a local anesthetic agent into the tissue on either side of the cervix. It blocks the inferior hypogastric plexus (see Fig. 17–1) and anesthetizes the cervix and upper two thirds of the vagina.

The initial dose is most commonly given at 4 cm cervical dilation with the presenting part at a +1 station. It is administered by the physician in the labor or birthing room, with the patient in a lithotomy position. A needle guide is used to prevent penetration of the needle more than 0.2 cm into tissue. Aspiration for blood is done before and during injection to prevent accidental intravascular administration. Relief of pain is felt within 3 to 5 minutes and lasts 1 to 3 hours. The block may be repeated as necessary.

Paracervical block relieves the pain of uterine contractions and decreases cervical stretching sensations. It may cause more rapid cervical dilation by promoting cervical relaxation.

Maternal complications include damage to uterine vessels, hematoma formation, and infection. Systemic toxic reactions may also occur from sensitivity to the anesthetic agent, too rapid absorption, or inadvertent intravenous administration. With inadvertent intravenous injection or rapid absorption of large doses there may be a direct maternal toxic effect, leading to dizziness, syncope, and vascular collapse.

The anesthetic agent may be accidently injected into the fetal scalp. Owing to the rapid absorption in the vascular paracervical area, the fetus may be affected, leading to fetal bradycardia, depression, and even death. The initial bradycardia is caused by the direct anesthetic effect on the fetal myocardium, the central nervous system, or both. If the bradycardia is moderate, the insult to the fetus is minimal. With marked and prolonged bradycardia, the fetus may become compromised due to hypoperfusion of tissues and placental insufficiency.

Nursing Responsibilities

Assessment for history of anesthetic allergy is done on admission to the labor room. Thorough explanation of the anesthesia is provided to the client and the support person. Maternal vital signs are monitored before, during, and after paracervical block. If maternal resuscitation is needed, airway maintenance, treatment of hypoxia and hypertension, cardiac massage, and control of convulsions may be necessary.

The fetal heart rate is monitored closely after injection of the anesthetic agent. Nursing interventions are instituted for bradycardia or distress patterns (see Chapter 16).

Uterine contraction patterns are monitored and cervical dilation is assessed at frequent intervals. The patient may not notice signs of impending delivery.

Nerve Root Blocks

Nerve root blocks, which are administered by trained anesthesia personnel, relieve uterine contraction and perineal pain. An anesthetic agent is injected into the appropriate nerve root and blocks pain pathways.

All regional anesthetics tend to alter the fetal environment and inhibit the client's ability to push effectively in the second stage of labor. Indirect effects may include maternal hypotension, caused by vasodilation below the level of anesthesia, and fetal bradycardia following uncorrected maternal hypotension. Direct effects result from maternal reaction to the anesthetic agent used and include acidosis and convulsions.

Some basic contraindications are shared by all nerve root blocks: (1) a known allergy to the anesthetic solution; (2) preexisting and active neurologic disease; (3) coagulation and platelet defects; (4) uncontrollable hemorrhage owing to blockage of reactive vasoconstriction; (5) infection of the proposed injection site; and (6) patient fear and refusal of nerve root block anesthesia.

CAUDAL ANESTHESIA

Caudal anesthesia is obtained by blocking nerves in the peridural space at the sacral hiatus (see Fig. 17–1). The caudal space is located within the sacrum at the lowest part of the bony spine.

For administration, the client is placed in a modified Sims' or knee-chest position. After the needle is inserted, attempts to aspirate spinal fluid are made. If spinal fluid is obtained, the procedure is discontinued. Anesthesia of short duration is obtained with a single injection of anesthetic. A continuous caudal anesthesia may be obtained by leaving a special polyethylene tube in place for further injections.

Caudal anesthesia provides pain relief in the first and second stages of labor. Continuous caudals are instituted at about 4 or 5 cm cervical dilation. Effects are obtained in 5 to 30 minutes following injection. The client remains awake and can take an active part in the birth.

Patients with metabolic diseases, pregnancy-induced hypertension, and respiratory or cardiac diseases benefit from the decreased amount of narcotic analgesia given for pain relief.

If analgesia or anesthesia is satisfactory, pelvic sensations are lessened and uterine contraction pain is relieved. The lower extremities are tingly and numb, and motor weakness develops. There is little inhibition of uterine contractions. Good perineal relaxation occurs.

Maternal hypotension may occur following administration. There is little fetal effect unless maternal hypotension occurs and goes uncorrected.

Nursing Responsibilities

On admission a history of allergy to anesthetic agents is obtained, as well as previous spinal or neural injury, and attitude toward anesthesia. The client's back is checked to ensure that no skin infection exists. Nursing actions during and after administration are discussed with lumbar epidural block.

LUMBAR EPIDURAL BLOCK

Lumbar epidural block is a versatile form of nerve root block. It can be used for many different operative and obstetrical situations. Injection of an anesthetic solution into the epidural space in the lumbar region provides extradural anesthesia (see Fig. 17–1). A needle is inserted between L2 and L3 or L3 and L4, and a small plastic catheter is threaded into the epidural space without puncturing the dura.

Before a lumbar epidural is initiated, the client must be in active labor, contractions must be regular and last a minimum of 40 seconds, the presenting part must be engaged, and cervical dilation must be at least 4 cm.

During the first stage of labor the epidural block can be limited to the lower thoracic and upper lumbar segments without involving the sacral segments, providing pain relief without interfering with Ferguson's reflex and internal rotation of the fetal head. During the second stage of labor the block is extended to the sacral segments to provide perineal anesthesia.

Advantages of a continuous epidural block include alertness and cooperativeness of the client. She feels little discomfort, and exhaustion is reduced. High levels of epinephrine are associated with longer labors. Abnormal fetal heart rate patterns and lower Apgar scores are associated with increased levels of epinephrine. Lumbar epidural anesthesia reduces maternal epinephrine levels by eliminating the psychological and physical stress associated with painful uterine contractions (Schnider, 1985). It may enhance labor and improve fetal outcome.

Maternal oxygen consumption during labor influences the development of metabolic acidosis. Painful uterine contractions are associated with hyperventilation, hypocapnia, an increase in oxygen consumption, decreased pH, and an increase in lactic acidosis. These all contribute to the development of maternal metabolic acidosis. Epidural anesthesia provides good analgesia and decreases maternal oxygen consumption.

Disadvantages of lumbar epidural anesthesia include both maternal and fetal effects. The most common complication is maternal hypotension. A slight degree of hypotension is expected, owing to the blockage of sympathetic nerve fibers with resulting vasodilation. A significant drop in maternal blood pressure will decrease uterine blood flow and may result in fetal hypoxia.

There is disagreement about uterine activity alterations following epidural anesthesia, with some studies supporting the prolongation of labor by decreased uterine activity (McDonald, 1982), while others find no prolonged or abnormal labor patterns (Schnider, 1985).

Accidental dural puncture, resulting in total spinal anesthesia, may occur with insertion of the epidural needle and catheter. Indications of total spinal anesthesia include respiratory depression, hypotension, circulatory collapse, and decreased uterine blood flow.

A seizure may occur following injection of the anesthetic agent from accidental intravenous injection, toxic blood levels of the medication, and total spinal anesthesia (Ralston and Schnider, 1979).

Other maternal disadvantages may also exist with epidural anesthesia. There may be an increased incidence of forcep deliveries. Bladder dysfunction may follow, owing to the loss of sensation of voiding. The catheter may break off or slip out of place. Psychological deprivation is reported by some women following epidural anesthesia.

Fetal effects include bradycardia, lack of FHR variability, and late decelerations resulting from uncorrected maternal hypotension that leads to decreased uterine blood flow.

Epidural anesthesia in obstetrics is versatile and has a wide margin of safety for the mother and the fetus when proper safety precautions are instituted before, during, and after administrations.

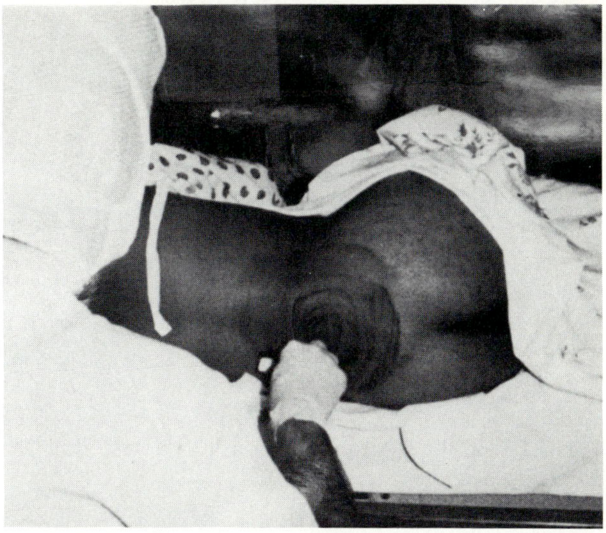

FIGURE 17-2. Cleaning the skin with antiseptic agent prior to epidural anesthesia.

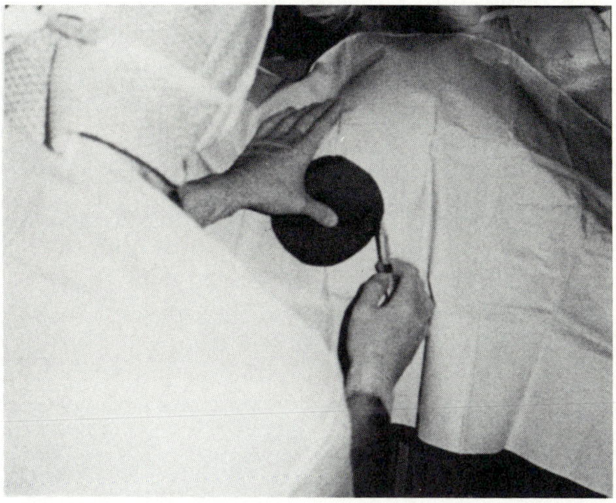

FIGURE 17-3. Identification of landmarks prior to infiltration with local anesthetic agent.

Nursing Responsibilities

Nursing responsibilities before lumbar epidural anesthesia include obtaining ordered laboratory tests, including a PTT and prothrombin time. The client should receive a thorough explanation to obtain her cooperation. She is asked to void before the catheter is inserted to avoid overdistention of the bladder as labor progresses. Baseline vital signs and fetal heart tones are obtained, and the client is assisted to the proper position (Figs. 17-2 to 17-5). Oxygen is administered per nasal cannula to maintain maternal and fetal oxygenation.

Following a lumbar epidural block, maternal vital signs and the fetal heart tone are assessed every 5 to 15 minutes. If hypotension develops, the client is turned to her left side, the legs are elevated, and the intravenous rate is increased. Uterine contraction status is monitored for labor progress.

SUBARACHNOID BLOCK

With a *subarachnoid block* (saddle block), a small amount of anesthetic is injected into the spinal fluid in the subarachnoid space (see Fig. 17-1). To administer the block, the patient sits up with the spine straight and the shoulders supported. When the needle is inserted, the patient should push the lumbar vertebrae out to widen the interspaces. After injection be-

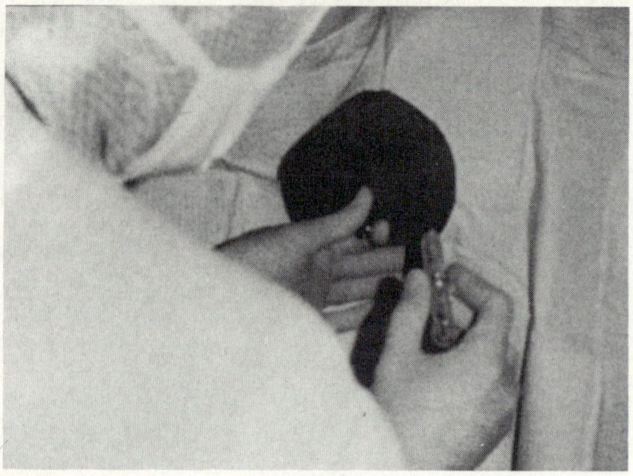

FIGURE 17–4. Preparing to inject 2 ml test dose of regional anesthetic.

tween uterine contractions, the client must remain upright for 30 to 60 seconds to assure descent of the anesthetic agent.

Subarachnoid blocks are quick, sure, and last about an hour. The anesthetic agent does not enter the fetal circulation. The patient is conscious and pain free, although the ability to push effectively is diminished.

It is possible to introduce contaminants into the spinal fluid and cause meningitis. If there is leakage of spinal fluid, postspinal headache may result. The level of anesthesia may ascend, causing respiratory difficulties.

Nursing Responsibilities

Aseptic technique is essential to avoid introduction of pathogens into the spinal fluid. Proper positioning of the client for injection is important. At a specified time following injection, the client is placed on her back with her head on a pillow to keep the neck sharply flexed. Trendelenberg position is not used following subarachnoid block to prevent ascent of the level of anesthesia.

To prevent and relieve postspinal headache, the client should remain flat for several hours after delivery. Fluids are encouraged, at least 3000 ml per 24 hours.

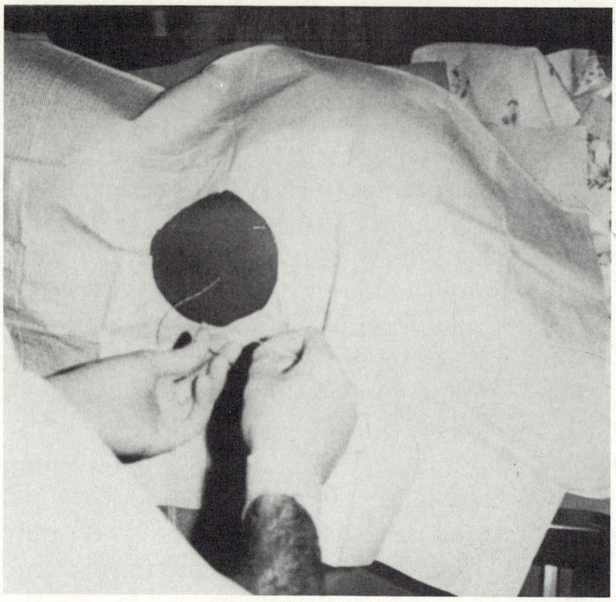

FIGURE 17–5. Plastic catheter in place for continuous epidural anesthesia.

An epidural injection of saline or a blood patch (10 ml of the client's blood is drawn) is injected into the epidural space, causing clot formation, which prevents further leakage of spinal fluid.

SPINAL ANESTHESIA

Spinal anesthesia is a form of regional anesthesia produced by injection of an anesthetic solution into the cerebrospinal fluid in the spinal canal. It is most commonly used for cesarean sections in obstetric patients.

With the patient on her side, a spinal needle is inserted into the cerebrospinal fluid at the L2, L3, or L4 interspace (see Fig. 17–1). This type of anesthesia has a rapid onset of action, certain block, and a low failure rate when performed properly. Hypotension and postspinal headaches are the two most common problems encountered with spinal anesthesia.

The choice of analgesia or anesthesia during labor and delivery should reflect the combined input of the client, the obstetrician, and the anesthetist or anesthesiologist. Whenever possible, the wishes and desires of the client concerning pain relief should be respected unless this choice is harmful to her or the fetus. Nursing assessments and interventions reflect a genuine interest in the client and the fetus, and in promotion of optimal maternal and fetal outcome.

BIBLIOGRAPHY

Basmajian, J.: *Biofeedback. Principles and practice for clinicians,* 2nd Ed. Baltimore: Williams and Wilkins, 1983.

Beck, N.C. & Siegel, L.J. Preparation for childbirth and contemporary research on pain, anxiety, and stress reduction: A review and critique. *Psychosomatic Medicine,* 1980, **42,** 429-447.

Brownridge, P.R., Taylor, G. & Ralston, D.H. Neural blockade for obstetrics and gynecology. In M.J. Cousins & P, O. Bridenbaugh (Eds.). *Neural blockade in clinical anesthesia and management of pain.* Philadelphia: Lippincott, 1980.

Brucker, M.C. Nonpharmaceutical methods for relieving pain and discomfort during pregnancy, *MCN,* 1984, **9,** 390-394.

Bundesen, P., et al. Pain relief in labor by transcutaneous electrical nerve stimulation. A prospective matched study. *ACTA Obstetrics & Gynecology Scandinavia,* 1981, **60,** 459-468.

Butani, P. & Hodnett, E. Mother's perceptions of their labor experiences. *MCN,* 1980, **9,** 73-82.

Dilts, P.V., Jr. Obstetric analgesia and anesthesia. *Clinical Obstetrics & Gynecology,* 1981, **24,** 519ff.

Gorvine, B., Hawkins, J.W., Fazekas, N. & Motti, S. *Health care of women. Labor and delivery.* Monterey, Calif.: Wadsworth, 1982.

Jiminez, S.L.M. Application of the body's natural pain relief mechanisms to reduce discomfort in labor and delivery. *NAACOG Update Series,* 1983, **1,** 1-6.

Lederman, R.P., et al. Relationships of psychological factors in pregnancy to progress in labor. *Nursing Research,* 1979, **28,** 94-97.

MacLaughlin, S.M. & Taubenheim, A.M. Epidural anesthesia for obstetric patients. *Journal of Obstetric, Gynecological & Neonatal Nursing,* 1981, **10,** 9-15.

McDonald, J.S. Obstetric analgesia and anesthesia. In R.C. Benson (Ed.). *Current obstetric and gynecologic diagnosis and treatment.* Los Altos, Calif.: Lange, 1982.

Melzack, R. & Wall, P.D. *The challenge of pain.* New York: Basic Books, 1983.

Morison, D.H. & Smedstad, K.G. Continuous infusion epidurals for obstetric analgesia. *Canadian Anaesthesiology Society Journal,* 1985, **32,** 101-104.

Nicolls, E.T., Corke, B.C. & Ostheimer, G.W. Epidural anesthesia for the woman in labor. *American Journal of Nursing,* 1981, **81,** 1826-1830.

Nigl, A.: *Biofeedback. Behavioral strategies in pain treatment* New York: Medical and Scientific Books, 1984.

Ralston, D.H. & Schnider, S.M. The fetal and neonatal effects of regional anesthesia in obstetrics. *Anesthesiology,* 1978, **48,** 34-64.

Roberts, J.E. Factors influencing distress from pain during labor, *MCN,* 1983, **8,** 62-66.

Schnider, S.M. Fetal and maternal benefits of obstetric anesthesia for labor. Presented at Changing Practice of Obstetrical Anesthesia for Normal and High Risk Pregnancy seminar., San Francisco, Calif., March 21, 1985.

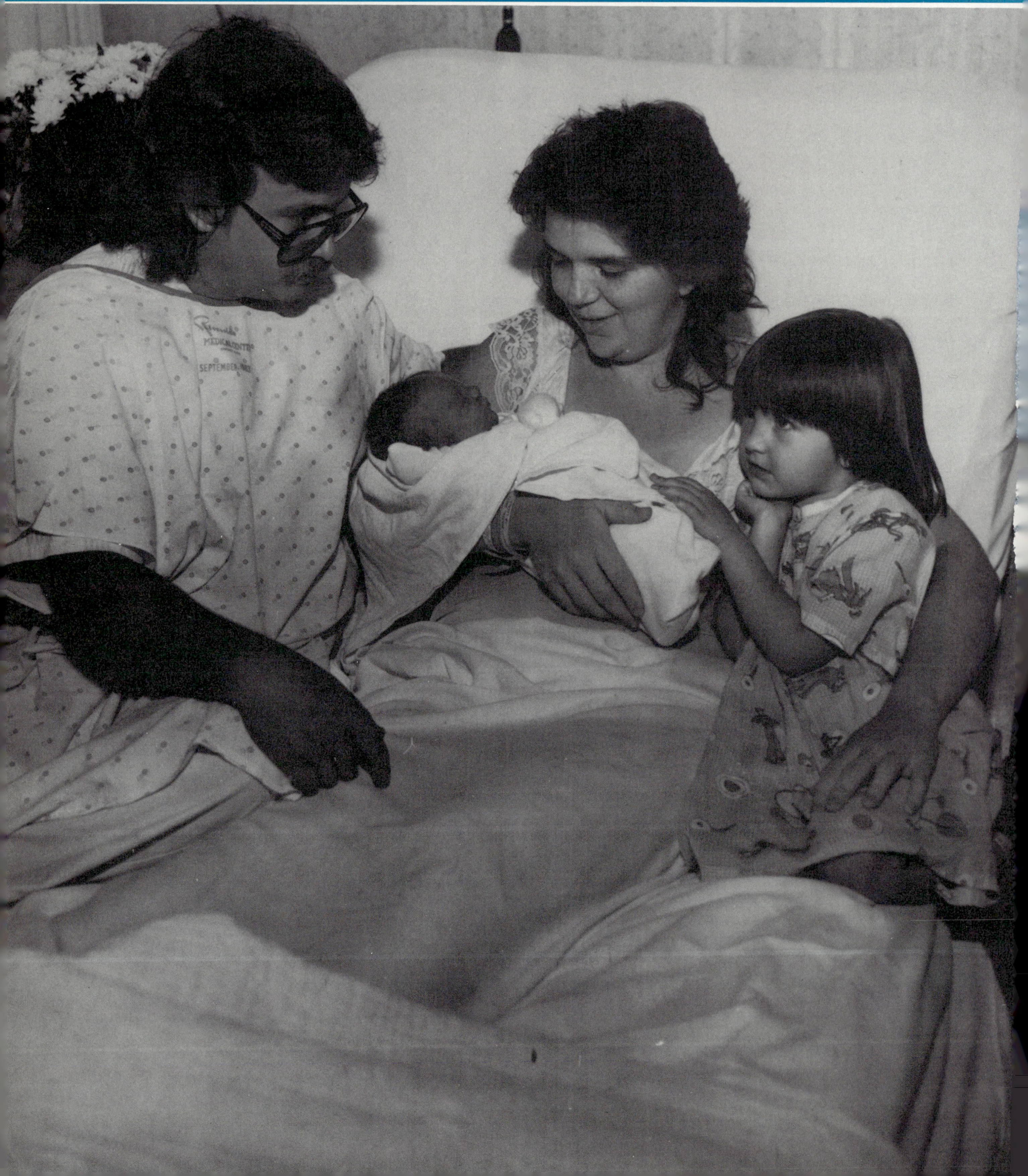
SEPTEMBER

UNIT V

THE POSTPARTAL FAMILY

UNIT V

THE POSTPARTAL FAMILY

chapter 18

PHYSIOLOGIC ASPECTS OF THE PUERPERIUM

OBJECTIVES

Upon completion of this chapter, the reader will be able to:

1. Define puerperium.
2. Describe the process of uterine involution.
3. Identify physiologic system changes that occur during the puerperium.
4. Describe progressive lochial changes that occur during the puerperium.
5. Identify the time interval following delivery for the return of ovulation and of menstruation.

KEY TERMS

Autolysis
Carunculae myrtiformes
Colostrum
Diastasis recti
Exfoliation
Involution
Lochia
Lochia alba
Lochia rubra
Lochia serosa
Morbidity temperature
Puerperal bradycardia
Puerperium

The *puerperium*, or postpartum period, is defined as the six-week period following the completion of the third stage of labor, during which the reproductive organs return to the prepregnant state. In the first few days following delivery, rapid physiologic changes take place to aid in restoration of maternal homeostasis. In the next few weeks, the changes that occur are more gradual.

In order to provide the nursing care needed to give the postpartum family a good start, an understanding of the physiologic changes that take place is needed.

REPRODUCTIVE ORGANS

Uterus

Immediately following delivery of the placenta and membranes, the contracted uterus can be felt at the level of the umbilicus or slightly lower. It is about the size of a grapefruit, with the fundus resting on the sacral promontory. At this time it is approximately 14 cm long, 12 cm wide and 10 cm thick (the size of a normal pregnant uterus at 16 weeks gestation), and weighs about 1000 gm or 2.2 pounds. The myometrial walls are collapsed together and are about 4 to 5 cm thick.

INVOLUTION

In the first minutes following placental expulsion, as uterine contraction takes place, the fundus of the uterus may be palpated through the abdominal wall approximately halfway between the umbilicus and the symphysis pubis. Within one hour after delivery it rises to the level of the umbilicus and remains at that level for the next 24 hours. From 24 hours postpartum on, the uterus will decrease a fingerbreath (approximately 1 cm) per day in size (see Fig. 18–1). In the average patient, the uterus cannot be palpated abdominally by the tenth day postpartum.

On palpation, the uterine fundus can usually be felt in the midline, but it may be palpated slightly to the right, owing to the rotation that took place during pregnancy. Uterine palpation is done shortly after voiding, because a full bladder may keep the uterus from contracting, push it upward, and give a false reading of uterine involution.

Decrease in uterine size following delivery takes place through the process of involution. The amount of cytoplasm in the myometrial cells of the uterus decreases. Uterine muscle protein is broken down into simpler compounds that are excreted in the urine. By the end of one week postpartum, the uterus weighs approximately 500 gm (1.1 pound), by two weeks postpartum 350 gm (11 ounces), and at six weeks 50 to 60 gm.

Uterine involution may be retarded in the presence of obstetric conditions such as multiple gestation, polyhydramnios, maternal exhaustion from prolonged labor, difficult delivery, grand multiparity, or excessive anesthesia. Uterine contraction may be delayed when pieces of the placenta or membranes are retained in the uterus or when the bladder is full.

Assessing the height and consistency of the uterine fundus following delivery will determine normalcy of involution. A well-contracted uterus feels firm and has the consistency of a grapefruit.

Postpartum uterine involution may cause alternate contraction and relaxation of the uterus, commonly called "afterpains." These occur more frequently in multiparas than in primiparas and in mothers who are breastfeeding.

FALLOPIAN TUBES

By two weeks after delivery the fallopian tubes are atrophic with deciliated epithelium

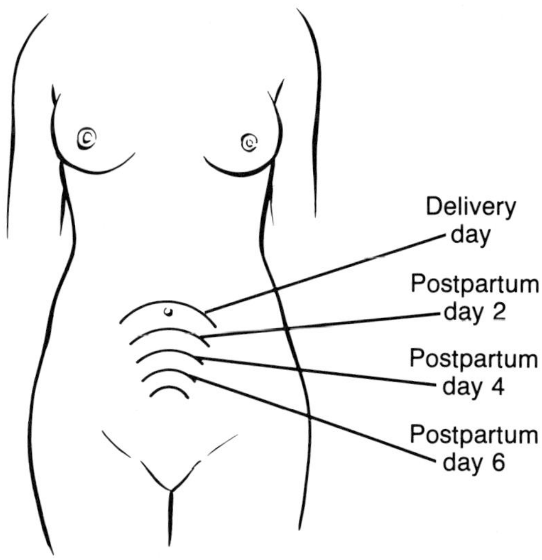

FIGURE 18-1. Normal heights of the uterus following delivery.

reflecting the low estrogen levels present following delivery.

ENDOMETRIUM

Within two to three days following delivery, the decidua that remains in the uterus differentiates into two layers. The superficial layer becomes necrotic and is cast off as lochia. The muscular layer remains intact and is the basis for the regeneration of new endometrium. This unique healing process enables the endometrium to resume its usual cyclic changes. Within 21 days the entire endometrium, with the exception of the placental site, is restored to the prepregnant state.

INVOLUTION OF THE PLACENTAL SITE

Immediately after delivery, the placental site is irregular and consists of thrombosed vascular areas. Involution of the site occurs through the process of *exfoliation,* in which the placental site is undermined by an ingrowth of new endometrial tissue. By six weeks postpartum the placental site has regenerated.

Failure of the placental site to heal completely is called *subinvolution of the placental site,* and symptoms include persistent lochial discharge with episodes of heavy, painless bleeding.

CERVIX

After a vaginal delivery, the cervix appears bruised, soft, and flabby, it may have small lacerations, and will admit two fingers. Within 18 hours it shortens and begins to regain its form as new muscle cells develop. By the end of a week, the cervical opening is about 2 cm, the lacerations heal, and new muscle cells form. At the end of the puerperium the internal cervical os is completely closed, while the external os remains slightly open and appears slitlike or stellate (star-shaped) where it was round before.

LOCHIA

Uterine discharge after delivery is called *lochia.* During the first few days postpartum it is called *lochia rubra,* which consists of blood and decidual debris, and is reddish in color. From the third to the eighth postpartum day, the lochia becomes pinkish in color, consists of erythrocytes, leukocytes, decidua, cervical mucus, and microorganisms, and is called *lochia serosa. Lochia alba,* seen from the eighth day until approximately three weeks after delivery, is creamy white in color, and contains serum, leukocytes, decidua, epithelial cells, mucus, and bacteria.

The amount of lochia discharged during the puerperium should approximate a menstrual flow and will vary from woman to woman. Mothers who breastfeed will have less lochial discharge than those who do not, owing to release of oxytocin from the anterior pituitary gland. Lochial flow will increase on exertion, especially with the first few ambulations following delivery, but will decrease with rest. This increase with ambulation is the result of pooling of lochia, not an increase in amount. Lifting heavy items or strenuous exercise will increase the amount of lochia. Saturating a perineal pad in less than 45 minutes is considered an abnormally heavy flow after the fourth stage of labor is completed, since a saturated perineal pad holds about 100 ml of blood.

Normally, lochia should contain no clots. If clotting is present, a portion of the placenta may have been retained, preventing closure of the uterine blood sinuses.

The pattern of flow from lochia rubra to lochia alba should not be reversed. If the pattern is reversed, placental fragments may have been retained or a decrease in uterine contraction may be present.

Lochial odor approximates that of menstrual flow and should not be offensive. If odor is offensive, a uterine infection may be present or increased hygiene measures may be needed. Absence of lochia may also indicate puerperal infection.

VAGINA

The vagina forms a spacious, smooth-walled cavity following vaginal delivery. During the puerperium, it gradually decreases in size, although it rarely returns to nulliparous dimensions. The mucosa is thin, owing to estrogen deprivation. Within three weeks, rugae begin to reappear. Carunculae myrtiformes, or hymenal tags, are often present at the vaginal outlet.

PERINEUM

The vaginal introitus may appear edematous and erythematous, especially if an episiotomy or laceration repair has been performed following delivery. During the puerperium, muscle tone is regained and healing occurs.

PELVIC MUSCULAR SUPPORT

Injury of the structures that support the uterus and vagina may occur during vaginal delivery and can cause gynecologic problems in later life if relaxation (lengthening and weakening of the fascial supports of pelvic structures) has taken place.

ABDOMINAL WALL

Because of the prolonged abdominal distention by the pregnant uterus and the rupture of elastic skin fibers, the abdominal wall is usually quite lax for several weeks after delivery. In the average puerperal patient, the abdominal wall returns to a nearly nonparous state by six to seven weeks postpartum, although some striae may remain. Abdominal muscles may remain separated from the midline (diastasis recti).

SYSTEMIC CHANGES

Urinary Tract

Immediately after delivery the bladder is edematous and hyperemic. The capacity is increased and there is a relative insensitivity to pressure from urine. Overdistention, incomplete emptying, and excessive amounts of residual urine are all common within the first few hours after delivery.

There is diuresis for two to five days after delivery, resulting from reversal of the increased blood volume, fluid retention, and increased glomerular filtration rate present during pregnancy. Glycosuria is common owing to lactose absorption from the mammary glands into the bloodstream. Acetonuria is also common, especially following a long labor. Proteinuria occurs in about 40 percent of postpartum women because of protein catabolism (autolysis) of the uterus. The dilated ureters and renal pelvis usually return to normal by six to eight weeks postpartum.

Circulatory System

CARDIAC OUTPUT

During the first few hours after delivery, the cardiac load is substantially increased owing to changes in the uterine blood vessels and the return of uterine blood to the general maternal circulation. Nonpregnant levels are attained within the first week postpartum.

BLOOD VOLUME

Changes in blood volume that occur postpartum depend on several factors: blood loss during labor and delivery and mobilization and excretion of extravascular water. By the third to fourth week after delivery the blood volume has returned to nonpregnant levels.

MATERNAL RESPONSE TO BLOOD LOSS

The majority of pregnant women can tolerate considerable blood loss during labor and delivery, owing to the hypovolemia that is normally present during pregnancy. Approximately 250 to 400 ml of blood are lost during a normal vaginal delivery.

During the early puerperium, three physiologic changes protect the woman from the effects of blood loss: (1) the elimination of uteroplacental circulation that reduces the size of the maternal vascular bed up to 15 percent; (2) the loss of endocrine functions of the placenta to remove the stimulus for vasodilatation; and (3) the mobilization of extravascular waste that has been stored during pregnancy.

VITAL SIGNS

Maternal vital signs measure the physiologic adaptations to the puerperium.

Temperature

A slight increase in maternal temperature may occur during the first 24 hours after delivery as a result of dehydration during labor and delivery. Temperature is taken orally because of the danger of vaginal contamination. A morbidity temperature during the puerperium is defined by the Joint Commission on Maternal Welfare as an oral temperature above 38°C (100.4°F), excluding the first 24 hours postpartum, with the temperature taken four times a day. On occasion, maternal temperature may be elevated on the third or fourth postpartum day in lactating mothers when the milk "comes in," but this temperature elevation should last only a short time.

Pulse

Puerperal bradycardia (50 to 70 BPM) occurs commonly during the early puerperium and is attributed to three causes: (1) the horizontal position commonly used for delivery; (2) the decreased fluid and nutritional intake during labor; and (3) the loss of fluids from the skin and uterus during labor and delivery.

Pulse rate should be evaluated carefully during the postpartum period. A rapid, thready pulse is a possible sign of hemorrhage. When assessing maternal pulse rate, it is important to remember the normal puerperal bradycardia that is present to identify rapid pulse rates.

Blood Pressure

Maternal blood pressure should remain within normal limits during the puerperium. Assessment of the blood pressure is important because of the information it gives about maternal bleeding. Blood pressure readings are compared with the predelivery readings rather than standard blood pressures, since normal variations in blood pressure occur.

Elevations in blood pressure of more than 30 mm Hg diastolic and 15 mm Hg systolic, or both, may indicate postpartal pregnancy-induced hypertension. Administration of oxytoxics may also cause temporary B/P elevation.

VARICOSITIES

Varicosities of the lower extremities that occur frequently during pregnancy often regress promptly after delivery. Vulvar varices also decrease following delivery.

CIRCULATION TO LOWER EXTREMITIES

Sluggish circulation to the lower extremities, a physiologic adaptation during pregnancy, continues during the early puerperium.

BLOOD CONSTITUENTS

Rather marked leukocytosis occurs during and after labor, with the white count sometimes reaching as high as 25,000 per mm^3. The increase is mainly in the granulocyte count. This, plus a normal increase in the erythrocyte sedimentation rate to 50 mm per hour or more, may confuse interpretation of acute infections during the early puerperium. These two changes help demonstrate that the body has mobilized its defense system against possible infection and is aiding in the many repairs taking place in the body.

The hemoglobin and hematocrit are often slightly over the prelabor values, reflecting a normal shift in body water that causes a greater decrease in plasma volume than in cellular components. These gradually return to normal within one week after delivery.

Coagulation factors I, II, VIII, IX, and X return to prepregnant levels within a few days after delivery. Fibrin split products are increased for the first seven to ten days following delivery, owing to their release from the placental site.

The total proteins and serum electrolytes return from their lower pregnancy levels to prepregnancy levels, as do the elevated plasma lipids.

Diaphoresis

Diaphoresis or excessive sweating is another way in which the body rids itself of excess fluid. This response is noticeable in the postpartum woman immediately after delivery.

Weight Loss

There is a loss of about 11 pounds at the time of delivery, with evacuation of the uterine contents. During the early puerperium, an additional six to eight pounds is commonly lost as a result of diuresis. The remainder of the weight gained during pregnancy is usually lost by the six-week checkup.

Postpartum Chill

A postpartum chill is not unusual in the first few hours following delivery. The exact cause is not known, but there are several factors that may contribute to its presence. Maternal nervous reaction and exhaustion as a result of labor can be manifest in chilling. Muscular exertion during labor and delivery can cause an imbalance in equilibrium of internal and external body temperature. Following the sudden release of intra-abdominal pressure with emptying of the uterus at the time of delivery the central nervous system is stimulated and may initiate a chill.

Postpartum chills may also represent maternal sensitization to elements of fetal blood and fetal/maternal transfusion at the time of delivery.

Respiratory System

During the early puerperium, many changes occur in respiratory function. An increase in residual volume, resting ventilation, and oxygen consumption occurs, with an accompanying decrease in vital capacity, inspiratory capacity, and maximum breathing capacity. Nonpregnant levels are reestablished by six months after delivery.

Lactation

During pregnancy, the breasts are exposed to high concentrations of estrogen, progesterone, and prolactin. Increased levels of insulin and human placental lactogen stimulate breast growth during the antepartal period.

The high estrogen levels present during pregnancy inhibit alveolar secretion in the breast by blocking prolactin binding, which in turn inhibits milk production.

Following delivery, estrogen, progesterone, HPL, and insulin levels decrease rapidly. By the second postpartum day, a modest amount of colostrum can be expressed from the nipples, and by approximately the third or fourth postpartum day the milk "comes in."

COLOSTRUM

Colostrum contains more protein in the form of globulin and more minerals than breast milk. Secretion of colostrum persists for about one week, with gradual conversion to mature breast milk. Colostrum contains antibodies in the form of immunoglobulins, in particular IgA, which offers protection against enteric infection. Colostrum also contains lactoferrin, lactoperoxidase, and lysozyme.

BREAST MILK

The major constituents of breast milk are protein, water, and fat. Major milk proteins are synthesized in the secretory cells of the alveoli. All vitamins except vitamin B_{12} are present in various amounts. There is little ascorbic acid, vitamin D, and iron.

ONSET OF LACTATION

With placental expulsion, an abrupt decrease in estrogen and progesterone levels aids in initiation of lactation. Prolactin is essential for lactation and a rise in prolactin levels is triggered by sucking. The neurohypophysis secretes oxytocin, which in turn stimulates expression of milk from the breast by causing myoepithelial cell contraction in the alveoli and small milk ducts. Once lactation is established, sucking is the most important stimulus to maintain milk production.

Endocrine System

PLACENTAL HORMONES

Plasma levels of placental hormones fall rapidly following delivery. Human chorionic somatomammotropin (HCS) (HPL) reaches undetectable levels within 24 hours after delivery. Human chorionic gonadotropin (HCG) levels also decline rapidly.

Estrogen levels in the maternal plasma fall to 10 percent of prenatal values within three hours after delivery, with lowest levels present by the seventh day. Progesterone levels fall below luteal levels by the third postpartum day and are not detectable in serum after one week. Resumption of progesterone production begins with the first ovulation following delivery.

PITUITARY HORMONES

Prolactin levels rise throughout pregnancy. Shortly after delivery in the mother who is not breastfeeding, these levels decline to pre-pregnancy ranges within two weeks. In the breastfeeding mother, high prolactin levels persist until cessation of breastfeeding.

RECURRENCE OF OVULATION AND MENSTRUATION

In the non-nursing mother, ovulation and menstruation usually return within four to six weeks after delivery. The exact time depends upon pituitary gland activity. The follicle-stimulating hormone produces a mature ovum within four to six weeks postpartum. Menstrual flow may be heavy for the first few menstrual periods following delivery.

Nursing mothers remain anovulatory for varying lengths of time. Some lactating mothers may have amenorrhea for as long as they nurse, even though ovulation has begun and pregnancy can occur.

OTHER ENDOCRINE CHANGES

Growth hormone secretion is depressed during late pregnancy and the early puerperal period. The low level of growth hormone and the decline in HCS, estrogen, cortisol, and insulinase, reduce the anti-insulin factors during the early puerperium. This alters insulin requirements for insulin-dependent diabetic mothers immediately after delivery.

Integumentary System

Following delivery, the striae gravidarum on the maternal abdomen still appear reddened and may even be more prominent than during pregnancy. These will gradually fade to a pale white in the Caucasian patient, and will be slightly darker in black patients. Chloasma and linea nigra will gradually disappear during the puerperium.

Gastrointestinal System

Digestion and absorption resume soon after labor and delivery. Hunger immediately following delivery is common.

Neurologic System

A reversal of maternal adaptations to pregnancy occurs in the neurologic system during the puerperium. Pregnancy-induced neurologic discomforts usually disappear shortly after delivery. Carpal tunnel syndrome that has been present during pregnancy abates with the diuresis that takes place.

A thorough knowledge of physiologic adaptations that occur in the normal postpartum patient will aid the nurse in planning effective care for mothers during the postpartum period.

BIBLIOGRAPHY

American Academy of Pediatrics and American College of Obstetricians and Gynecologists. *Guidelines for perinatal care*. Evanston, Ill., 1983.

Hathaway, W.E. & Bonnar, J. *Perinatal coagulation*. New York: Grune & Stratton, 1978.

Jennings, B. & Edmundson, M. The postpartum period after confinement. The fourth trimester. *Clinical Obstetrics & Gynecology*, 1980, **23**, 1093-1103.

Liu, J., Rebar, R.W., & Yen, S.S.C. Neuroendocrine control of the postpartum period. *Clinics in Perinatology*, 1983, **10**, 723-726.

Metcalfe, J., McAnulty, J.H. & Ueland, K. Cardiovascular physiology. *Clinical Obstetrics & Gynecology*, 1981, **24**, 693-708.

Monheit, A.G., Cousins, L. & Resnik, R. The puerperium—anatomic and physiologic readjustments. *Clinical Obstetrics & Gynecology*, 1980, **23**, 973-984.

chapter 19

PSYCHOLOGICAL ASPECTS OF THE PUERPERIUM

OBJECTIVES

Upon completion of this chapter, the reader will be able to:

1. List developmental tasks that confront all postpartum patients.
2. Describe taking in and taking hold; identify appropriate nursing interventions.
3. List symptoms commonly assessed in "postpartum blues."
4. State five conflicts that commonly occur in attainment of the parental role.
5. Describe maternal and paternal bonding behaviors.
6. Discuss nursing interventions that promote bonding.
7. Identify factors that influence parenting.
8. Discuss inclusion of siblings in the postpartum period.
9. Identify the importance of grandparents during the "fourth trimester."
10. Discuss adjustments needed during the "fourth trimester."

KEY TERMS

Bonding
"En face" position
Engrossment
Fourth trimester
Maternal task
Postpartum blues
Reciprocity
Rooming-in
Taking hold phase
Taking in phase

The puerperium is a time of many changes for the childbearing family. The delivery of a baby simultaneously expands and strains the family unit as the parents take on maternal and paternal roles.

During this period, which is often called the "fourth trimester" of pregnancy, the woman makes physiologic and psychological adjustments from being pregnant to being a mother, and the man becomes a father.

Loss During the Puerperium

Both the man and the woman experience losses following the birth of a baby. The father may feel isolated and of less importance to his partner. He may suffer from loss of sexual gratification and his comfortable patterns of daily living. The mother also experiences specific losses: the loss of the pregnant body, the temporary loss of control over bodily functions, the loss of self-control, and the loss of self-definition in social roles.

MATERNAL TASKS

Many developmental tasks must be completed during the fourth trimester (see Table 19–1). Certain factors influence maternal task attainment (see Table 19–2).

TABLE 19–1
MATERNAL DEVELOPMENTAL TASKS

Resolution of the pregnancy
Resolution of labor and delivery
Reconciliation of the real neonate with the antepartum fantasy infant
Continuance of acquaintance and attachment with the newborn
Replenishment of physical energy
Attainment of infant care skills
Reestablishment of the family unit to include the newest member

TABLE 19–2
FACTORS THAT INFLUENCE MATERNAL ATTACHMENT

Age
Labor and delivery perceptions
Separation from the neonate
Social stressors
Support system
Self-confidence
Maternal medical problems
Maternal obstetrical complications
Attitudes toward child raising
Neonatal temperament
Neonatal illness
Culture
Socioeconomic level

AGE

The young mother, under 20 years of age, is often not ready to assume the role of mothering. Insecurity in the maternal role compared with older mothers has been noted. The majority of adolescents continue to live with their extended families and maintain the already established support system. Women in their twenties and thirties are considered optimal both physically and psychologically to assume the mothering role.

LABOR AND DELIVERY PERCEPTIONS

The psychological impact of events during labor and delivery affect maternal task attainment. Complicated births are associated with significant delays in mothering.

SEPARATION FROM THE NEONATE

Prolonged separation from the neonate because of illness or prematurity delays maternal task attainment. Extended contact early in the puerperium is related to increased maternal attachment behaviors.

SOCIAL STRESS

Social stress may be related to pregnancy complications and thus to altered parenting.

SUPPORT SYSTEM

An established support system will have a positive influence on the development of mothering skills. Good marital relationships are linked with increased maternal warmth toward the neonate.

SELF-CONFIDENCE

Self-confidence and ego strength are considered basic determinants for attainment of maternal tasks and mothering. Highly impulsive women often have fussy neonates.

MATERNAL MEDICAL AND OBSTETRIC PROBLEMS

Maternal medical or obstetric problems during pregnancy or at the time of labor and delivery have a negative effect on self-esteem and drain energy that would otherwise be available for attainment of maternal roles.

CHILD REARING ATTITUDES

Attitudes toward child raising and child discipline influence interactions with the neonate.

NEONATAL TEMPERAMENT

Neonates that are easygoing add a positive influence to maternal attachment, whereas fussy neonates often create a negative reaction.

PHASES OF THE PUERPERIUM

Taking In Phase

The taking in phase of the puerperium is characterized by dependency needs and passivity. During this phase, which lasts from one to three days postpartum, the mother will take little initiative on her own. She takes in food, attention, and physical care. Every detail of the neonate is absorbed, although the mother may not initiate active caretaking. She has a need to talk about her labor and delivery in order to resolve the pregnancy.

NURSING INTERVENTIONS

Nursing interventions during the taking in phase include physical comfort measures such as backrubs and a sponge bath. Nonjudgmental listening to the client talk about her labor and delivery can aid in resolution. It is helpful if the nurse who cared for her during labor and delivery can be present to explain and offer positive reinforcement for behaviors exhibited during this time. Ample time is allowed with the neonate. A physical assessment of the neonate done in the mother's room, along with an explanation of findings, will point out the uniqueness of her baby.

Taking Hold Phase

The woman becomes more independent in both self and neonatal care, usually about the second or third postpartum day. She generally feels well, as physiologic stability is maintained. Lists of tasks to be done are made. Birth announcements are written. An active role in infant care is prevalent. She gains confidence in her own opinions about how things should be done.

NURSING INTERVENTIONS

The focus of nursing interventions during this phase changes to one of guidance and teaching of self and infant care skills. Positive reinforcement is necessary to encourage the move toward independence.

Postpartum Blues

Postpartum blues occur in the majority of postpartum clients on or about the third postpartum day. Predisposing factors include first pregnancy, pregnancy in the later child-bearing years, social isolation, ambivalence toward the woman's mother, prolonged or difficult labor, anxiety, marital disharmony, and crisis in the extended family unit.

Postpartum blues occur as the mother becomes aware of the gap between her aspirations and her actual capacities, between her self-expectations and her actual limitations, and between her drive and her actual available energy.

The depression in postpartum blues tends to occur in waves that last progressively longer, before disappearing. The first wave occurs on about the third postpartum day and lasts for several hours. In several days, another temporary wave of depression occurs.

MANIFESTATIONS

Manifestations of postpartum blues include fatigue, exhaustion, moodiness or mood swings, feelings of helplessness, feelings of inadequacy, feeling unloved and unlovable, feeling worthless, inability to concentrate, and lethargy.

NURSING INTERVENTIONS

The ability to listen in a nonjudgmental manner is essential when postpartum blues occur. Compassion is important in understanding the needs of the client. An understanding of the need to cry and express depression is necessary. Allowing the patient to cry is often more beneficial than attempting to provide diversion. The nurse must respect the patient's need to be alone or her need for company.

PARENTAL ROLE

A role is learned through the process of socialization. Roles are societal rituals that signify the change from one status to another and help to modify individual self-concepts to identify and integrate the new status.

DEVELOPMENT OF MATERNAL ROLE

The maternal role is a complex, culturally influenced, learned behavior in which the mother reorganizes, accepts, and meets her infant's dependency needs. Many conditions may affect mothering, including personality factors, environmental conditions, hormonal influences, childhood experiences, knowledge, and ignorance.

DEVELOPMENT OF PATERNAL ROLE

Fatherhood is complementary to the maternal role. The father sees in his newborn his hopes for self-realization and fulfillment. He often will become very involved in infant care as he acquires this role. Development of the paternal role is influenced by experiences in his own family and cultural norms, as well as by the extent of his participation in labor and delivery.

Conflicts in the Parental Role

A partner relationship is altered with the addition of a new family member. No longer can the man and woman belong only to each other. The established power relationship and division of labor are affected. Each parent may discover a different person in his or her partner. A sharp increase in role differentiation and role specialization occurs with infant care. The sexual relationship must be adapted to conform to the presence of a new family member. There may be difficulty in balancing the needs of the newborn with those of personal satisfaction. The opportunity for com-

TABLE 19-3
STRESSES OR CONFLICTS IN PARENTAL ROLE ATTAINMENT

Idealized vs. realistic role
Expectations vs. reality
Independence vs. dependence
Love vs. resentment
Self-realization through parenthood vs. self-realization through individual accomplishments

munication may be severely curtailed. There is often resentment by either or both partners caused by alterations in established family patterns.

Alterations in the partner relationship generate five main stresses or conflicts in attainment of the parental role (See Table 19–3).

IDEALIZED VS. REALISTIC ROLE

Early in life, little girls dream about being mothers. When a woman becomes pregnant, day dreams about ideal motherhood are common. A "good" mother will always be organized and will have all situations under control. Following delivery, she comes face to face with her newborn and reality. She is often unsure of her actions in caring for her newborn. The newborn makes demands when the mother is not physically or psychologically ready to meet them. If she feels inadequate in her mothering skills, a conflict occurs. Boys are taught early in life that the man is the provider, and that good fathers spend time with their children. When the reality of the newborn's schedule and pattern are realized and that this time is not available, he may feel inadequate, setting the stage for a conflict between the idealized and realistic father roles.

EXPECTATIONS VS. REALITY

Each parent dreams and fantasizes about his or her perfect newborn. The individual dreams and fantasies may be different, but the newborn is always perfect. Newborn infants are seldom beautiful; they may have blotchy skin, caput succedaneum, molding, and so on. The newborn makes demands and these must be met. When expectations and reality meet, conflict results.

INDEPENDENCE VS. DEPENDENCE

The mother's need to be dependent is very real in the early puerperium. At first she may be overwhelmed by birth, feeding her dependency needs. As she proceeds toward independence, decisions must be made. The neonate's needs take precedence over her own and those of her partner. Both parents must learn to cope with this conflict to successfully achieve the parental role.

LOVE VS. RESENTMENT

For both parents, time formerly spent with each other now must be divided with the newborn. This may be difficult to accept. Even though they love their newborn, resentment of time demands and physical and psychological energy may be created.

SELF REALIZATION THROUGH PARENTHOOD VS. SELF REALIZATION THROUGH INDIVIDUAL GOAL ATTAINMENT

When a newborn becomes a part of a family, a new role is created for both parents. Individual goal attainment may need to be postponed for a time. This creates conflicts for both parents.

With assumption of the parent role, the individual is now confronted, through the child, with repetition of earlier relationships to parents and a revival of the memories, feelings, and conflicts of childhood.

Parental behavior toward the infant is the result of a complex combination of genetic makeup, the response of the infant to the parents, interpersonal relationships within the family unit, past pregnancies, culture, and the way they were raised (see Table 19–4).

TABLE 19-4
INFLUENCES ON PARENTAL BEHAVIOR

Parent's care by his or her own parent
Genetic makeup
Cultural norms
Family relationships
Previous pregnancy
Course of this pregnancy
Behavior of health care personnel
Care and support during labor and delivery
First days following delivery
Separation from the newborn
Postpartum policies

TABLE 19-5
PRINCIPLES OF BONDING

A sensitive period that occurs immediately after birth when the mother, father, and newborn need close contact
A species specific response is present when a newborn is given to the parents
The attachment process is structured so that the parents attach to one infant at a time
The need for the infant to respond to the parents for attachment
The individual who witnesses birth becomes attached to the infant
There is difficulty in attaching to an infant while mourning the loss of another
Some events may have a long lasting effect on relationships

Phases

Parental-infant bonding may be divided into anticipatory and initial phases.

ANTICIPATORY PHASE

Pregnancy itself is the anticipatory phase to becoming a parent. Tasks are outlined during pregnancy, as the parents work through the psychological changes of pregnancy. Activities of family maintenance are assessed to identify task overload with the additional responsibilities of an added family member.

INITIAL PHASE

The postpartum period, during which an attachment with the child is achieved by the parents, is the initial phase of parent-infant bonding. This is an intense time, when the parents are exploring the new family member, as well as their relationships to each other. An emphasis is placed on the new forming relationship.

Bonding

Bonding, or the formation of a relationship with the newborn, is based on several principles (see Table 19-5). In the bonding process, the newborn is very adaptive. The child demonstrates the ability to habituate to different stimuli. If a light is flashed into its eyes, the infant startles the first two or three times, then settles down and no longer startles. A newborn also has auditory and visual orienting responses: it will follow a moving face, turn toward a female voice, and respond to human sounds. When the infant interacts or responds, it acts as a powerful reinforcer for the parents to continue the attachment process.

MATERNAL BONDING

Maternal bonding develops specifically in connection with certain events, including planning of the pregnancy, confirming of the pregnancy, accepting the pregnancy, feeling the fetus move, birth, seeing the newborn, touching the newborn, and taking care of the newborn.

The gravida's attitude toward the fetus has been found to correlate closely with her initial maternal-infant bonding. In a healthy relationship this response is an effort to satisfy the needs of the newborn, considering the newborn as an individual, and not according to the mother's own need for self-fulfillment.

Early bonding is not essential for survival of the newborn, but it appears to facilitate transition from the maternal-fetal synchrony during pregnancy to a positive maternal-fetal attachment.

The first interaction between mother and

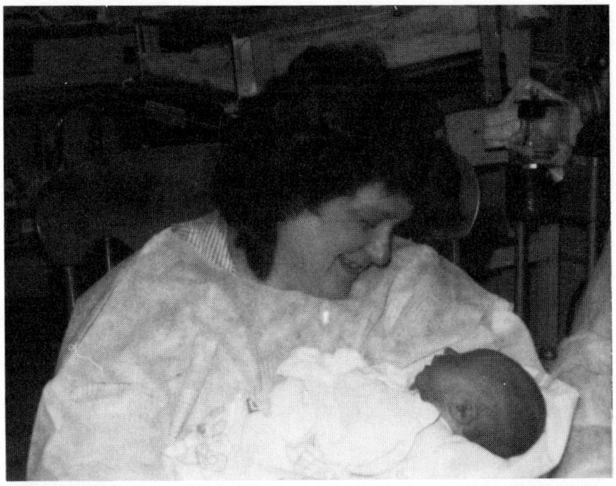

FIGURE 19–1. Initial bonding between parent and newborn.

TABLE 19–6
STAGES OF INFANT INTERACTION

Imitation: the infant's attention is attracted by the mother and the infant looks back at her
Orientation: the infant orients the body so that he or she faces the mother
Stage of attention: the infant alternately sends and receives cues
Acceleration: there are progressively fewer vacillations between inattention and attention
Vocalizing: vocal sounds by the mother cause body activity to begin
Peak of excitement stage: tension will cause jerky body activity
Deceleration: there is a gradual decrease in activity with eye contact and vocalization
Withdrawal: the infant withdraws after looking and interacting

newborn is one of exploration and examination. She will rapidly progress from touching the extremities with her fingertips to encompassing the trunk with her palm in a period of 4 to 8 minutes. In black mothers the progression is somewhat different, with reaching out for the newborn with both hands and arms immediately after delivery (Bampton et al., 1981).

The majority of all new mothers will hold their newborns closely to the left side of the chest where the heartbeat can easily be heard by the infant. The left side is preferred by mothers throughout the world, regardless of culture and ethnic variations (see Fig. 19–1).

For bonding to proceed, mother and infant are commonly in the "en face" position. When the newborn is held, the mother's face is rotated so that her eyes and those of the newborn are in the same vertical plane (see Fig. 19–2).

Infants normally exhibit a cycle that is characterized by eight stages of interaction (Table 19–6). The new mother gradually becomes aware of and accustomed to her infant's cycle. The maternal ability to respond to her infant's cycle is called *reciprocity*. As she becomes sensitized to the individual behaviors of her infant, she responds accordingly. The span of time required for the new mother to feel that the infant really belongs to her is called the *maternal time lag*.

DIFFERENCES BETWEEN MATERNAL-INFANT AND PATERNAL-INFANT BONDING

Mothering and fathering are separate entities. The maternal-child relationship is originally based on dependence and helplessness. The fetus is carried in the maternal body during pregnancy. The paternal-infant relationship revolves around caretaking activities. The father introduces and socializes the infant to the world outside the home. In the eyes of society, the father's role is to feed, protect, teach, and give the infant a place in the world. The relationship of each parent to the newborn is unique and depends on the sum total of the variables that make up the dynamics of the family unit.

PATERNAL-INFANT BONDING

Fathers go through the same progression in early bonding as mothers. Usually fathers who participate intimately in the birth experience find it fulfilling and have no difficulty in initiating bonding in the early minutes after delivery.

The link of the father to the newborn from the father's reference point is called *engrossment* (Table 19–7). Fathers are very active participants in interactions with their newborns when given the opportunity. They engage in more social and stimulating activities than do new mothers. Fathers are sensitive to signals

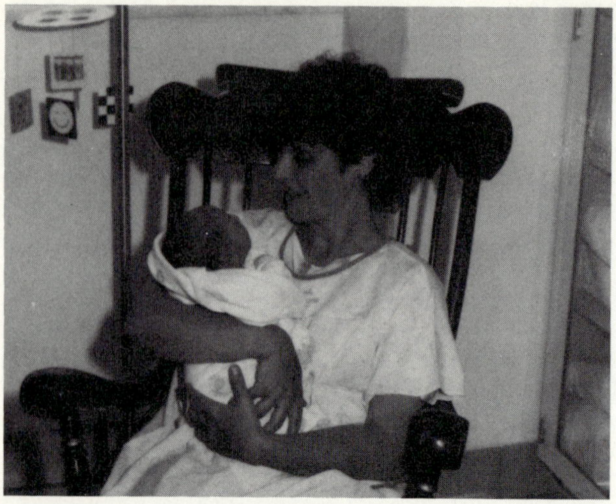

FIGURE 19-2. "En face" position.

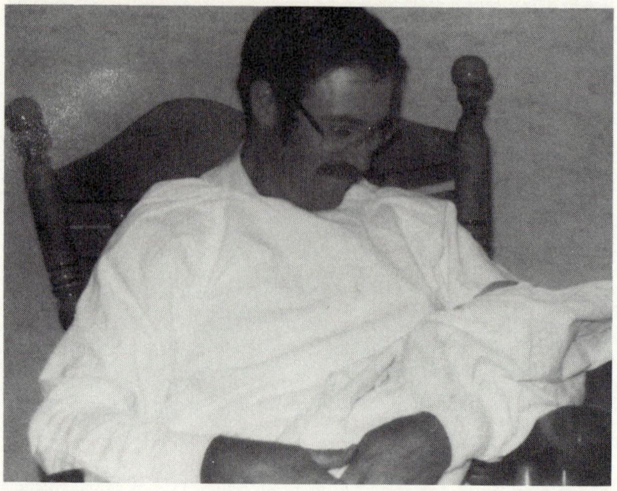

FIGURE 19-4. A relaxing moment between newborn and father.

TABLE 19-7
PATERNAL ENGROSSMENT CHARACTERISTICS

Visual awareness of the newborn
An awareness of the distinctive characteristics of the newborn
Tactile awareness of the newborn
Perception of the newborn as perfect
Paternal attraction to the newborn leads to a focusing of his attention on the infant
Experience of extreme elevation
Increase in self-esteem

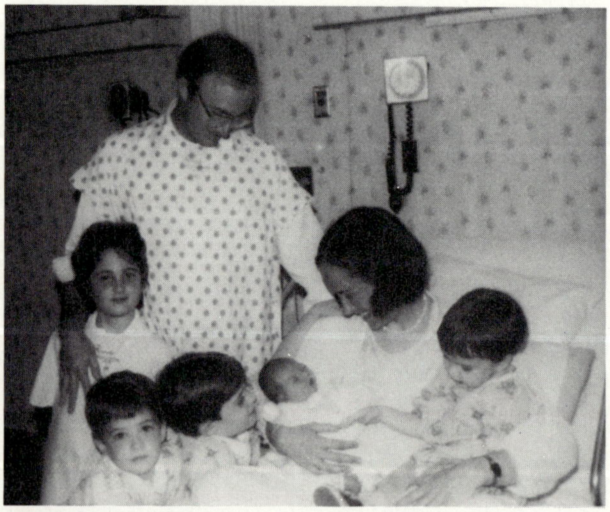

FIGURE 19-3. Interaction with the newborn.

from the newborn and respond appropriately (see Fig. 19–3). When the father is observed interacting with the newborn alone, there are no significant behavioral differences between his interactions and maternal interactions (see Fig. 19–4).

Nursing Interventions

INITIATION OF BONDING

Nurses must provide the opportunity for initial bonding to take place by encouraging holding, touching, examining, and establishing eye contact shortly after delivery. Newborn characteristics are explained to the parents as necessary.

Parental behaviors are assessed for clues to learning and teaching needs, support, and tension reduction. Parents will react individually to the newborn. Some respond by crying, some by laughing, and some will respond with silence. Behaviors noted with initial bonding are tempered by the level of energy of the parents, both physical and psychological, the level of anxiety, amount of discomfort present, and cultural and ethnic norms.

PROGRESSION OF BONDING

During this phase the parents develop a satisfactory level of competence in caring for the newborn. They evaluate realistically efforts in controlling infant responses, as they become accustomed to the infant's individual cycle of behavior.

Parental attachment behaviors are assessed during feeding and when other care is given. The mother's attitudes toward herself and mothering are assessed, as are infant care skills, and the need for teaching and support.

One way to encourage progression of bonding is by the use of rooming-in during the postpartum stay. Rooming-in is a hospital arrangement in which the mother has her newborn at her bedside and takes as much responsibility for the baby's care as she desires. The father can visit as much as he is able or wishes and can provide care as he desires. With rooming-in parental willingness to assume responsibility and capability for making intelligent decisions is recognized. Nursing staff assists the parents to assume responsibility and provides opportunities for parents to practice problem-solving during their hospital stay, with as much or as little supervision as they desire.

PSYCHOLOGICAL NEEDS OF CESAREAN BIRTH PARENTS

Couples who have experienced cesarean birth have special psychological needs during the early puerperium.

The mother who has had a cesarean birth will experience physical and psychological stresses related to her feelings of loss of control over the labor and delivery and anxiety for herself and for the infant. If the cesarean birth followed a particularly long and tiring labor, there is a sense of relief that it is finally over.

The father will experience loss, sadness, disappointment, and quite possibly anger. He is sometimes confused about the reason for the cesarean birth and may suffer a feeling of loss of control over the labor and delivery situation.

NURSING INTERVENTIONS

Nursing interventions pertinent to the needs of cesarean parents begin with assessment of responses to the entire cesarean experience. Assessment begins at the time the parents are informed that a cesarean birth is necessary. With an unplanned cesarean birth, explanations given prior to the cesarean are often brief and hurried. The mother is nervous and fatigued, as well as frightened by the prospect of surgery coupled with anxiety over the neonatal outcome. The father is worred about his partner and the infant, and he may feel helpless, powerless, and angry as he attempts to deal with an unplanned situation over which he has no control. With a planned cesarean birth, parents can be prepared for events that are to take place before, during, and after the cesarean. The cesarean experience can be made positive by the couple's active involvement in the cesarean delivery, including the father's presence at the cesarean birth.

Difficulty in attaining the maternal role is common with cesarean mothers. They need nursing support and guidance for a longer time than do mothers who deliver vaginally.

FAMILY INVOLVEMENT DURING THE PUERPERIUM

Maternity care should involve and include siblings and grandparents.

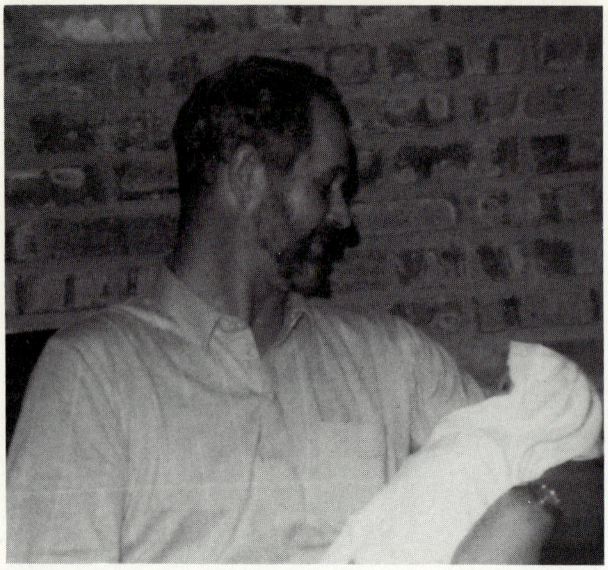

FIGURE 19–5. Grandparent interacting with newborn.

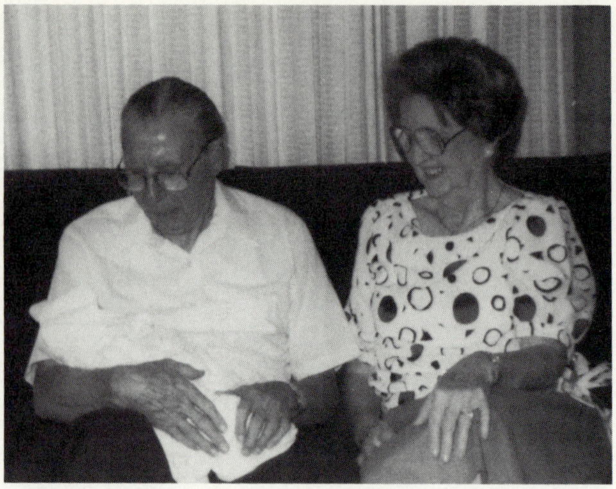

FIGURE 19–6. The presence of grandparents make infancy a valuable experience for both grandparents and baby.

Siblings

Inclusion of siblings during the puerperium is important in establishing new family relationships. There are many benefits to sibling inclusion. The older child will derive reassurance from the mother's presence, and anxiety will be alleviated. Feelings of abandonment are diminished. The trauma of maternal-child separation is lessened for the young child. Sibling visits help the mother to overcome loneliness and concern for the child or children at home. The child is made to feel a part of the family and of an important family event. The child is introduced to the new baby early.

Grandparents

Inclusion of grandparents during the early puerperium is important in sharing the experience of birth and greeting the newborn as a family member. Families are changing in today's society and need the closeness and support that is given by the extended family (see Fig. 19–5). Grandparents provide support, act as role models, and offer valuable information to the new mother who may be unsure of her abilities (see Fig. 19–6).

Intelligent and appropriate nursing interventions during the early puerperium can aid the childbearing family in dealing with the psychological stresses and adjustments following delivery.

BIBLIOGRAPHY

Anderson, C.J. Enhancing reciprocity between mother and neonate. *Nursing Research*, 1981, **30**, 89.

Bampton, B., et al. Initial mothering patterns of low income black primiparas. *Journal of Obstetric, Gynecological & Neonatal Nursing*, 1981, **10**, 174.

Brazelton, T.B. *Infants and mothers*. New York, Delacorte, 1983.

Bull, M.J. Changes in concerns of first-time mothers after one week at home. *Journal of Obstetric, Gynecologic & Neonatal Nursing*, 1981, **10**, 391.

———, & Lawrence, D. Mothers' use of knowledge during the first postpartum weeks. *Journal of Obstetric, Gynecological & Neonatal Nursing*, 1985, **14**, 315.

Hames, C.T. Sexual needs and interests of postpartum couples. *Journal of Obstetric, Gynecological, & Neonatal Nursing*, 1980, **9**, 313.

Hangsleban, K.L. Transition to fatherhood. An exploratory study. *Journal of Obstetric, Gynecological, & Neonatal Nursing,* 1983, **12,** 265.

Harrison, M.J. & Hicks, S.A. Postpartum concerns of mothers and their sources of help. *Canadian Journal of Public Health,* 1983, **74,** 325.

Heggenhougen, H.K. Fathers and childbirth. An anthropological perspective. *Journal of Nurse Midwifery,* 1980, **6,** 21.

Horn, M. & Manion, J. Creative grandparenting. Bonding the generations. *Journal of Obstetric, Gynecological & Neonatal Nursing,* 1985, **14,** 233.

Jennings, B. & Edmundson, M. The postpartum period after confinement. The fourth trimester. *Clinical Obstetrics & Gynecology,* 1980, **23,** 1093-1103.

Johnsen, M.M. & Gaspard, M.E. Theoretical foundations of a prepared sibling class. *Journal of Obstetric, Gynecological & Neonatal Nursing,* 1985, **14,** 237.

Klaus, M.H. & Kennell, J.H. *Parent-infant bonding* (2nd ed.). St. Louis: Mosby, 1982.

Kowba, M.D. & Schwiran, P.M. Direct sibling contact and bacterial colonization in newborns. *Journal of Obstetric, Gynecologic & Neonatal Nursing,* 1985, **14,** 412.

MacLaughlin, S. & Taubenheim, A. A comparison of prepared and unprepared first-time fathers' needs during the childbirth experience. *Journal of Nurse Midwifery,* 1983, **28,** 9.

Marecki, M., et al. Early sibling attachment. *Journal of Obstetric, Gynecological & Neonatal Nursing,* 1985, **14,** 418.

Philips, C.R. & Anzalone, J.T. *Fathering: Participation in birth.* St. Louis: Mosby, 1982.

Roberts, F.B. Infant behavior and the transition to parenthood. *Nursing Research,* 1983, **32,** 213.

Sears, W. *Creative parenting.* New York: Everest House, 1982.

Trevathan, W. Maternal "en face" orientation during the first hour after birth. *American Journal of Orthopsychology,* 1983, **53,** 92.

Weaver, R.H. & Cranley, M.S. An exploration of paternal-fetal attachment behavior. *Nursing Research,* 1983, **32,** 68.

Wranesh, B.L. The effect of sibling visitation on bacterial colonization rate in neonates. *Journal of Obstetric, Gynecological & Neonatal Nursing,* 1982, **11,** 211.

Young, D. *Changing childbirth. Family birth in the hospital.* Rochester, N.Y.: Childbirth Graphics, Ltd., 1982.

chapter 20

NURSING MANAGEMENT DURING THE PUERPERIUM

OBJECTIVES

Upon completion of this chapter, the reader will be able to:

1. Identify the steps of physical assessment of the puerperal patient and state pertinent observations for each.
2. Plan nursing care for the puerperal patient using the nursing process.
3. State the classification, action, route of administration, side effects, and nursing implications of medications given to suppress lactation.
4. Describe the needs of the postpartum patient for rest, nutrition, elimination, and hygiene.
5. Identify requirements for Rh (D) immunoglobulin administration.
6. Identify maternal self care skills that are stressed prior to postpartum discharge.
7. Identify infant care skills that are stressed prior to discharge from the hospital.
8. Identify assessments and observations during the postpartal checkup at the completion of the puerperium.

KEY TERMS

Afterpains
Diastasis recti
Discharge planning
Episiotomy care
Homan's sign
Kegal's exercises
Lochia
Luke's sign
Morbidity temperature
Oxytoxic
Perineal care
Puerperal bradycardia
Rh immunoglobulin
Sims' position

Nursing management during the puerperium is essential, whether a mother has a normal neonate or is separated from her neonate due to prematurity, illness, death, or adoption; whether she has a support system to assist her or not; and whether she delivers in the hospital setting or in a birthing center.

The postpartum mother is concerned about her own comfort and recovery, she desires contact with her neonate, she is motivated to learn about newborn care, and she is eager to share her birth experiences.

The nursing process is utilized in care of the postpartum mother. Once nursing diagnoses are formulated, appropriate nursing measures are identifed and priorities are set. Any implementations must take into account the care of the neonate and will usually revolve around the infant feeding and care times.

Two major nursing goals are identified during the puerperium: (1) to aid in normal physiologic changes; and (2) to aid in strengthening maternal-infant or paternal-infant bonding.

The nursing care plan will include assessments that detect deviations from the normal, comfort measures, safety measures, and teaching and counseling. Continuous evaluation is needed to provide appropriate, individualized care. A sample nursing care plan is found in Table 20–1.

INITIAL PATIENT ASSESSMENT

Within a short time after admission to the postpartum nursing unit, an assessment should be completed. This assessment of the physiologic and psychological state of the woman is necessary to identify both potential and actual problems.

Health History

Assessment begins with a health history. Specific data about pregnancy, labor, and delivery can be identified from the chart. In addition, this information is obtained from the client to determine her emotions and impressions.

FAMILY HISTORY

Information should include age, marital status, number of children, support systems, type of housing and community, occupation, education, husband's occupation and education, and socioeconomic level. These factors will aid in determining the impact of the newborn on the woman and her family, and provide the foundation for teaching of self-care and child care skills specific to the knowledge level of the parents.

Specific information about familial illnesses, especially hereditary diseases, is obtained.

PREGNANCY HISTORY

Information should include gravida and para, expected due date, nutritional status during pregnancy, and any problems that occurred during pregnancy. This information will aid in determining potential for bonding. Complications during pregnancy may interfere with bonding during the first few days postpartum.

LABOR AND DELIVERY HISTORY

Length of labor, fetal position at delivery, type of delivery, analgesics, anesthesic agents, and problems that occurred during labor can be obtained from the chart, but should also be obtained directly from the client to identify her reactions to the labor process.

NEONATAL DATA

The sex and weight of the neonate, any difficulties that occurred during labor and delivery, method of infant feeding chosen, and the presence of congenital abnormalities or neonatal illness are important data to know in planning care during the puerperium.

CULTURAL DATA

Identification of cultural norms that may influence dietary intake, dietary restrictions, and food preparation are assessments needed during the initial interview. Cultural differences in infant care are also identified in planning appropriate nursing interventions for the postpartal family. See Chapter 2 for a discussion of cultural influences during the postpartum period for the mother and the newborn.

ORIENTATION TO THE NURSING UNIT

Client Identification

Determination of client identity and the preferred form of address are important to planning individual nursing care for the patient.

Orientation

Upon transfer to the postpartum unit following completion of the fourth stage of labor, the client and her support persons are oriented to the nursing unit. If they are familiar with the unit and unit policies and routines, anxiety is reduced.

The call lights or call system are explained, as are services and supplies that can be expected and how to obtain these services or supplies. The client's usual activities of daily living are identified. If these vary from the routine on the nursing unit, the nurse and client work together to identify acceptable routines.

INFECTION CONTROL

Important to the care of the postpartum patient and the neonate are infection control policies and procedures within the nursing unit. Attention to personal hygiene is imperative.

Facilities such as kitchens, bathrooms, and bed units must be kept clean. A daily bed linen change is recommended, with draw sheet changes as needed. Prevention of cross contamination is necessary when facilities are shared by patients.

Nursing personnel must be conscientious about hand-washing techniques to prevent cross contamination. Personnel with colds, coughs, or skin infections are not allowed in contact with women during the postpartum period.

VITAL SIGNS

Following the fourth stage of labor, vital signs are monitored on a routine schedule during the postpartum stay.

Temperature

Maternal temperature is taken orally four times a day, unless elevations are noted. After the first 24 hours following delivery, the temperature should be normal. Temperature elevations above 38°C (100.4°F) on any two postpartum days, excluding the first 24 hours, after delivery are considered abnormal and are classified as *morbidity temperatures*.

If maternal temperature is elevated, more frequent assessments of temperature are needed. This opportunity may be used by the nurse to teach possible causes of temperature elevation and techniques for taking temperatures and reading thermometers. Signs of infections related to childbearing (e.g., mastitis, endometritis, thrombophlebitis) are assessed as are other possible causes of elevated temperatures, such as sore throat, nasal congestion, burning upon urination, and flank pain, which provide a database for diagnosis by the physician.

Physician-ordered therapies are implemented after explanation to the client, and responses to the interventions are documented.

TABLE 20-1
SAMPLE NURSING CARE PLAN: POSTPARTUM

Mrs. G.D., a 28-year-old gravida 2 para 2 delivered a live girl at 2200 on April 26. Delivery was spontaneous over a MLE. No maternal or fetal problems in labor and delivery.

Data Base:

Prenatal history negative
EDC 5/1
Type & Rh O+
RPR: non reactive
Family history negative
Obstetrical history: spontaneous vaginal delivery of live boy over MLE on 7/6/1980 following a 7 hour 42 minute labor. No prenatal or labor and delivery complications. Infant weight 6 lb 7 oz; no neonatal problems
Present labor: 4 hour 28 minutes
No analgesic or anesthetic medications, expect Carbocaine 1% for episiotomy repair
Placenta spontaneous expulsion, complete.
4th stage of labor completed without problem
Breastfeeding

Nursing Diagnosis	Goals	Nursing Interventions	Rationale	Evaluation
Potential alteration in tissue perfusion related to involution process	The client will have progressive uterine involution with no excessive bleeding The client's vital signs and other assessment data will remain within normal limits	Do complete assessment every shift Vital signs Breasts Fundus Bladder Bowel Lochia Perineum Homan's sign Psychological status	Doing a complete assessment will identify potential problems	Assessment within normal limits: TPR: 98-84-20 B/P: 122/74 Breasts slightly engorged Fundus 2,[1] in midline No bladder distention noted, voiding quantity sufficient. No BM since delivery MLE approximated. Moderate lochia rubra Homan's sign negative Cheerful, appropriate affect

Potential alteration in tissue perfusion related to puerperal infection	The client displays no signs of infection	Assess: Uterine tenderness Lochial odor, color Homan's sign Vital signs	Alteration in uterine tenderness or lochial progression may indicate an infectious process	Assessments within normal limits
Knowledge deficit related to altered nutritional needs during lactation	The client will verbalize understanding of nutrient needs during lactation	Assess understanding about nutrition needs during lactation Identify foods that client likes that will meet nutritional needs Assist in planning a typical day's menu	Nutrient needs during lactation are increased over pregnancy levels	Mrs. D. breast fed her first infant. She is aware of nutritional needs
Alteration in urinary elimination related to decreased bladder tone secondary to vaginal delivery	The client will resume normal bladder function	Assess bladder status for distention Assess output amounts	Incomplete emptying of bladder will predispose to postpartum urinary tract infections and abnormal involution patterns	Up and voiding without difficulties in sufficient amounts
Alteration in bowel elimination related to decreased gastric motility secondary to pregnancy	The client resumes normal bowel function	Assess bowel status: Administer stool softeners as ordered Give Fleets enema 3rd PP day as ordered by physician	Constipation is common in the puerperium	No BM on 2nd PP day Doxidan cap 1 at 6 pm
Potential for infection related to nosocomial infection	The client/family will demonstrate correct hand washing technique	Assess knowledge of importance of hand washing as prevention of infection	Good hand washing will prevent spread of micro-organisms	Verbalized and demonstrated throughout day
Potential for infection related to episiotomy	The client will display no evidence of infection in the episiotomy	Assess episiotomy for infection q shift Redness Swelling Tenderness Instruct on perineal care Sitz bath prn	Episiotomy infections can be prevented with appropriate teaching and assessment to identify deviations from normal	MLE clean, edges well approximated, no redness, etc. noted

TABLE 20-1 (continued)

Nursing Diagnosis	Goals	Nursing Intervention	Rationale	Evaluations
Alteration in comfort related to episiotomy and uterine involution	The client is comfortable The client reports relief from discomfort	Assess for presence of discomfort: Patient description Characteristics of pain Effect on ADL Anticipate need for analgesics Administer before breast feeding Administer pain medication as ordered Evaluate effectiveness	Uterine involution causes abdominal cramping. Episiotomy discomfort is noted for the first several days PP	c/o "afterbirth" cramping Fiorinal tab 2 given at 0800 and 1345
Potential alteration in comfort related breast engorgement	The client will demonstrate proper breast care The client will breast feed with minimal discomfort	Assess breasts q shift: Engorgement Redness Heat Instruct to wear supportive bra 24 hours a day	Assessing breasts and providing patient teaching will aid in prevening engorgement and decreasing the incidence of mastitis	Breasts slightly engorged Well fitting support bra on with breast pads in place Infant nursing well—getting 1/2 to 3/4 oz per feeding
Knowledge deficit related to infant care	The client/support person will verbalize and demonstrate infant care skills before discharge home	Assess learning needs of the family unit Implement teaching plans as needed Encourage questions Demonstrate infant care as needed	Evaluating learning needs will allow for individualized teaching	Mr. and Mrs. D. verbalized understanding of and demonstrated infant care skills with no apparent difficulty

Pulse and Respiratory Rate

Maternal pulse and respiratory rate are assessed four times a day at the same time as the temperature. Respirations should remain within normal limits. Puerperal bradycardia is common during the early puerperium and is to be expected. Any elevations in the pulse rate or respiratory rate indicate potential complications and need further assessment.

Blood Pressure

Blood pressure is measured twice a day during the puerperium. If oxytoxic medications are ordered by the physician, blood pressure is assessed before administration. If the blood pressure is elevated, the oxytoxic is held and the physician notified.

Orthostatic hypotension when the patient rises from a horizontal position to ambulate may occur during the postpartum period, especially for the first one or two ambulations following delivery. Supervision is needed for the first several ambulations. An explanation of this phenomenon is provided to the client, and she is instructed to call for assistance before attempting to ambulate, to rise gradually, to move slowly, how to use a call light and the emergency call system in the bathroom. She is instructed to sit on the floor if she begins to feel faint until someone arrives to assist her.

Postpartum blood pressure elevation is not normal and requires further assessment. Associated complaints of headache in the absence of spinal anesthesia for delivery may indicate development of postpartum pregnancy-induced hypertension. Postpartum headaches are always assessed further and are discussed later in this chapter. Assessments of elevated blood pressure are reported to the physician and ordered protocol is instituted and evaluated.

UTERINE ASSESSMENTS

Uterus

To accurately assess the uterus, have the patient lie flat on her back with her knees flexed to relieve tension on the abdomen.

Observe the abdomen for contour to detect distention. If diastasis recti is present, it is noted as a bluish-tinged, slightly indented groove in the abdominal midline. The width and length are measured in fingerbreadths and documented.

The uterine fundus is palpated by placing one hand on the base of the uterus just above the symphysis pubis and the other at the umbilicus. Press inward and downward with the hand on the umbilicus until you feel a firm, globular mass in the abdomen. This mass is the uterine fundus. Assess the fundus for consistency using the terms firm, soft, or boggy; is it in the midline? What is its height? Height is measured in fingerbreaths above or below the umbilicus and is recorded. If the bladder is distended, it may be noted as a rounded bulge in the suprapubic region that is dull to percussion and fluctuates in position during palpation. With bladder distention, the uterus may be felt upward and to the right of the umbilicus. Have the patient void and reassess the uterus.

Palpation of the uterine fundus should not cause pain. Pain present upon uterine manipulation suggests pelvic infection. If the uterus is not firm when palpated, gentle massage will cause it to contract and become firm.

During the postpartum period, lying on the abdomen will aid in uterine involution, since it tips the uterus into its normal forward position. If lying on the abdomen puts excessive pressure on sore breasts, a small pillow placed under the stomach will usually help. A knee-chest position is dangerous for the postpartum patient for at least three weeks following delivery owing to the natural opening of the vagina in this position. With this position, there is danger that air will enter the vagina and open cervix, penetrate the open sinuses in the uterus, and cause an air embolism. If this position has been used during pregnancy to relieve hemorrhoidal pressure, it should be discouraged.

Lochia

The amount, type, and character of the lochia are assessed twice a day as needed. During the first few days postpartum, the lochia, termed *lochia rubra*, consists of blood and decidual debris, and is reddish in color. From the third to the eighth postpartum day, the lochia becomes pinkish in color, consists of erythrocytes, leukocytes, decidua, cervical mucus, and microorganisms, and is called *lochia serosa*. *Lochia alba*, seen from day eight until approximately three weeks after delivery, is creamy white in color and contains serum, leukocytes, decidua, epithelial cells, mucus, and bacteria.

Amount is usually described using the terms scant, moderate, large, and excessive. Observations to aid in assessing normalcy in amount include the following:

Lochia usually occurs as a trickle from the vaginal opening

If the uterus is massaged at the same time as lochia is assessed, a gush of dark lochia may be observed following pooling in the relaxed vaginal canal

If oxytoxics are administered, lochia is scant until medication effect has decreased

A perineal pad saturated in 15 minutes or less indicates excessive lochial flow

Lochia has a characteristic fleshy odor. Foul odor indicates infection and requires further assessments.

Persistent lochia rubra or a return to lochia rubra from lochia serosa or alba indicates abnormal uterine involution. A consistent decrease in lochia occurs for about three weeks following delivery. This consistent decrease, as well as the occurrence of a "small period" about three weeks after delivery, is discussed as part of maternal education.

PERINEUM

Assessment and General Care

Following completion of the fourth stage of labor, the perineum is assessed at least twice a day. Daily cleansing should include a bath or shower in addition to careful cleansing after each voiding and defecation. Soap and water, warm water directed to the perineum from a peri-care bottle or medicated wipes may be used for routine perineal cleansing after voiding or defecation. Cotton balls should not be used for cleansing the perineum if it has been shaved or if an episiotomy has been done. Cotton sticks to the stubble of shaved hair on the suture line and leaves behind particles to invite lochial buildup.

Before beginning perineal care, wash hands to prevent contamination of the perineal area. Remove the perineal pad from front to back after placing a plastic-covered pad under the buttocks to protect the bed linen. When washing the perineal area, wash from front to back. Do not separate the labia when washing, to avoid accidental entry of the washing solution into the vagina.

Inspect the perineum to detect any stitches that are pulling out or any area that appears inflammed or reddened. It is often advantageous to turn the client to her side, so the episiotomy or perineal area can be thoroughly viewed.

If any cream or spray has been ordered for the perineum, it is applied after the area is dried. A clean pad is then applied from front to back.

SELF CARE INSTRUCTIONS

The client is instructed to cleanse from symphysis pubis to anal area to prevent vaginal and urethral contamination with fecal material. Sterile perineal pads are used until adequate healing has occurred (usually five to seven days). Hands should be washed before and after changing perineal pads. Perineal pads are applied from front to back without contamination of the portion of the pad that will be applied next to the perineum. Soiled pads are wrapped individually and placed in a specified waste container. The importance of using any ordered medications is emphasized. Caution the client against flushing the toilet before she is standing upright to prevent spraying of the perineum by the flushing water.

Even though most postpartum patients manage their own perineal care as soon as they are allowed up to the bathroom, the nurse is still responsible for assessing the perineum at least twice a day.

EPISIOTOMY CARE

If an episiotomy was performed during delivery to avoid perineal laceration, the closure is frequently a source of discomfort. Following suturing of the episiotomy there is a vasoconstriction of the area, followed by prolonged vasodilatation with hyperemia. Increased capillary permeability with fluid leaking into the injured tissue causes some localized edema. White blood cells migrate to the area in reaction to foreign bodies and cellular debris.

An incision in the perineal area can cause a great deal of discomfort to the postpartum patient. This discomfort is normal and should be explained. Many measures can aid in relieving episiotomy discomfort, including ice, exercises, heat lamps, anesthetic sprays, perineal care, witch hazel compresses, sitz baths, K-pads, and analgesic medications.

Ice

Ice may be used for the first 12 hours following delivery to decrease edema and reduce discomfort. A double walled ice bag wrapped in a sterile cloth to prevent tissue damage may be applied to the episiotomy site.

Perineal Exercises

Perineal exercises done three or four times a day may provide comfort. Kegal exercises, contracting and relaxing the perineal muscles five times in succession as if trying to stop a voiding, will improve circulation to the perineal area and help to decrease edema formation.

A postpartum client may need to sit a little differently until the perineum is healed to avoid stretching the perineal muscles. Before she attempts to sit, she should squeeze her buttocks together and sit with them squeezed together.

Heat Lamps

Dry heat to the perineum in the form of a perineal heat lamp will increase circulation to the perineal area, reduce edema, promote healing, and provide comfort. After the procedure is explained to the client, she should lie supine with her legs flexed and spread to expose the perineum. The perineal pad is removed from front to back. The perineum is cleansed to prevent drying of lochia during treatment. A heat lamp is then placed on the bed, positioned between the client's legs at a distance of 12 to 18 inches from the perineum. If an anesthetic spray is ordered, it is applied at this time. She is then covered with a sheet to provide privacy. The heat lamp should be left in place for approximately 20 minutes to provide optimal vasodilation to the area. At the end of the treatment, the light is removed, perineal care is administered, and a fresh perineal pad is applied from front to back. The procedure is documented, as is the client's response.

Anesthetic Sprays, Witch Hazel Compresses

Anesthetic sprays and anesthetic ointments may be applied two to four times a day. Witch hazel compresses may be applied directly to the perineum and should be changed with each urination and pad change.

Sitz Baths

A sitz bath may be used to soothe, promote healing, and increase circulation to the perineal area. A sitz bath is a small portable basin that fits on the toilet seat with water constantly circulating in the basin. The temperature of the water is maintained at 38° to 42°C (100°F) to prevent burning of the perineum. The treatment lasts about 20 minutes and may be repeated three or four times a day. Because of the soothing effects of the warm water and the sitting position, the client may be tired and unsteady on her feet and may need assistance in getting back into bed. Documentation includes that the sitz bath was taken, perineal condition, and tolerance of the procedure.

K-Pads

K-pads may also aid in bringing comfort to the perineal area. A long narrow pad is attached to a pump that circulates warm water. A cover should be placed on the K-pad before application to the perineum. Treatments are for 20 minutes, and are given three or four times a day.

Analgesic Medications

Analgesics are offered for relief of discomfort during the first several days postpartum.

HEMORRHOIDS

During delivery, pressure on the rectal veins may produce or aggravate existing internal or external hemorrhoids. Effective means of relieving discomfort include ice, cold witch hazel compresses, moist heat, anesthetic sprays, or suppositories. Assumption of a Sims' position while in bed will aid in increasing venous return of the rectal area and help in relieving discomfort. External hemorrhoids should be assessed for redness, swelling, and thrombosis.

LOWER EXTREMITIES

The lower extremities are assessed twice a day during the puerperium. The thighs are assessed for skin turgor by lifting a ridge of tissue and observing how readily it falls back into place. Edema at the ankle and over the tibia is assessed.

Indications of thrombophlebitis include assessment of Homan's sign and Luke's sign. *Homan's sign* is positive when calf pain is present following dorsiflexion of the foot. *Luke's sign* is positive when there is calf pain upon standing.

NEUROLOGIC STATUS

Neurologic assessment begins with observation of psychological status. Normal psychological status during the postpartum period has been discussed in Chapter 19.

Postpartum headaches require careful assessment. A constant throbbing or splitting headache that is frontal indicates potential pregnancy-induced hypertension (PIH). Stress headaches may be caused by anxiety, muscle tension, fatigue, or hunger. They are described as a consistent ache located as a band around the head, and are usually relieved by physical or psychological rest or food. Headaches may also follow subarachnoid or spinal anesthesia, caused by leakage of cerebrospinal fluid. They are usually located in the forehead, deep behind the eyes, and radiate to both temples. Treatment includes increase in oral fluids, intravenous fluids, analgesics, and extradural "blood patches."

Postnatal foot drop may occur with "normal" labor and delivery or following a prolonged labor with transverse arrest or a difficult forceps delivery. Symptoms include weak ankle dorsiflexion, weak toe extension, eversion of the foot, numbness, and decreased skin sensation.

URINARY TRACT ASSESSMENT

The postpartum patient is encouraged to void at least every four hours during the day. She is instructed to report the following symptoms:

pain or burning upon urination, voiding in small amounts, and an inability to void. Urinary output is monitored carefully for at least the first three voidings following delivery. Following each voiding, the uterine fundus is checked.

Nursing measures to enhance ability for spontaneous voiding are necessary, especially in the early puerperium, and include turning on the water in the bathroom, and pouring warm water over the vulva.

If catheterization becomes necessary, several alterations occur in the procedure. There is normally swelling of the vulva following delivery, and the urethral meatus may be difficult to locate. Perineal sutures are tender, making catheterization more uncomfortable. Some resistance may be encountered as the catheter is introduced owing to tissue trauma.

ABDOMINAL WALL ASSESSMENT

Following delivery, the abdominal wall and the uterine ligaments are stretched. The abdomen pouches forward and the client may feel fat and unattractive. If diastasis recti has occurred, the abdominal wall may remain weakened and not be supportive for subsequent pregnancies. Diastasis recti may be felt as a gap in the abdominal muscles felt on abdominal palpation. Documentation is in fingerbreadths of length and width. An abdominal binder is not usually recommended, even though it may make the client more comfortable because it hinders strengthening of the abdominal wall muscles. If a binder is ordered, it is applied from the top down, so that it pushes the uterus down and aids in uterine contraction. Teaching includes good body mechanics, good posture, rest, and exercises as ordered.

PERSONAL HYGIENE

Because of the normal diaphoresis that occurs in the early puerperium, frequent bathing is needed. A sponge bath is recommended for the first bath because it meets the normal dependency needs of the early puerperium, aids in establishing a trusting relationship between the client and the nurse, and allows an ideal opportunity to assess the client both physically and in terms of teaching needs.

Frequent gown changes may be needed to prevent chilling from diaphoresis. The client is cautioned against becoming chilled during this time.

PHYSICAL ASSESSMENT

During the early postpartum period, certain aspects of the physical examination are performed to determine client status. These aspects include nutritional and fluid status, energy level, presence or absence of pain, breast health, fundal height, lochial characteristics, perineal integrity, and circulatory adequacy.

General Appearance

A woman's general appearance during the early puerperium is a good indicator of energy level, self-esteem, and psychological state. Before assessment begins, ask the client to void so she has an empty bladder. Observe the energy level used to go to the bathroom, or for a cringing expression and hand pressure on the abdomen that suggests pain. Observe the presence or absence of makeup or hair combing. A woman who is extremely exhausted or depressed will not take pains with her personal appearance.

HAIR

Ask the client to lie in bed. Feel her hair to assess cleanliness. A good pregnancy diet will lend itself to firm, lustrous hair; a deficient diet causes listless, stringy hair. Not washing the hair may be a sign of depression. If concern is voiced about the loss of hair during the postpartum period, assure her that this is normal, as the body returns to normal following pregnancy.

FACE

The face is assessed for edema, which is more noticeable early in the morning as puffy eyelids. The conjunctiva of the eye is assessed for pinkness. Pale conjunctiva may indicate anemia. Dryness of the conjunctiva may indicate dehydration.

DIET AND HYDRATION

Nutrition

Oral fluids are given as soon as the mother is stable following delivery. A regular diet is begun as soon as tolerated. Postpartum nutrition should include 2,500 to 2,600 kcal per day, high in protein, vitamins, and minerals. An adequate supply of roughage is needed to help restore peristaltic action. If the patient is breastfeeding she needs 500 more calories and 500 ml additional fluids per day to encourage milk production.

The importance of maintaining an adequate nutritious diet at home is emphasized. Fatigue that occurs at home with the additional burden of caring for a newborn infant may lead to inadequate meal preparation. Neglecting proper nutrition leads to more fatigue and less nutrition.

Prenatal vitamins are continued until the prenatal supply is used up. Further vitamin supplements are ordered by the physician as needed.

Constipation

Constipation is common, owing to relaxation of the abdominal muscles and bowels, presence of hemorrhoids, and the presence of perineal sutures. To prevent constipation, many physicians order stool softeners, beginning on the first day after delivery. If no bowel movement has occurred by the third postpartum day, a cathartic or enema may be given. Measures that will aid in correcting constipation include early ambulation, adequate fluid intake, and a diet with adequate roughage.

Hydration

During the period of rapid diuresis postpartum, a woman often complains of thirst and requests additional fluids. Increased fluid intake is needed to increase excretion of nitrogen from the catabolism of uterine cells. At least three or four glasses of fluids are needed every day to maintain hydration.

ACTIVITY

Rest

Rest during the early postpartum period cannot be overemphasized. A time for naps should be provided as part of the nursing care plan. To facilitate rest periods for the new mother, visitors may need to be restricted. Adequate measures for relief of discomfort are important.

Bedrest

Most women are ambulatory by at least eight hours after delivery. Those who are confined to bed for a longer period include patients who received any type of spinal anesthesia. They should remain flat in bed with one pillow to align the head with the shoulders for at least eight hours before they are allowed to attempt ambulation. This prevents leakage of spinal fluid through the dural membrane at the site of the needle puncture. The nurse instructs the client not to raise her head until specifically allowed by physician order.

Clients who received epidural anesthesia for delivery may be ambulatory as soon as the numbness associated with the anesthetic is completely worn off. If restricted to bed for more than eight hours, leg exercises to promote circulation are initiated. These include alternate flexion and extension of both feet, rotation of the feet, alternate flexion and extension of the toes, and straight-leg raises.

Early Ambulation

For the majority of postpartum patients, early ambulation is advocated. Early ambulation has the benefit of decreasing the incidence of circulatory complications (thrombophlebitis or phlebothrombosis), as well as minimizing bladder and bowel problems. Early ambulation assists the new mother to regain her strength quickly.

Assistance is required for the first few ambulations after delivery. The new mother may feel dizzy and unsteady on her feet. She should dangle her legs over the edge of the bed for a few minutes before attempting to stand up. You should remain with her for the first ambulation and for later ambulations if needed.

She is usually allowed to be up on her own after the first several ambulations and begins to care for her own needs, including perineal care following proper instruction. The postpartum client should not sit in a chair for prolonged periods of time. She should lie with her legs stretched out when in bed, without crossing the legs at the knees.

BREAST CARE

Breast care during the postpartum period is directed at providing support of the breasts and cleanliness.

BREAST SUPPORT

A supportive bra to prevent undue ligament stretching is encouraged for at least the first week postpartum for both the bottlefeeding and breastfeeding mother. Good support will aid in positioning the breasts in good alignment and diminishes the amount of engorgement caused by blocked milk ducts. If no bra is available, a breast binder may be worn to provide needed support. If there is discharge of colostrum or milk from the breasts, a clean gauze square or breast pad should be inserted into the bra to absorb moisture; it is changed as often as necessary to keep the nipples dry. If the nipples remain moist and wet, the incidence of nipple fissures increases.

Nursing assessments include whether or not a bra is being used, and whether it is an adequate size for comfort. The straps should not leave red marks on the shoulders. The elastic on the bottom of the bra should not leave reddened areas on the breasts. If the client didn't bring an adequate bra, her family can purchase one for her to wear. Instruct them to purchase a bra that is one or two sizes larger than the prepregnancy size to allow for the increase in breast size as milk forms.

CLEANLINESS

The breasts should be washed daily at the time of the shower or bath. If the client is breastfeeding, no soap should be used on the breasts to prevent drying and cracking of the nipples. Products that have an alcohol base should not be used to clean the breasts because of their drying properties.

BREAST EXAMINATION

To properly assess the postpartum breast, the client should be asked to remove her bra. The breast is covered with a towel or sheet to preserve modesty. Breast tissue must be seen, not just palpated for accurate assessments. The size, shape, and color are observed. With the client's hand raised and tucked under her head, the breast tissue is stretched and thinned, making palpation easier. Firmness and warmth are assessed. For the first and second day after delivery, breast tissue should feel soft; by day three engorgement may occur and the breast will become firm, tense, and warm to touch. If a firm nodule is palpated, it is usually milk in a breast gland that has not started flowing toward the nipple. Note the location of the nodule, report it to the physician, and reassess it in 24 hours. If only one portion of the breast feels warm or appears reddened, mastitis or inflammation is suspected.

The nipple is assessed for erectness or inversion, as well as for cracks or fissures. It is not necessary to squeeze the nipple to assess it. To assess for the presence of colostrum, the thumb and forefinger are placed on the breast alveoli, light backward pressure is applied, followed by bringing the thumb and finger together. Colostrum is watery in appearance and is expressed for the first two days postpartum; breast milk that is white with a bluish tinge will be present on the third to fourth day. The mother who is bottlefeeding should not be assessed for the presence of colostrum to avoid stimulation of the mammary glands. Any colostrum or milk that is expressed is then wiped off the nipple.

The postpartum period is an ideal time to teach the patient breast self-examination or to reinforce breast self-examination techniques. The mother who is breastfeeding will normally not have a menstrual period for three or four months following delivery. She should select a specific day each month to do her breast self-examination until menses return.

MEDICATIONS

Afterpains

Uterine contractions that accompany normal uterine involution postpartum may cause cramping, commonly called "afterpains" or "afterbirth pains." These pains are caused by uterine ischemia as the uterus contracts. They are more common in clients who have had uterine overdistention by multiple pregnancies or polyhydramnios, have retained membranes or placental tissue, have retained blood clots within the uterus, are multiparas, and are breast feeding.

Clients are taught that this discomfort is normal and usually only lasts for three or four days. Lying on the abdomen with a pillow under the lower abdomen will often decrease the cramping sensation. If necessary, mild analgesics such as acetaminophen, propoxyphene (Darvon), or ibuprofen (Motrin) may be given every three to four hours to minimize discomfort. Heat applied to the abdomen should not be used to relieve discomfort from afterpains, since it may cause relaxation of the uterine muscle and increase uterine bleeding.

Suppression of Lactation

To suppress lactation, mechanical or pharmacologic means are employed. Mechanical means include discontinuing nursing of the neonate, milk expression, or breast pumping. A tight breast binder is applied for 48 to 72 hours, followed by use of a snug brassiere. Ice packs and analgesics may be used to relieve discomfort. Fluid restriction is not helpful in suppressing lactation.

Pharmacologic means to suppress lactation are administered in the form of medications. In the recent past, estrogens, androgens, or combinations of estrogens and androgens were given in an effort to prevent or suppress lactation. When these medications are prescribed, the client must give written informed consent to the use of these drugs, since they have been implicated in the etiology of uterine and endometrial cancer and have been shown to increase the incidence of thrombophlebitis.

An alternative to estrogens and androgens is bromocriptine mesylate (Parlodel). This medication is a dopamine receptor agonist and reduces high serum levels of prolactin that are needed for lactation, thus preventing milk secretion and breast engorgement in the postpartum client. Ordinarily, the medication is started no sooner than four hours after delivery. Ambulation is supervised because of the possible hypotensive effect of the medication. The recommended dosage for prevention of postpartum lactation is one 2.5 mg tablet two times a day with meals for 14 days. Patients who are sensitive to ergot preparations should not receive this medication; phenothiazines should be avoided while on bromocriptine mesylate. Possible side effects include hypotension, nausea, headache, dizziness, lightheadedness, and nasal congestion. The nurse emphasizes to the client the importance of reporting any of these symptoms. When the medication is discontinued, some women report rebound breast engorgement.

Immune Medications

Nursing assessment during the postpartum stay includes determining the client's need for prevention of Rh isoimmunization or rubella vaccination.

PREVENTION OF RH ISOIMMUNIZATION

A client is a candidate for Rh immunoglobulin if she is Rh negative, her neonate is Rh positive, and the neonatal Coombs test is negative. Occasionally Rh immunoglobulin is given when the Coombs test is weakly positive, especially when antepartal Rh immunoglobulin has been given. Injection of Rh immunoglobulin must be given to the mother within 72 hours of delivery. Prevention of maternal sensitization is by intramuscular administration of 300 μg of crossmatched Rh immunoglobulin to promote lysis of the fetal Rh positive red blood cells that may be circulating in the maternal blood stream.

Administration following delivery is made to any mother who meets these criteria:

1. The mother must be Rh negative with no Rh antibodies present (negative indirect Coombs' test)
2. The neonate must be Rh positive
3. The direct Coombs' test done on the cord blood must be negative

RUBELLA VACCINATION

For postpartum clients who have not had rubella or who are serologically negative (i.e., rubella titer of 1:10 or less), rubella virus vaccine is recommended in the immediate postpartum period to prevent problems with future pregnancies from exposure to rubella. Women who are allergic to ducks or duck eggs may have a hypersensitivity reaction to the vaccine. The vaccine is not administered until the mother can verbalize her understanding of the possible side effects: (1) a possible rash over the body in seven to ten days; (2) a possible slight temperature elevation in seven to ten days; (3) general malaise; and (4) anorexia. It must also be emphasized that pregnancy must be avoided for three months following immunization. The vaccine is not excreted through the breast milk and side effects are not communicable.

POSTPARTUM EXERCISES

Exercises to strengthen the abdominal and pelvic muscles may be started as soon as the first day after delivery, with the physician's consent. The client should begin with easy exercises and gradually progress to more difficult ones. They should be done daily until the end of the puerperium to derive maximum benefit. See Table 20–2 for common postpartum exercises that may be ordered.

Kegal Exercises

Kegal exercises may be started soon after delivery to aid in the recovery of the pubococcygeal muscle that has been stretched during delivery. These exercises do not require physician permission. They help to restore muscle tone and function and will facilitate healing by increasing circulation to the pubococcygeal area, as well as prevent urinary stress incontinence. Contraction of this muscle is described to the patient as picturing the

TABLE 20-2
COMMON POSTPARTUM EXERCISES

Exercise	Description
Abdominal breathing	This exercise may be started on the first postpartum day. Lie flat on your back. Take in and expel five breaths, breathing deeply from the abdomen.
Arm raises	Lie flat on your back, with your arms at your sides. Arm motions should be with elbows stiff out from the sides. Raise your arms over your head and bring your hands together. Return your arms to the original position at your sides. Rest. Repeat five times.
Chin to chest	Lie on your back with no pillow. Raise your head to touch your chin to your chest without moving any other part of your body. Repeat this exercise five times.
Kegal exercise	Tighten and relax your perineal muscles five times in succession, as if trying to stop urinary flow.
Leg raises	Lie on your back. Raise the right leg as high as possible, keeping the toes pointed in line with the leg. Do not bend the knee. Lower the leg slowly to the bed, using your abdominal muscles. Alternate with the right and left leg five times.
Situps	Lie on your back without pillows. Cross your arms on your chest and raise yourself to a sitting position while keeping your knees straight.

drawing of a string to pull the sides of the vagina together from the anus to the urethra. The muscle is firmly contracted and then slowly relaxed.

Advantages of Exercises

There are many benefits to be realized from progressive exercise. During pregnancy, normally increased fat deposits are acquired during the lipogenic state. These fat deposits are most commonly noticed in the abdominal and pelvic areas. As muscle tone improves with exercise, fat in these areas will also be reduced. Exercise improves venous return and prevents venous stasis. It also supplements the fibrinolytic response in the normal postpartum client, thereby decreasing the risk of thrombus formation. Healing of injured tissue is promoted through exercise. An improved ability to handle stress and to relax is also an important benefit of exercise.

EARLY POSTPARTUM DISCHARGE

The duration of hospital stay for the client and her neonate should be individualized. The majority of clients who have no labor, delivery, or postpartum complications return home within three days after delivery. In many institutions, programs exist in which the mother and her newborn can be discharged within 12 to 24 hours postpartum. These women and their neonates must meet certain criteria to be eligible for early discharge. They must live within a reasonable distance of the hospital. Childbirth preparation classes must have been taken prior to delivery. Assistance must be available at home. No major medical problems

TABLE 20-3
DISCHARGE TEACHING FOR THE POSTPARTUM FAMILY

Gravida ____ Para ____ Delivery Date ____ Time ____
Type & Rh ____ Pediatrician ____ Infant Sex ____ Weight ____
Address ____________________
Home Telephone Number ____________

MATERNAL SELF CARE SKILLS:
The patient/support person will verbalize understanding of the following:

a. Self care __
—Perineal
—Exercise
—Rest
—Nutrition
—Hemorrhoids
—Emotional changes

b. Warning signals ________

c. Rubella ________

d. Rhogam ________

INFANT FEEDING SKILLS:
The patient/support person indicates knowledge of the following:

a. Breast feeding
—Breast care
—Nipple care
—Nutritional needs
—Use of breast pump
—Expression of milk
—Milk storage
—Supplementary feedings

b. Bottle feeding
—Formula preparation
—Nipple care
—Engorgement
—Nutritional needs
—Feeding behaviors of infant
—Medications for suppression of lactation

INFANT CARE SKILLS:
The patient/support person will verbalize an understanding of the following:

____ a. Bathing skills
____ b. Cord care
____ c. Circumcision care
____ d. Cleansing the genitals
____ e. Dressing the infant
____ f. Infant safety
____ g. Evaluation of illness
____ h. Stool characteristics
____ i. Bulb syringe use
____ j. Car seat safety

can exist. The parents must agree to home visits by a nurse to assess progress.

Women who participate in these programs should be knowledgeable about self-care and infant care before discharge. After discharge, a telephone call is made to determine progress at home. Information assessed should include:

Maternal Health: Energy level
Adequate rest
Presence of discomfort
Lochia characteristics
Appetite
Difficulty in urination or defecation

Infant Health: Feeding pattern
Cord care
Cord characteristics
Difficulty in voiding or defecation
Sleeping pattern
Stool characteristics
Appearance of circumcision (if any)

Family Health: Is there help with household tasks?
How does she feel about being a mother?
How does the father feel?

How does the infant fit into the family structure?
What do the siblings think of the infant?

Future Health: Postpartum appointment made with physician
Checkup appointment for the infant
Any questions regarding sexuality or contraception
Any other concerns

DISCHARGE PLANNING

Discharge planning begins with the first contact with the client on admission to the postpartum nursing unit. The short postpartum stays of the typical delivered client stresses one of nursing's goals during this period: that of teaching care.

The client must learn how to care for herself both to attain physiological stability and to prevent complications. She must be aware of danger signs and what steps to take if they are noted. If there are gaps in the patient's knowledge, the nurse identifies and focuses on these points. All important points in caring for the infant should be identified and taught before discharge, ideally with both the mother and father (or support person). A sample teaching plan for discharge of the postpartum family is found in Table 20–3).

There is no one single way to teach the postpartum client and her partner. For some, individualized instructions are the most effective because they allow one-on-one discussion. Group classes are also of benefit for some clients, especially in covering material such as bathing of the infant, formula preparation, and sibling rivalry.

TABLE 20–4
POSTPARTUM PHYSICAL ASSESSMENT

Assessment Area	Expected Outcome
Interview	Identify chief concerns
	Review of appropriate systems—urinary, gastrointestinal, reproductive
	Assess nutritional status
General appearance	Note general appearance
Weight	Prepregnant weight achieved
Hair	Healthy looking hair
Eyes	Conjunctive pink and moist
Breasts	If nursing—full, firm to palpation
	If not nursing—return to prepregnant size with no palpable lumps or nodules
Abdomen	Muscle tone returning
	Striae fading
	No bowel or bladder distention
Perineum	Healing complete if laceration or episiotomy
Uterus	Unable to palpate abdominally
	Return to prepregnant size
	Cervix closed
	No abnormal uterine bleeding
Lower extremities	No varicosities present
Laboratory tests	Return to prepregnant laboratory values
	Pap smear normal

POSTPARTUM CHECKUP

Every client should have a checkup by her health provider at four to six weeks following delivery to assure good health without residual problems from childbirth (see Table 20-4). Along with a thorough physical examination, certain health teaching is done. Breast self-examination is emphasized, as is the necessity of a Papanicoloau smear for future health.

BIBLIOGRAPHY

Avery, M. et al. An early postpartum hospital discharge program: implementation and evaluation. *Journal of Obstetric, Gynecological & Neonatal Nursing,* 1982, **11,** 200.

Brooten, D.A., et al. A comparison of four treatments to prevent and control breast pain and engorgement in non-nursing mothers. *Nursing Research,* 1983, **32,** 225.

Carr, K.C. & Walton, V.E. Early postpartum discharge. *Journal of Obstetric, Gynecological & Neonatal Nursing,* 1982, **11,** 29.

Cranley, M.S., et al. Women's perceptions of vaginal and cesarean deliveries. *Nursing Research,* 1983, **32,** 10.

Goebel, J.B., et al. Infant car seat usage: Effectiveness of a postpartum educational program. *Journal of Obstetric, Gynecological, & Neonatal Nursing,* 1984, **12,** 33.

Gorrie, T.M. Postpartal nursing diagnosis. *Journal of Obstetric, Gynecological & Neonatal Nursing,* 1986, **15,** 52-57.

Hensleigh, P.A. Preventing rhesus isoimmunization. *American Journal of Obstetrics & Gynecology,* 1983, **146,** 749.

Ketter, D.E. & Sjelton, B.J. In-hospital exercises for the postpartal woman. *MCN,* 1983, **8,** 120.

Malinowski, J. Bladder assessment in the postpartum patient. *Journal of Obstetric, Gynecological & Neonatal Nursing,* 1978, **7,** 14.

Mansell, K.A. Mother-baby units; the concept works. *MCN,* 1984, **9,** 132.

McKenzie, C.A., et al. Comprehensive care during the postpartum period. *Nursing Clinics of North America,* 1982, **17,** 23.

Moss, J.R. Concerns of multiparas on the third postpartum day. *Journal of Obstetric, Gynecological & Neonatal Nursing,* 1984, **10,** 421.

Nurses Association of the American College of Obstetricians and Gynecologists: *Standards for Obstetric, gynecologic and neonatal nursing* (3rd ed.). Washington, D.C.: NAACOG, 1986.

Russell, T.R. Managing hemorrhoids during and after pregnancy. *Obstetrics & Gynecology,* 1983, **21** (special issue), 742.

Schwalb, R.B., et al. Preventing infection during pregnancy—and after. *RN,* 1984, **47,** 44.

Strelinck, E.G. Postpartum care: an opportunity to reinforce breast self-examination. *MCN,* 1982, **7,** 249.

chapter 21

ADAPTATIONS OF THE NEONATE

OBJECTIVES

Upon completion of this chapter, the reader will be able to:

1. Describe the role of surfactant in respiratory adaptations of the neonate to extrauterine life.
2. Describe the interaction of factors responsible for the establishment of neonatal circulation.
3. Discuss mechanisms of heat loss in the neonate and give an example of each mechanism.
4. Describe the mechanisms of thermogenesis in the neonate.
5. Describe the characteristics of normal neonatal respirations and cardiac rhythm.
6. Discuss the changes that occur in the gastrointestinal system of the neonate following birth.
7. Explain the relationship of bilirubin to neonatal physiologic jaundice.
8. Identify the major adaptations that occur in renal functions of the neonate and state their significance.
9. Describe the characteristics of the initial voidings of the neonate.
10. Discuss immunocompetency of the neonate.
11. Describe hormonal reactions that may occur in the neonate.
12. Explain the difference between caput succedaneum and cephalhematoma.
13. Discuss sensory adaptations occurring at birth.
14. Discuss the significance of trust in the psychologic development of the neonate.
15. Describe the sleep-wake pattern of the neonate.

KEY TERMS

Acrocyanosis
Bilirubin
Brown fat
Caput succedaneum
Cephalhematoma
Circumoral cyanosis
Conduction
Conjugated bilirubin
Convection
Evaporation
Glucuronyl transferase
Lecithin
Meconium
Physiologic jaundice
Radiation
Sphingomyelin
Surfactant
Unconjugated bilirubin

The neonatal period is defined as birth through the first 28 days of life. During this period the neonate undergoes transitions and adaptations from an intrauterine to an extrauterine existence. He is thrust from an environment where all his needs were met to an independent existence where he must make both immediate and ongoing adjustments in order to sustain life. Physiologic adaptations occur in all of his body systems. Success in adjusting to these changes is influenced by genetic inheritance, intrauterine factors, events and stressors during labor and delivery, and the care and management he receives from the moment of birth. Many of these factors are influenced and altered by medical and nursing management.

Nursing observations and assessments of the neonate as he undergoes transitional changes are vital to his well-being. The transitional period can be one of the most precarious periods of a neonate's life. Most neonates experience a minimum of stress, adapting to their new environments, while some find it difficult and require medical and nursing interventions. Knowledge of neonatal adaptations and characteristics is essential for the nurse to give optimal care to the neonate.

NEONATAL ADAPTATIONS OF THE RESPIRATORY SYSTEM

Establishment of respirations is crucial to survival of the neonate. Before birth, fetal oxygenation has been maintained by the functioning placenta and maternal host. Once the umbilical cord is cut, the "lifeline" from the placenta to the neonate is eliminated. Immediate and effective respirations must begin or physiologic homeostasis is jeopardized. The neonate must breathe or he cannot live without supportive mechanisms.

Respiratory development and maturation occur while the fetus is in utero, setting the stage for pulmonary functioning following birth. Highlights of these events include structural and vascular development, formation of lung fluid, and the production of surfactant.

The lung buds begin to develop at about four weeks gestation and by the end of the fourth week they are differentiated into the right and left bronchi. During the sixth and seventh week branches of the bronchi are present and by the 16th gestational week they are lined with epithelium. Shortly thereafter, vascularization of the bronchi and developing bronchioles begins. The capillaries extend and come into approximation with the alveolar ducts, which are terminal air spaces at the ends of the bronchioles destined to become the alveoli. Differentiation of the alveolar areas begins at 24 to 28 weeks gestation with the development of type I and type II cells. Type II cells participate in the formation of surfactant.

Surfactant

Surfactant is the surface tension–reducing substance of the lungs, which prevents alveolar collapse in extrauterine existence. It is composed of lipids (90 percent) and proteins (10 percent). Two of the major lipid components are the phospholipids *lecithin* and *sphingomyelin*. During the early weeks of surfactant production (24th week) there is a greater amount of sphingomyelin produced than lecithin. The level of sphingomyelin remains relatively constant throughout pregnancy, while the level of lecithin gradually rises. At the 35th week of gestation there is a sharp increase in lecithin, producing a ratio of lecithin to sphingomyelin (L/S ratio) of 2:1. When the L/S ratio is 2:1, the fetal lungs are considered mature and capable of supporting extrauterine respirations. Therefore, although surfactant is produced at 24 weeks gestation, the L/S ratio is not sufficient to support respirations until 35 to 36 weeks gestation.

An L/S ratio of 2:1 indicates that surfactant is capable of maintaining lung expansion by reducing surface tension of the alveoli. If surface tension of the alveoli were not reduced, the larger expanding alveoli would continue to get larger while the smaller alveoli would collapse during respiration. Surfactant increases the surface tension of those alveoli, which are larger, and decreases the surface tension in the smaller alveoli.

Continuous production of surfactant provides alveolar stability. In the immature lung, when the ratio of lecithin to sphingomyelin is 1:1 or less than 2:1, alveoli are not stable and will collapse after birth. However, certain factors will accelerate lung maturity and increase the L/S ratio before the 35th week of pregnancy. Accelerated maturation may be seen in the following conditions:

- Neonates of diabetic mothers with class D, E, F, and R diabetes
- Neonates of mothers with hypertensive disorders
- Neonates of mothers addicted to heroin
- Premature or prolonged rupture of the membranes (over 48 hours)
- Abruptio placentae
- Hyperthyroidism of the mother
- Placental insufficiency
- Neonates of mothers with sickle cell disease
- Neonates of mothers with severe infections
- Neonates of mothers receiving betamethasone

Conditions causing an early gestational increase in the L/S ratio are often associated with placental insufficiency (Gluck, 1978) and intrauterine stress, allegedly caused by the increase in the production of corticosteroids.

Delayed maturation of the L/S ratio is associated with the following conditions (Gluck, 1978):

- Neonates of mothers with class A, B, and C diabetes mellitus
- The smaller of fraternal twins
- Neonates of mothers with chronic glomerulonephritis (non-hypertensive)
- Neonates with hydrops fetalis (excessive edema of the neonate associated with Rh hemolytic disease)

Estimation of the L/S ratio may be made in utero to determine lung maturity and the neonate's chance for survival in the event of an early delivery. Samples of amniotic fluid are used for these determinations (see Chapter 24).

Lung Fluid

In utero the fetal lungs produce fluid responsible for the expansion of the air sacs in the latter part of pregnancy. This fluid is produced continuously at the rate of 250 ml per day (Strang, 1978), some of which contributes to the amniotic fluid via the fetal larynx and mouth, the remainder of which (80 to 100 ml) remains in the respiratory passages. The lung fluid, which passes to the amniotic fluid, provides the source of amniotic sampling necessary for determination of the L/S ratio.

Neonatal respiratory adaptations are affected by the change in lung fluid balance at birth. In order for the infant to establish effective respirations, elimination of the fluid from the lungs must occur, allowing the lungs to expand and functional residual capacity (the volume of gas in the lungs at the end of a normal expiratory movement) to be established. Compression of the fetal chest during a vaginal delivery forces about one third of the fluid out through the nose and mouth. The remainder is absorbed by the pulmonary, circulatory, and lymphatic systems.

Production of fluid must diminish after birth if air is to remain in the lungs. Suppression of fetal lung fluid production may begin in labor, owing to increased production of epinephrine.

Breathing Movements in Utero

Fetal breathing movements occur as early as 11 weeks gestation. At this time they are erratic and infrequent. Measurement of the respiratory rate by ultrasound denotes a range of 30 to 90 per minute with little regularity. Variations in central nervous system functioning will alter the respiratory pattern in the fetus, even at 34 weeks gestation. As the lungs continue to develop, the breathing pattern assumes a uniformity, simulating the normal neonatal respiratory pattern. Diminished fetal breathing movements late in pregnancy may, or may not, indicate fetal distress. Factors known to affect fetal breathing movements are: maternal smoking, hypoglycemia, hypoxia, hypercapnia, and exercise. Fetal distress is associated with gasping of the fetus in utero and usually indicates a poor prognosis.

Establishment of Neonatal Respirations

Following the biochemical, physical, and sensory changes that occur at birth (see Chapter 16), neonatal respirations begin. Continued neonatal respiratory efforts require:

- Open and clear respiratory passages
- Aeration of the lungs
- Expansion of the alveoli
- Establishment of functional residual capacity of the lungs
- Adequate amounts and composition of surfactant
- Decrease in pulmonary vascular resistance
- Increase in systemic pressure
- Increase in the pulmonary blood flow
- Closure of the foramen ovale and ductus arteriosus
- Diminished production of lung fluid

The first breath of the neonate is the most difficult. The establishment of lung volume requires a pressure of 40 to 80 cm of H_2O pressure. Following the first breath, functional residual capacity (FRC) is established, allowing some air to remain within the lungs after expiration. Since there is some air in the lungs, the next breath does not require as much pressure as the first. When surfactant is not present, surface tension of the lungs is not regulated and FRC is not established. Each successive neonatal breath becomes as difficult as the first, and normal respirations are not possible.

Continued respirations eliminate the transient asphyxia that occurs at birth. Ventilation of the lungs allows the accumulated carbon dioxide in the blood to be eliminated and restores the oxygen tension. The arterial PO_2 will range between 50 and 80 mm Hg, the PCO_2 between 33 and 45 mm Hg, and the pH 7.31 to 7.45.

As air enters the neonate's lungs resistance in the pulmonary vessels is decreased, affecting cardiovascular adaptations in the heart. Simultaneous adaptations of the pulmonary and cardiovascular system must also occur. One is dependent on the other for the successful transition from a fetal to a neonatal life. Relationships of these systems are explained in the discussion of cardiovascular adaptations.

Characteristics of Neonatal Respirations

During the first hour of life the neonate may exhibit periodic breathing (apnea of 5 to 10 seconds followed by an increased respiratory rate of 50 to 60 per minute for 10 to 15 seconds). The apnea does not exceed 20 seconds and there is no slowing of the heart rate (bradycardia). Flaring of the nares, expiratory grunt (sound heard when expirations occur against an occluded glottis), and chest retractions may also be noted. In most neonates these symptoms will subside within the first hour; however, they may be an indication of distress and continued observation is imperative.

Normal breathing following the initial transition is regular with a rate between 30 and 60 per minute. Diaphragmatic movements of the chest are noted and thoracic breathing is limited. *Circumoral cyanosis* (bluish appearance surrounding the mouth) and *acrocyanosis* (bluish discoloration of the hands and feet) may be present, especially in the first few hours of life. A few rales may be heard upon auscultation of the neonate's chest as the lung fluid dissipates; however, this finding is not normal in the subsequent hours of life. Frequently mucus is found in the oral and nasal passages, and if not removed, it may interfere with respirations. Gagging, spitting, and vomiting are efforts employed by the neonate to clear the mucus. Close observation and nursing interventions are often necessary to remove the mucus and prevent choking (see Chapter 22).

NEONATAL ADAPTATIONS OF THE CIRCULATORY SYSTEM

Early development and primitive functioning of the fetal cardiovascular system is necessary to insure distribution of nutritive materials to all the fetal cells.

Since oxygenation by the fetal lungs is not necessary, certain accommodations are made to bypass the lungs and facilitate circulation. The ductus venosus, ductus arteriosus, and foramen ovale are examples of structures that function in this capacity (see Chapter 7 for a complete discussion of fetal circulation). These fetal shunts also direct the more highly oxygenated blood to the cephalic areas where there is a greater demand by the brain for oxygen. Blood with a lower oxygen saturation is directed to the caudal areas, where oxygen requirements are less. The fetal shunts are vital for the development and survival of the fetus in utero; however, at birth their functions cease and a rapid transition from fetal circulation to neonatal circulation must occur.

Although the pulmonary and circulatory changes at birth are interrelated, certain factors appear to initiate the transitions. With the first breath, the lungs fill with air, the alveoli expand, and vasodilation of the pulmonary arterioles occurs. Pulmonary vascular resistance is lowered and pulmonary blood flow increases, resulting in increased pulmonary venous return to the left atrium and increasing the left atrial pressure. Meanwhile, elimination of the placenta causes decreased blood flow through the inferior vena cava, which decreases the right atrial pressure and raises the left atrial and systemic pressures. With lowered right atrial pressure and increased left atrial pressure the foramen ovale is forced shut.

Three factors interact to close the ductus arteriosus: rising systemic pressure, decrease in pulmonary pressure, and constrictive response of the muscle cells of the ductus arteriosus to the increased oxygen content of the blood. When the pulmonary pressure is less than the systemic pressure, the force for propulsion of the blood through the ductus arteriosus is diminished. At the same time the muscle cells of the ductus are constricting and affecting closure.

Closure of the ductus venosus appears to occur at the same time the other two shunts are closing. The mechanism for closure is unknown. Figure 21–1 depicts the interaction of factors responsible for establishment of neonatal circulation.

Functionally, closure of the shunts occurs within the first few hours of birth. They are not anatomically closed at this time, and when subjected to certain adverse conditions they may reopen. For example, hypoxia causes a lowered oxygen saturation of the blood and interferes with the constrictive response of the muscle cells of the ductus arteriosus, preventing closure. Alterations in systemic or pulmonary pressures caused by inadequate circulation may allow right atrial pressure to increase over that of the left atrium, forcing open the foramen ovale. In such circumstances normal neonatal circulation is not established and persistence of the fetal circulation (PFC) is encountered. A discussion of this condition can be found in Chapter 30.

Anatomic closure of the ductus arteriosus is

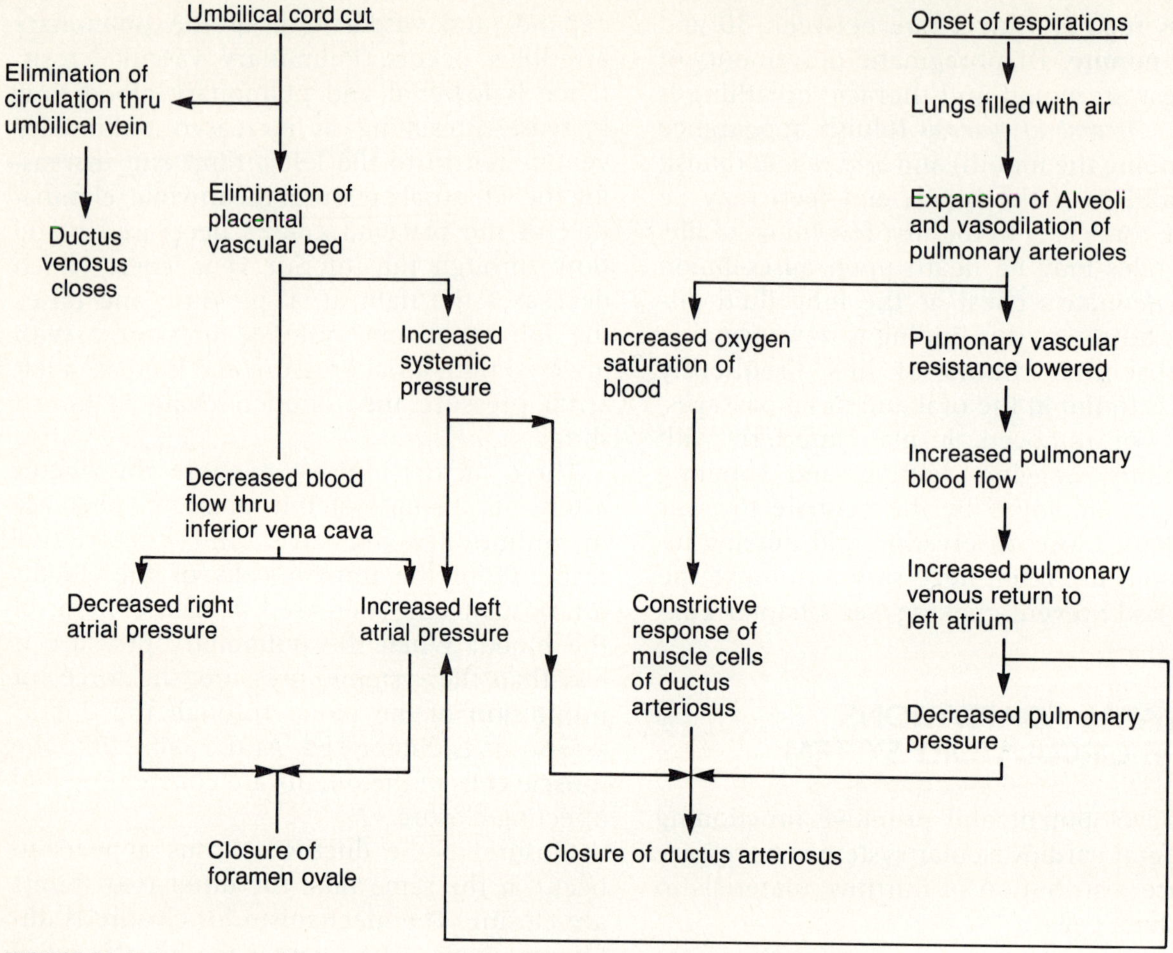

FIGURE 21-1. Interaction of factors responsible for establishment of neonatal circulation.

estimated to happen around the tenth day of neonatal life. The foramen ovale anatomically closes within several months or may remain partially open for several years. The ductus venosus closes anatomically within the first two weeks of life. Following anatomic closure, the ductus arteriosus becomes the *ligamentum arteriosum* and the ductus venosus becomes the *ligamentum venosum.*

Cardiac and Hematologic Characteristics of the Neonate

The normal heart rate of the neonate is between 120 and 160 beats per minute. Activity, stress, eating, eliminations, and crying will all affect the heart rate, and may accelerate it as much as 10 to 20 beats per minute. Sleeping may decrease the heart rate as low as 80 beats per minute.

The point of maximum intensity of the apical pulse (PMI) is located left of the midclavicular line at the fourth intercostal space. During the first week of neonatal life systolic murmurs may be heard when auscultating the heart sounds. They are usually benign and are related to the transitional changes in the cardiovascular system; however, they should be documented, assessed, and evaluated. Heart sounds are more distinct in the neonate than in the adult and may at times be irregular in rhythm.

BLOOD PRESSURE

Blood pressure elevations may be present in the neonate immediately after birth. At this time the blood pressure is approximately 80/45 mm Hg. Variations in weight and activity will alter the neonate's blood pressure. Normal pressures following the first 12 hours of life are:

Systolic	Diastolic	Weight of Neonate
50–80	30–45	2500 gm and over
45–65	25–35	1000–2500 gm

BLOOD VOLUME

At birth, before the umbilical cord is clamped, there is some transfer of blood from the placenta to the neonate while the uterus is still contracting and forcing blood through the umbilical vein. The amount of blood transferred depends on several factors:

The level the neonate is held when the cord is clamped in relationship to the level of the placenta. The neonate placed on the mother's abdomen receives less blood transfer than the infant held below the level of the placenta as the cord is cut.

The time interval between the delivery and the cord clamping. When there is late clamping of the cord there may be an additional 75 to 80 ml of blood added to the neonate's circulation, representing a blood volume increase of 50 percent. The neonate will thus, have an associated hypervolemia and elevated hematocrit and hemoglobin.

Type of delivery. Neonates delivered by cesarean section do not receive as great a transfer of blood as neonates delivered vaginally.

Complications may arise when there is an excessive amount of blood transfer at birth, resulting in the development of *polycythemia* (increased red blood cells) with increased viscosity of the blood and subsequent pulmonary edema and heart failure. When Rh sensitization is present, neonates who receive an additional volume of blood may be further jeopardized by the increase in Rh antibodies.

Some practitioners believe the additional blood received by late clamping of the cord increases the hemoglobin level and prevents anemia of the newborn. Others feel that clamping the cord after the onset of the first breath facilitates the absorption of lung fluid and decreases respiratory distress.

The normal blood volume at birth is 85 to 100 ml per kg of weight.

HEMATOLOGIC CHARACTERISTICS

In the immediate newborn period the red blood cell (RBC) count is approximately 5 million per mm^3. Thereafter, it drops to a level of 4 to 5 million per mm^3 for the next two to three months. Correspondingly, the hemoglobin and hematocrit will also be increased at birth, followed by a decrease in the next few months of neonatal life. The normal newborn hematocrit is 45 to 60 percent and the hemoglobin level is 15 to 18 g per 100 ml of blood. The drop in the RBC, hemoglobin, and hematocrit levels is described as "physiologic anemia." They are precipitated by the change from a fetal circulation, where higher numbers of RBCs are needed to insure oxygenation of the fetal blood, to a neonatal circulation, where oxygen is readily available from the pulmonary circulation.

The white blood count (WBC) is elevated in the immediate newborn period, with the increase mainly in neutrophils. The average WBC count of the neonate is 10,000 to 35,000 per mm^3. Elevation of the WBC in the early newborn period is not usually associated with pathology but is a response to the stress the neonate has experienced during labor and delivery. However, elevations of the WBC may be a response to infection and should always be carefully assessed.

Bilirubin (produced primarily by the breakdown of erythrocytes) may be elevated in the neonatal period. The increase in RBCs in the neonate contributes to the increased production of bilirubin, while immaturity of the neonate's liver lessens its ability to conjugate bilirubin. Since bilirubin may only be excreted in the conjugated form, there is a tendency for it to accumulate in the blood of the neonate. Total serum bilirubin levels will normally peak at 6 mg per 100 ml by the second or third day followed by a gradual decrease to 2 mg per 100 ml by the tenth day. A discussion of bilirubin and physiologic jaundice are found later in this chapter.

Table 21-1 summarizes the normal laboratory values found in the neonate.

TABLE 21-1
LABORATORY VALUES OF THE NEONATE

Test	Normal Range in Neonate
Hemoglobin g/dl (grams per deciliter) (1 dl = 100 ml)	15-18
Hematocrit vol %	45-60
Platelets mm^3	150,000-300,000
Reticulocytes %	3-7
White Blood Cells mm^3	10,000-35,000
Neutrophils %	46-80
Lymphocytes %	31
Eosinophils %	1-3
Monocytes %	5-10
Red blood cells mm^3	4,000,000-7,000,000
Bilirubin, direct mg/dl	0.5-1
Bilirubin, total mg/dl	5-12
Blood Sugar, mg/100 ml	40-80
Sodium mEq/liter	136-143
Potassium mEq/liter	4.0-7.0
Calcium mEq/liter	4-5
Chloride mEq/liter	95-105
Total protein g/dl	4.8-7.4
Iron $\mu g/dl$	100-200
Urea Nitrogen (BUN) mg/dl	5-15
Fibrogen mg/dl	150-300
Prothrombin time (sec)	12-18
Blood Gases	
Arterial	
pH	7.35-7.45
PO_2 mm Hg	50-80
PCO_2 mm Hg	33-45
Plasma bicarbonate mEq/liter	20-25
Base excess mEq/liter	+4 to −4

THERMOREGULATION OF THE NEONATE

Thermoregulation of the neonate during the first hours and days of life is one of the most critical aspects of effective neonatal adaptation. Thermal adaptations involve factors necessary for the maintenance of a balance between heat production and heat loss. When alterations in heat balance exist, either too warm or too cold, the metabolic processes of the infant are stressed. If the stressors are not modified or corrected, large amounts of energy are expanded by the neonate resulting in exhaustion, instability, and eventually death.

Heat Loss

Loss of heat in the neonate results from several factors that act alone or in combination.

RELATIONSHIP OF BODY SURFACE TO BODY WEIGHT

The relatively large body surface of the neonate, as compared with body weight increases the dissipation of heat from the neonate to his surroundings. This loss may be up to four times more per unit of body weight than the loss experienced by an adult (Korones, 1981).

SUBCUTANEOUS FAT

Normal neonates do not have substantial layers of subcutaneous fat to serve as insulators, preventing heat loss to the environment. The smaller the infant the greater the loss of heat. Premature infants and small-for-gestational-age infants are particularly vulnerable. Close proximity of blood vessels to skin surface, owing to the scarcity of subcutaneous fat, will cool the blood and influence hypothalamic temperature regulation.

MECHANISMS OF HEAT LOSS

Evaporation

Evaporation of amniotic fluid from the neonate begins at the moment of birth. Although this contributes to the initial drop in temperature, which stimulates respirations, if allowed to continue the neonate will be stressed. The rate of body temperature loss immediately after birth attributed to evaporation may be as much as 0.5°C per minute axillary or 0.3°C per minute rectally. Consideration of this mechanism is important when bathing the neonate, as exposure of the wet skin of the infant for even short periods of time can significantly decrease temperature.

Conduction

With conduction, heat is directly transferred from one surface to the other. Placing the neonate on cool surfaces will promote conduction and heat loss. Cool examining tables or weight scales are examples of surfaces that potentiate heat loss.

Radiation

Heat will radiate from a warm surface to cooler environmental air. Placing the neonate next to a cool outside wall or window will contribute to heat loss by radiation. The use of radiant warmers in the delivery room and wrapping the neonate in blankets will prevent heat loss by radiation.

Convection

Convection occurs when air currents carry heat away from the neonate's body. The temperature of the air in the nursery will determine the amount of heat loss through convection. A cool nursery will encourage heat loss by convection. Figure 21–2 demonstrates heat loss by all four of the mechanisms affecting the newborn.

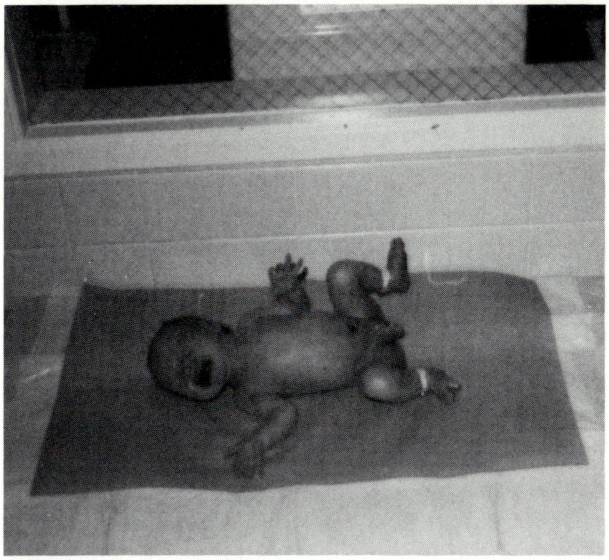

FIGURE 21-2. Examples of methods of heat loss in the newborn. Note heat loss by conduction of body heat to the examining table, radiation of heat to the wall, heat loss by convection as cool air passes over exposed surfaces of the neonate's body and evaporation as water from the moist surfaces and lungs is vaporized.

Heat Production

Thermogenesis is an important factor in maintaining body temperature in the neonate. Ideally, the temperature range is 36.6 to 37.0°C or 98 to 98.6°F. In an effort to balance heat loss, several different mechanisms are used to create and preserve heat.

MECHANISMS OF HEAT CONSERVATION

Peripheral Vasoconstriction

Vasoconstriction of the blood vessels in the skin is stimulated by the hypothalamus when skin or core temperature drops. Blood flow is directed toward circulation to the vital organs, thereby protecting their functions. Both full-term and preterm neonates are capable of utilizing vasoconstriction; however, lack of subcutaneous fat will cool the skin surface of the premature or small neonate and hasten the process.

Attitude of Flexion

In utero the fetus assumes an attitude of flexion. This same position is assumed by the normal neonate following birth. Although not as pronounced as in utero, there is flexion of the legs and arms, reducing the amount of body surface exposed to the environment. In this flexed position the neonate is able to conserve heat. When flexion is not present, as with the premature neonate, more body surface is exposed and rapid dissipation of heat occurs.

MECHANISMS OF HEAT PRODUCTION

The neonate at birth is capable of producing heat, depending on his degree of maturity and the stressors he encounters. Three known mechanisms are used by the neonate to increase his temperature.

Shivering

The neonate may or may not shiver when exposed to cold. This mechanism, by which heat is generated when the muscle fibers and muscles contract, is not well established in the neonate. Shivering may occur, but it appears to be a mechanism used only when the neonate is very cold. When it does occur, it indicates that the other mechanisms of heat production are stressed; immediate nursing interventions are needed to provide warmth.

Increased Metabolism

The neonate experiencing heat loss will attempt to increase his temperature by increasing metabolic activity. When he is cold, the hypothalamus is stimulated and the production of thyrotropin by the anterior pituitary, thyroxin by the thyroid gland, and epinephrine by the adrenal gland are increased, causing an increase in heat-producing cellular chemical activities. These hypermetabolic activities increase the consumption of neonatal oxygen and glucose. A neonate who is already hypoxic or has limited breathing capacity may be severely stressed by prolonged increases in metabolic activity.

Brown Fat Metabolism

The most readily available source of heat production in the neonate is nonshivering thermogenesis produced by metabolism of brown fat. This important and unique method of heat production is responsible for the largest percentage of total heat produced by the neonate (Brown, 1977; Davis, 1980). Brown fat cells are differentiated in the fetus at around 30 weeks gestation, with production continuing until the neonate is about three weeks old. This type of adipose cell has well-developed nerve and blood supply and venous drainage, making it quickly available for metabolism and heat distribution by the circulatory system. Although brown fat is produced during the first few weeks of neonatal life, deposits may diminish rapidly when large amounts are used for thermogenesis.

Deposits of brown fat are located in various areas of the body. Concentrations are found in the axillary region, midscapular region, posterior portions of the neck beneath the scapulae, surrounding the blood vessels of the neck and mammary arteries, and surrounding the kidneys and adrenal glands.

Utilization of brown fat for thermogenesis relies on the following factors:

Adequate deposits must be available. The preterm neonate will not have well-developed brown fat deposits.

An intact central nervous system. Release of norepinephrine from sympathetic nerve endings stimulates brown fat metabolism. Defects of the CNS or drugs given to the mother before delivery may suppress CNS functioning.

Adequate respiratory function. Metabolism requires oxygen utilization, and poor oxygenation reduces brown fat metabolism.

Adequate functioning of the endocrine system to stimulate production of epinephrine, thyrotropin, and thyroxin.

Adequate supplies of glucose to meet the caloric needs of metabolism. When the neonate is cold, there is rapid depletion of glycogen storage. Proper nutritional intake is vital to meet metabolic needs for glucose.

The effects of chilling on the neonate are discussed in Chapter 29.

NEONATAL ADAPTATIONS OF THE GASTROINTESTINAL SYSTEM

Both the sucking and swallowing reflexes are well developed at the time of birth. During the fetal period, swallowing has been evidenced by the presence of amniotic fluid in the intestinal tract. Intestinal peristalsis also occurs in utero, and meconium (the first stool of the neonate, which is black and tarry) is formed in the intestines. Air fills the small intestine by 12 hours after birth and within 24 hours there is air in the large intestine. Peristaltic movements are vigorous and occur frequently in the small intestines, while in the large intestines peristaltic movements are episodic and less frequent (Walker, 1977). Bowel sounds may be heard within one hour following birth. The intestinal tract is sterile at birth; however, within the first 6 to 12 hours bacteria are present. The bacteria are necessary for digestion and for the synthesis of vitamin K. Bacteria enter the gastrointestinal tract by both the oral and anal route during passage through the birth canal and from contact made when feeding and when examinations are performed.

Relaxation of the cardiac and pyloric sphincters is unpredictable, creating episodes of regurgitation. There is a tendency for air pockets to form in the stomach, and frequent burps are necessary. The stomach empties slowly, owing to irregularities in peristaltic movements and is greatly influenced by time, frequency, and amount of feedings. The capacity of the neonate's stomach is about 40 to 60 ml.

Preliminary digestion of milk in the stomach is influenced by gastric acidity and the enzyme pepsinogen. At birth gastric acidity is equal to that of the adult; however, after seven to ten days the level has dropped and remains low for the following two to three months, a factor which may contribute to episodes of gastric distress (colic) in the infant.

Energy requirements after birth are initially met by the use of glycogen stores; however, they are soon diminished. Within the first three hours after birth there is a rapid fall in blood glucose from a level of 70 mg per 100 ml to 50 mg per 100 ml, stabilizing at 60 to 70 mg per 100 ml at 72 hours. Glycogen stores in the liver are quickly depleted within two to three hours, while cardiac and skeletal muscle glycogen deposits are more slowly emptied. Both *glycogenolysis* (breakdown of liver glycogen) and *gluconeogenesis* (conversion of amino acids to glucose) are stimulated, producing glucose to meet the caloric needs. Free fatty acids formed from the breakdown of fats (*lipolysis*) are also available to the neonate as an energy source that spares glucose depletion. Shortly after birth there is a rise in free fatty acids and glycerol levels in the blood.

Additional sources of glucose must be supplied if hypoglycemia is to be averted. These sources include carbohydrates, fats, and proteins present in breast milk or formula. Carbohydrates from breast milk and formula containing simple sugars are easily digested and absorbed by the digestive tract of the neonate. The more complex starches are not easily digested because of the absence of the enzyme pancreatic amylase. Proteolytic enzymes from the intestinal mucosa make possible the digestion of proteins. Lipase, needed for the digestion of fats, is in short supply in the neonate, limiting the ability to digest fats.

Elimination is stimulated by the quantity, quality, and frequency of feedings. The first stool to be passed is sterile meconium, which has been formed in utero in the intestines of the fetus. Meconium formed from swallowed amniotic fluid, secretions from the digestive tract, and epithelial cells is usually passed within 24 hours after birth and several times thereafter. Passage of meconium indicates a patent rectum and its presence is documented. In the ensuing days, following feedings, the character of the stools will change from meconium to a loose brownish-green transitional stool and then to the traditional breastfed or formula-fed stool. The breastfed infant's stools will be more liquid in consistency and a bright yellow color. They reportedly have a more pleasant odor than the stool of the formula-fed baby. The stool of the formula-fed infant is pale yellow in color and has a pasty consistency. The neonate has four to six bowel movements daily during the first week of life. As the infant matures, the frequency of bowel movements will decrease and individual patterns will be developed.

NEONATAL HEPATIC ADAPTATIONS

Hepatic adaptations of the neonate following birth are related to earlier fetal hepatic events. During fetal life hepatic activities have resulted in:

Storage of iron in the liver

Formation of an ample supply of RBC's produced by the fetal liver and bone marrow

Storage of glucose in the fetal liver in the form of glycogen

All of the in utero hepatic events are important to the survival of the neonate. Since the neonate's diet of breast milk or formula is low in iron, the iron supply stored in the liver is very important for the production of hemoglobin during the first few weeks of fetal life. Also at birth there is a large demand for glucose to meet the increased energy needs created by labor and delivery, and physiologic adaptations. The liver of the neonate is immature, which hinders functions involving synthesis of glucose, proteins, and clotting factors, vitamin storage, metabolism of drugs, conversion of fatty acids to ketones, and conjugation of bilirubin.

Bilirubin

Bilirubin is formed when red blood cells are broken down to heme and globin. The heme portion is then catabolized to form *unconjugated* or *free bilirubin*. The unconjugated bilirubin in the blood combines with albumin and is transported to the liver where the enzyme *glucuronyl transferase* changes the unconjugated bilirubin to *conjugated bilirubin*. The conjugated bilirubin then enters the small intestine as a component of bile. Bilirubin in the intestine is changed to urobilinogen by bacterial flora. In this form it is water soluble and can be excreted.

Unconjugated bilirubin is fat soluble and cannot be excreted in the bile or by the kidneys; it can, however, be deposited in the tissues of the body, where it accumulates and the bilirubin pigment imparts a yellowish discoloration to the skin (*jaundice*) and sclera of the eye. In the neonate, physiologic jaundice (*icterus neonatorum*) does not become visible until the second or third day, when total serum bilirubin levels are 5 to 7 mg per 100 ml.

Several factors will alter the elimination of bilirubin by the neonate. First, the increased production of red blood cells and their shortened life span present a large volume of bilirubin for conjugation. Secondly, the liver is only capable of storing a limited amount of bilirubin for conjugation, owing to the presence of two liver proteins, *Y* and *Z*. In the neonate, sufficient amounts of these proteins are lacking and large loads of bilirubin cannot be accommodated by the liver.

The third factor responsible for physiologic jaundice is the relationship of bilirubin to albumin. Since bilirubin must bind with albumin for transportation to the liver, changes in this relationship may deter conjugation of bilirubin. Drugs such as aspirin, sulfonamides, heparin, sodium benzoate, novobiocin, and furosemide will compete with bilirubin for a binding site to albumin. Respiratory and metabolic acidosis diminish the attraction of bilirubin to albumin. Prematures and neonates with hypoproteinemia have low levels of albumin and therefore are unable to conjugate large amounts of bilirubin.

Fourth, because of the immaturity of the neonate's liver, production of the enzyme glucuronyl transferase, needed for conjugation, is limited. When moderate levels of bilirubin are delivered to the neonate's liver for conjugation, the level of glucuronyl transferase is sufficient, but when large amounts are presented it is not. Certain substances such as pregnanediol in breast milk may also inhibit the production of glucuronyl transferase, as will congenital or neonatal infection of protozoal, viral, or bacterial origin. Syndromes such as *Crigler-Najjar syndrome I and II* (autosomal disorders with absent or deficient glucuronyl transferase production) and *Gelbert's syndrome* (autosomal dominant benign hyperbilirubinemia) also alter levels of glucuronyl transferase (Frank, Turner, & Merenstein, 1985).

Neonatal jaundice is either of a physiologic or pathologic origin. Although nearly 50 percent of normal neonates will develop jaundice, when observed, it should be evaluated for cause and severity. Criteria for the evaluation of jaundice may be found in Table 21–2. Care of the neonate with pathologic jaundice is discussed in Chapter 31.

Glucose Metabolism

The liver is the organ that releases its glycogen stores for immediate glucose supply. Immaturity of the liver alters the release of liver enzymes and hormones needed for glycogenolysis and gluconeogenesis. Blood glucose levels are affected by stressors precipitated by cold, respiratory and digestive problems, activity levels, deficient nutrition, prematurity and gestational-age disorders, and central nervous system disorders.

TABLE 21–2
COMPARISON OF PHYSIOLOGIC JAUNDICE WITH PATHOLOGIC JAUNDICE

Criteria	Physiologic Jaundice	Pathologic Jaundice
First signs of jaundice	Appears 24 hours following birth on 2nd or 3rd day	Appears within the first 24 hours following birth
Duration of jaundice	Does not continue for more than a week	May continue beyond a week in full term neonate and 2 weeks in premature
Total serum bilirubin levels in first 24 hours	Below 5 mg/100 ml	Elevated beyond 6 mg/100 ml
Direct (conjugated) serum bilirubin level	Rarely present—not to exceed 0.5–1 mg/100 ml	Over 1–2 mg/100 ml
Daily increments of total serum bilirubin levels	Increases in total serum bilirubin less than 5 gm/100 ml in 24 hours	Increases in total serum bilirubin over 5 mg/100 ml in 24 hours
Total serum bilirubin level (combination of direct and indirect)	Below 12 mg/100 ml	Over 12 mg/100 ml

Coagulation Factors

Vitamin K–dependent coagulation factors are diminished in the neonate. These factors, II, VII, IX, and X, are present in the liver at birth but need vitamin K for synthesis. Sterility of the fetal bowel prevents the establishment of the normal intestinal flora needed for synthesis of vitamin K. Therefore, until feedings have begun and digestion is occurring, little or no bacteria are present in the bowel. Once these processes are instituted, the normal flora can be established and vitamin K will be produced. In order to enhance the activation of coagulation factors, vitamin K is administered to the infant within the first 24 hours following birth. This measure may temporarily increase coagulation factors, but levels remain low for several days or months.

NEONATAL ADAPTATIONS OF RENAL FUNCTION

Birth initiates changes in the renal system of the neonate that necessitate adaptations in kidney function. Before birth, the maternal-placental unit provides waste elimination and electrolyte balance for the fetus. Now, these functions must be assumed by the neonate. Minimal function of the fetal renal system produces urine voided into the amniotic fluid, but total renal function is limited in utero.

The neonate is born with the essential structures necessary for adequate renal functions. The kidneys are, however, immature for the first two years of life. Three basic differences may be noted: (1) although the full number of glomeruli are present they are small and capable of performing only 30 percent of the normal rate of glomerular filtration; (2) the tubular volume is reduced owing to underdevelopment of the proximal tubules; and (3) renal plasma flow is lowered. Some of the consequences of these changes are:

Glucose is absorbed slowly

Sodium and potassium reabsorption is low

Renal threshold for bicarbonate is reduced, resulting in a decreased ability to acidify urine and increasing the potential for acidosis

Decreased ability to excrete a sodium or water load

Decreased ability to excrete a solute load, limiting excretion of protein loads and contributing to dehydration

In the normal neonate renal adjustments occur with little difficulty; however, because of the immaturity of the kidneys, some conditions may jeopardize kidney function. Renal function may be stressed following prolonged labors or difficult deliveries, resulting in hypoxia or acidosis. Restricting fluids or oral intake for extended periods of time may create stress to the renal system. Alterations in electrolytes and fluid balance deter effective kidney function, as do any fluid losses associated with vomiting or diarrhea.

Voidings are small and infrequent in the first two days following birth, with the average output 30 to 60 ml per 24 hours. Thereafter, the frequency increases to 5 to 20 voidings per day with an average output of 150 to 250 ml per 24 hours. Variations in output are frequent and reflect the frequency, amount, and type of feedings.

Characteristics of the urine are:

First voiding: dilute and clear

Subsequent voidings: cloudy due to the presence of mucus

Voiding following feedings: pale or straw-colored urine

Occasional uric acid crystal: appears as red or pink spots on diaper called brick-dust

Odorless: odor does not develop until the ability to concentrate urine is established

ADAPTATIONS OF THE IMMUNE SYSTEM OF THE NEONATE

The immune system consists of a series of interrelated phenomena which contribute to the establishment of the neonate's biological individuality. Structured within the humoral and cellular components of the immune system are the mechanisms whereby cells recognize one another and reject those which are foreign. Immunocompetency relies on this recognition system to produce antibodies and manifest cellular reactivity.

The immune system originates as hematopoietic stem cells in the bone marrow which are then processed into three specialized divisions. One of the divisions, the promonocytes and monocytes, develops into phagocytic macrophages when stimulated by the presence of bacteria. The second division differentiates under the influence of the thymus gland into T lymphocytes responsible for cellular immunity. The third division is the B lymphocytes, responsible for the antibody-secreting plasma cells found in the gamma globulin fraction of the blood. The five classes of antibodies are: IgG, IgM, IgA, IgD, and IgE.

The antibody IgG comprises about 75 percent of the normal individual's antibodies and is the only antibody to cross the placenta. The neonate has a comparable level with the adult. However, the neonate's IgG levels fall steadily for approximately three to six months after birth, accounting for increased sensitivity to infection between three and six months of age. By age three, 75 percent of the adult level is reached. The IgG antibodies are specific to viral and bacterial organisms such as pneumococcus, streptococcus, diphtheria, *Haemophilus influenzae*, and tetanus, which have previously been encountered by the mother.

In contrast, IgM immunoglobulin is unable to cross the placental barrier (Speer and Dockhorn, 1973), although IgM synthesizing cells may be found in the fetus as early as ten weeks gestation. At birth, the neonate's IgM level is below the adult level, ranging from 20 to 30 mg per 100 ml, compared with the adult level of 75 to 150 mg per 100 ml. The IgM levels rise in the second or third week of life, followed by a drop from the fourth to the sixth week. Girls show higher levels of IgM than boys. Acute intrauterine infections give rise to high IgM cord serum levels. Disease such as toxoplasmosis, cytomegalovirus, congenital syphilis, and rubella also elevate cord IgM levels. Very severe fetal infections may cause the IgM level to drop. IgM antibodies are most important against gram-negative organisms such as E. coli and Pseudomonas, however IgM is initially produced in the presence of any infection.

Serum IgA is not capable of crossing the placental barrier and is absent in the neonate at birth, but develops by four weeks of neonatal life. It then continues to rise until puberty. The specific function of this immunoglobulin is not known. Mucosa of the intestinal and respiratory tract give rise to a different form of IgA called "secretory IgA." This antibody is present in breast milk and is significantly higher in colostrum. Unlike the other antibodies, it is not destroyed by gastric secretions and will afford immunity to the intestinal mucosa.

Immunoglobulin IgE does not cross the placenta and levels are very low at birth. It is present in nasal, bronchial, and gastrointestinal secretions. Elevated IgE levels are observed with allergic reactions and it is thought to be responsible for the release of histine (Nysather, Katz & Lenth, 1976). The exact function in the neonate is not known.

The IgD class of antibodies are found in low serum concentrations in the neonate as well as the adult. Their function has not been established.

The immunity of the neonate at birth is passive immunity, acquired by the passage of antibodies from the mother to the fetus. IgG is the only antibody capable of passing in this manner, since it is the only one to cross the placenta. The neonate may rely on his mother's IgG antibodies for a short period of time, thereafter he must establish his own immunity to infectious organisms. During the first few weeks of life, when the neonate's level of immunity is low, he is susceptible to infections. Efforts should be made to provide a pathogen-free environment.

NEONATAL ENDOCRINE ADAPTATIONS

The endocrine system is developed and functions adequately at birth. Some immaturity may be noted, but normal activity is achieved within the first few weeks following birth. The most apparent hormonal reactions at birth are associated with increased levels of estrogen and progesterone derived from the maternal circulation. Estrogen may cause breast engorgement of both male and female neonates. There may be a slight amount of milklike secretion from the breast ("witch's milk"). This reaction is transient and will disappear in a few days. Hormonal reactions may produce hypertrophia of the female labia and pseudomenstruation (slight, bloody, mucoid vaginal discharge).

Stimuli present at birth, such as cold, will influence the level of thyrotropin produced by the pituitary gland. During the first 30 minutes following birth there is a surge in thyrotropin followed by a return to normal in two to four days. Thyroxine progressively rises and serum T_3 rises during the first 24 hours of life. Production of parathyroid hormone (PTH) is minimal, decreasing renal excretion of phosphate and tubular reabsorption of calcium. Stimulation of the antidiuretic hormone (ADH) produced by the posterior pituitary gland is slow, promoting dehydration.

NEONATAL SKELETAL AND NEUROMUSCULAR ADAPTATIONS

Ossification of the skeletal system is not complete at birth, allowing passage of the fetus through the birth canal free from skeletal injuries. Cartilage is widely distributed throughout the skeletal system. The cranial bones are separated by suture lines and fontanels, which are open and palpable at birth. Overlapping of the suture lines may be noted in the first 24 hours following birth due to molding of the head during labor and delivery. Molding will give the head a very distorted, elongated appearance compared with the round head of the neonate delivered by breech or cesarean section.

Pressure on the presenting part of the fetal head against the cervix during labor may cause edema of the scalp, known as *caput succedaneum.* This diffuse swelling is temporary and will be absorbed within two to three days. Bleeding between the bone and the periosteum of the bone owing to rupture of a blood vessel may cause swelling over one of the cranial bones, most commonly the parietal bone. This type of swelling, called *cephalhematoma,* does not cross the suture lines and may vary a great deal in size (see Fig. 21–3). Swelling from a cephalhematoma is well defined and may impart a bluish discoloration to the area, much as in a black and blue mark. Disappearance of the swelling is not as rapid as that of the caput succedaneum, remaining for days or even weeks before it is absorbed. During the process of absorption of blood in the hematoma there is a significant release of indirect bilirubin, which contributes to neonatal jaundice.

Muscle tone of the neonate is good, with flexion of the extremities and random movement of the muscles and joints. A flaccid posture is not normal and may indicate prematurity, CNS disorders, trauma or depression from maternal drugs, and shock. Purposeful movements are not noted, although attempts at head lifting may be present.

Primitive reflexes are present in the neonate at birth (Chapter 22), reflecting the maturity and intactness of the nervous system. Movements are uncoordinated, and immaturity of the nervous system accounts for the slight tremors displayed as twitching of the extremities and quivering of the mouth. These

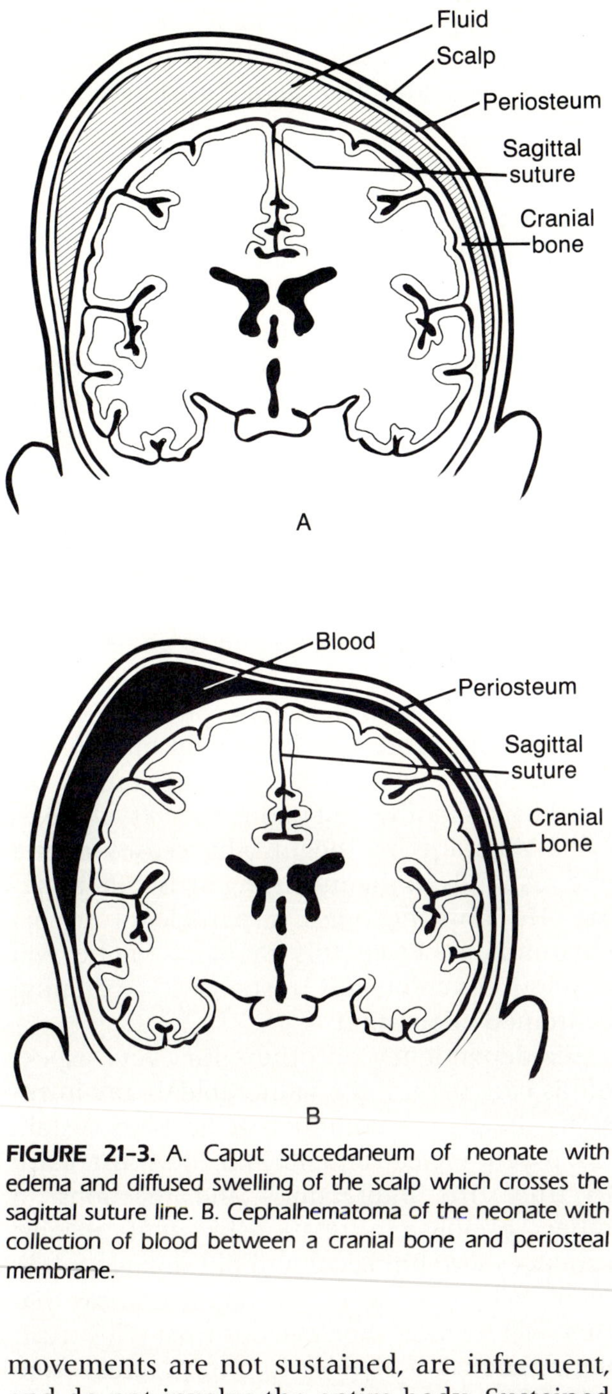

FIGURE 21-3. A. Caput succedaneum of neonate with edema and diffused swelling of the scalp which crosses the sagittal suture line. B. Cephalhematoma of the neonate with collection of blood between a cranial bone and periosteal membrane.

movements are not sustained, are infrequent, and do not involve the entire body. Sustained tremors of the entire body may be indicative of pathology such as central nervous system disorders or hypoglycemia.

Myelination of the neural pathways is substantially developed, facilitating transmission of nerve impulses. Sensory areas involved in smelling, tasting, and hearing appear to have the most well-developed myelination of the neural pathways. These senses are acutely developed in the neonate.

A full complement of brain cells is present at birth; however, their growth and development continues throughout most of life. Rapid growth occurs in the first years of life, with cerebral and cortical development influenced by genetics and environment. Adverse conditions such as improper nutrition, injury, deficient metabolic and hormonal functions, and lack of environmental stimulation can alter brain development at birth and throughout the entire life span.

NEONATAL SENSORY ADAPTATIONS

Vision

At birth, the development of the eye is not complete. Myelination of the optic nerve has not been achieved and the muscles of accommodation (ciliary muscles) are immature. The newborn is able to fixate on an object at a focal distance of 8 inches (Ludington-Hoe, 1983), but beyond this range focusing is impaired. Visual acuity is developed within a range of 9 to 12 inches. The neonate is unable to distinguish color but has the ability to discriminate shades of light and dark. Eye movements are uncoordinated, producing transient *strabismus* (cross-eyed) and *nystagmus* (rapid, involuntary movements of the eyeball).

Epicanthal folds on the upper eyelids obscure the inner canthus, producing a pseudostrabismus. The sclera has a bluish tint and the iris of all newborns is a grayish-blue. Eye color is established at 6 to 12 months. Salt and pepper speckling of the iris (*Brushfield spots*) may occur in normal infants but it is also frequently seen in infants with Down's syndrome.

The protective blink reflex is not present, but the neonate will blink when a bright light is directed toward his eye. The pupils are equally reactive to light. The red reflex may be elicited when light from an ophthalmoscope falls on the retina and produces a small orange-red spot.

Smell

Research lacks confirmation of the ability or inability of the neonate to distinguish smells. There is some indication that breastfed infants are more sensitive to the smell of the milk from their own mother than that from another. Very pungent odors will elicit a response in the newborn.

Taste

Taste buds, on the tip of the tongue, are developed in the neonate at birth and different responses are evoked by different substances. Grimacing is seen when the neonate tastes a bitter substance and an expression of satiety is rendered when a sweet substance is offered.

Hearing

The neonate is capable of hearing at birth following drainage of the amniotic fluid from the ear and the removal of vernix caseosa from the outer ear passages. Reactions to various sounds may produce a range of responses. Loud and high-pitched sounds will alarm the neonate and may stimulate a startle response. Soft, low-pitched sounds are soothing and may be used to comfort the neonate. The neonate will respond to the human voice and appears to follow that sound more readily than other sounds.

Tactile

Tactile stimulation of the infant is essential to his development. At birth the neonate is acutely sensitive to touch, contact which produces pain, soothing contact, and stroking. Areas with increased sensitivity are the soles of the feet, and the area surrounding the mouth and the lips.

NEONATAL PSYCHOLOGICAL ADAPTATIONS

The nonstressed neonate responds to the world into which he is thrust at birth with a loud objecting cry. Bright lights in the delivery room, a complexity of sounds and an uncomfortable environmental temperature greet him as he enters the world. His reflexes are stimulated by measures to secure his welfare. Even as he objects to the turn of events which forced him into the world, his physiologic adaptations urge him to continue his existence.

Comfort is afforded him, at last, when warmth and protective arms hold him closely and securely while soft soothing sounds uttered by his mother fall on his ears. Psychological adaptation has begun—he ceases crying and responds to the nurturing he is experiencing. He now becomes a participant in his environment. From this moment on he will develop psychological responses, facilitating continued adaptation.

His dependency on others for every aspect of his care makes him vulnerable to any intrusions on his environment. If he is to sustain his psychological equilibrium, he must learn to trust. His interactions and reactions to others establish a relationship that, ideally, produces psychological and physiologic fulfillment. When he has needs, he must know that they will be met—he develops trust. This trusting relationship enables him to progress from one developmental task to the other. He develops means of effectively communicating his needs—he cries, he smiles, he coos. At the same time he learns to depend on his nurturing caregiver, generally his mother, to provide for him. Provision of this care becomes a time of satisfaction and he associates mothering with pleasurable experiences.

Adjustment to his environment includes his ability to habitate. As he trusts, he learns to accept those environmental factors such as noise that were previously threatening or disruptive. He becomes selective when responding to his environment. He will visually explore his environment when satisfied but will cry loudly when hungry or cold.

He develops his own preferences for comforting as well as stimulation. Some infants prefer to be cuddled and rocked while others are more easily comforted by the sound of their mother's voice. He responds to his own biological timing and will develop periods of wakefulness alternating with sleep periods. His sleep periods may involve 75 percent of his total day, averaging about 15 to 20 hours per day. During his sleep states he progresses through several patterns of deep and light sleep. Interruption of his sleep in any one of the stages is disruptive to him. He is more comfortable in the presence of those who are familiar with his sleep patterns and who plan his care accordingly.

While awake, the neonate may respond in several ways. When he first awakens, he responds in a quiet, passive way. Reactions to stimuli are limited and he is not interested in his environment. As his level of wakefulness increases, he becomes more alert and will react to and interact with others. Eye contact will be maintained and, as he grows older, smiles may be offered. Hunger pains are more noticeable to him during this period and he may react by crying. Once in the crying state, he is not comforted until his needs are met. When satisfied, the cycle may begin all over as he again enters the sleep state.

Gradually, patterns of behavior based on trust in those who nurture him and harmony with his environment develop. The foundations have been laid and psychological adaptation is underway.

BIBLIOGRAPHY

Brown, B. Brown adipose tissue as an effector of nonshivering thermogenesis. *Experientia* 1977, **33,** 1124-1126.

Bushness, I.W.R. Discrimination of faces by young infants. *Journal of Experimental Child Psychology,* 1982, **33,** 288-308.

Davis, V. The structure and function of brown adipose tissue in the neonate. *Journal of Obstetric, Gynecological & Neonatal Nursing,* 1980, **9,** 368-372.

Frank, C. Turner, B. & Merenstein, G. Jaundice. In G. Merenstein & S. Gardner. *Handbook of neonatal intensive care.* St. Louis: Mosby, 1985.

Gould, J. Gluck, L. & Kulovich, M. The acceleration of neurological maturation in high stress pregnancy and its relation to fetal lung maturity. *Pediatric Research,* 1972, **6,** 335.

Korones, S. *High risk newborn infants* (3rd ed.). St. Louis: Mosby, 1981.

Liggins, G. & Howie, R. A controlled trial of antepartum glucocorticoid treatment for prevention of the respiratory distress syndrome in premature infants. *Pediatrics,* 1972, **50,** 515.

Ludington-Hoe, S. What can newborns really see? *American Journal of Nursing,* 1983, **83,** 1286-1289.

Nysather, J., Katz, A. & Lenth, J. The immune system: Its development and functions. *American Journal of Nursing,* 1976, **76,** 1614-1618.

Strang, L. Fluid transfer across capillary and alveolar walls: The surfactant system and the neonatal lung. *Monograph of Mead Johnson Symposium on Perinatal and Developmental Medicine, No. 14,* 1978, pp. 50-51.

Walker, W. Development of intestinal host defense mechanisms and the passive protective role of human milk. *Monograph of Mead Johnson Symposium on Perinatal and Developmental Medicine, No. 11,* 1977, pp. 39-48.

chapter 22

NURSING MANAGEMENT OF THE NORMAL NEONATE

OBJECTIVES

Upon completion of this chapter, the reader will be able to:

1. Describe the initial nursing assessment of the neonate, assessments following stabilization and during the transitional period, and assessments used when giving daily care.
2. Describe the clinical behavior of the neonate in the first period of reactivity, rest and sleep, and second reactivity period.
3. Discuss the components of the neonatal physical examination, normal and abnormal findings, and their significance.
4. Explain the Dubowitz method of assessment of gestational age and describe the criteria used.
5. Discuss the Brazelton Neonatal Behavioral Assessment Scale.
6. Identify the essential parameters of nursing care during the transitional period.
7. Discuss nursing assessments and interventions employed when giving daily care to the neonate.
8. Identify methods of infection control within the neonatal nursery.
9. Describe the components of neonatal screening and explain why they are necessary.
10. Formulate a teaching plan for the parents of a normal neonate, including aspects of neonatal care and development.
11. List measures that can be undertaken by the parents to insure the safety of the neonate.
12. List immunizations necessary for the infant and know the recommended scheduling.

KEY TERMS

Ballard Maturity Rating
Brazelton behavioral assessment
Circumcision
Epstein's pearls
Erythema neonatorum toxicum
Galactosemia
Gestational age—SGA-AGA-LGA
Harlequin skin changes
Inclusion cyst
Lanugo
Milia
Mongolian spots
Nevi
Phenylketonuria
Telangiectatic nevi
Transitional period
Vernix caseosa

Nursing management is one of the key factors in neonatal adaptation to extrauterine life. Foundations of care are based on the nursing process, which is the core of neonatal nursing care. Skillful use of the nursing process enables the nurse to deliver care to the neonate which is individualized and eclectic in scope. Neonatal nursing management is not based on the delivery of routine care, but on careful initial and ongoing assessments and evaluations of all dimensions of the neonate. Appropriate nursing interventions may then be instituted to provide holistic care.

NEONATAL MANAGEMENT DURING THE FIRST TWENTY FOUR HOURS

The first 24 hours of neonatal life are critical determinates for continued survival. Assessments of all parameters affecting adaptations necessary for survival are important. Continuous monitoring determines normal physiologic adaptations and any deterioration in health status. A thorough understanding of prenatal and intrapartal factors influencing the neonate is also necessary for prevention of complications.

Initial assessment of the neonate is undertaken immediately following birth (see Chapter 16). At this time, assessments are directed toward determination of Apgar scores, observation for anomalies, and evidence of alterations in thermoregulation. Continued care is based on evaluation of these assessments and measures needed to meet the physiologic needs of the neonate. Priorities of care are established and medical and nursing interventions instituted accordingly. Neonates who are experiencing difficulty maintaining homeostasis are directed to high-risk nurseries where more intensive care is provided. If it is determined that normal neonatal physiologic adaptations are occurring, nursing care is directed toward continued assessments and evaluations as a basis for individualized care.

Neonatal care following delivery may be given in the nursery or at the bedside of the mother, depending on the policies of the individual hospital. However, provisions are made for continued observation of the neonate until stabilization has taken place. Although the neonate may appear normal at birth and respond with good Apgar scores, he may still experience difficulty during the transition to extrauterine life. Not all abnormalities are apparent at birth and discrimination must be used by the nurse when assessment of physiologic adaptations indicate deviations from the normal. During the first 24 hours observation of the neonate is the main focus of care, with attention directed toward assessments of physical and neurologic status, estimation of gestational age, and behavioral assessment. Other aspects of care which are important and are included at this time are: maintenance of thermo stability, identification of the neonate, provision for a safe environment, administration of medications, and provision for proper nutritional intake.

Identification

When the neonate is received from the delivery area, identification bands are checked with the delivery room personnel and with the records of the neonate. Mother's name, hospital number, date and time of delivery, and physician are verified. Any discrepancies are clarified and corrections made.

Communication of Data

Communication between the personnel involved in the delivery of the neonate and those who will be giving nursery care is essential. A brief summary of the events that took

TABLE 22-1
GUIDE FOR PERINATAL ASSESSMENT OF THE NEWBORN—IDENTIFICATION OF RISK FACTORS BY MATERNAL COMPONENTS
(Risk significance: 3=High risk, 2=Moderate risk, 1=Slight risk)

Factor	Risk
GENERAL INFORMATION	
Age: <18 or >40	2
Marital status	
Single, separated, divorced	
Widow	2
Socioeconomic level	
Low	2
Low-middle	1
Ethnic-cultural group:	
Minority	2
Educational level: 10th Gr.	1
Hereditary disorder: genetic	3
Familial health history	
Diabetes	2
Chronic hypertension	1
Prepregnancy weight:	
<100 or >200	2
History of infertility	
Para 0, >35 yr	2
Problem conceiving	1
Pregnancy interval >4 yr	1
Rx for infertility	2
OBSTETRICAL HISTORY	
Gravida: ≥6	2
Parity: ≥5	2
Abortions	
≥1 (≤20 wk)	3
Gravida <1 + Para	3
Stillbirths: ≥1 (≥37 wk)	3
Prematurity: <37 wk	3
SGA	
<37 wk	3
37–41 wk	2
≥42 wk	2
LGA	
<37 wk	3
37–41 wk	2
≥42 wk	2
Neonatal death: ≤4 wk	3
History of congenital anomalies	2
History of neonatal asphyxia	2
Previous prenatal history	
Preeclampsia	2
Eclampsia	3
PROM	2
Ectopic pregnancy	2
Placenta previa	2
Placenta abruptio	2
CPD	2
Uterine dystocia	3
Cesarean section	2
Induction	1
Rh sensitization	3
ABO incompatibility	2
PRESENT PREGNANCY ANTEPARTAL COURSE	
General prenatal information	
Prenatal care: little or none	3
Weight gain: ≤15 lb or ≥35 lb	2
Medications other than dietary supplement	3
Maternal medical/surgical problems	
Diabetes	3
Heart disease	2
Chronic hypertension	2
Thyroid disease	2
Other endocrine disorders	2
Anemia	
Iron deficiency	2
Sickle cell	3
Other	3
Pulmonary disease	2
Chronic renal disease	2
Neurologic disease	2
PID	2
Pelvic surgery	2
Habits/Present pregnancy	
Heavy smoker: ≥ 20/day	2
Alcohol	
Moderate use	1
Heavy use	2
Abuse	3
Drug abuse	3
Complications	
Preeclampsia	2
Eclampsia	3
Hyperemesis gravidarum	3
Early bleeding ≤ 20 wk	2
Late bleeding ≤ 20 wk	3
Bleeding with pain	3
Hydramnios	2
Oligohydramnios	3
Rubella infection (8–12 wk)	3
Venereal disease	3
Other infections	2
Maternal FUO	2
Rh sensitization	3
Antepartal diagnostic tests	
Estriol level: no rise > 36 wk	3
Ultrasonography: growth retardation > 2 wk	3

TABLE 22-1 (continued)

Factor	Risk	Factor	Risk
Amniocentesis		Fetal heart monitoring	
L/S ratio < 2:1	3	Base line FHR <100 or >160	3
Billirubin present	3	Bradycardia >30 min	3
Meconium present	3	Tachycardia ≥30 min	3
Other evidence of immaturity	3	Poor beat-to-beat variability	3
NST: nonreactive	3	Increasing number of variables (decelerations)	3
OCT: positive	3	Late decelerations	3
Duration of pregnancy		Analgesia	
< 37 wk	3	Total Demerol >200 mg	3
> 42 wk	2	Demerol >25 mg. I.V. within ½ hr of delivery	3
PRESENT PREGNANCY INTRAPARTAL COURSE		Demerol >25 mg. I.M. within 1 hr of delivery	3
Onset of labor		Course of delivery	
Early labor: <37 wk	3	Presentation	
PROM	3	Breech	3
Induction	2	Transverse lie	3
Cesarean section	2	Position: vertex other than OA	2
Duration of labor		Forceps	
1st stage >16 hr	2	Outlet	1
2nd stage >2 hr	3	Low	2
2nd stage <10 min	3	Mid or >	3
Total >20 hr	2	Vacuum extraction	2
<3 hr	2	Identified problems	
Identified intrapartal problems:		Shoulder dystocia	3
CPD	2	Nuchal cord × 1	1
Preeclampsia	2	≥ × 2	3
Eclampsia	3	Short cord	2
Rx $MgSO_4$ >25 g	3	Cesarean section	
Meconium staining	3	Repeat	2
Placenta previa	3	Emergency	3
Abruptio placentae	3	Episiotomy: none with laceration	1
Cord compresion	2	Anesthesia	
Prolapsed cord	3	General	3
Uterine inertia	3	Spinal 15 min before delivery	2
Uterine tetany	3	Maternal bonding	
Multiple birth	3	No bonding	2
Maternal fever ≥100°F	3	Inappropriate affect	2

Source: Brodish, M. Perinatal assessment. **Journal of Obstetric, Gynecological & Neonatal Nursing,** 1981, **10,** 42–46.

place during maternal prenatal and intrapartal periods that may influence the neonate's condition is given. Fetal responses to labor and delivery, conditions of the neonate at birth and immediately following, and any resuscitative measures are also communicated. This information is included in the written record of the neonate, but the brief verbal report provides the basis for immediate care by nursery personnel. Following observations of the neonate, the nurse then thoroughly reviews the written records. Factors that may alter neonatal physiologic adaptations to extrauterine life are noted. Table 22–1 provides a guide for perinatal assessment of the neonate with identification of risk factors by maternal components.

Neonatal General Assessments

Before a systematic assessment is begun the nurse observes the general appearance of the neonate, relating it to the information communicated by the delivery nurse. Evaluation of the present status of the neonate is made and the need for therapeutic interventions is determined. Assessments are made in the following areas:

Respiratory Effort	No indications of distress such as tachypnea, sternal retractions, flaring nostrils, grunting or stridor. Rate between 30 to 60/minute.
Heart	Rate above 100
Color	Pink with some acrocyanosis of extremities No evidence of pallor or cyanosis
Size	No extremes in size. Appears well nourished and hydrated. No edema.
Posture & Muscle Tone	Flexed posture. Flexion of arms and legs. No limpness.
Activity	Responsive to stimuli. Good cry.
Umbilical Cord	Clamped with no bleeding. Normal vessels
Injuries & Anomalies	None apparent.

Any indications of respiratory distress or depression of the infant preclude the systematic assessment at this time. These neonates are transferred to an area of more intensive care. If the neonate is not experiencing difficulties, continuation of the assessment process is undertaken.

Physical Assessment of the Neonate

A warm, safe environment is provided, and all equipment is assembled before the examination is begun (see Table 22–2 for necessary equipment). The examination is conducted as swiftly as possible to avoid stressing the neonate. Every effort is made to allow the parents an opportunity to bond with the neonate before the examination is conducted and, when possible, they may desire to participate in or observe the examination. Ideally, the first examination is performed when the neonate is in the reactive stage and is responsive to his environment.

WEIGHT

The neonate is weighed on a scale that has protective paper or a liner on its surface to prevent chilling and contamination. Adjustment of the scale is made to allow for the weight of the protective sheet before the neonate is placed on the scale (see Fig. 22–1).

TABLE 22–2
EQUIPMENT UTILIZED FOR ASSESSMENT OF NEONATE

Warm table surface or crib
Infant scale (calibrated with protective covering in place)
Disposable measuring tape
Stethoscope
Thermometer
Tongue blade
Flashlight
Alcohol wipes
Ophthalmoscope
Nipple or pacifier
Neonatal blood pressure cuff

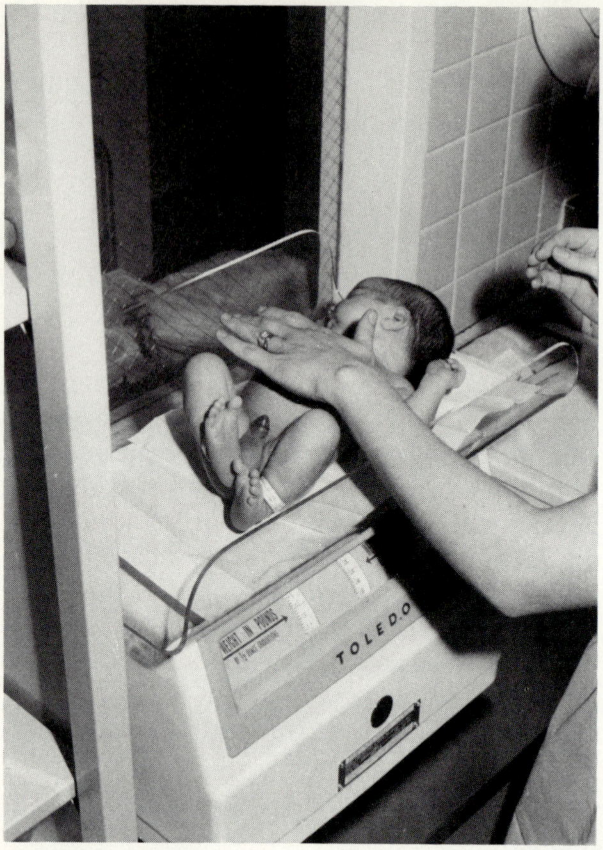

FIGURE 22-1. Weighing the neonate.

The average neonate weighs 3400 g (7.5 pounds) at birth. Variations within the normal range of 2500 to 4000 g may occur because of ethnic influences, gestation, and prenatal factors. Weights falling outside of the normal range may indicate abnormalities or disorders and are therefore noted and evaluated. The initial weight of the neonate serves as a data base for subsequent daily weight. Most neonates normally lose approximately 10 percent of their birth weight within the first three to four days following birth owing to excretion of the relatively large fluid volume present in utero. Delays in feeding or inability to feed will increase the fluid loss and consequently the weight loss.

LENGTH

The average length of the normal neonate is 48.3 cm (19 in) to 53.3 cm (21 in). Measurements are made using a disposable tape measure extended from the heel of the neonate and following the contours of the body to the crown of the head (see Fig. 22-2).

TEMPERATURE

Assessment of the neonate's temperature is undertaken early in the examination, before environmental factors influence it. The temperature may be taken rectally or axillary, depending on hospital policies. Some institutions feel that the initial temperature should be taken rectally in order to assess the patency of the rectum. Most hospitals do not rely on the rectal route as a routine measurement of temperature for subsequent examinations, since irritation and damage to the rectal tissue may occur with repeated rectal temperatures.

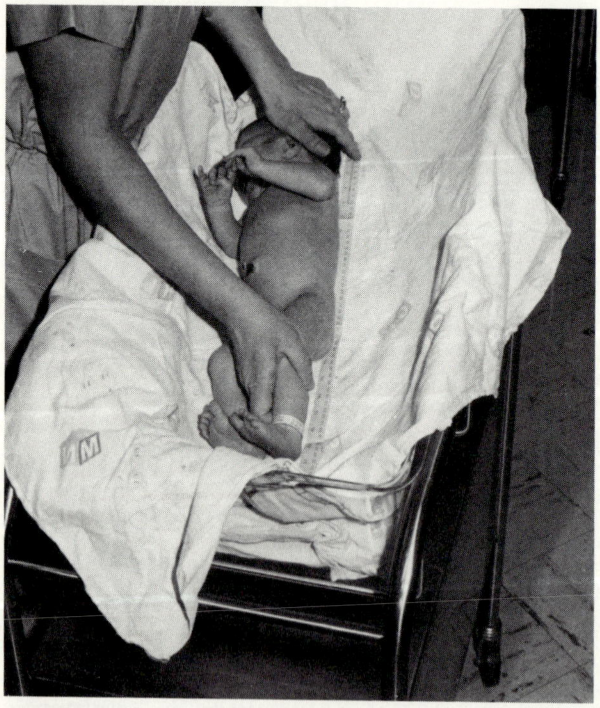

FIGURE 22-2. Heel to crown measurement of length of the neonate.

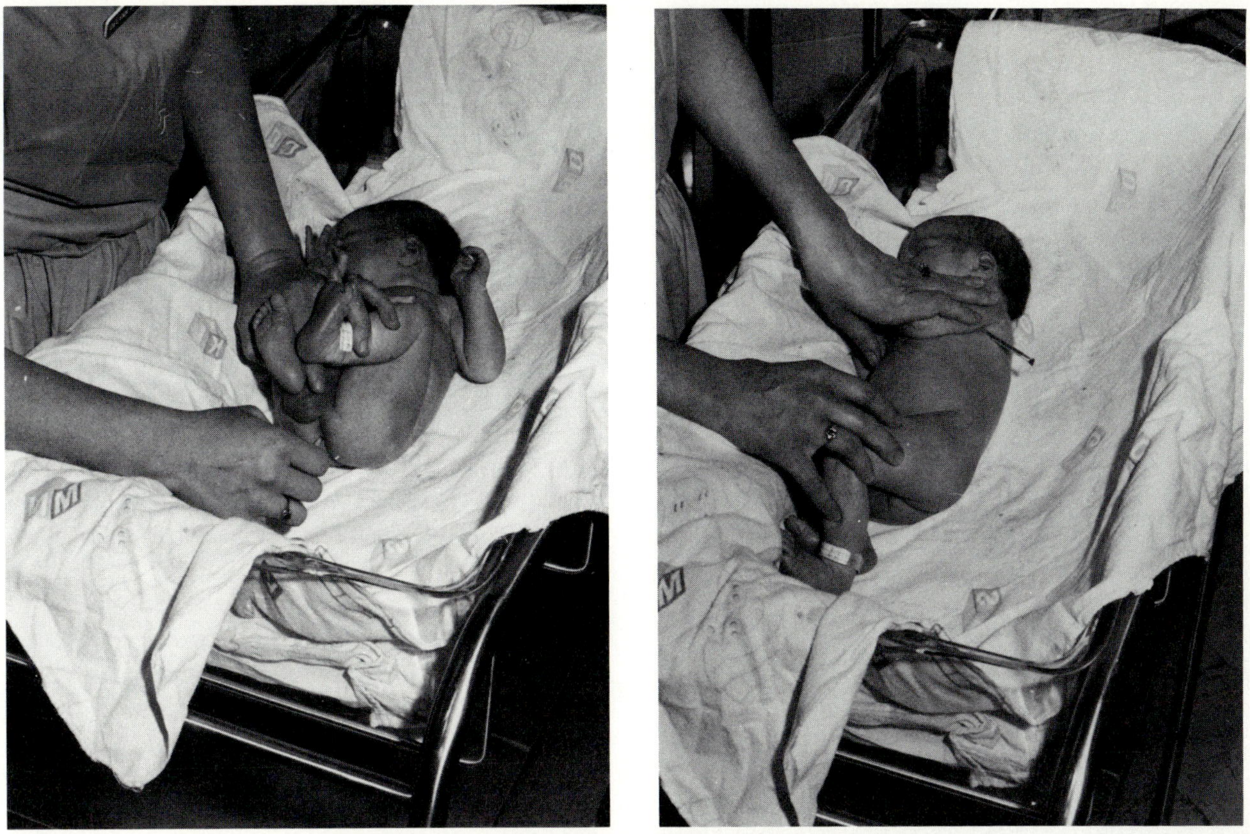

FIGURE 22-3. Methods of temperature assessment in neonate utilizing rectal and axillary assessments.

The rectal thermometer is always well lubricated before insertion into the anus. Normal rectal temperature, taken for 3 minutes, is 36.4° to 37.5°C (97.5° to 99.5° F).

Axillary temperatures will give an indication of skin surface temperature and will be close to the oral temperature reading because of the lack of subcutaneous fat. The normal temperature range for axillary temperature, taken for at least 3 minutes, is 36.5° to 37° C (97.7° to 98.6° F). Neonates whose temperatures fall below 36.7° C (98° F) are experiencing heat loss and measures should be taken to promote warmth. Axillary temperatures should be taken every hour until the temperature has stabilized. Figure 22-3 demonstrates methods of temperature assessment in the neonate. The method used to assess the temperature should always be noted when the temperature is recorded.

If it is determined that the temperature of the neonate is below the normal range and the infant is experiencing heat loss, the remainder of the examination is postponed and measures are taken to prevent further heat loss and to warm the neonate. Radiant warmers with temperature probes (see Fig. 22-4), incubators, or simply wrapping the neonate in warmed blankets may be used to increase the temperature.

HEAD

The head is symmetrical, with possible molding or mild caput succedaneum. Some bruising may occur, but a cephalhematoma is not usually evident until the second or third day. Upon palpation of the head, the fontanels and suture lines may be felt. The anterior fontanel is diamond-shaped and measures approximately 3 cm in length and 2 cm in width,

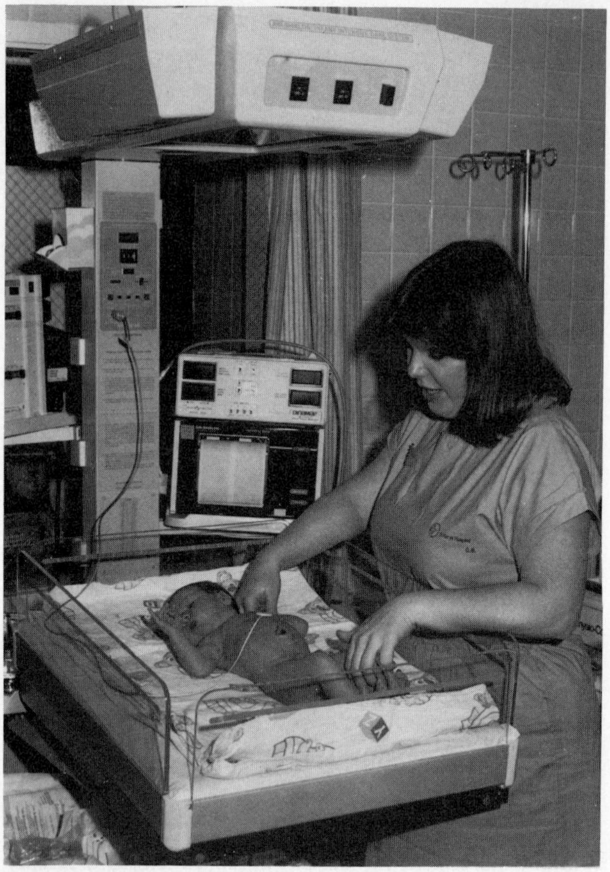

FIGURE 22-4. Use of the radiant warmer.

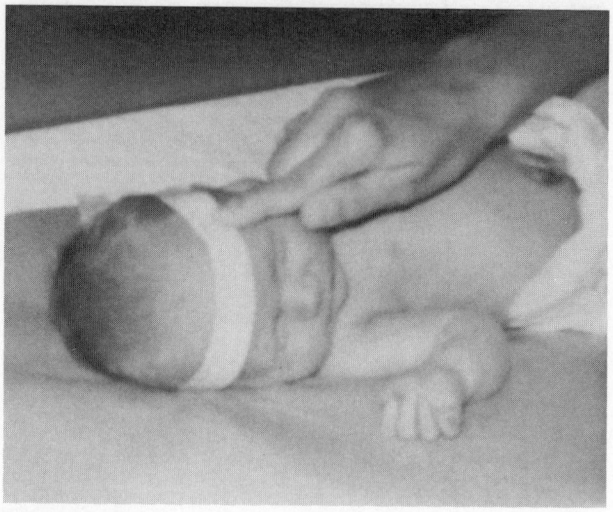

FIGURE 22-5. Measuring the head circumference of the neonate.

while the posterior fontanel is triangular in shape and measures 1 cm in width. Fontanels should be flat with no evidence of bulging or tenseness, which are indicative of intracranial pressure. Depressed fontanels are associated with dehydration. The suture lines are palpated and some overlapping may be noted. Neonates who have been malnourished in utero may have suture lines over 1 cm in width. Wide suture lines and very large, flat fontanels suggest the possibility of hypothyroidism, *osteogenesis imperfecta* (inherited disorder manifested by brittle bones), and *cleidocranial dystosis* (a rare hereditary disease with defective ossification of the cranial bone and absent clavicles).

Measurement of the head is made using a disposable measuring tape (see Fig. 22-5). The tape measure should be placed so that it is directly above the ears, across the occiput, and slightly over the eyebrows. Head circumference normally measures between 33 and 35 cm. Molding may account for some variations in size and, therefore, the head should be measured in the following days when the head has assumed a more normal shape. Very large heads are associated with *hydrocephalus* (enlarged head due to fluid in the cranial vault) or *hydranencephaly* (cerebral hemispheres absent caused by the presence of large amounts of cerebrospinal fluid). *Microcephaly* (small head) is associated with mental retardation related to chromosomal abnormalities and in utero diseases such as cytomegalovirus and toxoplasmosis. Neonates with Apert's syndrome (acrocephalosyndactylism) will have pointed heads with accompanying *syndactylism* (webbing of the fingers and toes).

Facial asymmetry may be present if in utero the fetal head was in a lateroflexed position causing the shoulder to place pressure on the mandible and neck just beneath the ear. This condition is not permanent and will disappear in a few weeks.

HAIR

The hair of the neonate is silky and fine with varying amounts present. The normal growth pattern is toward the face and a few swirls may be noted. Abnormal growth patterns, an excessive amount of swirls, a low-set hairline and coarse hair may be associated with a genetic or endocrine disorder. The amount of hair varies from neonate to neonate and is not related to the prenatal heartburn of the mother, as often stated in old wive's tales. Hair color may change as the infant grows older and it is difficult to determine at birth. Vernix caseosa and bloody mucus are often present in the hair following birth. If the vernix caseosa is meconium stained, the vernix caseosa on other parts of the body should be inspected. Stained vernix caseosa on the hair or any part of the body indicates in utero distress and alerts the nurse to the possibility of neonatal complications. When removing the vernix caseosa from the hair the nurse should avoid vigorous rubbing or strong soaps.

EYES

The eyes of the neonate should be symmetrical and the pupils equally reactive to light. An ophthalmoscope may be used to elicit the red reflex. If this reflex is not present, the eyes are examined for cataracts. Corneal opacities may be noted in the presence of a bright light. The cornea will have a cloudy, rough appearance. Cataracts, usually not seen until several days after birth, are generally bilateral and may be associated with a cytomegalovirus or rubella infection of the mother during the prenatal period.

Subconjunctival hemorrhages of the sclera are normal, related to increased vascular tension during birth. Rupture of a conjunctural capillary causes a red crescent-shaped band to appear adjacent to the iris. It is very noticeable not only to the nurse but to the parents as well. This situation may interfere with bonding if the parents are concerned about the hemorrhages and unable to sustain eye contact with the baby. The nurse should explain to the parents that this condition is normal and the hemorrhages will disappear within a few weeks.

Neonates whose eyes have been prophylactically treated with 1 percent silver nitrate in the delivery room may show signs of chemical conjunctivitis and lid edema; these are temporary and will disappear within a few days. Ideally, prophylactic treatment of the eyes for the prevention of *ophthalmia neonatorum* (infection of the neonate's eyes caused by the Neisseria gonorrhoeae) with eye instillations of silver nitrate or antibiotic ointment should be delayed until the parents have had an opportunity to bond with the baby. Eye examinations are also altered by the presence of these medications. A more thorough examination of the eye is needed when effects of the medications have diminished.

The *doll's eye phenomenon* is present at birth and for the next two or three months. This phenomenon is characterized by the inability of the eyes to adjust to the position of the head when the head is turned from one side to the other. The eyes will lag, appearing like dolls' eyes.

The *setting-sun sign* is caused by neuromuscular immaturity, in which case it may be transitory, or by sensitivity of the brain stem. The iris appears to vanish below the lower eyelids when the neonate is rapidly changed from a sitting posture to a supine posture.

Stork beak marks are areas of *telangiectasia* (a grouping of small dilated blood vessels) that are red in color and may appear on the upper eye lid, nape of the neck, or across the glabella. They have no clinical significance and usually disappear within the first year.

Eye characteristics that may be associated with chromosomal abnormalities are: eyes unusually far apart or too close, very long eyelashes, presence of cataracts, unusual slant to the eye, and the absence of ocular tissue. Wide set eyes (4.5 cms apart, called *hypertelorism*) are frequently seen with Apert's syndrome. They may also be associated with Cri-du-Chat (cat cry) syndrome (chromosomal deletion), in which heart defects and mental retardation are also common. Other abnormalities are a lack of eye movements and pupillary response, and jaundice discoloration of the sclera. A fixed eye state is indicative of seizure behavior, even when there are no spasmodic movements of the extremities. Brushfield's spots (white or yellow pinpoint areas on the iris) may indicate Down's syndrome.

EARS

The ears are examined for anomalies, size, set, shape, and auditory capabilities. Variations may exist in the ears as familial characteristics, and minor deviations may be normal. The pinna of the full-term neonate's ear is firm with well developed cartilage, while that of the preterm neonate is flabby and minimally developed. The set of the ears should be consistent with a line from the top of the ear across the outer and inner canthi of the eyes (see Fig. 22-6). Abnormally low-set ears are associated with renal abnormalities such as bilateral renal agenesis and with neonates who have Down's syndrome. Neonates with low-set ears should be observed for kidney problems and voidings should be monitored.

The posterior and superior margin of the ear (*helix*) is rounded and curved inward. A very large, flat, and flaccid helix may be associated with unilateral renal agenesis and renal obstructions.

The internal ear is examined by pulling the pinna downward and back. Amniotic fluid and vernix caseosa may be seen in the internal auditory passages and may interfere with examination of the inner ear. Drainage of these substances occurs naturally and attempts at removal are unnecessary. The vernix may be removed from the outer ear when present in large amounts. Clapping the hands directly above the neonate's head will cause a startle reflex if normal auditory capabilities are present. However, if the ear passages are blocked, this response may not occur until later.

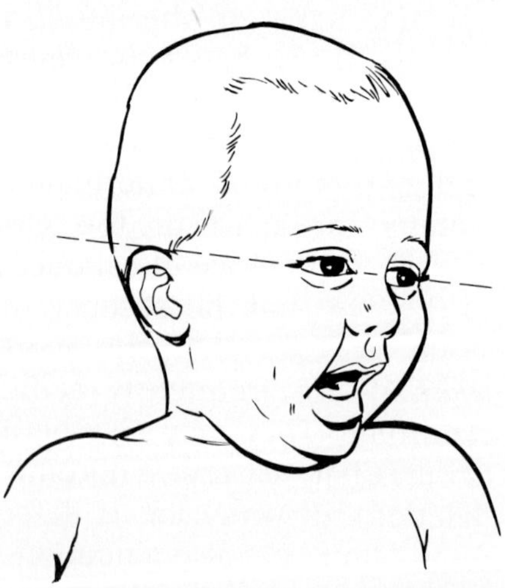

FIGURE 22-6. Normal set of ear as indicated by straight line drawn from top of ear across the outer and inner canthi of the eyes.

Preauricular skin tags may be found on the skin adjacent to the ear and occasionally in a line extending from the base of the ear across the jaw line. These are of little clinical significance but are noted and may be ligated by the physician, allowing the tags to drop off.

NOSE

Alignment and placement of the nose are noted upon inspection of the face. The nose is centered in the middle of the face and may appear very flat. Amniotic fluid and mucus present in the nasal passages are removed when sneezing occurs or with a bulb syringe. Patency of the nasal passages is assessed in either of two ways: (1) a small catheter may be inserted into the nares and passed through the passages, or (2) since neonates are obligatory nasal breathers, occluding one side of the nose and then the other while the mouth is closed will interfere with breathing if patency is not present. If the nasal passages are not patent, *choanal atresia* (membrane or bone occluding the nares) is suspected and, if confirmed, corrective surgery may be needed to prevent respiratory distress.

The neonate's need to sneeze is explained to the parents, since they often believe the baby to have a cold when he sneezes frequently. They are also told not to try to clean the nasal passages with cotton swabs, since the delicate nasal membranes can be injured.

Flaring of the nares may be present with respiratory distress, and a thorough assessment of respiratory status is done immediately.

MOUTH

The lips and mucous membranes of the mouth are inspected to detect any bluish discoloration or paleness that may indicate respiratory difficulties. Normally, the lips and mucous membranes are pink, but, circumoral pallor may be seen in the first few hours after birth. A cleft lip may be immediately apparent and notations are made of the location, the extent of the cleft, and whether it is unilateral or bilateral.

The hard and soft palates are examined by placing a clean index finger into the mouth and running the finger over the entire palate. A cleft palate can easily be missed when the mouth is inspected only visually. If it is noted, the extent of the cleft is assessed, i.e., clefts of both the hard and soft palate, clefts of the lip and hard and soft palate, cleft of the hard palate only.

The gums are pink, smooth, and without visable teeth. Occasionally a lower incisor may be found. It may be one of two types, predeciduous or true deciduous. Predeciduous teeth are loose and must often be removed to prevent them from being swallowed. True deciduous teeth are more frequently found and do not usually require removal. Small, round, grayish cysts on the gums (*inclusion* or *retention cyst*) may be mistaken for teeth. They are of little clinical significance and will disappear in a few weeks.

Excessive amounts of saliva, drooling, and choking are symptoms of *tracheoesophageal fistula* (a defect with the tracheal and esophagus connected) or esophageal atresia. In this instance, as the neonate is fed he may begin to choke, cough, and experience respiratory difficulties as the feeding is aspirated into the lungs. When this condition is suspected, diagnostic measures should be undertaken before feedings are given.

Multiple grayish-white lesions called Epstein pearls, may be found on the hard and soft palates. These very small epithelial cysts are often confused with the lesions of *thrush* caused by *Candida albicans.* Thrush lesions have a curdled-milk appearance and are found on the hard palate, tongue, and buccal mucosa. Thrush is contracted by the neonate as he passes through the birth canal and is exposed to vaginal monilia infection. The lesions of thrush will break off and bleed when rubbed, whereas Epstein pearls may not be dislodged.

The tongue of the neonate is freely moveable and not limp or protruding. The frenulum of the tongue is an extension of the mucous membrane at the base of the tongue that attaches to the floor of the mouth. In some neonates the frenulum is attached more anteriorly, near the tip of the tongue, and is commonly referred to as "tonguetie." Previously, this tissue was snipped in an effort to prevent speech problems. However, more recently, this practice was discontinued, as few speech problems appear to be related to this condition.

Very large protruding tongues may be present in neonates with Down's syndrome, cretinism, and hyperpituitarism. The mandible is assessed when a tongue appears to be large, since a short mandible will cause the tongue to appear larger than it really is.

NECK

The neck of the neonate is examined for range of motion, abnormal masses, injuries, and excessive tissue. The neck appears short and blends into the skin folds, making examination difficult in the supine position. Holding the infant and allowing the head to fall back slightly will provide a better position for examination. Movement of the neck in all directions should not be restrained. Inability to move the neck freely is an indication of injury to the sternocleidomastoid muscle (*torticollis*).

Palpation of the clavicles will reveal any masses, positional abnormalities, and *crepitus* (crackling sound when fragments of bone are in apposition) indicative of a fractured clavicle. Broken clavicles are not uncommon, especially when shoulder dystocia has occurred during delivery. Palpation also includes the thyroid gland, assessments of any masses, lymph nodes, brachial cleft cyst (muscle cyst), and webbing of the neck. Congenital chromosomal abnormalities such as Turner's syndrome (X chromosome monosomy with gonadal dysgenesis), Down's syndrome, or trisomy 18 are associated with webbing of the neck.

CHEST

Inspection, auscultation, and measurements are employed to assess the chest. The respiratory rate and characteristics are noted while the infant is in a quiet state and not crying. Respirations are diaphragmatic, with equal movements of both sides of the chest and no retractions. The normal respiratory rate is between 30 and 60 per minute, with the average being 40 per minute. Some irregularity and brief apneic spells (see Chapter 21) may be seen in the early neonatal period; however prolonged apnea with expiratory grunting, nasal flaring, and retractions of the sternal or intercostal spaces is not normal and indicates respiratory distress.

The chest appears round with a prominent sternum and xiphoid process. Chest circumference, measured at the nipple line (see Fig. 22-7), is 30 to 33 cm, 1 to 2 cm smaller than the head circumference. Asymmetry of the chest may suggest severe problems such as pneumomediastinum, pneumothorax, and diaphragmatic hernia (see Chapter 29).

The breast nodules measure from 3 to 10 mm. The nipples may be engorged, with a slight amount of secretion on the second or third day following birth. Supernumerary nipples (extra nipples) are occasionally found below the nipple line.

Auscultation of the chest provides information regarding both the pulmonary and cardiac status. Bilateral breath sounds should be present, although they may be difficult to assess immediately following birth. Often breath sounds may be absent in some areas of the chest until the lung fluid is absorbed. Rales may be heard in the immediate period following birth but are not normal on the second or

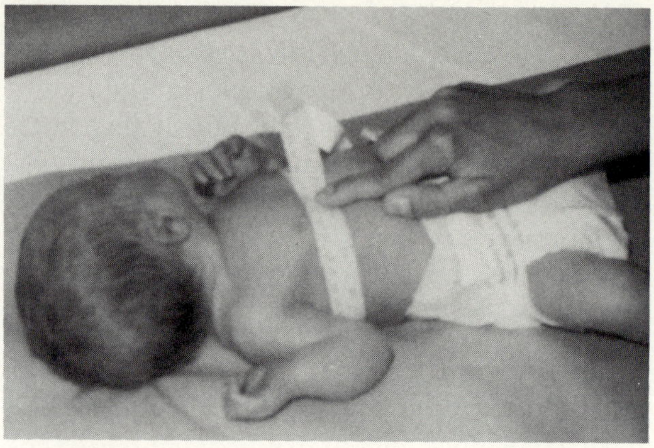

FIGURE 22-7. Measurement of chest circumference.

third day. Breath sounds are auscultated on both the anterior and posterior aspects of the chest.

When auscultating the heart, the point of maximum intensity [(PMI) heart apex] may be heard at the fourth intercostal space in the midclavicular line (see Fig. 22-8). The first and second heart sounds may be clearly heard and differentiated. Murmurs in the first hours of life are not abnormal; however, their presence is reported and recorded. During the transitional period the heart rate may be somewhat irregular, varying from the normal 120 to 160. Persistant bradycardia (rate below 120) or persistant tachycardia (rate over 160) may indicate respiratory or cardiac problems. Abnormal placement of the PMI may be associated with a diaphragmatic hernia or *dextrocardia* (heart located on the right side in reverse).

ABDOMEN

The abdomen is round and protuberant, with the umbilical stump located in the midline. The stump is inspected to determine if there are two umbilical arteries, one vein and Wharton's jelly, as well as the size and placement of the vessels within the cord. Absence of one of the arteries may be associated with congenital deformities while very small vessels may indicate inadequate in utero nourishment. The cord is moist, soft, and a creamy-

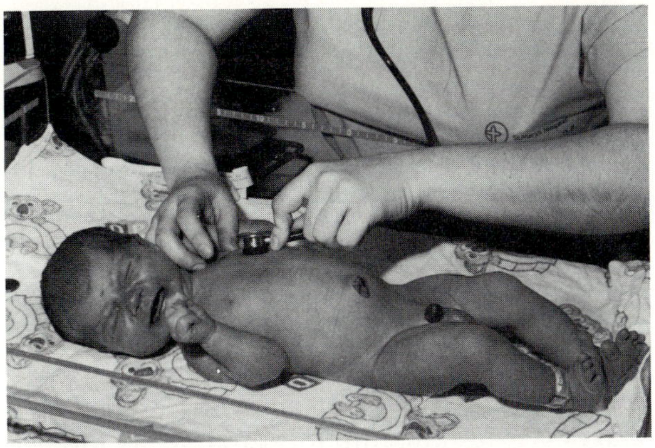

FIGURE 22-8. Auscultation of heart sound.

white color following delivery. It should be securely tied or clamped, with no evidence of bleeding. In the ensuing days, the cord begins to dry and becomes dark shriveled, and black, eventually falling off around the third to seventh day. A meconium-stained cord at birth is indicative of in utero distress, and the neonate should be observed carefully for possible complications. Umbilical hernias appear more frequently in black neonates, and are noted as a slight outpouching of the umbilicus.

Ascultation of bowel sounds is done before the abdomen is palpated or percussed. The sounds may be heard as a tinkling sound occurring every 10 to 30 seconds; absence of sounds may indicate obstruction of the bowel. The circumference of the abdomen is measured to serve as a baseline for future assessments in the event of intestinal blockage.

Abdominal palpation is begun in the upper right quadrant of the abdomen. The finger tips are used to gently palpate the liver, which is located 1 to 3 cm below the right costal margin. An upward cupping motion is used to prevent depressing the organ, which would make it difficult to distinguish borderlines. The liver margins are well defined and sharply demarcated. Experience is necessary for accurate assessment of the liver by palpation.

The tip of the spleen is felt 1 to 2 cm below the left costal margin. It is difficult to locate and often is not felt until the neonate is six to seven days old.

Hepatomegaly may indicate congestive heart failure, and hepatosplenomegaly may be found in neonates who have encountered toxoplasmosis, syphilis, sepsis, and erythroblastosis in utero.

The kidneys are more easily examined immediately after birth when the intestines are not filled with air (Corones, 1981). Attempts are made to palpate both kidneys to determine size and location. Flexing the neonate's knees onto his chest will relax the abdominal muscles and facilitate palpation. The lower aspect of the right kidney is felt in the posterior flank approximately 1 to 2 cm above the level of the umbilicus. The right kidney is more easily felt than the left and often only the extreme tip of the left kidney can be felt.

Inspection of the abdomen may reveal severe abnormalities. Absence of the abdominal musculature ("prune-belly syndrome") gives a wrinkled appearance to the extremely protuberant abdomen. The lateral aspects of the abdomen bulge and the anterior portion appears concave. This condition is associated with renal abnormalities.

A scaphoid abdominal appearance suggests a diaphragmatic hernia. The intestinal contents protrude through the hernial opening and enter the thoracic cavity, placing pressure on the lungs and resulting in respiratory difficulties. A history of polyhydramnios is also consistent with diaphragmatic hernia and displacement of the PMI is either to the right (most common) or the left.

Diastasis recti (separation of the rectus muscle of the abdomen) is a congenital weakness seen in some neonates. Protrusion of the intestines through the muscle separation may be felt when the neonate is crying. This condition is of no clinical significance and usually disappears within a month.

Inguinal hernias may be unilateral or bilateral and are most frequently found in male neonates but may also be present in females. Abdominal contents protrude into the inguinal canal, producing a swelling noted when the neonate cries.

Femoral pulses are palpated simultaneously

in the inguinal area. Absence of the femoral pulse suggests coarctation of the aorta (stenosis or narrowing of the aorta). Radial, brachial, and dorsal pedis pulses are assessed at the same time to note any differences indicating the location of the interruption in circulation. Bounding pulses on the third or fourth day following birth may indicate patent ductus arteriosus.

FEMALE GENITALIA

At birth the labia majora are pink and, in the full-term neonate, larger than the labia minora. Some edema may be present following breech delivery. The clitoris is prominent but not greatly enlarged. When enlargement is excessive, *adrenogenital syndrome* may be suspected. This condition significantly alters the physiology of the neonate, resulting in electrolyte disturbances and dehydration.

Hormonal influences may cause a *pseudomenstruation* (bloody mucus discharge), which is not significant. Vaginal hymenal tags may also be present and are, likewise, insignificant. Vernix caseosa may be abundant between the folds of the labia; its removal is not necessary, as it will disappear within a few days.

MALE GENITALIA

The scrotum of the full-term male is rugated and pendulous, often appearing large in relationship to the size of the neonate. When examining the testes, slight pressure is applied with one hand in the inguinal area while the testis is felt with the thumb and forefinger of the other hand. Failure to apply pressure in the inguinal area will allow withdrawal of the testis into the inguinal area. Palpation should reveal a testis in each scrotal sac. *Hydrocele* (fluid around the testis) may be present at birth but will generally disappear without treatment in a few weeks. *Cryptorchidism* (undescended testicle) is difficult to diagnose in the first few days of life when just a slight stroke to the inner side of the thigh causes the testicle to withdraw into the inguinal area (cremasteric reflex).

The glans penis is covered by the prepuce, making it difficult to observe the urinary meatus. The prepuce of most male infants is not completely retractable until two to three months of age and injury may occur if attempts are made to completely retract the prepuce before this time. *Phimosis* (stricture of the prepuce, causing it to be tight and nonretractable) may occur, but this is difficult to diagnose until the infant is three to six months old. *Hypospadias* (urethral opening on the underside of the penis) and *epispadias* (urethral opening on the anterior penile surface) is seen in a small percentage of infants. There is usually no treatment for hypospadias. Epispadias is often associated with other genitourinary abnormalities and corrective surgery is performed during childhood. When either of these two conditions is present, careful inspection of the genitalia will determine if there is ambiguity of the genitalia.

ANUS

The anal opening is checked for patency and to rule out an imperforate anus. This assessment may be made when the temperature is taken rectally or by digital examination. Regardless of the method, pressure is not exerted during examination, as injury to the rectal mucosa may occur. The first meconium stool is often passed during examination. Passage of meconium indicates that the bowel is functioning and its presence is recorded.

BACK

Examination of the back is done by placing the neonate on his abdomen and palpating the spine. The normal curvature of the neonate's spine is "C"-shaped, since only the thoracic and pelvic curves are developed at this time. The complete length of the spine is palpated, noting any openings, or tufts of hair at the base of the spine; these are indications of *spina bifida occulta.* This condition occurs during fetal development if the posterior vertebral arches fail to fuse, causing a small opening in the lumbar-sacral area. The opening is usually not visible and may be covered with tufts of hair. Twenty percent of neonates with this condition will have little or no effects.

Dimpling in the sacral area does not always indicate spina bifida occulta but may be an indication of either a closed or fistulated pilonidal cyst.

Spinal bifida cystica is noted as an external herniation of the spinal contents into a saclike cyst. If the herniation contains only meninges, it is called a *meningocele*. When the sac contains meninges, cerebrospinal fluid, and spinal cord it is defined as a *meningomyelocele*.

EXTREMITIES

Examination for dislocated hips is done while the neonate is prone. The neonate with a dislocation will exhibit asymmetry and an increase in the number of gluteal and popliteal skin folds on the affected side (see Fig. 22-9). Further assessment may be accomplished by placing the neonate in the supine position and performing Ortolani's maneuver (see Fig. 22-10), which assesses the movement of the head of the femur in the acetabulum. With both of the neonate's legs in a flexed position, the nurse rotates the legs a full 90 degrees while applying downward pressure. If a dislocation is present, the head of the femur can be felt to slip in and out of position and a clicking noise may be heard.

The legs should be of equal length and there should be no evidence of extra toes or syndactylism (webbing). *Phocomelia* (absence of a proximal portion of a leg or arm) should be noted if present and further assessments for congenital abnormalities done. The legs commonly have a bowed appearance, which is not significant at this time but should be noted for future assessment.

The feet are examined for indications of congenital clubfoot, which are of several varieties, the most common being talipes equinovarus (95 percent occurrence). Although either sex may have this condition, it is more common in boys. Direction of the foot is turned inward and downward. If the foot can

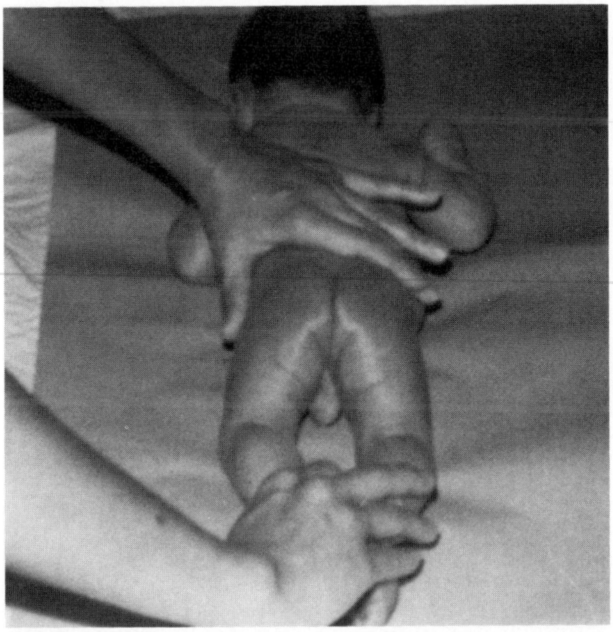

FIGURE 22-9. Examination for dislocation of hips. Note symmetry of gluteal and popliteal skin folds in normal neonate.

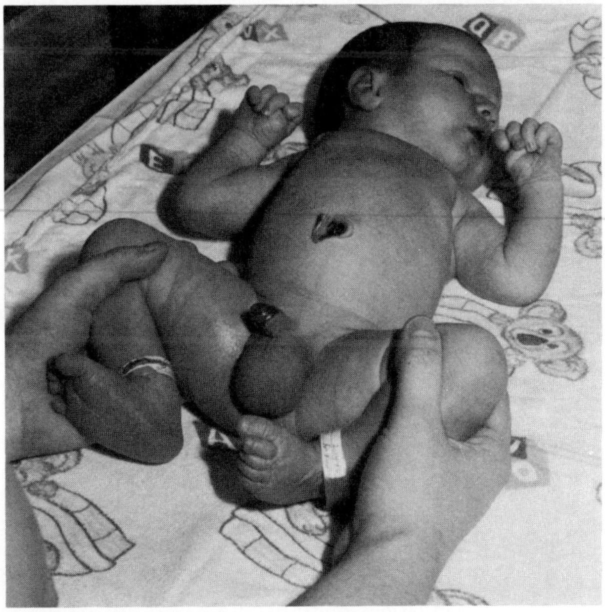

FIGURE 22-10. Ortolani's maneuver.

be placed in the normal position, the condition is less severe and may not require treatment. Examination of the feet also includes an assessment of the creases on the sole of each foot, noting if plantar creases cover the entire foot. Preterm infants will have creases located primarily in the anterior portion of the foot with a smooth appearance to the heel. Full-term neonates will show creases over the entire foot (see Fig. 22–11). The arch is not developed at this time, giving the foot a flat appearance.

The arms appear long in comparison with the legs of the normal neonate. They should be symmetrical and freely moveable, with a normal range of motion. If the arm falls limply at the side with no flexion and little response to stimuli, brachial plexus injury may be suspected. This type of injury is called *Erb's paralysis* and is usually seen when there has been a difficult delivery involving shoulder dystocia or with a breech presentation. Another type of brachial plexus injury involves lower spinal nerves influencing the brachial plexus and is characterized by a dropping of the wrist (wrist-drop). Brachial plexus injuries require treatment in order to prevent muscular contractures. Each hand is inspected for syndactylism and polydactylism (extra digits). The fingernails of the neonate are somewhat long and sharp; however, if they are very long and/or yellowish, postmaturity is suspected. The palms are inspected, noting the creases. A single simian crease, broad flat hands, and short stubby fingers are often associated with Down's syndrome.

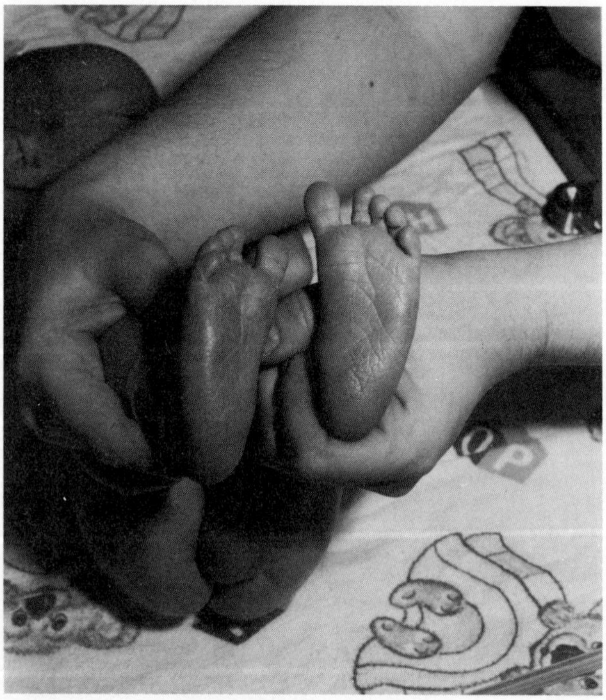

FIGURE 22-11. Sole creases.

MUSCLE TONE

All of the joints are put through the normal range of motion and assessments are made of muscle tone. When the extremities are straightened and released they should return to a state of flexion. Hypotonicity is related to prematurity, central nervous system disorders, and intrauterine hypoxia. Muscles involved in head lifting are not well developed at birth.

SKIN

After birth, large amounts of vernix caseosa may be seen, with accumulations in the hair, genital area, and arm and leg creases. Some of the vernix caseosa may be removed during the neonate's first bath; however, complete removal is not necessary. Scrubbing the vernix-laden areas will only cause irritation of the skin and provide a portal of entry for bacterial organisms.

The skin tone is pink in neonates of Caucasian descent. Black neonates have creamy tan appearance at birth much the same as neonates of Latin and Asian descent. However, black infants will darken in the days following delivery. Many variations exist in skin color, even among neonates of the same race.

Acrocyanosis and Circumoral Pallor

Sluggish peripheral circulation following birth is responsible for the bluish discoloration characteristic of acrocyanosis of the extremities and circumoral pallor around the mouth. These findings are normal in the first 24 to 48 hours but may also be an indication of hypothermia. Generalized cyanosis or pallor is not normal, and immediate measures are taken to determine the cause.

Mottling and Harlequin Skin Changes

Mottling (*cutis marmorata*) is a patchy, purplish discoloration of the skin seen when the neonate is cold. It is considered normal if the neonate is chilled when exposed; however, if present when the neonate is warm and the temperature normal, it is an indication of hypoxia and further respiratory assessments are necessary.

Harlequin skin changes appear frequently in the early days of life owing to the immaturity of the circulatory system. The neonate will appear to have a sharply demarcated color difference, varying from a deep red to a pale pink. The most dependent areas, such as the back, will appear red, while the abdomen will be pale. If the neonate is placed in a prone position, the back will be pale and the abdomen red. Generally, these changes are episodic, do not last long, and will disappear in a few days without consequence.

Milia

Milia, appearing on the nose and chin, are small, white spots caused by the accumulation of sebum in the ducts of the sebaceous glands. Parents will often believe their infant has "pimples" and will try to break them open. They should be informed that milia are normal, they will go away in a few weeks, and that attempting to break them open may cause harm to the skin.

Lanugo

Lanugo is the very fine, soft hair that is formed during uterine development. It is most abundant on the forehead, shoulders, and back of prematures and may be found to a lesser extent on fullterm neonates.

Erythema Neonatorum Toxicum

A reddish-pink papular rash with small (1 to 4 mm) vesicles and pustules resembling flea bites are frequently seen on the face, trunk, and genital areas after the first 24 hours. These lesions are not bacterial, contain many eosinophilic cells, and are of unknown origin. They come and go at random in different locations, have no accompanying symptoms, and require no treatment.

Telangiectatic Nevi (Stork Beak Marks)

As described earlier, stork beak marks are clusters of dialated blood vessels found on the nape of the neck, nose, and eyelids. They appear as red or pink marks that blanch with pressure and disappear within the first year of life.

Nevus Vasculosus (Strawberry Marks)

Capillary hemangiomas, formed from dilated capillaries in the dermal and subdermal tissue, create a raised, rough, well-defined area resembling a strawberry. They are seldom present at birth but will develop shortly afterwards and continue to grow until the seventh or eighth month of life. Thereafter, they will regress and disappear by the time the child is eight or nine years old.

Nevus Flammeus ("Port Wine Stain")

These capillary angiomas are concentrated in the epidermis of the skin. Their surface is smooth with no elevation on the skin. They are a very deep red or purple color and may involve either small or very large areas of the skin. Blanching does not occur when pressure is applied and they do not disappear as the child grows older. When they appear on the face they may be associated with Sturge-Weber syndrome (intracranial calcification, glaucoma, and muscular weakness on one side of the body).

Mongolian Spots

Areas of bluish discoloration resembling bruises may appear on the buttocks and sacral area of the neonate. These areas, called *Mongolian spots,* are most frequently found in black and Oriental neonates. They may easily be mistaken for areas of injury and their presence is always explained to the parents. They are insignificant and will disappear in the first few years of life.

Petechiae

Pinpoint areas of hemorrhage under the skin called petechiae may be caused by pressure on the presenting part during delivery. If wide-spread and noted in areas other than pressure areas, systemic infections and thrombocytopenia may be suspected. Petechiae do not blanch when pressure is applied which differentiates them from newborn rashes.

Café-au-lait Spots

Areas of increased pigmentation resembling brown "birth marks" may be present. If more than six are observed, it may indicate neurofibromatosis (von Recklinghausen's disease), an autosomal dominant neurologic disorder.

Subcutaneous Fat Necrosis

Well-delineated, hard masses of varying size, found in the subcutaneous tissue and fixed to the skin are the result of trauma. These masses are usually found on either the face, back, buttocks, and thighs, appearing on the second or third day following birth. They will dissolve without incidence within a few weeks.

Sclerema

Large areas of thick, rigid, cold skin involving the cheeks, buttocks, and eventually all the skin areas is indicative of *sclerema.* This condition may be seen in conjunction with infections, *marasmus* (malnourished condition) and severe cold stress. Its appearance denotes a poor prognosis.

Jaundice

Jaundice prior to 24 hours following birth is considered abnormal (see Chapter 31). The sclera of the eye, buccal mucosa, and skin may be assessed for jaundice. Blanching of the skin on the abdomen may help to determine if jaundice is present.

Causes of Birth Marks

Birth marks are not related to the prenatal activities of the mother. Although mothers will often blame themselves, fearing that they have marked the baby, the cause of birth marks is for the most part unknown. This should be discussed with parents and any guilt feelings resolved.

Neurologic Assessment

A complete neurologic assessment is usually not done immediately after birth; however, certain assessments may be undertaken during the initial nursery examination. A more thorough examination is completed after the transition period when the neonate is stabilized. Table 22–3 lists and describes reflexes of the normal neonate that may be assessed.

Prematurity and immaturity will alter many of the reflex responses and muscle tone; gestational age must be considered when performing a neurologic examination.

During the first few days of life the neonate may exhibit fine tremors, normally seen at times when the neonate is stimulated, crying, or as he is first falling asleep and suddenly jerks (*myoclonis*).

Jitteriness may also be noted with hypoglycemia, and assessment of glucose levels is needed (normal glucose is 40 to 80 mg per 100 ml). Tremors or jitteriness accompanied by other neurologic symptoms may indicate

TABLE 22–3
GUIDE TO ASSESSMENT OF NORMAL REFLEXES OF THE NEONATE

Reflex	Method of Assessment & Response	Illustration	Alteration
Rooting	When the corner of the mouth is gently stroked the neonate will turn his head in the direction of the stroking and will open his mouth attempting to suck Present at birth Disappears between 4–12 months	Figure 22–12	May be weak or absent in premature or depressed neonate
Sucking	A nipple, finger or object placed in the mouth will elicit sucking motions		When absent, prematurity or neurologic disorders; possible barbituate depression
Gag	Stimulated when the back of the throat is touched by object such as catheter, bulb syringe, tongue depressor, or finger		Absent when there is nerve damage to the nerves of the neck or extreme prematurity
Swallow	During episodes of sucking the neonate is continually swallowing		Immature neonate wil suck for short period and then swallow increasing possibility of aspiration
Extrusion	Tongue protrudes when touched with finger or object	Figure 22–13	Tongue protruding without stimulation may indicate Down's syndrome
Optical blink	Suddenly shining a bright light directly in the neonate's eyes will cause him to blink accompanied by dorsal flexion of the head		Absence indicates poor light perception and possible damage to 3rd, 4th, and 5th cranial nerves
Masseter	Index finger is placed on lower chin and a sharp rap is applied by the index finger of the other hand. The masseter muscle will contract lifting the chin slightly Present for first ten days		When absent may indicate brain stem or 5th cranial nerve lesion
Glabellar	A brisk tap on the bridge of the nose will cause the eyes to close tightly or blink		Lack of symmetry may possibly indicate paralysis of eye muscle
Auditory	The hands are held about 15 inches over the neonate's head and clapped. He will blink or respond with a startle reflex		If no response auditory problems suspected
Tonic neck	"Fencing position." When neonate's head is turned, the leg and arm of the corresponding side will extend and the opposite side will flex Partial disappearance by 3–4 months Complete disappearance by 2–3 years	Figure 22–14	If the complete response may be elicited after 6 months neurologic dysfunction may be present

TABLE 22-3 (continued)

Reflex	Method of Assessment & Response	Illustration	Alteration
Arm recoil	Both of the arms are pulled outward simultaneously and then quickly released. Both arms should return to a state of flexion		If absent neonate may have nerve damage, apathy from drugs, or prematurity
Grasp	When an object is placed in the palms the neonate will grasp the object (Palmer grasp reflex). Present for 3-6 months. When an object is placed on the sole of the foot near the toes, the infant will curl his toes around the object (Plantar grasp reflex) Present for 8 months	Figure 22-15 Figure 22-16	When absent may be due to prematurity or depressed from drugs
Galant's trunk (incurvation reflex)	A sharp object such as a pin is run alongside the spinal column about 3 cm from the spine from shoulder to the sacrum. The trunk of the neonate will curve toward the stimulation. May not be present until 5th or 6th day. Disappears after 1 month	Figure 22-17	When a lesion of the spinal cord is present, the response will be negative at the site of the lesion
Moro	Sudden jarring of the crib or allowing the head to fall back unsupported while the trunk is supported will elicit the following response: abduction and extension of arms fanning out of fingers formation of a C with forefinger and thumb adduction of the arms resembling an embrace Disappears at 3-4 months	Figure 22-18	If persistent after 6 months brain and neurologic dysfunction possible. Lack of symmetry may indicate paralysis or birth injury, especially to the brachial plexus
Babinski's	Stroke the sole of the foot along the outside from the heel to the toes and across the ball of the foot. The big toe will dorsiflex and the other toes will fan out and hyperextend. Disappears at 1 yr of age	Figure 22-19	If present after 1 yr, suspected neurologic involvement
Magnet	With the neonate in a supine position, the lower limbs are semiflexed and pressure is applied to the sole of both feet. The legs will extend toward the direction of the pressure	Figure 22-20	Absent where there is lower spinal cord damage and weak following a breech delivery in which the legs were flexed. A breech with extended legs may demonstrate an exaggerated response
Crossed extension	One leg is extended and pressure is placed on the knee. At the same time, the sole of the foot is pricked with a pin. In response, the other leg will flex, slightly adduct and then extend		If absent may indicate lesions of the spinal cord or if very weak response there may be peripheral nerve damage

TABLE 22-3 (continued)

Reflex	Method of Assessment & Response	Illustration	Alteration
Stepping	With the neonate in an upright position, the soles of the feet are allowed to just touch the top of the table surface. The neonate will make stepping motions. May be difficult to elicit in the first 2 or 3 days of life Disappears by 3-4 weeks	Figure 22-21	May be absent with breech deliveries, when neonate is apathetic or paralysis is present
Crawling	When newborn is placed on abdomen crawling movements are made Disappears at 6 weeks		Absent when neonate is depressed from drugs or neurologic impairment

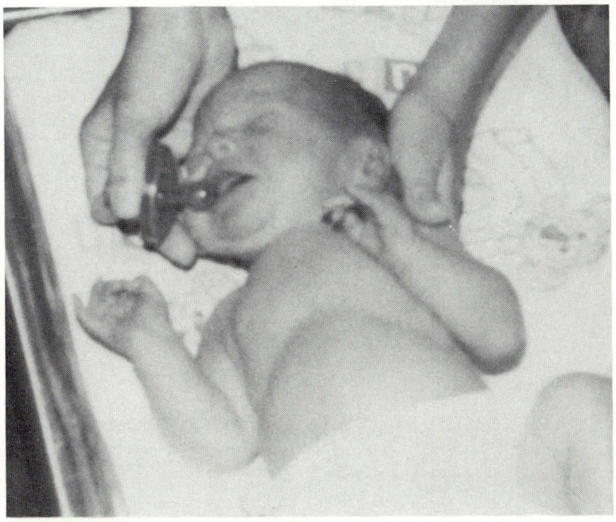

FIGURE 22-12. Rooting reflex.

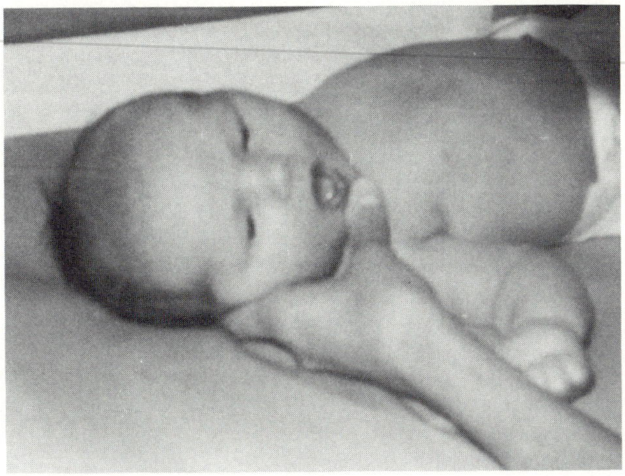

FIGURE 22-13. Extrusion reflex.

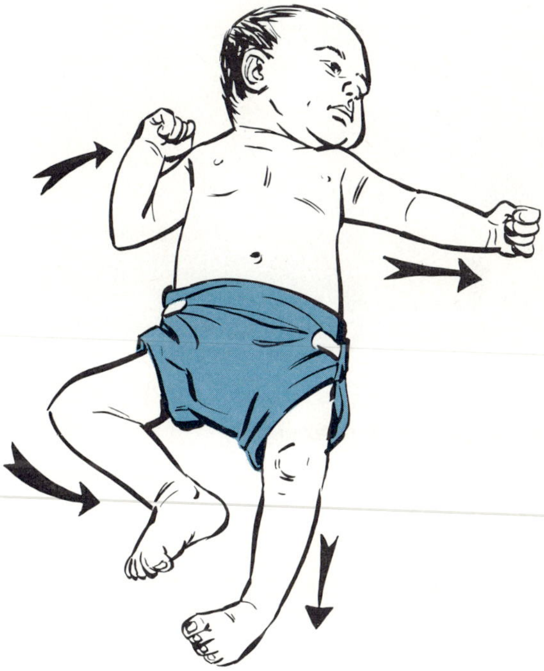

FIGURE 22-14. Tonic neck reflex.

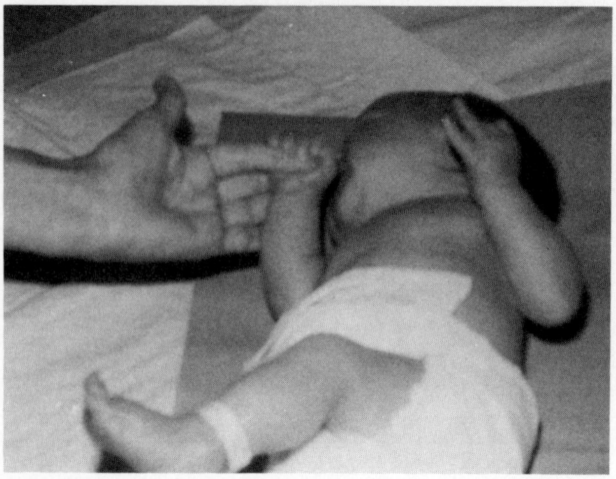

FIGURE 22-15. Grasp reflex.

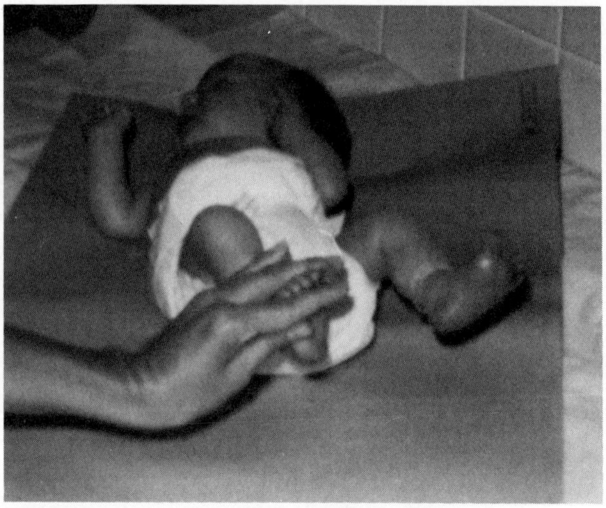

FIGURE 22-16. Plantar reflex of foot.

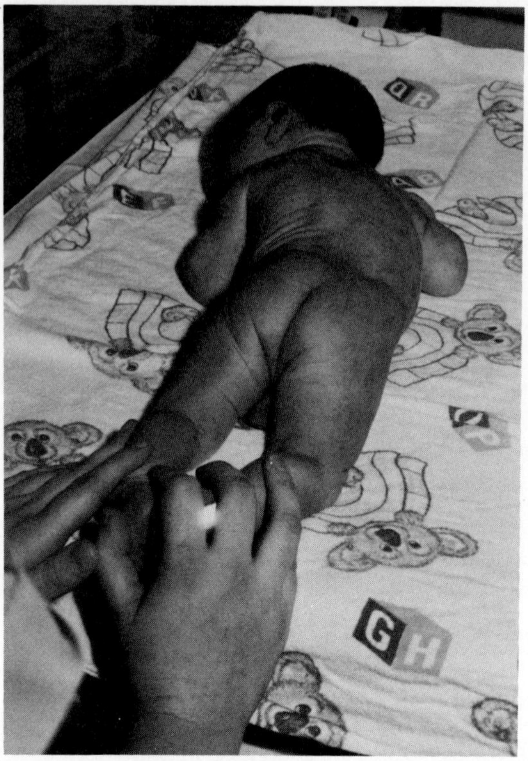

FIGURE 22-17. Galant's reflex.

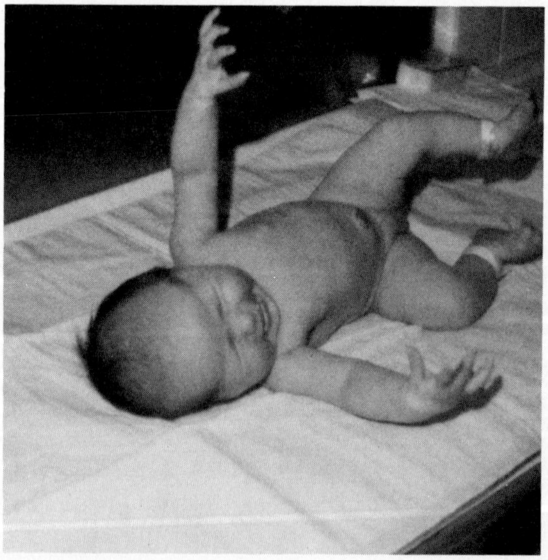

FIGURE 22-18. Moro reflex.

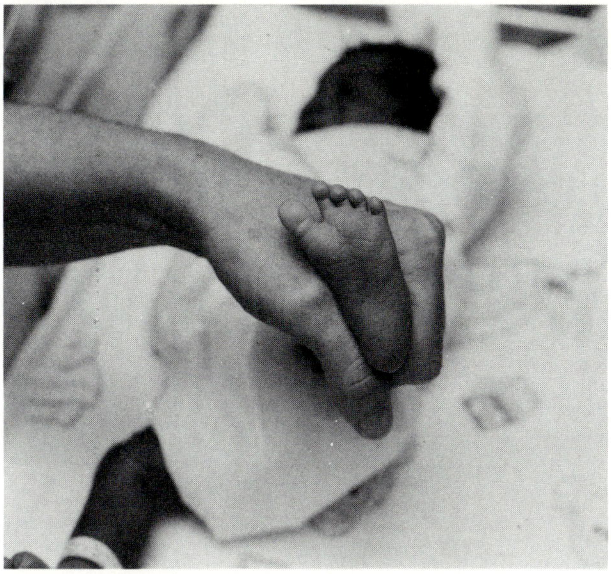

FIGURE 22-19. Babinski reflex.

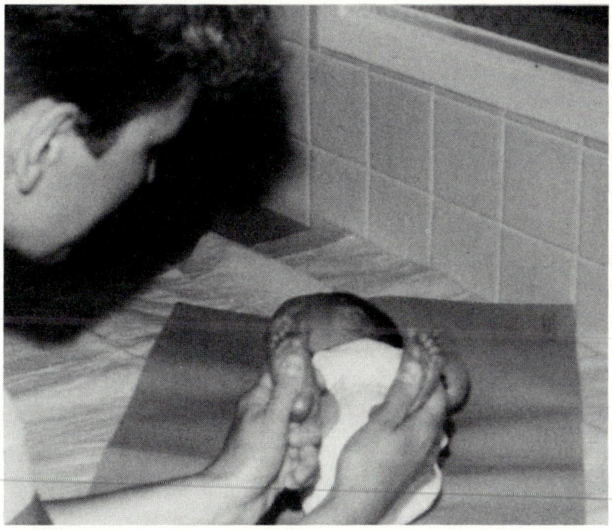

FIGURE 22-20. Magnet reflex.

abnormalities. Observation of any of the following warrant careful examination and assessment:

- Lack of response to stimuli
- Hypotonia
- Extreme irritability
- Absent blink reflex to light
- Fixated pupils
- Opisthotonos
- Unresolved jitteriness
- Seizures

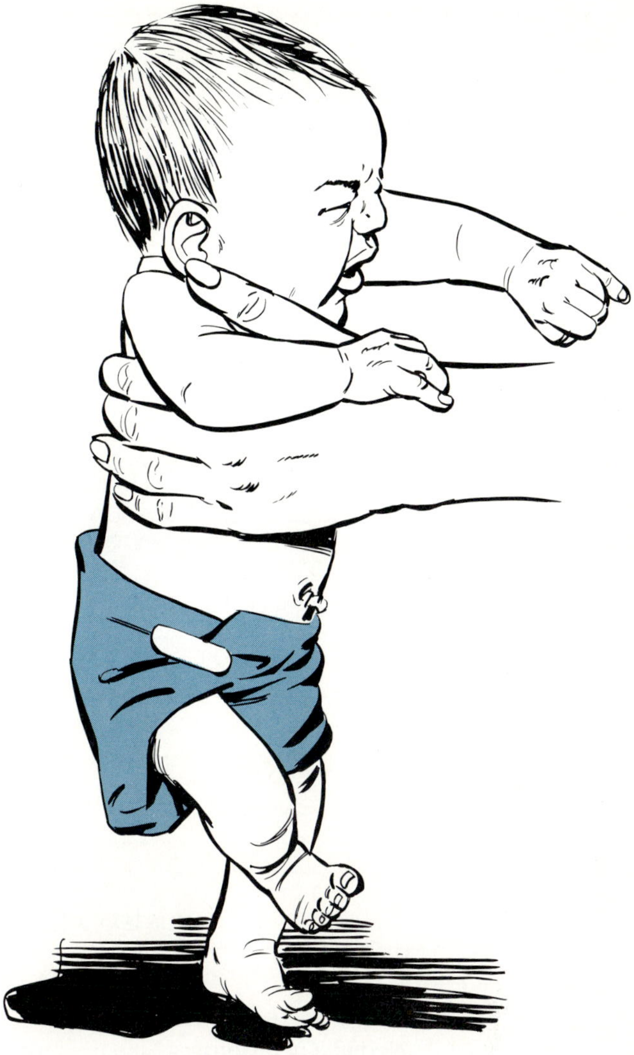

FIGURE 22-21. Stepping reflex. When soles of the feet are allowed to barely touch the top of the table surface, the neonate will make stepping motions.

Table 22-4 provides an assessment guide for performing a neonatal physical examination.

Gestational Age Assessment

Correlation of birth weight, gestational age, and intrauterine growth is a valuable tool when planning care for the neonate and iden-

TABLE 22-4
NEONATE ASSESSMENT TOOL

Name ______________________ Sex __________ Date of Birth ______________
ID No. ______________ Del. Time ______________ Method of Del. __________

Delivery Assessment:

Apgar Score 1 minute __________ 5 minutes __________
Respirations ______________ Heart Rate ______________ Muscle Tone __________
Reflex ______________________________ Color ______________________________
Resuscitation ____
Drugs Administered ____
Comments ____
____

Mother's History:

Mother's Name ______________ GRAVIDA __________ PARA __________ EDC __________
Age ______________ Blood type and Rh factor ______________________________
Titre ______________ VDRL ______________ Duration of labor ______________
Rupture of membrane (date & time) ____
Character of amniotic fluid ____
Medications administered (date & time) ___________________________________
____
Character of FHT ____
____
Anesthesia ____
Antepartal complications ____
Intrapartal complications ____
Comments ____

NURSERY ASSESSMENT

Date ______________ Time ______________ Examiner ______________
Circle Observed Characteristics:

	Normal Characteristics	**Deviations or Risk Factors**	**Comments**
Respirations	Respiratory		
	Rate for full minute ______	<40 or >60	
	Diaphragmatic breathing	Retractions	
	Transient tachypnea	Flaring nares	
		Grunting	
		See-saw respiration	
		Chin tug	
		Stridor	
		Rales	
	Apnea <20 seconds	Apnea >20 seconds	
Color	Pink	Pallor	
	Circumoral pallor	Generalized cyanosis	
	Acrocyanosis of extremities	Jaundice	
		Plethoric	
		Cracked or peeling skin	
Size	Weight ______	<2700 g [6 lb]	
		>4082 g [9 lb]	
	Length ______	<45.7 cm [18 in]	

NURSERY ASSESSMENT (continued)

	Normal Characteristics	Deviations or Risk Factors	Comments
Posture & Reactivity	Crying Flexed posture Resist extension of extremities Fist clenched Reactive to stimuli	Weak cry Shrill cry Rigid posture Flaccid posture No flexion of extremities Opisthotonos Weak movements Unresponsive to stimuli	
Cord	Clamped—no bleeding Two arteries and one vein Creamy-white color	Bleeding Two vessels Meconium stained Small in diameter Herniation of abd. contents thru cord (omphalocele)	
Vital Signs	Heart rate ________ B/P ________ Temperature ________	<120 or >160 Systolic <60 or >80 Diastolic <40 or >50 Axillary <36.7° or >37°C (98°–98.6F) Rectal <36.4° or >37.5°C (97.5°–99.5°F)	
Head	Circumference ________ Cephalhematoma (2nd & 3rd (day) Caput Succedaneum Molding Fontanels Anterior—3 cm length ◇ 2 cm width Posterior Δ -1 cm width Pulsation felt Suture lines some overlapping	<32 cm or >36 cm (12½ in–14 in) Bulging Fontanels Depressed Fontanels Large, flat fontanels Wide suture lines Closed suture lines	
Eyes	Symmetrical Doll's eye phenomena Pupils equally reactive to light Red reflex present Subconjunctival hemorrhages Blink reflex Strabismus (transient)	Pupils fixated unequal dilated constricted Nonreactive pupils Eyes wide set Very long eye lashes Corneal opacity Sclera jaundice Setting sun sign Brushfield's spots	

NURSERY ASSESSMENT (continued)

	Normal Characteristics	Deviations or Risk Factors	Comments
	Lid edema	Purulent drainage	
	Epicanthal folds (orientals)	Epicanthal folds in non-oriental	
	Chemical conjunctivitis		
Ears	Pinna	Pinna	
	firm & well developed	flat-soft-poor recoil	
	good recoil	little cartilage	
	Set	Low-set ears	
	Top of ear in line with outer canthus of eye		
	Helix round & curved inward	Helix lg, flat, flaccid	
	Internal ear		
	amniotic fluid & vernix caseosa in auditory canal		
	Preauricular skin tags		
	Reacts to sound	No reaction to loud noise	
Nose	Symmetrical & centered	Flaring nostrils	
	Broad & flat (1st 48 hrs)		
	Patent nares	Nares not patent	
	No discharge	Snuffles (copius discharge)	
	Sneezing occasionally	Frequent episodes of sneezing	
Mouth	Mucus membranes pink	Mucus membranes pale cyanotic	
	Circumoral pallor		
	Gums smooth	Predeciduous teeth	
	Inclusion cyst on gums	Dropping of mouth to one side	
	Tongue freely moveable	Frenulum short	
		Large tongue	
		Protruding tongue	
	Epstein pearls	Small white patches on tongue & back of throat	
		Cleft lip	
		Cleft palate	
	Gag reflex	Gag reflex absent	
	Sucking & swallowing reflex present	Excessive salivation	
		Sucking reflex absent	
Neck	Thick and short with skinfolds	Webbing	
	Freely moveable from side to side	Restricted movement	
		Crepitus	
	Clavicles palpated and intact	Fractured clavicle	
		Masses felt	
	Muscle symmetry	Sternocleidomastoid muscles not equal	
	Some head control	Head floppy	
		Brachial cleft cyst	

NURSERY ASSESSMENT (continued)

	Normal Characteristics	Deviations or Risk Factors	Comments
Chest	Chest circumference ________ about 2 cm (3/4 in) smaller than head circumference	<30.5 mm (12 in) or > 33 cm (13 in)	
		Funnel shaped	
	Round	Bulging	
	Symmetrical	Asymmetry of chest	
	Movements symmetrical	Asymmetry of chest movements	
	Rib-cage developed	Retractions frail rib-cage	
	Breast nodules 3–10 mm	Little or no breast tissue palpable	
	Nipple prominent	Flat nipples	
	Breast engorgement (24–48 hrs. after birth)		
	Sm. am't discharge from nipples (witch's milk)		
	Supernumerary nipples		
	Auscultation of lungs Bilateral breath sounds Distinct & loud (after 1st 8 hrs)	Rales (after 24 hrs) Rhonchi Wheezes Grunting	
	Few rales (1st 24 hrs)		
	Auscultation of heart		
	PMI at 4th intercostal	Shift of PMI to right or left	
	Distinct 1st & 2nd heart sounds	Persistent tachycardia	
	Rhythm regular	Persistent bradycardia	
	Transient murmurs	Arrhythmias	
		Persistent murmurs	
Abdomen		Scaphoid abdomen	
	Round protuberant	Distended abdomen	
	Umbilicus in midline cord moist & soft	Shiny abdomen	
		Prune-belly appearance to abdomen	
		Cord meconium stained	
		Prurulent drainage from cord	
		Foul odor to cord	
		Red at base of cord	
		Umbilical hernia	
	Liver: 1–3 cm below right costal margin	Hepatomegaly	
	Spleen: 1–2 cm below left costal margin (difficult to feel)	Hepatosplenomegaly	
		Diastasis recti	
		Gastroschisis (fissure in abdominal wall)	
	Kidney palpated in posterior flank (difficult to feel)		
	Bowel sounds present	Bowel sounds absent after 1st 2 hr of life	
		Meconium stool not passed in 1st 24 hr	
		Inguinal hernia unilateral bilateral	

NURSERY ASSESSMENT (continued)

	Normal Characteristics	Deviations or Risk Factors	Comments
	Femoral pulses present and equal	Faint or absent femoral pulse Bounding pulses Unequal pulses	
Genitalia	Female		
	Labia majora prominent covering most of labia minora	Prominent labia minora Enlarged clitoris	
	Edema of labia		
	Vaginal hymenal tags		
	Small amount of bloody discharge		
	Vernix caseosa in folds of labia	Ambiguity of genitalia	
	Voiding	No voidings within 1st 24 hr	
	Uric acid crystal (red-rust stain on diaper)		
	Male		
	Scrotum rugated & pendulous	Smooth scrotum	
	Testis present in each scrotal sac	Undescended testicle Hydrocele	
	Cremasteric reflex present	Inflammation of scrotum (orchitis)	
	Urinary meatus at end of penis	Hypospadias Epispadias	
	Prepuce covering glans penis	Ambiguity of genitalia	
	Anus patent	Imperforate anus	
	Meconium stool	Meconium stool not present in 1st 24 hr	
	Contraction of anal sphincter when perineal area stimulated	Condylomas (wartlike lesion)	
Back	C-shaped spine		
	Able to raise head slightly	Tufts of hair in pilonidal dimple	
	Dimple in pilondial area (no opening)	Spina bifida	
Legs	Hips	Hips	
	Symmetrical gluteal and popliteal skin folds	Asymmetrical gluteal and popliteal skin folds	
	Ortolani's maneuver negative	Positive Ortolani's maneuver (femur slipping in and out of position clicking heard	
	Length of legs equal		
	Bowed appearance	Phocomelia Polydactylism Syndactylism Talipes equinovarus	
	Acrocyanosis of feet		
	Full plantar creases on sole of foot	Heel creases covering less than half of sole	
	Flat feet		

NURSERY ASSESSMENT (continued)

	Normal Characteristics	Deviations or Risk Factors	Comments
Arms	Arms equal in length	Limpness of arm	
		Restrained movement	
	Acrocyanosis of hands	"Wrist-drop"	
		Syndactylism	
		Polydactylism	
	Fingernails: sharp, soft	Nails yellowish stained	
		Extra long nails	
		Simian crease on palm	
		Broad, flat hands	
		Short stubby fingers	
Skin	Vernix caseosa	Vernix caseosa stained yellow or with meconium	
	Pink skin tone: Causcasian	Pallor	
	Tan skin tone: Black-Asian	Generalized cyanosis	
	Mottling	Mottling when neonate warm	
	Harlequin skin changes	Ecchymoses	
	Milia: nose, chin	Abrasions	
	Lanugo: scant amount on shoulders, forehead back	Abundant lanugo	
	Erythemia neonatorum toxicum	Generalized rash	
	"Stork beak marks" (Telangiectatic nevi) on nape of neck on eyelid	"Port wine stain" (Nevus flammeus)	
	"Strawberry mark" (Nevus vasculosis)	Sclerema Cafe-au lait spots (6)	
	Mongolian spots on buttocks and sacral area	Maculopapular lesions on palms, soles of feet	
	Pressure petechiae	Wide-spread petechiae	
	Subcutaneous fat necrosis (face, buttocks, back, thigh)	Severe edema (hydropic)	
Muscle Tone	Muscles		
	Good muscle tone	Hypotonicity	
	Flexion following extension	Limp extremities	
	Symmetrical movements	Asymmetrical movements	
	Full range of motion	Limited motion	
		Paralysis	
Neurologic	Fine tremors	Jitteriness (unresolved)	
	Myoclonis	Lack of response to stimuli	
		Extreme irritability	
		Seizures	
		Lethargic	
	Reflexes		
	Rooting	Rooting reflex absent	
	Sucking	Sucking reflex absent	
	Gag	Gag reflex absent	
	Swallow	Swallow reflex absent	
	Extrusion	Extrusion reflex absent	
	Optical blink	Optical blink absent	

NURSERY ASSESSMENT (continued)

Normal Characteristics	Deviations or Risk Factors	Comments
Masseter	Masseter reflex absent	
Moro	Moro reflex absent	
Glabella	Glabella reflex absent	
Magnet	Magnet reflex absent	
Auditory	Auditory reflex absent	
Grasp	Grasp reflex absent	
Tonic neck	Tonic neck reflex absent	
Arm recoil	Arm recoil reflex absent	
Crawling	Crawling reflex absent	
Stepping	Stepping reflex absent	
Galant's	Galant's reflex absent	
Crossed extension	Crossed extension reflex absent	
Babinski	Babinski reflex absent	

tifying those at risk. Previously, birth weight was the only criteria used to determine prematurity. Neonates of less than 2500 gm were considered prematures regardless of their gestation time. This method failed to identify the needs of many neonates; for example, the neonate who was full-term but small or the neonate who was preterm but weighed more than 2500 gm. Consequently, a system evaluating physical and neurologic characteristics related to birth weight and gestation was developed, providing a classification of neonates according to their maturity.

Upon admission of the neonate to the nursery, a quick assessment will identify neonates who are obviously premature and in need of specialized care. However, gestational age assessment of all neonates is necessary to determine maturity and plan individualized care. Consideration is given, not only to the gestational age determined by the mother's last menstrual period (LMP), but also to the maturity of the neonate as determined by neurologic and physical examination. As the initial physical examination is being done, the physical characteristics may be classified. Because neonates experience nervous system instability in the first 24 hours of life, the neurologic examination may be delayed, or completed and reevaluated at a second examination 12 hours later.

Several methods of classifying neonatal characteristics have been designed. In 1961 the World Health Organization developed standards used for estimations of gestation according to the number of weeks gestation. The following classifications were determined:

Gestation of 37 weeks or less: preterm neonate

Gestation of 38 to 41 weeks: full-term neonate

Gestation of 42 weeks or more: postterm neonate

The University of Colorado Medical Center Intrauterine Growth Charts graphically plot the birth weight of the neonate against the gestational weeks to determine the classification within nine categories, as shown in Figure 22–22. The neonate would be classified in one of the following categories:

Preterm
- Small for gestational age (SGA)
- Appropriate for gestational age (AGA)
- Large for gestational age (LGA)

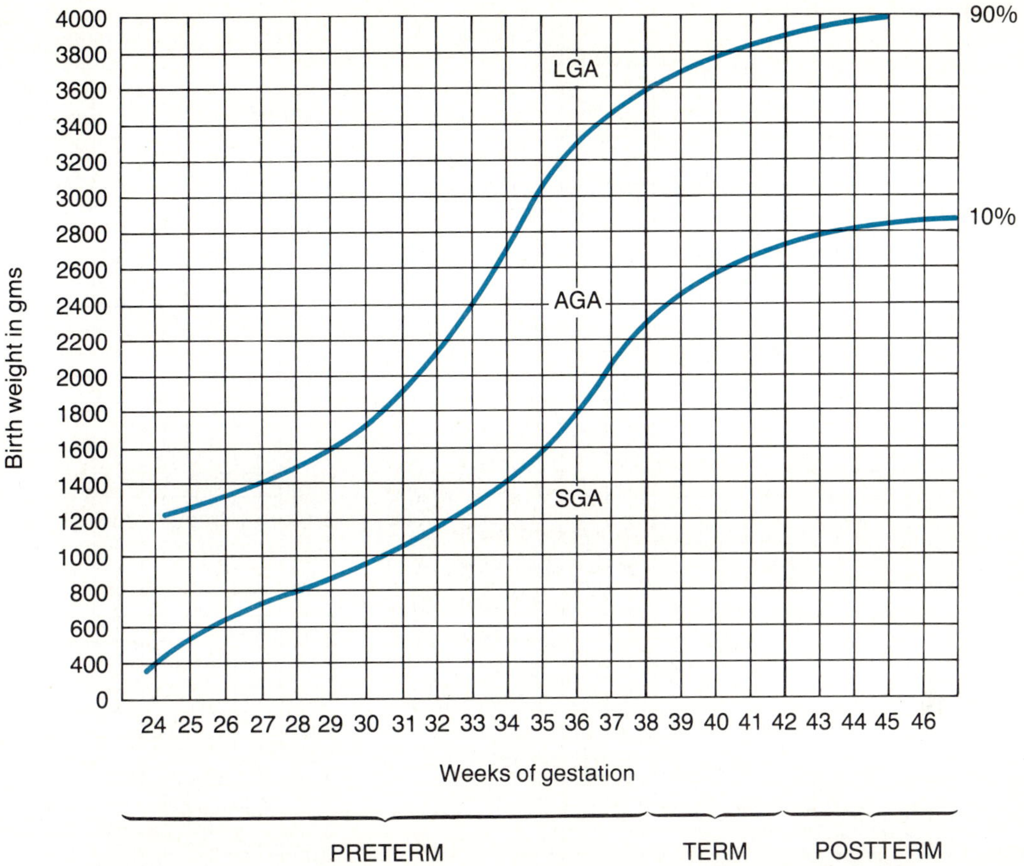

FIGURE 22-22. Distribution of birth weight according to gestational age among neonates. Adapted and reprinted with permission. Lubchenco, L., Hansman, C., Dressler, M. & Boyd, E.: Distribution of birth weights according to gestational age among neonates. Pediatrics, 1963, **32,** 793.

Full term SGA
AGA
LGA
Postterm SGA
AGA
LGA

Neonates falling in or above the 90th percentile are large for gestational age (LGA), those between the 10th and 90th percentile are AGA and those below the 10th percentile are SGA. Further classifications graphically evaluate weight, length, head circumference, and weight–length ratio (see Fig. 22–23). These parameters provide a more accurate evaluation by discriminating assessments that identify intrauterine growth retardation (small head circumference and weight-length ratio) from conditions affecting only weight or length, e.g., maternal smoking.

The Dubowitz scoring system may be used to evaluate neurologic and physical determinants of maturity (see Figs. 22–24 and 22–25). Although lengthy, it provides a valuable screening method for identification of gestational maturity. Both physical and neurologic characteristics are observed, scored, and indicated on the guide. The scores are then combined, the total score is identified on the

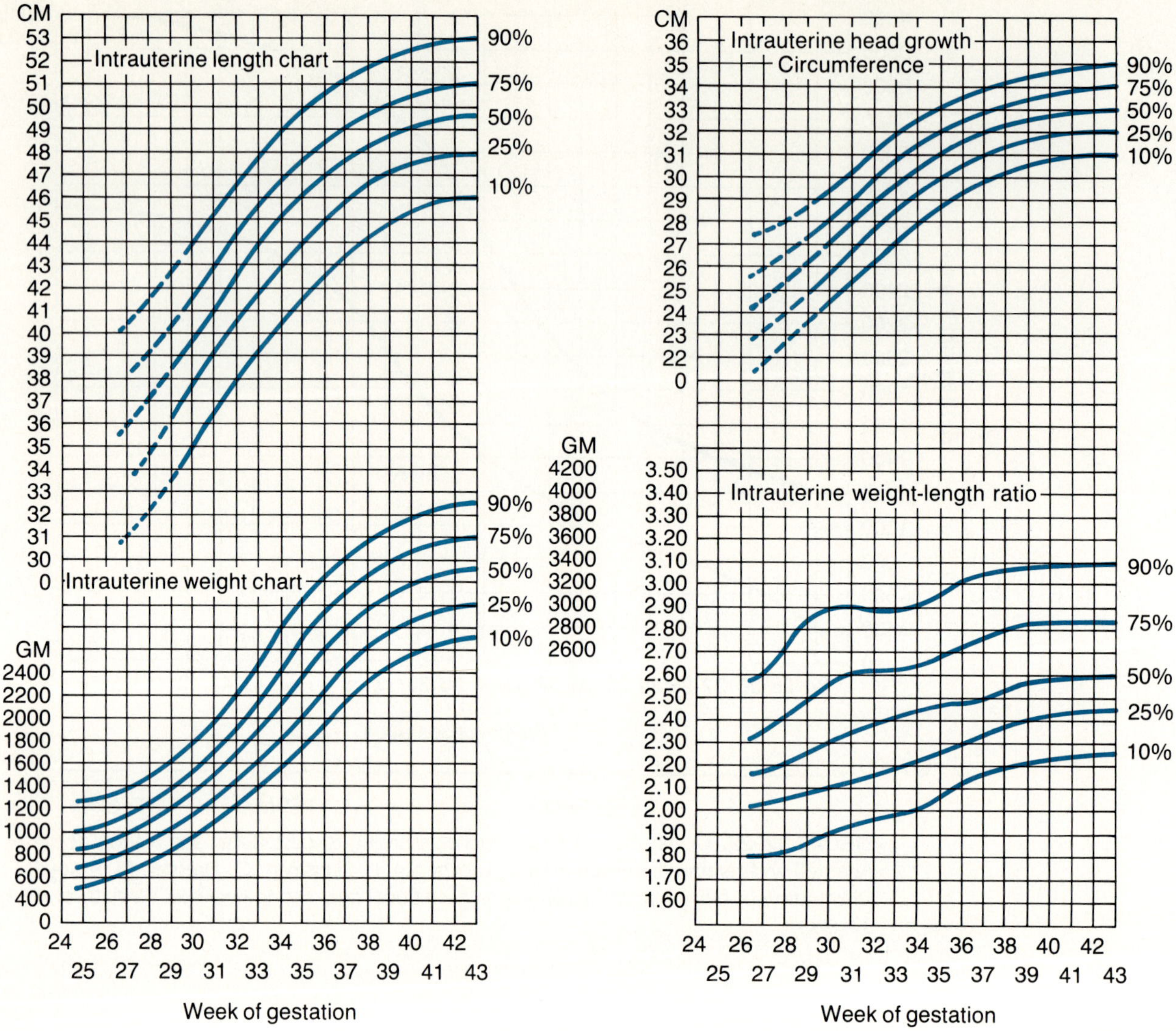

FIGURE 22-23. Percentiles of intrauterine growth in weight, length, head circumference and weight-length ratio. Reproduced by permission. Lubchenco, L., Hansman, C. & Boyd, E.: Classification of newborns based on maturity and intrauterine growth. Pediatrics, 1966, **37,** 403.

Maturity Rating Chart (see Fig. 22-26), and it is related to the number of weeks gestation.

An abbreviated form of gestational age assessment is provided by Ballard et al. (see Fig. 22-27). This method utilizes six neuromuscular and six physical criteria, which are:

Neuromuscular

Posture: 0-4 (see Fig. 22-27)

The posture of the quiet neonate is observed while he is in a supine position.

0 Indicates extension of both the arms and legs without flexion.

1 Indicates slight amount of flexion of the knees and hips.

2 Indicates moderate amount of flexion of the knees and hips.

3 Indicates legs and arms moderately flexed.

4 Indicates complete flexion of the arms and legs.

Square Window: 0-4 (see Fig. 22-28)

The wrist is firmly flexed on the forearm.

0 Indicates a 90° angle between the base of the palm and the forearm (wrist angle).

1 Indicates a 60° angle between the base of the palm and the forearm (wrist angle).

External sign	*Score**				
	0	*1*	*2*	*3*	*4*
Edema	Obvious edema of hands and feet; pitting over tibia	No obvious edema of hands and feet; pitting over tibia	No edema		
Skin texture	Very thin, gelatinous	Thin and smooth	Smooth; medium thickness. Rash or superficial peeling	Slight thickening. Superficial cracking and peeling especially of hands and feet	Thick and parchment-like; superficial or deep cracking
Skin color	Dark red	Uniformly pink	Pale pink; variable over body	Pale; only pink over ears, lips, palms, or soles	
Skin opacity (trunk)	Numerous veins and venules clearly seen, especially over abdomen	Veins and tributaries seen	A few large vessels clearly seen over abdomen	A few large vessels seen indistinctly over abdomen	No blood vessels seen
Lanugo (over back)	No lanugo	Abundant; long and thick over whole back	Hair thinning especially over lower back	Small amount of lanugo and bald areas	At least ½ of back devoid of lanugo
Plantar creases	No skin creases	Faint red marks over anterior half of sole	Definite red marks over > anterior ½; indentations over < anterior ⅓	Indentations over > anterior ⅓	Definite deep indentations over > anterior ⅓
Nipple formation	Nipple barely visible; no areola	Nipple well defined; areola smooth and flat, diameter < 0.75 cm.	Areola stippled, edge not raised, diameter < 0.75 cm.	Areola stippled, edge raised, diameter > 0.75 cm.	
Breast size	No breast tissue palpable	Breast tissue on one or both sides, < 0.5 cm. diameter	Breast tissue both sides; one or both 0.5 - 1.0 cm.	Breast tissue both sides; one or both > 1 cm.	
Ear form	Pinna flat and shapeless, little or no incurving of edge	Incurving of part of edge of pinna	Partial incurving whole of upper pinna	Well-defined incurving whole of upper pinna	
Ear firmness	Pinna soft, easily folded, no recoil	Pinna soft, easily folded, slow recoil	Cartilage to edge of pinna, but soft in places, ready recoil	Pinna firm, cartilage to edge; instant recoil	
Genitals Male	Neither testis in scrotum	At least one testis high in scrotum	At least one testis right down		
Female (with hips ½ abducted)	Labia majora widely separated, labia minora protruding	Labia majora almost cover labia minora	Labia majora completely cover labia minora		

*if score differs on two sides, take the mean

FIGURE 22-24. Scoring system for gestational age external criteria. Reprinted with permission. Adapted from Dubowitz, L.M.S., Dubowitz, V. & Goldberg, C.: Clinical assessment of gestational age—Scoring system for external criteria. Journal of Pediatrics, 1970, **77**(1), 7. Modified from Farr, V. et al. Develop Med Child Neurol, 1966, **8,** 507.

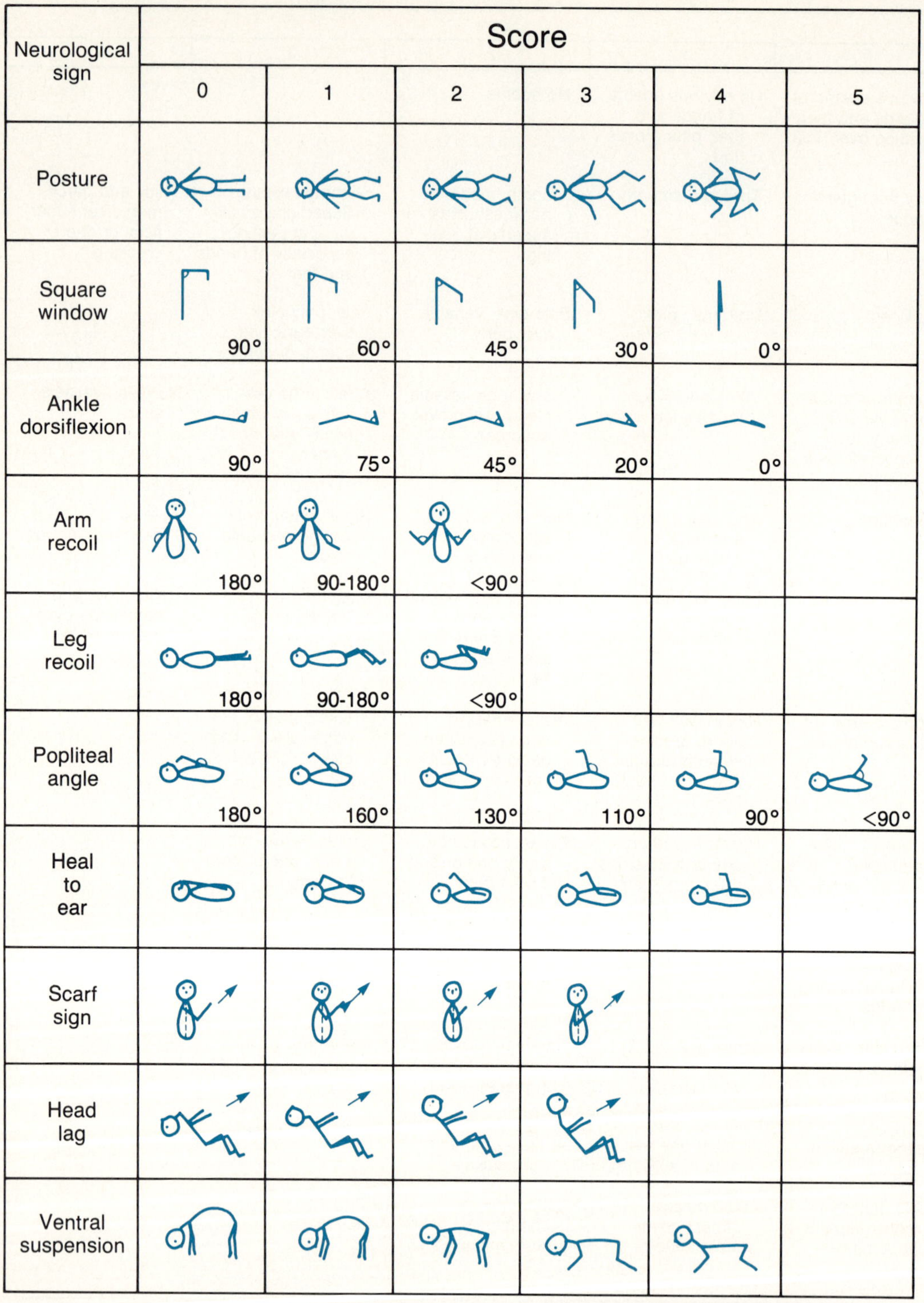

FIGURE 22-25. Scoring system for gestational age neurologic criteria. Reprinted with permission. Adapted from Dubowitz, L.M.S., Dubowitz, V. & Goldberg, C.: Clinical assessment of gestational age—Scoring system for neurologic criteria. Journal of Pediatrics, 1970, **77**(1), 7.

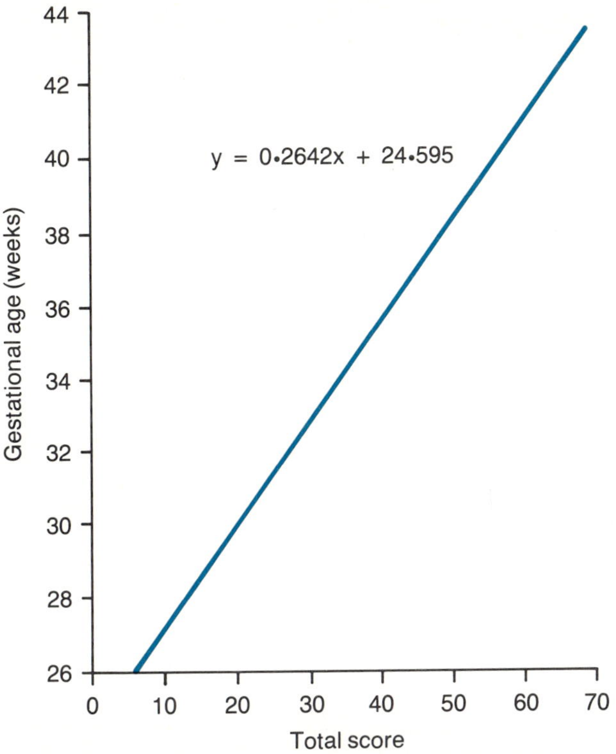

FIGURE 22-26. Graph for reading gestational age from total score. Reprinted with permission. Adapted from Dubowitz, L.M.S., Dubowitz, V. & Goldberg, C.: Clinical assessment of gestational age—Graph for reading gestational age from total score. Journal of Pediatrics, 1970, **77**(1), 7.

2 Indicates a 45° angle between the base of the palm and the forearm (wrist angle).
3 Indicates a 30° angle between the base of the palm and the forearm (wrist angle).
4 Indicates 0° angle between the base of the palm and forearm (wrist angle).

Arm Recoil: (see Fig. 22-27)
With the neonate in a supine position, the arm is flexed at the elbow for four to five seconds and then extended.
0 Indicates 180° less than full return to flexion, remaining complete extended.
2 Indicates 100° to 180° less than full return to flexion, exhibiting some flexion.
3 Indicates 90° to 100° less than full return to flexion, exhibiting moderate flexion.
4 Indicates less than 90° from full flexion.

Popliteal Angle: (see Fig. 22-27)
The neonate is supine and his hips are flat on the table. The thigh is flexed on the abdomen and efforts are made by the examiner placing one finger behind the ankle, to extend the leg. The angle of resistance is measured.
0 Indicates only little resistance with a 180° popliteal angle.
1 Indicates small amount of resistance with a 160° popliteal angle.
2 Indicates slight resistance with a 130° popliteal angle.
3 Indicates a moderate amount of resistance with a 110° popliteal angle.
4 Indicates good resistance with a 90° popliteal angle.
5 Indicates strong resistance with less than a 90° popliteal angle.

Scarf Sign: (see Fig. 22-29)
While the neonate is in a supine position the arm is extended across the chest, reaching as close as possible to the opposite shoulder. Placement of the elbow is then noted.
0 Indicates no resistance and the elbow will reach the opposite shoulder.
1 Indicates elbow is between the opposite axilla and the midline.
2 Indicates the elbow will not reach beyond the midline.
3 Indicates the elbow is between the nipple line and the midline.
4 Indicates the elbow is not to the nipple line.

Heel to Ear (see Fig. 22-27)
With the neonate in the supine position, pressure is placed on the foot, directing it toward the ear until resistance is met. The distance the foot will reach is graded and the degree of extension of the knee is graded.
0 Indicates the foot will touch or almost touches the ear.
1 Indicates the foot will not reach the ear but is between the neck and the nipple line.
2 Indicates the foot is between the nipple line and the umbilicus and the knee flexed.
3 Indicates the foot does not extend beyond the umbilicus and the knee flexed.
4 Indicates the foot does not reach to the level of the umbilicus and the knee flexed.

Physical Characteristics

Physical characteristics (skin, lanugo, plantar creases, breast, ear, genitals) are rated from 0 to 4 or 5, as described in Figure 22-27.

Brazelton Neonatal Behavioral Assessment Scale

Assessment of the neonate includes not only his physical and neurologic characteristics, but also his behavioral characteristics. Dr. T. Berry Brazelton (1973) was one of the first to focus on the neonate's behavioral responses to his environment and his interactive abilities. Development of the Brazelton Neonatal Behavioral Assessment Scale provided insight into the behavioral individuality of the neonate as well as his neurologic capabilities.

The scale includes 27 behavioral items and 20 reflex responses that require a minimum of 20 minutes to assess by an experienced examiner. A score ranging from 1 to 9 may be obtained on the behavioral items and from 1 to 3 on the reflex items, with the norm at midpoint. During examination of each of the categories, the state of consciousness is noted. Although the learner is referred to the original source (Brazelton, T., 1973) for the complete assessment scale, a brief summary of the scale follows:

1. Deep sleep. Undisturbed by sound and minimal stimuli, regular breathing, eyes shut, no activity, a few uncoordinated movements.
2. Light sleep. Slight arousal from sounds and stimuli, irregular breathing, eyes closed but some rapid eye movements can be detected, a few sucking motions and some startle responses, with return to sleep or advance to next state.
3. Drowsiness. Responds to noise and stimuli slowly, irregular breathing, eyes open but heavy, some movements which are not jerky.
4. Quiet alert. Minimal movement, eyes open with attempts at focusing, quiet and not fussy, regular breathing.
5. Active alert. Eyes open with increased movement, may be fussy, irregular breathing, movements of the extremities and active response to stimuli.
6. Crying. Vigorous movements, eyes open or tightly closed, irregular breathing, loud cries.

The different levels of consciousness will alter neonatal responses to stimuli. The method of adapting in each of the six categories describes neonatal behavioral and reflex response. These categories are:

1. Habitation. Assessed during deep and light sleep and drowsy state (1, 2, 3). Refers to the ability of the neonate to moderate his reaction to repeated stimuli. When first confronted with the stimuli, such as a ringing bell or light in his eyes, he will react with a startle or blink response, but if repeated many times, the response diminishes and little reaction is seen.
2. Orientation. Assessed in quiet or active alert state (4, 5). Presented with an auditory or visual type stimuli, the neonate will respond by turning his head toward the stimuli or attempting to focus his eyes on it, indicating his awareness of the stimuli and the ability to attend to it.
3. Motor maturity. Assessed in the quiet alert state (4). Determines the control and coordination of motor response and body tone as the neonate is manipulated throughout the examination. Head righting, hand to mouth coordination, and startle movements are examples of measures used to make this assessment.
4. Variation. Assessed in the quiet alert state (4 only). As the examination is conducted, the variations in the alert states and peak of excitement state are noted. Concurrent with these responses are autonomic nervous system responses inducing color changes.
5. Self-quieting abilities. May be assessed in all states with emphasis on and progression away from the more active states (6, 5, 4, 3, 2, 1). Observations are made of the neonate's ability to console himself and the length of time needed. Measures he may use include sucking on hand or fist, or involvement in an auditory or visual distraction.
6. Social behavior (cuddliness). Assessed in the quiet and active alert states (4, 5). This category speaks to the neonate's response

Neuromuscular maturity

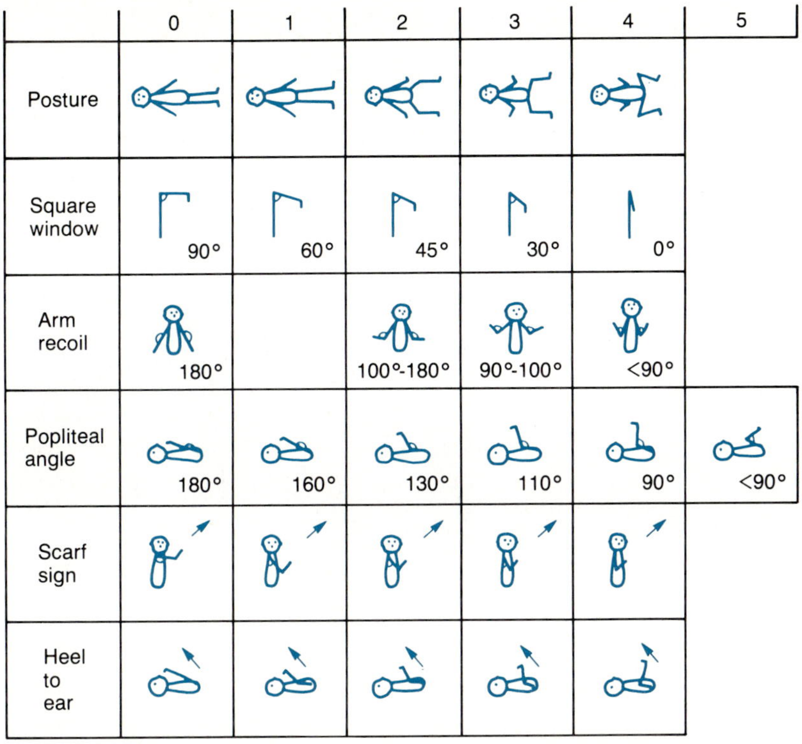

Physical maturity

Skin	Gelatinous red, trans-parent	Smooth pink, vis-ible veins	Superficial peeling, &/or rash few veins	Cracking pale area rare veins	Parchment deep cracking no vessels	Leathery cracked wrinkled
Lanugo	None	Abundant	Thinning	Bald areas	Mostly bald	
Plantar creases	No crease	Faint red marks	Anterior transverse crease only	Creases ant 2/3	Creases cover entire sole	
Breast	Barely percept	Flat areola no bud	Stippled areola 1-2 mm bud	Raised areola 3-4 mm bud	Full areola 5-10 mm bud	
Ear	Pinna flat, stays folded	Sl curved pinna; soft c slow recoil	Well-curv. pinna; soft but ready recoil	Formed & firm c instant recoil	Thick cartilage ear stiff	
Genitals ♂	Scrotom empty no rugae		Testes descend-ing, few rugae	Testes down good rugae	Testes pendulous deep rugae	
Genitals ♀	Prominent clitoris & labia minora		Majora & minora equally prominent	Majora large minora small	Clitoris & minora completely covered	

Maturity rating

Score	Wks.
5	26
10	28
15	30
20	32
25	34
30	36
35	38
40	40
45	42
50	44

FIGURE 22-27. Ballard maturity rating and classification. Reprinted with permission. Ballard, J.L.: Scoring system for simplified clinical assessment of maturation in newborn infants. Journal of Pediatrics, 1979, **95,** 769.

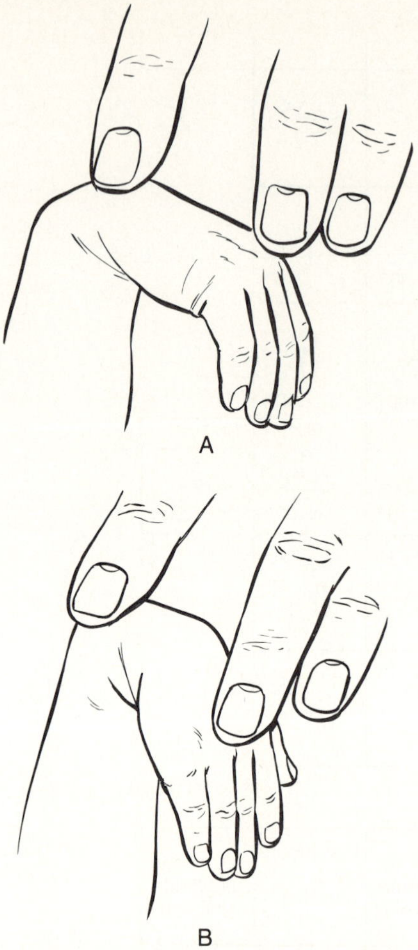

FIGURE 22-28. Assessment of square window sign: A. Assessment of 90° angle consistent with 28–32 weeks gestation. B. Assessment of 0° angle as seen in the neonate of 40–42 weeks gestation.

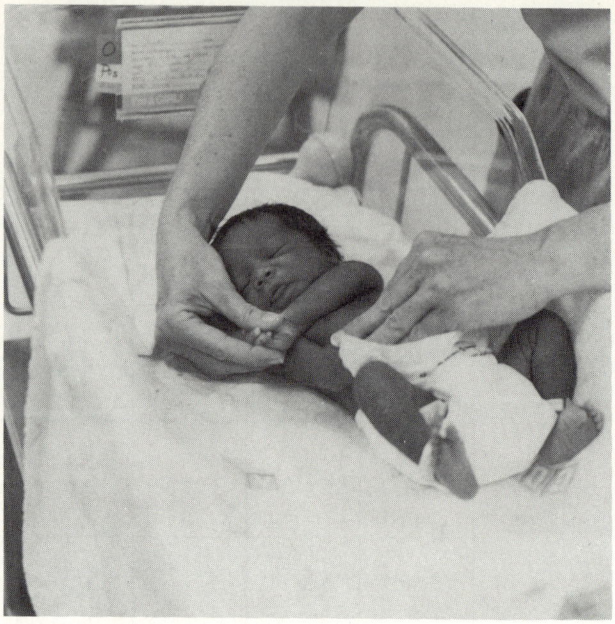

FIGURE 22-29. Assessment of scarf sign.

as he is being held, his need for being held, and his smiles, which initially may only be grimaces but which engender a reaction by parents and caregivers.

The test is preferably administered on the third day of life, following the transitions from fetal to extrauterine life when there is less central nervous system irritability. Other factors that will influence the neonate's responses to the test are:

Environmental influences (temperature of room, stimuli such as noises or bright lights)

Medications (administered to the neonate or mother during labor which are still influencing the neonate)

Disruptive procedure (circumcision, bathing, footprinting)

Time of the last feeding

State of consciousness

Ethnic influences

Test results are indicators of the neonate's behavioral responses and do not determine whether he is a "good" or "bad" baby. The tests simply indicate how he reacts to and copes with certain stimuli during various levels of consciousness. The test, or elements of the test, may be repeated in an effort to elicit the best responses. A complete explanation of the test may be found in Brazelton (1973).

Many therapeutic implications are derived from the Brazelton test. Caregivers, specifically parents, become aware of the manner in which their neonate is striving to interact with his environment. Cues given by the neonate may be interpreted by the parents, enabling them to respond in the manner best suited to meet the needs of the infant. Frustrations and guilt feelings are minimized as parents realize that a particular behavior is normal for their individual baby and not caused by parental or neonatal inadequacies.

Awareness of the behavioral characteristics of their neonate also helps parents to plan his care. When parents understand the cyclic attention patterns of their neonate they are not as likely to overstimulate him during nonattention periods. Yet, when he is responsive they find great satisfaction in interacting with him. Knowledge of variations of state enables the parents to be more keenly attuned to specific needs. Test results may show that their infant has limited self-quieting abilities and needs calming activities such as a pacifier or rocking. Knowing that their baby is a social being, even at birth, will encourage parents to communicate with him in both verbal and nonverbal ways. Although these are but a few of the benefits that can be derived from the test, they serve as examples of the advantages realized when parents have an understanding of their neonate as an individual.

Nurses are responsible for communicating neonatal responses to the parents before the mother and the newborn are discharged from the hospital. The nurse who states only, "the baby is a good baby and doing just fine" has not provided the mother with sufficient insights into her baby's needs. An elaborate explanation of the care of the neonate may be given by the nurse but frequently little is said about the response of the neonate to the care or caregiver. Often the mother returns home and when confronted with a crying or fussy baby, feels she is incapable since he was such a "good baby" while in the hospital. She feels she is doing something wrong because he is fussy and yet, she has done everything the nurse told her to do. Guilt feelings such as these might be prevented if the nurse provides insights into neonatal behavior before discharge. This awareness enables the mother to realize that her neonate's fussy behavior is normal and can be expected at times, rather than being the result of poor mothering.

Parents' expectations and responsibilities to the neonate are discussed before discharge. Unrealistic expectations may exhaust both the mother and father as they strive to give perfect care to the baby. Frustrations are encountered and anxiety develops. However, if they are aware of the realities of parenting, their expectations may not be so magnanimous and confidence develops in their ability to assume a parenting role.

Neonatal Periods of Reactivity

The first 12 hours following birth are designated as the transitional period. The highest percentage of neonatal mortality is seen in this period, as adaptations to extrauterine life rapidly occur and increase the vulnerability of the neonate. Therefore, knowledge of these changes and the characteristics of the transitional period is important for the nurse in planning care for the neonate.

The *first period of reactivity* occurs within the first 30 minutes of life. During this time the neonate who has not been influenced by maternal drugs or anesthesia during labor will be alert and responsive. The first initial response in the healthy neonate is a vigorous cry followed by an increase in erratic movements as muscle tone and activity increase. The eyes appear bright, as if the neonate were exploring his new environment. His color at this time may vary from an initial brief period of cyanosis to a generalized pink, ruddy color with some acrocyanosis of the extremities.

Respirations during the first period of reactivity are irregular and shallow at a rate of 60 to 90 per minute. There may be some brief periods of tachypnea, apnea, nasal flaring, retractions, and grunting as respiratory stability is established. Small amounts of fluid remaining in the lungs may be responsible for the rales and rhonchi heard during initial lung assessments.

Mucus present in the oral and nasal passages of neonates may be obstructive if not removed. Suctioning of the mouth and air passages prevents aspiration of secretions. The mouth is suctioned first, as suctioning of the nasal passages may evoke a gasp, causing aspiration of the oral mucus. A bulb syringe is usually employed to remove secretions before more extensive methods are initiated. When using the bulb syringe, the bulb is compressed before insertion into the mouth (Fig. 22–30). Both sides of the mouth are suctioned gently, avoiding vigorous suctioning that may cause episodes of neonatal bradycardia and laryngospasm.

The heart rate is irregular, with periods of tachycardia reaching up to 180 beats per minute for short intervals. The tachycardia is only transient and should not continue beyond the first period of reactivity.

Bowel sounds may not be heard in this period of reactivity and usually are not present until one hour following birth. Neonates who have experienced distress in utero and early passage of meconium may have peristaltic movements that can be auscultated.

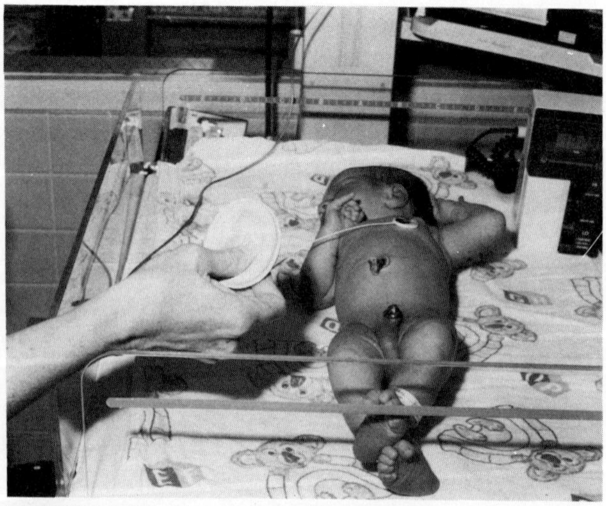

FIGURE 22–30. Use of the bulb syringe.

The responsiveness of the neonate during these first few moments following birth fosters parental-infant bonding. His alert expression coupled with his reaction to a soothing voice and protective fondling makes him a participant in the bonding process. Measures that alter this process, such as the instillation of neonatal eye medications in the delivery room, are not recommended as they interfere with eye contact between the mother and baby. When normal Apgar scores are present and the mother is responsive without complications, there is no reason to delay the mother and father from holding the infant and initiating bonding. Priorities of care during this period are found in Chapter 16.

After the first 30 minutes of life, and for approximately the next two hours, the neonate enters the *resting and sleeping period.* During this time, activities are minimized as he undergoes a period of drowziness and sleep. The respiratory and heart rates decrease. The sleep interval may be short or extended, but he remains basically quiet during this phase. Characteristics of the first period, such as barreling of the chest, tachypnea, and retractions, disappear and are replaced by regular respiratory movements. While in periods of light sleep, episodes of twitching and responsiveness to stimuli may occur; however, the neonate will generally fall back to sleep and remain inactive.

Disruption of the neonate during this period is not recommended. Care should be planned to allow him to recover from the effects of stimulation incurred during the birth. Ideally, the neonate will fall asleep in his mother's arms and will be observed by nursing personnel while at her bedside.

The *second period of reactivity* follows the rest and sleep period, lasting two to six hours. Characteristics of the first period of reactivity are present and varying levels of activity are seen. Stimuli presented to the neonate at this time may induce an inordinate response. Fluctuation in heart rate is responsible for episodes of bradycardia and tachycardia. Apneic episodes are present and normal but require close observation. The flushed appearance observed during the resting stage may abruptly change to a mild pallor with evidence of circumoral pallor and acrocyanosis.

Attention is given to oral mucus, which may be present in large amounts and cause choking. Some neonates will become fussy, make swallowing movements, gag, and spit out the mucus. Others are "quiet chokers" and may experience respiratory difficulties before the nurse is aware they are choking. All neonates must be carefully observed for mucus difficulties, especially during this period. When a neonate's respiratory passages are obstructed, immediate suctioning is necessary and a bulb syringe is always kept in the crib for this purpose. The neonate is held with his head down, allowing gravity to aid in the removal of the mucus while the nurse suctions the mouth with the bulb syringe. If the mucus is thick and cannot be removed with a bulb syringe, a catheter (French-size 12 or 14) attached to a wall suction may be used.

Bowel activity is frequently noted during the second period of reactivity, with passage of the first meconium stool. Notations are made of the characteristics of the first stool and those thereafter. The characteristics of any voiding are also noted and recorded.

Care During the Transitional Period

During this very sensitive period of extrauterine life assessment and supportive nursing care of the neonate is essential. The initial nursery assessment will provide information needed to determine priorities of care for the neonate as he progresses through the transitional stage. Physiologic parameters that are monitored include:

- Respirations
- Cardiac status
- Temperature
- Oral intake
- Evaluation of blood glucose levels

RESPIRATIONS

Respiratory assessments are made every 15 minutes during the first hour following birth and every 30 minutes for the next two hours or until stable. Routine oxygen administration is not recommended to enhance respirations unless there are indications of respiratory distress, such as nasal flaring, sustained apnea, grunting, pallor, continued retractions, and cyanosis.

Brief periods of apnea may be interrupted by stimulation such as positional change or gently rubbing the spinal column (Perez maneuver). Oxygen administered directly to the neonate's face (free flowing) may stimulate breathing. It is used for short periods only, as the facial areas are more sensitive to temperature drops and a pseudohypothermia will result.

CARDIAC STATUS

The apical pulse is assessed with the same frequency as respirations. As previously noted, some variations and irregularities may be present. Displacement of the PMI, sustained tachycardia (over 160), or bradycardia (under 100) are abnormal.

TEMPERATURE

Fluctuations in the temperature may be expected during the transitional period. Assessment of the temperature is made every hour for the first four hours and then every four hours during the remainder of the first 24 hours. The temperature is maintained at 36.4° to 37.0°C (97.6 to 98.6°F). Axillary temperatures are taken unless otherwise ordered.

Frequently, a radiant warmer is used to increase or maintain neonatal temperature in a neutral thermal range. The unit should be calibrated, the control point set at 98°F, the unit prewarmed, and the alarms set before using. Sensory probes are placed on a fleshy part of the abdomen midway between the sternum and the umbilicus (see Fig. 16–26), avoiding bony areas that would interfere with the accuracy of the probe. The probe is covered with an insulator strip to prevent the warmer from heating the probe and causing false readings. Temperatures are taken every hour while the neonate is under the warmer. He will remain in this environment until the temperature is stable (about one to four hours).

If thermoregulation is adequate, the neonate may be wrapped in prewarmed blankets to prevent heat loss by conduction and a cap may be placed on his head, preventing heat loss by radiation. Temperature checks are important to prevent hyperthermia.

All surfaces used to weigh or examine the neonate should be warm or covered with a warm covering. The first bath is not given until physiologic stability is achieved with temperature and vital signs within the normal ranges. The initial bath is given quickly, avoiding unnecessary exposure. When the bath is completed, the temperature is again rechecked and if low, corrective measures are instituted.

ORAL INTAKE

Within the first few hours after birth, signs such as lip-smacking, sucking, and swallowing, indicate readiness to feed. The initial feeding consists of only sterile water to prevent aspiration of irritating substances in the event that abnormalities, such as tracheoesophageal fistula, are present. Glucose water is not recommended for the first feeding since, if aspirated, it is very irritative to the lungs. Many facilities will give glucose water in subsequent feedings during the transition period in order to prevent hypoglycemia. Other institutions prefer to begin formula feedings at the next feeding following the sterile water.

When breastfeeding is the chosen method, the neonate may be put directly to breast while in the delivery room. If there are no problems, breastfeeding may be continued at subsequent feedings. A discussion of nutrition of the neonate is found in Chapter 23.

EVALUATION OF BLOOD GLUCOSE LEVELS

A blood sugar level is determined in the first hour following birth to detect the presence of hypoglycemia. Neonates with hypoglycemia are at risk for respiratory problems and alterations in physiologic homeostasis. SGA neonates, preterm infants, infants of diabetic mothers, neonates with intrauterine growth retardation, those with *erythroblastosis fetalis* (hemolytic disorder of the newborn), and those with cold stress are candidates for the development of hypoglycemia.

Glucose levels in the neonate are obtained before the first glucose water, formula, or breast feeding. The Dextrostix test may be used by obtaining a small amount of blood from a heel stick (see Fig. 22-31). Following cleansing of the heel with alcohol, the stick is performed in the lateral aspect of the heel. The first drop of blood is wiped away with a clean gauze strip and the second drop of blood is placed on the Dextrostix test strip; after 1 minute the strip is rinsed with clear, free-flowing water. Comparisons of the strip are made with the accompanying chart. A reading of 40 mg per dl or below is indicative of hypoglycemia and the physician is notified. Glucometers may also be used to assess glucose levels.

MEDICATIONS

Vitamin K injections are given within the first four hours of birth in order to enhance activation of coagulation factors and prevent hemorrhage. A single dose of 0.5 to 1.0 mg is given in the lateral aspect of the vastus lateralis muscle or the rectus formis muscle of the thigh (see Fig. 22-32). Although either of these two sites is relatively void of large blood vessels or nerves, the preferred site is the vastus lateralis, the larger of the two muscles. The injection site is determined using the knee and the greater trochanter as landmarks. The area between these two points is divided

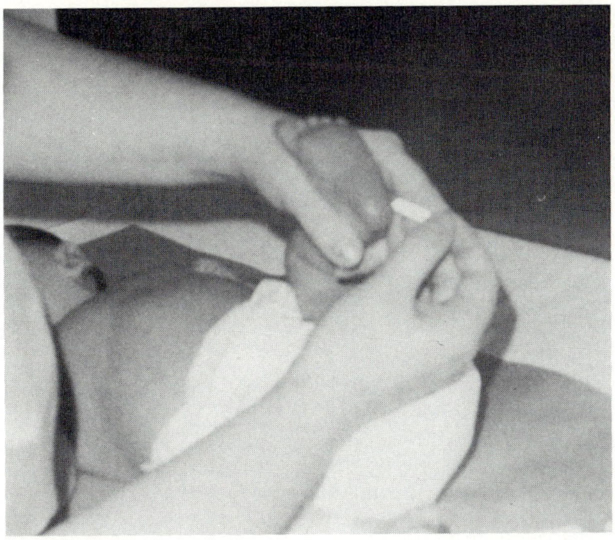

FIGURE 22-31. Heelstick.

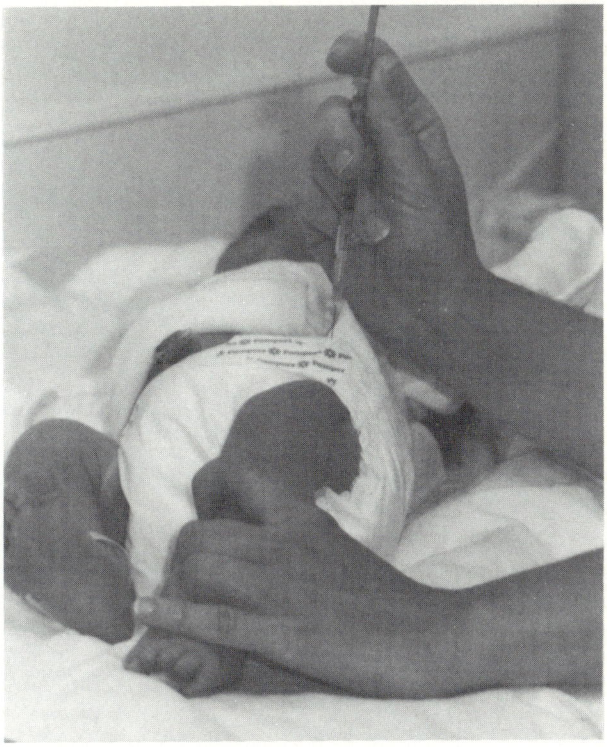

FIGURE 22-32. Injection of Vitamin K.

into thirds, with the injection given in the middle third.

Eye instillations of prophylactic medications to prevent ophthalmia neonatorium may be done in the delivery room but preferably are not done until bonding of the neonate and parents has occurred. An antibiotic ointment or silver nitrate may be used (see Chapter 16). Table 22-5 provides a summary of nursing responsibilities during the transitional period.

ASPECTS OF DAILY CARE

Environment

The environment of the neonate ideally fosters family-centered maternity/newborn care. The Interprofessional Task Force on Health Care of Women and Children (1978) recommends that emphasis be placed on "the provision of maternity/newborn health care which fosters family unity while maintaining physical safety."

Many nurseries prefer to designate one area as an observation area for the first 24 hours of the neonate's life. The neonate is then transferred to a different level if he is stable and without major complications.

Rooming-in facilities provide opportunities for optimal mother-infant interaction. Following a period of observation, the neonate is cared for by the mother at her bedside with guidance and observations by the nurse. If the mother is tired and prefers to rest, the neonate is returned to the nursery and cared for by nursery personnel until the mother wishes to resume care. An explanation of the concepts and procedures of rooming-in is found in Chapter 20.

All nurseries should be well lighted, free from drafts, thermostatically controlled to promote neutral thermoregulation of the neonate, and well ventilated. Safety of the neonate is considered when using any electrical equipment. Each nursery is equipped with facilities for handwashing and each neonate should have his own crib, basic supplies, and clean linens.

TABLE 22-5
NURSING RESPONSIBILITIES DURING THE TRANSITIONAL PERIOD

Protocol	Nursing Intervention
Verify identification of neonate	Check: Hospital number-date-time of delivery-sex-physician-name
Communication of data	Briefly review: Synopsis of maternal prenatal, labor, and delivery record Fetal responses to labor and delivery resuscitation efforts Neonatal Apgar scores at 1 and 5 minutes
Assess vital signs	Auscultate heart and lung sounds Count and assess respirations and pulses every: 1st hour—every 15 minutes 2nd hour—every 30 minutes 3rd hour—every 30 minutes 4th–11th hour—every 2 hours 12th–24th hour—every 4 hours
Maintain respirations	Suction oral and nasal passages as needed Observe for respiratory distress Institute resuscitative measures when necessary Position on side to allow draining of mucus
Maintain temperature in neutral thermal range	Initial assessment of rectal temperature, followed by axillary temperature every hour for first 4 hours and then every 4 hours for 20 hours Utilize warmed blankets or radiant warmer to provide warmth when needed Maintain room temperature between 75° and 78°F (24.0°C–25.5°C) Place cap on head
Assess general appearance of neonate	Note: Skin color Reflex responses Muscle tone Cry Movement Size
Observe umbilical stump	Count vessels and check for bleeding

Personnel are well trained before and during their assignment to the nursery. A registered nurse, prepared to handle any emergency situation, is present in the nursery at all times. All personnel are well prepared in emergency evacuation procedures in the event of a fire or disaster.

Infection Control

Fetal life is passed in a sterile environment. As the neonate enters the extrauterine environment he is confronted with many microorganisms, some pathogenic and others compatible with his existence. The neonate's

TABLE 22-5 (continued)

Protocol	Nursing Intervention
Weigh and measure neonate	Determine relationship of weight and length to gestation
Determine gestational age	Assess for gestational age if condition of neonate is satisfactory
Head-to-toe assessment of neonate	Perform physical examination of neonate if condition allows
Administer medications	Give vitamin K injection IM in vastus lateralis muscle Do prophylactic eye treatment after interaction with parents
Assess blood glucose levels	Perform Dextrostix test in the first hour after birth Report levels below 40 mg/dl
Bathe and dress neonate	Delay bath until vital signs stable Sponge bathe face and head with warm water. Cleanse remainder of body as necessary Do not expose and chill neonate unnecessarily
Assess eliminations	Record meconium stools and voidings
Provide for parent–infant interaction	Allow parents to observe bath and provide time for parents to hold and interact with neonate during 1st period of reactivity
Provide for recovery period of neonate	Provide safe, quiet environment with attention to asepsis and protection from infection Limit amount of handling when neonate is in resting and sleeping period
Provide nutritional intake	Assess feeding capabilities by offering sterile water feeding after second period of reactivity If no abnormalities feed 5% glucose water, formula or breast feeding
Provide data base for continued care	Record all assessments and nursing interventions
Develop nursing care plan for neonate	Determine neonate's individualized needs, priorities of care and evaluation criteria

defenses are not complete at this time and susceptibility to infections remains a danger. Protection from infection becomes a priority when giving nursing care to the neonate.

The rate of nosocomial infections in the neonatal nursery ranges from 1.7 to 24 percent. These infections are often transmitted from equipment and nursery personnel. It is the responsibility of each individual involved in the care of the neonate to employ infection control measures in an effort to decrease nosocomial infections and improve the health of the neonate.

HEALTH STANDARDS

Standards may vary among institutions but commonly include current immunizations, rubella titers, and tuberculosis tests on all personnel. Restrictions are placed on individuals with suspected infections such as sore throat, skin rashes, open lesions, sores, diarrhea, flulike symptoms, communicable diseases, and elevated temperatures. Throat cultures are not routine but may be required when there are repeated infections within nursery personnel or clusters of infection.

PERSONNEL PRACTICES

Personnel are required to change into hospital scrub uniforms before entering the maternity department. Shoes worn in the department are not to be worn outside of the hospital. When leaving the department for other areas of the hospital a covergown is worn over the scrub uniform. Scrub uniforms are to be laundered after each use and a clean scrub uniform is put on for the next tour of duty. Covergowns are used for individuals not normally caring for the neonates such as physicians, x-ray personnel, or laboratory personnel. Supplies for each neonate include a covergown that is put on before holding the neonate in order to prevent cross-contamination. Personnel who have been working in medical areas or pediatrics areas may not be assigned to the nursery area for at least eight hours following completion of their medical assignment.

Handwashing

All personnel are required to complete an initial 3-minute scrub at the beginning of each shift. Fingernails are to be kept short and cleansed well while scrubbing. The hands are washed before administering care to any neonate and before touching another. Care is taken not to touch contaminated objects such as the hair or face of the caregiver or equipment used by another neonate. When personnel leave the department for other areas of the hospital and then return to the nursery they must rescrub. Hand lotions are not used in the nursery, as they favor the growth of gram-negative organisms.

EQUIPMENT

Housekeeping policies include a thorough daily cleansing of the nursery and washing of each bassinet and isolette following usage. Equipment that is jointly used, such as scales, stethoscopes, and monitors, should be cleansed after each use. Clean linens are labeled with sterility dates and rotated. Separate areas are designated for storage of clean linen and disposal of dirty linens.

Bassinets are placed at least three to four feet apart, with handwashing facilities available for every six neonates. It is recommended that there be no more than 12 neonates in each cohort area.

All electrical equipment is checked daily for proper functioning and grounding. No equipment may be used in the nursery that has not been properly inspected for safety.

ISOLATION

Isolation procedures are employed when caring for a neonate having or suspected of having an infection or communicable disease. Symptoms that may indicate infection are:

- Conjunctivitis
- Cough
- Diarrhea
- Purulent drainage
- Pustular lesions
- Rash
- Temperature elevation

When an infection is confirmed, the neonate is cared for in a separate area with handwashing and isolation facilities. Mask and gloves are worn according to policy.

Neonates with mothers exhibiting the following disorders or conditions are isolated according to departmental policies.

Aids
Chickenpox (varicella)
Delivery outside of the hospital
Diarrhea
Enterovirus
Foul odor of amniotic fluid
Herpes simplex II
Influenza
Streptococcus (A)
Syphilis

VISITORS

When the neonate is present, visitors are required to scrub (3 minutes) and put on a clean cover gown before holding him.

If a visitor, parent, or employee has an upper respiratory infection they must wear a mask when handling the infant. Masks are changed every 30 minutes and discarded. An area for siblings to view the neonate and visit with the mother is provided.

Safety Provisions for the Neonate

Beyond the control of infections in the nursery, safety is of primary concern when handling the neonate, providing for warmth, and positioning of the infant.

HANDLING

Whenever the neonate is handled by either the nurse or the parents, it is important that he feels secure. The method of handling is not as important as the feeling of security the infant experiences. Support of the head is essential and should be maintained while the infant is held. When lifting the neonate, it is helpful to place one arm behind the head with the hand grasping the far arm of the baby. The other hand is then placed under the buttocks grasping the far leg. In this manner both the head and the buttocks are supported while the individual has a firm grip on the baby (see Fig. 22-33). The "football hold" may also be used to keep the neonate in a secure position. The neonate's back is supported by the arm while his head is supported by the hand (see Fig. 22-34). While using this position, the nurse has one free hand, as the neonate is securely tucked under her arm. Neonates should be transported in their bassinets with the head of the bassinet down.

WARMTH

The nursery must be thermostatically controlled to provide warmth for the neonate. The increased temperature gradient of the neonate allows rapid exchange of body heat from the neonate to the environment, subjecting him to cold stress if chilling occurs. Heat loss from radiation, conduction, evaporation, and convection should be minimized. Bassinets are not placed next to cold walls or windows,

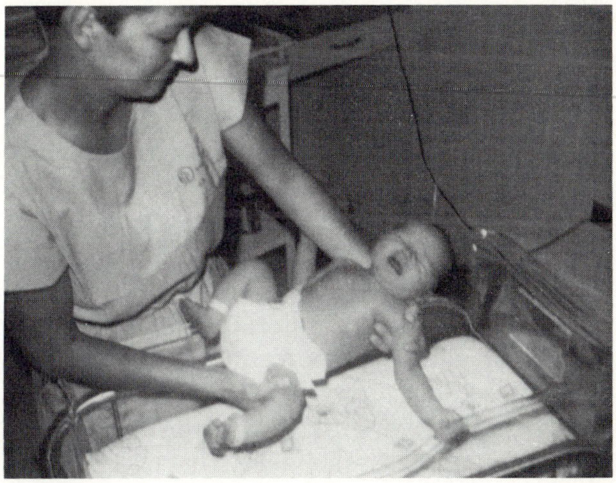

FIGURE 22-33. Method of picking up neonate.

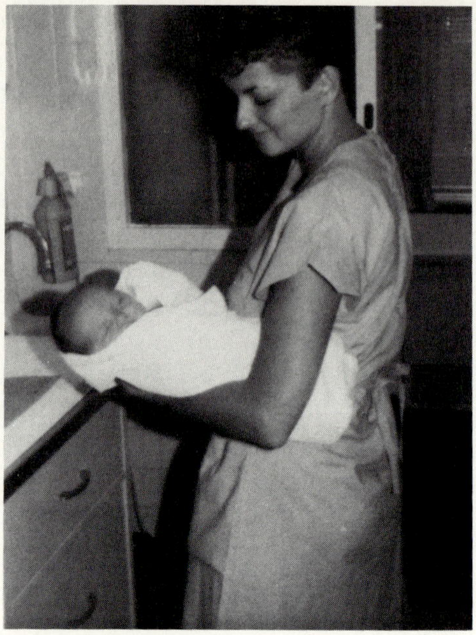

FIGURE 22-34. Football hold.

drafts from open windows are prevented, exposure when bathing or examining is minimized, temperature checks should be frequently performed, and infants are warmed when needed. Normally, wrapping the infant securely in a receiving blanket and one additional blanket is sufficient to maintain warmth and gives the neonate a sense of security. Stocking caps are utilized during the transition phase but are not usually necessary following thermal stability.

POSITIONING

The neonate is placed on his side with a blanket rolled and placed along his back to help maintain a side-lying position. This position will help to facilitate drainage of mucus and assist in preventing choking. Bassinets are not placed with the head down, as was formerly done, as this position places pressure on the head and diaphragm, increasing the risk of intracranial pressure and respiratory difficulties. Following feedings, the neonate is positioned on his side with the head of the bassinet elevated.

Daily Care

Daily care and observation are based on the database obtained during the initial physical assessments and care during the transitional periods. Daily care should never be considered routine, but should reflect the individual needs of the neonate.

ASSESSMENTS

Each neonate receives a head-to-toe assessment daily. This may be done once a day or at the beginning of each shift, noting any changes in general appearance or homeostasis. Vital signs are assessed on each shift and when indicated. Respirations and pulses are counted for a full minute. Weight is measured daily, noting any losses or gains. A loss of 5 to 10 percent of the neonate's weight is normal within the first two days owing to increased metabolic activity and insensible water loss. Table 22-6 provides a list of daily assessments used when caring for the neonate.

Neurological behavior as well as activity and rest states are assessed and noted. (Table 22-7 is a sample nursing care plan for a 24 hour old neonate.)

ELIMINATION

Characteristic changes occur in the stool of the neonate during the first days of life. The first stool passed during the early transition period is meconium, which is formed in the intestines during fetal life. This black, tarry stool will continue to be seen for one or two days. Failure to pass meconium within the first 24 hours is abnormal and may indicate imperforate anus or a *meconium ileus* (a blockage of the intestines caused by very thick meconium). Meconium is very sticky and may be difficult to remove from the buttocks. A small amount of petroleum jelly or a diaper cream may be applied to the buttocks at each diaper change to facilitate removal of meconium. Continued use of diaper lubricants on

TABLE 22-6
DAILY ASSESSMENT OF THE NEONATE

Vital signs	Check and record vital signs every 8 hours Count respirations and pulses for a full minute Auscultate heart and breath sounds every 8 hours Record characteristics and rate of respirations and pulses. Record temperature and method of assessing
Weight	Daily weight observed and recorded at the same time each day
Eyes	Check and record any discharge, inflammation or jaundice
Skin	Note presence of jaundice, rashes, mottling, pallor and assess level of jaundice Assess for signs and symptoms of hypothermia, hypoglycemia, and infection
Feedings	Note: Type of feeding Amount taken Response to feeding Frequence of feedings
Elimination	Record character and frequency of each stool. Record each urination, note unusual characteristics
Cord	Record characteristics of cord (moist-drying-bleeding-odor-inflammation at base), apply alcohol at each diaper change
Circumcision (if present)	Check for bleeding and signs of infection. Apply vaseline dressings until healed if needed
Activity	Note frequency and characteristics of cry and behavioral states (deep or light sleep, drowsy, quiet alert, active alert) Note muscle tone and reflexes
Parent-infant interaction	Note and record any indications of abnormal bonding or rejection of neonate

the buttocks is controversial, with some believing that it increases the possibility of infections.

Generally, the stools following the meconium stools are yellowish-brown or greenish-black transitional stools. These stools are loose, sticky, and messy, and will be present for two to three days.

Stools following transitional stools are characteristic of the feeding substance received by the neonate. Breastfed stools are a yellowish-orange color, partially formed, and with a somewhat sweet-sour odor. The stools of the formula-fed neonate are yellow, pasty, and have a rancid odor.

The characteristics and frequency of stools are noted and recorded following each diaper change. Many neonates become fussy before a stool is passed while others are not bothered

TABLE 22-7
SAMPLE NURSING CARE PLAN: CARE OF THE NEONATE 24 HOURS OLD

Neonate girl V. was born on 5/19 at 6:00 a.m. She is the second child and first girl born to Lisa (age 28) and Jon (age 28) V. Twenty-four hours after birth on 5/20 at 7:00 a.m. the following data base was obtained and utilized to plan continued care for girl V.

Admission Data:
- Maternal prenatal, labor and delivery history normal
- Delivery spontaneous LOA
- Apgar score at 1 minute—8; at five minutes—9
- Birth weight—3856 gm: Length—50.8 cm
- Physical assessment at birth within normal limits
- Voidings normal ×3 and meconium stool on 5/19.
- Feedings—Sterile water taken well @ 9:00 a.m. on 5/19—¼ ounce intake
  - Breast feed @ 1:00 p.m.—no measurable intake
    - 5:00 p.m.—no measurable intake—¼ ounce of 5% glucose water as supplement
    - 9:00 p.m.—no measurable intake—½ ounce of 5% glucose water as supplement.
  - 5/20 @ 1:00 a.m.—no measurable intake—½ ounce of 5% glucose water as supplement.
    - 2:00 a.m.—¼ ounce—nursing well
    - 5:00 a.m.—¼ ounce—nursing well

Assessment Data 5/20 @ 7:00 a.m.:
- Temperature 96.6° F.
- Apical pulse—120
- Respirations—40
- Weight—3799 gm
- Heart sounds—no murmurs; regular rhythm
- Lung sounds—clear
- Cord—moist and no bleeding noted
- Head-to-toe examination within normal limits
- Frequent episodes of gagging and choking with excessive amounts of mucus.

Nursing Diagnosis	Goals	Nursing Intervention	Rationale	Evaluations
Alteration in tissues perfusion related to hypothermia	Neonate will: Maintain temperature in neutral thermal range Demonstrate improved peripheral circulation	Wrap neonate in warm blankets Cover head with cap Assess axillary temperature q 1 hour for 4 hours	Neonate with hypothermia has decreased tissue perfusion, increasing oxygen demands, and subjecting to hypoglycemia Warm blankets and cap will decrease heat loss by conduction and radiation	Axillary temperature: 5/20— 8:00 am 98°F 9:00 am 98°F 10:00 am 98.6°F 11:00 am 98.6°F
Ineffective airway clearance related to inability to remove excessive mucus	Demonstrate effective air exchange Maintain open airway	Position neonate on side	Side-lying position facilitates drainage of mucus	Maintained in side-lying position 5/20

		Closely observe and gently suction oral and nasal passages with bulb syringe when necessary	Close observation necessary to prevent silent aspiration of mucus	Respirations 8:00 am 40 9:00 am 52 10:00 am 48 11:00 am 48 3:00 pm 42
		Observe adequacy of gag and swallowing reflex	Gentle suction to prevent damage to mucosa	
		Assess respirations and breath sounds every hour for 4 hours, then q 4 hours	Inadequate gag or swallowing reflex increases risk of aspiration	Breath Sounds 8:00 am few rales 9:00 am clear 10:00 am clear 11:00 am clear 3:00 pm clear
		Assess skin color for pallor, or cyanosis	Mucus could block air passage creating ineffective air exchange causing pallor or cyanosis	Oral & nasal suctioning 8:15 am large amount of mucus 9:30 am small amount of mucus 10:45 am small amount of mucus 2:45 pm small amount of mucus Color remained pink
		For sustained spells of choking use nasopharyngeal catheter with wall suction for 10 seconds	Catheters more effective when deeper suctioning needed. Periods of suctioning over 10 seconds creates possibility of oxygen deprivation	N/A
		If in respiratory distress: Administer O_2 Resuscitate (CPR) if necessary	 Increase cellular perfusion	
		Offer 5% glucose water between feedings	Liquefy secretions	5% glucose H_2O 11:00 am ¼ oz. 2:00 pm ¼ oz.
Self-care deficit related to immaturity of neonate	Demonstrate and maintain physiologic homeostasis	Assess & maintain Nutrition: plan & assist mother with feedings	Inadequate nutritional intake will alter homeostasis causing hypoglycemia & fluid volume deficit	Breast fed 9:00 am ¼ oz 12:15 pm ½ oz 2:00 pm ½ oz
		Elimination: assess characteristic of stools & voiding	Determine adequacy of digestive & renal functioning	Stools 12:00 pm yellowish brown
		Maintain aseptic technique	Reduces risk of infection allowing physiologic well-being	Urination: 10:00 am 12:00 pm

and will give no indication of discomfort. Three to six stools a day are normal during the first week of life. Loose, watery stools that are greenish in color may indicate an intestinal infection, and the cause should be determined. Occasionally, mucus and a small amount of blood may be seen in the stool during the first few days after birth.

The normal neonate usually voids shortly after birth and may continue to void small amounts (30 to 60 ml per 24 hours) for the first two days. By the time the neonate is four to five days old, urine output has increased to 150 to 250 ml per 24 hours of straw-colored urine with occasional uric acid crystals present. The number of voidings range from 5 to 20 per day. Failure of the neonate to void within the first 24 hours may be an indication of urinary tract abnormalities and should be reported to the physician.

Diapers used in the nursery are sterile disposable or cloth diapers. A supply of diapers is provided for each neonate. The nurse must wash her hands following each diaper change before she touches any other area of the neonate or any other baby.

FEEDINGS

Following the initial sterile water feedings, which establish feeding capabilities, formula or breast feeding is begun. The following recommendations may be used when assessing the nutritional needs of the neonate.

Recommendations for daily (24 hours) caloric intake are:
120 calories per kg of body weight
(55 calories per pound of body weight)

Recommendations for daily (24 hours) fluid intake are:
200 ml per kg of body weight
(3 ounces per pound of body weight)

Rigid schedules for feedings are not adhered to, as each neonate has individual nutritional needs and will develop a feeding pattern suitable to his needs. Self-demand feedings are the most acceptable method of addressing the feeding habits of the neonate. The following characteristics are assessed at each feeding.

Type of feeding (formula or breast)
Time of feeding
Amount taken
Response to feeding

CORD CARE

The cord may serve as a portal of entry for and colonization of bacteria if meticulous care and assessment are not provided. Following birth the cord appears moist, soft, and creamy-white in color. It gradually begins to dry and atrophy, and by the third day it appears as a black, atrophied stump. At this stage it is sufficiently dried to allow removal of the clamp. Observations of the cord include assessments for the presence of a discharge, odor, or an irritation at the base of the cord indicating the possibility of a cord infection. The cord will usually drop off between the seventh and the tenth day of life.

Cord care consists of cleansing the cord with an antiseptic solution each time the diaper is changed and after each bath. Agents that may be used are alcohol, triple dye, or an antimicrobial. Use of triple dye generally consists of painting the cord with the bacteriostatic agent at the time of birth and then utilizing alcohol (70 percent) for routine care. Many institutions prefer to use alcohol for initial and continued care. The nurse's hands are washed and an alcohol swab or wipe is used to cleanse around the base of the cord. This treatment is continued for several days after the cord has dropped off and until the navel is healed.

The undershirt is folded above the umbilicus and the diaper below in order to avoid moisture on the cord from a wet diaper or undershirt. When bathing the infant, care is taken to prevent the cord from becoming wet. Parents are advised to give only sponge baths to the infant until the cord is healed.

SKIN CARE

Daily bathing of the neonate is no longer considered necessary. Many hospitals prefer to bathe the neonate only upon admission to the nursery and at the time of discharge. The use of hexachlorophene preparations to reduce staphylococcal infections is not recommended owing to neurologic toxicity caused by skin absorption of the hexachlorophene. Soaps that have an alkaline base change the pH of the skin, decreasing bacteriostatic skin properties. Warm water bathing of the face and head is usually sufficient for the initial admission bath. Removal of the vernix is not necessary and any large accumulations over the other areas of the body may be gently rubbed off. The genital area and buttocks are also cleansed as necessary when changing the diaper.

Oils, creams, and lotions are not routinely applied, as they increase the risk of infections by encouraging the growth of certain microorganisms. However, areas with cracked or peeling skin may provide a portal of entry for bacteria and an application of a moisturizing cream may be necessary.

CIRCUMCISION CARE

Throughout history circumcision of male infants has been performed for religious and cultural purposes. It has not been until modern times that circumcisions were performed for medical reasons such as phimosis and the prevention of penile carcinoma. The American Academy of Pediatrics Committee on Fetus and Newborns (1975) stated, however, that there are no valid medical reasons for routine circumcisions of neonates. Yet, circumcisions remain a common minor surgical procedure.

Ritualistic circumcision of the Jewish male infant may not be performed until the eighth day of life and is done in a ceremonial manner. A Jewish man called the *Mohel* is trained in the surgical and religious performance of the circumcision. The ceremony is called the *bris* and is usually performed following discharge from the hospital at the home of the infant with family and friends present to witness the fulfillment of the command to Abraham.

Circumcisions performed at home and in the hospital involve the removal of the distal end of the foreskin, resulting in exposure of the glans penis. The procedure is performed under sterile technique using instruments such as the *Plastibell* and *Gomco* clamps. Following the procedure the neonate is observed for signs of bleeding or evidence of urinary retention. Observations of the surgical site are made every 15 minutes for the first hour and every 30 minutes for the next 4 hours. The first voiding following circumcision is recorded. Aseptic technique is an important aspect of postoperative care, as efforts are made to keep the surgical site as clean as possible. A liberal amount of sterile petroleum jelly or an antibiotic ointment such as Neosporin is placed on a sterile gauze square and used to cover the circumcision. The dressing is changed following each diaper change until healing has occurred. Individual supplies for circumcisions are provided for each circumcised neonate and are not shared with other neonates in order to prevent cross-contamination. When a Plastibell is used, ointments or lubricants are not necessary.

Although rare, hemorrhage, infection, and trauma are the most common causes of complications following circumcision. When bleeding is observed, pressure is applied to the site with a sterile gauze. If bleeding does not subside, one to two drops of a 1:1000 Adrenalin solution may be applied to the site. Signs of infection may be indicated by severe inflammation and are treated with antiseptic solutions or antibiotic ointments.

To prevent cold stress, the neonate must be 24 hours old before a circumcision is done. Permission slips validating consent of the parents must be signed before the procedure is performed. The decision for circumcision is the right of the parents and should not be made without a thorough understanding of the current medical opinion regarding circumcisions as well as the procedure involved. A frequent question asked by the parents is "Will the circumcision be felt by the baby and if so, is an anesthetic given?" The common reply has been, "The baby cannot feel anything at this time and there is no real need for an anesthetic." This answer is insufficient, as research has indicated that the neonate does experience stress, as evidenced by increased cortisol levels (Talbert, Kraybill & Potter, 1976). The degree of discomfort or stress has not been determined; but the nurse may explain to the parents that comfort measures are employed during the procedure to relieve the discomfort.

Conditions and abnormalities that prohibit circumcisions include: prematurity, elevated bilirubin (over 13 mg percent), hypospadias, neonatal infections, undetermined sex, blood dyscrarasias and infections (Iffy & Charles, 1984).

PREPARATION FOR DISCHARGE

The normal neonate may be discharged from the hospital when physiologic homeostasis is established, nutritional intake is adequate, neonatal screening has been done, and guidelines for infant care have been discussed with the parents.

Neonatal Screening

The neonate is screened for inborn errors of metabolism before discharge. Many of these disorders are transmitted by heterozygous parents, each being a carrier of an autosomal recessive gene. The neonate is homozygous for the trait and will have characteristic manifestations of the disorder. Most states require screening for two disorders, phenylketonuria (PKU) and galactosemia. Some hospitals will also test for maple syrup urine disease (MSUD) and hypothyroidism.

PHENYLKETONURIA (PKU)

This disorder is characterized by the inability of the neonate to metabolize the essential amino acid phenylalanine to tyrosine, owing to a deficiency of the enzyme phenylalanine hydoxylase. Phenylalanine accumulates in the blood, altering brain development and causing mental retardation. Phenyl acids produced by abnormal metabolism are present in the urine, giving it a slightly stale, musty odor.

The effects of the disorder can be prevented if a diet limiting the amount of phenylalanine is provided for the infant before brain damage has occurred (about three weeks) and until brain growth is completed. Detection of the disorder while the neonate is in the hospital ensures early treatment and greatly reduces the risk of complications. The *Guthrie* blood test, obtained from a heel stick, is used to determine the presence of phenylalanine levels over 4 mg per 100 ml. This test is performed after the neonate has received protein feedings (formula or breast milk) for three to four days.

False negative results may be obtained if the test is performed earlier than 72 hours after birth or when feedings have been delayed or regurgitated. False positive results occur when levels are in a borderline range, especially with the preterm neonate. If the reliability of the first test is questioned, the test is repeated at four weeks of age. When the neonate is discharged before 72 hours following birth, the mother is instructed to have the baby tested at the physician's office or clinic within the first ten days following discharge.

GALACTOSEMIA

When galactosemia is present, the liver enzyme galactose-l-phosphate uridyl transferase is absent, preventing conversion of galactose to glucose, which encourages accumulations of galactose in the blood. Symptoms of vomiting, lethargy, diarrhea, and eventually mental retardation will develop. If discovered and treated within the first few weeks of life, however, the condition may be corrected.

Treatment consists of eliminating milk and milk products from the diet and by giving a galactose-free formula such as a soybean or meat-based formula.

Diagnostic testing consists of a blood test to detect elevated levels of galactose in the blood or levels of galactose-1-phosphate uridyl transferase reduced below 18.5 μ per g hemoglobin.

MAPLE SYRUP URINE DISEASE (MSUD)

This genetic disorder involves the accumulation of the amino acids leucine, isoleucine, and valine in the blood and urine. Failure to metabolize these amino acids produces a maple syrup odor to the urine, hypoglycemia, feeding problems, seizures, and, if untreated, death. Special formulas may be given that contain limited amounts of these amino acids. A diagnostic blood test is used to determine the disorder.

HYPOTHYROIDISM

Congenital hypothyroidism may be detected in neonates who have been deprived of maternal iodine. At birth noticeable symptoms such as hypotonia, large fontanels, large tongue, low hair line, weak cry, and jaundice may be present. The NeoT_4 test may be used to screen all infants with or without symptoms. A drop of blood obtained from a heel stick is needed to perform the test. This condition may be reversible if prompt treatment with thyroid medication is instituted.

Parent Instruction

Aspects of infant care are discussed with parents before discharge, either in individual teaching sessions or in group sessions. These sessions may be offered at different times throughout the patient's hospitalization, but they are always individualized to meet parental learning needs. Ideally, sessions are planned when the parents are receptive, relaxed, and interested. Explaining cord care to the mother on the first day following delivery may evince little interest; however, the day before she is discharged she may be very receptive to any information concerning the care of her infant. Likewise, presenting all the information in one long session before she goes home may be overwhelming and does not offer her the opportunity to assimilate the information and formulate questions.

INFANT BATHING

Newborn infants do not need to be bathed daily, however parents may find the bath a pleasant time for both the baby and themselves as they are becoming acquainted. All babies cry when they are given their first baths, but the cries soon turn to laughs and coos as the baby begins to enjoy the bath.

Sponge baths are recommended until the cord and circumcision are healed, usually within eight to ten days after discharge from the hospital. Tub baths may then be instituted, using a large basin, baby bath tub, or even the sink. Safety is of prime importance, requiring the bathing surface to be firm and secure. Drafts and unnecessary exposure of the infant should be eliminated. All equipment is assembled before the bath is begun. The infant is never left unattended while on a surface such as a table or counter top.

Suggested equipment used for the bath includes:

- Cotton balls
- Mild soap
- Shampoo
- Clean washcloth and towel
- 70% alcohol for cord care and swab
- Ointment or vaseline for diaper area
- Infant clothing: diaper, undershirt, sleeper
- Clean receiving blanket

Once the equipment has been assembled, the bath is begun by cleansing the eyes. A clean cotton ball is dampened and the eye is cleansed with clear water using one stroke from the inner corner of the eye outward, never wiping back and forth across the eye. If any discharge or matter remains in the eye, another clean cotton ball is used and the procedure repeated. A clean cotton ball is used for each eye. The face may then be wiped with warm water using a cloth or cotton ball. The ears are cleaned externally but nothing is introduced into the ear canal. If the parent feels it is necessary to clean inside the ears, he or she is told to consult a physician or nurse.

The head is shampooed using a mild baby shampoo or plain soap. Parents are told about the soft spots (fontanels) and assured that gently washing over them will cause no harm. They may be shown the football grip as a method of securely holding the baby. Following the shampoo, the hair is gently dried with a clean towel.

The infant's clothing is removed and a mild soap is used for lathering, starting with the neck and working downward to the genital area. It is important to remind parents to wash thoroughly all the skin folds, such as the creases of the neck, arms, and legs. The female genital area is washed from the front to the back, avoiding rectal contamination of the urethra. The infant may be rolled to the side to lather the back and buttocks. He is then securely and gently picked up and placed in the infant tub, which is half filled with warm (98° to 100°F) water. He may be held in the manner shown in Figure 22–33, with his head supported and a firm grasp on his arm.

Quite often the baby objects and cries vigorously as he is first placed in the water; however, as he adjusts to the water the crying stops and the baby appears to be more comfortable. Parents are told that crying is normal and not an indication of discomfort or wrong technique. They are encouraged to allow the baby a few minutes to enjoy the water, but to avoid chilling the baby. Following removal from the tub, the baby is thoroughly dried, clothed, and wrapped in the receiving blanket.

If the cord is not healed and a sponge bath is given, only the undershirt is removed while the chest, back, and upper extremities are washed and dried. This area is then covered with a light blanket while the diaper is removed and the lower portion of the body is washed.

Cord care is provided until the stump has dropped off. An alcohol wipe or a cotton ball saturated with 70 percent alcohol is used to cleanse around the base of the cord. The mother is assured that the procedure will not sting the baby because there are no nerve endings in the cord stump. She is told to observe the cord for a yellowish or green discharge, redness surrounding the base of the cord, or a distinct odor. If any of these symptoms are noted, they are reported to the physician. The diaper is positioned below the cord stump and the undershirt above it. Cord care is given after each bath and diaper change.

Lotions and powders are not recommended unless specified for cracked and peeling skin. If powders are used, they are kept out of reach of the baby. A small amount of powder is placed in the parent's hand and then applied to the baby. Sprinkling the baby with powder may allow him to inhale it, creating respiratory problems. Infants have been known to grasp an open powder can and spill it on their faces, resulting in suffocation.

A small amount of vaseline or ointment may be applied to the genital area and buttocks before diapering. The lubricant is applied from front to back, proceeding from the genitals to the rectum. If the circumcision has not completely healed, parents are told to place a liberal amount of sterile vaseline on a gauze square and place it over the head of the penis. It should not be taped or pinned but just laid over the head of the penis and the diaper then placed over it. Parents are reminded to report to the physician if there are any signs of infections such as inflammation, swelling, or discharge. The dressing is changed following each bath and diaper change.

After the infant is dressed, he is swaddled in a warm blanket and held securely. Often the mother will find feeding the infant is appropriate at this time as he is hungry following the stimulation and activity of the bath. A quiet nap is generally in order for the infant after he is fed.

DEVELOPMENT

Parents are made aware of the initial 5 to 10 percent weight loss following birth. Daily weights are not necessary but, for the most part, infants can be expected to double their birth weight by six months of age. The average weight gain is 4 to 6 ounces per week for about the first five months, with a slight reduction to 1 to 2 ounces per week in the following months. At one year of age the infant will have tripled his birth weight.

Developmental patterns are individualized, with emphasis on the sequence rather than the age of or time of occurrences. Developmental milestones may be used by the parents as guidelines, but the rate of development may fluctuate. Parents are made aware that each infant develops in a unique pattern and that to compare one infant with another is not advisable unless there are obvious deviations from the normal patterns.

ACTIVITY

Parents are encouraged to view the infant as a social being having needs for communication and interaction with others. Discussion of the results of the Brazelton Behavioral Assessment enables parents to plan and coordinate activities specific to their infant's needs.

Sleep is an important part of the infant's life. Yet, his days are not completely devoted to sleep. The average infant may be expected to sleep nearly 16 hours a day during the first two weeks, distributed in short naps at varying intervals. Some infants will sleep 16 hours during a 24-hour period one day and only 12 hours the next day. Other infants will appear to be more placid and sleep most of the day, waking only for feedings. By the time he is three months old, the infant will be sleeping for longer intervals and perhaps through the night. Allowing the infant to develop his own sleeping patterns is the most satisfactory policy.

Crying is an activity the infant engages in frequently. He may cry when he is uncomfortable, hungry, or ill, or for myriad other reasons. Crying is one of the most effective means of communication and parents will soon learn to recognize some of the baby's needs by his cry. Cries should not be ignored for fear of spoiling the baby. When the baby cries he is expressing a need, and when that need is met he develops trust in those he depends on.

Stimulating activities are just as important to the infant as are sleeping and eating. Since newborns are capable of focusing their eyes at a distance of eight inches, brightly colored mobile or crib toys attached to or near the crib within this distance may provide visual activity. Talking and smiling at the baby stimulates his interaction with others, and it will not be long before he will try to imitate his mother's speaking gestures by cooing and opening and closing his mouth as she speaks. Tactile stimulation is experienced by the infant as he is bathed, fed, and held. Holding the infant securely and closely imparts to him a feeling of trust and security.

SAFETY

The environment of the infant should be made as safe as possible. Safety in the home includes consideration of potential hazards that may be avoided or eliminated. Furniture used for the infant should be well made, serviceable, and safe. Cribs should be sturdy with bars spaced no more than 2 3/8 inches apart to eliminate the possibility of the baby's head being caught between the rails. Mattresses and crib guards should be abuted directly against the sides of the crib with no opening between the mattress and the crib borders. Railings are at least 26 inches above the level of the mattress to prevent the infant from falling over the side of the crib as he learns to stand. Pillows are not used in the crib.

Blankets are lightly laid over the baby but are not pinned or tied down.

All painted surfaces with which the infant will come in contact are painted with child-approved paints. Lead-based paints are not used and may be particularly dangerous when the infant begins to chew on surfaces or objects.

Poisonous substances, medicines, and household cleaning material may be dangerous and are kept locked and inaccessible to the infant as he learns to crawl and walk. Consideration is also given to plants or foilage in the home that may be poisonous.

Car safety begins the moment the neonate is placed in the car for his ride home from the hospital. At this time the infant is placed in a car seat that meets federal vehicle safety standards. Holding babies or infants on the lap is dangerous and has resulted in serious injury and death. All 50 states in the U.S. require car seats for infants. Parents are made aware that all children under the age of five or less than 40 pounds must be in a car seat when riding in an automobile. Many hospitals provide a car seat program that offers parents the opportunity to buy or rent a car seat at a minimal price.

ILLNESS

No matter how conscientious or devoted the parents may be to the care of the infant, all babies will experience some illness. When parents are informed of the signs and symptoms indicating illness they become more secure in their ability to handle the situation. Signs and symptoms that parents should be aware of are:

- Poor feeding or refusal of nourishment
- Fussiness
- Diarrhea
- Coughing and sneezing
- Rash
- Elevated temperature
- Lethargy
- Vomiting

As parents become accustomed to their infant's behavior, they may be able to detect subtle changes indicating illness. All of the previously mentioned symptoms may or may not be present; however, when observed they should be reported to the physician.

Assessment of the infant's temperature is an important diagnostic aid when illness is suspected. The proper method of assessment of axillary or rectal temperatures should be demonstrated by the nurse. Parents are reminded to always shake the thermometer down before each use and to lubricate the tip of the rectal thermometer with vaseline before inserting it. The rectal thermometer is placed about 0.5 inch into the rectum for 5 minutes. The infant's feet and the thermometer are securely held while the thermometer is in place. The normal rectal temperature is 36.4° to 37.5°C (97.5° to 99.5°F).

Axillary temperatures are taken for 5 minutes with the thermometer placed in the armpit. The normal axillary temperature will range from 36.5° to 37°C (97.7° to 98.6°F). Axillary temperatures may be assessed, but rectal temperatures will provide the most accurate assessment of temperature elevations at the onset of illness.

If the temperature is elevated, the reading is communicated to the physician along with the method used. Parents should not begin treatment for fever without consulting the physician. The indiscriminate use of medications such as aspirin to treat temperature is not recommended.

IMMUNIZATIONS

Immunization of infants has eliminated many of the infectious diseases that plagued and threatened the lives of babies and small children in past years. Protection from these diseases has resulted in increased health of children in all age groups. The benefits derived from immunizations should be stressed to the parents before the neonate is discharged. At that time a review of the recommended

TABLE 22-8
IMMUNIZATION SCHEDULE FOR NORMAL INFANTS

Age	Immunization
Two months	TOPV (Trivalent Oral Polio Vaccine)
	DTP (Diphtheria-Tetanus-Pertussis)
Four months	TOPV
	DTP
Six months	DTP
Fifteen months	Measles
	Mumps
	Rubella
Eighteen months	TOPV
	DTP
Four to six years	TOPV
	DTP
Fourteen to sixteen years	Td (Adult type Tetanus & Diphtheria)
Every ten years	Td

schedule for immunizations may be described (Table 22-8).

HEALTH MANAGEMENT

Instructions for continued health care of the neonate are given before discharge. These instructions include the arrangements for medical supervision of the infant and the scheduling of the first well-baby checkup with the physician or at the clinic. Information concerning resources to use if problems or questions arise is provided.

Followup care by the nurse often includes a telephone call to inquire about the health of the baby and to offer suggestions or answers to concerns or questions. It is important for parents to know that the nurse offers her help and guidance not only within the hospital setting but as a member of the health team in the community.

BIBLIOGRAPHY

Bernard K., Blackburn, S., Kang, R. & Spietz, A. Early parent infant relationships. In *Series I, The first six hours of life, module 3.* White Plains, N.Y.: The National Foundation March of Dimes, 1978.

Brodish, M. Perinatal assessment. *Journal of Obstetric, Gynecological & Neonatal Nursing,* 1981, **10,** 42.

Brazelton, T.: The neonatal behavioral assessment scale. Philadelphia, J.B. Lippincott, 1973.

Buckner, E. Use of Brazelton neonatal behavioral assessment in planning care for parents and newborn. *Journal of Obstetric, Gynecological & Neonatal Nursing, 1983,* **12,** 26–30.

Copobianco, J. Keeping the newborn warm: How to safeguard the infant against life-threatening heat loss. *Nursing 80,* 1980, **10,** 64–67.

Center for Disease Control. *Guidelines for isolation precautions* (4th ed.). Washington D.C.: U.S. Government Printing Office, 1983.

Center for Disease Control. *Guidelines for the prevention and control of nosocomial infections.* Washington, D.C.: U.S. Government Printing Office, 1981.

Committee on Environmental Hazards. Infant radiant warmers. *Pediatrics,* 1978, **61,** 113.

Committee on Fetus and Newborn. Report of the ad hoc task force on circumcisions. *Pediatrics,* 1975, **56,** 610.

Committee on Fetus and Newborn. *Standards and recommendations for hospital care of newborn infants* (6th ed). Evanston, Ill.: American Academy of Pediatrics, 1977.

Dahl, N. & Frazier, S. Neonatal thermoregulation. In *Series I, The first six hours of life, module 1.* White Plains, N.Y.: The National Foundation/March of Dimes, 1976.

Doyle, N. & Sinclair, J.C. Insensible water loss in newborn infants. *Clinics in Perinatology,* 1982, **9,** 453.

Funke, J. & Irby, M. An instrument to assess the quality of maternal behavior. *Journal of Obstetric, Gynecological & Neonatal Nursing,* 1978, **7,** 19–22.

Grimes, D.A. Routine circumcision of the newborn: A reappraisal. *American Journal of Obstetrics & Gynecology,* 1978, **130,** 125–129.

Harpin, V. & Rutter, N. Barrier properties of the newborn infant's skin. *Journal of Pediatrics,* 1983, **102,** 419–425.

Hazuka, B. Prevention of infection in the nursery. *Nursing Clinics of North America, 1980,* **15,** 825.

Iffy, L. & Charles, D. *Operative perinatology.* New York: Macmillan, 1984.

Joint Position Statement on the Development of Family Centered Maternity/Newborn Care in Hospitals, Interprofessional Task Force on Health Care on Women and Children, June, 1978.

Krozy, R. & McColgan, J. Auto safety and the newborn. *Journal of Obstetric, Gynecological & Neonatal Nursing,* 1985, **14,** 11.

Labson, L.H. Newborn exam: Evaluation in the nursery. *Patient Care,* 1983, **17,** 95–98, 100, 102.

Larrow, L. & Noe, J. Port wine stain hemangiomas. *American Journal of Nursing,* 1982, **82,** 786–790.

Lepley, C. Assessment of risk in the newborn: Evaluation during the transitional period. White Plains, N.Y.: March of Dimes Birth Defects Foundation, 1978.

McBride, A.B. *Growth and development of mothers.* New York: Noble Books, 1974.

McCabe, E. Principles of newborn screening for metabolic disorders. *Perinatology/Neonatology, 1982,* **6,** 63.

NAACOG. *Infection control for the obstetric patient and the newborn infant.* Technical Bulletin No. 9, 1981.

NAACOG, *Standards for obstetric, gynecologic and neonatal nursing* (3rd ed.) Washington, D.C., 1986.

Reid, T. Newborn cyanosis. *American Journal of Nursing,* 1982, **82,** 1230–1234.

Scharping, E.M. Physiological measurements of the neonate: Methods of accurately measuring vital signs are constantly being refined. *MCN,* 1983, **8,** 70–73.

Sholder, D. Portrait of a newborn. *Journal of Obstetric, Gynecological & Neonatal Nursing,* 1981, **10,** 98–101.

Stranik, M.K. & Hogberg, B. Transition into parenthood. *American Journal of Nursing,* 1979, **79,** 90–93.

Talbert, L.M., Kraybill, E.N. & Potter, H.D. Adrenal cortical response to circumcision in the neonate. *American Journal of Obstetrics & Gynecology,* 1976, **48,** 208.

chapter 23

INFANT NUTRITION

OBJECTIVES

Upon completion of this chapter, the reader will be able to:

1. Discuss growth and development needs of infants during the first year of life.
2. List caloric requirements needed for an infant to achieve ideal weight gain.
3. Identify nutritional requirements for the normal infant for the following: calories, protein, fat, carbohydrates, water, vitamins, and minerals.
4. Discuss the first feeding after birth.
5. State advantages of breastfeeding.
6. Describe the process of lactation.
7. Discuss nursing interventions for the breastfeeding mother.
8. Identify learning needs of the breastfeeding mother.
9. Identify common problems with breastfeeding and possible solutions.
10. Describe sources and effects of contaminants in breast milk.
11. Discuss drug excretion in breast milk.
12. State advantages of bottlefeeding.
13. Describe correct bottlefeeding techniques.
14. Compare the protein, fat, and carbohydrate contents of the major types of standard commercial infant formulas.
15. Differentiate nutritional components of special formulas and human milk for the full-term infant.
16. Explain methods of formula preparation.

KEY TERMS

Acini cells
Breast milk jaundice
Colostrum
Demand feeding
Engorgement
Lactation
Lactiferous duct
Lactiferous sinus
Lactoferrin
Let down reflex
Lobule
Nutrient requirements
Prolactin
RDA
Test feeding

Good nutrition is necessary throughout life for maintenance of health and prevention of disease. The period of rapid growth in infancy requires careful nutritional support to continue the growth and development that began at conception. The key to good nutrition is effective balance of the right nutrients.

The normal full-term infant may be either breast- or bottle-fed. The method chosen is based on psychological, sociological, and physical factors. Approximately 70 percent of mothers choose a feeding method before pregnancy (Mackey & Fried, 1981) and more than 80 percent have selected a method by the end of the second trimester (Beske & Garvis, 1982).

Some mothers are very eager to breastfeed their infants; others find breastfeeding undesirable. Books and pamphlets influence feeding decisions. Additional influences include opinions of their own mothers and friends, as well as the attitude of the father of the baby toward breastfeeding.

GROWTH AND DEVELOPMENT NEEDS

Growth and development in the human organism is a specific, highly individualized process. There are wide variations in requirements for normal healthy infants.

Physical Growth

The first year of life is one of the most intense periods of rapid growth. During this year many changes in form and function take place. By six months of age, the infant will have doubled his birth weight. Full-term infants have the ability to digest and absorb proteins, moderate amounts of fats, and simple carbohydrates. They are unable to digest starches because amylase is not yet produced. The renal system functions adequately, but infants need more water in relation to their size than adults. During this period of life, measurements of physical growth as well as assessments of nutritional status (see Table 23–1), laboratory data, and dietary analysis provide evidence of adequate physical growth.

Psychosocial Growth

Parameters of psychosocial growth include the ability of the infant to respond to care. Emotional growth is measured in the increased capacity for love and affection shown to parents and in the ability to deal with frustration and anxiety. For psychosocial growth to take place, physical needs must be met and satisfied in a supportive environment. Food and the process of eating meet not only essential requirements for physical growth but also serve to foster psychological growth.

NUTRITIONAL REQUIREMENTS

The infant diet should provide adequate amounts of calories, protein, fluid, vitamins, and minerals for health and normal growth. These nutrients should be easily digestible. The composition of breast milk is usually used as the standard for preparation of infant formulas that meet nutritional requirements.

Nutrient requirements are the least amount of a particular nutrient that will maintain ideal nutritional health. Advisable intake of particular nutrients are usually set at levels higher than the nutrient requirements to allow for individual variations in infants. *Recommended dietary allowances* (RDA) set by the Food and Nutrition Board, National Academy of Science, and National Research Council are usually higher than actual nutrient requirements and advisable intakes, and are intended to serve

TABLE 23-1
ASSESSMENT OF NUTRITIONAL STATUS

Assessment Parameter	Expected Data
Appearance	Alert and responsive
Hair	Lustrous, shiny
Skin	Smooth, good color, mucus membranes pink and moist
Eyes	Clear, bright
Lips	Good color
Tongue	No lesions present, good color
Teeth (if present)	Straight, no discoloration
Skin	Smooth, good color
Abdomen	Flat
Extremities	No weakness or swelling
Weight	Within normal range for height, age
Posture	Erect
Muscles	Firm, well developed
Nervous system	Attention span normal for age No irritability
GI function	Appetite good, regular elimination

as guides to adequate nutritional intake for healthy individuals.

Calorie Requirements

Energy needs are high in relation to body size during the first year of life. Calories are required to cover basal metabolic needs and provide growth and development. The normal full-term neonate needs 110 to 120 kilocalories per kilogram of body weight or 50 to 55 calories per pound per day. Calorie requirements will vary for different infants of the same size and age. The infant who is active or who cries a lot requires more energy than the quiet infant. The needs of a particular infant are based on normal weight gain, satiety, and general well-being.

A rule of thumb used for sufficient growth of the normal infant is 120 kcal per kg per 24 hours. Weight gain of 15 to 30 grams per day (0.5 to 1 oz) is considered satisfactory.

Of the total calorie requirement, 7 to 16 percent should be from protein, 30 to 55 percent from fat, with the remainder from carbohydrates. A minimum of 1 percent of calories should be supplied by linoleic acid (an essential fatty acid). Human milk provides approximately 7 percent calories as protein, 55 percent as fat, and 38 percent as carbohydrates. Most commercially prepared formulas supply 9 to 15 percent of calories as protein, 45 to 50 percent as fat, and the rest as carbohydrate. For good infant nutrition, protein intake must be more than 6 percent to prevent deficiency, and fat content should not be excessive to prevent ketosis.

Protein Requirement

Protein supplies the growth element for the body. Essential amino acids needed for body tissue synthesis and tissue maintenance should come from high biologic value protein sources. Proteins also supply needed amino acid elements for enzyme, hormone, lymph, and plasma.

Actual protein requirements are determined by overall growth. During the first six months of life, the average infant requires 2.2 gm per kg per 24 hours. The necessary amount of protein is provided in human milk and in commercial formulas.

Fluid Requirements

Fluid requirements are greater in the full-term infant per kilogram of body weight than in the adult. The infant has increased muscular activity, increased calorie intake, and a higher basal metabolic rate, which accounts for the increase in requirements. Even though the normal full-term infant has a greater percentage of body water than the adult, infants cannot concentrate urine to decrease fluid loss, nor can they withstand inadequate fluid intake.

The normal newborn requires 150 to 200 ml per kg per day (2.5 to 3 oz per lb). When expressed in relation to calorie intake, fluid intake is 1.5 ml per kcal according to the RDA. The minimal water requirement for the normal full-term infant is 70 to 90 ml per kg per day (1.2 to 1.2 oz per lb) to guard against dehydration.

Mineral Requirements

All major minerals are essential for metabolism. For the normal full-term infant, two basic minerals are of particular importance in maintaining adequate nutrition.

CALCIUM

Calcium is essential for the rapid bone mineralization that takes place during the first year of life. In the newborn, mineralization has taken place only in the center sections of the large bones. Calcium is also needed for muscle contraction, blood coagulation, nerve irritability, tooth development, and heart muscle action. Milk satisfies the need for calcium in the newborn during the first six months of life.

IRON

Iron is an essential element needed for synthesis of hemoglobin and cell metabolism. Normally, a six-month supply of iron is stored in the fetal liver before birth. Human milk and commercial formulas are low in iron but have high bioavailability. When an infant is breastfed, about 50 percent of available iron is absorbed, while in commercial formulas only about 10 percent is absorbed.

Vitamin Requirements

When the mother is well nourished throughout pregnancy, the full-term neonate can be expected to have adequate vitamin stores at birth. Infant vitamin requirements are high owing to rapid growth; therefore, vitamins are required for development of growing tissues and bones during infancy. Table 23–2 lists some of the RDA for vitamins during the first six months of life.

VITAMIN A (RETINOL)

Vitamin A is needed for visual purple of the retina to adapt to light and dark, as visual adaptation progresses throughout infancy. It is also needed for bone mineralization and development of teeth, as well as formation and maintenance of epithelial tissues.

VITAMIN B COMPLEX

The vitamins of the B complex are important coenzyme factors in energy and protein me-

TABLE 23–2
RDA OF SELECTED NUTRIENTS

Nutrient	Advisable Intake	RDA
Calories	110–120/kg	115/kg
Water	150–200 ml/kg	1.5 ml/kcal
Protein	1.9 g/ml00 kcal	2.2 gm/100 kcal
Minerals		
Calcium	360 mg	360 mg
Iron	7 mg'	10 mg
Vitamins		
A	500 IU	1400 IU
Thiamine	0.2 mg	0.3 mg
Niacin	5 mg	6 mg
C	20 mg	35 mg
D	400 IU	400 IU

tabolism, especially thiamine, niacin, and riboflavin.

Thiamine is used in carbohydrate metabolism. The need for thiamine increases as the calorie need increases. During the rapid growth that occurs in infancy, thiamine is required for anabolic activity increases and to meet increased energy demands.

Niacin is an important part of protein and energy metabolism, and is required for cellular oxidation of tissue growth materials.

Riboflavin is a coenzyme factor in metabolism, especially reactions that involve amino acids and fatty acids.

VITAMIN C (ASCORBIC ACID)

During the growth spurt that occurs during infancy, vitamin C plays several important roles. It provides an essential material for the formation of cement substance in all tissues. It aids in the absorption of essential iron by helping to change the ferric iron found in foods to ferrous iron for absorption. Vitamin C is an active participant in bone mineralization and enzyme systems needed for growth.

VITAMIN D

Vitamin D prevents rickets. It is present in only small amounts in breast milk and unfortified cow's milk. Supplements are often given when the infant is breastfed.

VITAMIN E

Vitamin E is used as an antioxidant to protect polyunsaturated fatty acids from oxidative degeneration. This is particularly important when special formulas are prescribed for infants.

THE FIRST FEEDING

The normal healthy neonate with good Apgar scores who appears hungry is often ready for the first feeding shortly after birth. Newborns should be fed according to individual needs rather than according to an established routine. Some neonates are ready to eat shortly after birth, while others are not ready for several hours.

To determine the time of the first feeding, several factors must be considered. The neonate must be healthy and in good condition. Vital signs should be within normal limits. Signs of hunger are demonstrated by a search for food, sucking motions, and crying.

If the mother plans to breastfeed, her condition is stable, and she desires to feed the neonate, breastfeeding may begin. In many neonates, the sucking reflex is at its height for 20 to 30 minutes after birth. Initiation of early breastfeeding soon after delivery aids in placental expulsion, helps to control excessive maternal blood loss, decreases the amount of mucus in the neonate, has a laxative effect on the meconium, and helps to establish early bonding.

Colostrum has many benefits for the neonate. It is rich in vitamins A and E, high in protein, and contains immune factors. The antibody content of colostrum is at its maximum during the first 12 hours postpartum. Its laxative effect on the neonate encourages early evacuation of meconium, making the baby hungry. The hungry baby will nurse more vigorously and stimulate the onset of lactation. In addition, early evacuation of meconium will decrease resorption of bilirubin from castoff red cells present in the meconium, and decrease the incidence of physiologic jaundice.

If the neonate is to be bottle fed, the first feeding is usually postponed until the second period of reactivity, unless signs of hypoglycemia are present or the neonate appears hungry. The first feeding is often called a test feeding and is used to assess neonatal ability to swallow fluid. It consists of sterile water, followed by a glucose solution if the water is tolerated without distress. When the water feeding is regurgitated, or if the neonate cannot swallow the feeding, there is less irritation to the respiratory tract. When it has been determined that the neonate can successfully tolerate water and glucose feedings, formula feedings are started.

FREQUENCY OF FEEDINGS

For the normal full-term neonate, rigid feeding schedules are unsatisfactory. The neonate wants to be fed when hungry, not when a schedule dictates that feeding should take place. Some neonates need to be fed every 2 hours, while others are satisfied for 5 or 6 hours between feedings.

Demand Feedings

A *demand feeding schedule* allows the neonate to eat when he is alert and hungry. It also allows the neonate to take the amount of food needed. Intervals between feedings may be from 2 to 6 hours, according to individual needs.

The normal neonate is the best judge of his need for food. When hungry, he will wake and begin crying. Feeding becomes a pleasureable experience, because when he is hungry, needs are met. When scheduled feedings are given regardless of the neonate's state of alertness and hunger, feedings have an unpleasant connotation.

Self-demand schedules are especially important for the breastfed baby. If the baby is not hungry, there is no desire to grasp the nipple and attempt to suck. This apparent lack of interest in feeding is not only unpleasant for the neonate, but will cause undue concern for the mother about her ability to successfully breastfeed.

The normal newborn will eat about 6 to 8 times in a 24-hour period during the first several weeks of life. Occasionally there may be a day when more frequent feedings are desired and needed. After 3 or 4 days of age, the normal newborn will usually have several days in succession where he wishes to eat more frequently, sometimes as frequently as every 2 hours. This frequency will not continue, and a fairly regular schedule will usually be established by the neonate within a week or two, with feedings usually desired every 3 to 4 hours of about 3 to 4 ounces of milk.

BREASTFEEDING

Breast milk is the ideal food for the neonate and infant. Each species has formulated within itself the substance called milk which satisfies the nutritional requirements of that species until babies triple their weight. Human milk is ideally suited for the adaptation of the human during early life.

Advantages of Breastfeeding

During the first 2 or 3 days of life, the breasts produce colostrum, a premilk that has increased antibody content. Colostrum is sterile as it leaves the breast, and breastfeeding decreases the likelihood of the neonate contracting a bacterial infection. Colostrum and breast milk contain active white blood cells to defend against bacteria and viruses.

Breast milk meets the nutritional needs of the neonate. Its protein is more digestible than is cow's milk. Enzymes that aid in digestion of fats are present in breast milk. The fat present in human milk is almost completely digested and absorbed by the neonate; it is rich in essential fatty acids needed for brain growth. The predominant sugar in human milk is lactose, which is efficiently absorbed and used by the infant. Lactose favors the development of bacteria in the intestines that serve a protective function during infancy. The lower calcium-to-phosphorus ratio of breast milk is ideal for the absorption of calcium needed for bone growth. There is also a lower amount of salt in breast milk, which also contains factors that favor absorption of iron.

Powerful agents to fight bacterial infection are present in breast milk. Among these is lactoferrin, which prevents bacteria from getting the iron they need to grow, helps absorb iron into the bloodstream, and works directly to kill some bacteria.

Breastfeeding provides immunity for the newborn by the presence of antibodies that specifically protect against certain diseases. These antibodies inactivate bacteria within the digestive tract to prevent harm, and they appear in the bloodstream to protect against certain diseases.

Other factors present in breast milk include certain enzymes, such as RNAase, lipoprotein lipase, and lysozyme. A factor that enhances absorption of folacin is also present, as are several hormones (thyroid hormone, prostaglandins) and lipids. Breastfeeding appears less likely to produce an obese child, promotes better tooth and jaw alignment, and protects against allergy development during infancy.

Breastfeeding allows easier bonding between mother and newborn. The oxytocin produced by breastfeeding helps increase maternal uterine involution following delivery and decreases the incidence of postpartum bleeding. The hormone prolactin, produced by continued breastfeeding has been associated with an increase in mothering abilities, and is thought to be a part of the "radiance" described in breastfeeding mothers. It also decreases the incidence of postpartum depression.

Breastfeeding is convenient and eliminates formula preparation. The breastfed baby is usually healthy, so an incidental advantage is fewer medical bills. Breastfeeding is more economical, there is no need to purchase formula and related equipment. There is also a decreased incidence of breast cancer in women who have breastfed their infants.

Anatomy and Physiology of Lactation

The body of each breast is contained within the layers of the superficial fascia of the anterior chest wall, and is composed of the glandular tissues of the breast and the fibrous tissue and fat which supports it.

Each breast is composed of 15 to 20 separate branching ducts (see Fig. 23–1). Each of these forms a separate lobe and branches to form *lobules* from clusters of alveoli. These alveoli are lined with a single layer of cells, called *acini cells*. These acini cells are the milk-secreting cells.

Each lobule is drained by a duct connected to the ducts of the other lobules. The main ducts are called the *lactiferous ducts* and converge toward the areola of the breast. Just prior to opening in the nipples, there is a dilated portion to the duct called the *lactiferous sinus* that serves as a reservoir for milk.

Throughout pregnancy, large amounts of estrogen secreted by the placenta cause the ductile system of the breasts to grow. The connective tissue increases in quantity and fat deposits are established. Progesterone causes additional growth of the lobules, budding of the alveoli, and development of secretory characteristics in the alveolar cells.

SECRETION OF COLOSTRUM

During the first several days after birth, the breasts secrete a thin yellowish fluid called colostrum. This fluid contains less fat and

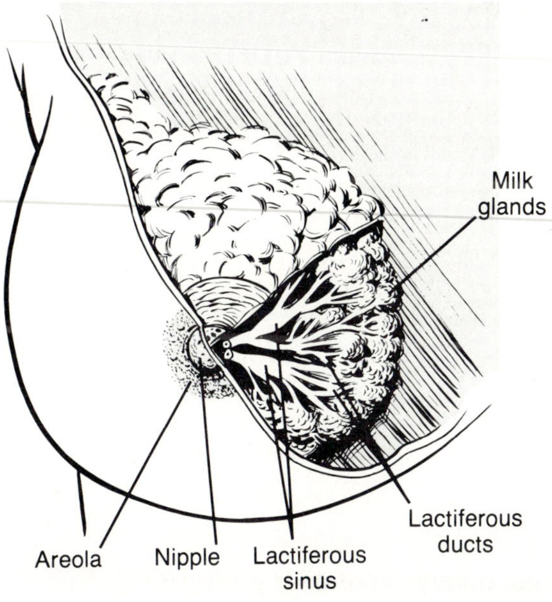

FIGURE 23–1. Schematic drawing of the female breast.

sugar and more protein and salts than breast milk, as well as large amounts of antibodies and vitamin and fat cells.

The neonate receives colostrum from the breasts at the first few feedings following delivery in amounts varying from several milliliters to 0.5 ounces.

INITIATION OF LACTATION

Breast milk begins to replace colostrum on about the third day after delivery. At this time, the breasts secrete large amounts of fluid that change the composition of colostrum to that of breast milk. This change is caused by hormones, biochemical changes in the alveolar cells, and circulatory changes in the breasts.

When the placenta is delivered at the end of the third stage of labor, the influence of hormones produced by the placenta ceases. Estrogen and progesterone levels fall, causing an accompanying secretion of anterior pituitary hormones. The blood flow to the breasts increases and brings more hormones and milk precursors to the breasts. A complex of hormones that includes prolactin, somatotropin, ACTH, and TSH causes the beginning of milk secretion.

Further milk production is caused by the sucking of the infant, which empties the breasts. As the alveoli are emptied, they secrete more milk. When the breast milk comes in, the breast become heavy, full, and firm. This filling of the breasts may be accompanied by engorgement that may last for several days. Following initiation of milk secretion, milk supply increases to meet the demands of the infant.

Mechanisms of Lactation

For adequate lactation to occur, milk must be secreted and expelled from the breast.

MILK SECRETION

Approximately three days after delivery secretion of milk begins. Frequent and complete emptying of the breasts stimulate milk production.

Prolactin is responsible for milk secretion following sucking by the neonate. Increasing frequency of feedings and nursing at both breasts will increase the secretion of milk.

MILK EXPULSION

The let down reflex is necessary for expulsion of milk from the breast. The reflex is initiated by sucking or psychological factors and causes release of oxytocin from the posterior pituitary gland. Oxytocin is produced in response to impulses along the nerve endings in the breasts and is released into the maternal circulation. Upon reaching the breast, the oxytocin causes the tissue surrounding the alveoli to contract and propel the milk from the alveoli to the ducts that open in the nipple. Compression and suction then remove the milk from the breasts.

Psychological factors also influence the let down reflex. Anticipation of infant feeding or hearing an infant cry may cause dripping of milk from the breasts. Worry, anxiety, fatigue, and pain may decrease the let down reflex and cause less production of milk.

Nursing the Neonate

Before the infant nurses, the mother should wash her hands and assume a comfortable position. Some mothers will prefer a side-lying position, with the head of the bed elevated slightly; others prefer to sit up either in bed or in a chair. If she wishes to lay on her side, the mother should turn enough that the infant does not have to reach to grasp the nipple. If the infant is held in the curve of her arm, she needs to take care that he is not held in a cramped position.

When the mother is comfortable and the breast is exposed, no immediate attempts should be made to make the infant nurse. Normally, within a few minutes, the infant will root and find the breast or will smell the milk and hunt for it. Touching the nipple to

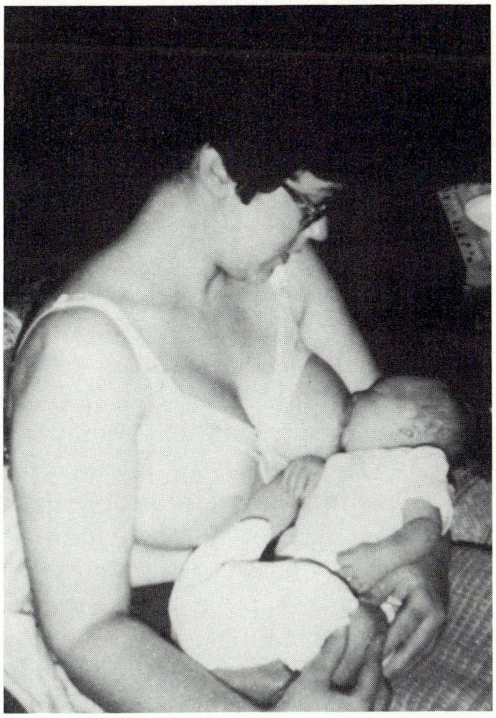

FIGURE 23–2. Breastfeeding.

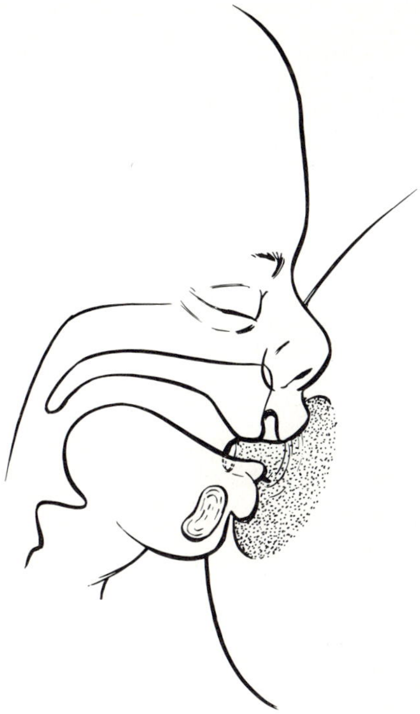

FIGURE 23–3. Position of baby's mouth on breast.

the infant's cheek will cause him to turn his head, open his mouth, and grasp the nipple (see Fig. 23–2).

Many newborns will easily grasp the nipple and start sucking, but some may need a little prodding. Expressing a few drops of colostrum or milk may prompt sucking.

For satisfactory nursing, the infant needs to suck the nipple well back in the mouth with the tongue pressing the nipple against the palate. The gums will press on the areolar area of the breast and the lips will close tightly around breast tissue to permit suction. The breast is emptied by compression and suction. The combination of tongue action and suction will completely remove milk from the nipple and the infant will swallow. This action is repeated for a short period of time, the infant will rest, and repeat the sequence (see Fig. 23–3). Nursing will usually slow as hunger decreases. Breast tissue should not impede the infant's breathing during nursing, since infants are obligate nose breathers.

Some newborns do not nurse well in the first week of life. The newborn should not be forced to take the breast or to nurse longer than desired. If the infant becomes upset and cries while attempting to persuade nursing, efforts should stop, the infant should be comforted until quiet, and then start again. If he is crying, he will not take the nipple, even though his mouth is wide open and the nipple can be placed inside. If the infant is sleepy, efforts to awaken and stimulate him are not appropriate. These will usually only result in a resistant crying infant who will not nurse.

After feeding, the infant should be burped to raise the air bubble in the stomach (see Fig. 23–4).

LENGTH OF NURSING

The length of nursing periods is usually limited to about 5 minutes for the first few feedings, owing to the sensitivity of the nipples. If the period of nursing is less than 5 minutes, the let down reflex may not have begun to function and the milk ducts may not be emptied

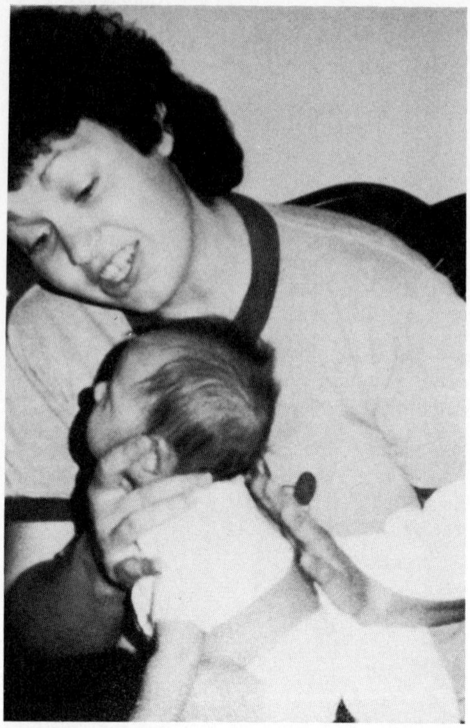

FIGURE 23-4. Bubbling the infant by holding the infant upright and gently patting the back.

during nursing. If the milk ducts are not emptied, milk production is not stimulated and engorgement may result.

Nursing periods are gradually lengthened as tolerated by the mother's nipples. When lactation is well established, nursing periods will usually average about 20 minutes, although there are variations in individual infants.

Nursing may be accomplished from only one breast at a feeding, or both breasts may be used. Maternal preference and the condition of the nipples are determining factors in using one or both breasts. If both breasts are used at each feeding, nursing on each side is usually done for approximately 5 to 10 minutes, alternating the starting breast.

DETERMINING INTAKE

In most hospitals, the infant is weighed before and after each feeding to determine the amount of breast milk received. Weighing is done without changing the infant's clothing or diapers. Once lactation is well established, weighing is omitted.

PUMPING THE BREASTS

On occasion, the breasts will need to be emptied artificially to relieve discomfort, maintain milk secretion when an infant cannot nurse, or allow nipples that are fissured to heal with minimal irritation. If an infant cannot breastfeed owing to preterm status or illness, the breasts may be pumped to maintain lactation until the infant is able to nurse. The pumped milk is saved and then fed to the infant.

The breasts can be pumped manually or with a pump. Manual expression may be used before nursing periods to soften the areolar area so the infant can grasp the nipple or to relieve maternal discomfort when the breasts are full and the infant cannot nurse (see Fig. 23-5). Pumping can be done with a hand or electric pump. A hand breast pump is not satisfactory when pumping will be done for a prolonged period of time and is usually used when only a small amount of milk is to be expressed. When an electric pump is used, it normally takes about 15 to 20 minutes to empty the breast.

CARE OF THE BREASTS

The nipples and breasts are protected from pathogenic organisms. Meticulous handwashing before touching the breast is of paramount importance. During lactation, the breast is very vascular and is prone to infection. If nipples are abraded or cracked from nursing, the risk of pathogen entry is increased.

Antiseptic solutions are not used on the breasts. The breasts and nipples are washed once a day using water and a clean washcloth.

Breast pads used inside the brassiere to absorb milk that leaks must be changed frequently. A brassiere that offers good support without pressure is worn during the day and

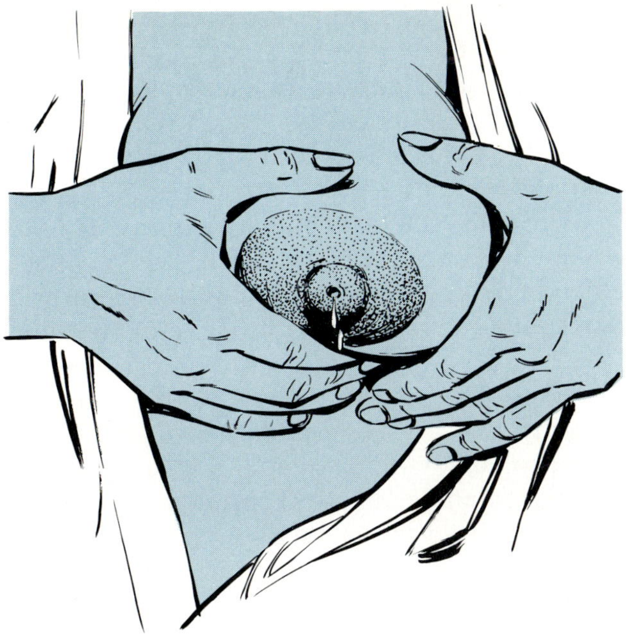

FIGURE 23-5. Manual expression of milk.

at night to provide support to full breasts and to prevent discomfort from the weight of the breasts.

Breastfeeding Supplements

Breast milk provides optimum nutrition for the first six months of life. There are, however, several supplements that may be suggested:

Iron. The use of iron supplements during breastfeeding is controversial. For many breastfed infants, a supplement of 7 mg of iron daily is recommended.

Vitamin K. Vitamin K is given to all neonates shortly after birth. The content of vitamin K in breast milk is low compared with standard infant formulas.

Vitamin D. A supplement of 400 IU of vitamin D daily is normally recommended for breastfed infants to prevent the possibility of rickets, especially when exposure to sunlight will be minimal.

Fluoride. A daily supplement of 0.25 mg fluoride is recommended by the American Academy of Pediatrics beginning at about two weeks of age, because of the relatively low concentration of fluoride in breast milk.

Common Breastfeeding Problems

Common breastfeeding problems that may occur include delayed milk production, sore breasts, engorgement, maternal anxiety, leaking breasts, sore, cracked, or fissured nipples, flat or inverted nipples, breast milk jaundice, breast infections, thrush, inadequate milk supply, and persistently hungry babies.

DELAYED MILK PRODUCTION

Delayed milk production is usually the earliest of breast feeding problems. During the first few days after delivery, colostrum is secreted by the breasts and provides nutritional needs. Milk production may be delayed if the infant is not breastfed within a short time after birth. If the infant is not breastfed early, milk production will often be set back several days.

If the infant and mother are well and healthy, delayed milk production may be the result of not letting the infant suck early enough, not allowing flexibility in infant feeding, and giving supplemental feedings.

SORE BREASTS

Occasionally the breastfeeding mother will complain of breast soreness in the first few weeks of nursing, most commonly related to the let down reflex not functioning properly. This is not an unusual complaint and reassurance should be given that the situation is temporary. When the mother becomes more relaxed and self-confident with nursing her infant, the pain will disappear.

ENGORGEMENT

Engorgement normally occurs on about the third postpartum day and results from an increase of milk into the milk ducts, combined with increased blood and lymph supply to the breast, making the breast hard and painful. Engorgement is usually more common in the first-time breastfeeding mother. It usually begins at the top or outer aspect of the breast and extends into the axillary area, where a small nodule may be palpated.

When the breast becomes engorged, the angle of the nipple-areola will flatten, so that the infant cannot grasp the areola properly for sucking. Even though the breasts are not emptied, milk production continues, suppressing the milk ejection reflex, and allowing the milk to stagnate.

Engorgement can often be prevented by manual expression of milk if the breasts are full but the infant is not ready to nurse, and by wearing a supportive bra that is comfortable without being too tight. A too-tight brassiere will aggravate engorgement.

When the breasts are engorged, a small amount of milk is manually expressed before attempting to breastfeed, allowing the infant to properly grasp the areola and completely empty the breast. Heat or ice to the breasts and administration of a mild analgesic may aid in relieving maternal discomfort. Immersing the engorged breasts in comfortably warm water for approximately 10 minutes will facilitate emptying of the breasts. The severity of engorgement is lessened by frequent nursing to decrease fullness of the breasts and to clear the ducts to allow passage of milk.

LEAKING BREASTS

Leakage is a common annoyance for the breastfeeding mother. A conditioned response will occur when she sees or hears the baby that causes milk to let down. Instructing the mother to fold her arms across her breasts and press them firmly against the chest wall will aid in stopping milk leakage. It is common for the second breast to leak as the baby nurses on the first, because milk will let down in both breasts at the same time.

MATERNAL ANXIETY

Maternal anxiety or emotional upset will decrease milk production and the let down reflex. Often the infant's behavior may provide the clue to maternal anxiety. When the mother is relaxed and not anxious or upset, the infant will take the breast readily, suck steadily, and become drowsy as satiation occurs. An infant reacting to maternal anxiety will usually act in one of two ways: (1) the infant will suck, stop, cry, suck, stop, cry, and then may regurgitate; or (2) the infant will suck, stop, cry, refuse to nurse, and continue to cry.

Determination of the cause of maternal anxiety will aid in formulating a solution to this problem. Often explanations of the cause of poor infant feeding will correct the problem. As the mother understands the importance of relaxation and avoiding emotional upsets, her anxiety will decrease.

SORE, CRACKED, OR FISSURED NIPPLES

Five factors will cause problems with the nipples during breastfeeding. If the infant does not have the nipple and areola properly in the mouth, friction of the baby's gums on the nipple will cause problems. When the infant is allowed to suck on an empty breast for a period of time, the sustained negative pressure will cause sore or cracked nipples. Washing the nipples with soap will dry the nipple and deplete it of natural oils that prevent cracking. The infant may be improperly positioned at the breast, creating traction on the nipples. When removing the infant from the breast, failure to break suction can cause nipple problems.

Cleansing of the nipple with plain water daily and omission of soap and any astringents will prevent removal of protective natural oils. Following feedings, air drying of the breasts for 10 to 15 minutes with the flaps of the nursing brassiere open will be helpful. Avoiding plastic-covered pads in the brassiere will prevent moisture retention. Following air drying, application of a lanolin ointment to the nipples promotes healing and toughens the skin. Nursing time is gradually increased, and alternate breasts used first. Prevention of engorgement will help to prevent sore, cracked, or fissured nipples. A change of position during breastfeeding will sometimes aid in improvement of sore, cracked nipples.

Exposure of the breasts to the sun for short period of time is very effective in healing cracked and fissured nipples. If outdoor privacy is unavailable, sitting in the direct sunlight near an open window is beneficial. When used properly, an ultraviolet lamp is also a good substitute for direct sunlight.

FLAT OR INVERTED NIPPLES

In order to breastfeed, the nipple must be able to be drawn to the back of the baby's mouth. Without this flexibility, the nipple is considered inverted or flat and the baby may not be able to keep it in his mouth. In addition, the lacteal sinuses under the areola will not be brought within reach of the baby's jaws so that the breast can be milked effectively.

Ideally, flat or inverted nipples are corrected by prenatal nipple preparation. Nipple exercise will improve protractibility during the prenatal period. During the postpartum period, wearing a nipple shield will aid in improving nipple position. Using a cold wet washcloth on the nipple immediately before offering the breast increases nipple erectibility.

BREAST MILK JAUNDICE

Some breastfed infants develop hyperbilirubinemia between the fifth and fourteenth day of life. This is characterized by elevated indirect (unconjugated) bilirubin levels for a prolonged period of time in an otherwise healthy neonate. It occurs in 1 to 2 percent of all breastfed babies.

Treatment consists of three approaches: continuance of breastfeeding while monitoring bilirubin levels, temporarily withholding breastfeeding and substituting formula feedings, and alternating breast and formula feedings.

BREAST INFECTION

Mastitis and abscesses of the breast require medical intervention. Most commonly, the causative organism is *Staphylococcus aureus*, with entry gained through a cracked or fissured nipple. The infection is usually interstitial and not intraductal, so the infection will not harm the baby. Treatment consists of application of moist heat, forcing fluids, antibiotics, rest, and continuance of breastfeeding.

THRUSH

When sore nipples are persistant, oral thrush in the baby should be suspect. Oral thrush thrives in the warm moist environment of the baby's mouth and the mother's nipples. When nursing has been proceeding without difficulty, and the mother suddenly develops sore nipples, the baby's mouth should be examined for white patches surrounded by redness, and the breast should be examined for redness and inflammation. Treatment of the thrush will correct the problem.

INADEQUATE MILK SUPPLY

When the mother has an inadequate milk supply for nourishment of the baby, she may not be nursing often enough. The complaint of inadequate milk is most frequently heard at six weeks and again at three months after delivery. These two periods coincide with rapid growth periods in the infant. If the mother continues to nurse, her milk supply will increase to meet infant demands.

PERSISTENTLY HUNGRY BABY

Babies sometimes seem to want to nurse all the time—they seem constantly hungry. When babies go through this phase, the mother becomes fatigued and less able to cope. Human milk is digested more easily and rapidly than formula, leading to more frequent feedings for the breastfed baby. Babies will also have days in which they need to be fed more frequently, commonly in response to a growth spurt.

Explanations to the mother of the normalcy of this infant response are of utmost importance. She needs to be assured that the baby is getting enough milk, as evidenced by six to eight wet diapers a day, several stools per day, weight gain, generally happy disposition, and vigorous sucking. She should be encouraged to nap when her baby is napping to keep from becoming fatigued. Feeding in a pleasant environment may also help.

Drug Excretion in Breast Milk

In order for drugs to enter the breast milk, they must cross capillary endothelium, extracellular tissue spaces, and cell membranes of the alveoli. Transfer occurs by simple passive diffusion, facilitated diffusion, and active transport. As a general rule, water-soluble drugs with molecular weights below 200 can enter breast milk.

The amount of drug excreted into the breast milk depends upon several factors: the pharmacology of the drug itself; the dosage, frequency of administration, and method used to administer the drug; and the maternal ability to metabolize and excrete the drug from her body.

There are possible adverse neonatal effects of maternal drugs excreted in breast milk. If the drug is stored in proteins, a cumulative effect may occur. Metabolism of the drug in the liver may be increased or decreased. Hereditary metabolic conditions may cause increased sensitivity in some infants. The drug taken can alter normal physiologic functions. Hypersensitivity reactions may occur, most commonly from maternal ingestion of antibiotics.

Before any medication is ordered for the breastfeeding mother, the benefits should clearly outweigh the hazards. The safety of ordered medications should be clearly explained to the mother so she can make an informed decision about taking the medication. Certain medications are contraindicated for the breastfeeding mother (see Table 23–3). Other medications are to be used with extreme caution.

TABLE 23–3
MEDICATIONS CONTRAINDICATED DURING LACTATION

Medication
Lithium
Antimetabolites
Radioactive medications
Hexachlorophene
Phenindione
Chloramphenicol
Isoniazid (INH)

Environmental Contaminants

Two groups of chemicals are present in breast milk in varying amounts. Agricultural chemicals include chlorinated hydrocarbons such as DDT, aldrin, and benzene hexachloride (BHC). Exposure to these chemicals leads to accumulation in the fat cells, with carcinogenicity. Pesticides are present in breast milk in large amounts. Chlorinated hydrocarbons used for industrial purposes have also been found in breast milk in varying amounts. Breast milk concentrations are proportional to concentrations in the body. Polychlorinated biphenyls (PCBs), chlorinated hydrocarbons, are found in bullheads, catfish, and other fresh water fish. Pesticides are found in foods of animal origin.

The mother who is breastfeeding must be aware of environmental contaminants that may be excreted to her infant through breast milk. Some dietary modifications may need to be made.

Storage of Breast Milk

If there is a need to store breast milk at home, there are certain general guidelines:

Hand express breast milk after breastfeeding

Use a sterile plastic container to express the milk

Pour breast milk into plastic disposable liner bottle

Collect the milk over a 24-hour period, keeping the milk refrigerated

Breast milk can be refrigerated for up to 48 hours

If the breast milk is not to be used within 48 hours, place a wire twist tightly around the top of the liner bag.

Label the bag with the date the milk was pumped, and place in the freezer

Breast milk can be frozen for two weeks

To thaw frozen breast milk, place it under running cold water, and gradually warm the water until the milk is liquid. Place the milk in a container under hot running water until body temperature is reached.

Do not thaw the milk too quickly

Breast milk that has been thawed cannot be reused; if it is not taken, discard the remainder

Weaning the Infant

Weaning the infant refers to the transitional period of time during which a mother gradually discontinues all nursing.

Usually, replacing one breast feeding at a time with another type of feeding is the easiest way to wean. After a few days of substituting one feeding, substitute a second feeding. Continue with this process until the baby is no longer breastfeeding.

A logical feeding to substitute is one when the breasts feel least full, or to substitute a feeding in which the baby seems less interested. The feeding that is the most satisfying for the baby and mother should be the last one given up. If the breasts become uncomfortable when skipping feedings, manual expression of a small amount of milk using a hand or electric breast pump can be suggested. Care must be taken not to express too much milk, since that will stimulate more milk production.

BOTTLE FEEDING

Formula feeding by bottle may be preferred by some mothers. The substitution of formula feeding for breastfeeding involves copying nature as closely as possible. The majority of these mothers will use a commercially prepared formula for infant feeding.

Advantages of Bottle Feeding

The mother who chooses to bottle feed her infant should be supported in her choice. Nurturing of an infant involves much more than feeding the baby. The mother who wishes to bottle feed has valid reasons for making her choice, and her feelings and choice should be honored. There are benefits for her and the baby.

An advantage of formula feeding is that gained by the mother whose attempts at breastfeeding have been frustrating. If she doesn't want to breastfeed, or if she wants to breastfeed and can't, continuing to try is as hard on the baby as it is psychologically difficult for her. Following the frustration of attempting to breastfeed, bottle feeding may be accompanied by the onset of peace and the first real mothering.

There are other advantages. The mother can be sure the baby is getting enough milk for nutrition. She can offer the same closeness, warmth, and stimulation as the breastfeeding mother can. There is also the opportunity for other members of the family unit to get close to the baby and develop a warm relationship during feeding times with the baby. Formula feeding will allow the mother to give more of her time to other children or allow more flexibility to return to work.

Many mothers choose to breastfeed for a period of time after delivery and wean the baby within the first six months. Even a few weeks of breastfeeding will reduce the likelihood of allergy development in the infant, and increase immunologic protection for the infant. When the switch is made from breast to bottle feeding, the baby must be weaned to formula, not cow's milk.

Bottle Feeding the Baby

The formula chosen for infant feeding must meet the standards established by the American Academy of Pediatrics, which allows for various choices in formula. If the mother mixes or bottles formula for feeding, she needs to learn the rules of safe formula preparation and administration. Until the baby is stronger and resistant to infection (about two to three months of age), formula should be prepared with care, using safe pure water and following prescribed preparation methods. Sterilization of formula is recommended until two to three months of age.

FORMULAS

A formula must satisfy infant requirements for water, calories, vitamins, and minerals; it must have an appropriate distribution of calories from carbohydrates, fats, and protein, and be easily digestible. Commercially prepared formulas are made according to established standards. Most infant formulas provide 7 to 16 percent protein, 35 to 55 percent fat, and 35 to 65 percent carbohydrate. The established standards designate 20 kcal per oz.

A commercially prepared modification of cow's milk is the basic constituent of milk-based formula feedings. The protein is modified for easy digestibility and is "whey-based," or similar to human milk, or "casein-based." In addition to the milk-based formulas, there are formulas with vegetable proteins as their major protein source, used for infants who are sensitive or allergic to cow's milk protein or who have difficulty in digesting lactose. Table 23–4 compares major nutrients in breast milk, cow's milk, goat's milk, commercially prepared milk-based formulas, and commercially prepared soy-based formulas.

Commercially Prepared Formulas

Several different commercially prepared milk-based formulas are available for infant feeding

TABLE 23–4
COMPARISON OF BREAST MILK, COW'S MILK, GOAT'S MILK, COMMERCIAL MILK-BASED FORMULA, AND COMMERCIAL SOY-BASED FORMULA

Parameter	Breast Milk	Cow's Milk	Goat's Milk	Milk-Based Formula	Soy-Based Formula
Energy (kcal/100 ml)	74	67	76	68	68
Protein (gm/100 ml)	1.1	3.5	3.3	1.5–1.6	1.5–1.6
Whey/casein ratio	80/20	20/80	18/82	20/80	60/40
Carbohydrate (gm/100 ml)	7.2	5.0	4.7	7.1	7.0
Fat (gm/100 ml)	2.7–4.6	3.5	4.7	3.6–3.7	3.6–3.8
Minerals					
Calcium (mg/l)	340	1200	1300	540	400–440
Phosphorus (mg/l)	140	955	1060	410	200–330
Iron (mg/l)	0.2–1	0.5	0.5	1.5	13 or 2.6
Sodium (mEq/l)	7	25	18	11–12	6–7
Potassium (mEq/l)	13	35	46	19	14–15
Renal solute load	74	220	—	106	91–92
Vitamins					
Vitamin A (IU)	200	103–190	207	169–250	250–264
Thiamin (mcg)	15	44	40	53–65	65–70
Riboflavin (mcg)	36–37	175	184	63–100	100–110
Folacin (mcg)	2–5	0.3	0.2	5–11	5.0–5.3
Vitamin C (mg)	5.0	1.1	1.5	5.5	5.5–5.8
Vitamin D (IU)	2.2	1.3–38	2.4	41	40–42

in either powdered or liquid form. They have a composition basically similar to that of breast milk and have added vitamins. Commercially prepared cow's milk–based formulas available include Enfamil and Similac.

Formula Prepared At Home

For some mothers, the cost of commercially prepared formulas is prohibitive. These mothers may instead choose to use formula that is completely made at home, most commonly by combining three ingredients—evaporated milk, water, and sugar. Proportions of each of these ingredients is determined by the infant's calorie and fluid requirements.

The kind of milk used in formula will depend on its safety and digestibility by the infant. Unmodified cow's milk is not used, owing to its high bacterial content and undigestibility. Evaporated milk is most commonly used. With evaporated milk the cow's curd is altered, making it more digestible by the infant. Evaporated milk is readily available, relatively inexpensive, and easy to use to make infant formula.

The milk used is diluted with water to supply the amount needed in a 24-hour period. Sugar is added to furnish needed calories. When the evaporated milk is diluted, the calorie content is decreased, making it necessary to add additional calories to meet infant requirements. Many sugars can be used in formula preparation, but corn syrup is the most common addition. Honey is not used as a sugar source in formula because of the possibility of contamination. The amount of sugar to be added varies, but general guidelines are: add 0.5 oz to a 24-hour supply of formula for the first two weeks of life, then 1 oz for four to six months, with a maximum of 0.2 oz per 24-hour formula supply. The amount of sugar needed can be altered according to the infant stool pattern. If the infant has loose stool, the amount of sugar in the formula may be decreased.

TABLE 23-5
EQUIPMENT NEEDED FOR FORMULA PREPARATION

A regular bottle sterilizer or a large kettle with lid
A wire rack (comes with commercial sterilizer) or clean dish towel
A mixing bowl
A measuring cup
A punch-type can opener for liquid or a rotary-type opener for powder
Mixing spoon
Seven baby bottles with nipples, caps, collars
Bottle brush
Nipple brush
Tongs

Cow's Milk Feeding

Whole cow's milk is not recommended for feeding infants under six months of age. Undiluted cow's milk has a high solute load that cannot be handled by the kidneys; this may lead to illness from dehydration. Cow's milk contains approximately three times more protein, four times more calcium, six times more phosphorus, and three times more ash than does human milk.

Formula Preparation

Infant formula may be prepared by terminal heating, aseptic, or single-bottle method. Factors to be considered in choosing a method include the type of formula used, safety of the home water supply, availability of adequate refrigeration, ability to utilize the method, and the amount of formula needed each day.

Regardless of the method chosen, avoidance of contamination is important in preventing infection. Before any formula preparation is begun, hands should be washed thoroughly and dried with a clean towel. The work area and sink must be cleaned thoroughly with hot water and detergent and rinsed well.

Labels on the cans of formula should be checked when purchasing and before preparing formula to identify formulas that are ready-to-use and those that need to be diluted with water. Expiration or "use before" dates are checked. Opened cans of liquid formula

TABLE 23-6
TERMINAL HEATING METHOD OF FORMULA PREPARATION

Measure the required amount of water into a clean pitcher or mixing bowl
Measure the amount of formula needed to mix the formula as ordered
With concentrated liquid, standard dilution is equal parts of liquid and water
With powder, add 1 level scoop of powder for every 2 oz of water and stir until completely mixed. Warm water will give the best results
Pour specified ounces of mixed formula into the number of clean nursing bottles needed for one day's feedings. Fill one or two extra bottles with tap water for drinking water. Put nipples, caps, and collars loosely on the bottles
Place filled bottles on a wire rack or towel in the sterilizer or deep kettle. Add 3 inches of water to the sterilizer. Place over heat
When the water starts to boil, cover and boil for 25 minutes
Remove the sterilizer from the heat, but leave it covered until it is cool to the touch. Do not cool the bottles too quickly
When the bottles are cool enough to handle, remove them from the sterilizer, tighten the caps, and store in the refrigerator until bottles are needed
Use prepared bottles within 48 hours
Shake the bottle well before feeding
Discard any formula left in the bottle after the baby has been fed
Rinse bottles and caps after use

TABLE 23-7
ASEPTIC METHOD OF FORMULA PREPARATION

Place the bottles, nipples, collars, caps, mixing spoon, can opener, measuring pitcher and tongs on a rack or on a clean cloth in the bottom of a sterilizer or large covered pan. Cover these items with water and place the sterilizer over heat
Place the specified amount of water needed to make formula in a clean pan. Place over heat
When the water in the sterilizer and pan come to a boil, cover both and boil for 5 minutes. Let cool to room temperature while covered
Measure the amount of formula you need to mix as ordered. Add to sterilized water in the pan
With liquid, standard dilution is equal parts of liquid and water
With powder, add 1 level scoop of powder for every 2 oz of water. Stir until completely dissolved
Pour the desired ounces of formula per feeding from the pan into nursing bottles. Put the nipples, collars, and caps on the bottles, using tongs to avoid touching them with your hands
Store in the refrigerator until needed
Use within 48 hours
Shake the bottle well before feeding
Discard any formula left in the bottle after the baby has been fed
Rinse bottles and nipples after use

are covered and stored in the refrigerator and used within 48 hours. Opened cans of powdered formula are covered and stored in a cool, dry place.

Regardless of the method of sterilization used, equipment (see Table 23-5) must be washed and rinsed before using. Bottles, nipples, collars, and caps are scrubbed with a bottle brush, detergent, and hot water. Water is squeezed through the nipple holes during washing and rinsing, and the nipple is inverted to cleanse both sides. Bottles and

TABLE 23-8
SINGLE-BOTTLE METHOD OF FORMULA PREPARATION

To prepare a full day's supply of bottles, add a specified amount of water to each nursing bottle
Put the nipples and caps loosely on the bottles. Place the bottles on a wire rack or clean cloth in the bottom of a sterilizer or a large covered kettle. Add water to the level of water in the bottles. Place over heat
After the water has come to a boil, cover and boil for 25 minutes
When the sterilizer is cool to touch, remove the bottles, tighten the caps, and store at room temperature. Use within 48 hours
At feeding time, remove the cap and nipple from one bottle. Add the proper amount of liquid or powder to the bottle. Replace cap. Shake well to mix, and feed
Discard any formula left in the bottle after the baby has been fed
Rinse bottles and nipples after use

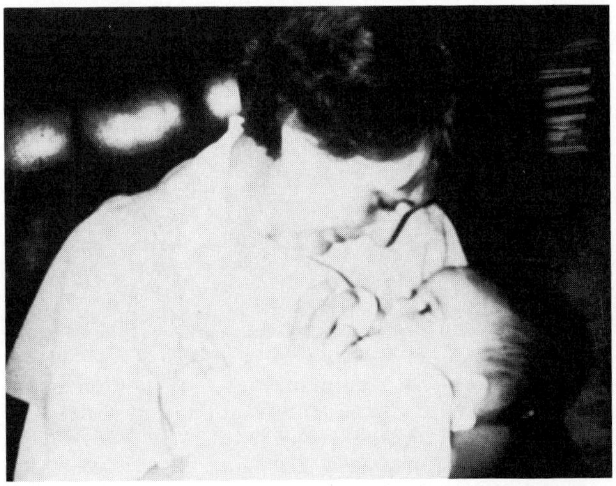

FIGURE 23-6. Mother bottle feeding the baby.

nipples are rinsed with hot, running water. The top of the can is washed with soap and hot water, rinsed, and dried. If liquid is used, shake the can well and punch two holes in the top with a clean punch-type opener. If powder is used, remove the lid with a clean rotary-type opener. Maternal instructions for the terminal heating method of formula preparation are found in Table 23-6; for the aseptic method, see Table 23-7; and for the single-bottle method, see Table 23-8.

FEEDING THE INFANT

It is best to feed the bottle fed infant on demand as with the breastfed infant. Formula at room temperature usually is well-tolerated by the infant. The temperature is not important unless it is too hot or too cold, but feedings are best given at approximately the same temperature at each feeding. Commercially prepared formulas that are sterile and do not require refrigeration allow storage at room temperature. With use of these formulas, warming is not needed before feeding. If refrigerated formula is used, the bottle can be placed in a pan of warm water or in the microwave to remove the chill. The bottle should not be placed under running water in the sink to avoid contamination.

Feeding should take place in a comfortable setting and be given in an unhurried manner (see Fig. 23-6). Always hold the infant when feeding with a bottle. Propping a bottle is dangerous because of the danger of choking and aspiration, as well as the increased amount of air that may be sucked in during feeding when lying flat. When the infant is held during feedings, he gets more enjoyment from the closeness and security that accompany holding. The infant should be held in a semireclining position (see Fig. 23-7) while eating, so that air swallowed is kept at the top of the stomach contents. The bottle should be tilted to keep the nipple filled with milk at all times.

The infant usually sucks well after he has had a satisfactory start on feeding. If the in-

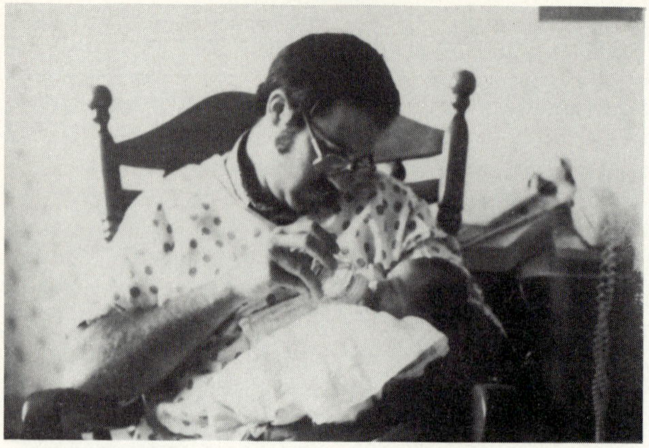

FIGURE 23-7. Father bottle feeding the baby.

fant is getting formula, air bubbles can be seen going up into the bottle during feeding. Feeding usually takes 15 to 20 minutes for the average infant.

Air is swallowed during sucking. To prevent regurgitation of formula, the infant should have air bubbles raised from the stomach. To bubble the baby, hold in an upright position to allow the air to rise to the top of the stomach. Support the body against the arm or shoulder and gently pat or rub the back of the baby. As the bubble comes up, a belching noise will be heard. Most commonly the baby should be bubbled or burped several times during a feeding.

SUPPLEMENTS FOR THE FORMULA FED INFANT

Normally, supplements of vitamins or minerals are not required for the formula fed infant under six months of age who takes a commercially prepared formula. Infants fed a home prepared evaporated milk formula usually require a supplement of vitamin C, most commonly administered in a multivitamin combination along with vitamins A and D.

BIBLIOGRAPHY

Aberman, S. & Kirchhoff, K.T. Infant feeding practices. Mother's decision making. *Journal of Obstetric, Gynecological & Neonatal Nursing*, 1985, **14**, 294.

Anderson, S.A., Chinn, H.I. & Fisher, K.D. History and current status of infant formulas. *American Journal of Clinical Nutrition*, 1982, **35**, 381.

Balkam, J.A. Guidelines for drug therapy during lactation. *Journal of Obstetric, Gynecological & Neonatal Nursing*, 1986, **15**, 65.

Beske, E.J. & Garvis, M. Important factors in breast feeding success. *MCN*, 1982, **7**, 174.

Brooten, D.E., et al. Breast-milk jaundice. *Journal of Obstetric, Gynecological & Neonatal Nursing*, 1985, **14**, 220.

Cadwell, K. Improving nipple graspability for success at breastfeeding. *Journal of Obstetric, Gynecologic & Neonatal Nursing*, 1981, **10**, 227.

Committee on Nutrition, American Academy of Pediatrics. Soy-protein formulas. Recommendations for use in infant feeding. *Pediatrics*, 1983, **72**, 359.

Committee on Nutrition, American Academy of Pediatrics. The use of whole cow's milk in infancy. *Pediatrics*, 1983, **72**, 253.

Committee on Nutrition, American Academy of Pediatrics. Vitamin and mineral supplement needs of normal children in the United States. *Pediatrics*, 1980, **66**, 1015.

Lambert-Lagace, L. *Feeding your child.* New York: Beaufort Books, 1983.

Mackey, S. & Fried, P.A. Infant breast and bottle feeding practices. Some related factors and attitudes. *American Journal of Public Health*, 1981, **72**, 312.

Paige, D.M. (Ed.). *Manual of clinical nutrition.* Pleasantville, N.J.: Nutrition Publications, 1983.

Pipes, P.L. *Nutrition in infancy and childhood* (3rd ed.). St. Louis: Mosby, 1984.

Ream, S., et al. Infant nutrition and supplements. *Journal of Obstetric, Gynecological & Neonatal Nursing*, 1985, **14**, 371.

Riordan, J. & Riordan, M. Drugs in breast milk. *American Journal of Nursing*, 1984, **84**, 328.

Roy, S., III. Perspectives on adverse effects of milks and infant formulas used in infant feeding. *Journal of the American Dietetic Association*, 1983, **82**, 373.

Sears, W. *Creative parenting.* New York: Everest House, 1982.

Sunshine, P. Advantages of breastfeeding in infant nutrition. *Nutrition and the MD*, 1983, **9**, 1.

Suskind, R.M. (ed.). *Textbook of pediatric nutrition.* New York: Raven Press, 1981.

Wiles, L.S. The effect of prenatal breastfeeding education on breastfeeding success and maternal perception of the infant. *Journal of Obstetric, Gynecological & Neonatal Nursing*, 1984, **13**, 253.

Wink, D.M. Getting through the maze of infant formulas. *American Journal of Nursing*, 1985, **85**, 388.

UNIT VI

ASSESSMENT AND MANAGEMENT OF MATERNAL DISORDERS

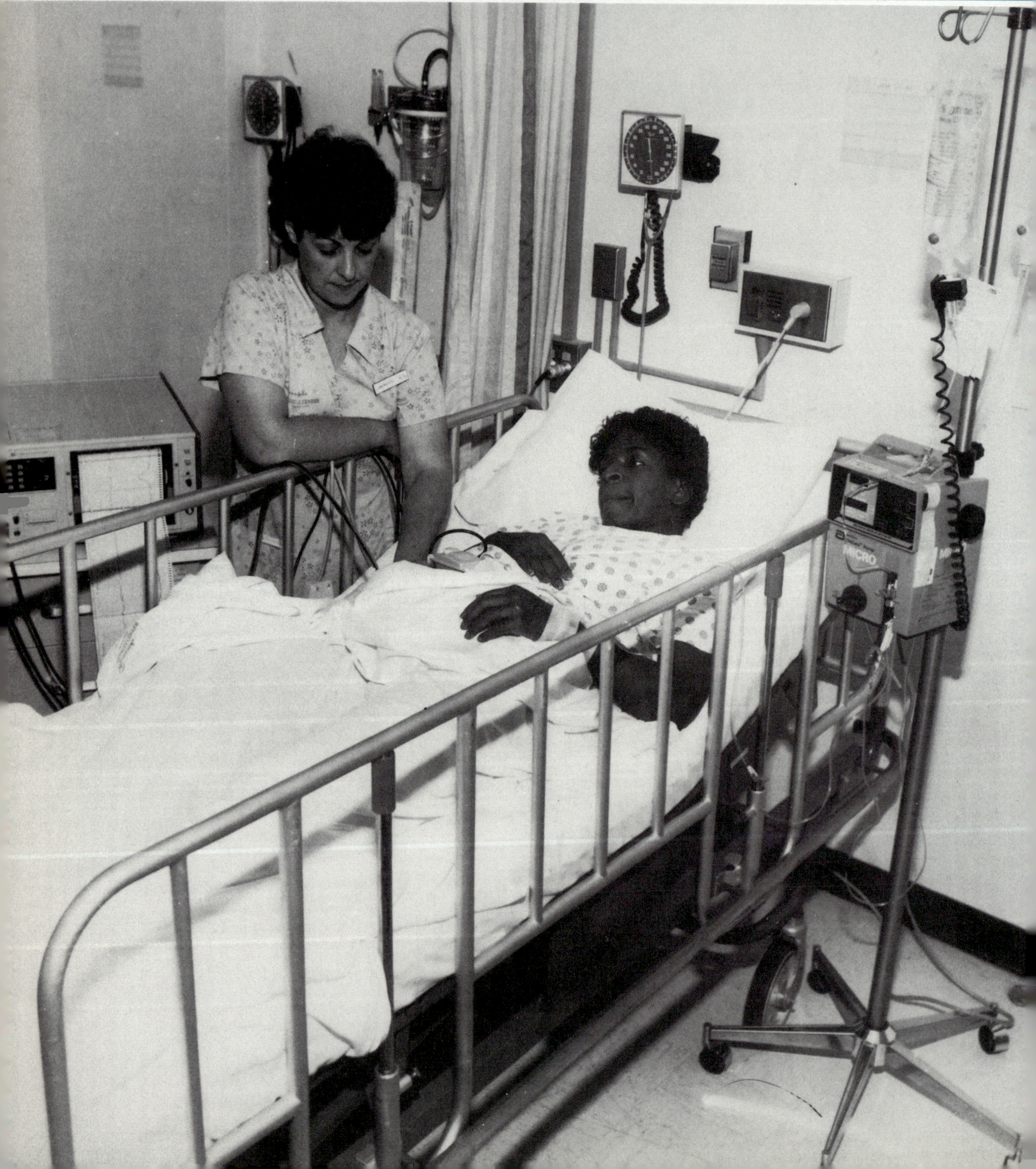

UNIT VI

ASSESSMENT AND MANAGEMENT OF MATERNAL DISORDERS

UNIT VI

ASSESSMENT AND MANAGEMENT OF MATERNAL DISORDERS

chapter 24

CONCEPTS OF HIGH-RISK PREGNANCY

OBJECTIVES

Upon completion of this chapter, the reader will be able to:

1. Define high-risk pregnancy.
2. Identify maternal, paternal, and fetal factors that may be present in a high-risk pregnancy.
3. Discuss nursing interventions appropriate during high-risk pregnancy.
4. Describe biochemical testing to evaluate fetal well-being.
5. Identify biophysical monitoring techniques utilized in high-risk pregnancies.
6. Define amniocentesis.
7. Discuss tests that can be done on amniotic fluid to evaluate fetal status.
8. Differentiate between nonstress testing and contraction stress testing in terms of purpose, procedure, and interpretation.

KEY TERMS

Amniocentesis
Amniography
Amnioscopy
Biochemical testing
Biophysical testing
Chorionic villi sampling
Contraction stress test
Fetoscopy
High risk pregnancy
Magnetic response
Nonstress testing
Ultrasonography

A *high-risk pregnancy* is one in which the mother has a significantly increased chance of morbidity or mortality before, during, or after birth for her or the fetus.

Innumerable factors can cause a pregnancy to be classified as high-risk; these can be maternal, paternal, fetal, or neonatal (see Table 24–1). Neonatal factors are discussed in Chapter 29.

It is rare for just one factor to create a high-risk pregnancy; most commonly, three or more factors present increase the risk for the mother and the fetus.

Normal pregnancy is a maturational crisis in the life cycle. Each woman brings to pregnancy her total cultural, societal, and familial expectations. If high-risk factors are superimposed, pregnancy becomes both a maturational and a situational crisis.

INITIAL SCREENING

Before pregnancy or early in pregnancy, initial screening should identify families at increased reproductive risk. Factors specifically queried at the initial assessment are summarized in Table 24–2.

Diagnostic Measures

Certain laboratory tests are essential to detect or confirm risk factors. Laboratory screening tests that should be obtained as early as possible in pregnancy include hemoglobin and hematocrit, white blood count, differential, urinalysis, urine culture, serologic testing for syphilis, rubella antibody titer, toxoplasmosis antibody titer, blood group and Rh determination, screening for isoimmunization, Papanicolaou smear, culture for Neisseria gonorrhoeae, and test for sickle cell trait or disease (if appropriate). Pregnant women over 35 years of age are offered chorionic villi sampling or amnio-

TABLE 24–1
IDENTIFICATION FACTORS IN HIGH-RISK PREGNANCY

MATERNAL

Physical Factors

- Teratogenic viral illness
- Parity >5
- Conception within 2 to 3 months of previous delivery
- Small stature—height <60 inches
- Prepregnant weight 20% over or under desired weight
- Minimal or no weight gain
- Obstetrical complications
  - PIH
  - Abruptio placentae
  - Placenta previa
  - Multiple pregnancy
  - Pyelonephritis
  - Polyhydramnios
- Abnormal presentations
- Postterm gestation
- High altitude
- Irradiation
- Anatomic defects
- Visual or hearing impairments
- Current medical condition

Psychosocial Factors

- Age
  - Under 17 years
  - Primigravida over 35 years
  - Over 40 years
- Race
  - Native American
  - Negro
- Occupation
- Cigarette smoking
- Stressful life situations
- Extreme anxiety
- Poor nutritional status
- Lack of education
- Suboptimal housing and sanitation
- Irresponsible pregnancy
- Treatment for psychosis or neurosis
- Noncompliance
- Alcohol intake
- Lack of support persons
- No childbirth preparation

Historical Factors

- Hereditary anomaly
- Previous preterm or SGA infant
- Illicit drug intake
- Delayed antepartal care

TABLE 24–1 (continued)

Infertility
Previous poor obstetrical outcome
Inappropriate coping mechanisms
Prior abortions
Previous neurosis or psychosis
Medical illness
PATERNAL
Increased age
Inheritable disorders
FETAL
Congenital anomalies
Short umbilical cord
Cord compression
Hydramnios
Abnormal presentation
Abnormal position
Immaturity
Prematurity
Infection

centesis to identify chromosomal anomalies in the fetus. Pregnancies complicated by medical illnesses may require testing to evaluate fetal status and growth during pregnancy. These are discussed later in this chapter.

TABLE 24–2
INITIAL ASSESSMENT FACTORS

MATERNAL PHYSICAL FACTORS
Maternal age <15 years
Maternal age >35 years
Massive obesity
Nonwhite
Single
Malnutrition
Short stature
Visual or hearing impairment
Pelvic inadequacy or anomaly
Major medical illness
Poor gynecologic or obstetric history
Previous poor pregnancy outcome
Two previous preterm deliveries
Two previous LGA neonates
Maternal malignancy
Uterine leiomyomata
Ovarian masses
Parity >5
Previous isoimmunized infant
History of PIH
Previous infant with congenital anomalies
Medical indications for termination of previous pregnancy
MATERNAL PSYCHOSOCIAL FACTORS
History of drug dependence
History of abusive behavior
Cigarette smoking
History of mental illness
History of poor coping mechanisms
Mental retardation
Hazardous occupation
Environmental contamination
Lack of support system
Lower socioeconomic status
High altitude
Mobile life style
Poor housing

ONGOING SCREENING

Following the initial assessment with identification of high-risk factors, ongoing assessments further delineate other factors of importance in early pregnancy (see Table 24–3), in late pregnancy (see Table 24–4), intrapartum (see Table 24–5), and in the postpartum period (see Table 24–6).

Nursing Responsibilities

Employing a screening system to identify high-risk pregnancies will enable the nurse to recognize these patients as having an increased tendency for perinatal problems. Nursing goals will then focus on reducing or preventing problems. The focus will be on both the patient and her support system.

Appropriate nursing interventions include:

- Development of a trusting relationship
- Recognizing nonverbal cues
- Provision of continuity of care

TABLE 24-3
EARLY PREGNANCY ASSESSMENT FACTORS

Failure of intrauterine growth
Exposure to teratogens
Isoimmunization
Need for antenatal genetic diagnosis
Severe anemia
Urinary tract infection
Suspected ectopic pregnancy
Severe hyperemesis gravidarum
Positive VDRL
Positive gonorrhea screening
Viral illness
Vaginal bleeding
Poor acceptance of pregnancy

TABLE 24-4
LATE PREGNANCY ASSESSMENT FACTORS

Failure of uterine growth
Severe anemia
Postterm gestation
PIH
Isoimmunization
Placenta previa
Polyhydramnios or oligohydramnios
Antenatal fetal death
Thrombophlebitis
Threatened preterm labor
Premature rupture of the membranes
Abruptio placenta
Multiple gestation
Decreased placental function
Loss of support person
Illness of family member
Poor pregnancy acceptance
Neglected prenatal care
Decrease in economic status

TABLE 24-5
INTRAPARTAL ASSESSMENT FACTORS

Severe PIH
Polyhydramnios or oligohydramnios
Amnionitis
PROM
Hemorrhage
Meconium staining of amniotic fluid
Abnormal presentation
Multiple gestation
Fetal weight <2000 gm or >4000 gm
Fetal distress
Prolapsed cord
Dystocia
Fluid and electrolyte imbalance
Induction of labor
Precipitous labor
Cesarean birth
Excessive anxiety/fear about labor and delivery
No childbirth preparation classes
Lack of support persons

TABLE 24-6
POSTPARTAL ASSESSMENT FACTORS

Hemorrhage
Infection
Abnormal vital signs
Traumatic delivery
Family history of vulnerability
Preexisting major medical problem
Poverty
Lack of support system
Family disruption
Role changes and/or conflicts
Maturational crisis
Situational crisis
Noncompliance with expected norms
Poor coping behaviors

Anticipatory guidance
Appropriate teaching
Encouragement of communication
Appropriate nursing assessments
Acceptance of behaviors
Awareness of available community resources
Support

FIRST TRIMESTER

During the first trimester, the nurse helps the client to face realistically and understand the factors that make her pregnancy high risk. Emphasizing the woman's strengths, ability to adapt to changes, knowledge level, religious beliefs, cultural background, support system, risks are discussed. Information about probable pregnancy outcome is related. If the client makes the decision to terminate pregnancy, understanding and a nonjudgmental manner are important to minimize guilt and ambivalence. If the pregnancy is maintained, realistic optimism is appropriate.

SECOND TRIMESTER

During the second trimester, the nurse should be alert to certain factors that may increase the patient's high-risk status. These include ambivalent or negative feelings about the pregnancy, negative attitudes about mothering skills, inappropriate positive feelings about the present pregnancy, inadequate support systems, and psychological or psychiatric problems.

THIRD TRIMESTER

During this trimester, fantasies surrounding pregnancy are common. Anxieties and conflicts in relationships with others occur. Anticipatory guidance is given from clues assessed. Preparation for the arrival of the baby usually takes place during this time; however, the high-risk mother may avoid any preparation for delivery by refusing to allow baby showers or purchasing baby items. The nurse continuously appraises the client and her support person of the medical and obstetrical situation.

FETAL ASSESSMENT

The goals of antepartal fetal assessment are (1) to determine the presence of genetic anomalies, (2) to monitor fetal growth and development, and (3) to document the ability of the fetus to adapt to extrauterine life. Fetal assessment during pregnancy includes physical examination, biophysical monitoring, biochemical monitoring, amniotic fluid assessment, and fetal heart rate monitoring.

Physical Examination

Physical examination of the fetus is done during antepartal visits to the clinic or office and includes assessment of the fetal heart tones and palpation of the uterus.

FETAL HEART TONES

With a standard stethoscope, the fetal heart tones can be heard by 18 to 20 weeks gestation. With a Doppler unit, the FHT can be heard by 10 to 12 weeks gestation. Normally, the FHR is rapid early in pregnancy and stabilizes at about 120 to 160 beats per minute by term. The area in which the fetal heart tones are heard will aid in determining position and presenting part of the fetus (see Fig. 24–1).

PALPATION OF THE UTERUS

Careful palpation of the uterus beginning in the second half of pregnancy by using

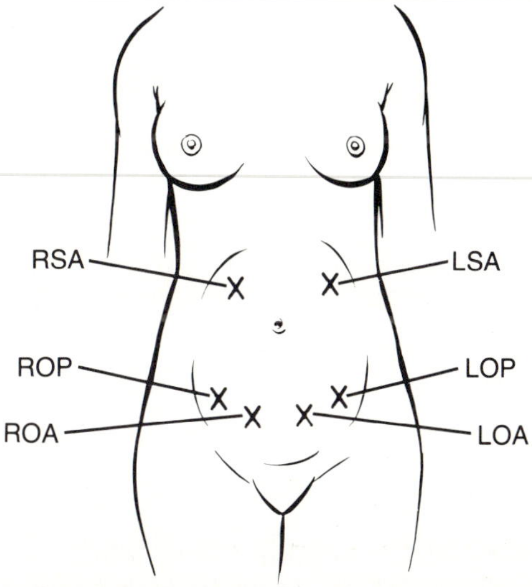

FIGURE 24–1. Areas of maximum intensity of FHT.

Leopold's maneuvers (see Chapter 16) will aid in ascertaining the lie, presenting part, and position. Uterine size and contour are assessed. If the uterine size is not appropriate for the length of gestation, alterations in fetal growth may be suspected. A small-for-date uterus suggests inaccurate dating of the length of gestation or intrauterine growth retardation. Sudden uterine growth may indicate hydatidiform mole, multiple gestation, or polyhydramnios. Unusual contours may indicate fetal malpresentations or anomalies.

Biophysical Assessment

Biophysical assessment of the fetus includes ultrasonography, magnetic response, fetoscopy, amnioscopy, amniography, roentgenography, and chorionic villi sampling.

ULTRASONOGRAPHY

Ultrasonography involves sending very short pulses of low-intensity, high-frequency sound waves into the body and receiving any echoes which return. These sound waves are at a frequency higher than that of normal human hearing and are usually within the range of 1 to 10 mHz. Owing to the high frequency of the sound waves directed into tissue and fluids, echoes are reflected back onto a screen whenever there is a change in relative tissue density.

Two types of basic equipment may be used. Static scanners use a single transducer and produce a static image of the structures that are under the transducer as it is moved across the skin. These scanners are large and require considerable expertise. Real-time scanners are smaller, portable, and use a multiple-transducer head to produce a continuous moving picture of structures.

Indications for Ultrasonography in Pregnancy

Ultrasonography is usually performed for specific clinical indications to aid in diagnosis and followup of the fetus at increased risk (see Table 24-7).

TABLE 24-7
INDICATIONS FOR OBSTETRICAL ULTRASOUND

- Estimation of gestational age for patients with uncertain menstrual dates
- Verification of EDC for patients who are to have elective Cesarean section
- Evaluate fetal growth
- Vaginal bleeding of undetermined etiology
- Diagnose fetal presentation
- Suspected multiple gestation
- Aid before amniocentesis
- Uterine size/clinical date discrepancy
- Pelvic mass
- Diagnosis of hydatidiform mole
- Timing for cervical cerclage
- Diagnosis of ectopic pregnancy
- Aid before special procedures
  - Fetoscopy
  - Intrauterine transfusion
  - In vitro fertilization
  - Chorionic villi sampling
- Suspected fetal death
- Locate intrauterine device
- Surveillance of ovarian follicle development
- Assess fetal well-being after 28 weeks
- Suspected polyhydramnios/oligohydramnios
- Suspected abruptio placenta
- Aid before external version
- Placental localization
- History of previous congenital anomaly
- Serial evaluation of fetal growth
- Evaluate fetal condition
- Placental grading
- Estimate fetal weight
- Abnormal serum alpha fetoprotein value
- Identification of fetal anomalies

Assessment of Fetal Viability

Activity of the fetal heart can be demonstrated as early as 6 weeks gestation by real-time scanners. By approximately 10 weeks, molar pregnancy can be diagnosed.

Assessment of Gestational Age

Assessment of gestational age is indicated when menstrual dates are uncertain or when

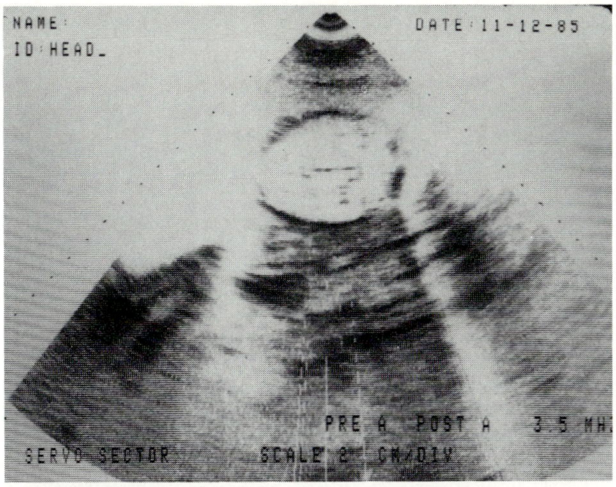

FIGURE 24–2. Ultrasonography. Biparietal diameter of 4.6 cm, consistent with a 20.4 week gestation.

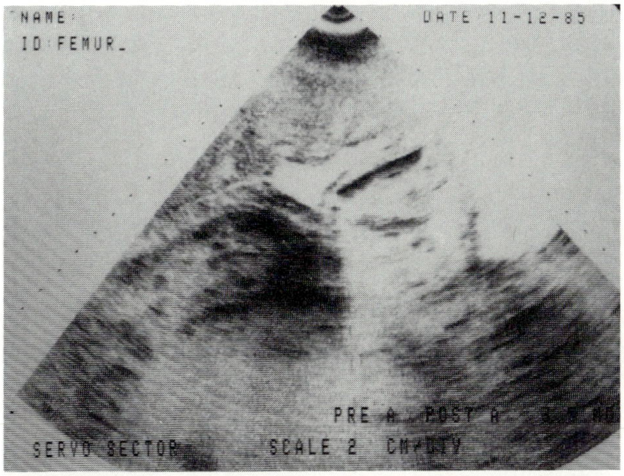

FIGURE 24–3. Ultrasonography. Femur length is 3.3 cm, consistent with a 20 week gestation.

there is a discrepancy between uterine size and gestational age. The *diameter of the gestational sac* can be used to assess gestational age when the crown-rump length is unobtainable. The *crown-rump measurement* is best obtained prior to the 13th week of gestation by measuring the distance from the upper part of the cephalic pole to the lower portion of the fetus (rump) and adding 6.5 to the measurement in centimeters to give the gestational age in weeks. Measurement of the *biparietal diameter* (BPD) can be utilized from the 12th week of gestation (see Fig. 24–2). The accuracy of this measurement diminishes with advancing gestational age. At 36 weeks gestation the biparietal diameter should be approximately 8.7 cm. *Abdominal circumference* is obtained by identifying the long axis of the fetus and measuring a transverse section just below the fetal heart. *Fetal limb measurement* is obtained by scanning the femur to determine its length (see Fig. 24–3).

Assessment of Fetal Growth

When the mother has an abnormal pattern of weight gain, a history of previous intrauterine growth retardation (IUGR), chronic infections, diabetes mellitus, pregnancy-induced hypertension (PIH), or other medical complications, serial evaluations of the BPD and limb length can aid in differentiating between incorrect dates and IUGR.

Aid Prior to Amniocentesis

Before performing amniocentesis, identification of the exact location of the fetus, placenta, and pockets of amniotic fluid will increase the safety of the procedure and avoid inadvertent risk to the fetus.

Diagnosis of Fetal Anomalies

Fetal structures can be identified to diagnose congenital anomalies prior to delivery (see Figs. 24–4 and 24–5).

Fetal Breathing Movements

Fetal breathing movements may be detected by ultrasound and are used to evaluate fetal health in utero. These movements may be observed as early as 11 weeks gestation.

Placental Position

The location of the placenta can be clearly defined throughout pregnancy, to aid in guiding amniocentesis and in diagnosing placenta previa. In approximately 40 percent of gravidas

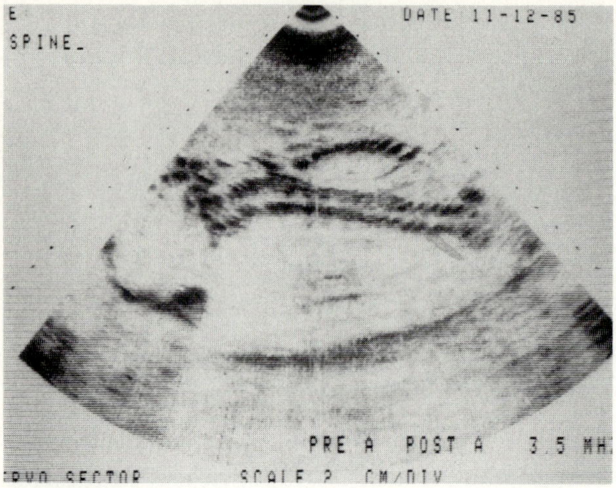

FIGURE 24-4. Ultrasonography. Visualization of the fetal spine to identify anomalies.

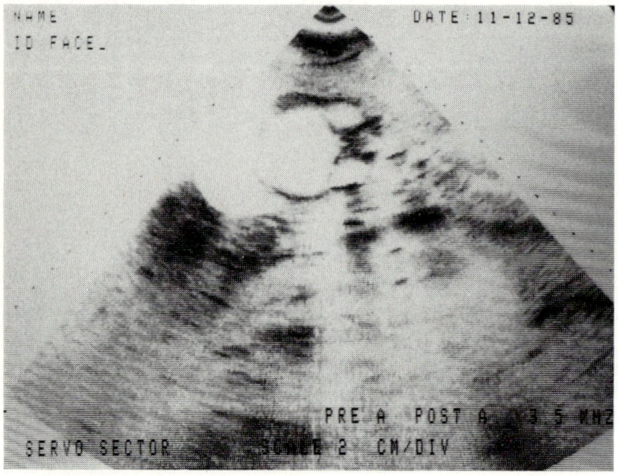

FIGURE 24-5. Ultrasonography. Fetal skull and eye orbits are identified.

the placenta covers the anterior uterine wall. By using ultrasound guidance, avoidance of placental perforation is possible (see Fig. 24-6).

Placental Grading

Placental maturational changes may be noted on ultrasound as early as 12 weeks gestation, and increasing changes throughout pregnancy can be documented. The placental grade is described according to the degree of calcification. Grade III placentas appear to be corre-

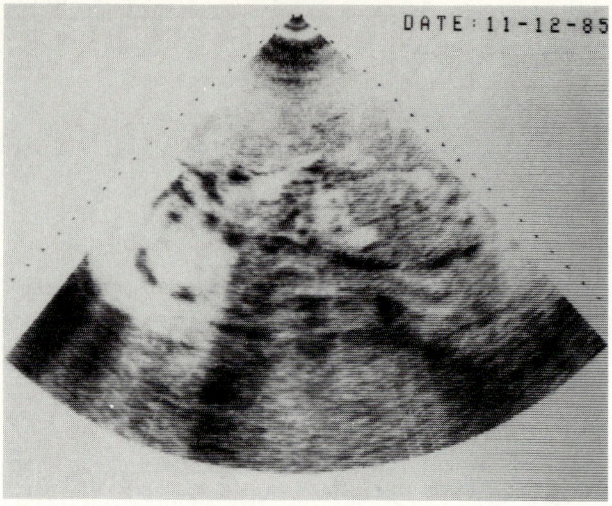

FIGURE 24-6. Ultrasonography. Note the anterior placenta.

lated with L/S ratios greater than 2:1, denoting lung maturity. Placental grading is used as an adjunct to determine fetal maturity when amniocentesis is difficult or impossible to perform.

> **Nursing Responsibilities in Patient Preparation for Ultrasound**
>
> An explanation of the procedure that includes the reason for the study, that it is not uncomfortable, and that there is no radiation or x-ray harm to the fetus is provided. An ultrasound takes about 15 minutes, and involves putting a gel on the abdomen to increase efficiency of the transducer. A full bladder helps to obtain accurate pictures and is achieved by having the client drink four or five cups of water, by intravenous infusion, or by filling the bladder through an in-dwelling bladder catheter.

MAGNETIC RESONANCE

A noninvasive tool used for obstetric imaging, magnetic resonance tracks the distribution and motion of the body's hydrogen nuclei in water to obtain cross-sectional images. It provides excellent pictures of fetal and maternal soft tissues and can be used to identify pelvic masses, pelvic blood flow, placental location, and placental infarctions.

FETOSCOPY

With fetoscopy, the fetus can be directly visualized through a tiny endoscope introduced through the abdominal wall into the uterus under local anesthesia (see Fig. 24–7). A tiny sample of fetal skin or blood is obtained for further testing. Before the fetoscope is introduced, an ultrasound is done to accurately identify a pocket of amniotic fluid, and then is used to direct the endoscope for viewing and sampling.

This procedure can diagnose many fetal defects, including skin conditions such as ichthyosis and epidermolysis bullosa, blood hemoglobinopathies, cleft lip, cleft palate, limb dysplasias, and spina bifida.

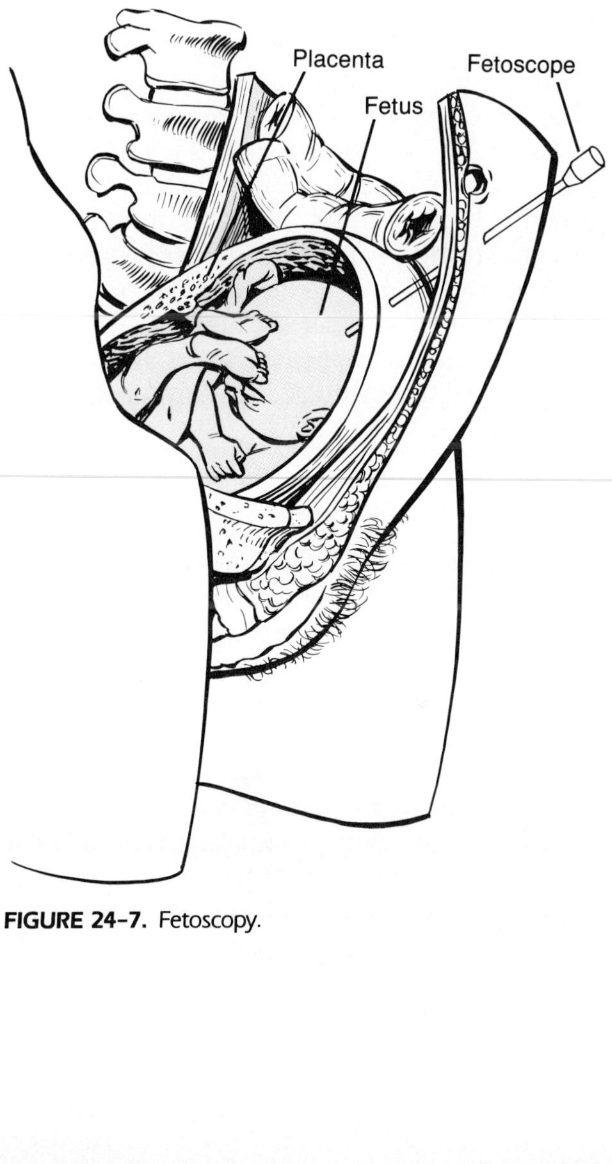

FIGURE 24–7. Fetoscopy.

There are significant risks, specifically fetal mortality of 7 to 8 percent, preterm labor in 10 percent of patients, and leakage of amniotic fluid in 7 percent of patients.

AMNIOSCOPY

This technique can show meconium staining of the amniotic fluid before rupture of the membranes to identify the fetus at increased risk for intrauterine hypoxia. Amnioscopy is used in patients with documented placental insufficiency, postmaturity, and PIH. An amnioscope is placed in the vagina against the fetal presenting part and the amniotic fluid is visualized to determine if meconium staining has taken place.

Potential problems include accidental rupture of the membranes, intrauterine infection, difficulty in identifying the color of the amniotic fluid, and inability of the client to maintain the proper position for the examination.

AMNIOGRAPHY

Amniography is a radiologic procedure in which the amniotic fluid is injected with a contrast material to identify the fetus and uterine cavity. It is occasionally used for placental localization, to diagnose placenta previa, and to diagnose intrauterine fetal demise, but has been largely replaced by other more accurate methods.

X-RAY EXAMINATION

Simple x-ray studies can identify skeletal system abnormalities at about 16 weeks gestation. Fetal age can be estimated by visualization of ossification centers. The distal femoral epiphysis is seen by 36 weeks gestation. Due to the radiation hazard to the mother and to the fetus, x-ray examination has largely been replaced by ultrasound for fetal age assessment.

CHORIONIC VILLI SAMPLING

Chorionic villi sampling involves removing a small portion of tissue from the fetal portion of the placenta (the chorion frondosum or chorion laeve) to determine the genetic makeup of the fetus. It can be used at about 8 weeks gestation as a part of a genetic workup for couples at increased risk for genetic defects in their offspring.

Biochemical Testing

Biochemical testing of the fetus includes human chorionic gonadotropin (HCG) determinations, progesterone evaluation, urinary estriol determinations, and maternal plasma tests for estriols, human placental lactogen (HPL), alkaline phosphatase (HRAP), diamine oxidase (DAO), and oxytocinase.

HUMAN CHORIONIC GONADOTROPIN (HCG)

HCG is produced by the trophoblast and normally peaks in early pregnancy, falling off to low levels in the second and third trimesters. The presence of HCG is the basis of pregnancy tests. Extremely high levels of HCG are present in trophoblastic disease (hydatidiform mole) during the second trimester of pregnancy. Increased levels of HCG near term in patients with diabetes mellitus, Rh isoimmunization, or PIH suggest impending intrauterine fetal demise.

PROGESTERONE

Progesterone, a steroid hormone, is produced by the placenta in increasing amounts during pregnancy. It may be measured as serum progesterone or urinary pregnanediol. The normal ranges of progesterone vary widely, making determinations of little value in evaluating fetal well-being.

URINARY ESTRIOL LEVELS

The amount of estriol excreted in the urine of a pregnant woman is used as an indicator of placental function and as a predictor of possible fetal jeopardy in high-risk pregnancies. The majority of the dehydroisoandrosterone sulfate that is secreted by the fetal adrenals is converted to estriol by a healthy placenta and excreted in the maternal urine. Estriol levels rise progressively during normal pregnancy.

Urinary estriol determinations are of value in pregnant patients with hypertension, PIH, diabetes mellitus, renal disease, placental insufficiency, IUGR, and postmaturity to evaluate placental function.

The range of normal values is broad, and serial determinations are needed to accurately determine placental function. The production of estriol will fluctuate from day to day. Creatinine in the urine is also measured to allow calculation of the estriol/creatinine ratio. As a general rule, a decrease in 50 percent from the previous level indicates fetal jeopardy. A decrease up to 30 percent can be caused by laboratory variation or normal fluctuation. Estriol values indicating fetal jeopardy usually fall gradually, except in the gravida with diabetes mellitus. At term urinary estriols measure 12 to 50 mg per 24 hour. Fetal jeopardy may be indicated by values between 4 and 12 mg per 24 hour, or a fall of 35 percent from the mean of the three previous consecutive values. Critical levels of estriol excretion are 7 mg per 24 hours at 30 weeks gestation and 12 mg per 24 hours at 40 weeks gestation. If the values are chronically low, IUGR may be present.

Procedure

A clear explanation of the test and procedure to be followed is presented to the client. She needs to understand why all urine must be saved, why it must be refrigerated, when to bring the specimen to the laboratory, and what the results indicate.

The first specimen of the morning is discarded. All urine is then collected for the next 24 hours in a clean container that is kept refrigerated to prevent bacteria formation or breakdown of estrogen. The specimen is taken to the laboratory to be processed the same day.

Serial Determinations

Serial determinations are needed to evaluate the pattern of estriol excretion, beginning at approximately 32 weeks of gestation, and are done once or twice a week.

Alterations in Results

Accurate results may be altered owing to problems in collection of specimens or maternal renal disease. If the gravida is taking corticosteroids, ampicillin, aspirin, phenolphthalein, or methenamine mandelate, false readings may be obtained. Gravidas with pyelonephritis may have false low values.

PLASMA ESTRIOLS

Plasma estriol determinations have several definite advantages over urinary estriol. There are fewer difficulties in processing results, less time is needed to collect specimens, and fewer errors are made in collection. However, many laboratories are not equipped to process plasma estriol specimens. The levels of serum estrogen are subject to variation and should be collected at the same time on each occasion.

HUMAN CHORIONIC SOMATOMAMMOTROPIN (HCS)

Human chorionic somatomammotropin (HCS), also called human placental lactogen (HPL), is synthesized by the syncytiotrophoblast of the placenta in increasing amounts throughout pregnancy. HCS can be detected in maternal serum from 6 to 36 weeks gestation. When fetal compromise is the direct result of impaired placental function, HCS levels will fall to critical levels of less than 4 mg per ml. HCS determinations are useful in evaluation of pregnancies complicated by PIH, placental insufficiency, and postdates.

ALKALINE PHOSPHATASE

Heat stable alkaline phosphatase (HSAP) is an enzyme that originates in the placenta. Values normally rise gradually throughout pregnancy. A sudden rise in late pregnancy indicates placental damage and potential fetal death.

PLASMA DIAMINE OXIDASE (DAO)

Plasma diamine oxidase is produced by the retroplacental decidua during pregnancy. The exact function is not known, but it is thought to protect the gravida against histamine produced by the fetus. It normally rises at a rapid linear rate throughout pregnancy and plateaus in the third trimester. Alterations in the rate of increase indicate potential fetal jeopardy.

PLASMA OXYTOCINASE

Oxytocinase, an aminopeptide enzyme, is produced by the syncytiotrophoblast layer of the placenta and functions to inactivate oxytocin during pregnancy. It gives an indirect assay of placental function. Values normally rise steadily from 11 weeks gestation until term and decrease in postterm gestations.

Assessment of Amniotic Fluid

Amniocentesis is a withdrawal of amniotic fluid by insertion of a needle through the abdominal and uterine walls. The fluid withdrawn is then examined for antepartal fetal assessments.

INDICATIONS

There are many indications for amniocentesis including genetic diagnosis and estimation of fetal maturity (see Table 24–8).

RISKS

Both maternal and fetal risks are associated with amniocentesis, although occurrence is

TABLE 24-8
INDICATIONS FOR AMNIOCENTESIS

- Prenatal detection of genetic disorders
  - Cell cultures for karotype
  - Sex chromatin
  - Cell cultures for biochemical studies
  - Alpha fetoprotein for diagnosis of neural tube defects
- Assess fetal maturity
- Monitor isoimmune disease
- Abnormal amniography
- Intrauterine fetal transfusion
- Second trimester elective abortions

less than 1 percent. Maternal risks include the possibility of amniotic fluid embolism, hemorrhage secondary to perforation of uterine or other abdominal blood vessels, infection, preterm labor, abruptio placentae, puncture of the intestine or bladder, or Rh isoimmunization. Potential fetal risks include injuries from the needle, leakage of amniotic fluid, amnionitis, bleeding, abortion, preterm delivery, or fetal death.

PROCEDURE AND NURSING RESPONSIBILITIES

Amniocentesis is performed on an outpatient basis, usually in a labor or delivery area. Written consent for the procedure is obtained after explanation and verbalization of understanding of the procedure. The client is asked to empty her bladder to avoid accidental puncture. She lies on her back with a pillow under her head and shoulders. Ultrasonography is used to locate the placenta, fetus, and an adequate pocket of amniotic fluid. The abdominal skin is cleansed with an appropriate solution and a local anesthetic may be used before needle insertion into the amniotic fluid pocket. A spinal needle is used for insertion into the uterine cavity. About 15 to 20 ml of amniotic fluid are withdrawn into a syringe, placed in a dark-colored container to prevent breakdown of bilirubin and other pigments,

TABLE 24-9
NURSING RESPONSIBILITIES WITH AMNIOCENTESIS

- Patient preparation
  - Schedule the amniocentesis
  - Explain procedure to decrease anxiety
  - Offer reassurance
  - Sign consent form
  - Empty bladder
  - Obtain baseline maternal vital signs
  - Obtain baseline FHR
  - Answer any questions
- Equipment preparation
  - Obtain needed supplies, including
    - Syringe with 25 g needle
    - Local anesthetic
    - Spinal needle with stylet
    - 10 ml syringe
    - 20 ml syringe
    - Dark colored container
    - Drapes
- Assist with location of fetus and placenta
- Provide assistance to physician during palpation
- Assist with ultrasonography
- Cleanse abdomen with prescribed solution to decrease incidence of infection
- Collect specimen
  - Obtain dark colored container from physician
  - Identify specimen
  - Send to laboratory after making out requisitions
- Assess vital signs
  - Assess maternal B/P, pulse, respirations
  - Assess FHR
  - Assess uterus
  - Fetal monitoring is preferred for 15 to 30 minutes
- Documentation
  - Record pertinent data
    - Type of procedure done
    - Date
    - Time
    - Physician performing test
    - Maternal response
    - Fetal response
    - Disposition of specimen
    - Appearance and amount of fluid
- Discharge instructions
  - Explain when and how results will be obtained
  - Instruct to report any of the following
    - Unusual fetal hyperactivity
    - Lack of fetal movement
    - Vaginal discharge
    - Uterine contractions
    - Abdominal discomfort
    - Elevated temperature
    - Chills
- Prevention of Rh isoimmunization
  - If Rh negative, administration of Rh(O) immunoglobulin recommended to eliminate the possibility of antibody formation

and sent to the laboratory for testing (see Fig. 24-8). The needle is withdrawn and the FHT and maternal vital signs are assessed. After observation of the gravida for about 30 to 45 minutes, discharge instructions are given and she may leave. Nursing responsibilities with amniocentesis are listed in Table 24-9.

GENETIC DIAGNOSIS

Amniotic fluid analysis for genetic diagnosis is accomplished by examining cells floating in amniotic fluid or cultures of floating cells.

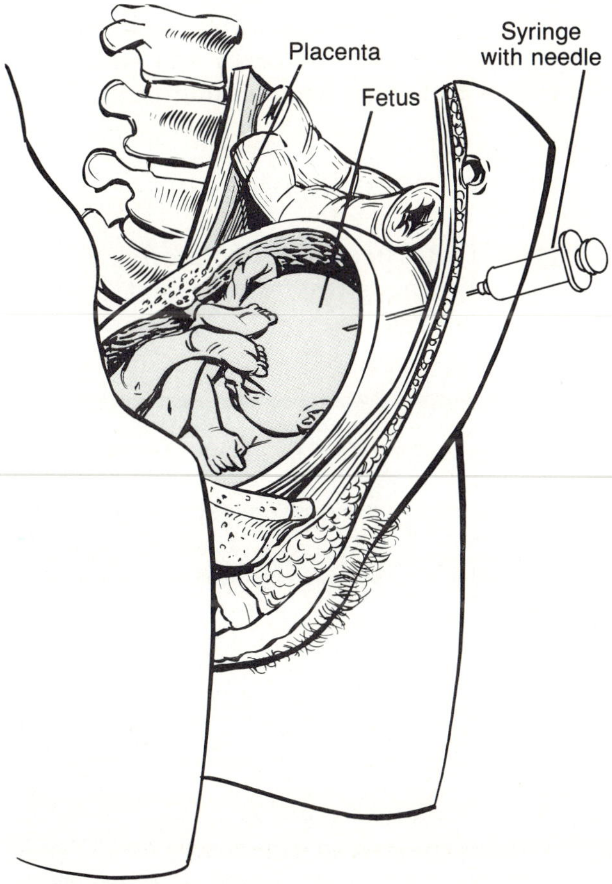

FIGURE 24-8. Schematic drawing of amniocentesis.

Genetic amniocentesis is done at about 14 to 16 weeks gestation (see Chapter 5).

Amniotic fluid can also be assessed for the amount of alpha fetoprotein present. Alpha fetoprotein is produced by the fetal liver and yolk sac. The amount present normally begins to decrease by about the 14th week of gestation. If the fetus has an open neural tube defect, the amount of alpha fetoprotein may be up to eight times normal.

FETAL MATURITY

Fetal maturity is a functional term that reflects the ability of the neonate to adapt to extrauterine existence. Several parameters of amniotic fluid indicate fetal maturity and ability to adapt to extrauterine life. They include creatinine, cytology, lung profile, microviscosity, and bilirubin.

Creatinine Concentration

The fetal kidneys begin to function as early as 12 to 14 weeks gestation. By 24 weeks, tubular function develops, creatinine is filtered by the kidney and appears in the fetal urine. As pregnancy progresses, the level of creatinine in the urine rises. From 34 weeks gestation to term, the level rises rapidly. Amniotic fluid creatinine in late gestation reflects fetal muscle mass and renal function. Levels of less than 1.5 mg per 100 ml indicate a preterm fetus, while those greater than 2 mg per 100 ml indicate a fetus of 37 weeks.

Cytology

Fetal cells are shed into the amniotic fluid from both the fetus and the fetal membranes. As pregnancy nears term, lipid-containing cells from the fetal epidermis increase in number. These cells are identified by staining with Nile blue sulfate. When the lipid-containing cells exceed 20 percent, the fetus is considered mature.

Lung Profile

The major challenge facing the neonate at birth is switching from oxygen obtained from the placenta to oxygen obtained through the lungs. If the neonate is unable to convert from one source to the other, the result is respiratory distress. For adequate respirations to be maintained after birth, surfactant must be present in sufficient amounts. Pulmonary surfactant consists primarily of two surface-active phospholipids, lecithin and sphingomyelin. It functions to lower the surface tension in the fluid lining of the lung that comes in contact with alveolar air.

In order to determine the lung maturity of the fetus before delivery, a fetal lung profile is often created. This profile consists of a lecithin/sphingomyelin (L/S) ratio and percentages of disaturated lecithin, phosphatidyl inositol (PI), and phosphatidyl glycerol (PG).

Lecithin/Sphingomyelin Ratio (L/S Ratio)

In a normal pregnancy, the concentrations of lecithin and sphingomyelin closely approximate each other until approximately 32 weeks gestation, after which the lecithin concentration rises rapidly and the fetal lung matures. The amount of sphingomyelin present changes little. By recording the ratio of lecithin to sphingomyelin, fetal lung maturity can be determined prior to delivery. Results are interpreted as follows:

L/S Ratio >2=mature lungs
L/S Ratio 1.5 to 1.9=transitional lung
L/S Ratio 1.0 to 1.5=immature lung
L/S Ratio <1.0=severe RDS if delivered

Foam Test

A rapid bedside test for the presence of surfactant in the fetal lungs is the foam test. It is based on the principle that an emulsion will stay stable in the presence of surface active materials. Amniotic fluid diluted in saline is placed in a clean test tube. One ml of 90 or 95 percent ethanol is added to the amniotic fluid and shaken vigorously for 15 seconds. The test tube is placed where it will not be disturbed, but at room temperature. In 15 minutes the test tube is observed. If there is a complete ring of small bubbles at the air-liquid interface, the fetal lungs are mature.

Microviscosity

Another test for the presence of surfactant is the measurement of the viscosity of the amniotic fluid. Both surface tension and viscosity are affected by surfactant concentration.

Bilirubin

The quantity of bilirubin in the amniotic fluid can be used to determine fetal maturity, as well as the severity of hemolytic disease in the isoimmunized fetus. Normally, the amount of bilirubin in the amniotic fluid reaches a maximum at 20 to 24 weeks gestation, and then decreases. In the isoimmunized fetus, the amount of bilirubin increases and will determine fetal condition while in utero.

Fetal Heart Rate Monitoring

Antepartal fetal heart rate monitoring is done in two ways: nonstress testing, and contraction stress testing.

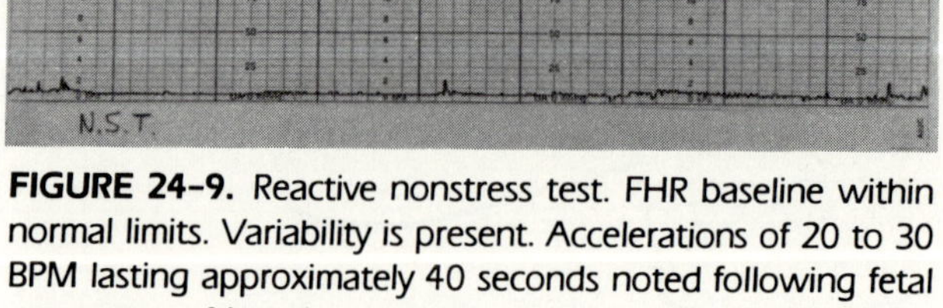

FIGURE 24-9. Reactive nonstress test. FHR baseline within normal limits. Variability is present. Accelerations of 20 to 30 BPM lasting approximately 40 seconds noted following fetal movements. No other periodic changes noted. No uterine contractions noted.

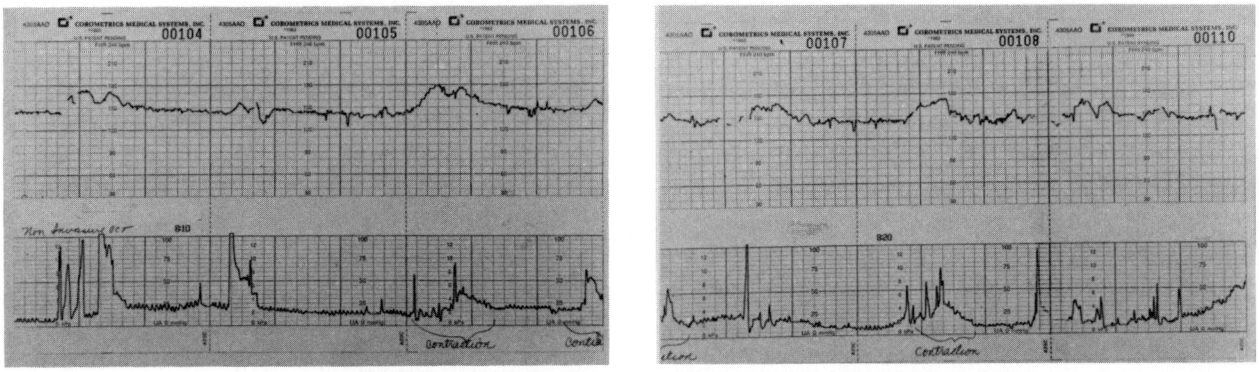

FIGURE 24–10. Negative noninvasive oxytocin challenge test. FHR baseline 140 to 150 BPM. Variability present. Accelerations of 20 to 30 BPM noted at frequent intervals. No other periodic changes noted with three uterine contractions.

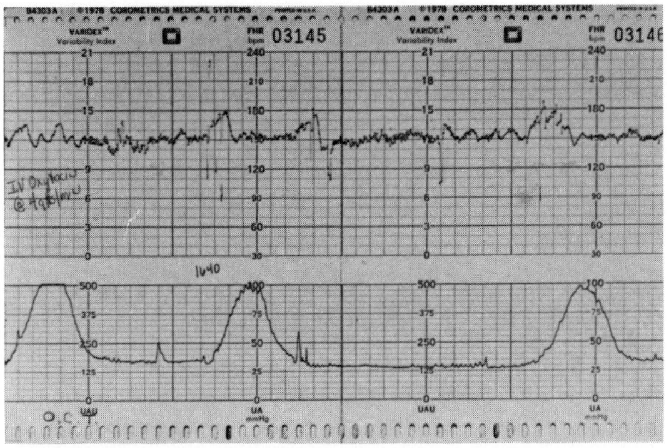

FIGURE 24–11. Negative OCT. FHR baseline 146-152 BPM. Variability present. Accelerations of 10 to 20 BPM noted without other periodic changes identified during three uterine contractions within 10 minute period.

The results of nonstress testing are interpreted as reactive or nonreactive. A *reactive nonstress test* has a baseline FHR of 120 to 160 BPM, beat-to-beat variability of 10+ BPM, at least five fetal movements accompanied by FHR accelerations of at least 15 BPM for 15 seconds in a 20-minute period (see Fig. 24–9). A *nonreactive nonstress test* has a baseline FHR of 120 to 160 BPM, variability less than 10 BPM, and no fetal movements accompanied by accelerations or fewer than five accelerations in a 20-minute period. A reactive nonstress test indicates no further testing is needed at this time. A nonreactive test may indicate the need for contraction stress testing.

NONSTRESS TESTING

Nonstress testing ascertains the integrity of the fetal reflex mechanisms that control the heart rate, thus reflecting the central nervous system status of the fetus. The integrity of the uteroplacental unit is assessed by observing fetal heart rate patterns when stressed by fetal movement.

There are several advantages to nonstress testing. There are no contraindications precluding use of this test. The average time needed for the testing is about 30 minutes. It is noninvasive and does not require the presence of the physician.

CONTRACTION STRESS TESTING

Contraction stress testing is based on the principle that late decelerations following intermittent fetal hypoxia from induced or spontaneous uterine contractions measures uteroplacental reserve. Contraction stress testing can be accomplished in one of two ways: with intravenous oxytocin or by nipple stimulation.

Oxytocin challenge tests are done with a physician's order to determine fetal response to the stress of labor and intravenous oxytocin. The intravenous oxytocin is used in conjunction with an infusion pump and an electronic fetal monitor. After obtaining a baseline FHR strip for at least 10 minutes, intravenous oxytocin is started via piggyback in the same manner as for induction of labor (see Chapter 26).

Nipple stimulation stress tests are performed under a physician's order to stimulate uterine contractions without intravenous oxytocin, to determine fetal response to the stress of labor.

All stress tests must record three uterine contractions within a 10-minute period. More frequent uterine contractions will make results invalid. In a *positive stress test,* late decelerations are present with each uterine contraction and the results identify the fetus unable to tolerate uterine contractions. In an *equivocal stress test* there are decelerations with one or two contractions. In a *negative stress test* no decelerations are noted with any of the three uterine contractions. An example of a nipple stimulation stress test is seen in Figure 24–10, while an oxytocin challenge test is seen in Figure 24–11.

Antepartal testing of the gravida and the fetus are imperative for optimal outcome in the high-risk pregnancy. The members of the health care team, working with parents, will achieve the goal of a healthier mother and neonate.

BIBLIOGRAPHY

A natural oxytocin contraction stress test. *American Journal of Nursing,* 1984, **84,** 707.

Bishop, E.H. Fetal acceleration test. *American Journal of Obstetrics & Gynecology,* 1981, **141**, 905.

Castle, B.M. & Turnbull, A.C. The presence or absence of fetal breathing movements predicts the outcome of preterm labour. *Lancet,* 1983, **2**, 471.

Cetrulo, C.L., et al. Amniotic fluid optical density and neonatal respiratory outcome. *Obstetrics & Gynecology,* 1980, **55**, 262.

Chatterjee, M.S. Paternal age and Down's syndrome. *Contemporary Obstetrics & Gynecology,* 1983, **21**, 171.

Curet, L.B. & Olson, R.W. Oxytocin challenge tests and urinary estriols in the management of high risk pregnancies. *Obstetrics & Gynecology,* 1980, **55**, 296.

Fletcher, J.C. The fetus as patient: Ethical issues. *Journal of the American Medical Association,* 1981, **246**, 772.

Freeman, R.K., et al. Postdate pregnancy: Utilization of contraction stress testing for primary fetal surveillance. *American Journal of Obstetrics & Gynecology,* 1981, **140**, 128.

Gabbe, S.G. Amniotic fluid indices of maturity. In J.T. Queenan & J.C. Hobbins. *Protocols for high risk pregnancies.* Oradell, N.J.: Medical Economics, 1982.

Gelman, S.R., et al. Fetal movement in response to sound stimulation. *Obstetrics & Gynecology,* 1982, **143**, 484.

Graham, D., et al. The role of ultrasound in the diagnosis and management of the obstetrical patient. *Journal of Obstetric, Gynecological & Neonatal Nursing,* 1983, **12**, 307.

Harrison, M.R., Golbus, M.S. & Filly, R.A. Management of the fetus with a correctable congenital defect. *Journal of the American Medical Association,* 1981, **246**, 774.

Hobbins, C.W. Cross-checking pregnancy landmarks by ultrasound. *Contemporary Obstetrics & Gynecology,* 1982, **20**, 169.

Hohler, C.W. & Quetal, T.A. Comparisons of ultrasound femur length and biparietal diameter in late pregnancy. *American Journal of Obstetrics & Gynecology,* 1981, **141**, 761.

Horwell, D.H. Assessment of transcervical aspiration technique to chorionic villus biopsy in the first trimester of pregnancy. *British Journal of Obstetrics & Gynaecology,* 1983, **90**, 196.

Inturrisi, M., Perry, S.E. & May, K.A. Fetal surgery for congenital hydronephrosis. *Journal of Obstetric, Gynecological & Neonatal Nursing,* 1985, **14**, 271.

Kazy, A., et al. Chorionic biopsy in early pregnancy: A method of early prenatal diagnosis for inherited disorders. *Prenatal Diagnosis,* 1982, **2**, 39.

Kremkau, F.W. How safe is obstetric ultrasound. *Contemporary Obstetrics & Gynecology,* 1982, **20**, 182.

Kulovich, M.V., et al. The lung profile. I. Normal pregnancy. *American Journal of Obstetrics & Gynecology,* 1979, **135**, 57.

———, & Gluck, L. The lung profile. II. Complicated pregnancy. *American Journal of Obstetrics & Gynecology,* 1979, **135**, 64.

NIH Report. Reasons to consider diagnostic ultrasound. *Contemporary Obstetrics & Gynecology,* 1984, **23**, 168–169.

Platt, L.D. & DeVore, G.R. Detecting fetal malformations. *Contemporary Obstetrics & Gynecology,* 1983, **21**, 203.

Ward, R.H., et al. A method of chorionic villus sampling in the first trimester of pregnancy under real time ultrasound guidance. *British Medical Journal,* 1983, **1**, 1542.

chapter 25

COMPLICATIONS DURING THE ANTEPARTUM PERIOD

OBJECTIVES

Upon completion of this chapter, the reader will be able to:

1. Identify the two classifications of abortion.
2. Identify the characteristics of the types of spontaneous abortions.
3. List the causes of spontaneous abortions.
4. Given a client with a spontaneous abortion, identify appropriate interventions.
5. Given a method of inducing abortion, state the gestational period in which it is used.
6. List characteristics of a hydatidiform mole.
7. Identify nursing interventions when the client has a hydatidiform mole.
8. Identify factors that predispose to the development of ectopic pregnancies.
9. Identify classic symptoms of a tubal rupture.
10. Define hypertension; state the level of B/P indicative of PIH.
11. Describe the three cardinal signs of PIH.
12. Given a specific patient with PIH, identify appropriate interventions.
13. Discuss nursing interventions with magnesium sulfate administration.
14. Given a client with chronic hypertension, state signs and symptoms, and appropriate nursing interventions.
15. Discuss management of urinary tract infections during pregnancy.
16. Given a pregnant patient with a respiratory, autoimmune, or vascular disorder, identify appropriate interventions.
17. State the most common cardiac problems seen during pregnancy.
18. Identify functional categories of heart disease.
19. Identify appropriate interventions for the cardiac patient antepartum, intrapartum, and postpartum.
20. Discuss management of the client with thyroid disease.
21. Explain how diabetes alters the maternal state; how pregnancy alters diabetes.
22. Know White's classification of diabetes in pregnancy.
23. Discuss nursing assessments and interventions appropriate for the diabetic mother.
24. Given a client with multiple gestation, discuss interventions that improve maternal or fetal outcome.
25. Discuss maternal and fetal effects of postterm pregnancy.
26. Identify considerations when caring for a client with acquired immune deficiency syndrome (AIDS).
27. Given a pregnant client with a gastrointestinal or neurologic disorder, discuss appropriate interventions.
28. Given a pregnant client with a specified anemia, state appropriate nursing interventions.
29. Discuss fetal effects of diseases in the TORCH complex.
30. Identify two common vaginal infections seen during pregnancy.
31. Identify the factors that produce Rh and ABO incompatibility.
32. Know the effects of Rh incompatibility on the fetus.
33. Identify methods of antepartum diagnosis and treatment for Rh negative patients.
34. State the dosage, route of administration, action, and requirements for Rhogam administration.
35. Given a pregnant client with a psychiatric disorder, identify characteristic symptoms.
36. Know the signs and symptoms of hyperemesis gravidarum.
37. Given a client with hyperemesis gravidarum, identify appropriate medical and nursing interventions.

KEY TERMS

ABO incompatibility
Abortion
Asymptomatic bacteriuria
Chronic hypertension
Eclampsia
Ectopic pregnancy
Hydatidiform mole
Incompetent cervix
Induced abortion
Mild preeclampsia
Missed abortion
Pregnancy-induced hypertension
Rh incompatibility
Severe preeclampsia
Spontaneous abortion
Therapeutic abortion
Tocolytic
Viability

BLEEDING PROBLEMS

Abortion

Abortion may be defined as the termination of pregnancy before viability. *Viability* is the state of fetal development theoretically compatible with extrauterine survival. Interpretations of the term viability have varied between a fetal weight of 400 gm (20 weeks gestation) and 1000 gm (28 weeks gestation). For reporting perinatal statistics in the majority of states, viability is defined as 20 weeks gestation.

Abortions are generally classified as *spontaneous* (occurring naturally) and *induced* (termination of pregnancy by artificial means).

TABLE 25-1
CAUSES OF SPONTANEOUS ABORTIONS

Embryonic or fetal abnormalities—50 to 60 percent
Defective ovum or sperm
Blighted ovum (no zygote development)
Chromosomal abnormalities
Faulty implantation
Defective placental development
Maternal factors—15 to 20 percent
Uterine anomalies
Tumors
Incompetent cervix
Smoking
Acute infections
Endocrine dysfunction
Coincidental systemic diseases
Poor maternal nutrition
Accidental trauma
Radiation
Psychogenic factors
Rh sensitization
Intrauterine herpes infection
Unknown factors—20 to 25 percent

SPONTANEOUS ABORTIONS

The incidence of spontaneous abortion varies from 10 to 23 percent of all pregnancies, but has been reported as high as 43 percent of all postimplantation pregnancies before 20 weeks gestation (Miller et al., 1980), with the greatest percentage in the first trimester.

Causes

Embryonic or fetal abnormalities account for 50 to 60 percent of spontaneous abortions. Maternal factors are responsible for 15 to 20 percent, and 20 to 25 percent occur from unknown factors (see Table 25-1).

Types and Manifestations

Six types of spontaneous abortion have been identified (see Table 25-2). Signs and symptoms assessed with spontaneous abortion include vaginal bleeding, uterine cramping, and passage of the products of conception.

When abortion is *threatened,* there is some vaginal spotting or bleeding with mild uterine cramping. The cervix is usually closed, but it may be slightly dilated. Heavier vaginal bleeding, cervical dilatation, and more intense uterine cramping are present with an *inevitable abortion.*

Expulsion of the fetus with retention of the placenta and membranes and continued vaginal bleeding occurs with an *incomplete abortion.*

TABLE 25–2
TYPES OF SPONTANEOUS ABORTION

Type	Description
Threatened abortion	There is uterine cramping and some vaginal bleeding. The possibility of abortion exists, but the pregnancy may continue
Inevitable abortion	The cervix is dilated and the pregnancy cannot be salvaged
Incomplete abortion	A portion of the conceptus is expelled from the uterus, while a portion remains within the uterus
Complete abortion	All products of conception are expelled from the uterus
Missed abortion	The fetus dies in utero but is not expelled
Habitual abortion	Spontaneous abortion in three or more successive pregnancies

A woman with a *missed abortion* may have no symptoms, but complains of malaise, headache, and anorexia. The products of conception are retained in the uterus following fetal death. Estrogen deprivation decreases the contractility of the myometrium. As fetal autolysis occurs following demise, a hypercoagulability of the blood and a decrease of clotting factors occurs, increasing the chances of disseminated intravascular coagulation (DIC).

Nursing Interventions

Nursing interventions are based on four main goals: (1) provision of nursing surveillance; (2) relief of pain and anxiety; (3) provision of emotional support; and (4) monitoring for developing complications.

Using interviewing skills, a nursing history is obtained that includes length of gestation, onset and type of bleeding, presence or absence of cramping, and expulsion of clots or tissue.

Laboratory tests are requested as ordered by the physician. Complete bed rest, decreased environmental stimulation, and reduction of anxiety and stress are important. Vital signs are monitored, the amount of vaginal bleeding is estimated (usually by perineal pad count), and all clots or tissue passed are saved for examination. If bleeding is profuse, an IV is started and intake and output are assessed.

Analgesics are administered, with close monitoring of blood pressure, pulse, and respirations after administration. Intelligent reassurance without false hope is given. Explanations are important in relieving anxiety.

If this is the first pregnancy, the woman is likely to question her ability to bear children, and guilt feelings related to a real or imagined failure may predominate interactions. If the pregnancy is unwanted, guilt feelings are further increased. Realistic and unrealistic fears should be sorted out and dealt with.

Factors that are taken into account in dealing with the spontaneous loss of pregnancy include interactions and relationships of the couple, available support systems, the response to the loss, and socioeconomic and cultural data. See Table 25–3 for a sample nursing care plan.

Incompetent Cervix

Spontaneous termination of pregnancy may be caused by an incompetent cervix. After 20 weeks of pregnancy, the cervix dilates without accompanying uterine contractions. The membranes rupture, labor begins, and a nonviable or preterm fetus is delivered. The exact etiology is not known, but previous cervical trauma is occasionally a factor.

When repeated pregnancies are terminated during the second trimester because of an incompetent cervix, surgical treatment may be used to maintain pregnancy. Treatment consists of reinforcing the cervix with a nonabsorbable purse-string suture by either the Shirodkar or McDonald technique (see Fig. 25–1).

TABLE 25-3
SAMPLE NURSING CARE PLAN: SPONTANEOUS ABORTION

M.G., a 22-year-old, gravida 1 para 0, LNMP 8-24 (12 weeks ago) was admitted to labor and delivery per cart from Emergency Room. She states she started bright red vaginal bleeding about one hour ago. Denies any passage of clots or tissue. Has saturated two perineal pads since onset of bleeding. Complaining of lower abdominal pain, "like menstrual cramps." Moderate bright red vaginal bleeding with no clots on perineal pad worn in. To bed and initial assessment done.

Data Base:

Gravida 1 para 0
LNMP: 8-24 (12 weeks ago)
Religion: Methodist
Height 5'4"
Weight 124 lb
A negative
No known allergies
No medical problems
On no medications

Apprehensive, frightened
No prostheses
Ate at 2100 (5 hours ago)
Vital signs: Temperature 98.6° F
Pulse 92
Respirations 20
B/P 116/74
Dr. V. notified of status—orders received

Nursing Diagnosis	Goals	Nursing Interventions	Rationale	Evaluation
Alteration in tissue perfusion related to excessive vaginal bleeding	Diagnosis is established and appropriate interventions instituted to prevent or control hemorrhage	Maintain bed rest Maternal vital signs q hour and prn	Nursing interventions will prevent or control excessive vaginal bleeding	Bed rest instituted and maintained as ordered Maternal vital signs at 0200: 98.6°F -92-20 B/P 116/74 0230: 90-16 B/P 116/76 0300: 92-16 B/P 110/74 0330: 88-16 B/P 110-74 Remained within normal limits
Potential fluid volume deficit related to excessive vaginal bleeding	No fluid volume deficit will exist	Assess vaginal bleeding by peri pad counts Save all clots or tissue passed Laboratory tests as ordered		Vaginal bleeding assessments: 0200: moderate bright red 0230: moderate bright red 0300: moderate bright red 0330: large bright red CBC, PTT, prothrombin time within normal limits

		Assess cramping for increase or decrease Medicate prn for pain per physician's orders Institute intravenous fluids as ordered Monitor intake and output Offer complete explanations Encourage expression of feelings		Meperedine 75 mg IM at 0300 per physician order 0200: cramping mild 0300: cramping more intense 0330: cramping decreased Clean catch mid stream urine to lab at 0230 for urinalysis and pregnancy test AZ positive Urinalysis within normal limits 1000cc D5LR started at 0220 and maintained at 8 hour rate M.G. crying and expressing guilt over "causing this problem." Denies heavy lifting, excess activity, intercourse within last 24 hours 0345 passed fetus and placenta intact Vital signs stable Small amount dark vaginal bleeding immediately following expulsion. 10U oxytocin added to intravenous already infusing (850 ml) 0350 Dr. V. here. Speculum and vaginal examination done Fetus shown to parents
Potential for injury related to possible Rh isoimmunization with next pregnancy	Rh isoimmunization is prevented	Rh immune globulin given IM before discharge	Rh immune globulin will prevent Rh isoimmunization	Rh immune globulin given IM at 0900 after explanation to parents
Grieving related to pregnancy loss	The grief process is progressing at a normal pace	Offer emotional support Answer questions honestly	The grief process needs to be resolved for psychological stability	Upset. Crying Minister called per parents' request

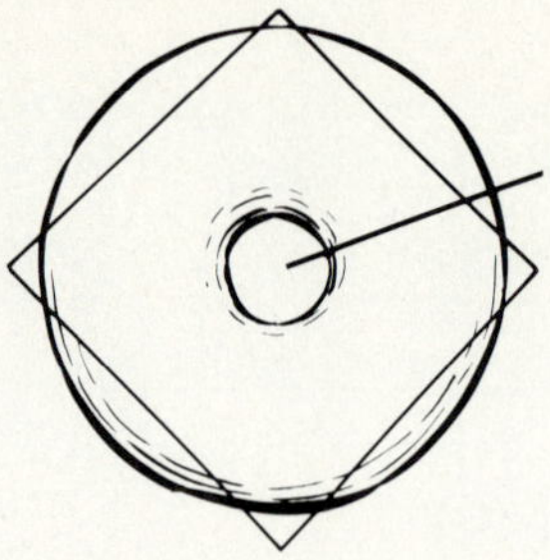

FIGURE 25-1. McDonald technique for suturing incompetent cervix.

Either procedure can be done between pregnancies if there is a definite diagnosis of incompetent cervix, or during pregnancy at about 12 to 18 weeks gestation. General anesthesia is used for the procedure, and the gravid woman is usually hospitalized for at least 24 hours postoperatively.

Major concerns postoperatively are rupture of the membranes and uterine contractions. If membranes rupture, the suture is removed and the uterus emptied to decrease the incidence of infection. If uterine contractions begin, tocolytic medications are prescribed to decrease uterine contractility.

Postoperative client teaching includes recognition of signs and symptoms of membrane rupture and labor. Some cervical spotting may be noted but bright red vaginal bleeding should be reported immediately. The client should abstain from intercourse and douching until after the followup visit to the physician approximately two weeks postoperatively. Tiny pieces of suture material may be noted on the perineal pad from the absorbable suture used to close the cervix.

INDUCED ABORTION

Induced abortions are of three types: therapeutic, criminal, and legal. *Therapeutic abortions* are performed when the mental or physical health of the mother is endangered by the continuation of pregnancy. *Criminal abortions* are those done without legal sanction. *Legal abortions* are those done within the framework of the law.

The legal parameters of abortion were defined by the U.S. Supreme Court on January 22, 1973 (*Roe* v. *Wade*). Abortions were divided into three categories:

1. For the stage of gestation prior to the end of the first trimester, the abortion decision is left to medical judgment
2. For the stage of gestation after the end of the first trimester, the state may regulate abortion procedures
3. For the stage of gestation after viability, the state may regulate and prohibit abortion except where medically necessary to preserve maternal health and life

Incidence in the United States

Abortions by instrumental evacuation accounts for the majority of all induced abortions.

Approximately 30 percent of abortions are obtained by teenagers, 35 percent by women 20 to 24 years of age, and 35 percent by women 25 years of age and over (Henshaw and O'Reilly, 1982). The total number of abortions has increased each year, with no reversal of the trend noted. The highest abortion rates are for nonwhite, unmarried, under 30-year-old women.

Abortion Counseling

Abortion counseling includes identification of perceptions of pregnancy, information about choices available, and information about the different types of abortion procedures.

Abortions are ideally performed in the first trimester to decrease maternal risk (Grimes et al., 1983). The decision for abortion may be delayed until the second trimester for many reasons: irregular menses which may lead to underestimation of the length of pregnancy, denial, ambivalence about having an abortion, lack of access to abortion services, lack of funds, or detection of fetal anomalies with genetic amniocentesis.

The goal of abortion counseling is to assist the woman to make a decision that is her own, not that of the nurse. The decision to terminate a pregnancy is neither casual nor easy. Women seeking abortion may view it as a difficult but necessary alternative.

The decision for or against abortion is influenced by the woman's relationship with the father, her own mechanisms for decision making, her extramarital aspirations, and her self-concept. A calm, matter-of-fact approach by the nurse is helpful in establishing an open accepting environment and in helping the woman to make and solidify the decision that is right for her.

Abortion counseling of adolescents includes identification and expression of the client's behavior and reactions. Ideally, significant family members are included in the counseling process. Cultural, ethnic, religious, and socioeconomic considerations must be balanced against the adolescent's attitudes and reactions to the pregnancy. Interruption of the pregnancy should not be forced on her.

Preabortion Procedures

Once the reproductive decision of elective abortion is made, pregnancy evaluation begins. Pregnancy evaluation includes a pregnancy test, a pelvic examination, and screening for gonorrhea.

Immediately before the abortion procedure, laboratory testing including hemoglobin, hematocrit, Rh(D) screening, serology, and a repeat pregnancy test is done. Nursing assessments include a current medical history, onset of last normal menstrual period, contraceptive history, and drug allergy or sensitivity. Preexisting medical conditions such as cardiac or renal problems, asthma, and epilepsy require medical evaluation prior to the abortion procedure.

Abortion Procedures

Three procedures are used during the first trimester of pregnancy: menstrual extraction, dilatation and curettage, and suction curettage (see Table 25-4). From 14 to 16 weeks prostaglandin, saline, and urea instillations are the procedures of choice, and after 16 weeks, hysterotomy may be done (see Table 25-5).

Postabortion Care

Immediately after abortion, bleeding, uterine cramping, and vital signs are monitored. If the

TABLE 25-4
FIRST TRIMESTER ABORTION PROCEDURES

Method	Advantages	Disadvantages
Menstrual extraction: forced endometrial extraction through undilated cervix by vacuum	Done up to 14 days after missed menstrual period Outpatient procedure	Complications: cervical trauma, hemorrhage
Dilatation & curettage (D&C): cervix dilated with metal sounds; endometrium scraped with a spoon-shaped instrument	Can be done up to 12 to 14 weeks of gestation Outpatient procedure	Complications: uterine perforation, cervical tears, hemorrhage, infection
Suction curettage: cannula suction used following cervical dilatation	Local anesthesia Outpatient procedure Can be done up to 12 to 14 weeks of gestation	Complications: uterine perforation, hemorrhage, cervical tears, infection

TABLE 25-5
SECOND TRIMESTER ABORTION PROCEDURES

Method	Advantages	Disadvantages
Saline induction: abdominal extraction of amniotic fluid and replacement with equal amount of hypertonic saline Fetus dies within one hour Deliver fetus within 30 to 40 hours	Readily available Inexpensive Outpatient procedure	Incidence of complications increases with length of gestation Saline reactions: extreme thirst tinnitus tachycardia headache numb extremities Complications: water intoxication hemorrhage retained placenta infection DIC
Prostaglandin induction: abdominal extraction of amniotic fluid and replacement with 40 to 45 mg prostaglandin F_2 or E_2	Outpatient procedure Shorter labor than with saline No water intoxication No hypernatremia Abortion occurs in about 36 hours	Fetus may be born alive May cause nausea, vomiting, diarrhea, elevated temperature Intravascular injection may cause vomiting, flushing, hypertension, bronchospasm Complications: hemorrhage retained placenta infection Contraindicated in asthma, epilepsy, hypertension, glaucoma
Urea induction: abdominal extraction of amniotic fluid and replacement with equal amounts of 30% urea in D_5W	Outpatient procedure Urea decreases the circulating progesterone levels and increases prostaglandin release	Complications: hemorrhage DIC infection water intoxication

patient is Rh negative, Rh immunoglobulin is to be given to prevent Rh sensitization. Written instructions and an emergency 24-hour telephone number are given to the client. Any written instructions should be explained thoroughly. Signs of possible complications are included in all written instructions. For two to three weeks following the abortion, she is instructed to avoid coitus, tampons, and douching. Contraceptive methods are discussed. Menses usually resumes in four to six weeks.

Psychological support must be available. The postabortion patient commonly experiences a range of emotions, from relief to guilt and depression. The type of reaction is often determined by the method of abortion: curettage procedures are associated with more favorable psychological reactions. The level of support available to the woman greatly influences her reaction. Women at increased risk for psychological difficulties following induced abortion are those who are ambivalent, were coerced into obtaining the abortion, or have a current severe psychological or psychiatric problem.

Complications

Complications of induced abortion are related to the method of pregnancy termination and the length of gestation. Potential complications include infection, uterine perforation, hemorrhage, laceration of the cervix, incomplete removal of the products of conception, and an occasional viable fetus.

Postabortion infection can be caused by hemolytic streptococcus, Neisseria gonorrhoeae, Chlamydia trachomatis and Staphylococcus aureus. Rarely, Clostridium perfringens is the causative organism. The incidence of postabortion infection can be decreased by preabortion screening for gonorrhea and Chlamydia, treatment of cervicitis, and complete emptying of the uterus at abortion. When asymptomatic Chlamydia is present in the cervix, the increase in postabortion infection is increased (Westergaard et al., 1982).

Trauma to the cervix may be caused by the use of laminaria and by forced mechanical dilatation. It may produce a degree of cervical incompetence following repeated cervical trauma.

Hemorrhage following induced abortion may be caused by retained products of conception, incomplete uterine involution, lacerations, or uterine perforations.

Delayed menses following abortion can be caused by either missed abortion, repeat pregnancy, hormonal imbalance, or emotional factors.

Future Pregnancies

There is no increased risk with subsequent pregnancy following suction curettage. There does seem to be a direct relationship between the number of previous abortions and the loss of subsequent pregnancies. Two or more induced abortions place the client at increased risk for future abortions or preterm deliveries (Schoenbaum et al., 1980).

Hydatidiform Mole

Hydatidiform mole is a placental development anomaly that results in a grapelike swelling of the chorionic villi from accumulation of fluid within the villi. The fertilized ovum degenerates and is retained within the uterus.

The cause is unknown, but hydatidiform moles occur more frequently in women over 40 years of age who have had three or more pregnancies. Incidence is approximately 1:2000 pregnancies. Moles are the most common condition preceding choriocarcinoma.

SYMPTOMS

Hydatidiform mole should be suspected when the following symptoms are noted:

The uterus is enlarged out of proportion to gestational age

Intermittent or continuous dark vaginal bleeding at about 12 weeks gestation

Excessive nausea and vomiting

No FHT

Elevated human chorionic gonadotropin (HCG) levels 100 days or more after the LNMP (normally, HCG should peak at 10 weeks gestation and remain at lower levels after 14 weeks)

Albuminuria, hypertension, or edema before 20 weeks gestation

Decreased hemoglobin and hematocrit levels

Vaginal expulsion of vesicular tissue

Diagnosis is confirmed with ultrasonography

MEDICAL AND NURSING INTERVENTIONS

If the woman does not wish to have more children, a hysterectomy is the treatment of choice, owing to the increased risk of choriocarcinoma development. If another pregnancy is desired, the uterus is evacuated with suction curettage.

Thorough explanations of the hydatidiform mole are given. Grief over the loss of the pregnancy is expected and must be worked through. Nursing assessments for ketosis or electrolyte imbalance from excessive nausea and vomiting, symptoms of toxemia, and blood loss are important.

Followup care following mole removal is essential and includes thorough explanations. HCG is measured weekly with 24-hour urine collections until the titers are negative for three consecutive weeks. HCG is measured once a month for six months, then once every six months. If HCG titers rise three to four months after termination of the pregnancy, chemotherapy is begun using either methotrexate or dactinomycin. Chest x-rays may be taken every month until HCG titers are negative, then every two months for one year. The woman must understand the importance of avoiding pregnancy until tests are negative for one year. Oral contraceptives are not usually used owing to the suppression of luteinizing hormone that could distort HCG titers.

Ectopic Pregnancy

Ectopic pregnancy is implantation of the blastocyst outside of the uterine cavity. About 95 percent of all ectopic pregnancies occur in the ampulla of the fallopian tube, although implantation can occur in the cervix, cornua, ovary, or abdomen (see Fig. 25–2).

INCIDENCE

The incidence of ectopic pregnancy has nearly tripled during the last decade, from about 17,800 cases in 1970 to about 52,000 cases in 1980 (Dorfman, 1980). This rise may be due to an increase in associated risk factors.

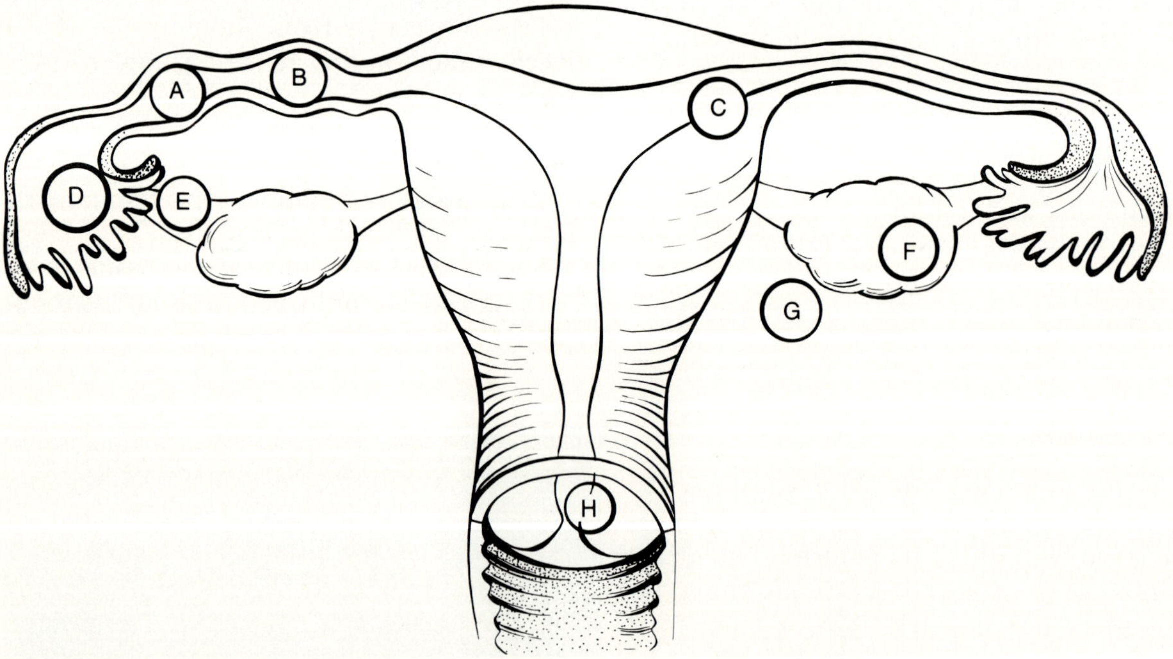

FIGURE 25–2. Sites of ectopic pregnancy implantation. A. Ampulla. B. Isthmus. C. Interstitial. D. Fimbria. E. Tuboovarian ligament. F. Ovary. G. Abdominal cavity. H. External cervical os.

RISK FACTORS

Anything that interferes with the normal transfer of the fertilized ovum into the endometrial cavity will increase the chances of ectopic pregnancy. A history of pelvic infection, previous abdominal or pelvic surgery, infertility, and use of a progestin-only oral contraceptive are all factors. Infantile fallopian tubes and congenital defects of the fallopian tubes also increase the incidence of ectopic pregnancies.

The use of intrauterine devices (IUD) has been implicated in ectopic pregnancies, especially use of the Dalkon shield (Lee et al., 1983), which is associated with pelvic inflammatory disease. Current IUD users have 0.8 times the risk, and past IUD users have 1.4 times the risk of having an ectopic pregnancy, compared with women who have never used an IUD (Ory, 1981). About 7 percent of ectopic pregnancies occur in women who have had previous tubal ligations (Snyder, 1983), possibly due to recanalization and reformation of a tubular structure over the passage of time.

SYMPTOMS IN TUBAL PREGNANCY

Before rupture of the tubal pregnancy, early pregnancy symptoms are usually present. The gravida may have breast tenderness, nausea, a positive pregnancy test, and an enlarged uterus. Decidual cells that are enlarged (Arias-Stella phenomenon) may be passed vaginally. Abdominal pain will be of a crampy or dull nature. Vaginal examination may reveal pain on cervical movement.

The classical picture of ectopic pregnancy—pain, vaginal bleeding, adnexal mass, and amenorrhea—is absent in more than half the patients. Other conditions may produce these same signs or symptoms, such as pelvic inflammatory disease, threatened abortion, incomplete abortion, ovarian cyst rupture, torsion of an ovarian cyst, and appendicitis.

When the tube ruptures, pain is sudden, severe, and unilateral. Pain may radiate to the shoulder and neck if internal bleeding has reached the level of the diaphragm. Nausea and vomiting may occur. Tachycardia and hypotension may be manifest. Temperature is usually normal or low. Leukocyte counts may be normal if only leakage is occurring, but they may be elevated following sudden hemorrhage. A vaginal examination reveals a tender adnexal mass and a full cul-de-sac. When the cervix is manipulated on vaginal examination, pain is present. Syncope occurs in about half of patients, as the so-called "bathroom sign" that is present when the patient strains to defecate, resulting from pressure on perineal nerves.

MEDICAL AND NURSING INTERVENTIONS

The first step in treatment of an ectopic pregnancy is to establish a diagnosis. A thorough history includes risk factors, recent medical or gynecologic problems, and symptoms.

Physical examination may or may not be helpful. An adnexal mass may be present from an ectopic pregnancy or the corpus luteum of a normal pregnancy.

Continual nursing assessments are needed to monitor any change in physical condition. Vital signs are taken and recorded at frequent intervals, and vaginal bleeding is assessed frequently with perineal pad counts.

A pregnancy test is performed. Rapid urine tests may not be sensitive enough to detect low hormone levels associated with an ectopic pregnancy, so blood should be drawn for radioimmunoassay testing. A positive pregnancy test will not identify the location of the pregnancy. Ultrasound will be helpful in diagnosis after the fifth week following the last menstrual period.

An intravenous line is established with a large bore needle. Laboratory studies including complete blood counts, and type and crossmatching of blood are ordered. The informed consent permits are signed and witnessed. Analgesics are administered as ordered for pain, since extremes of pain can precipitate shock.

Support and explanations of all activities and procedures are needed to reduce fear and anxiety. The client is prepared for surgery as appropriate. *Culdocentesis* (aspiration of fluid from the cul-de-sac of Douglas) will indicate intraperitoneal bleeding if bloody fluid is obtained. *Culdoscopy* will allow visualization of the pelvic organs. *Colpotomy,* incision through the posterior fornix, may be done to remove the fallopian tube. *Laparoscopy* is done when signs and symptoms suggest ectopic pregnancy. *Laparotomy* is the definitive treatment for ectopic pregnancy.

The choice of procedure varies with the location of the pregnancy, the length of gestation, and the patient's feelings about future fertility. If the ectopic pregnancy has not ruptured, surgery may be avoided if monitoring of beta-HCG levels shows a continuous decrease in values and symptoms resolve as the patient spontaneously aborts (Mashiach et al., 1982).

Postoperative nursing care is the same as for an abdominal laparotomy, including helping the patient and her support person to work through the grieving process following the loss of the pregnancy.

OTHER ECTOPIC SITES

Abdominal Pregnancy

Abdominal pregnancy probably results when a tubal pregnancy ruptures without loss of the pregnancy and without symptoms dramatic enough to indicate surgery. As the placenta develops, it can form over the peritoneum, into the bowel, or over the uterus. The greatest danger occurs after delivery, with placental removal. If the placenta is removed, there is no homeostatic mechanism to stop maternal bleeding. Most commonly, the placenta is left where it is and allowed to degenerate.

Cervical Pregnancy

About 1 percent of ectopic pregnancies implant in the cervix. Cervical pregnancies are frequently misdiagnosed because symptoms are similar to those of an incomplete abortion, with tissue present at the cervical os. If the tissue is removed, the cervical surface will bleed uncontrollably because the cervix does not contract. Hysterectomy may be necessary with a cervical pregnancy.

Cornual Pregnancy

Cornual or interstitial pregnancy does not usually rupture until after 12 weeks gestation because the cornual portion of the tube is more distensible. Owing to the longer length of gestation, rupture can involve the entire side of the uterus.

HYPERTENSIVE DISORDERS

Hypertensive disorders of pregnancy have been classified as follows:

- Pregnancy-induced hypertension
  - Mild preeclampsia
  - Severe preeclampsia
  - Eclampsia
- Chronic hypertension preceding pregnancy
- Chronic hypertension with superimposed pregnancy-induced hypertension
- Late or transient hypertension

Pregnancy-Induced Hypertension (PIH)

Pregnancy-induced hypertension (PIH) is a broad term for hypertensive disorders peculiar to pregnancy and includes mild preeclampsia, severe preeclampsia, and eclampsia.

DEFINITION

PIH appears after 20 weeks gestation and is characterized by three main signs or symptoms: hypertension, edema, and proteinuria. The degree of hypertension, edema and proteinuria present determine the degree of preeclampsia (mild or severe).

INCIDENCE

PIH occurs in approximately 5 percent of all pregnancies in the United States, and accounts for about 25,000 fetal and neonatal deaths per year. It is the second leading cause of maternal mortality in the United States today.

PREDISPOSING FACTORS

Many factors predispose to the development of PIH (see Table 25-6). A large number of these predisposing factors relate to exposure to chorionic villi for the first time, an excess of chorionic villi in certain complications of pregnancy, or the presence of a compromised maternal or fetal vascular system.

TABLE 25-6
PREDISPOSING FACTORS FOR PIH

PREPREGNANCY FACTORS
Preexisting hypertensive disease
Preexisting vascular disease
Preexisting renal disease
Low socioeconomic status
Family history of preeclampsia/eclampsia
Nulligravida
Diabetes mellitus
Age extremes: under 18 years
over 35 years
Black
PIH in previous pregnancies
Underweight
Obesity
Dietary deficiencies, especially iron deficiency anemia
ANTEPARTUM FACTORS
Hydatidiform mole
Fetal hydrops
Polyhydramnios
Primigravida
Multiple gestation
Poor nutritional status
Excessive weight gain
Glomerulonephritis
Large fetus
Emotional conflicts
Poor prenatal care

CLINICAL RISK FACTORS

Currently, two tests can aid in early diagnosis of PIH by predicting the risk of developing this complication in the primigravida.

Angiotensin II Test

The angiotensin II test is based on the fact that normal pregnant women are resistant to the pressor effect of angiotension II. Women at increased risk for PIH become progressively more sensitive to the pressor effects of infused angiotensin II after the 18th week of gestation.

Women who are identified as having predisposing factors for PIH are given angiotensin II by infusion during the 28th to 32nd weeks of gestation: If less than 8 mg per kg per minute of angiotensin II is needed to raise the diastolic pressure 20 mm Hg, the client has a 90 percent chance of developing PIH. Increased sensitivity to angiotensin II appears several weeks before any symptoms of PIH are noted.

This test is a fairly reliable clinical predictor of PIH, but requires highly specialized equipment and laboratory facilities.

Roll-Over Test

The Roll-Over test is another clinical tool used on selected primigravidas at 28 to 32 weeks gestation (Gant et al., 1980). The client is positioned in a left lateral recumbent position and the blood pressure is taken every 5 minutes until a baseline is obtained, usually about 20 minutes. The patient is then turned supine, and the blood pressure is taken every 5 minutes until stable. If the diastolic pressure rises 20 mm Hg, a positive response is obtained. Some 93 percent of women with a positive test develop PIH, while 91 percent with a negative test do not develop PIH.

Both the Roll-Over test and the angiotensin II test are useful clinical risk predictors for PIH, but have limited use. Early detection of PIH still depends upon client education and frequent antepartum evaluations of weight and blood pressure changes.

ETIOLOGY

The exact cause of PIH is unknown. There are many proposed theories as to etiology, but none are proven. The more commonly accepted etiologic theories include uteroplacental ischemia and an autoimmune process.

Uteroplacental ischemia is the result of vascular spasm. The placenta provides a mechanism for the regulation of B/P throughout pregnancy. If placental perfusion is decreased, there is less efficient inactivation of physiologic hypertensive agents and hypertension will result.

PIH is sometimes considered an autoimmune disease. The placenta is antigenic and reacts immunologically to the maternal organism.

FETAL EFFECTS

The risk to the fetus in PIH increases. Death before labor may occur owing to intrauterine hypoxia. There is an increased incidence of IUGR and congenital malformations. At the time of delivery, the neonate may appear pale and dehydrated, may exhibit signs of acute or chronic hypoxia, and may require resuscitation. In the neonatal period there is increased risk of jaundice, hypoglycemia, hypocalcemia, polycythemia, and respiratory distress.

Monitoring of fetal well-being is essential to ensure an optimal fetal outcome. Tests most commonly used to evaluate fetus status are discussed in Chapter 24 and include fetal movements, nonstress tests, contraction stress tests, ultrasonography, estriol and creatinine determinations, and amniocentesis.

PATHOPHYSIOLOGY

PIH is characterized by vasospasm with arteriolar vasoconstriction and increased peripheral resistance. These in turn affect almost all body organs and systems (see Table 25–7).

SYMPTOMS

The symptoms of PIH are traditionally considered a triad of hypertension, edema, and proteinuria. A diagnosis of PIH may be made without all three being present.

Hypertension is caused by arteriolar vasospasm that manifests itself by an elevated systolic and diastolic pressure. Hypertension may be defined as: (1) a B/P of 140/90 mm Hg taken on two occasions at least six hours apart; or (2) a 30 mm Hg systolic rise and/or a 15 mm Hg diastolic rise from the baseline parameters on two occasions at least six hours apart.

Edema is most commonly reflected in a sudden excessive weight gain. It is caused by retention of water and impairment of sodium excretion that results from impaired renal function. A weight gain in excess of 1 pound per week before 32 weeks gestation or more than 2.5 pounds per week after 34 weeks suggests preeclampsia.

TABLE 25-7
PATHOPHYSIOLOGIC CHANGES IN PIH

Placenta
- Small degenerative infarcts that release thromboplastin
- Increased number of retroplacental hematomas
- Cytotrophoblastic proliferation
- Thickened trophoblastic membrane
- Autolysis and clumping of nuclei of synctial cells
- Atherosclerosis of decidual arterioles
- Premature degenerative aging

Kidney
- Glomerular lesions with marked swelling of endothelial cells, narrowed capillaries, and fibrin deposits (glomerular endotheliosis)
- Kidney lesions responsible for proteinuria, decreased renal blood flow, and decreased glomerular filtration rates

Enlarged kidneys

Tubular changes include swelling, hyaline droplet degeneration, fatty changes, necrosis

Edema
- Plasma volume is lost to interstitial space and causes hypovolemia and a rise in hematocrit
- Fluid moves into interstitial and intracellular spaces with resultant facial, finger, and abdominal edema

Liver
- Irregular small areas of hemorrhage
- Local hemorrhages in periportal areas which may later be replaced by fibrin
- Various grades of ischemic lesions ranging from very small to large infarcts

Brain
- Edema
- Cerebral hemorrhage
- Vasospasms cause scotoma, diplopia, blurred vision, headache, and retinal spasms

Heart
- Small petechial hemorrhages

Lungs
- Small petechial hemorrhages
- Pulmonary congestion or edema

Adrenals
- Extensive petechial hemorrhages
- Thrombi
- Necrosis of cortex

Reflexes
- Hyperreflexia due to increased intracellular sodium and decreased intracellular potassium levels

Proteinuria is usually the last of the three symptoms to appear. Vasoconstriction of the afferent glomerular arterioles alters the permeability of the glomerular membrane and allows protein to escape into the urine. A concentration of 500 mg per liter or more in a clean catch urine specimen on two or more occasions at least six hours apart indicates proteinuria.

Differentiation of mild and severe preeclampsia is based on the severity of the symptoms (see Table 25-8).

MEDICAL AND NURSING INTERVENTIONS: MILD PREECLAMPSIA

Mild preeclampsia is most commonly treated conservatively and may be treated at home.

Bedrest in the left lateral recumbent position is advocated to improve uterine blood flow and increase the glomerular filtration rate. Blood pressure is monitored at specific intervals with an appropriate sized cuff at the same time of day on the same arm and in the same position. Arterial blood pressure varies with maternal position, with the lowest reading obtained in the left lateral recumbent position and the highest in the sitting position. Family members can be taught to take the B/P. If this is not feasible, home visits by the nurse will be needed to obtain B/P measurements.

Weight restriction, low sodium diets, and diuretics are no longer ordered for the client with PIH. Low maternal weight gain has been associated with low birth weight and fetal compromise. Sodium restriction and diuretic usage decreases blood volume when hypovolemia is already present and may further decrease placental perfusion.

The patient is weighed each day before breakfast and the weight recorded. The urine is tested for protein twice a day with reagant strips. Instructions include doing the evaluation in a room with a good light source. The bottle containing the strips is kept tightly closed.

TABLE 25-8
COMPARISON OF MILD AND SEVERE PREECLAMPSIA

	Mild Preeclampsia	Severe Preeclampsia
Blood pressure	>140/90 but <160/110 OR 30 mm Hg rise systolic 15 mm Hg rise diastolic on 2 occasions at least 6 hours apart	>160/110
Edema	+1 or +2 +1 = edema of pedal and pretibial areas +2 = edema of lower extremities	+3 or +4 +3 = edema of face, hands, lower abdominal wall, sacrum +4 = anasarca with ascites
Weight gain	1 to 5 pounds/week	Up to 11 pounds/week
Proteinuria	+1 or +2 500 mg/24 hours	+3 or +4 5 gm/24 hours
Oliguria	Absent	Present
Retinal changes: spasm ischemia edema	Some	Moderate
Reflexes: 4+ hyperactive 3+ brisk 2+ average response 1+ diminished response 0 no response	Hyperreflexia	Increasing hyperreflexia
Cerebral symptoms: headache scotoma diplopia	Occasional	Persistent with alteration of LOC
Epigastric distress	None	May be present
Temperature	Normal	Normal
Pulmonary edema	None	None
Peripheral resistance	Increased	Increased
Blood volume	Normal pregnancy levels	Decrease to prepregnancy levels
Hematocrit	Rises	Rises
Blood urea nitrogen	Normal	Normal or moderately elevated
Uric acid	Increased	>5 mg%
Creatinine	Increased	Increased
Thrombocytes	Decreased	Decreased
Prothrombin time	Slightly prolonged	Prolonged
Platelets	Normal	Decreased
Serum protein	Reversal of albumin/globulin ratio	Reversal of albumin/globulin ratio
Sodium	Slight hyponatremia	<120 mEq
SGOT	Increased	Increased
SGPT	Increased	Increased
Alkaline phosphatase	Increased	Increased

A high protein (75 to 80 gm) diet is recommended to replace protein lost in the urine. Excessive dietary salt is limited to 2 to 7 gm per day. Foods such as potato chips, prepared luncheon meats, and peanuts, which are high in sodium, should be avoided. Water intake of six to eight glasses per day is adequate.

Fetal status is assessed at frequent intervals to assure maintenance of adequate fetal oxygenation.

Areas of concern for the client are identified and discussed. She may feel well and not understand the importance of increasing rest periods. Even if she does not find resting in bed difficult during the initial days of treatment, as blood pressure stabilizes, she will experience a general sense of well-being and find it increasingly difficult to stay in bed. Provision of diversional activities to ease restlessness is important at this time. Sedation is not without its effects on the fetus and should not be used to combat boredom. The availability of help for the family is determined. Homemaker services may be needed to help with child care and housekeeping.

Significant symptoms to be reported to the physician immediately are taught and verbalized. These include increases in B/P, weight gain over 3 pounds in one week, 2+ or greater urine protein, headaches, scotoma, and diplopia.

MEDICAL AND NURSING INTERVENTIONS: SEVERE PREECLAMPSIA

Medical and nursing interventions in the care of the client with severe preeclampsia involve seven primary considerations: prevention of convulsions, reduction of vasospasm, identification and treatment of complications, prevention of ischemia of vital organs, delivery of an uncompromised neonate, provision of psychological and supportive care, and thorough explanations to the client and support persons.

The gravida with severe preeclampsia is hospitalized. If severe preeclampsia is not treated, it may progress to fetal death in utero from asphyxia and maternal death from disseminated intravascular coagulation, liver rupture, cerebrovascular accident, and abruptio placentae.

Bedrest in the left lateral recumbent position is highly encouraged. The left side lying position will prevent supine hypotension and improve renal function and urinary output. Up to 4 pounds may be lost in 24 hours from bedrest alone. Visitors may be restricted, and a quiet private room is ordered.

TABLE 25-9
PIH TRAY

EQUIPMENT
Ophthalmoscope
Syringes
Needles
Tourniquet
Alcohol wipes
Padded tongue blade
Plastic airway
Reflex hammer
Fetoscope
Oxygen
Suction
MEDICATIONS
Magnesium sulfate 50%
Sodium bicarbonate
Hydralazine
Heparin sodium
Diazepam
Chlordiazepoxide
Epinephrine
Atropine sulfate
Sterile water
Sterile saline
Calcium gluconate 10%
Phenytoin
Barbiturates

Fluids and electrolytes are monitored to keep a balance between correcting hypovolemia and preventing circulatory overload. The amount of fluid intake needed can be estimated by using 1000 ml plus the amount of urinary output of the previous 24 hour period. Electrolytes are replaced as needed.

A PIH tray is kept in the client's room (see Table 25-9). Laboratory values are obtained on admission and at frequent intervals (often every two to four hours). The hematocrit is assessed for elevation because of intravascular volume depletion. Determinations of the blood urea nitrogen (BUN) and serum creatinine are done to assess kidney function. Uric acid levels are watched to assess the severity of the PIH. Clotting studies are done to note the presence of DIC. Thrombocytopenia may be present, as may low platelet values.

Nursing responsibilities in caring for the patient with severe preeclampsia are outlined in Table 25-10.

TABLE 25-10
NURSING RESPONSIBILITIES IN SEVERE PREECLAMPSIA

Initial patient assessment
Bed rest in left lateral recombent position
Laboratory testing as ordered
Weigh daily at same time
Accurate intake and output (Foley catheter may be ordered with hourly outputs)
PIH tray in patient room
Temperature every 4 hours or prn
B/P, pulse, respirations every 2 to 4 hours or prn
Urine for protein and specific gravity
Assess edema
Auscultate lungs
Check deep tendon reflexes
Assess uterine contraction status
Assess for CNS symptoms
Side rails up
Daily fundoscopic examinations
Administer medications as ordered
Thorough explanation to patient and support persons
NPO
Intravenous fluids as ordered by infusion pump
Continuous FHR and uterine contraction monitoring
Assist with tests for fetal well-being
Maintain quiet environment

Drug Therapy

The two most commonly prescribed medications for PIH are magnesium sulfate and hydralazine (see Table 25-11). Other medications may be prescribed in an effort to improve PIH and prevent progression to eclampsia. Barbiturates act by decreasing catecholamine output and conserving oxygen utilization by their calming effects. They are sometimes given to help relax the client and aid in maintenance of bedrest.

Reserpine (Serpasil) is a potent antihypertensive agent, but it is usually avoided during pregnancy because it freely crosses the placental barrier. Neonates will have symptoms of nasal stuffiness, bradycardia, respiratory distress, hypothermia, and abnormal muscle tone.

Aldomet is primarily used for the PIH client with acute hypertension who has been brought under control with vasodilators and requires maintenance therapy to prevent blood pressure elevations. Propranolol has no role in PIH management because of the increased fetal hazards of hypoglycemia, bradycardia, and respiratory depression at birth.

Delivery

Delivery is the definitive treatment for PIH. If the client's condition is stable, oxytocin induction is attempted. If the induction fails or if the maternal or fetal condition is deteriorating, a cesarean section is performed.

TABLE 25-11
DRUG THERAPY IN SEVERE PREECLAMPSIA

MAGNESIUM SULFATE

Action: Anticonvulsant
Acts as a central nervous depressant by blocking neuromuscular transmission and decreasing the amount of acetylcholine liberated
Not an antihypertensive
Relaxes smooth muscle, thus decreases B/P and induces uterine relaxation

Dosage and Administration:
IM Regimen: 10 gm 50% solution as loading dose then 5 gm IM q 4 hours
Combined Regimen: 2 to 4 gm 10% solution slowly IV **then** 10 gm 50% solution IM
IV regimen: 4 gm of 10% solution IVPB as loading dose over 20 minutes **then** 1 to 3 gm/hour IV solution via infusion pump
Therapeutic Plasma levels: 3 to 9 mg/dl

Adverse Reactions: Drowsiness, flushing, diaphoresis, decreases reflexes, oliguria, respiratory paralysis, circulatory collapse. Adverse reactions most commonly develop at plasma levels over 10 mg/dl (8.3 mEq/L)

Elimination: Via the kidneys
Do not give if severe renal impairment is present

Fetal Effects: FHR tracing will show decreased or increased variability and tachycardia
Fetal magnesium levels are 96% of maternal levels
Assess neonate for magnesium toxicity: hypotonia, respiratory distress

Nursing Implications: Continuous electronic fetal monitoring
Do not leave alone
Left side-lying position
Quiet nonstimulating environment
Have injectable calcium gluconate [1 gm (10 ml of a 10% calcium gluconate solution) administered IV over 3 minutes] drawn up as antidote
Accurate intake and output
Have resuscitation equipment available
B/P, P, R q 5 to 15 minutes
Assess patellar reflexes q hour and prn
Assess LOC
Assess symptoms
PIH tray at bedside
Offer explanations to patient and support person
Withhold dose and notify physician if:
- respirations $<$ 12 to 14/minute
- urine output $<$ 30 ml/hour
- decreasing patellar reflexes
- hypotension

Magnesium sulfate will be continued for at least 24 hours postpartum

HYDRALAZINE (APRESOLINE)

Actions: Antihypertensive that directly relaxes vascular smooth muscle
Reduces peripheral vascular resistance
Increases renal and cerebral blood flow
Decreases diastolic pressure more than systolic

Dosage and Administration: IV: 100 mg in 1000ml normal saline titrated at 6 to 12 mg/hour via infusion pump to maintain the desired B/P
IV Push: 5 to 10 mg slow IV
IM: 5 to 10 mg

Adverse Reactions: Headache, palpitations, anginal pain, tachycardia, nausea, vomiting, diaphoresis, diarrhea

Fetal Effects: Hypotonia in the fetus if the maternal blood pressure falls precipitously

TABLE 25-11 (continued)

	HYDRALAZINE (APRESOLINE) (continued)
Nursing Implications:	Monitor B/P q 2 to 3 minutes until B/P stabilized, then every 15 minutes Continuous electronic fetal monitoring Assess mental status: note anxiety, depression Monitor intake and output Assess for edema Contraindicated in hypersensitivity, rheumatic heart disease, tachycardia, lupus erythematosus

ECLAMPSIA

If left untreated or inadequately treated, preeclampsia will often progress to eclampsia. The symptoms that indicate eclampsia development are: (1) epigastric pain, indicating ischemia in areas served by the major abdominal vessels; (2) oliguria progressing to anuria, indicating increasing renal impairment; (3) hyperactive reflexes, indicating increasing cerebrovascular resistance; (4) increasing CNS symptoms, indicating increases in cerebral edema; and (5) restlessness.

Eclamptic convulsions usually begin with facial twitching, progress to tonic-clonic convulsive activity, and are followed by a comatose period lasting a variable length of time. Nursing interventions during an eclamptic convulsion include: (1) insert a padded tongue blade to protect the tongue; (2) protect the client from injury by using padded siderails or placing a pillow between her and the rails; (3) release or loosen restraints to prevent injury; (4) insert an oral airway after the convulsion to maintain a patent airway; (5) position client on her side to facilitate drainage of secretions and prevent aspiration; (6) suction as needed; (7) restrict oral intake and maintain IV line; and (8) monitor maternal and fetal status.

Intravenous diazepam (Valium) may be used as an anticonvulsant in eclampsia. A central nervous system depressant, it acts on parts of the limbic system, thalamus, and hypothalamus. The drawback is that the fetus cannot metabolize the medication and decreased sucking ability, hypotonia, and impaired thermoregulation may be present for several days after birth.

Following a convulsion, amnesia is common. Respirations may increase to 50 per minute and cyanosis is usually present. Poor prognostic signs include hyperthermia, pulmonary edema, or tachycardia.

Approximately 25 percent of eclampsia occurs antepartum, 50 percent intrapartum, and 25 percent postpartum. To prevent postpartum eclampsia, magnesium sulfate is continued for 24 to 48 hours after delivery. Particular care must be taken to avoid excessive blood loss. A moderate blood loss may be devastating to the patient with PIH owing to the reduced circulating blood volume before delivery.

Medical and nursing management of the eclamptic patient includes the following: (1) treat the convulsions with magnesium sulfate, thiopental sodium, amobarbital sodium, or diazepam; (2) control the blood pressure; (3) stabilize maternal condition in a non-stimulating environment; (4) monitor maternal vital signs with central venous pressure (CVP) and/or pulmonary artery wedge pressure (PAWP) catheters; (5) assess lungs for the development of pulmonary edema; (6) monitor urinary output; (7) support client and support persons; and (8) deliver the fetus.

Chronic Hypertension Preceding Pregnancy

Chronic hypertension is defined as a blood pressure of 140/90 before pregnancy, or a blood pressure of 140/90 before 20 weeks gestation that persists indefinitely following delivery.

SYMPTOMS

Blood pressure elevations are present without proteinuria or edema. Retinopathy with arteriovenous nicking (constriction of retinal vessels) and torturous arterioles is usually present.

MATERNAL PROGNOSIS

Five groups of patients with chronic hypertension have a poor prognosis during pregnancy, including those having: (1) accompanying cardiac enlargement; (2) decreased renal function; (3) old retinal changes; (4) initial systolic pressure of 180 mm Hg or more; and (5) a history of superimposed preeclampsia with the previous pregnancy.

FETAL EFFECTS

About 33 percent of chronic hypertensive patients have previable preterm infants or stillborns. Infants born alive commonly suffer from intrauterine growth retardation (IUGR).

MEDICAL AND NURSING INTERVENTIONS

During the antepartal period, these clients are seen every two to three weeks until 32 weeks gestation, then weekly. Teaching includes the importance of increased rest periods in bed lying in the left lateral recumbent position. The client is encouraged to stop working and to stop smoking.

Antihypertensive agents are avoided, if at all possible, since they further reduce placental perfusion and increase fetal risks. Antihypertensive drugs of choice are hydralazine and methyldopa, if medication must be given to control the blood pressure. If diuretics only are used prior to pregnancy for blood pressure control, they are usually continued. Thiazides are the diuretics of choice, even though they may raise serum uric acid and urea levels and mask early PIH symptoms.

The gravida with chronic hypertension is admitted to the hospital when: (1) there is evidence of superimposed preeclampsia; (2) there is sustained or severe B/P elevation; (3) retinal hemorrhage or exudates are detected; (4) proteinuria is noted in the absence of urinary tract infection; (5) blood urea or uric acid levels increase; (6) there is a history of previous intrauterine fetal death; (7) intrauterine growth retardation is present; (8) placental function tests decrease; and (9) weight gain abnormality indicated by change in the rate of gain, no weight gain, or excessive weight gain occurs.

Fetal status is monitored regularly. An ultrasound examination is undertaken prior to 30 weeks gestation and again at 34 weeks to assess for intrauterine growth retardation. Beginning at 32 weeks gestation, fetal maturity studies are done. Nonstress testing is done weekly, starting at 30 to 32 weeks. The fetus is delivered if intrauterine growth retardation is present and the fetal lungs are mature, if fetal distress develops, or if maternal hypertension is worsening.

Chronic Hypertension with Superimposed PIH

When preeclampsia is superimposed on chronic hypertension, fetal mortality approaches 20 percent. There is a rapid progression to eclampsia, often before 30 weeks gestation.

MEDICAL AND NURSING INTERVENTIONS

When PIH is diagnosed, the client is admitted to the hospital and placed on bed rest in the left lateral recumbent position.

Phenobarbital may be ordered for sedation. Laboratory tests include complete blood count, BUN, creatinine, uric acid, peripheral blood smear, platelet count, SGOT, urine protein, and 24-hour urine for total protein and creatinine on admission and repeated as the client's condition warrants.

Magnesium sulfate is administered intravenously to aid in controlling maternal B/P and is continued until 24 to 48 hours after delivery. If the blood pressure exceeds 160/110, hydralazine may be administered by intermittent bolus.

If the preeclampsia is mild, the fetus is monitored with serial ultrasounds and nonstress testing, and delivery is accomplished as soon as possible. With severe preeclampsia, labor is induced as soon as the mother's condition has been stabilized.

Late or Transient Hypertension

This category includes patients with transient hypertension during labor or early puerperium that returns to normal within 10 days postpartum.

URINARY TRACT DISORDERS

Urinary Tract Infections

It is estimated that 5 to 10 percent of all gravidas have a urinary tract infection at some point during pregnancy. The predominant organism in the majority of these infections is Escherichia coli. Urinary tract infections most commonly seen are asymptomatic bacteriuria, acute cystitis, and acute pyelonephritis. Many urinary tract infections go undiagnosed during pregnancy because the symptoms are unrecognized or unreported.

Contributing factors in the development of urinary tract infections are the same as the normal alterations that occur during pregnancy. Relaxation of smooth muscle allows urine to accumulate in the urinary system and to become stagnant. As the enlarging uterus compresses the ureters, stagnation and obstruction result. The increased nutrient content of the urine during pregnancy creates a good culture medium.

Certain women are at increased risk for developing urinary tract infections during pregnancy: those with a history of prior infections, diabetes mellitus, sickle cell trait, urinary tract anomalies, anemia, renal stones, and prior oral contraceptive usage.

Fetal effects from urinary tract infections range from none, to preterm deliveries related to activation of prostaglandins by bacterial wall enzymes or underlying renal pathology, to the effects of the various antibiotics used to treat the maternal infection.

ASYMPTOMATIC BACTERIURIA

Asymptomatic bacteriuria is defined as a colony count of 100,000 microorganisms per ml in a clean catch midstream voided urine specimen; it is found in 3 to 12 percent of all pregnant women. Women with asymptomatic bacteriuria have an increased incidence of anatomic anomalies of the upper urinary tract and previous urinary tract infections. About one-fourth of these women develop a symptomatic urinary tract infection during pregnancy. There is a relationship between asymptomatic bacteriuria, preterm labor, and intrauterine growth retardation.

Medical and Nursing Interventions

A clean catch midstream voided urine specimen is obtained at the first prenatal visit. Urine is cultured for colony count and increased white cell content. If bacteriuria is present, treatment is a single dose regimen of either amoxicillin

(Larotid) or sulfamethoxazole/trimethoprim (Bactrim, Septra) (Ronald, 1984).

Client education is of prime importance. She is taught symptoms (fever, chills, urgency, burning upon urination, nausea, vomiting) that are to be reported immediately. Good personal hygiene, which includes wiping the perineum from front to back after voiding or defecation, proper cleansing of the genitalia, and wearing of clean cotton underwear, is stressed. An increase in fluid intake exclusive of those fluids high in sugar to avoid urinary stasis is emphasized, as is a well-balanced diet with sufficient protein and carbohydrates. Daily vitamin C to promote healing, a glass of cranberry juice at bedtime to acidify the urine, foods high in iron, and avoidance of coffee, tea, alcohol, and spices are all recommended.

Followup urine cultures are obtained to identify gravidas with bacteriuria. If bacteriuria is found, a longer regimen of drug therapy may be required with ampicillin or nitrofurantoin (Macrodantin). The importance of completing the full course of medication ordered is emphasized.

CYSTITIS

Cystitis is diagnosed by the presence of clinical symptoms of urgency, frequency of urination, dysuria, and positive urine cultures. Temperature is not elevated and costovertebral angle is not tender. Cystitis occurs in 1.3 percent of pregnant women (Harris and Gilstrap, 1981), most commonly during the second trimester.

Diagnosis

Diagnosis of acute cystitis is confirmed by the presence of white cells, bacteria, and red cells in the urine. Culture and sensitivities tested in a catheterized specimen often reveal E. coli as the predominant organism.

Medical and Nursing Interventions

Oral antimicrobial and antibacterial medications are ordered, pending the results of the urine culture and sensitivity. Client education includes the importance of taking all medication prescribed. When the results of the culture and sensitivity are completed, the gravida is notified of any change in the medication.

An increase in fluid intake and a well-balanced diet are important. Instructions are given regarding personal hygiene measures: good perineal hygiene, clean cotton underpants, emptying the bladder frequently, and avoidance of tight underwear.

Repeat urine cultures are obtained upon completion of the prescribed medication and at specified intervals during the remainder of pregnancy.

ACUTE PYELONEPHRITIS

Acute pyelonephritis occurs in approximately 2 percent of all pregnant women (Gilstrap et al., 1981). Onset of symptoms is usually sudden, with a high temperature (104+°F), chills, and costovertebral angle pain that extends into the flank. The client may complain of anorexia, malaise, nausea, vomiting, and abdominal distention.

Pyelonephritis has a greater incidence in primigravidas, women with an obstetrical history of difficult labors, diabetes mellitus, and sickle cell trait. It usually occurs after 12 weeks gestation and is most commonly caused by E. coli.

Signs of uterine hyperirritability that stimulate preterm labor may exist. Decreased urinary output related to edema of the renal parenchyma or ureteral obstructions may be noted and a catheterized urinalysis will show proteinuria and numerous red blood cells, white blood cells, and bacteria. A complete blood count will show an increase in the white blood cells.

Medical and Nursing Interventions

Clients with pyelonephritis are hospitalized. A catheterized urine specimen is obtained for urinalysis, culture, and sensitivity. Antibiotics are started immediately, with the antibiotic order changed if necessary after sensitivities are reported.

Complete bedrest in a left lateral position is ordered to increase uterine and fetal perfusion. Adequate hydration with strict intake and output monitoring is imperative to prevent dehydration and decreased renal perfusion. Analgesics are administered as needed to keep the client comfortable. Maternal vital signs and fetal heart tones are monitored frequently.

If the pyelonephritis fails to respond to therapy after 72 hours, an ultrasound or a one-film excretory urogram may be ordered to rule out other pathology.

The incidence of repeated pyelonephritis during the same pregnancy has been reported as high as 23 percent (Gilstrap et al., 1981). Clients with persistent or recurrent urinary tract infection are evaluated after 12 weeks postpartum for further renal problems.

Other Urinary Tract Disorders

ACUTE GLOMERULONEPHRITIS

Acute glomerulonephritis is relatively uncommon during pregnancy, occurring once in every 40,000 pregnancies. When it occurs in early pregnancy, fetal loss is common. Later in pregnancy, it is sometimes mistaken for PIH.

CHRONIC GLOMERULONEPHRITIS

During pregnancy, maternal treatment is based on laboratory and clinical findings, which are carefully monitored. A high-protein, low-sodium diet is usually ordered. Antihypertensive agents are prescribed to control rising blood pressure. Renal function is monitored frequently. The disease process is irreversible, and maternal condition will not improve following pregnancy.

The primary risk is to the fetus, however. If there is no hypertension or renal failure, 90 percent of neonates will survive. There is increased risk of spontaneous abortion, preterm labor, or intrauterine death. Maternal uterine vascular changes and placental lesions occur with chronic glomerulonephritis and lead to placental insufficiency and IUGR.

PREEXISTING RENAL DISEASE

Pregnancies in women with preexisting renal disease usually are completed successfully if renal dysfunction is minimal and no hypertension exists. Overall, pregnancy does not affect the natural course of the renal disease. When renal insufficiency exists prior to conception, complications occur more frequently, and there is association with spontaneous abortions, PIH, preterm labors, and an increase in intrauterine and neonatal deaths.

URINARY CALCULI

Urinary calculi occur in 1 in 1500 pregnancies (Lattanzi & Cook, 1980). Signs and symptoms are comparable to those seen in the nonpregnant client and occur more frequently during the second and third trimester. Spontaneous passage occurs in more than 50 percent of cases, so conservative therapy is usually indicated.

RESPIRATORY DISORDERS

Influenza

Influenza is an acute viral infection characterized by respiratory and constitutional symptoms. It is one of the most common viral infections that complicate pregnancy. Influenza may take a mild self-limiting course or may take a severe course, with reduction in the vital capacity of the lungs and tracheobronchitis or pneumonia.

Management of uncomplicated influenza is symptomatic, with close observation for development of complications. When complications occur, hospitalization is needed for intravenous antibiotics, and close monitoring of pulmonary function and blood gases. Annual vaccination is recommended only for high-risk individuals. Active immunization with an attenuated vaccine should not be injected during pregnancy because of potential teratogenic effects. Inactivated virus preparations are commonly used and are considered safe for pregnancy use.

FETAL EFFECTS

Fetal effects include an increased incidence of spontaneous abortions and preterm labor. Occasional association of influenza with congenital defects, specifically anencephaly and meningomyelocele have been reported.

Bronchial Asthma

Pregnant asthmatics have a slightly increased incidence of hyperemesis gravidarum, pregnancy-induced hypertension, hemorrhage, and complicated labors. The major concern in pregnant asthmatics is maintenance of maternal and fetal oxygenation. Treatment of asthma includes relief of hypoxemia by oxygen administration, decrease in airway obstruction with bronchodilators, and providing adequate hydration.

Asthma symptoms may improve, not change, or worsen during pregnancy. Typically, improvement will occur early in pregnancy, with exacerbations seen most frequently during the second and third trimesters. Gravidas with chronic asthma need to identify and avoid factors that may precipitate attacks: inhaled allergens, irritants, emotional stress, steroid withdrawal, and smoking. Desensitization may be started or may continue throughout pregnancy. Bronchoconstricting medications should be avoided. Serial ultrasounds can detect IUGR. Respiratory infections are treated vigorously to prevent acute asthma attacks that may threaten the fetus.

DRUG THERAPY

If the client is already taking medications and has the asthma under control, the regimen is normally maintained throughout pregnancy, unless there are specific contraindications to the medications.

If control of asthma is necessary during pregnancy, a stepwise program may be instituted (Hernandez, Angella, Johnson, 1980). Each agent is added separately and the dosage gradually increased until the maximum therapeutic effect is obtained. Dosage is titrated to desired blood levels.

Adrenergic drugs are useful in controlling asthma through the bronchodilation they produce. Theoretically, these drugs should be avoided during pregnancy because the associated peripheral vasodilatation may shunt blood from the fetus, but the significance of this is not known (Whipkey et al., 1984). Epinephrine should be avoided during pregnancy owing to its teratogenic effects. Isoproterenol, terbutaline, metaproterenol, aminophylline, and theophylline are not associated with adverse fetal effects (Berkowitz et al., 1981), although theophylline toxicity in neonates (tachycardia, irritability, jitteriness, gagging, and vomiting) have been reported. Corticosteroids can also be given for short intervals during pregnancy when indicated.

FETAL EFFECTS

The increase in perinatal mortality and morbidity rates depend on the severity of the maternal disease. There is a higher incidence of spontaneous abortion, preterm delivery, stillbirth, perinatal mortality, and infant mortality (Turner et al., 1980). Neurologic abnormalities are noted twice as often, and neonates of asthmatic mothers have a higher incidence of asthma and severe respiratory distress.

Tuberculosis

Tuberculosis is an infectious disease caused by *Mycobacterium tuberculosis*. The incidence of tuberculosis in the United States varies with geographic and socioeconomic situations. A higher risk of tuberculosis exists in low-income overcrowded urban areas, on Indian reservations, and among Middle Eastern and Asian immigrants.

A careful initial assessment will aid in identifying the gravida at risk. Risk factors include a previous history of tuberculosis, pleural effusion, contact with known tuberculosis clients, chronic liver disease, and severe psychological stress. If recognized and treated promptly, tuberculosis does not have a deleterious effect on pregnancy, nor does pregnancy worsen tuberculosis. All prenatal clients should be given the skin test for tuberculosis unless they have a prior history of the disease. If the test is negative, no further testing is needed. If the test is positive, a chest x-ray is done with proper shielding, and cytologic evaluation of sputum is undertaken to rule out fungal infections or carcinoma of the lung. If these are negative, no further testing is done.

When tuberculosis is inactive in the gravida under 35 years of age, treatment with isoniazid and pyridoxine is begun following delivery and continued for one year. If active tuberculosis is present, the gravida is hospitalized and chemotherapy is started with isoniazid, ethambutol, and pyridoxine. If cultures are negative after eight weeks of therapy, chemotherapy can be discontinued.

NURSING INTERVENTIONS

Appropriate nursing interventions for the patient with tuberculosis include explanations of the causative factors of the disease and the importance of compliance with the medical regimen. The client is taught the importance of covering her nose and mouth while sneezing or coughing. Undue stresses are reduced or eliminated. Good nutrition during pregnancy is important for maternal and fetal health. All active cases are reported to the Board of Health.

Pneumonia

The significance of pneumonia as a risk during pregnancy has been minimized by appropriate treatment with antibiotics. The hazards to the mother and fetus occur as a result of cyanosis, reduced oxygen content of the maternal blood, bacteremia, and transplacental infection.

Prenatal education of the gravida includes the importance of avoiding contact with individuals with respiratory infections. If pneumonia does develop, hospitalization and antibiotics are needed. When antibiotics are prescribed, special attention to fetal effects is important. Nursing care during pneumonia is the same as in the nonpregnant client, with the additional monitoring of fetal status.

AUTOIMMUNE DISEASES

Systemic Lupus Erythematosus

Systemic lupus erythematosus (SLE) is a diffuse multisystem autoimmune disease characterized by the production of antibodies by an affected individual against her autologous DNA. It occurs in two or three individuals per 100,000 and affects young females.

MATERNAL EFFECTS

Pregnancy itself probably exerts no consistent influence on the course of SLE, although there is an increased incidence of exacerbation during the puerperium. Effects of SLE on pregnancy include an increased incidence of spontaneous abortions and pregnancy-induced hypertension.

FETAL EFFECTS

There is an increased incidence of stillbirth, preterm delivery, and low birth weights. Congenital heart block has also been associated with SLE.

MEDICAL AND NURSING INTERVENTIONS

Most clients are counseled to postpone conception until at least two years after diagnosis of SLE. During pregnancy, serum complement levels (C_3 and C_4) are monitored at monthly intervals. A fall in the complement levels may signify the onset of an exacerbation. The 24-hour urine protein excretion and creatinine clearance tests are performed at monthly intervals to monitor renal status. Careful monitoring of the uterine height at each prenatal visit is important. Ultrasound examinations are done at 18 to 22 weeks, 30 to 32 weeks, and 36 to 38 weeks, to monitor fetal growth. The mainstay of therapy is corticosteroid administration in the lowest doses compatible with control of the disease. The importance of taking the prescribed medication is emphasized to the client. At about 32 weeks gestation, weekly fetal heart rate testing with nonstress tests are started to monitor fetal status in utero.

During labor and delivery, continuous fetal heart rate and uterine contraction monitoring is necessary. A fetal heart rate of 60 to 80 beats per minute may indicate congenital heart block with hypoxia, but fetal blood sampling is done to verify the diagnosis. Intravenous hydrocortisone is given to limit the chance of exacerbation.

Rheumatoid Arthritis

For a large percentage of women with rheumatoid arthritis, symptoms will dramatically improve during pregnancy, possibly related to increased free cortisol blood levels associated with normal pregnancy. Rheumatoid factors (IgM antibodies against autologous IgG) do not cross the placenta. There is usually no fetal or neonatal involvement.

Medical and nursing interventions during pregnancy are aimed at maintaining adequate rest and exercise, heat, physical therapy, and salicylates as tolerated. Aspirin is the most common therapy used, even though mild hemostatic changes in the neonate and slightly prolonged length of gestation may be noted.

Myasthenia Gravis

Myasthenia gravis is a chronic autoimmune neuromuscular disorder characterized by fatigue and weakness, especially of the facial, pharyngeal, and respiratory muscles.

MATERNAL EFFECTS

During pregnancy regular rest periods and limited physical activity are important. Anticholinergic medications are used for control of symptoms. Signs and symptoms of infection are aggressively treated to prevent exacerbation, with avoidance of the aminoglycosides to prevent precipitation of myasthenic crisis.

Labor often progresses normally since smooth muscle is not affected by the disease process. Assisted ventilation must be readily available in the event of sudden respiratory difficulty. The established medication regimen is maintained in parenteral form. The gravida with myasthenia gravis is very sensitive to sedatives, analgesics, tranquilizers, and narcotics. Magnesium sulfate is contraindicated because of the decrease in the effect of acetylcholine, which may precipitate a crisis.

NEONATAL EFFECTS

Approximately 20 percent of neonates born to women with myasthenia gravis exhibit neonatal myasthenia (Plauchi, 1979). Symptoms usually do not develop until the first or second day of life and are caused by transplacental transfer of acetylcholine-blocking factor. The neonate will exhibit muscular weakness, hypotonic extremities, and appear limp with a weak Moro reflex, a feeble cry, and an inability to suck, swallow, and breathe for several days.

Idiopathic Thrombocytopenic Purpura

Idiopathic thrombocytopenic purpura (ITP) is an autoimmune hemolytic disorder characterized by an abnormally low platelet level, owing to production of antiplatelet antibodies that shorten the platelet life span.

MATERNAL EFFECTS

Maternal problems include petechiae and bleeding from various body sites, especially from episiotomies and abdominal or uterine incisions.

FETAL EFFECTS

The antiplatelet antibody can cross the placenta and cause thrombocytopenia (platelet count <100,000 mm^3) in approximately half of neonates. Clinical manifestations of bleeding are noted as hematuria or intracranial hemorrhage.

MEDICAL AND NURSING INTERVENTIONS

All gravidas should have a platelet count as part of their initial prenatal laboratory work. If ITP is diagnosed, steroids are used to bring platelet counts to normal and to maintain the maternal platelet count above 100,000 per mm^3. In rare instances, a splenectomy may be needed if there is no response to steroids and the disease becomes life-threatening.

Client education during the prenatal period focuses on the importance of taking medications exactly as prescribed. Scrupulous hygiene to avoid infection caused by decreased antibody production is necessary. In gravidas with a family history of diabetes, hyperglycemia and glycosuria may occur. Corticosteroids may be prescribed during the later weeks of pregnancy to help prevent thrombocytopenia (Karpatkin et al., 1981), but the results are not always predictable (Cines et al., 1982). Infusions of high-dose gamma globulin have been found to increase platelet counts in gravidas with ITP (Tchernia et al., 1984) late in pregnancy or during labor and delivery.

During labor, a fetal scalp blood platelet count is obtained to help determine the optimal method of delivery. According to the fetal platelet count, labor can be allowed to proceed, or cesarean section may be done to prevent fetal intracranial hemorrhage during vaginal delivery.

VASCULAR DISORDERS

Thromboembolic Disorders

Thromboembolic disease in the gravida may develop in the pelvic veins and femoral system, and occurs as a thrombosis associated with *thrombophlebitis* (vessel wall inflammation) or as a *phlebothrombosis* (clot without vessel involvement).

Development occurs most often in the puerperium secondary to pelvic cellulitis or a traumatic delivery, but may also occur during the second trimester of pregnancy at about 26 weeks gestation. Despite the normal increase in clotting factors and decrease in fibrinolytic activity during pregnancy, about 0.18 to 2.9

antepartum women per 1,000 develop thromboembolic disease. Predisposing factors include obesity and advancing maternal age.

MEDICAL AND NURSING INTERVENTIONS

The gravida with thromboembolic disease should be hospitalized with complete bed rest ordered. The lower extremities are elevated, avoiding the use of pillows and without flexing the knees. Temperature, pulse, respirations, and B/P are monitored every four hours. FHT are measured and recorded every shift. She is assisted to turn, cough, and breathe deeply every two hours, and the chest is auscultated every four hours. Moist heat is applied as ordered, and circulation in the affected extremity is assessed every four hours.

Anticoagulant Therapy

Anticoagulants are administered as ordered. Warfarin sodium crosses the placenta readily and increases the risk of fetal hemorrhage in utero. Dicumarol has been implicated in fetal eye anomalies, incomplete nasal development, respiratory distress, mental retardation, and blindness.

Subcutaneous or intravenous heparin is prescribed for treatment of thromboembolic disease during pregnancy. Subcutaneous heparin doses are usually ordered individually after coagulation studies are assessed. Onset of action is seen in about two to four hours. Intravenous heparin has an onset of action within minutes of administration. Baseline blood coagulation tests and a complete blood count are done before therapy is initiated, and one half hour before each scheduled subcutaneous or intermittent intravenous dose and every four hours with continuous intravenous administration.

CARDIAC DISEASE

The incidence of cardiac disease during pregnancy is about 2 percent in the United States, with the majority of the gravidas having established cardiac disease at the time of conception.

Rheumatic heart disease and congenital heart disease account for the largest percentage of cardiac disease complicating pregnancy. Other forms include arteriosclerotic heart disease, hypertensive heart disease, and coronary artery disease. Although each of these requires specific medical and nursing management, general principles of management apply to all pregnant cardiac clients.

Significance

Pregnancy outcome for the gravida with cardiac disease is usually favorable, as long as a balance between cardiac load and cardiac reserve is maintained. Certain burdens on the heart cannot be altered during pregnancy (see Table 25–12). These physiologic changes impose an increased burden on the already compromised heart. Labor adds an additional strain, with an increase in cardiac output, pulmonary capillary wedge pressure, and peripheral blood pressure during uterine contractions. Immediately following delivery there is remobilization of extravascular fluid into the maternal blood stream and a significant increase (about 60 percent) in cardiac output.

TABLE 25–12
ANTEPARTAL PHYSIOLOGICAL CHANGES THAT AFFECT CARDIOVASCULAR FUNCTION

Cardiac output increases by 35 percent (peaks at about 28 weeks gestation)
Plasma volume increases 40 to 50 percent
Oxygen requirement increases 20 to 25 percent
Sodium retention increases up to 900 mEq
Water retention
Red cell volume increases 20 to 32 percent
Pulse rate increases an average of 10 to 15 BPM
Weight gain

Classification

Maternal outcome for the pregnant cardiac client depends on maternal age, duration of the cardiac problem, and the functional capacity of the heart at the beginning of pregnancy.

Prior to pregnancy, the client is assigned to a class of cardiac disease. She is reevaluated for change in classification during antepartal care.

Class I. Cardiac disease without limitations on physical activity. Ordinary activity does not cause undue fatigue, dyspnea, palpitations, or angina.

Class II. Cardiac disease with some limitation of physical activity. Ordinary activity results in some fatigue, dyspnea, palpitations, or anginal pain.

Class III. Cardiac disease with marked limitation of physical activity. Less than ordinary activity results in fatigue, dyspnea, palpitations, or angina.

Class IV. Cardiac disease with inability to carry on any physical activity without discomfort.

Maternal Mortality

Certain factors affect maternal mortality. Adequate medical and nursing supervision is the most important factor, since classification can change rapidly as pregnancy progresses. Age is a factor—women with cardiac disease are more prone to cardiac failure as they get older. The incidence of heart failure is directly related to the interval between the first symptoms of cardiac disease and the onset of pregnancy. The cardiac client with minimal heart enlargement is a better risk than the patient with an enlarged heart. Pregnant clients with a class I or class II functional classification rarely undergo decompensation during pregnancy, completing pregnancy without excessive risk. Scarring of the mitral value from rheumatic endocarditis produces mitral stenosis and increases the risk of pulmonary edema. A history of prior heart failure will also increase maternal mortality.

The pregnant cardiac client may have a favorable or unfavorable prognosis during pregnancy. Favorable prognoses include; absence of diastolic murmur with or without cardiac enlargement, no history of heart failure, no significant heart conduction abnormality, and freedom from other medical diseases. An unfavorable prognosis during pregnancy exists for those who have a diastolic murmur and/or cardiac enlargement, a history of previous heart failure, severe abnormalities in cardiac rhythm, and associated medical noncardiac complications.

Symptoms

The normal stresses of pregnancy may cause cardiac symptoms in a woman with undiagnosed heart disease, but a diagnosis of heart disease is often difficult to establish during pregnancy. Signs in normal pregnancy that mimic findings in organic heart disease include hyperventilation that is not accompanied by decreased vital capacity, elevated jugular vein pressure, decrease in exercise tolerance, edema of the lower extremities, prominent apical pulse, extracardiac murmurs caused by increased blood flow in the internal mammary artery and breast veins, changes in heart sounds, sinus tachycardia, and ejection systolic murmurs.

Certain detectable signs are considered reliable indicators of organic heart disease, including diastolic murmurs, cardiac enlargement, systolic murmurs grade III or IV, cardiac arrhythmias other than sinus tachycardia and paroxysmal atrial tachycardia, the presence of distended neck veins, central cyanosis, pericardial friction rub, and/or asymmetrical peripheral pulses.

The most common complication in the pregnant cardiac client is congestive heart failure due to the increased burden superimposed on a diminished cardiac reserve. Congestive heart failure is most likely to occur from 24 to 32 weeks gestation and may be precipitated by infection, severe anemia, or PIH. Signs of congestive heart failure (see Table 25-13) may appear without warning or may be gradual in onset, beginning as persistent rales at the lung bases.

Subacute bacterial endocarditis is also associated with cardiac disease in pregnancy. Bacteria lodge in the aortic and mitral valve endocardium and multiply. Fibrin and platelet thrombi are deposited, forming vegetations called verrucae, which may embolize to other organs and tissues. Symptoms noted are weight loss, fatigue, elevated temperature, joint pains, and splenomegaly. Antibiotic prophylaxis for subacute bacterial endocarditis must be given when the pregnant cardiac client undergoes any procedure, including dental fillings, amniocentesis, and delivery. Prophylaxis consists of penicillin and an aminoglycoside such as gentamicin.

TABLE 25-13
SIGNS OF CONGESTIVE HEART FAILURE IN THE PREGNANT CARDIAC

Severe orthopnea
Exertional dyspnea
Paroxysmal nocturnal dyspnea
Distended neck veins
Moist basal pulmonary rales
Hemoptysis
Tachycardia
Increasing edema
Cough

Fetal Effects

There is an increased incidence of congenital cardiac defects and a threefold increase in perinatal mortality. The risk of perinatal death increases when maternal decompensation is present with a resultant decrease in fetal oxygen supply.

Medical and Nursing Interventions

ANTEPARTUM

Medical and nursing interventions during the antepartum period revolve around the following goals: (1) constant pregnancy monitoring; (2) promotion of rest; (3) limitation of physical activities; (4) psychological support; (5) maintenance of adequate nutritional status; (6) maintenance of maternal hemodynamic stability; (7) maintenance of drug therapy; (8) prevention and treatment of infections; (9) prevention and treatment of anemia; and (10) fetal surveillance.

Constant Pregnancy Monitoring

Pregnancy management in cardiac disease is a joint venture between the obstetrician, cardiologist, and nurse. The client is seen prenatally every two weeks to evaluate the heart's capacity to tolerate the stresses imposed by pregnancy. The functional capacity of the gravida is determined at the first prenatal visit and again at 28 to 32 weeks gestation. Alertness for signs of cardiac decompensation is mandatory (see Table 25-13) and the client and support person are taught to report immediately any signs of congestive heart failure.

Promotion of Rest

Adequate rest prevents fatigue in cardiac function and is a vital part of management. Sleep patterns of eight to ten hours minimum per night and at least a half-hour nap after meals are recommended.

Limitation of Physical Activities

Pregnancy increases the cardiac work load and heart disease decreases cardiac activity, so physical activity is limited in an effort to decrease demands upon the heart. Household activities are limited, with restrictions on housework, shopping, and laundry.

Psychological Support

Anxiety elevates the basal metablic rate. Anxiety is kept to a minimal level during pregnancy to decrease the workload upon the heart. Client teaching that includes a thorough understanding of her condition and its impact upon pregnancy can greatly reduce maternal concern.

Maintenance of Adequate Nutritional Status

A diet high in protein, iron, and other essential nutrients is especially important to meet the increased demands for oxygen and blood plasma volume. Excessive weight gain is avoided to prevent an increased load on the already overburdened heart. Moderate sodium restriction is usually indicated for the pregnant cardiac client. Rarely is it necessary to limit the sodium intake to under 2 gm per day.

Maintenance of Maternal Hemodynamic Stability

Changes in maternal position can result in fluctuations in maternal hemodynamics owing to obstruction of the vena cava by the enlarged uterus and peripheral pooling of blood. Wearing of pressure-graded pantyhose helps to decrease this dependent pooling of blood and to maintain hemodynamic status.

Maintenance of Drug Therapy

Medications in use at the beginning of pregnancy are evaluated. Many women are aware of the teratogenic effects of medications; this may create anxiety. The reason for each medication and for medication changes is explained, with reassurance about fetal effects given.

Diuretics. Diuretics are used occasionally to prevent excessive fluid retention and congestive heart failure. Fluid and electrolyte balance are carefully monitored. Intake of foods high in potassium is stressed.

Digitalis. Digoxin or digitoxin is given to improve the mechanical efficiency of the myocardium and to increase the work capacity of the heart. The drug does cross the placenta, but there is no known harm to the fetus. The associated expansion of body water may lower the circulating level of the medication and necessitate increasing the dosage to maintain therapeutic levels.

Anticoagulants. If the woman is taking coumarin anticoagulants, she is changed to heparin, since heparin does not cross the placenta. When heparin is given, client teaching includes administration of the medication subcutaneously and avoidance of foods high in vitamin K (raw deep green leafy vegetables), since these act as antagonists to heparin. An alternate source of folic acid is prescribed.

Prophylactic Antibiotics. Prophylactic antibiotics are continued throughout pregnancy.

Propranolol. If the gravida is taking propranolol, it is discontinued during pregnancy. Propranolol has the potential for initiating preterm labor and may increase uterine tone to the point that uterine circulation may be compromised, thus compromising the fetus.

Quinidine. Quinidine usage is not contraindicated during pregnancy.

Prevention and Treatment of Infections

Infections are the most important precipitating cause of heart failure in the pregnant woman with rheumatic heart disease. Crowds are to be avoided. At the first sign of an infection, antibiotics are started.

Prevention and Treatment of Anemia

Anemia is to be avoided during pregnancy. Iron supplementation is important, since diet alone cannot meet the increased requirements of pregnancy. If anemia does occur, it must be treated to prevent congestive heart failure. If transfusions are needed, packed cells are used to avoid overloading the maternal circulation.

Fetal Surveillance

Serial ultrasound scans, weekly nonstress testing beginning at 32 weeks gestation, and triweekly estriols are recommended for the pregnant cardiac client.

INTRAPARTUM

Labor and delivery is a time of maximum risk for the pregnant cardiac client. Goals of care include noting current medications, continuous monitoring, assessing respiratory status, positioning, supportive care, medical assistance for delivery, and psychological support.

Note Current Medications

Initial assessment includes a current medication history. If the gravida is on heparin maintenance therapy, it will be discontinued during labor.

Continuous Monitoring

Maternal and fetal physiologic status are monitored during labor and delivery. Maternal vital signs are assessed frequently, noting especially tachycardia (pulse over 100 BPM) and hyperventilation (respirations over 25 per minute). A cardiac monitor may be used to continuously assess cardiac rhythm. Continuous fetal heart rate and uterine contractions monitoring are accomplished with a fetal monitor to evaluate labor status and monitor fetal welfare.

Assess Respiratory Status

The lungs are auscultated at frequent intervals for rales. The presence of cough or dyspnea is noted and reported.

Positioning

A side-lying position, with the head and shoulders elevated and the body parts supported, or a mid-Fowler's position, is optimal to assure proper oxygenation and cardiac emptying during labor. The client may also deliver in a side-lying position.

Supportive Care

Elastic stockings are worn during labor to help prevent venous congestion in the lower extremities. An intravenous line is established, usually of 5 percent D/W, at a keep-open rate or a rate of 50 ml per hour to decrease the incidence of heart failure. Prophylactic antibiotics are administered to prevent valvular damage. Oxygen by mask is given for tachycardia, dyspnea, or chest pain.

If cardiac decompensation occurs, digitalis, diuretics, and oxygen by intermittent positive pressure are usually administered.

Adequate analgesia is provided early in labor to limit the cardiac workload associated with pain and anxiety. Regional anesthesia is preferred for delivery to minimize discomfort, decrease the bearing down reflex, and decrease peripheral resistance, venous return, and cardiac output. Low forceps are commonly used for delivery to circumvent maternal bearing down efforts during the second stage of labor.

If stirrups are used for delivery, the legs are lowered immediately after delivery. Ergot preparations are avoided owing to the incidence of elevated blood pressure associated with their use.

Psychological Support

The nurse should remain with the client and her partner during labor and delivery. The couple is informed of labor progress and any proposed interventions. A calm atmosphere is important to decrease anxiety.

Hypovolemic shock following delivery associated with visceral engorgement is anticipated and appropriate interventions implemented.

POSTPARTUM

The postpartum period is also a time of concern for the cardiac client. Early in the puerperium there is an increase in the incidence of decompensation, collapse, and maternal death. The cardiac output rises significantly immediately after delivery, with rapid mobilization of fluid from the extravascular spaces and release of blood from the lower extremities as the gravid uterus is emptied, and vena caval obstruction is released.

During the several days following delivery, extravascular fluid is returned to the blood stream for excretion, placing a strain on the heart, as excessive interstitial fluid has accumulated. The cardiac client may decompensate up to six days postpartum.

Goals of postpartum care include monitoring maternal physiologic status, proper positioning, resumption of activity, psychological support, and preparation for discharge.

Monitoring Maternal Physiologic Status

The condition of the fundus and the amount of blood lost are assessed frequently to avoid anemia. Ergotrate is not administered, because of its effect on the circulatory system. Edema and changes in the apical pulse and respiratory rate are assessed frequently. If intravenous fluids are infusing, the rate of flow is determined by the physician and carefully monitored to prevent fluid overload. Intake and output are monitored. If the client elects to bottle feed, estrogens are not given because of the associated fluid retention. When the cardiac client requires blood, packed cells are given to prevent overloading of the circulatory system.

Diuresis during postpartum days 2 through 5 helps to establish physiologic equilibrium of the cardiovascular system. The nonpregnant cardiac output level is not usually reached until two weeks postpartum.

Assessments for infection are important during the postpartum period. The cardiac client who develops puerperal infections and mastitis is also in danger of developing bacterial endocarditis. Slight infections can trigger congestive heart failure.

Stool softeners are given to avoid straining. Bladder overdistention followed by rapid emptying causes a rapid drop in intra-abdominal pressure and visceral engorgement, and results in uterine relaxation.

Proper Positioning

A semi-Fowler's or side-lying position, with the head and shoulders elevated, is preferred to aid in cardiac and respiratory functioning.

Resumption of Activity

Gradual activity progression during the postpartum period is determined by maternal pulse and respirations. Initially, bed rest with complete care is ordered. A gradual resumption of activities of daily living determined by pulse and respiratory rate comes next. Progressive ambulation follows.

Psychological Support

Keep the client and support person informed of progress and proposed interventions. Encourage bonding by arranging frequent contact with the neonate with no maternal caretaking activities. When she is allowed caretaking activities, assistance with care of the neonate is essential. Breastfeeding for the class III and class IV cardiac client is not usually recommended, owing to maternal medications and fatigue.

Preparation for Discharge

Before discharge, the home situation and the availability of assistance for the mother are assessed and any necessary provisions made.

Eisenmenger Syndrome

Eisenmenger syndrome consists of pulmonary hypertension caused by high pulmonary vascular resistance with reversed or bidirectional shunts. It is associated with a decrease in oxygen saturation in the systemic circulation and cyanosis. It includes certain atrial septal defects, ventricular septal defects, and patent ductus arteriosus.

ANTEPARTUM MANAGEMENT

The focus of antepartum management is to prevent complications, specifically congestive heart failure and to decrease the workload of the heart during the last trimester.

A well-balanced diet with mild sodium restriction is usually ordered. Calories may be controlled to prevent excessive weight gain. Medications are given as necessary for control of arrhythmias, treatment of congestive heart failure, and hypertension. Prophylactic antibiotic therapy with penicillin is given throughout the antepartum period. Heparin therapy is initiated 12 to 24 hours before delivery.

INTRAPARTUM MANAGEMENT

Intrapartum medical and nursing management is similar to that in other clients with cardiovascular disease, with the addition of Swan-Ganz catheter insertion, measurement of cardiac output, and electrocardiographic monitoring. Vaginal delivery is indicated unless severe cardiac compromise occurs. Epidural anesthesia without epinephrine is the method of choice.

POSTPARTUM MANAGEMENT

The client is assessed carefully for circulatory collapse and reversal of the cardiac shunt. Increasing periods of cyanosis and episodes of syncope are frequently followed by sudden death from fatal arrhythmias. Anticoagulants are administered to prevent pulmonary thrombosis. Oral contraceptives are contraindicated in clients with Eisenmenger syndrome.

ENDOCRINE DISORDERS

Hyperthyroidism

Thyroid disease is not uncommon during pregnancy. When it occurs, it requires care by the obstetrician, internist, pediatrician, and nurse. Pregnancy can obscure the signs and symptoms of thyroid disease and make diagnosis difficult.

Symptoms of nervousness, palpitations, heat intolerance, a resting pulse of over 100 BPM, goiter, and weight loss are common initial complaints. Many early symptoms are similar to normal alterations during pregnancy. Weight loss or failure to gain weight during pregnancy is suggestive of hypothyroidism, as is an enlarged thyroid gland and eye signs (lid lag and exophthalmos). When suspicious symptoms are noted, hyperthyroidism should be either diagnosed or ruled out, since newborn hyperthyroidism can result without maternal treatment.

MEDICAL AND NURSING INTERVENTIONS

There are three treatments for hyperthyroidism: radioactive iodine, surgery, and antithyroid medications.

Radioactive Iodine Therapy

Radioactive iodine therapy is contraindicated during pregnancy because it freely passes across the placenta and can concentrate in the fetal thyroid.

Surgery

Surgery is reserved for gravidas who experience severe side effects from antithyroid medication, who do not comply with a prescribed regimen, and who are unresponsive to medical therapy. If surgery is required, it is usually done during the late second or early third trimester to decrease fetal effects.

Antithyroid Drugs

Antithyroid drugs are the treatment of choice in management of hyperthyroidism during pregnancy. Untreated hyperthyroidism is related to increased frequency of preterm deliveries and preeclampsia. The goal of treatment with antithyroid medication is to keep the gravida euthyroid (normal thyroid function) with the minimum amount of medication. Overtreatment with antithyroid medications may result in deficient fetal development, especially of the central nervous system, and fetal hyperthyroidism. Methimazole or prophythiouracil are usually used for treatment. Clients who become pregnant while on antithyroid medication are usually continued on their medication in amounts that will maintain a euthyroid state. Maternal risks with antithyroid medication are low. Minor adverse reactions include skin rashes, fever, arthralgia, nausea, vomiting, diarrhea, loss of taste, jaundice, lymphadenopathy, and vertigo.

Client Teaching

Client teaching for hyperthyroid gravidas includes the importance of taking prescribed medication in the proper dosage and at the proper time. Side effects and toxic effects need to be understood. Over-the-counter medications are avoided. Planned rest periods are important, and stressful events are avoided. A high-calorie, high-protein, high-carbohydrate, high-vitamin diet is usually ordered.

THYROID STORM

The greatest maternal danger with hyperthyroidism is thyroid storm. It usually follows a precipitating stress such as infection, labor, or cesarean section. Treatment of thyroid storm is aimed at blocking the effects of thyroid storm, inhibiting synthesis and release of thyroid hormone, and providing supportive care.

FETAL AND NEONATAL EFFECTS

Spontaneous abortion and stillbirths are increased when maternal hyperthyroidism is poorly controlled.

About 2 percent of neonates are born with

hyperthyroidism owing to transplacental passage of the thyroid-stimulating immunoglobulins. If the mother is treated with antithyroid medications up until delivery, symptoms of newborn thyrotoxicosis may be delayed.

Fetal goiter is present in approximately 13 to 15 percent of neonates exposed to antithyroid medication in utero (Mestman, 1980). The presence of a goiter may prevent normal flexion of the head and lead to abnormal presentations during labor. A large goiter may obstruct the trachea and necessitate intubation of the neonate after delivery.

On occasion transient hypothyroidism may be present in the neonate following maternal antithyroid medication administration during pregnancy. The neonate will exhibit poor sucking, hypotonia, hypothermia, mottled and cyanotic skin, and wide fontanels. Careful control of maternal medications during pregnancy will decrease the incidence.

POSTPARTUM CARE

Breastfeeding should be avoided if the mother is taking antithyroid medications, since these drugs are excreted in breast milk.

Hypothyroidism

Hypothyroidism is not commonly seen during pregnancy, because severely hypothyroid women have a tendency towards anovulation. A greater incidence of preterm deliveries and thyroid disturbances is seen with maternal hypothyroidism. Congenital hypothyroidism occurs in approximately 1 in 5000 live births (Mestman, 1980).

Addison's Disease

Addison's disease is caused by hypofunction of the adrenal gland, owing to destruction or atrophy of the adrenal cortex. Characteristics include asthenia, skin and mucus membrane pigmentation, anorexia, gastrointestinal disturbances, hypotension, and nervous symptoms.

MATERNAL EFFECTS

The principal hazards to the gravida arise during the first trimester of pregnancy when vomiting is present. During the last two trimesters improvement of symptoms occurs, probably due to the hyperplasia of adrenal tissue. Infections are more common and response to trauma and blood loss is diminished.

Adrenal crisis is most likely to occur immediately following delivery. To compensate for the stress of labor, hydrocortisone is given IM every six hours until labor is completed. Labors should be as short as possible, and outlet forceps may be used to shorten the second stage of labor. Morphine and other opiates are not well tolerated, so use should be avoided. Cortisone is continued during the puerperium, with the dosage gradually being decreased to the usual maintenance level.

FETAL EFFECTS

On the average, neonates of gravidas with Addison's disease weigh about 500 gm below normal. These neonates usually do well after birth. There is an increased incidence of minor congenital defects with maternal steroid administration.

Pheochromocytoma

Pheochromocytoma is a tumor of the sympathoadrenal system that causes increased secretion of norepinephrine and epinephrine. When this tumor is present during pregnancy, the risk is 1 in 3 that the gravida will die during pregnancy or immediately postpartum, following a prolonged episode of hypertension.

Hyperparathyroidism

Hyperparathyroidism is not commonly seen in conjunction with pregnancy. Characteristics seen in the gravida include excessive urinary loss of phosphorus, loss of calcium from bone, hypercalcemia, and calciuria. Calciuria may lead to renal changes. The outcome of pregnancy is influenced by the extent of functional impairment. The perinatal death rate is approximately 35 percent and may be caused by increased maternal serum calcium or parathyroid hormone.

Hypoparathyroidism

Hypoparathyroidism, with its accompanying deficiency of parathyroid hormone, may be caused by accidental removal of, or damage to, the parathyroid glands. During pregnancy, symptoms may become exaggerated. If adequate calcium/phosphorus balance is maintained during pregnancy, fetal outcome is good.

DIABETES MELLITUS

Diabetes mellitus is a chronic systemic disease characterized by carbohydrate, fat, and protein metabolism disorders and disorders in the structure and function of blood vessels. It complicates 1 of every 100 to 500 pregnancies. Maternal mortality is approximately 0.5 percent and perinatal mortality averages about 10 percent.

Pathophysiology

The primary pathology in diabetes lies in deficient insulin secretion. There are three major effects of this lack of insulin: (1) decrease in glucose use by body cells; (2) marked increased mobilization of fats that causes abnormal fat metabolism and deposit of lipids in blood vessel walls; and (3) decrease in the deposit of protein in body tissues.

Diabetogenic Effect of Pregnancy

During pregnancy, significant metabolic changes occur that have an influence on the course of diabetic pregnancies. The fetus is dependent for an uninterrupted supply of fuel. Maternal adaptations help to meet these needs. Pregnancy is characterized by maternal hyperinsulinemia associated with resistance to insulin. Three physiologic responses create this diabetogenic effect: (1) human chorionic somatomammotropin (HCS), also known as human placental lactogen (HPL), is produced by the placenta and exerts its most profound effect in the last trimester of pregnancy by increasing the mobilization of free fatty acids and diminishing the effect of maternal insulin; (2) estrogen and progesterone increase as gestation advances and act as insulin antagonists; and (3) cortisol may cause maternal hyperglycemia by increasing gluconeogenesis.

In a pregnancy not complicated by diabetes, the maternal pancreas responds to the need for insulin while maintaining maternal homeostasis, as discussed in Chapter 9. During pregnancy in the Class B through F diabetic, hyperglycemic episodes occur and result in fetal hyperglycemia. The elevated fetal glucose stimulates the fetal pancreas and results in fetal beta cell hyperplasia and elevated blood glucose.

Maternal Morbidity

The greatest risk during diabetic pregnancy is for women with vascular involvement and/or unstable diabetes. Pregnancy does not shorten the lifespan of women with diabetes, although concurrent coronary artery disease increases the risk of death.

Diabetic nephropathy will not deteriorate permanently with pregnancy. Retinopathy may worsen as the pregnancy advances, but will usually regress following delivery.

There is commonly difficulty in maintaining diabetic control during pregnancy because of the normal physiologic changes that occur with pregnancy. Maternal deaths related to hypoglycemia most often occur during the first trimester and the early puerperium.

Maternal complications associated with diabetes are summarized in Table 25–14.

TABLE 25-14
MATERNAL COMPLICATIONS IN THE PREGNANT DIABETIC

Spontaneous abortion
Monilial vaginitis
Urinary tract infections
Pregnant headache
Ketoacidosis
Pregnancy-induced hypertension
Polyhydramnios
Preterm labor
Psychiatric problems
Postpartum hemorrhage
Progression of diabetic complications
Generalized artherosclerosis
Nephropathy
Retinopathy
Coronary artery disease

Diagnosis

A complete history to identify risk factors for diabetes mellitus is obtained as part of the initial assessment at the first prenatal visit. Risk factors that are indications for glucose tolerance evaluations include: a family history of diabetes in siblings, parents, or grandparents; history of large babies (greater than 4000 gm); history of poor fetal outcome—term stillborn, term neonate with respiratory distress syndrome, congenital anomalies, repeated miscarriage, or prematurity; maternal obesity (20 percent over standard weight for height); maternal age (over 35 years); polyhydramnios; glycosuria (less than two episodes); repeated monilial vaginal infections; grand multiparity; or hypertension.

Diabetes mellitus is suspected in any client who has sugar in the urine. Glycosuria occurs in about 50 percent of normal pregnancies owing to lowered renal threshold. It is significant when present in two successive specimens or in the second-voided specimen before breakfast. The presence of glycosuria is an indication for further testing. Tests include fasting blood sugar, postprandial blood sugar, oral glucose tolerance test, and intravenous glucose tolerance test. Some physicians advocate glucose tolerance testing done on every woman early in pregnancy and repeated at 24 to 28 weeks gestation.

Classification of Diabetes During Pregnancy

Gestational diabetes occurs during pregnancy and is significant, owing to the possibility of permanent diabetes and greater risks of fetal morbidity and mortality than in the non-diabetic pregnant woman. This temporary state results from the hormonal changes of pregnancy. *Chemical diabetes* identifies the stage of an asymptomatic client who presents with an abnormal glucose tolerance test or an increase in the fasting blood sugar. These tests remain abnormal following pregnancy. *Overt diabetes* is the end point in the development of diabetes. Clients present with classical symptoms of polyuria, polydipsia, and polyphagia.

White (1974) classified diabetes during pregnancy according to the severity and duration of the disease (see Table 25-15). As a general rule, the earlier the onset of diabetes, the longer its duration, and the greater the degree of vascular involvement present, the worse the prognosis during pregnancy.

Pederson et al. (1974) identified four prog-

TABLE 25-15
WHITE'S CLASSIFICATION OF DIABETES DURING PREGNANCY

Class	Characteristics
A	Chemical diabetes; asymptomatic; abnormal GTT
B	Diabetes of less than 10 years' duration; onset after age 20; no detectable vascular changes; insulin needed for control
C	Diabetes of 10 to 20 years' duration; onset between age 10 and 20; no detectable vascular changes; insulin needed for control
D	Diabetes of 20 years of longer duration; onset before age 10; calcification of vessels of legs; retinopathy; insulin needed for control
E	Calcification of the pelvic vessels present; insulin needed for control
F	Diabetic retinopathy; diabetic nephropathy; insulin needed for control

nostically bad signs in pregnancy that are associated with a three- to four-time increase in perinatal mortality: clinical pyelonephritis, ketoacidosis, pregnancy-induced hypertension, and neglect (pregnant diabetics who first seek care 60 days or less before delivery).

Effect of Pregnancy on Diabetes

INSULIN REQUIREMENTS

Fluctuation in insulin requirements is a primary problem in diabetic management during pregnancy. During the first trimester, there is usually improvement in carbohydrate tolerance owing to the transfer of glucose to the fetus, creating lowered insulin requirements.

By the third trimester, hyperinsulinemia is present. The decrease in insulin effectiveness influences maintenance of blood sugar levels. When the pancreas cannot meet the needs for insulin, intolerance to glucose develops and insulin requirements are increased.

KETOSIS

Ketosis is more common during pregnancy. There is a diminished carbon dioxide combining power of the blood. This, coupled with the elevation of the basal metabolism rate during pregnancy, increases the occurrence of ketosis. Fetal use of carbohydrates and increased metabolism lower antiketogenic substances, while maternal lipids are augmented and alkali reserve is reduced, favoring the production of ketosis. When maternal complications such as hyperemesis gravidarum occur, they are very difficult to treat.

HYPOGLYCEMIC REACTIONS

Hypoglycemic insulin reactions occur more frequently in the pregnant diabetic. These are often characterized by the absence of the normal warning symptoms.

OXYGEN CONSUMPTION

One fairly predictable occurrence in the diabetic client is the fall in oxygen consumption that begins around the 34th week of gestation, in contrast to the normal gravida whose oxygen consumption continues to rise until term. This decrease in oxygen consumption supports the theory that physiologic maturation of the fetus may occur several weeks earlier in the diabetic than in the normal gravida.

STATUS OF DIABETES

The status of diabetes changes because of the differing metabolic needs of pregnancy. There is an increase in skin and urinary tract infections. Sensory neuropathies may appear during pregnancy. Development of macrovascular disease often intensifies. Latent nephropathy may increase in severity.

Effect of Diabetes on Pregnancy

In the well-controlled diabetic, fertility is usually unaffected. Diabetes mellitus does have a negative effect on pregnancy, accounting for increased perinatal morbidity and mortality.

SPONTANEOUS ABORTIONS

Spontaneous abortion occurs more frequently in the pregnant diabetic owing to compromised placental circulation with diabetic vascular complications.

HYPERTENSIVE DISORDERS

Hypertensive disorders of pregnancy occur in approximately 25 percent of all pregnant diabetics, possibly caused by the vascular changes that occur with longstanding diabetes.

INFECTIONS

Skin and urinary tract infections are often aggravated during pregnancy. Frequent screening for urinary tract infections is necessary to prevent pyelonephritis. Monilial vaginitis is common, owing to the altered vaginal environment during pregnancy.

POLYHYDRAMNIOS

Excess accumulation of amniotic fluid occurs in about 10 to 25 percent of pregnant diabetics. Theories for the etiology include increased osmotic pressure, increased secretion of amniotic fluid, and diuresis from fetal hyperglycemia.

Fetal Effects

ALTERED FETAL GROWTH

The combination of fetal hyperglycemia and hyperinsulinemia during pregnancy leads to excessive fetal growth. Excessive fetal growth (*macrosomia*) has been associated with an increased incidence of traumatic complications during vaginal delivery. Shoulder dystocia may also occur, leading to perinatal asphyxia and brachial plexus injuries. Small-for-gestational-age (SGA) neonates are more common in diabetic women with vascular complications, where there is uterine or placental blood flow compromise.

STILLBIRTH

After 35 weeks gestation, the frequency of intrauterine fetal death in diabetic pregnancies is ten times that of the normal pregnant population. The increased incidence may be caused by fetal hyperglycemia and hyperinsulinemia, especially in poorly controlled patients. Patients who have a history of prior stillbirth, pregnancy-induced hypertension, or vascular involvement also have a higher incidence of intrauterine fetal death. Arbitrary termination of pregnancy between 35 and 38 weeks gestation is still advocated by some obstetricians to prevent stillbirths.

CONGENITAL ANOMALIES

Infants of diabetic mothers have a two to three times greater frequency of severe congenital malformations involving many organ systems than do infants born to nondiabetic mothers. The incidence of congenital malformations approaches 6 to 8 percent of all live neonates, with the most common anomalies involving the cardiac, renal, and central nervous systems.

NEONATAL PROBLEMS

Neonatal problems such as respiratory distress syndrome, hypoglycemia, hypocalcemia, hyperbilirubinemia, and electrolyte imbalance are frequent in neonates born to diabetic mothers.

Medical and Nursing Interventions: Gestational and Class A Diabetics

The gestational diabetic can be detected through past health or obstetrical history. Fasting blood sugars, two-hour postprandial blood sugars, and glucose tolerance tests are used for diagnosis in women who have identified risk factors. These patients are seen biweekly until 32 weeks gestation and weekly thereafter to closely monitor the pregnancy.

DIET

A diet low in concentrated carbohydrates and moderate in protein is recommended to avoid stressing the pancreas from excess insulin production. A diet of 35 to 40 kcal per kg actual body weight is usually ordered with a desired weight gain of 25 to 30 pounds. Composition of the diet is 45 percent carbohydrate, 20 to 25 percent protein, and 30 to 35 percent fat. Calories are divided as follows: 24 percent at breakfast, 30 percent at lunch, 33 percent at dinner, and 13 percent for snacks. The goal of the diet is to prevent fasting hyperglycemia with rebound (the *Somogyi effect*) and postprandial hyperglycemia.

PROPHYLACTIC INSULIN THERAPY

Insulin therapy may be ordered prophylactically either in an effort to decrease potential morbidity or to maintain blood glucose levels in an acceptable range. If insulin is used, both regular and intermediate-acting (NPH) are used before breakfast and supper.

GLUCOSE MONITORING

Urine is tested for glucose at each prenatal visit. Positive results are followed with blood glucose testing.

FETAL SURVEILLANCE

Risk of intrauterine fetal death dictates accurate determination of gestational age. Ultrasound assessment of fetal growth is done at intervals, beginning at 17 to 20 weeks gestation, to identify macrosomia or intrauterine growth retardation (IUGR). Antepartum testing with nonstress or contraction stress tests is done weekly, beginning at about 36 weeks gestation.

Medical and Nursing Interventions: Other Classes of Diabetes

ANTEPARTUM

Ideally, diabetics who are Class B, C, D, E, and F are followed throughout pregnancy by an obstetrician, internist, nurse, and dietitian. The initial visit should come early in pregnancy with a thorough history and complete physical examination to determine medical and obstetrical status, assess individual client needs, and plan management with the client and her support person. Assess to determine knowledge of diabetes, diet, and urine and blood tests.

Medical and nursing interventions revolve around certain goals: (1) supervision; (2) determination of dietary requirements; (3) glucose determinations; (4) insulin requirements; (5) physical activity; (6) monitoring for complications; and (7) fetal surveillance.

Supervision

Diabetic clients require close supervision during pregnancy to control the disease and prevent complications. They are seen weekly or biweekly until 26 weeks gestation, then weekly until delivery. Hospitalization is appropriate during pregnancy to assess diabetic status and to treat complications that may arise.

At each prenatal visit, in addition to the routine assessments, blood is drawn for glucose, carbon dioxide level, and urea nitrogen determination. Eyegrounds are examined routinely. Between visits, the client keeps a daily record of urine sugar and acetone and glucometer readings.

Determination of dietary requirements

Diet is individualized to allow increased maternal and fetal metabolic requirements. The goal is normal weight gain during pregnancy while minimizing ketosis. Usually calories are 30 to 40 kcal per Kg ideal body weight, with 40 to 50 percent of the total calories carbohydrates, 30 to 35 percent fats, and 20 to 25 percent proteins. Calorie distribution is usually 25 percent at breakfast, 30 percent at lunch, 30 percent at supper, and 15 percent for snacks.

Glucose Determinations

Blood glucose should be in optimum control throughout pregnancy. Maternal glucose ideally is maintained at less than 100 mg per dl. Clients are instructed to monitor blood glucose values at home four times a day (before meals and at bedtime) and to report glucose readings of greater than 180 mg per dl or less than 80 mg per dl. Urine testing four times a day for glucose and ketones is done and documented.

Glycosolated hemoglobin determinations are made every one to two weeks to evaluate average blood sugars. To assess the degree of diabetic control, the following parameters are usually used:

less than 7.5 percent = good control
7.6 to 8.9 percent = fair control
greater than 9.0 percent = poor control

Insulin Requirements

Oral hypoglycemia agents are not given during pregnancy. In addition to the teratogenic effects, oral agents may not control diabetes during pregnancy. They cross the placental barrier and may induce hypoglycemia in the fetus/neonate.

Insulin requirements frequently decrease during the first trimester, owing to the utilization of glucose by the fetoplacental unit. During the second and third trimester, insulin requirements usually increase, due to the insulin-antagonist state that results primarily from the placental production of hormones as the placenta enlarges. It also results from a slight elevation in the free thyroxine and cortisol. If insulin requirements decrease during the second or third trimester, it may indicate a failing placental unit and fetal compromise.

Adequate control usually requires split dosages of insulin. Most clients require an intermediate-acting insulin (NPH) and a short-acting insulin (Regular) before breakfast and supper. As a general guideline, the NPH:Regular ratio is 2:1 in the morning and 1:1 before supper.

Portable, battery-powered subcutaneous infusion pumps may be used in selected clients to maintain glucose control, especially during the third trimester of pregnancy.

Physical Activity

Exercise must be regular. The client needs to recognize the effects of exercise on dietary and insulin requirements and be able to make adjustments if the exercise pattern is altered.

Complications

Education of signs and symptoms of frequent complications is an important aspect of care. Unusual symptoms that should be reported to the physician immediately are taught: headaches, blurred vision, scotoma (blind gaps in the visual field), swelling in the face or fingers, sudden weight gain, or abdominal pain.

Symptoms of insulin overdosage and underdosage are reviewed with the client. Diabetics are prone to infections. Precautions that are reviewed with the client include the following: (1) stay away from persons with colds or other infections; (2) avoid drinking or eating from utensils others have used; (3) wipe from front to back after urination or defecation; (4) urinate as soon as the urge is felt; (5) drink eight glasses of water a day; (6) brush teeth frequently and floss; (7) take proper care of the feet.

Fetal Surveillance

At about 14 weeks gestation, ultrasonography will estimate gestational age. From 20 to 34 weeks, serial ultrasonography documents fetal growth by measurement of the fetal biparietal diameter and abdominal circumference, as well as femur length.

During the third trimester, various tests assess fetal status and well-being. Amniocentesis determines fetal lung maturity. Tests usually ordered are L/S ratio, phospholipid creatinine, acetone precipitate fraction, PI (phosphatidylinositol), and PG (phosphatidylglycerol). Fetal lung maturity is considered present and the risk of respiratory distress minimal with the following results:

L/S ratio greater than 2.0
Acetone precipitate greater than 50 percent
PI small
PG 3 percent

Weekly estriols are done from 26 weeks gestation on to determine the adequacy of placental functioning. Nonstress testing is done weekly from 34 weeks until delivery to determine placental reserve. If the results are nonreactive, contraction stress testing is done to determine fetal response to labor. These tests are explained in Chapter 24.

INTRAPARTUM

The results of fetal surveillance testing determine the timing of delivery. Often a combination of test results, such as a positive oxytocin challenge test (OCT) and falling estriol levels, dictate an early delivery date. Induction of labor by oxytocin infusion with vaginal delivery is preferred if conditions are favorable. Repeated attempts at induction over several days is not recommended because maternal glucose control will deteriorate.

Labor Care

During labor, continuous fetal heart rate monitoring will assure fetal well-being. If fetal distress is confirmed, a cesarean section is performed. Labor is allowed to progress as long as cervical dilatation and fetal descent follow the normal labor curve. Any evidence of arrest in labor progress is an alert to the possibility of cephalopelvic disproportion owing to fetal macrosomia.

Nursing care during labor is as for any other client having labor induction by oxytocin infusion (see Chapter 26), with the addition of observation for hypoglycemia. Supportive care is especially important to prevent anxiety-produced hypoglycemia. Information about labor progress and fetal status is essential for the laboring client and her support person.

A neonatologist in attendance at delivery is mandatory. The neonate of a diabetic mother is prone to problems resulting from hypoxia, respiratory distress, prematurity, hypoglycemia, and congenital anomalies.

Insulin Requirements

Prior to labor, insulin dosage is altered to a short-acting type to allow easier control during labor and delivery. Regular insulin is given with glucose intravenously by infusion pump, and blood glucose levels are determined every one-half to one hour. Intravenous infusions should not exceed 200 ml per hour. All voidings are tested for sugar and ketones.

POSTPARTUM

There are four main goals of care during the puerperium: (1) maintenance of normal blood glucose levels; (2) prevention of postpartum complications; (3) development of a positive parent-infant relationship; and (4) discharge planning.

Maintenance of Normal Blood Glucose Levels

Important factors in controlling blood glucose levels are diet and insulin. Immediately following delivery, a blood glucose level is drawn. Urine is tested for sugar and acetone every two hours for the first 24 hours postpartum. Insulin coverage is usually on a sliding scale according to blood glucose or urine testing results.

When the placenta is expelled after delivery and insulin antagonists (HCS, estrogen, progesterone) are removed, insulin requirements are greatly decreased. Some clients require no insulin for the first day or so.

Anabolic activity of the prenatal period changes to catabolic activity during the puerperium. Catabolism lowers the fasting blood sugar level and causes frequent insulin reactions early in the puerperium. Intravenous fluids are usually continued for 24 hours postpartum, with resumption of predelivery ADA diets after the first postpartum day.

Prevention of Postpartum Complications

The nurse must be aware of the most common postpartum complications in the diabetic—PIH, hemorrhage, and puerperal infections.

PIH develops in about one-third of postpartum diabetics, possibly due to the cardiovascular degeneration present in longstanding diabetes. Vital signs are assessed frequently for at least 48 hours after delivery. Assessment for symptoms is done frequently.

Hemorrhage resulting from uterine atony and excessive amniotic fluid is more common in the diabetic. Assessments for postpartum hemorrhage (see Chapter 27) are an intergral part of postpartum nursing care.

Infections can be a major hazard to the diabetic during the puerperium. Even a mild postpartum infection complicates diabetic regulation and increases the risk of acidosis. Prevention of infections is a major goal. The significance of meticulous personal hygiene is stressed and assessment for signs of puerperal infection (see Chapter 27) is a part of nursing care.

Development of a Positive Parent-Child Relationship

The infant of the diabetic mother is often in the special care nursery. Flexible family-centered policies are needed, and scheduling of maternal care around opportunities to interact with her neonate are important. Communication between nursery personnel and parents is necessary to maintain contact with the neonate.

Breastfeeding is not contraindicated. When the insulin-dependent diabetic client breastfeeds, calorie intake is increased by about 400 to 500 kcal per day, of which at least 20 percent is protein. Insulin dosage needs to be adjusted accordingly.

Discharge Planning

Discharge teaching for the diabetic mother includes the usual information for self-care plus instruction for infant care. Review of dietary and insulin requirements for the remainder of the postpartum period and of symptoms of hypoglycemia is needed. Ongoing medical attention and adequate instructions regarding diabetic regulation prior to future conception are stressed.

Genetic counseling is often included as part of the discharge teaching. The infant of a diabetic mother does have an increased chance of developing diabetes.

Family planning information is also included. Oral contraceptives are not usually recommended for the diabetic because of the associated diabetogenic effect. Intrauterine devices are controversial because of the increased risks of infection. Mechanical barriers are effective and have no adverse systemic effects. Women with associated renal disease are advised of the risks of future pregnancies and informed of sterilization procedures.

MULTIPLE GESTATIONS

Incidence

The incidence of multiple gestation is:

Twins 1:1000 births
Triplets 1:10,000 births
Quadruplets 1:750,000 births

Occurrence of twin gestations tends to vary among racial groups. Twins are most common in blacks and less common in whites, with the least incidence among Orientals. The frequency of twins is associated with maternal age, reaching a maximum incidence at about 39 years, then falling abruptly. Multiple births increase with paternal age, up to 34 to 48 years of age. They occur with increased frequency with administration of the ovulation-stimulating drugs.

Twin Gestations

Twin pregnancies may be monozygotic or dizygotic. Monozygotic or identical twins arise from a single fertilized ovum that develops into two embryos at an early stage. There is one placenta, one chorion, and one or two amniotic sacs (see Fig. 25–3). The blood circulation of the two fetuses interconnect in the common placenta. If there is incomplete division of the blastoderm, anomalies such as cojoined twins may result. The two children are genetically identical (isogenic). They are of the same sex, of similar appearance, and have identical blood groups. Monozygotic twins have the highest mortality, usually related to entangling of their umbilical cords, with resultant interruption of circulation.

Dizygotic or fraternal twins result from the fertilization of two ova by two separate sperm. Each twin has its own placenta, chorion, and amniotic sac (see Fig. 25–3). The placentas may seem to fuse if the ova implant near each other, but the circulations remain separate. These children may be of the same or different sex and are no more similar genetically than are other brothers and sisters.

On rare occasion, superfetation or superfecundation may occur. *Superfetation* is the fertilization of a second ovum at a later ovulation. *Superfecundation* is the fertilization of two ova expelled at the same ovulation but fertilized at separate copulations.

Triplet Gestations

Triplets may be monozygotic, dizygotic, or trizygotic. Monozygotic triplets derive from one fertilized ovum that splits twice. Dizygotic triplets derive from two ova from one or both ovaries, one of which splits after fertilization. Trizygotic triplets result from fertilization of three ova from one or both ovaries.

Quadruplet Gestations

Quadruplets derive from one, two, three, or four ova. Symmetrical monozygotic quadruplets result when monozygotic embryos each split again. Asymmetrical monozygotic quadruplets are formed from monozygotic embryos, each of which split twice.

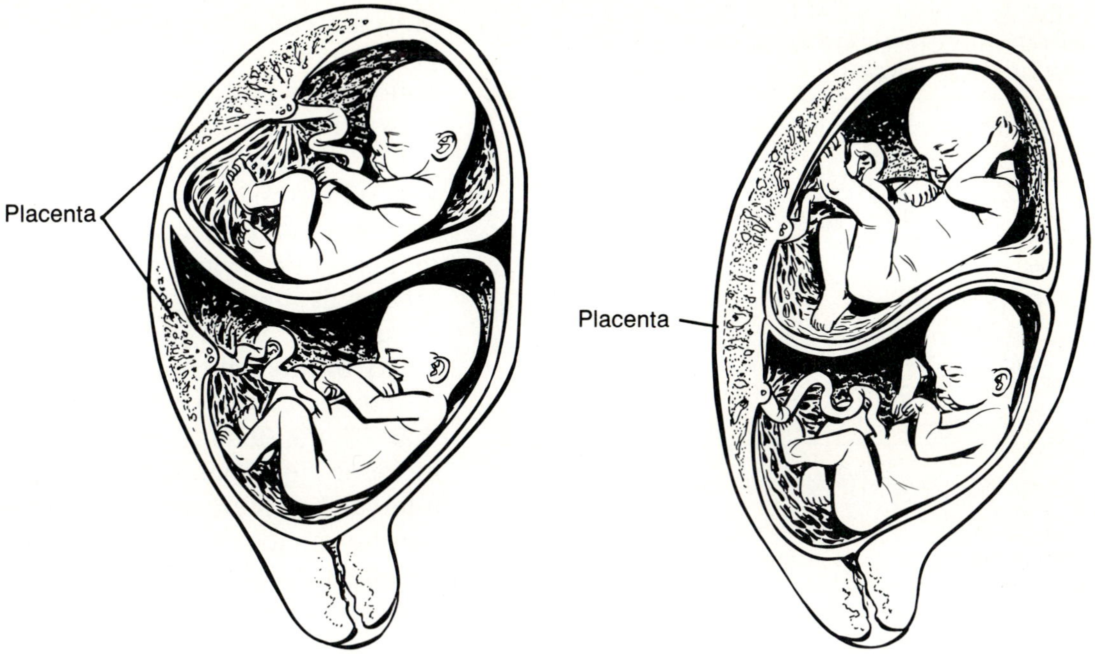

FIGURE 25-3. Placenta and membranes in twin pregnancy: A. Binovular. B. Uniovular.

Diagnosis of Multiple Gestation

Multiple pregnancy is suggested by a history of dizygotic twins in the family, use of ovulation-inducing fertility drugs, a uterus that is at least three weeks larger than expected for gestational date, rapid uterine growth, or an excessive weight gain. There may also be increased levels of human chorionic gonadotropin (HCG), human chorionic somamammotropin (HCS), and alpha fetoprotein.

Diagnosis of multiple gestation is confirmed by abdominal palpation, auscultation of multiple heart beats, roentgenography, or ultrasonography. When the examiner can palpate more than one head, breech, and back, the diagnosis of multiple gestation can be made. A difference of more than 10 beats per minute upon auscultation of the fetal heart rates is diagnostic for multiple gestation. X-ray of the maternal abdomen will show two or more skeletons, but the presence of a second skeleton cannot be definitely ascertained until the 25th week of gestation. Ultrasonography done at 12 to 16 weeks gestation will demonstrate the presence of two or more fetal skulls.

Complications in Multiple Pregnancy

Many maternal and fetal complications are more prevalent in multiple gestations than in single gestations (see Tables 25-16 and 25-17).

MATERNAL COMPLICATIONS

Multiple gestations are associated with increased pressure on the ureters, bladder, intestines, vena cava, renal veins, and diaphragm. Increased fetal demands for folic acid and for iron lead to the development of megaloblastic and iron deficiency anemias. The incidence of pregnancy-induced hypertension and polyhydramnios are significantly increased. Preterm labor is common in multiple gestations. Placenta previa occurs more frequently because of the increased area of placental attach-

TABLE 25-16
MATERNAL COMPLICATIONS ASSOCIATED WITH MULTIPLE GESTATIONS

Severe nausea and vomiting in the first trimester
Pressure symptoms
Anemia
Pregnancy-induced hypertension
Polyhydramnios
Preterm labor
Placenta previa
Amniotic fluid infection
Uterine dystocia
Complicated delivery
Postpartum hemorrhage

TABLE 25-17
FETAL COMPLICATIONS ASSOCIATED WITH MULTIPLE GESTATIONS

Preterm delivery
Congenital anomalies
Stillbirth
Increased mortality rate
Intrauterine growth retardation
Malpresentations
Cord entanglement
Velamentous insertion of umbilical cord
Twin-to-twin transfusion syndrome
Fetus papyraceus
Disseminated intravascular coagulation
Acardia
Cojoined twins
Locking of twins

ment. An increased risk of amniotic fluid infections is present, and other labor and delivery complications occur more frequently. Postpartum hemorrhage is more frequent owing to uterine overdistention that predisposes to uterine atony.

FETAL COMPLICATIONS

The incidence of preterm deliveries is increased in multiple gestations. Average gestation for twins is 260 days, for triplets 246 days, and for quadruplets 236 days.

Intrauterine growth retardation also complicates the fetal and neonatal period. Multiple fetuses tend to have a decreased rate of growth after 30 weeks gestation, when the majority of body cells are increasing in size rather than in number.

The incidence of congenital malformations and stillbirths increase in multiple gestations. A higher fetal mortality rate occurs in monozygotic twins, probably caused by the greater likelihood of communication between circulations and a decrease in the functional ability of the placenta.

The risk to the second twin is almost twice that of the first, owing to: (1) the greater incidence of operative deliveries; (2) a long interval between deliveries; (3) reduction of uterine capacity after delivery of the first fetus leading to altered placental function; (4) occupation by the second twin of a less favorable position in the uterus; and (5) increased incidence of malpresentation in the second twin.

Cord entanglement that sometimes occurs in monochorionic, monoamniotic twins leads to an interruption of circulation. Velamentous insertion of the cord may cause fetal demise during delivery.

Twin-to-twin transfusion syndrome may complicate multiple gestations. During development of a single placenta, some blood vessels may anastomose. This anastomosis can be artery to artery, artery to vein, or vein to vein. The recipient twin is heavier and polycythemic. Because of the polycythemia, there is a tendency to develop jaundice. Polyhydramnios is more frequent in the recipient twin. The donor twin will appear anemic, pallid, dehydrated, growth-retarded, and hypovolemic. In *fetus papyraceus*, the donor twin succumbs from transfusion syndrome prior to birth. Gradually, the donor twin's fluid constituents are reabsorbed and become a shriveled, compressed appendage. DIC can occur when thromboplastin material from a dead fetus passes through vascular shunts in a monochorionic placenta.

When an artery-to-artery and a vein-to-vein anastomosis occur simultaneously in monochorionic twins, a rare condition called *acardia*

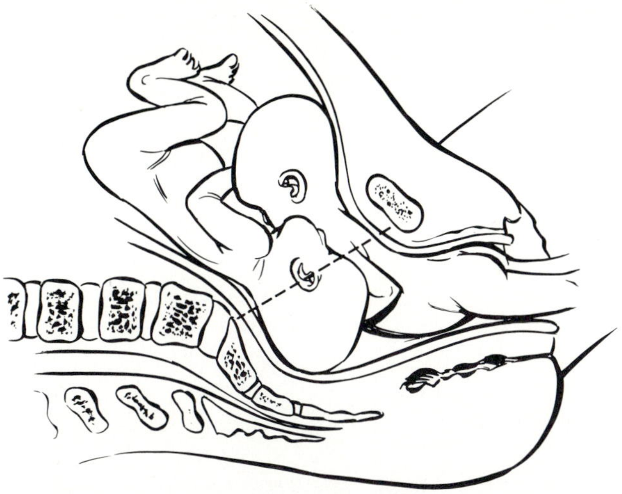

FIGURE 25-4. Interlocking of twin fetuses.

may occur. Early in embryonic development one twin reverses blood flow into the other. The latter fails to develop a heart and is nourished during intrauterine development as an appendage to the donor.

The incidence of cojoined twins is 1:50,000 to 1:100,000 births (Hubinot et al., 1984). Cojoined twins are unioval twins with an embryonic area that failed to split completely and the two individuals remain attached. The most common site of union is the thoracopagus or anterior thoracic and abdominal fusion (Appuzio et al., 1984). The majority are female.

Locking of twins occurs when one baby impedes the descent and delivery of the other. The most common presentations are breech-vertex (see Fig. 25-4).

Medical and Nursing Management

Medical and nursing management of multiple gestations is based on certain goals (see Table 25-18).

CONTROL NAUSEA AND VOMITING

Nausea and vomiting may be severe during the first trimester, owing to the high levels of HCG. Decreasing fatty and fried food intake and eating two or three crackers upon awakening, before getting out of bed, may help to decrease nausea. Eating six small meals rather than three regular meals may also be of benefit in control of nausea and vomiting.

FREQUENT PRENATAL VISITS

Because of the increased incidence of maternal and fetal complications, prenatal visits are more frequent. Careful assessments by the nurse and physician will help to detect potential or developing complications.

SUPPLEMENT IRON AND FOLIC ACID STORES

The increased fetal demands for folic acid and iron lead to development of megaloblastic anemia in the presence of dietary deficiency and iron deficiency. As soon as a diagnosis of multiple pregnancy is made, a high-protein diet is ordered, plus a prenatal multivitamin and iron supplement. Counseling by the nurse or dietitian is

TABLE 25-18
MEDICAL AND NURSING MANAGEMENT IN MULTIPLE PREGNANCIES

Control nausea and vomiting
Frequent prenatal visits
Supplement iron and folic acid stored
Increased periods of rest
Relief from pressure symptoms
Monitor polyhydramnios
Evaluate fetal growth and well-being
Maternal teaching
Evaluate maternal psychological status
Careful conduct of labor and delivery
Observation for postpartum hemorrhage

needed to attain nutritional goals—a mother with adequate nutrient stores and two or more fetuses receiving adequate nutrients for growth and development.

REST

Rest is important for maternal and fetal well-being. Rest periods during the day and a minimum of eight hours of sleep at night are needed. The client's partner is included in discussions when planning increased rest periods. From 30 to 36 weeks gestation, longer periods of bed rest in the left lateral position will improve placental circulation and decrease the incidence of pregnancy-induced hypertension and preterm delivery.

RELIEF FROM PRESSURE SYMPTOMS

The rapidly enlarging uterus causes increased pressure on the ureters, bladder, intestines, vena cava, renal veins, and diaphragm. Increased pressure on the venous circulation predisposes to rectal and vulvar varicosities.

Constipation and digestive disturbances are accentuated during the second and third trimesters. Urinary stasis and chronic urinary tract infection may occur following prolonged pressure on the ureters. In the third trimester, polyhydramnios and increasing pressure on the diaphragm cause abdominal discomfort and dyspnea.

Suggestions to relieve pressure symptoms include frequent position changes, small frequent feedings, and positioning of pillows to support the uterus during rest periods.

MONITOR POLYHYDRAMNIOS

Polyhydramnios, an excessive amount of amniotic fluid, can precipitate preterm labor and cause maternal discomfort and distress. Normally the amnion circulates and reabsorbs approximately 350 ml of amniotic fluid per hour in late pregnancy. When an imbalance in the amount of amniotic fluid occurs, the buildup in pressure can be quite dramatic. The uterus enlarges rapidly and maternal symptoms may be severe. If maternal distress and dyspnea become pronounced, amniocentesis may be required to relieve the pressure.

EVALUATE FETAL GROWTH AND WELL-BEING

Women with diagnosed multiple gestation should have serial ultrasonography at three to four-week intervals to verify symmetrical intrauterine growth of each fetus, beginning at about 24 weeks gestation. Intrauterine growth retardation is suspected when oligohydramnios is present, unequal growth is noted, a difference in the biparietal diameters is seen, or placental infarctions are identified. Routine nonstress testing is started at about 36 weeks gestation and is repeated weekly until delivery.

MATERNAL TEACHING

In addition to the normal teaching required during the antepartum period, signs and symptoms of pregnancy-induced hypertension, placenta previa, and preterm labor are emphasized.

EVALUATE MATERNAL PSYCHOLOGICAL STATUS

Multiple gestations place an added stress on the mother, creating anxieties about the potential problems that frequently complicate multiple gestations. She may feel incapable of caring for more than one infant at a time. Financial needs are increased by her inability to work outside the home until delivery, antepartum testing, antepartum hospitalizations, potential increased length of stay in the hospital for the infants, and the cost of raising more than one infant at a time.

Discussions encouraging maternal verbalization will aid in identification of concerns specific to her family and financial situation. Information about community support groups will provide parents with an additional support system. Referral to an appropriate source for financial counseling and assistance is helpful.

The effect of the multiple gestation on internal family relationships should be determined and important support persons identified. These persons are included in discussions of prenatal needs, anticipatory guidance, and postpartum planning.

CONDUCT OF LABOR AND DELIVERY

Overstretching of the uterus by the combined weights of the fetuses, placentas, and amniotic fluid may lead to preterm labor, early rupture of the membranes, or uterine inertia with weak and inefficient uterine contractions. Continuous monitoring of fetal heart rates and uterine contractions is essential. Two units of blood must be typed and crossmatched to be used in the event of postpartum hemorrhage.

If labor is preterm or if the fetuses are small, analgesia administration will be decreased, and teaching or reinforcing breathing and relaxation techniques is important throughout labor.

In twin gestations, there are six possible combinations of presentations (see Fig. 25–5). The most common combination is two vertices. Other combinations include vertex and breech, two breeches, vertex and transverse lie, breech and transverse lie, and two transverse lies.

During delivery, maternal vital signs, fetal heart rates, and uterine contractions are monitored. The delivery room is

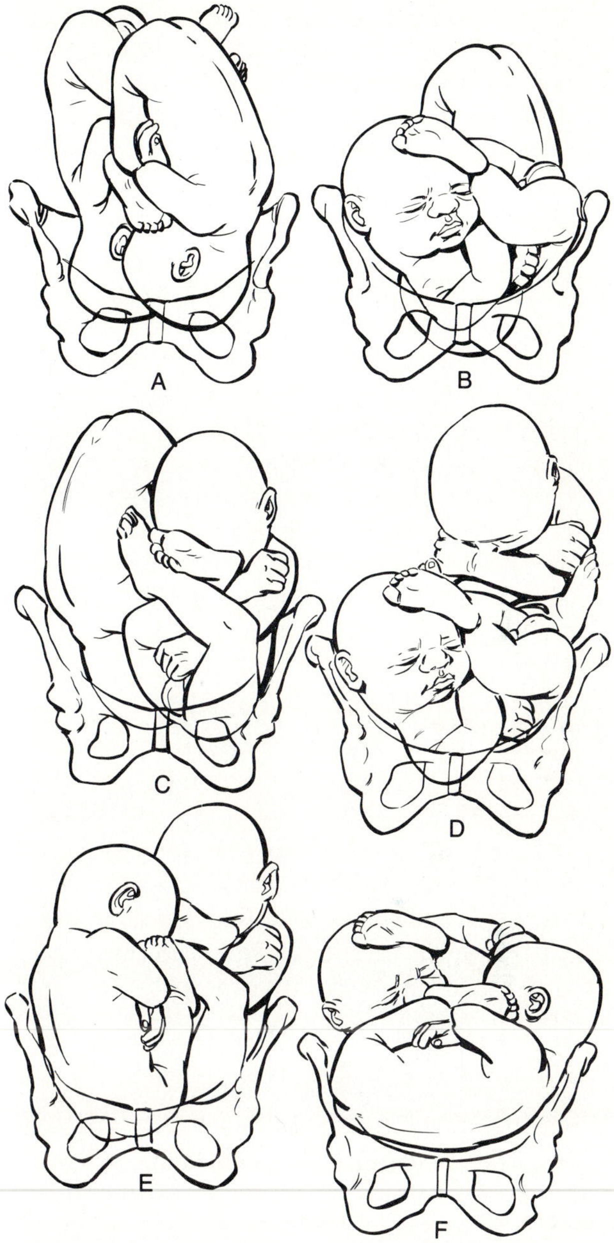

FIGURE 25–5. Types of twin presentations: A. Two vertex. B. Vertex and transverse lie. C. Vertex and breech. D. Breech and tranverse lie. E. Two breech. F. Two transverse lie.

equipped with the appropriate number of cord clamps, neonatal warmers, resuscitation equipment, neonatal identification tags, and records. The high-risk nursery and pediatrician are notified of impending delivery.

After delivery of the first fetus, the umbilical cord is double-clamped to prevent the possibility of the second baby bleeding through the cord of the first if placental circulations communicate. Care of the neonates depends on condition at birth, i.e., Apgar scores. Oxytocic drugs are withheld until after all fetuses are delivered. Fetal heart rate and uterine contraction monitoring is essential. Placental expulsion occurs after all fetuses are delivered.

OBSERVATIONS FOR POSTPARTUM HEMORRHAGE

Incidence of postpartum hemorrhage is increased, owing to the larger placental site and the uterine atony that may result from uterine overdistention. Maternal vital signs, fundus, and lochia are assessed at frequent intervals for symptoms of shock or excessive blood loss. If the uterine fundus is boggy, it is gently massaged until firm, taking care not to overmassage and cause further relaxation of the uterine muscle. Oxytoxic drugs may be administered intravenously or intramuscularly to contract the uterus and help maintain uterine contraction.

PROLONGED (POSTTERM) PREGNANCY

Pregnancy normally lasts 280 days from the first day of the last normal menstrual period. Only a small percentage of women deliver on their estimated due date. Some deliver earlier, and others deliver later. Approximately 7 percent of pregnancies reach 42 weeks, and 3 percent extend beyond 42 weeks gestation. Pregnancies that extend beyond 42 weeks are classified as postterm. One-third of these will have a postmature neonate, characterized as malnourished with an alert, apprehensive appearance, cracked and peeling skin, and meconium staining of the skin, nails, and umbilical cord. As a group, postterm neonates weigh the same as neonates delivered at term, but may be larger than average or have growth retardation.

The incidence of prolonged pregnancy appears to be slightly higher in primigravidas and will tend to recur in subsequent pregnancies. Perinatal deaths from birth asphyxia, meconium aspiration, and congenital anomalies are increased as the length of gestation increases and when maternal hypertension is present.

Etiology

PROLONGED PREGNANCY

The causes of prolonged pregnancy are obscure, because the factors responsible for the initiation of labor at term are not clearly understood. The administration of prostaglandin synthetase inhibitors such as aspirin and indomethacin can delay the onset of labor. Women with low levels of estriol in serum and urine may be postterm. Pregnancies complicated by *anencephaly* (congenital absence of the brain and spinal cord) are associated with fetal adrenal insufficiency and postterm delivery.

POSTMATURITY

Postmature neonates seem to result from a gradual decline in placental function as the placenta ages. Placentas from postterm pregnancies often exhibit thickened vascular membranes, calcification, and fibrin deposits in the intervillous spaces.

Effects

MATERNAL EFFECTS

Physiologically, the mother demonstrates few, if any, effects. The major effects are psychological. When pregnancy is prolonged, its positive qualities are lost to feelings of fatigue and frustration. The expectant mother may generate critical and negative perceptions of herself in terms of body image and degree of self-confidence. Relationships with others may become stressed. Fears and concerns regarding the baby's well-being and normalcy are created as the pregnancy progresses past the expected due date.

NEONATAL EFFECTS

Three stages of postmaturity are observed in the neonate. In the first stage, the skin is cracked and peeling and the neonate appears open-eyed and alert but malnourished. The second stage includes characteristics of stage one plus green-stained membranes and umbilical cord. In the third stage, the skin and nails are stained a yellow-green color.

Prolonged pregnancy is associated with a two-fold to seven-fold increase in perinatal mortality (Khouzami et al., 1981). Postmature neonates often tolerate labor poorly and are at increased risk for intrauterine death. Meconium aspiration at birth may lead to neonatal demise. Cold stress, caused by reduced fat stores, and hypoglycemia, caused by reduced glycogen stores, are common. Postmature neonates suffer higher mortality rates up to the age of two years.

Medical and Nursing Management

AVOIDING PROLONGED PREGNANCY

Probably the most important part of management of prolonged pregnancy is accurate dating of pregnancy.

Menstrual Dates

Nursing assessment includes the date of the last menstrual period, whether the period was normal, whether it began on time, and the usual length of time between periods. If normal length of time between periods is one or two months or is irregular, the expected due date may be inaccurate. Oral contraceptive history is obtained, since amenorrhea can occur following discontinuance.

Pelvic Examination

The length of gestation can be estimated with accuracy during a pelvic examination done between six to seven weeks and three months.

Auscultation of the Fetal Heart

When the fetal heart can be auscultated with a Leffscope, DeLee-Hillis stethoscope, or regular stethoscope (not a Doppler-type instrument), the pregnancy is 20 weeks gestation.

Quickening

All pregnant women should be instructed to note and record the date of quickening. Quickening should occur at approximately 19 to 20 weeks in a primigravida and 17 weeks in a multipara.

Ultrasound Cephalometry

The uterine size compared with gestational age is recorded at each prenatal visit. Any discrepancy between uterine size and gestational age is investigated with ultrasonography. Between 20 and 26 weeks an ultrasound cephalometry is performed if there is a question of length of gestation. A second scan is taken at 31 to 33 weeks. These two measurements can predict gestational age within a five-day range.

PHYSICAL EXAMINATION

Physical examination can be helpful in determining postterm pregnancy. Serial measurements of maternal abdominal girth may be of some benefit. The normal girth at term is 38 to 40 inches, although this is subject to variations. Positive signs of decreasing maternal weight in the last weeks of pregnancy and decreased amniotic fluid on palpation of the uterus will help to establish the diagnosis of postterm pregnancy.

VAGINAL EXAMINATION

A vaginal examination is performed weekly from 42 weeks to establish a baseline of cervical effacement and dilation and to judge whether the cervix is favorable for labor induction.

SURVEILLANCE FOR FETAL COMPROMISE

Surveillance for fetal compromise can be accomplished by a combination of ultrasound, estriol determination, serum human placental lactogen levels, fetal heart rate testing, and amniocentesis.

Ultrasound

Late in pregnancy, ultrasound is not helpful in determining age by biparietal diameter measurements, but it can assess placental aging and amniotic fluid volume. Term placentas exhibit indentations of the chorionic plate that separate the placenta into echo-free compartments. The volume of amniotic fluid slowly declines to 150 to 200 ml at 42 weeks gestation. A mature placenta and reduced amount of amniotic fluid documented by ultrasound support the diagnosis of prolonged pregnancy and confirm the need for further testing and/or monitoring.

Estriols

A baseline estriol determination is made at 41 weeks and again at 42 weeks. After 42 weeks estriols are measured biweekly. Biweekly estriol levels that continue to rise suggest that placental function is not decreasing and that the fetus is not postmature, even if it is postterm. If estriol values fall 30 percent or more from the preceding value, fetal heart rate testing is indicated. Serial estriol determinations that remain the same are not significant.

Human Chorionic Somatomammotropin

HCS levels may be measured twice weekly after 42 weeks gestation to aid in assessing fetal status. Decreasing levels suggest serious fetal jeopardy.

Fetal Heart Rate Testing

An initial nonstress test is done at 42 weeks and repeated twice weekly thereafter (Barrett et al., 1982). Nonstress tests that gradually display decreasing reactivity, a changing baseline, or less frequent, smaller accelerations are followed with contraction stress testing.

Amniocentesis

Amniocentesis is sometimes recommended to determine meconium staining of the amniotic fluid.

INTRAPARTUM

If the conditions for induction of labor, i.e., cervix soft, thin, anterior, dilated or dilatable, vertex presentation, and the presenting part engaged, are present the membranes are usually ruptured to induce labor. If labor does not begin within a short period of time, an oxytocin infusion is started to stimulate uterine contractions.

Fetal monitoring, preferably using internal methods, is maintained in all postterm patients in labor. As a group, these fetuses are at greater risk for fetal distress and lower Apgar scores.

Elective cesarean section may be performed if the cervix is unripe, the oxytocin challenge test is suspicious or positive, or if a breech presentation is noted. If abnormalities of labor progression or fetal distress occur, a cesarean section is performed.

Complete explanations of procedures and options are presented throughout antepartum and intrapartum care.

GASTROINTESTINAL DISORDERS

Cholestasis

Many pregnant women complain of itching, which is most commonly caused by a subclinical cholestasis. In a few gravidas, a marked cholestasis can occur during pregnancy. The symptoms of pruritis and icterus are estrogen-dependent and therefore difficult to treat. Cholestasis has been associated with an increased incidence of pregnancy-induced hypertension and urinary tract infections. Vitamin K absorption may be impaired, so prothrombin levels are monitored near term. Beginning at 32 weeks gestation, nonstress testing is done to monitor fetal status. There is an associated increase in the incidence of preterm labor, low birth weight neonates, meconium staining, fetal distress, and fetal death in utero.

Viral Hepatitis

Hepatitis may be caused by at least two viruses: hepatitis A virus and hepatitis B virus. Hepatitis A virus is transmitted orally or fecally with an incubation period of 15 to 40 days. Symptoms include fever, nausea, and vomiting. The virus does not cross the placenta and has not been shown to cause any fetal or neonatal disease. If exposure occurs, immune serum globulin is given in an effort to modify the disease.

Hepatitis B virus is transmitted by close contact and by puncture with contaminated needles. The incubation period is 50 to 180 days, and the onset is usually insidious. It is more common than hepatitis A and occurs in younger age groups, possibly owing to the higher incidence of parenteral drug abuse. There is a slight risk of transplacental transmission to the fetus during early pregnancy. The fetus may acquire hepatitis at the time of delivery since both maternal blood and vaginal secretions are infectious.

MATERNAL COURSE

An important prognostic factor is maternal nutritional status when the infection occurs. Basic interventions include a diet high in protein, carbohydrates, and vitamins. No obstetric interference is needed, since pregnancy has no influence on the course of the disease.

During labor, sedation, analgesia, and anesthesia are kept to a minimum, owing to the decreased ability of the liver to metabolize. Blood must be available, since even mild anemia or hemorrhage may be disastrous. The prothrombin time is determined and vitamin K is administered.

FETAL EFFECTS

Hepatitis B is associated with a high incidence of fetal wastage, including spontaneous abortion and stillbirth. Neonates born to mothers with acute or chronic hepatitis B are at increased risk of becoming chronically infected with the hepatitis B virus. If the neonate acquires the infection during vaginal delivery, symptoms of jaundice, hepatosplenomegaly, and liver damage may result. In an effort to prevent the disease, hepatitis B immune globulin may be given on the first day of life. Mothers are carefully instructed in precautions necessary to handling the neonate. Handwashing and gloves are usually indicated.

About 90 percent of neonates born to carrier mothers are infected with hepatitis B virus. As chronic carriers, these neonates are infectious and needle precautions must be taken. These neonates have a life-long predisposition to chronic liver diseases. A combination of hepatitis B immune globulin (HBIG) and hepatitis B virus (HBV) vaccines has been used in an effort to prevent transmission (Kanai et al., 1985).

Acute Appendicitis

Acute appendicitis complicates pregnancy in about 1 in 1000 pregnancies, but is associated with a high maternal and perinatal mortality. The greatest risk is during the third trimester, when the large uterus interferes with localization of the infection.

Initial symptoms usually involve anorexia, nausea, vomiting, and abdominal pain. The pain is usually mild, dull, or crampy and either constipation or diarrhea may be present, as are tenderness to palpation and guarding. In the third trimester of pregnancy the cecum is displaced upward and into the right flank by the enlarged uterus, possibly interfering with accurate diagnosis. Gastrointestinal symptoms may be difficult to ascertain owing to discomfort associated with uterine contractions. Without accurate diagnosis and treatment, the appendix may perforate and peritonitis and secondary abscesses may result.

Ulcerative Colitis

Ulcerative colitis has an unpredictable course during pregnancy. Preexisting colitis may be reactivated or aggravated, particularly during the first trimester. If signs and symptoms of inflammatory bowel disease first appear during pregnancy, the diagnosis is made by ultrasonography rather than with x-ray.

Medical and nursing interventions revolve around controlling the disease with emotional support, adequate rest, and dietary modifications. These patients should not eat fruits and vegetables or any food containing lactose, especially milk, ice cream, and cottage cheese. A calcium supplement is given three times a day. Drug therapy must be approached with caution. Pregnancy outcome is usually successful.

ACQUIRED IMMUNODEFICIENCY SYNDROME

Acquired immunodeficiency syndrome (AIDS) is a sexually transmissible infection caused by a retrovirus currently known as human T-cell lymphotropic virus type III/lymphadenopathy-associated virus (HTLV-III/LAV) (Center for Disease Control, 1985b). It appears to be transmitted by intimate sexual contact or by blood and blood-products.

The high-risk group for AIDS includes homosexual men, bisexual men, intravenous drug users, Haitians, and hemophiliacs. Previously healthy women who are steady sexual partners of men in the high-risk AIDS group have developed infections that are typical of the AIDS spectrum (Center for Disease Control, 1983a). This syndrome can be passed on to the newborn although the method of transmission is uncertain (Center for Disease Control, 1983a).

ANTEPARTAL CARE

Women who are in the high-risk group for developing HTLV-III/LAV infection are counseled to refer their sexual partners for testing. If the sexual partner is unaffected, teaching of modifications of sexual practice are needed to reduce the risk of transmission to the unaffected partner. If infected, women are advised to delay pregnancy because of the unavailability of information about perinatal transmission. If the woman is already pregnant, the psychological impact of the disease will affect well-being during pregnancy.

Due to the low survival rate of both the mother and infant, the gravida will often expend little psychological energy toward meeting the emotional tasks of pregnancy. One of the most important roles of the nurse is that of communicator. Availability to listen, and referral to the appropriate agencies for help, whether that help be financial or psychological, is important.

NURSING INTERVENTIONS

On admission to the hospital, the gravida with AIDS is placed on blood and secretion precautions to minimize the possibility of transmission to other patients, visitors, or staff. Disposable gloves and a plastic protective apron are to be worn by anyone coming in contact with bodily fluids (lab specimens, dressings, excretions, dishes, linens, trash). The hospital should have established guidelines for cleaning or disposing of contaminated material. Explanations to the client and her visitors include the importance of the precautions.

Labor and Delivery

Blood and secretion precautions are maintained. Special care is taken to avoid contact with amniotic fluid, blood, and stools. Labor and delivery should take place in one room. Psychological support during labor and delivery is especially important. Provisions for infant bonding are made available unless there are open skin lesions. Decontamination of the room and equipment following delivery is done according to protocol.

Postpartum

All precautions are continued. A private room is recommended with rooming-in highly encouraged to avoid potential contamination of other neonates. If rooming-in is not desired or advisable, the neonate is placed in strict isolation within the nursery. The psychological needs of the family are a high priority of nursing care during this period.

NEUROLOGIC DISORDERS

Carpal Tunnel Syndrome

Carpal tunnel syndrome is transient paresthesia of the hands in the area of the median nerve distribution in the palm. Pain and paresthesia of the hand and forearm with decreased sensations and muscle weakness are symptoms noted. The disorder occurs in the second and third trimesters and is associated with edema, hypertension, and PIH. Spontaneous remission of symptoms occurs with delivery. Treatment for relief of symptoms includes restricting sodium intake, increasing rest periods, splints, and arm exercises.

Epilepsy

Epilepsy is a complex of symptoms characterized by attacks of unconsciousness that may or may not be associated with convulsions, sensory phenomena, or alterations in behavior. The frequency of seizures may increase, decrease, or remain the same during pregnancy. Nearly half of epileptic pregnant women have increased seizure activity during pregnancy, most commonly caused by a decrease in drug levels of anticonvulsants. Reasons for changes in drug levels include fluid retention, electrolyte changes, and hormonal influences that occur during pregnancy. In addition, the decreased motility of the gastrointestinal tract may change the bioavailability of medication taken orally. Normal increases in glomerular filtration rate will influence renal clearance rates of many medications. When seizure activity increases, potential fetal damage secondary to hypoxia may occur.

The incidence of seizures does not increase the risk of spontaneous abortion, pregnancy-induced hypertension, or preterm delivery. The major fetal effect is due to the teratogenic effects of the anticonvulsants administered to the mother.

MEDICAL AND NURSING INTERVENTIONS

Treatment of the pregnant epileptic ideally begins before pregnancy. Seizure status is assessed to evaluate the need for anticonvulsants. The smaller the dose and number of anticonvulsant medications used, the less potential for teratogenic effects.

During pregnancy, anticonvulsants are administered to keep the gravida seizure-free. Blood anticonvulsant levels are monitored every three to four weeks and the medication dosage adjusted accordingly. Folic acid deficiency is common with anticonvulsant medication so folic acid supplementation is given.

Following delivery, vitamin K is administered to the neonate to prevent coagulation defects. Reduction of anticonvulsant medication may be needed during the puerperium, as maternal physiologic status gradually returns to prepregnancy norms. Many anticonvulsant medications are transferred to the neonate through breast milk, so breastfeeding is evaluated individually.

Meralgia Paresthetica

Meralgia paresthetica is compression and stretching of the lateral femoral cutaneous nerve. Beginning at about 13 weeks gestation, there is tingling and numbness in the lateral third of the thigh, which is aggravated by the lordosis of pregnancy and obesity.

Interventions include client education about avoiding excess weight gain, maintaining good posture, and wearing low-heeled shoes. Reassurance that the symptoms usually resolve within three months after delivery is given.

Neuralgia and Neuritis

PERIPHERAL NERVE DISORDERS

Peripheral nerve disorders may appear during pregnancy from many causes, the most common causes of which are nutritional deficiencies and trauma. Vitamin B deficiency is associated with polyneuritis. Traumatic injuries to the nerves may occur during labor and delivery following injury to the lumbosacral plexus or to the peripheral nerves by improper forceps placement, incorrect positioning of the legs in stirrups, and faulty attempts at regional anesthesia. Most of the injuries cause temporary sciatic pain and muscle spasms, although paralysis may be seen. During the last trimester of pregnancy, pressure on the nerve as the fetal head engages may produce similar symptoms.

FACIAL PALSY

Facial palsy may be caused by many conditions, including hemorrhage, tumors, and otitis media. Late in pregnancy or early in the puerperium, Bell's palsy may be seen in association with edema that causes increasing tissue pressure and compression of the facial nerve. The left side of the face is usually involved, with complete recovery in about 85 percent of patients.

Poliomyelitis

An increased susceptibility to poliomyelitis exists during pregnancy, although immunization has decreased occurrence. Labor proceeds normally in spite of the associated paralysis, although outlet forceps may be needed. If the client is not immunized prior to pregnancy, routine immunizations are not recommended.

Polio virus can cross the placenta and cause spontaneous abortion or neonatal problems. The fetus may contract polio during delivery. If the mother has severe paralytic poliomyelitis, the fetus may exhibit growth retardation.

THE ANEMIAS

Anemia

Anemia is defined as a reduction below normal limits in the concentration of red blood cells and hemoglobin, resulting in a decrease in the amount of oxygen-carrying pigment of the blood. In the nonpregnant woman, a hemoglobin below 12 gm per 100 ml denotes anemia. A hemoglobin below 10 gm per 100 ml and/or a hematocrit less than 30 percent defines anemia during pregnancy.

CAUSES

Causes of anemia include nutritional deficiency, chronic blood loss, chronic infections, metabolic disorders, or genetic defects (see Table 25-19). The incidence varies greatly, but occurs most commonly in the malnourished and in those who receive inadequate medical care.

TABLE 25-19
CAUSES OF ANEMIAS DURING PREGNANCY

ACQUIRED ANEMIAS
Iron deficiency anemia
Acute blood loss anemia
Anemia associated with chronic disorders
Folate deficiency anemia
Acquired hemolytic anemia
Aplastic anemia
Vitamin B_{12} deficiency anemia
HEREDITARY ANEMIAS
Sickle hemoglobinopathies
Hemoglobin SS disease
Hemoglobin SC disease
Sickle-B thalassemia
Thalassemia
Other

DIAGNOSTIC STUDIES

Hemoglobin and hematocrit determinations are made at the initial prenatal visit, at approximately 26 weeks gestation, and several weeks before delivery. A venous blood sample taken without stasis should be used: stasis with a tourniquet or blood pressure cuff may cause hemoconcentration in the specimen. Other diagnostic studies may be ordered to evaluate anemia during pregnancy (see Table 25-20). The type of testing ordered is determined by maternal symptoms.

TABLE 25-20
DIAGNOSTIC STUDIES TO EVALUATE ANEMIA

Complete blood count
Serum iron
Total iron binding capacity
Hemoglobin electrophoresis
Glucose-6-phosphate dehydrogenase
Stool cultures for ova and parasites
Sickle cell test
Serum ferritin
Peripheral blood smear examination
Bone marrow aspiration

FETAL EFFECTS

There is an association between maternal anemia and perinatal mortality. Urinary estriols are typically lower than normal. Fetal anoxia follows severe untreated maternal anemia and may increase the risk of damage to fetal nervous tissue or cause fetal death.

Iron Deficiency Anemia

Iron deficiency anemia, a condition in which the total body iron content is below normal levels, is the most common anemia of pregnancy and occurs in 1 of every 5 pregnancies in the United States.

The amount of iron needed during pregnancy exceeds that available from iron stores and a well-balanced diet. Over the course of pregnancy the additional requirement imposed by the fetus, placenta, maternal hemoglobin, and red cell mass is a minimum of 600 mg.

MATERNAL EFFECTS

When iron deficiency anemia is untreated and progresses to severe anemia, with the hemoglobin level below the minimum level for safety (greater than 9 gm per 100 ml), intolerance of even moderate blood loss at delivery, predisposition to infection, and even cardiac failure may occur.

FETAL EFFECTS

Late spontaneous abortions and preterm labor are more common with severe iron deficiency anemia. Anemia of the neonate is rarely a problem because the transfer of iron to the fetus is not significantly impaired even though the mother has severe anemia.

MEDICAL AND NURSING INTERVENTIONS

Oral iron supplementation is usually adequate treatment. Iron is absorbed in the upper duodenum which has a limited capacity, so iron (180 mg) is given in divided doses three times a day with meals. Side effects expected with most iron preparations including heartburn, black stools, and constipation are reviewed with the patient. The importance of taking the medication as prescribed with water or fruit juice (not milk) to aid in absorption is stressed. Blood work is repeated in three weeks to monitor response to therapy. Iron treatment is continued throughout pregnancy and for three to six months after delivery.

Nutritional counseling is needed to encourage intake of a well-balanced diet with emphasis on iron-rich foods. Parenteral iron may be ordered if the anemia is diagnosed late in pregnancy. Blood transfusions are seldom indicated unless hypovolemia from blood loss is present or surgery must be performed.

Folic Acid Deficiency Anemia

Folic acid deficiency anemia (pernicious anemia, megaloblastic anemia) occurs in women who do not eat fresh vegetables or foods with high protein content. During pregnancy there is increased utilization of ingested folic acid caused by the presence of the fetus and decreased absorption of folic acid. When combined with low intake, folic acid deficiency anemia may result.

MATERNAL EFFECTS

Maternal pregnancy-induced hypertension is possibly associated with megaloblastic anemia.

FETAL EFFECTS

Impairment of brain function and fetal malformations have been noted in neonates whose mothers have uncorrected anemia. Rarely will the neonate have megaloblastic anemia because the fetus and placenta efficiently extract folate from the mother.

MEDICAL AND NURSING INTERVENTIONS

The nursing data base includes several pertinent items. Is the gravida malnourished or alcohol-dependent? Does she have a chronic infection? Is she a drug-controlled epileptic? What other symptoms are present?

Treatment consists of administration of folic acid. The usual dose is 1 mg per day or more. Oral iron is given at the same time because iron stores are used to fill newly produced red blood cells. A high vitamin, high protein diet is recommended, with emphasis on foods high in folacin (liver, yeast, and deep green leafy vegetables).

This type of anemia tends to recur in subsequent pregnancies, owing to dietary inadequacies or diminished absorption of folic acid. The use of combination estrogen/progestin oral contraceptives has been associated with folate deficiency.

Glucose-6-Phosphate Dehydrogenase Deficiency (G6PD)

In approximately 10 to 15 percent of black women, G6PD deficiency is present. The disease is an X-linked red blood cell enzyme deficiency. The pentose shunt (G6PD is the initial enzyme needed) is an aerobic bypass for glycolysis used by the liver and adipose tissue to synthesize ribose (constituent of RNA) and essential fatty acids, and to use lactic acid in muscular work.

Hemolysis may be caused by drugs, infection, and acidosis. Common drug classifications that can cause a hemolytic reaction include nitrofurans, antimalarials, analgesics, antipyretics, sulfonamides, and vitamin K.

Anemia in these women can be successfully treated with iron, folic acid, and a nutritional diet. The greatest maternal risk is the increased incidence of urinary tract infections that are difficult to treat owing to the limited number of medications available. Perinatal risks include jaundice, hydrops fetalis, and intrauterine death.

Aplastic Anemia

Severe bone marrow depression accompanied by reduced erythrocytes, leukocytes, and platelets characterize aplastic anemia. Causative agents include x-ray, radioactive materials, and medications. When aplastic anemia is present prior to conception, pregnancy interruption will not improve client status. Pregnancy termination often results in remission if aplastic anemia first develops during pregnancy.

Sickle Cell Disease

The most common sickle cell hemoglobinopathies are sickle cell anemia (Hb SS), hemoglobin SC disease (Hb SC), and hemoglobin S-thalassemia disease (Hb S-Thal). All are generally referred to as sickle cell disease.

Sickle hemoglobin (S) differs from normal (A) hemoglobin as a result of the mutation from glutamic acid to valine in the hemoglobin olypeptide chain. This single mutation is the direct cause of the physiochemical alterations in the hemoglobin molecule that are responsible for clinical problems. When the level of oxygen in the tissues decreases, erythrocytes containing hemoglobin S lose their normal shape and become sickled forms that are unable to migrate successfully to the microvasculature of various organs.

The clinical manifestations of the various sickle cell diseases are determined by the amount of hemoglobin S present in the red cells, the type and amount of any other hemoglobin in the same red blood cells, the presence of any additional red cell abnormalities, and modifying factors.

SICKLE CELL TRAIT

Sickle cell trait affects approximately 10 to 20 percent of all blacks in the United States. It is a benign condition with rare signs and symptoms. Blood counts, red blood cell morphology, and red blood cell life span are all normal. Since it is a heterozygous manifestation of sickle cell disease, only a portion of hemoglobin S is present.

The main concern in reproduction with sickle cell trait is the potential for transmission of the sickling gene to the child. If both parents have the trait, each of the children has a 1 in 4 chance of having sickle cell anemia. There are no alterations in fertility, pregnancy, and labor and delivery. An increased incidence of urinary tract infections, especially pyelonephritis, during pregnancy is common. There is no documented increase in spontaneous abortion rates, preterm deliveries, stillbirths, or neonatal death.

SICKLE CELL ANEMIA

Sickle cell anemia occurs in approximately 0.2 to 1.2 percent of the black population. Pregnancy imposes a serious burden on women with sickle cell anemia.

A hereditary condition, sickle cell anemia is a disease in which erythrocytes contain an abnormal hemoglobin (Hemoglobin S) and assume a sickle shape upon deoxygenation. Sickle cell anemia is characterized by chronic hemolytic anemia and intermittent crises of varying frequency and intensity.

Maternal Effects

There is an increased incidence of anemia, infections, sickle cell crisis, pregnancy-induced hypertension, pulmonary infarctions, congestive heart failure, and preterm labor in the gravida with sickle cell anemia.

Fetal/Neonatal Effects

One-fourth to one-half of pregnancies end in spontaneous abortions, stillbirth, or neonatal death. Preterm deliveries and intrauterine growth retardation are increased. Live-born

TABLE 25-21
ANTEPARTUM NURSING RESPONSIBILITIES FOR THE GRAVIDA WITH SICKLE CELL ANEMIA

Initial assessment, including:	Past medical and surgical history
	Family history
	Review of support systems
Obtain laboratory testing as ordered	
Assess client perceptions of her disease	
Assess feelings about pregnancy	
Encourage medications as ordered:	Folic acid
	Iron
	Antibiotics if infection is present
Nutrition education:	Well-balanced diet
	High iron and folic acid
	Adequate fluid intake
Include support persons in all discussions	
Assess for complications	
Interaction with same nurse throughout the antepartal period will allow continuity	
Anticipatory guidance:	Avoid exposure to infectious diseases
	Avoid excessive chilling
	Avoid high altitudes
	Avoid excessive dampness
	Get adequate rest
Return visits:	1st trimester: q 2 weeks
	2nd trimester: q 2 weeks
	3rd trimester: q week
Fetal surveillance:	Testing for fetal well-being from 34 weeks until term
Refer for genetic counseling as necessary	

neonates have a sufficient amount of fetal hemoglobin to postpone sickling. By the age of four to six weeks, the red blood cells will contain predominantly sickle hemoglobin, and symptoms may be seen.

Medical and Nursing Interventions

Close medical and nursing monitoring of gravidas with sickle cell anemia is mandatory for a favorable outcome. Early in pregnancy, planning and implementing physical and psychosocial care as well as counseling and health education are begun (see Table 25-21). Frequent and systematic evaluation is important throughout the antepartal period. Vaginal delivery is preferred, with cesarean section indicated only for obstetrical reasons. Nursing responsibilities are many and varied (see Table 25-22).

HEMOGLOBIN SC DISEASE

Hemoglobin SC disease is a hereditary, chronic, hemolytic anemia that occurs in approximately 1 of every 2400 black pregnant women. When not pregnant, the woman with SC disease seldom experiences serious illness. Pregnancy increases morbidity and mortality. Episodes of joint and bone pain are frequent,

TABLE 25-22
INTRAPARTUM NURSING RESPONSIBILITIES FOR THE GRAVIDA WITH SICKLE CELL ANEMIA

- Inpatient client assessment with focus on sickle cell status
- Laboratory testing as ordered: minimum of CBC
  - Type and crossmatch for 4 U packed cells
- Initiate intravenous fluids as ordered
- Maintain adequate hydration: dehydration may precipitate crisis
- Monitor intake and output
- Maintain support system
- Continuous FHR and UC monitoring
- Minimal analgesia, but keep comfortable
  - Encourage breathing and relaxation techniques
- Regional anesthesia preferred
  - General anesthesia usually avoided because of compromised oxygenation that may occur, followed by an increased sickling rate
- Assess for complications: Monitor hemoglobin and hematocrit
  - Infection
  - Sickle cell crisis
  - PIH
  - Thrombophlebitis
  - Congestive heart failure
  - Pulmonary infarction
- Monitor labor progress
- Maintain warmth: hypothermia may precipitate crisis
- May use prophylactic transfusion with packed red blood cells
  - Avoid circulatory overload
- Assess for edema
- Auscultate lungs
- Maintain semirecumbent or lateral position
- Oxygen usually given by mask to maintain oxygenation
- Maternal vital signs every hour
- Obtain a cord blood specimen at delivery

especially during the third trimester. Pneumonitis related to embolization of necrotic bone marrow is also encountered. There is an increased incidence of low birth weight neonates and perinatal mortality.

HEMOGLOBIN S-THALASSEMIA DISEASE

When one parent has a gene for hemoglobin S and the other has a gene for β-thalassemia, the result is hemoglobin S-thalassemia disease. Maternal and fetal effects are similar to those of sickle cell anemia.

Thalassemia

The thalassemias are a genetically determined group of disorders characterized by decreased production of one or more of the globin chains in human hemoglobin. The anemia is a hypochromic microcytic variety, with abnormally shaped erythrocytes, that results from both inadequate globulin production and an excessive breakdown of erythrocytes. It is most often seen in persons of Mediterranean, Central African, and Asian descent.

THALASSEMIA MAJOR

Thalassemia major or Cooley's anemia is homozygous with inheritance from both parents. Chronic severe anemia and hemachromatosis lead to death before age 30 years.

THALASSEMIA MINOR

Many patients with thalassemia minor, a heterozygous form of thalassemia, are asymptomatic until pregnancy. With the onset of pregnancy there are recurrent acute hemolytic crises and severe anemia. There is an increased incidence of maternal pyelonephritis, pneumonia, and pulmonary emboli. Blood transfusions are rarely indicated, except to treat hemorrhage. Iron and folic acid supplements are given, although the anemia is usually unresponsive to therapy. Infections should be avoided. Fetal mortality is approximately 15 percent.

INFECTIONS

The list of maternal infections that have a real potential for causing detrimental effects on the fetus or neonate is increasing. Maternal infections occur in approximately 15 percent of all pregnancies. The effects of these maternal infections fall into five broad categories: (1) no effect; (2) spontaneous abortion; (3) fetal death in utero; (4) teratogenic effects; and (5) neonatal infection (see Table 25-23).

TORCH Infections

The TORCH group of infections present a serious threat to the fetus and neonate. They include: TO–toxoplasmosis, R–rubella, C–cytomegalovirus, and H–herpes virus. The O in TORCH is often designated as other.

TOXOPLASMOSIS

The etiologic agent of toxoplasmosis is the protozoan *Toxoplasma gondii.* When contracted during pregnancy, the disease frequently affects the fetus and neonate. Ingestion of infected cysts in meat or in other contaminated food or by oocysts from animal feces is followed by an incubation period of 10 days.

Screening by serologic methods during pregnancy is recommended. Pregnant women are tested before 10 weeks gestation, retested at 20 to 22 weeks, and again at term. Prevention of infection during pregnancy is accomplished by hygienic measures, i.e., cooking meat well, avoiding touching mucous membranes of the mouth and eye while handling raw meat, washing hands thoroughly after handling raw meat, washing fruits and vegetables before consumption, avoiding contact with or wearing gloves when handling materials potentially contaminated with cat or dog feces, and disinfection of cat litter boxes.

TABLE 25-23
MATERNAL INFECTIONS AND THEIR EFFECTS

Infection	Maternal Effects	Mode of Transmission	Fetal/Neonatal Effects
TORCH INFECTIONS			
Toxoplasmosis	Transmission by hand-to-mouth transfer of oocysts Headache, lethargy, rash Acute chorioretinitis	Transplacental	Spontaneous abortion Preterm delivery Chorioretinitis, IUGR, hydrocephaly, rash, microcephaly, psychomotor retardation, jaundice, immune deficiencies, hepatosplenomegaly
Rubella	Transmission by droplet Maculopapular rash, arthralgia, low-grade fever, lymph gland enlargement	Transplacental	Spontaneous abortion Cataracts, deafness, cardiac defects, IUGR, retinopathy, pneumonia, encephalitis, mental retardation, jaundice, microcephaly, glaucoma, microophthalmia
Cytomegalovirus	Maternal contact with virus by contaminated saliva, urine, semen Asymptomatic Mononucleosis type symptoms	Transplacental Vaginal secretions Breast milk	IUGR, mental retardation, jaundice, hepatosplenomegaly, petechiae, pneumonia, microcephaly, anemia, chorioretinitis, hydrocephaly, deafness, seizures, cerebral calcifications
Herpes virus	Sexual contact Herpetic lesions, fever, headaches, adenopathy, node tenderness	Ascending infection infection after ROM Direct contact with lesion	Spontaneous abortion Preterm delivery IUGR, localized lesions, microcephaly, patent ductur arteriosus Disseminated infection: lethargy, febrile episodes, mottled skin, hepatosplenomegaly, poor feeding, seizures, lesions 50% mortality with disseminated infection
OTHER INFECTIONS			
Brucellosis	Enters through GI tract or droplet Weakness, chills, fever, headache, myalgia, arthralgia, cough, lymphadenopathy, tender abdomen	Transplacental	Spontaneous abortion Preterm delivery SGA neonate

TABLE 25–23 (continued)

Infection	Maternal Effects	Mode of Transmission	Fetal/Neonatal Effects
OTHER INFECTIONS (continued)			
Chickenpox	Droplet transmission Vesicular rash, shingles	Transplacental Direct contact with infected areas	Spontaneous abortion Fetal death Asymptomatic Cerebral atrophy, mental retardation, limb hypoplasia, IUGR, hydrocephaly, chorioretinitis Neonatal chickenpox
Cholera	Profuse diarrhea with electrolyte imbalance, acidosis	Transplacental	Intrauterine fetal death
Coccidiomycosis	Fungus infection by inhalation Self-limited pulmonary infection May have secondary dissemination to other organs	Transplacental	Spontaneous abortion Intrauterine fetal death
Hepatitis B	Serum innoculation Intimate contact Jaundice, lethargy, vomiting, anorexia	Contact with vaginal secretions and blood during delivery	Asymptomatic Carrier status Acute hepatitis Preterm delivery Fetal intrauterine death
Influenza	Flulike symptoms	Transplacental	Spontaneous abortion Preterm delivery Intrauterine fetal death
Listeriosis	Influenza symptoms, vaginitis, UTI, meningitis May be harbored in cervix	Direct contact at birth Transplacental	Spontaneous abortion Preterm delivery Intrauterine fetal death Neonatal infection: skin rash, meningitis, pneumonia
Malaria	Chills and fever	Transplacental	Spontaneous abortion Preterm delivery SGA neonate Intrauterine fetal death Neonatal malaria rare
Mumps	Viral Malaise, fever, pain at jaw angle, swollen parotid glands	Transplacental	Spontaneous abortion Preterm delivery Intrauterine fetal death Endocardial fibroblastosis

TABLE 25-23 (continued)

Infection	Maternal Effects	Mode of Transmission	Fetal/Neonatal Effects
OTHER INFECTIONS (continued)			
Poliomyelitis	Virus	Transplacental	Spontaneous abortion Congenital anomalies Flaccid paralysis
Scarlet fever	Scarlet fever	Transplacental	Spontaneous abortion
Smallpox	Viral Dermal lesions, fever	Transplacental	Spontaneous abortion Intrauterine fetal death Preterm delivery Intrauterine infection Neonatal smallpox
Typhoid fever	Typhoid symptoms	Transplacental	Spontaneous abortion Fetal death Preterm delivery
SEXUALLY TRANSMITTED DISEASES			
Beta B Strep	Asymptomatic Septicemia, fever, cellulitis, UTI, impetigo, chorioamnionitis	Direct contact after ROM	Neonatal death Blindness, deafness, meningitis, mental retardation, learning problems
Condyloma accuminata	Viral Venereal warts	Direct contact	Laryngeal problems
Gonorrhea	Sexual contact Asymptomatic Leukorrhea, dysuria, low backache, nausea	Direct contact	Ophthalmia neonatorum
Syphilis	Primary chancre Various manifestations of the disease	Transplacental Direct contact with lesions	Spontaneous abortion Preterm delivery Intrauterine fetal death May be asymptomatic Congenital syphilis
Vaginitis			
Candida albicans	Overgrowth of fungus Cheesy, curdy discharge White patches on cervix and vaginal mucosa Vulvar pururitis, edema Dyspareunia	Direct contact	Neonatal thrust
Chlamydia	Asymptomatic Cervical congestion, edema, urethritis	Direct contact	Spontaneous abortion Inclusion conjunctivitis Pneumonia, septicemia, chronic follicular conjunctivitis

TABLE 25-23 (continued)

Infection	Maternal Effects	Mode of Transmission	Fetal/Neonatal Effects
Vaginitis (continued)			
Hemophilus vaginalis	Minimal creamy yellow, gray vaginal discharge	Direct contact	Intrauterine fetal death Septicemia
Trichomonas vaginalis	Copious, frothy thin yellow-green vaginal discharge Pruritis, dysuria, dyspareunia	Direct contact	None reported

Treatment is by administration of a combination of pyrimethamine and sulfadiazine. A drug called spiramycin has been used with some success, but is not available in the United States at this time.

RUBELLA

Rubella is a viral infection that carries an ominous prognosis for the fetus or neonate if maternal disease occurs during the first 20 weeks gestation. The risk of fetal damage varies with the time of maternal infection: 50 percent if infection manifest during the first four weeks of gestation, 22 percent if during weeks 5 through 8, 10 percent during weeks 9 through 12, and 6 percent during weeks 13 to 20.

The best approach to rubella is early immunization. Vaccine should be administered to children at 15 months of age. All women of childbearing age should be tested for antibody to rubella; if antibody levels are not sufficient, vaccine is given.

CYTOMEGALOVIRUS

Maternal intrauterine infection with cytomegalovirus (CMV) occurs in 1 to 5 percent of pregnancies in the United States. Women infected with CMV are often asymptomatic, but may have mononucleosis-type symptoms. Primary CMV infections carry a 30 percent chance that the fetus or neonate will be affected, particularly if active infection occurs late in pregnancy.

HERPES VIRUS

Herpes may be of the nongenital type (HSV_1) or genital variety (HSV_2) with HSV_2 more often implicated in neonatal disease. Antibody to either type of herpes does not protect against the other.

Herpes simplex infections complicate about 1 percent of gestations. The risk to the fetus is higher with primary genital herpes because: (1) virus titers are higher; (2) there is greater risk of an infected cervix; and (3) the neonate lacks herpes antibodies at birth.

There is no known cure for herpes. Symptomatic relief can be achieved with hot sitz baths, antibiotic and anesthetic ointments, analgesic medications, and pyridium to decrease dysuria.

If a gravida has a history of herpes, or if her partner has herpes, she is at risk for developing genital herpes. Cervical cultures are taken every two weeks during the last trimester of pregnancy to detect active herpes virus. If active virus is detected, delivery by cesarean section before the membranes rupture or within four hours of spontaneous rupture of the membranes is preferred.

Postpartum, the client is placed in a private room and contact isolation procedures are instituted. Breastfeeding is permissible provided careful handwashing procedures and prevention of contact with infected sites or secretions is maintained.

Neonates at risk of herpes infection are isolated to prevent horizontal transmission of infections within the nursery.

ISOIMMUNE DISEASE

Isoimmune disease is a disorder of the fetus or neonate caused by maternal sensitization to fetal red cell antigens. Sensitization is followed by transfer of resultant antibodies to the fetus. During gestation some fetal blood cells pass into the maternal circulation. If the cells are incompatible, antibodies are produced by the mother in response. These antibodies are returned to the fetus where they destroy red blood cells, causing hemolytic disease of the newborn.

ABO Incompatibility

One form of hemolytic disease of the newborn occurs when there is an incompatibility between ABO blood groups of the mother and the fetus. Most commonly it occurs when the mother is type O and the fetus is type A, although other combinations may also cause incompatibility.

Hemolytic disease from ABO incompatibility has several characteristics: (1) it can occur in any pregnancy; (2) it does not increase in severity with subsequent pregnancies; (3) it does not require intrauterine therapy; and (4) neonatal symptoms are usually mild.

Rh Incompatibility

The Rh factor is an antigen present in the red blood cells of 85 percent of whites and 95 percent of blacks, American Indians, and Orientals in the United States. Those who have the antigen are Rh positive and those who do not are Rh negative.

Rh isoimmunization occurs when the mother is Rh negative, the father is Rh positive, and the fetus is Rh positive. Positive fetal cells cross the placenta and cause antibody production in the mother which then return to the fetus through the placenta and attack fetal red blood cells. The destruction of fetal blood cells causes anemia that may be mild or severe enough to produce *hydrops fetalis* (edema and circulatory collapse) in the fetus. Bilirubin, a breakdown product of red blood cells, may rise and cause jaundice. If the bilirubin levels rise to a toxic level (18 mg per 100 ml in the term neonate), *kernicterus* (jaundice of the nuclear masses of the brain) may result. Once maternal antibodies are present, all subsequent pregnancies with an Rh positive fetus will have hemolytic disease.

MEDICAL AND NURSING INTERVENTIONS

There are two objectives of medical and nursing interventions in Rh incompatibility: prevention of isoimmunization, and monitoring of maternal antibodies and fetal condition.

At the initial prenatal visit a blood group and Rh type are tested. If the mother is Rh negative, an indirect Coombs' test will also measure the amount of antibodies present in maternal serum. An antibody screen aids in identification of the mother as a potential Rh immune globulin candidate.

At 28 weeks gestation, the indirect Coombs' test is repeated. If no Rh antibodies are detected, Rh immune globulin (300 μg) is given IM to prevent the occasional antibody development that may occur during gestation.

The precise mechanism of action of Rh immune globulin is not clear, but it seems to depend on the coating of circulating Rh positive fetal cells by the passively administered antibody. A full dose provides protection for about 12 weeks of pregnancy and will be effective until a postpartum dose is needed. Client teaching should alleviate fear and anxiety. The gravida is told that reactions to Rh immune globulin are rare and generally local in nature, but that a slight elevation in temperature may develop. The absence of adverse effects on the fetus is emphasized.

At the time of delivery, cord blood is obtained for blood group, Rh type and direct Coombs' test. The direct Coombs' test will measure the number of fetal cells coated with maternal antibodies. Weak anti-D antibodies may be present if the mother received antepartal Rh immune globulin owing to the residual immunoglobulin present in the maternal blood serum. If the neonate is Rh positive, 300 μg of Rh immune globulin are administered intramuscularly to the client after crossmatch with maternal red cells.

Rh immune globulin is administered following delivery of each successive Rh positive fetus, following spontaneous or induced abortion, ectopic pregnancy, and amniocentesis. For pregnancies terminated prior to 12 weeks gestation and following amniocentesis, a 50 μg dose of Rh immune globulin is administered.

If the client is Rh negative, the father is Rh positive, and antibodies are detected with an indirect Coombs' test, titration determines the degree to which antibodies are present. Titers are done every three to four weeks to determine the level of antibodies. If the titer remains negative or below the critical level (1:8), pregnancy can continue without further intervention.

If the antibody titer goes above 1:8, significant sensitization is present and fetal evaluation is necessary. Amniocentesis evaluates the amount of bilirubin present. The amniotic fluid is placed in a light-resistant container to prevent false bilirubin levels. The optical density of the amniotic fluid is analyzed to measure light absorption. The optical density of normal amniotic fluid plotted on a graph will resemble a straight line. When bilirubin is present, a bulge will appear in the line. The bulge is measured and plotted against gestational age to assess severity of hemolytic disease.

The Liley graph is divided into three zones, indicating disease severity. If the optical density is in zone I, the fetus is mildly affected. Zone II indicates moderate fetal disease, and zone III indicates a severely affected fetus who requires immediate treatment.

The amniocentesis is repeated at one- to three-week intervals and the serial optical density values evaluated to determine a trend. If the trend is downward, pregnancy is allowed to continue until fetal lung maturity is documented. If the trend is rising between 23 and 31 weeks, an intrauterine fetal transfusion with type O negative packed red cells is instituted to enable the fetus to survive in utero until sufficiently mature enough to deliver.

Erythrocyte membrane oral therapy may be initiated in selected clients in an attempt to alter antibody production (Gold et al., 1983). This therapy attempts to alter established antibody production by the oral administration of the Rh antigen located on the erythrocyte membrane.

PSYCHIATRIC DISORDERS

Mental illness complicates about 1 in 400 to 1000 pregnancies, the majority of these being postpartum psychosis (see Chapter 27). Psychiatric disorders during pregnancy are not considered separate and distinct from psychoses that occur at other times. Most women who develop psychiatric disorders during pregnancy have a history of maladjustment, immature behavioral patterns, and matrimonial difficulties. Prepregnancy psychological testing can help to identify some of these women, but behavior patterns can be identified without testing each and every woman before conception.

During the prenatal period, assessments are made for symptoms that warn of potential psychiatric problems. Awareness of the client's personal and family history, social and marital adjustments, psychological maturity, and attitudes toward pregnancy and child rearing aids in assessing her reactions to the present pregnancy. Early recognition of symptoms and prompt referral for treatment will help reduce the severity of psychiatric disorders concurrent with pregnancy. Removing the client from the current situation and placing her in a favorable environment is recommended.

Psychiatric medications should be carefully selected. Antidepressants are avoided. If lithium is used, careful monitoring of blood levels is needed owing to the normal changes in blood volume as pregnancy advances. Recovery rate is about the same as for the nonpregnant population.

Pseudocyesis

In pseudocyesis there is a strong biologic, economic, or sociologic need for children that creates the symptoms of pregnancy in the mind and body of a woman. The etiology is hypothetical, but it is generally accepted that the occurrence of pseudocyesis originates from two related components: an awareness of body changes associated with pregnancy and a fantasy about some aspect of pregnancy. Women with a strong desire for, or fear of, pregnancy will miss a period and then experience symptoms of early pregnancy because they assume they are pregnant.

Characteristic symptoms include menstrual disturbances of varying duration, abdominal enlargement, assumed lordosis, breast changes, and weight gain. The client may describe fetal movements.

Nursing interventions are based on these goals: (1) acceptance of the woman's claim to encourage her to see the physician; and (2) appreciation of the interrelationship between pseudocyesis and feelings of fear and depression.

SUBSTANCE ABUSE

Substance abuse during pregnancy is an increasing problem in our society today. If the pregnant client is a chronic substance abuser, not only will she be more prone to complications, but the incidence of complications for the fetus will also increase. History during the prenatal period and counseling should be geared to increasing maternal awareness of potential problems. Maternal and fetal complications are summarized in Table 25–24.

HYPEREMESIS GRAVIDARUM

Excessive or pernicious vomiting of pregnancy occurring before 20 weeks gestation that is severe enough to require admission to the hospital, and is not associated with coincidental conditions, is designated *hyperemesis gravidarum.*

It occurs in approximately 1 of 300 pregnancies. The exact cause for the excessive vomiting is not known, although several theories have been proposed: the high levels of chorionic gonadotropin present in early pregnancy create endocrine imbalances; the decreased secretion of free hydrochloric acid present during early pregnancy; reduced gastric motility present during pregnancy; psychological factors, e.g., symbolic rejection of pregnancy and maternal ambivalence toward the developing fetus.

The incidence of hyperemesis gravidarum is increased in multiple pregnancies and primigravidas. It is relatively infrequent among blacks and will tend to recur with subsequent pregnancies.

Clinical Manifestations

Clinical manifestations observed in hyperemesis gravidarum correlate closely with manifestations noted in starvation state and include: weight loss due to anorexia, nausea and vomiting, hiccups, thirst, dehydration, alkalosis, acidosis, hypokalemia, tachycardia, oliguria, hemoconcentration, withdrawal, and depression.

TABLE 25-24
SUBSTANCE ABUSE DURING PREGNANCY

Substance	Maternal Effects	Fetal/Neonatal Effects
Alcohol	Poor nutritional status Bone marrow suppression Increased incidence of infections Liver disease Delerium tremens Withdrawal seizures 12–48 hours after cessation of drinking	IUGR Immature motor activity Increased incidence of cardiac anomalies Decreased muscle tone Poor sucking response Stillbirth Decreased placental weight Increased structural brain anomalies Fetal alcohol syndrome Withdrawal symptoms within 8–12 hours after delivery
Amphetamines	Agitation Malnutrition Vasculitis Psychological dependence	Learning disabilities Poor motor coordination Transposition of great vessels Cleft palate Low birth weight
Barbiturates	Malnutrition CNS depression Hypertension Anxiety	Neonatal depression Increase in anomalies Withdrawal symptoms Convulsions Neonatal hyperactivity Hyperreflexia Vasomotor instability Vitamin K deficiency Neonatal jaundice
Caffeine	Nervousness Diuresis Dependence	Spontaneous abortion IUGR Increased incidence of cleft palate Preterm deliveries Increased incidence of limb anomalies
Cannabis	None known	IUGR Bradycardia EEG changes
Cocaine	Excitation Euphoria Decreased sensation of fatigue	Learning disabilities ?? increase in cardiac anomalies
Diazepam	Dependence	Hypotonia Hypothermia Low Apgar scores Respiratory depression Poor sucking reflex

TABLE 25-24 (continued)

Substance	Maternal Effects	Fetal/Neonatal Effects
Heroin	Maternal malnutrition Increase in alcohol intake Pulmonary disease Poor prenatal care 2-6 time increase in PIH Increased malpresentations Increase in third trimester bleeding Increased puerperal morbidity PROM Hepatitis	IUGR Preterm deliveries Increased perinatal mortality Withdrawal symptoms Convulsions Respiratory alkalosis Hyperbilirubinemia
Methadone	see Heroin	Fetal distress Meconium aspiration Irritability Hyperactivity Sleep problems Withdrawal symptoms
Nicotine	Poor nutrition Increase in abruption Placenta previa Cardiovascular disease	Reduced gestational length Preterm delivery SGA infants Increased spontaneous abortion Small head circumference Increased perinatal mortality

Medical and Nursing Interventions

Initially, other diseases are ruled out, specifically gastroenteritis, hepatitis, cholecystitis, peptic ulcer, or brain tumor.

If the hyperemesis gravidarum is mild, interventions revolve around support of the client. She is encouraged to verbalize concerns. Morning nausea may be prevented by instructing the client to eat two or three crackers and remain in bed for 15 minutes after awakening. Dry carbohydrates have an antiemetic action. Approximately one half hour after arising, a small, dry breakfast may be tolerated. Prochlorperazine or another antiemetic may be prescribed to be taken on awakening and every six or eight hours.

When hyperemesis gravidarum is severe and requires hospitalization, medical and nursing measures are based on three main goals (see Table 25-25): (1) protection from dehydration and starvation; (2) provision of physiologic support; and (3) psychological support.

Therapeutic abortion is sometimes recommended for the client with hyperemesis gravidarum. The presence of retinal hemorrhages is considered a grave sign, resulting from changes in the permeability of the retinal vessel walls due to profound avitaminosis. A persistent elevation in temperature despite adequate hydration, persistent tachycardia, jaundice, profound depression, and delerium are considered indicators for induced abortion.

TABLE 25-25
NURSING RESPONSIBILITIES IN SEVERE HYPEREMESIS GRAVIDARUM

Protection from dehydration and starvation
- Hospitalize
- Private room
- Decrease stimuli
- Complete bed rest
- NPO for at least 24 hours
- Provide parenteral fluids as ordered
- Obtain laboratory tests as ordered
- Evaluate laboratory test results
- Monitor intake and output
- Administer other medication as ordered: Antihistamines, Antiemetics, Anticholinergics, Sedatives
- Vital signs every 4 hours
- Institute small frequent feedings as tolerated after NPO status lifted

Provision of physiologic support
- Oral hygiene every 2 to 3 hours
- Remove emesis promptly
- Change linens prn
- Special attention to temperature and appearance of foods when ordered
- Provide rest and sleep
- Restrict visitors for first 24 hours
- Provide same personnel to care for client

Psychological support
- Same personnel to care for client
- Listen
- Nonjudgemental attitude
- Help to identify her feelings
- Help to initiate problem-solving approach if problems identified
- Psychological or psychiatric evaluation may be needed

TRAUMA DURING PREGNANCY

Accidents associated with trauma are not uncommon during pregnancy, occurring as a result of normal maternal adaptations to pregnancy. Syncope and loss of balance are responsible for accidents, especially during the last trimester. It is estimated that approximately 7 percent of women sustain an accidental injury during pregnancy (Smith & Payne, 1984), although the incidence of severe trauma is rare.

Abdominal trauma includes potential injuries to the fetus, pelvic organs, and abdominal organs. Fetal injury may result from penetrating instruments and projectiles. Injury to pelvic organs can result in damage to the uterus, membranes, cord, or placenta. Blunt trauma may result in injury to the abdominal organs.

Automobile injuries account for the major portion of severe maternal injuries during pregnancy. The degree of maternal and fetal damage is related to the force of the accident and the resistance of the maternal abdominal wall. Wearing seat belts greatly reduces maternal and fetal injuries. If a lap belt only is worn in the car, it should be worn low over the iliac crests to prevent injury to the uterus and bladder. If a three-point harness is worn, it should be placed high over the chest to prevent uterine compression on impact.

Immediate care of trauma during pregnancy consists of the ABCs: airway, breathing, and circulation. When hypoxia is present, the mother attempts to maintain homeostasis at the expense of the fetus. Hypotension has a deleterious effect on the fetus. Emergency personnel must remember the potential for vena cava syndrome and position the woman on her side or in a position that displaces the uterus laterally. The maternal cardiovascular and respiratory changes that occur during pregnancy must be considered. The normal maternal increase in blood volume will prevent the usual observations of hypovolemia from being noted. A significant blood loss (about 30 percent) may be present before the usual signs and symptoms are observed. Usual signs of organ rupture may not be noted because of the stretching of the abdominal wall. Decreased gastrointestinal motility may mask signs of severe bowel trauma.

If the mother has expired and a postmortem cesarean section is necessary, fetal outcome is often good if the time elapsed after maternal death is less than 20 to 25 minutes.

TRANSPLANT PATIENTS

With the numbers of patients successfully surviving transplants increasing, the incidence of pregnancy in the posttransplant patient is increasing. Early diagnosis of pregnancy is important in these women, so meticulous medical and nursing care can be given during the antepartal period.

During pregnancy, prenatal visits are at least every three weeks until 28 weeks gestation, then weekly. During these visits, general health is evaluated. The weight, blood pressure, urinary protein and glucose, fundal height and fetal heart tones are assessed. Ultrasound is used to assess placental localization and biparietal diameter during the first trimester, and is repeated at 32 and 36 weeks. Periodic creatinine clearance and urine cultures are tested. Cervical cultures for viruses are taken at 28 weeks gestation, repeat blood counts and cervical cytology are done at 32 weeks, and the client is hospitalized as needed to evaluate maternal or fetal condition.

OBESITY

Pregnancy in the obese woman poses specific problems during the antepartal, intrapartal, and postpartal periods. The fetus is also subject to increased risks.

During the antepartum period, there is an increased incidence of hypertension, hyperglycemia, and decreased urinary estriol excretion. During labor, there is an increase in prolonged labor and operative deliveries. Postpartum hemorrhage is more common in the obese client. There is also an increase in asphyxia in the fetus.

BIBLIOGRAPHY

ABORTION

A toxic way to abort. *Emergency Medicine*, 1984, **16**, 75.

Blum, R.W. & Resnick, M.D. Adolescent sexual decision making: Contraception, pregnancy, abortion, and motherhood. *Pediatric Annals*, 1982, **11**, 797.

Goldsmith, M.F. Possible herpesvirus role in abortion studied. *Journal of the American Medical Association*, 1984, **251**, 3067.

Grimes, D.A., Cates, W., Smith, J.C. & Rochat, R.W. Mortality from abortion and childbirth. *Journal of the American Medical Association*, 1983, **249**, 194.

Henshaw, S.K. Abortion services in the United States, 1979-1980. *Family Planning Perspective*, 1982, **14**, 5-15.

Hern, W.M. Midtrimester abortion. *Obstetrics & Gynecology Annual*, 1981, **10**, 375.
Kline, I., Shot, P., Stein, Z., et al. Drinking during pregnancy and spontaneous abortion. *Lancet*, 1980, **2**, 176.
———, et al. Smoking: A risk factor for abortion. *New England Journal of Medicine*, 1977, **297**, 793.
Late abortions linked to education, age and irregular menses. *Family Planning Perspective*, 1981, **13**, 86.
Levin, A.A., Schoenbaum, S.C., Stubblefield, P.G., Zimicke, S., Monson, R.R. & Ryan, K.J. Ectopic pregnancy and prior induced abortion. *American Journal of Public Health*, 1982, **72**, 252.
Miller, J.F., et al. Fetal loss after implantation. *Lancet*, 1980, **2**, 554.
Sasso, S.C. Prostaglandin for ob-gyn. *MCN*, 1983, **8**, 107.
Schneider, T.B.: Voluntary termination of pregnancy. *Journal of Obstetric, Gynecological & Neonatal Nursing*, 1984, **13**, 775.
Schoenbaum, S.C., Monson, R.R., Stubblefield, P.G., Darney, P.D. & Ryan, K.J. Outcome of delivery following an induced or spontaneous abortion. *American Journal of Obstetrics & Gynecology*, 1980, **136**, 19.
Westergaard, L., Philipsen, T. & Schiebel, J. Significance of cervical Chlamydia trachomatis infection in postabortal pelvic inflammatory disease. *Obstetrics & Gynecology*, 1982, **60**, 322.
Wetzel, S.K. Are we ignoring the needs of the woman with a spontaneous abortion? *MCN*, 1982, **7**, 258.

HYDATIDIFORM MOLE

Celeste, S.M. & Smith, M.D. Gestational trophoblastic neoplasms. *Journal of Obstetric, Gynecologic & Neonatal Nursing*, 1986, **15**, 11-16.
Pardue, S.F. Hydatidiform mole: A pathological pregnancy. *American Journal of Nursing*, 1977, **77**, 863.
Smith, E.B., Weed, J.C., Tyrey, L. & Hammond, C.B. Treatment of nonmetastic gestational trophoblastic disease. *American Journal of Obstetrics & Gynecology*, 1982, **44**, 88-92.

ECTOPIC PREGNANCY

Dorfman, S.F. Deaths from ectopic pregnancy, United States, 1979 to 1980. *Obstetrics & Gynecology*, 1983, **62**, 334.
Freeman, J. & Goldberg, L. Ectopic pregnancy. *Annals of Emergency Medicine*, 1984, **13**, 339.
Kadar, N., Caldwell, B.V. & Romero, R. A method of screening for ectopic pregnancy and its indications. *Obstetrics & Gynecology*, 1981, **58**, 162.
LeBolt, S.A., Grimes, D.A. & Cates, W. Jr. Mortality from abortion and childbirth: Are the populations comparable? *Journal of the American Medical Association*, 1982, **248**, 188.
Lee, M.C., Rubin, G.L., Ory, H.W., et al. Type of intrauterine device and the risk of pelvic inflammatory disease. *Obstetrics & Gynecology*, 1983, **62**, 1.
Mashiach, S., Carp, H.J. & Serr, D.M. Nonoperative management of ectopic pregnancy. *Journal of Reproductive Medicine*, 1982, **27**, 127.
Ory, H.W. Ectopic pregnancy and intrauterine contraceptive devices. The Women's Health Study. *Obstetrics & Gynecology*, 1981, **27**, 127.
Piiroinen, O. & Pannonen, R. The use of ultrasonography in the diagnosis of ectopic pregnancy. *Clinical Radiology*, 1981, **32**, 331.
Rubin, G.L., Peterson, H.B., Dorfman, S.F., et al. Ectopic pregnancy in the United States, 1970 through 1978. *Journal of the American Medical Association*, 1983, **249**, 1725.
Snyder, J.R. Defusing the deadly ectopic. *Emergency Medicine*, 1983, **15**, 92.

HYPERTENSIVE DISORDERS

Cavanaugh, D. & Knuppel, A. Preeclampsia and eclampsia. In L. Iffy & H.A. Kaminetzky (Eds.). *Principles and practice of obstetrics and perinatology.* New York: Wiley, 1981.
Cockbum, J., Moar, V.A., Ounsted, M., et al. Final report of study on hypertension during pregnancy: The effects of specific treatment on the growth and development of the children. *Lancet*, 1982, **1**, 647.
Dennis, E.J., McFarland, K.F. & Hester, L.L. The preeclampsia-eclampsia syndrome. In D.N. Danforth, et al. (Eds.). *Obstetrics and gynecology.* New York: Harper & Row, 1982.
Ferris, T.F. How should hypertension during pregnancy be managed? *Medical Clinics of North America*, 1984, **68**, 491.
———. Toxemia and hypertension. In G.N. Burrow & T.F. Ferris (Eds.). *Medical complications during pregnancy* (2nd ed). Philadelphia: Saunders, 1982.
Fidler, J., Smith, V., Fayers, P., et al. Randomized controlled comparative study of methyldopa and oxprenolol in treatment of hypertension in pregnancy. *British Medical Journal*, 1983, **286**, 1927.
Gant, N.F. & Worley, R. *Hypertension in pregnancy: Concepts and management.* New York: Appleton-Century-Crofts, 1980.
Harris, B.A., Jr. Pregnancy with complications. *Emergency Medicine*, 1984, **16**, 29-32.
Kassar, N.S., Aldridge, J. & Quirk, B. Roll over test. *Obstetrics & Gynecology*, 1980, **55**, 411-413.
Kelley, M. & Mongiello, R.: Hypertension in pregnancy: Labor, delivery, and postpartum. *American Journal of Nursing*, 1982, **82**, 813.
Lueck, J., et al. Observation of an organism found in patients with gestational trophoblastic disease and in patients with toxemia of pregnancy. *American Journal of Obstetrics & Gynecology*, 1983, **145**, 15.
Liebowitz, H.A. & Hall, P.E. Cortical blindness as a complication of eclampsia. *Annals of Emergency Medicine*, 1984, **13**, 365-367.
Lindheimer, M.D. & Katz, A.I. Pathophysiology of preeclampsia. *Annual Review of Medicine*, 1981, **32**, 273-289.
Lison, A.E. & Marx, M. Proteinuria in relation to toxemia of pregnancy, *Contemporary Nephrology*, 1981, **25**, 128-131.
Ogle, M.E. & Sanders, A.B. Preeclampsia. *Annals of Emergency Medicine*, 1984, **13**, 368–370.
Sibai, B.M., Graham, J.M. & McCubbin, J.H. A comparison of intravenous and intramuscular magnesium

sulfate regimens in preeclampsia. *American Journal of Obstetrics & Gynecology,* 1984, **150,** 727-733.

Sibai, B.M., Lipshitz, J., Anderson, G.D., et al. Reassessment of intravenous $MgSO_4$ therapy in preeclampsia-eclampsia. *Obstetrics & Gynecology,* 1981, **57,** 199.

Wheeler, L. & Jones, M.B. Pregnancy-induced hypertension. *Journal of Obstetric, Gynecological & Neonatal Nursing,* 1981, **10,** 212.

Willis, S.E. Hypertension in pregnancy: Pathophysiology. *American Journal of Nursing,* 1982, **82,** 792.

———, & Sharp, E.S. Hypertension in pregnancy: Prenatal detection and management. *American Journal of Nursing,* 1982, **82,** 798.

URINARY TRACT DISORDERS

Cumming, D.C. & Taylor, P.J. Urologic and obstetric significance of urinary calculi in pregnancy. *Obstetrics & Gynecology,* 1979, **53,** 505-508.

Evans, D.A., Kass, E.H., Hennekens, C.H., et al. Bacteriuria and subsequent mortality in women. *Lancet,* 1982, **1,** 156.

Gilstap, L.C., III, Cunningham, F.G. & Whalley, P.J. Acute pyelonephritis in pregnancy: An anterospective study. *Obstetrics & Gynecology,* 1981, **57,** 409.

Harris, B.A., Jr. Pregnancy with complications. *Emergency Medicine,* 1984, **57,** 22.

Harris, R.E. & Gilstap, L.C., III. Cystitis during pregnancy: A distinct clinical entity. *Obstetrics & Gynecology,* 1981, **57,** 578.

Katz, A.I., Davison, J.M., Hayslett, J.P., et al. Pregnancy in women with renal disease. *Kidney International,* 1980, **18,** 192.

Lattanzi, D.R. & Cook, W.A. Urinary calculi in pregnancy. *Obstetrics & Gynecology,* 1980, **56,** 462.

Pritchard, J.A. & MacDonald, P.C. Medical and surgical diseases complicating pregnancy. In Pritchard, J.A. *Williams obstetrics* (16th ed.). New York: Appleton-Century-Crofts, 1980.

Ronald, A.R. Current concepts in management of urinary tract infections in adults. *Medical Clinics of North America,* 1984, **68,** 335-349.

Walt, R.B. Urinary tract infection during pregnancy. *Postgraduate Medicine,* 1984, **75,** 153.

RESPIRATORY DISEASES

Arwood, L.L., Dasta, J.F. & Friedman, C. Placental transfer of theophylline: Two case reports. *Pediatrics,* 1979, **63,** 844.

Berkwiz, R.L., Coustan, D.R. & Michizuki, T.L. (Eds.). *Handbook for prescribing medications during pregnancy.* Boston: Little, Brown, 1981.

Greenberger, P.A. & Patterson, R. Beclomethasone dipropionate for severe asthma during pregnancy. *Annals of Internal Medicine,* 1983, **98,** 478.

Griffiths, P.D., Ronalds, C.J. & Health, R.B. A prospective study of influenza infections during pregnancy. *Obstetric & Gynecologic* Survey, 1981, **36,** 73.

Harris, B.A. Pregnancy with complications. *Emergency Medicine,* 1984, **16,** 22.

Hernandez, E, Angell, C.S. & Johnson, J.W.C. Asthma in pregnancy: Current concepts. *Obstetrics & Gynecology,* 1980, **55,** 739.

Holbreich, M. Care of the asthmatic during pregnancy. *Contemporary Obstetrics & Gynecology,* 1984, **21,** 155.

Turner, E.S., Greenberger, P.A. & Patterson, R. Management of the pregnant asthmatic patient. *Annals of Internal Medicine,* 1980, **6,** 905.

Whipkey, R., Paris, A. & Stewart, T. Drug use in pregnancy. *Annals of Emergency Medicine,* 1984, **13,** 5, 349-354.

AUTOIMMUNE DISEASES

Baum, J. Arthritis and pregnancy. *Contemporary Obstetrics & Gynecology,* 1984, **23,** 97.

Carloss, H.W., McMillan, R. & Crosby, W.H. Management of pregnancy in women with immune thrombocytopenic purpura. *Journal of the American Medical Association,* 1980, **244,** 2754.

Cines, D.B., Dusak, B., Tomaski, A., Mennut, M. & Schreiber, A.D. Immune thrombocytopenic purpura and pregnancy. *New England Journal of Medicine,* 1982, **306,** 826.

Fine, L.G., Barnett, E.V., Danovitch, G.M., et al. Systemic lupus erythematosus in pregnancy. *Annals of Internal Medicine,* 1981, **94,** 667-677.

Galea, P., Patrick, M.J. & Goel, K.M. Isoimmune neonatal thrombocytopenia. *Archives of Diseases of Children,* 1981, **56,** 112.

Harris, C.J. Pregnancy can offer a welcome reprieve from the chronic inflammation of arthritis. *American Journal of Nursing,* 1985, **85,** 415-417.

Karpatkin, M., Forges, R.F. & Karpatkin, J. Platelet counts in infants of women with auto-immune thrombocytopenia. Effect of steroid administration to the mother. *New England Journal of Medicine,* 1981, **305,** 937.

Laros, R.K. & Kagan, R. Route of delivery for patients with immune thrombocytopenic purpura. *American Journal of Obstetrics & Gynecology,* 1984, **148,** 901.

Mizunuma, H., Takahashi, Y., Taguchi, H., Arai, A., Igarashi, M., Morita, K., Omine, M. & Maekawa, T. A new approach to idiopathic thrombocytopenic purpura during pregnancy by high-dose immunoglobulin G infusion. *American Journal of Obstetrics & Gynecology,* 1984, **148,** 218.

Noriega-Suerra, L., Aviles-Miranda, A., de la Cadena, O.A., Espinosa, L.M., Chavez, F. & Pizzuto, J. Pregnancy in patients with autoimmune thrombocytopenic purpura. *American Journal of Obstetrics & Gynecology,* 1979, **133,** 439.

Ostensen, M. & Husby, G. A prospective clinical study of the effect of pregnancy on rheumatic arthritis and ankylosing spondylitis. *Arthritis & Rheumatology,* 1983, **26,** 1155-1159.

Plauché, W.C. Myasthenia gravis in pregnancy: An update. *American Journal of Obstetrics & Gynecology,* 1979, **135,** 691.

Pope, R.M., et al. Effect of pregnancy on immune complexes and rheumatoid factors in patients with rheumatoid arthritis. *American Journal of Medicine*, 1983, **74**, 973.

Scott, J.R., Rote, N.S. & Cruikshank, D.P. Antiplatelet antibodies and platelet counts in pregnancies complicated by autoimmune thrombocytopenia purpura. *American Journal of Obstetrics & Gynecology*, 1983, **145**, 932.

Tchernia, G., Dreyfus, M., Laurian, Y, Derycke, M., Mirica, C. & Kerbat, G. Management of immune thrombocytopenia in pregnancy: Response to infusions of immunoglobulins. *American Journal of Obstetrics & Gynecology*, 1984, **148**, 225.

Thurnan, G.R. Rheumatoid arthritis. *Clinics in Obstetrics & Gynecology*, 1983, **26**, 558.

Varver, M.W., et al. Pregnancy in patients with systemic lupus erythematosus. *American Journal of Obstetrics & Gynecology*, 1983, **148**, 1025.

VASCULAR DISORDERS

Govoni, L.E., & Hayes, J.E. *Drugs and nursing implications* (4th ed.). Norwalk, Conn.: Appleton-Century-Crofts, 1982.

Loebel, S., Spratto, G. & Heckheimer, E. *The nurse's drug handbook* (2nd ed.). New York: Wiley, 1980.

CARDIAC DISEASE

Burrow, G.N. & Ferris, G.F. *Medical complications during pregnancy* (2nd ed.). Philadelphia: Saunders, 1982.

Canobbio, M.M. The eisenmenger syndrome. *Nursing Clinics of North America*, 1984, **19**, 545.

Chesley, L.C. Severe rheumatic cardiac disease and pregnancy; the ultimate prognosis. *American Journal of Obstetrics & Gynecology*, 1980, **136**, 552.

Graham, T.P. The eisenmenger reaction and its management. *Cardiovascular Clinics*, 1980, **10**, 531-542.

Harris, B.A., Jr. Pregnancy with complications. *Emergency Medicine*, 1984, **16**, 22.

Leman, R.B. & Assey, M.E. Heart disease and pregnancy. *Southern Medical Journal*, 1981, **74**, 944.

Miller, L.D. Eisenmenger's syndrome and the pregnant patient. *Journal of Obstetric, Gynecological & Neonatal Nursing*, 1983, **12**, 175.

McAnnulty, J.H., Metcalfe, J. & Ueland, K. General guidelines in the management of cardiac disease. *Clinics in Obstetrics & Gynecology*, 1981, **24**, 773-787.

ENDOCRINE DISORDERS

Harris, B.S., Jr. Pregnancy with complications. *Emergency Medicine*, 1984, **16**, 48.

Mestman, J.H. Management of thyroid diseases in pregnancy. *Clinics in Perinatology*, 1980, **7**, 371.

Thyroid dysfunction in pregnancy. Diagnosis can be difficult. *Clinical Aspects of High Risk Pregnancy*, 1983, **1**, 4-5.

DIABETES MELLITUS

Burns, E.M. Diabetes mellitus and pregnancy. *Nursing Clinics of North America*, 1983, **18**, 673-685.

Cruikshank, D.P., et al. Calcium metabolism in diabetic mother, fetus, and newborn infant. *American Journal of Obstetrics & Gynecology*, 1983, **148**, 1010.

Ferroni, K.M., Gross, T.L., Sokol, R.J. & Chik, L. What affects pulmonary maturation during diabetic pregnancy? *American Journal of Obstetrics & Gynecology*, 1984, **150**, 270.

Golde, S.H., Montoro, M., Good-Anderson, B., et al. The role of nonstress tests, fetal biophysical profile, and contraction stress tests in the outpatient management of insulin-requiring diabetic pregnancies. *American Journal of Obstetrics & Gynecology*, 1984, **148**, 269.

Good-Anderson, B. Home blood glucose monitoring in the pregnant diabetic. *Journal of Obstetric, Gynecological & Neonatal Nursing*, 1983, **12**, 89-92.

Harris, B.A., Jr. Pregnancy with complications. *Emergency Medicine*, 1984, **16**, 22.

Jorge, C.S., Artral, R., Paul, R.H., et al. Antepartum fetal surveillance in diabetic pregnant patients. *American Journal of Obstetrics & Gynecology*, 1981, **141**, 641.

Miller, J.M., Jr. Antenatal fetal heart rate testing in diabetic pregnancy (Class B-F). Proceedings of the Third Annual Scientific Meeting of the Society of Perinatal Obstetricians, San Antonio, Tx., 1983.

Metzger, M.J. A new test for blood sugar. *American Journal of Nursing*, 1983, **83**, 763.

Moore, D.S., Bingham, P.R. & Keesling, O. Nursing care of the pregnant woman with diabetes mellitus. *Journal of Obstetric, Gynecological & Neonatal Nursing*, 1981, **10**, 188.

White, N.E. & Miller, B.K. Glycohemoglobin: A new test to help the diabetic stay in control. *Nursing 83*, 1983, **13**, 55.

White, P. Diabetes mellitus in pregnancy. *Clinics in Perinatology*, 1974, **1**, 340.

MULTIPLE PREGNANCY

Appuzio, J.J., Ganesh, V., Landau, I. & Pelosi, M. Prenatal diagnosis of cojoined twins. *American Journal of Obstetrics & Gynecology*, 1984, **148**, 343.

Daw, E. Triplet pregnancy. *British Journal of Obstetrics & Gynecology*, 1978, **85**, 505.

Evrand, J.R. & Gold, E.M. Cesarean section for delivery of the second twin. *Obstetrics & Gynecology*, 1981, **57**, 581.

Gray, C.M., et al. Thoracopagus twins; prenatal diagnosis. *Radiology*, 1950, **54**, 398.

Hubinont, C., et al. Dicephalus: Unusual report of cojoined twins and its prepartum diagnosis. *American Journal of Obstetrics & Gynecology*, 1984, **149**, 698.

Leonard, L.G. Twin pregnancy: Maternal-fetal nutrition. *Journal of Obstetric, Gynecological & Neonatal Nursing*, 1982, **11**, 139.

Padilla, M., Chin, A.J. & Padilla, T. Cardiovascular abnormalities in thoracopagus twins. *Teratology*, 1981, **23**, 101.

Ron-El, R., et al. Triplet and quadruplet pregnancies and management. *Obstetrics & Gynecology,* 1981, **57,** 458.

PROLONGED (POSTTERM) PREGNANCY

Affonso, D.D. & Harris, T.R. Postterm pregnancy implications for mother and infant, challenge for the nurse. *Journal of Obstetric, Gynecological & Neonatal Nursing,* 1980, **9,** 139.

Barrett, J.M., Salyer, S.L. & Boehm, F.H. Nonstress test: Evaluation of 1000 patients. *American Journal of Obstetrics & Gynecology,* 1982, **143,** 243.

Khouzami, V.A., Johnson, W.C., Hernandez, E., Rotmensch, J., Erye, R. & Daikoku, N. Urinary estrogens in postterm pregnancy. *American Journal of Obstetrics & Gynecology,* 1981, **141,** 205.

Shime, J., Gare, D.J., Andrews, J., Bertrand, M., Salgado, J. & Whillans, G. Prolonged pregnancy: Surveillance of the fetus and the neonate and the course of labor and delivery. *American Journal of Obstetrics & Gynecology,* 1984, **148,** 547.

Yeh, S.Y. & Read, J.A. Management of postterm pregnancy in a large obstetrical population. *Obstetrics & Gynecology,* 1982, **60,** 282.

GASTROINTESTINAL DISEASES

Harris, B.A., Jr. Pregnancy with complications. *Emergency Medicine,* 1984, **16,** 22.

Kanai, K., et al. Prevention of perinatal transmission of hepatitis B virus (HBV) to children of antigen-positive HBV carrier mother by hepatitis B immune globulin and HBV vaccine. *Journal of Infectious Disease,* 1985, **151,** 287-290.

ACQUIRED IMMUNODEFICIENCY SYNDROME

Advisory Committee on Infections within the Hospital. A hospital-wide approach to AIDS. American Hospital Association, 1985.

Bennett, J. AIDS epidemiology update. *American Journal of Nursing,* 1985, **95,** 968-972.

Center for Disease Control. Acquired immunodeficiency (AIDS). Precautions for health care workers and allied professionals. *Morbidity and Mortality Weekly Report,* 1983a, **32,** 450.

Center for Disease Control. Immunodeficiency among female sexual partners of males with AIDS—New York. *Morbidity and Mortality Weekly Report,* 1983b, **32,** 698.

Center for Disease Control. 1985 STD treatment guidelines. *Morbidity and Mortality Weekly Report,* 1985a, **34,** 45.

Center for Disease Control. Current trends. Recommendations for assisting in the prevention of perinatal transmission of human T-lymphotropic virus type III/lymphadenopathy-associated virus and acquired immunodeficiency syndrome. *Morbidity and Mortality Weekly Report,* 1985b, **34,** 48.

Jensen, L., et al. Acquired immunodeficiency (AIDS) in pregnancy. *American Journal of Obstetrics & Gynecology,* 1984, **148,** 1145.

Loveman, A., Colburn, V. & Dobin, A. AIDS in pregnancy. *Journal of Obstetric, Gynecological & Neonatal Nursing,* 1986, **15,** 1ff.

Mason, J. Public health service plan for the prevention and control of acquired immune deficiency syndrome. *Public Health Reports,* 1985, **100,** 453ff.

NEUROLOGIC DISORDERS

Harris, B.A., Jr. Pregnancy with complications. *Emergency Medicine,* 1984, **16,** 22.

Voitk, A.J., Mueller, J.V., Farlinger, D.E. & Johnston, R.U. Carpal tunnel syndrome in pregnancy. *Canadian Medical Association Journal,* 1983, **128,** 277.

Weisz, R.R. Facial paralysis in a pregnant woman. *Clinical Pearls,* 1984, **7,** 5.

ANEMIAS

Charache, S., Scott, J., Niebyl, J. & Bonds, D. Management of sickle cell disease in pregnant patients. *Obstetrics & Gynecology,* 1908, **55,** 407-410.

Luff, J. Pregnancy and sickle cell disease. *Nursing Clinics of North America,* 1983, **18,** 164-171.

Milner, P.F., Jones, B.R. & Dobler, J. Outcome of pregnancy in sickle cell anemia and sickle cell-hemoglobin C disease. *American Journal of Obstetrics & Gynecology,* 1980, **138,** 239.

Ship-Horowitz, T. Nursing care of the sickle cell anemic patient in labor. *Journal of Obstetric, Gynecological & Neonatal Nursing,* 1983, **12,** 381-386.

INFECTIONS

Adler, M.W. ABC of sexually transmitted diseases: Pregnancy and the neonate. *British Medical Journal,* 1984, **288,** 624-627.

Boehm, F.H., Estes, W., Wright, P.F., et al. Management of genital herpes simplex virus infection occurring during pregnancy. *American Journal of Obstetrics & Gynecology,* 1984, **141,** 735-740.

Gennaro, S. Listerial infection: Nursing care of mother and infant. *MCN,* 1980, **5,** 390.

Haggerty, L. TORCH: A literature review and implications for practice. *Journal of Obstetric, Gynecological & Neonatal Nursing,* 1985, **14,** 124-129.

Handsfield, H.H. Nongonococcal urethritis. *Cutis,* 1981, **27,** 269.

Holmes, K.K. The chlamydial epidemic. *Journal of the American Medical Association,* 1981, **245,** 1718.

Jeffries, D.J. Management of herpes simplex infection

during pregnancy and in the neonate. *Journal of Hospital Infections*, 1983, **4**, 217-220.

Kibrick, S. Herpes simplex infection at term. *Journal of the American Medical Association*, 1980, **243**, 157-160.

McCoy, M.J., Ellenberg, J.F. & Killam, A.P. Coccidiomycosis complicating pregnancy. *American Journal of Obstetrics & Gynecology*, 1980, **136**, 739.

Miller, E., Cradock-Watson, J.E. & Pollock, T.M. Consequences of confirmed rubella at successive stages of pregnancy. *Lancet*, 1982, **2**, 781-784.

Morgan-Capner, P. & Griffiths, G. Fetal and neonatal infection. *Nursing Times*, 1984 (Nov. 7), **12**, 28–32.

Nankervis, G.A., Klumar, M.L., Cox, F.E. & Gold, E. A prospective study of maternal cytomegalovirus infection and its effect on the fetus. *American Journal of Obstetrics & Gynecology*, 1984, **149**, 435.

Peckham, C.S., Coleman, J.C., Hurley, R., et al. Cytomegalovirus infection in pregnancy: Preliminary findings from a prospective study. *Lancet*, 1983, **1**, 1352-1355.

Rapp, F. Herpes simplex virus type 2 and cervical cancer. *Current Problems in Cancer*, 1981, **6**, 5-18.

Stagno, S., Pass, R.F., Dworsky, M.E., et al. Congenital cytomegalovirus infection. *New England Journal of Medicine*, 1982, **306**, 945.

RH ISOIMMUNIZATION

American College of Obstetrics and Gynecology. Prevention of Rho(D) isoimmunization. *ACOG Technical Bulletin, No. 79*, 1984.

Berger, G.S. & Keith, L. Utilization of RH prophylaxis. *Clinics in Obstetrics & Gynecology*, 1982, **25**, 267-275.

Gold, W.R., Jr., Queenan, J.T., Woody, J. & Sacher, R.A. Oral desensitization in RH disease. *American Journal of Obstetrics & Gynecology*, 1983, **146**, 980-981.

Hammer, R.M., Bower, E.J. & Messina, L.J. The prenatal use of Rho(D) immune globulin. *MCN*, 1984, **9**, 29-31.

Hensleigh, P.A. Preventing rhesus isoimmunization: Antepartum RH immune globulin prophylaxis versus a sensitive test for risk identification. *American Journal of Obstetrics & Gynecology*, 1983, **146**, 749-755.

Riley, E.N. Rh immunoglobulin prophylaxis. NITA, 1983, **6**, 420-422.

Scott, J.R., Kochenour, N.K., Larkin, R.M. & Scott, M.J. Changes in the management of severely Rh-immunized patients. *American Journal of Obstetrics & Gynecology*, 1984, **149**, 226-241.

PSYCHIATRIC DISEASES

Carmack, B.J. & Corwin, T.A. Nursing care of the schizophrenic maternity patient during labor. *MCN*, 1980, **5**, 107.

SUBSTANCE ABUSE

Danis, R.P. & Keith, L. Fetal alcohol syndrome: Insurable but preventable. *Contemporary Obstetrics & Gynecology*, 1983, **21**, 57.

Jhaveri, R.C., et al. Effects of methadone on thyroid function in mother, fetus, and newborn. *Pediatrics*, 1980, **65**, 557.

Lindor, E., et al. Fetal alcohol syndrome. *Journal of Obstetric, Gynecological & Neonatal Nursing*, 1980, **9**, 222.

Little, R.E., et al. Decreased brain weight in infants of alcoholic women who abstained during pregnancy. *Journal of Pediatrics*, 1980, **96**, 974.

Scialli, A.R., Toxicology: Safe medications during pregnancy. *Contemporary Obstetrics & Gynecology*, 1983, **22**, 39.

Worthington-Roberts, B. & Weigle, A. Caffeine and pregnancy outcome. *Journal of Obstetric, Gynecological & Neonatal Nursing*, 1983, **12**, 21.

Zuspan, F.P. When drugs and alcohol complicate pregnancy. *Contemporary Obstetrics & Gynecology*, 1984, **24**, 35.

HYPEREMESIS GRAVIDARUM

Bouillon, R. Thyroid function in patients with hyperemesis gravidarum. *American Journal of Obstetrics & Gynecology*, 1982, **144**, 922.

TRAUMA

Buchsbaum, H.J. Accidental injury in pregnancy: *Contemporary Obstetrics & Gynecology*, 1982, **20**, 26.

Smith, L.C. & Payne, T. Pregnant trauma victims. *American Journal of Nursing*, 1984, **84**, 14.

OBESITY

Calandra, C., et al. Maternal obesity in pregnancy. *Obstetrics & Gynecology*, 1981, **58**, 8.

chapter 26

COMPLICATIONS DURING LABOR AND DELIVERY

OBJECTIVES

Upon completion of this chapter, the reader will be able to:

1. Identify danger signs during labor.
2. Know the three types of placenta previa.
3. Identify four etiologic factors that may lead to abruptio placentae.
4. Differentiate between signs and symptoms of placenta previa and abruptio placentae.
5. Given a client with placenta previa or abruptio placentae, identify appropriate nursing interventions.
6. Explain the pathophysiology and management of DIC.
7. Define dystocia.
8. Discuss dysfunctional labor patterns.
9. Differentiate between hypotonic and hypertonic uterine contraction patterns.
10. Given a fetus in an abnormal presentation or position, describe the position and identify appropriate nursing interventions.
11. Define inlet, midplane, and outlet pelvic contractions.
12. Discuss preterm labor.
13. State indications, dosage, complications, and nursing responsibilities when administering a tocolytic agent.
14. Given a client in preterm labor, identify appropriate nursing assessments.
15. Identify maternal and fetal effects of PROM.
16. Define oligohydramnios and polyhydramnios.
17. Discuss nursing interventions appropriate with prolapse of the umbilical cord.
18. Given a client having an induction of labor, identify appropriate nursing interventions.
19. State the prerequisites for a forceps delivery.
20. Use the nursing process to plan and provide nursing care for a client with an intrapartal complication.
21. State the indications for a primary cesarean section.
22. Discuss nursing interventions following a cesarean birth.
23. Describe the four degrees of perineal lacerations.

KEY TERMS

Abruptio placentae
Amniotomy
Breech presentation
Brow presentation
Cervical dystocia
Cesarean section
Compound presentation
Couvelaire uterus
DIC
Dystocia
External version
Face presentation
Induction of labor
Internal version
Occiput posterior
Oligohydramnios
Placenta previa
Polyhydramnios
Primary inertia
Secondary inertia
Transverse arrest
Transverse lie
Uterine rupture
Vasa previa

Interruptions in health that occur during the intrapartal period can cause injury or even death of a mother and fetus. Prevention of complications is a primary goal for the maternity nurse. When complications do occur, early detection and appropriate interventions become the goals. During the labor and delivery process, the nurse must constantly employ assessment skills to plan appropriate nursing care. Certain observable danger signs that may be noted during labor are indicative of specific alterations in the labor and delivery process (see Table 26–1).

BLEEDING PROBLEMS

Placenta Previa

Placenta previa is the implantation and development of the placenta in the lower uterine segment, adjoining or covering the internal cervical os and preventing fetal descent.

CLASSIFICATION

The amount of cervical os that is covered by the placenta determines the classification (see Fig. 26–1). In *total placenta previa*, the placenta completely covers the internal cervical os. In *partial placenta previa*, a portion of the os is covered by the placenta. In *marginal placenta previa* the placenta is implanted near but does not extend over the internal os. A marginal placenta previa is also referred to as a low-lying placenta or low implantation.

INCIDENCE

Placenta previa occurs in approximately 1 in 200 deliveries, with 3 of 4 cases in multigravidas. The total incidence is decreasing, possibly due to the decline in the number of high parity women.

During the second trimester, half of all placentas are low-lying. By the time the upper uterine segment elongates and the lower uterine segment unfolds at term, only 1 placenta in about 200 will remain as a placenta previa. The greatest chance of remaining a placenta previa occurs in placentas that completely cover the internal os in the second trimester.

ETIOLOGY

The specific cause of placenta previa is not known. There are, however, certain predisposing factors (see Table 26–2). It has been proposed that at the stage of the chorion frondosum, the vascular development of the uterine fundus is deficient, increasing the probability that attachment will be in the lower uterine segment. Early or late fertilization and variability in the implantation potential of the blastocyst may also play a role. Multiple pregnancy may predispose to placenta previa because of the increased placental surface. Previous uterine surgeries may increase the incidence, owing to the higher rate of implantation at the site of the previous uterine scar. The shape and size changes in the uterus following normal pregnancy may influence development of placenta previa with successive pregnancies. It is known that the greater the parity, the more frequently placenta previa occurs. A rapid succession of pregnancies may cause atrophic changes and endometrial deficiencies as well as decreased muscularity in the uterine fundus. The presence of fibroid tumors also increases the incidence, possibly because of the decreased amount of endometrium available for implantation.

MANIFESTATIONS

The most characteristic symptom is *painless* vaginal bleeding. In more than half of clients with placenta previa, the initial episode of

TABLE 26-1
DANGER SIGNS IN LABOR

Assessment	Possible Significance
Rapid, slow, or irregular FHT	Fetal hypoxia
Greenish-brown amniotic fluid in a cephalic presentation	Fetal distress
Port-wine stained amniotic fluid	Abruptio placentae Ruptured vasa previa
Unengaged presenting part	Fetopelvic disproportion Malpresentation
Failure of progress in cervical dilation	Prolonged labor Increased danger of fetal demise
Failure of descent of the presenting part after complete cervical dilation	Fetopelvic disproportion
Vaginal bleeding	Placenta previa Abruptio placentae Maternal lacerations
Rising blood pressure	PIH Extreme anxiety
Low maternal B/P	Shock Supine hypotension syndrome Reaction to medication
Elevated temperature	Amnionitis Chorioamnionitis Extrauterine infection
Maternal tachycardia	Fever Impending shock
Foul or purulent vaginal discharge	Amnionitis Potential fetal sepsis
Abnormal abdominal pain and tenderness	Abruptio placentae Ruptured uterus Nonobstetrical abdominal pathology
Uterine tetany	Abruptio placentae with intrauterine bleeding Injudicious use of oxytocin
Excessive discomfort or pain	Anxiety Hysteria Undetected complications Reaction to medication
Prolapsed umbilical cord	Fetal death if no intervention
Uterine contractions decreasing in frequency, duration, and intensity after the onset of true labor	Uterine inertia Maternal overmedication
Pallor, clammy cool skin, air hunger	Bleeding Maternal shock
Decreasing level of consciousness	Impending eclampsia Shock Heavy sedation Hysteria
Cyanosis	Aspiration Cardiac decompensation

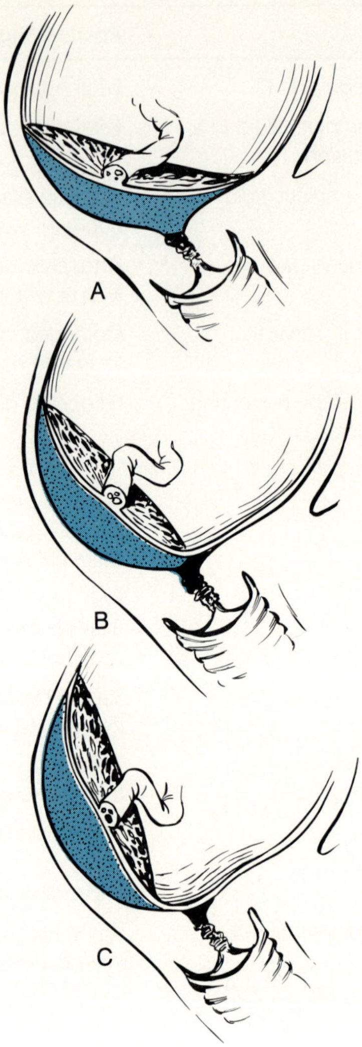

FIGURE 26-1. Types of placenta previa: A. Total placenta previa. B. Partial placenta previa. C. Marginal placenta previa.

vaginal bleeding occurs between 34 and 40 weeks gestation (see Table 26-3).

During late pregnancy the lower uterine segment normally stretches and thins as the softening cervix begins to efface and dilate. If the placenta is implanted in the lower uterine segment, separation occurs at the placental site, causing vaginal bleeding. The lower the placenta, the earlier the bleeding episodes begin.

The bleeding is usually bright and occurs whether the client is active or in bed. The initial episode is often small, with the amount

TABLE 26-2
PREDISPOSING FACTORS IN PLACENTA PREVIA

Deficient decidua in the uterine fundus
Early or late fertilization
Multiple pregnancy
Previous uterine surgery
Multiparity
Advancing maternal age
Rapid succession of pregnancies
Fibroid tumors

of vaginal bleeding increasing with each successive episode. A constant seepage of blood-tinged serous vaginal drainage is sometimes present.

PATHOGENESIS

The pathogenesis of placenta previa concerns three possible altered mechanisms: defective endometrial vascularization, altered transport mechanism, and development of the placenta in the decidua capsularis.

Defective Endometrial Vascularization

The endometrium may be poorly vascularized because of atrophic and inflammatory changes. When there is inadequate or insufficient endometrium in the upper uterine segment, the ovum may continue to descend and implant in an area of healthy endometrium located in the lower uterine segment, or it may implant in the inadequate upper segment with development of a large placental surface to provide adequate maternal-fetal exchange. In these situations, marginal insertion of the umbilical cord is common, owing to the eccentrical development of the placenta.

Altered Transport Mechanism

The fertilized ovum normally remains free in the uterine cavity until implantation. During this three- or four-day period the ovum can be displaced to the lower uterine segment for

TABLE 26-3
COMPARISON OF PLACENTA PREVIA AND ABRUPTIO PLACENTAE

Placenta Previa	Abruptio Placentae
Painless vaginal bleeding	Pain associated with vaginal bleeding
Bright red vaginal bleeding	Vaginal bleeding is often dark
Vaginal bleeding and signs of shock are comparable	Shock symptoms may be out of proportion to visible vaginal bleeding
Initial bleeding episode often slight	Initial bleeding episode often profuse
Uterus soft, not tender, and uterine contractions may or may not be present	Uterus firm, tender, tetanically contracted
Fetus is easily palpated	Fetus is difficult to palpate
FHT present	FHT irregular or absent
Usually no blood clotting defect	Blood clotting defect often present

implantation by altered uterine motility, deviations in uterine shape or size, or fluid in the uterine cavity.

Development of the Placenta in the Decidua Capsularis

The chorionic membrane in the lower uterine segment fails to atrophy and the villi develop in the decidua capsularis. When this surface adheres to the decidua vera on the opposite uterine wall, the villi become incorporated into the developing placenta and impinge upon the lower uterine segment.

DIAGNOSIS

Diagnosis of placenta previa may be made by indirect or direct methods.

Indirect Methods

If the initial episode of vaginal bleeding has stopped and delivery is to be delayed until the fetus is more mature, indirect methods of diagnosis are employed to confirm or rule out the diagnosis of placenta previa. About half of clients with painless vaginal bleeding have placenta previa. Indirect methods of diagnosis include direct placentography, indirect gravitational placentography, cystography, placental localization, and ultrasonography.

Differential Diagnosis

Differential diagnosis includes identification of vaginal bleeding as being of maternal or fetal origin. Causes of vaginal bleeding of maternal origin include rupture of a placenta marginal sinus, abruptio placentae, circumvallate placenta, ruptured uterus, local lesions of the cervix, vaginal lesions, and clotting disorders. Causes of vaginal bleeding that are of fetal origin include vasa previa, in which one or more fetal vessels lie across the internal cervical os.

Direct Diagnosis

A definitive diagnosis of placenta previa is made by palpating the placenta through the cervix. Direct diagnosis is only undertaken if all is in readiness for an instant cesarean section and if conservative treatment is not appropriate because of the danger of profuse bleeding.

Incidential Diagnosis

Occasionally, an ultrasound examination during pregnancy for estimations of gestational age or for other purposes may lead to a diagnosis of placenta previa before an episode of vaginal bleeding has occurred.

MEDICAL MANAGEMENT AND NURSING INTERVENTIONS

Second Trimester

Usually, the gravid woman arrives at the hospital with active vaginal bleeding in varying amounts. Upon arrival, she is placed on bed rest. An initial assessment is completed (see Chapter 16), with special emphasis on the vaginal bleeding. The client's estimation of the bleeding is assessed by the nurse: the amount, the number of perineal pads used in a specified time, and the amount, size and number of any clots (see Table 26–4). Unless the bleeding has stopped, intravenous fluids are started, and laboratory studies, including a complete blood count and a type and crossmatch for possible blood transfusion, are begun. External fetal monitoring is explained and instituted to monitor the fetal heart rate and uterine contraction status. Maternal vital signs are monitored closely. An accurate intake and output is needed.

Vaginal bleeding is assessed continuously. The initial episode of vaginal bleeding usually occurs at a time in pregnancy when the circulating blood volume is normally increased 20 to 40 percent, and vaginal bleeding may not be in proportion to changes in the maternal pulse and blood pressure.

All vaginal or rectal examinations and enemas are deferred, since manipulation of the lower uterine segment may precipitate massive maternal hemorrhage.

The uterus remains soft and not tender. The fundus may be higher than expected for the length of gestation, owing to the presenting part remaining high in the uterus, with the placenta occupying the lower uterine segment (see Table 26–4). Indirect methods are used to localize the placenta and make an accurate diagnosis.

When the bleeding decreases or stops, as is often the case with an initial bleeding episode, conservative management is followed to prolong gestation and increase the chances of neonatal survival. Slow progressive ambulation is begun, with constant supervision for the reoccurence of vaginal bleeding.

The importance of thorough explanations to the client and her partner cannot be overemphasized. When vaginal bleeding occurs, the anxiety level will be high. Explanations should be brief but complete, with an understanding of the explanations verbalized. Questions are encouraged.

Medications to inhibit uterine contractions called tocolytic agents are given to selected clients to decrease the possibility of the onset of preterm labor. Amniocentesis may help to determine fetal lung maturity.

If the gravida is to be discharged home before delivery, she will need referral to a homemaker service to help with household tasks, since activity at home will likely be curtailed. She must have

TABLE 26–4
NURSING RESPONSIBILITIES IN PLACENTA PREVIA

Initial patient assessment
Maintain bed rest
No rectal or vaginal examinations
Start IV fluids with a large bore (18G or larger) needle
NPO
Obtain laboratory studies as ordered
Type and crossmatch for at least 2 U blood
Monitor maternal vital signs
Monitor intake and output
Test urine for glucose and protein
Monitor FHR
Monitor uterine contractions
Evaluate blood loss
Offer psychological support
No enemas
Provide thorough explanations at an appropriate level for understanding
Prepare for testing, if ordered
Notify operating room personnel of possible surgery
Notify high-risk nursery and pediatrician

ready access for return to the hospital, since successive episodes of bleeding are usually greater than previous episodes.

It is important to emphasize adequate nutritional intake and the cessation of smoking, because of the increased incidence of associated intrauterine growth retardation. The frequency of followup appointments in the physician's office or clinic is explained. A repeat ultrasound is normally taken at 35 or 36 weeks gestation if no further bleeding has occurred to determine if the placenta previa is still present. Nine of ten placenta previas are no longer present by term gestation, owing to the uterine changes concurrent with normal pregnancy.

37+ Weeks Gestation

If vaginal bleeding occurs at 37+ weeks gestation, the gravida is admitted to the labor unit and placed on complete bed rest. Intravenous fluids are started with a large bore needle, and laboratory tests, including type and crossmatch for blood, are ordered. The initial client assessment (see Chapter 16) is made as thoroughly as the maternal condition allows. Maternal vital signs are monitored closely. The fetal heart rate and uterine contraction status are continuously monitored with an external fetal monitor. Accurate intake and output and assessment of vaginal bleeding is necessary. Explanations to the client and her partner must be complete and at an appropriate level of understanding. For a sample nursing care plan for a client with a placenta previa, see Table 26-5.

If vaginal bleeding continues, bed rest is maintained with the head of the bed elevated to allow the fetal presenting part to exert pressure against the placenta and possibly help control bleeding. The client remains NPO, intravenous fluids are continued, and an accurate intake and output record is maintained. Blood replacement may be necessary. Maternal, fetal, and uterine status are constantly monitored.

An amniocentesis may be carried out to determine fetal lung maturity if the maternal physiologic status remains stable. If the fetal lungs are mature, delivery by either vaginal or abdominal route is indicated.

If the maternal physiologic status is not stable or is deteriorating, immediate intervention is needed, regardless of fetal maturity. An emergency cesarean section may be performed or a double setup may be used.

Double Setup

A double setup is prepared in the operating room. All equipment, physicians, and staff are scrubbed and ready for either an immediate vaginal delivery or an immediate cesarean section. Two intravenous lines are infusing, a minimum of two units of blood are ready, and sterile equipment is set up and opened before an examination is begun.

When all is ready, including psychological preparation of the client, a gentle sterile vaginal examination is done. If the cervix is dilated 3 cm or more and the placenta previa is marginal, an amniotomy will permit the presenting part to tamponade the placenta and control vaginal bleeding. If bleeding is controlled, labor may be allowed to proceed. Care of the mother and fetus are described in Chapter 16. When the placenta previa is complete or partial, an immediate cesarean section is performed.

COMPLICATIONS

Maternal complications result from both the placenta previa and its treatment. Antepartum

TABLE 26-5
SAMPLE NURSING CARE PLAN: PLACENTA PREVIA

Monica F., a 30-year-old gravida 2 para 1 who is at 32 weeks gestation is brought to the labor area with "bright red vaginal bleeding." She is put to bed and an initial assessment is conducted.

Data Base:

Gravida 2 para 1, 32 weeks gestation
Moderate amount bright red vaginal bleeding present
States saturated 2 perineal pads in last 20 minutes, no clots noted
Denies trauma or recent intercourse
Denies abdominal pain or uterine contractions
Abdomen soft, not tender
Uterus approximately 33 cm fundal height
FHT 136 in LML

Maternal vital signs: temperature 98.4° F (0)
pulse 98
respirations 16
B/P 104/72
Vaginal examination deferred at this time
Blood type and Rh: AB+
No known allergies
No current medical problems
On no medications, other than prenatal vitamins
Prenatal history uneventful

Nursing Diagnosis	Goals	Nursing Interventions	Rationale	Evaluation
Potential for injury to mother related to excessive vaginal bleeding	Maternal physiologic status will remain stable: Vital signs stable Decreased vaginal bleeding No uterine contractions	Assess for vaginal bleeding: Amount Color Clots Perineal pad count	Potential for injury to mother is minimized by appropriate nursing assessments and interventions	On 15 minute checks: moderate bright red vaginal bleeding Peri pads changed q 30 minutes for first 3 hours, then bleeding decreased in amount to scant red
Potential fluid volume deficit related to excess vaginal bleeding	Vaginal bleeding will decrease in amount	No vaginal examinations	Massive maternal bleeding may be precipitated with vaginal examinations	VE deferred
		Monitor B/P P, & R q 15 minutes until stable Obtain laboratory tests as ordered	Frequent assessments will help to identify hypovolemic shock	Vital signs remained within normal limits Urinalysis, CBC, PTT, prothrombin time, Type & crossmatch done for 2 U. packed cells. All results were within normal limits

		Maintain NPO status IV fluids as ordered to maintain hydration Accurate intake and output	Client should remain NPO until vaginal bleeding decreased, in the event OR necessary	NPO status maintained 100 ml D5/LR at 125 ml/hr maintained Intake—1000 ml/8 hours Output—845 ml/8 hours No uterine contractions or uterine irritability noted
		Monitor uterine contraction status with external fetal monitor Maintain complete bed rest with head of bed elevated Assess abdomen q 15–30 minutes	Fetal PP may exert pressure to control maternal bleeding	Bed rest maintained after explanation of importance Abdomen remained soft, no tenderness noted
Potential for injury to fetus related to decreased utero-placental function secondary to maternal fluid volume deficit	The fetus will exhibit no signs of fetal distress: FHR baseline 120–160 BPM No periodic changes	Monitor FHT with external fetal monitor Assess for fetal distress and institute appropriate interventions if noted (see Table 16–14) Alert nursery and neonatologist of potential compromised preterm neonate	Fetus will become compromised as maternal blood loss continues or increases	FHR tracing documented q hour Baseline 120–140 BPM Average variability noted on external tracing No identifiable periodic changes Nursery informed of maternal and fetal status
Knowledge deficit related to nursing care and hospital procedures	The client and support person will verbalize understanding of procedures	Orient to environment Provide explanations (at appropriate level) of all nursing procedures Provide additional explanations of medical procedures ordered or planned Encourage verbalization of concerns for self and fetus	An unplanned admission to the hospital will increase stress and anxiety levels	Monica & Roger were oriented to the unit and staff as well as planned nursing care Ultrasound done: partial placenta previa confirmed Amniocentesis done: fetal lungs immature No concerns verbalized at this time
Knowledge deficit related to outcome of pregnancy secondary to vaginal bleeding	The client will verbalize an understanding of placenta previa and possible maternal/fetal outcomes	Assess knowledge of placenta previa Assess informational needs Provide explanations at appropriate level of understanding Provide information re: Placenta previa Expected pregnancy outcome Expected fetal outcome	Adequate information given at a level understood by the client will aid in decreasing anxiety and acceptance of prescribed regimen of treatment	Explanations given to Monica & Roger with understanding verbalized

TABLE 26-5 (continued)

Nursing Diagnosis	Goals	Nursing Interventions	Rationale	Evaluation
		Prepare for double setup if vaginal bleeding increases or does not decrease	Delivery and operating room must be ready for **immediate** cesarean delivery before vaginal examination is done	Double setup not utilized: conservative management indicated at this time
		If conservative management indicated: Prepare for administration of tocolytics	Tocolytics may help to inhibit preterm labor	No tocolytic medication ordered
		Slow progressive ambulation		Monica allowed up to bathroom after vaginal bleeding stopped—no further bleeding noted
Activity intolerance related to activity limitations secondary to risk of recurrent vaginal bleeding episodes	No further bleeding episodes will occur with appropriate self-care	Specific discharge instructions re: Activity limitations Nutrition No smoking Followup appointments Return to hospital	Each bleeding episode is usually greater than the previous one There is an increased incidence of IUGR	Discharge instructions given and understanding verbalized re: BRP only No housekeeping chores Adequate dietary intake To return to obstetrician office in 1 week Symptoms indicating need to return to the hospital
Anxiety related to uncertain maternal and fetal outcome	The client will verbalize fears or concerns for herself and neonate	Assess client's perception of current status of self and fetus/neonate Assess nonverbal signs of anxiety: Trembling Restlessness Encourage verbalization	Verbalization of fears and concerns will aid in dealing with these fears	Monica freely talked about current status of herself and the fetus She felt that if she followed doctor's orders, outcome would be positive for both her and the fetus
Anticipatory grieving related to possible loss of fetus	The family will adjust to the stress of the situation	Provide realistic information to the parents		A tour of the high-risk nursery was taken and she asked many questions about possible neonatal care

hemorrhage may be massive enough to be fatal. Prolonged maternal hypotension that may accompany massive bleeding can cause cerebral or renal ischemia. Clotting defects may also develop.

Postpartum uterine atony may be caused by lessened muscle content in the lower uterine segment following delivery. Natural mechanisms to control postpartum bleeding are lessened owing to the decreased muscle content. If postpartum hemorrhage occurs, the usual method of control (uterine massage and oxytoxic medications) is of little use. Bleeding control may require ligation of the hypogastric arteries or hysterectomy. The incidence of placenta accreta is increased with placenta previa and may require hysterectomy to control bleeding.

Complications associated with treatment include hemorrhage following vaginal examination, blood transfusion reactions, sepsis, anesthesia-related problems, operative trauma, thrombophlebitis, and air embolism.

MORTALITY

Maternal mortality from placenta previa is approximately 1 percent. Perinatal mortality is decreasing, in part because of conservative treatment, increasing use of cesarean section for delivery, and more sophisticated neonatal intensive care. Major problems for the neonate are those associated with prematurity and fetal hypoxia. Mortality still ranges from 10 to 15 percent.

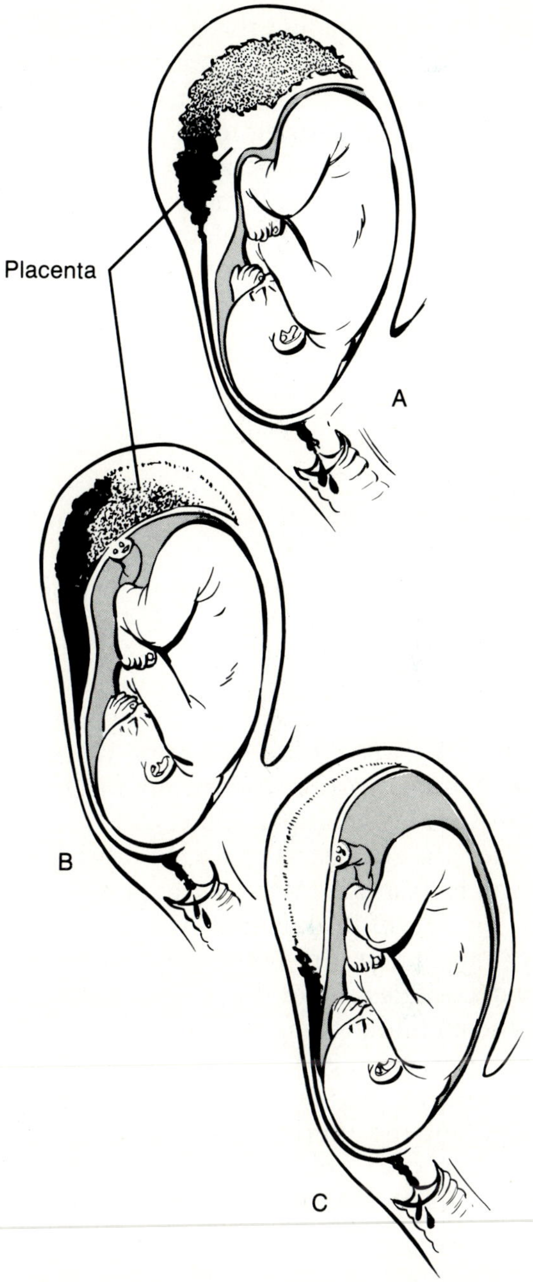

FIGURE 26-2. Degrees of abruptio placentae: A. Partial separation. B. Complete separation with concealed hemorrhage. C. Marginal separation.

Abruptio Placentae

Abruptio placentae is the premature separation of a normally implanted placenta after 20 weeks gestation. The separation may be complete, partial, or marginal (see Fig. 26-2). A marginal abruptio placentae is sometimes called marginal sinus rupture or marginal sinus bleeding. The amount of placental separation will determine maternal blood loss, severity of symptoms, decrease in oxygenation of the fetus, and the degree of coagulation defects present in the mother.

Bleeding from the placental site may be seen externally as blood escapes from between the chorion and the decidua vera and exits through the cervix, or it may remain trapped between the placenta and the uterine decidua if the placental margins do not separate. A combination of external and concealed bleeding may also occur. Symptoms noted vary according to the degree of detachment. In marginal abruptio placentae, symptoms are often minor. Complete placental detachment may be quickly fatal if there is no intervention.

INCIDENCE

Abruptio placentae occurs once in every 85 to 250 deliveries.

ETIOLOGY

The specific cause of abruptio placentae is not known, but certain factors predispose to its occurrence. Abruptio placentae occurs more frequently in multiparas, especially those over 35 years of age. Pregnancy-induced hypertension, especially with underlying renal vascular disease, and chronic hypertension also predisposes to abruptio placentae.

Another factor implicated in abruptio placentae is trauma. A direct blow to the uterus or forceful external version may produce abruption. In polyhydramnios, the sudden decompression of the uterus after rupture of the membranes may cause the placenta to separate prematurely.

When the gravida is in the supine position, the weight of the uterus may compress the inferior vena cava and increase intrauterine pressure, causing a portion of the placenta to detach. When the pressure in the uterine veins is increased, retroplacental bleeding and placental separation may result.

Fifteen percent of all placentas that abrupt are circumvallate placentas. Other factors also seem to affect the occurrence of abruptio placentae (see Table 26–6).

TABLE 26–6
PREDISPOSING FACTORS IN ABRUPTIO PLACENTAE

Pregnancy-induced hypertension
Chronic hypertension
Inferior vena cava compression
Trauma
Prior abruptions
Sudden uterine decompression
Uterine anomalies
Traction on the placenta by a short umbilical cord
Injudicious use of oxytocin
Multiparity
Advancing maternal age
Circumvallate placenta
Multiple gestation
Diabetes mellitus
Postmaturity
Low socioeconomic status
Folic acid deficiency

PATHOPHYSIOLOGY

Degenerative changes occur in small intervillous space arteries and cause thrombosis, decidual degeneration and rupture of the vessels. The vessel rupture is compounded by the fact that the uterus cannot contract sufficiently to close off the vessels, owing to its distention by the fetus.

Blood from the ruptured vessels may flow beneath the placenta, shearing it off completely or partially, and may separate the membranes from the uterine wall, eventually exiting through the cervix into the vagina.

If the blood cannot escape, a large amount of blood may be stored under the placenta, resulting in necrosis of the decidua and local clotting. Retroplacental clotting will cause depletion of fibrinogen from the general circulation. If the blood fibrin falls below 100, bleeding may occur from all mucosal surfaces into the uterus and result in the formation of a Couvelaire uterus with increased tone, irritability, and decreased ability to relax.

GRADES

Abruptio placentae can be classified into four grades of severity: grade 0, grade 1, grade 2, and grade 3.

Grade 0

Grade 0 is usually a retrospective diagnosis made by examination of the placenta after delivery. A large dark adherent clot is found over a segment of the placenta. There are no specific symptoms. About 30 percent of all abruptions are grade 0.

Grade 1

About 45 percent of abruptions are classified as grade 1. Some external bleeding occurs and uterine tetany may or may not be present. There is no associated maternal shock and no fetal distress. Placental attachment is usually in the lower portion of the upper uterine segment.

Grade 2

With a grade 2 abruption, there is concealed hemorrhage with or without external bleeding. The uterus is tender, and contractions may become tetanic in nature with little relaxation between them. Maternal vital signs usually remain within normal limits, but fetal distress is commonly present and may result in fetal death. Grade 2 abruptions account for 15 percent of all abruptio placentae. If delivery does not occur quickly, this abruption will progress to grade 3.

Grade 3

Ten percent of abruptio placentae are of this grade. Extensive hemorrhage occurs with or without external vaginal bleeding. The uterus is tetanic and has a boardlike consistency. Maternal shock and fetal death are common, with maternal mortality approaching 11 percent (Burchell et al., 1985).

DIAGNOSIS

Diagnosis of abruptio placentae is made by assessment and observation of clinical symptoms (see Table 26–3): uterine tenderness, increased uterine muscle tone, vaginal bleeding in varying amounts, fetal tachycardia (under 50 percent abruption), no FHT (over 50 percent abruption), and maternal shock. Ultrasonography may be of value if the abruption is concealed, but is of little or no value if there is substantial evidence of external bleeding.

MILD ABRUPTIO PLACENTAE

Symptoms

In mild or marginal abruptio placentae, symptoms are minimal. There is usually no effect on the fetus during labor and the fetal heart rate remains within normal limits with no excessive fetal movement. Since there is only minimal blood loss, maternal vital signs are within normal limits. Scant to moderate *dark* vaginal bleeding may be seen. The uterus is irritable and may fail to relax completely between uterine contractions. Complaints of vague lower abdominal discomfort and tenderness are vocalized by the gravida. It is difficult to effect Leopold's maneuvers, because uterine contractions will result from the external manipulations needed to outline the fetus.

Medical and Nursing Interventions

When vaginal bleeding is slight or moderate, uterine relaxation is present between contractions, and no fetal distress is noted, abruption must be differentiated from placenta previa (see Table 26–3).

Pregnancy of Less Than 36 Weeks Without Labor

No rectal or vaginal examinations should be attempted. Indirect diagnostic tests are initiated to rule out placenta previa. If placenta previa is ruled out and vaginal bleeding does not recur after a period of intensive observation and slow progressive ambulation, the gravida may be allowed to go home with specific instructions.

If placenta previa is definitely ruled out but vaginal bleeding continues, a speculum examination will rule out vaginal or cervical sources of bleeding. If there are no vaginal or cervical sources of bleeding, the client remains in the hospital to await the onset of labor or the onset of new symptoms. Maternal and fetal status are monitored for changes in parameters.

Explanations are necessary to alleviate anxiety and fears. The enforced inactivity will be difficult for the client and diversional activities are often needed. Verbalization of fears and concerns is encouraged.

Pregnancy of Less Than 36 Weeks in Labor

If the client is already in labor and placenta previa has been ruled out, the membranes are ruptured. Amniotomy will usually accelerate labor and decrease uterine bleeding, as the uterus contracts to adjust to the smaller contents. If the uterine contractions are ineffective, an oxytocin infusion will augment labor. Nursing care during labor has been discussed in Chapter 16. Nursing interventions during oxytocin infusion are discussed later in this chapter.

Pregnancy of 37+ Weeks

If gestation is 37 weeks or more, the gravida is admitted to the labor area and placed on bed rest. Intravenous fluids are started, laboratory testing is ordered, NPO status is maintained, and an accurate intake and output is recorded. Maternal and fetal physiologic status are monitored closely. The amount of vaginal bleeding is assessed for an increase or decrease in amount. The uterus is assessed for contractions and increases in tone and tenderness. Fundal height is monitored for increases (see Table 26–7).

A double setup examination is conducted to rule out placenta previa. If no placenta previa is found, an amniotomy is performed to induce labor. If labor does not begin promptly, an oxytocin infusion is started, following established guidelines. Meticulous fetal monitoring is essential during labor.

A cesarean section is performed if fetal distress occurs, vaginal bleeding continues and increases, or the uterus fails to relax between contractions.

TABLE 26–7
NURSING RESPONSIBILITIES IN ABRUPTIO PLACENTAE

Initial patient assessment
No vaginal or rectal examinations until placenta previa is ruled out
No enemas
NPO
Intravenous fluids with a large bore needle
Laboratory tests as ordered
Type and crossmatch for a minimum of 2 U blood
Monitor maternal vital signs
Monitor intake and output
Test urine for glucose and protein
Monitor FHR
Monitor uterine status
Evaluate blood loss
Notify high-risk nursery and pediatrician
Alert surgery of the possibility of a cesarean delivery
Offer emotional support to the gravida and her support person
Maintain bed rest
Measure fundal height and monitor for changes
Offer explanations as appropriate

MODERATE ABRUPTIO PLACENTAE

The separation of one-fourth but less than two-thirds of the placental surface from the uterine wall is considered moderate abruptio placentae.

Symptoms

Symptoms may be gradual or abrupt, with onset of continuous abdominal pain followed by dark vaginal bleeding. The external vaginal bleeding is usually moderate in amount, although up to 1000 ml of blood may be lost by the time the gravida arrives at the hospital. Fetal distress may or may not be present, depending upon the length of time elapsed since the abruption.

The uterus is tender to touch and manifests a sustained firm contraction with little relaxation between uterine contractions. The fetal heart rate may be difficult to hear, owing to increased uterine tone. If the client is not in labor, it will usually begin within two hours following the abruption. Clotting deficiencies and renal problems may occur, but are most common with the severe form.

Medical and Nursing Interventions

When moderate abruptio placentae is present, the objectives of intervention are: (1) to replace maternal blood lost; (2) to allay anxiety; (3) to expedite delivery; (4) to monitor fetal condition; (5) to monitor maternal physiologic status; and (6) to anticipate and deal with clotting defects.

When the gravida arrives at the hospital with abdominal pain and vaginal bleeding, she is placed on complete bed rest and is made NPO (see Table 26–8). An initial assessment determines maternal vital signs, amount of vaginal bleeding present, and fetal and uterine status. The attending physician is notified. Intravenous fluids are started with a large bore needle and laboratory testing is ordered, including type and crossmatch for three or more units of blood and a coagulation profile (platelet count, fibrinogen level, prothrombin time, partial thromboplastin level, and fibrin split products).

Maternal vital signs are monitored frequently, if necessary with central venous or pulmonary wedge pressure monitoring. A Foley catheter is inserted to obtain accurate urinary output for appraisal. Continuous fetal monitoring is done.

Uterine status is assessed continuously with a fetal monitor, and changes in tone, tenderness, and relaxation ability are monitored. To measure increases in uterine size that may occur with a concealed hemorrhage, a line may be drawn at the top of the uterine fundus and evaluated frequently for changes in the fundal height (see Table 26–8).

A vaginal examination is conducted by the physician and an amniotomy performed regardless of maternal shock and whether vaginal or abdominal delivery is anticipated. If labor does not begin within a short time, an oxytocin infusion may be used to initiate uterine contractions. Coagulation studies are repeated at frequent intervals, usually every two to three hours.

A cesarean section is performed if fetal distress occurs, if effective labor is not established within two to six hours, or if delivery cannot be anticipated within six to eight hours.

SEVERE ABRUPTIO PLACENTAE

In severe abruptio placentae, more than two-thirds of the placenta has separated from the uterine wall.

Symptoms

The onset of symptoms is usually very sudden, with little or no warning. The clinical symptoms are classic: (1) severe uterine pain described as tearing, knifelike, unremitting; (2) uterus is boardlike and tender; (3) external bleeding is small or moderate in amount; (4) fetus is almost always dead; (5) maternal shock is out of proportion to external vaginal bleeding; and (6) maternal oliguria and coagulation defects develop.

Medical and Nursing Interventions

For severe abruptio placentae treatment is basically the same as for the moderate

TABLE 26–8
SAMPLE NURSING CARE PLAN: MODERATE ABRUPTIO PLACENTAE

M.J., a gravida 4 para 3 of 36 weeks gestation was admitted to the labor unit with complaints of severe abdominal pain and a small amount of dark vaginal bleeding. She was put to bed and an initial assessment was conducted.

Data Base:

Gravida 4 para 3
36 week gestation
Small amount dark vaginal bleeding on perineal pad
Denies trauma to abdomen
Abdomen slightly firm between uterine contractions, not tender to touch
Uterine contractions every 2 minutes, lasting 90 seconds
States "My uterus doesn't relax between pains"
Uterine fundal height 37 cm

FHT 132 and irregular LLQ
VE done—3 cm cervical dilation at +1 station
cervix 80% effaced
PP cephalic
Blood type and Rh—A+
No known allergies
Denies any medical problems
On no medications, other than prenatal vitamins
Prenatal history uneventful
Last prenatal visit two weeks ago

Nursing Diagnosis	Goals	Nursing Interventions	Rationale	Evaluation
Potential fluid deficit related to vaginal bleeding	The effects of fluid volume deficit are decreased, as evidenced by: Normal laboratory values Adequate urinary output Maternal hydration Stable maternal vital signs	Assess and document vaginal bleeding	Vaginal bleeding in abruptio is usually dark	Small dark vaginal bleeding noted. Perineal pad applied for further assessment
		Measure and record abdominal girth on admission Mark fundal height and document Assess and record these parameters q ½ hour	With concealed bleeding, the uterus will enlarge and bleed into itself	Not done due to active labor status Fundal height 37 cm
		Monitor maternal vital signs including level of consciousness	Maternal shock is often out of proportion to amount of external bleeding	98.4°F-104-24 B/P 100/64 Alert and oriented
		Obtain laboratory tests as ordered	Coagulation defects occur in abruptio placentae frequently Blood replacement may be needed to replace maternal blood loss	CBC, Coagulation profile done, results within normal limits Stat type & crossmatch 4 U packed cells
		Assess hydration status Intake & output Skin turgor Mucous membranes		Hydration status normal IV of 1000 ml lactated Ringer's started RFA with 18 G Angio-cath to infuse at 168 ml/hour

		Urine specific gravity IV fluids as ordered		
		Document client perception of pain	Abdominal pain is sudden, severe, knifelike with a complete abruption	Stated, "This is my worst labor yet"
		Continuous monitoring of uterine contractions with fetal monitor: Frequency Duration Intensity Complete bed rest	With abruption, uterine tone is increased and uterine tenderness is present	Uterine contractions q 2 min, 90 seconds, severe intensity Little relaxation noted between contractions with external fetal monitor Abdomen slightly tender to touch
		Prepare for delivery	The longer the delay before delivery the greater the incidence of maternal complications	In active labor—vaginal delivery expected within 2 hours
Potential for injury to fetus related to decreased oxygenation secondary to abruptio placentae	The fetus will exhibit no fetal distress Injury to the fetus is minimized with appropriate nursing interventions	Continuous FHT monitoring with external monitor Assess and document: Baseline FHR Variability Periodic changes If alterations indicating fetal distress are noted, institute interventions as in Table 16–14	Fetal distress may or may not be present, depending on degree of abruption. With complete abruption, FHT are absent As maternal-fetal oxygen exchange becomes more compromised, fetal distress will develop	External fetal monitor instituted according to OB policy and procedure after explanation to client and husband FHR baseline 124 to 128 BPM, decreased variability on external tracing, no periodic changes at this time
		Prepare for delivery of compromised neonate Notify nursery Notify neonatologist		High-risk nursery and Dr. R. notified
Alteration in comfort related to inadequate uterine relaxation secondary to placental separation	The client verbalizes an understanding of why she has an alteration in comfort	Assess client understanding of pain associated with abruptio placentae	Patient understanding of causes of pain will help client to cope	Brief explanations of reasons for increased pain given to client and husband Client states "Pains are so hard"
		Assess client discomfort: Frequency of contractions Duration of contractions Quality of contractions Location of pain Intensity of pain Uterine relaxation Backache	Complaints of severe backache can indicate an increase in retroplacental bleeding	No complaints of backache
		Offer explanations to the client		

TABLE 26–8 (continued)

Nursing Diagnosis	Goals	Nursing Interventions	Rationale	Evaluation
	The client verbalizes that the discomfort is less	Minimize or eliminate factors that may contribute to pain Provide Positive reinforcement Personal contact Relaxation techniques Breathing modifications Distraction techniques		
Anxiety related to uncertain outcome for self and fetus	The client and support person are adapting to the situation as evidenced by: Lack of morbid grief Participation in self-care Decreased verbal/non-verbal anxiety	Encourage verbalization of fears and concerns for self and fetus Explain all procedures at appropriate level	Verbalizing concerns will aid in dealing with them	M and H very anxious about fetal outcome—verbalizing "Is the baby too small to live?"
Knowledge deficit related to bleeding cause, hospital environment	The client will verbalize an understanding of abruptio placentae	Assess client knowledge of abruptio placentae Assess the influence of anxiety or level of discomfort will have on the ability to understand explanations Provide information re: Abruptio placentae Effects of labor Possible maternal outcome Possible fetal outcome	The more advanced labor is, the less able the client is to retain information	Knowledge of abruptio was minimal Explanations very brief due to active labor status
Anxiety related to unfamiliarity with nursing procedures	The client will verbalize understanding of nursing or medical procedures done	Assess client knowledge of nursing interventions Explain all actions taken Available options Expected outcomes Reinforce physician's explanations Simplify Repeat prn Utilize calm approach in nursing interventions Begin teaching plan for type of anticipated delivery	Knowledge decreases	All interventions explained and understanding verbalized Dr. R. in to see client and examine—expected maternal and fetal outcome explained Not implemented due to active labor, multiparity, vaginal delivery expected

form, with the following additions: greater amounts of blood are needed for replacement, close vigilance is maintained for clotting deficiencies, and little or no consideration needs to be given to the fetus.

Upon admission, the gravida is placed on bed rest. The initial assessment will need to be brief, owing to maternal physiologic instability. The physician is notified immediately of the results of the initial assessment. Intravenous fluids are started, the client is NPO, and an accurate intake and output is recorded. A Foley catheter is inserted to obtain accurate assessment of urinary output. Laboratory testing is ordered, including type and crossmatch for a minimum of four units of blood and coagulation studies.

A primary objective of medical and nursing interventions is to control hemorrhage and overcome the effects of shock. Maternal vital signs are monitored constantly. The shock is almost always out of proportion to the external vaginal bleeding. Fetal heart tones are usually not present. Maternal blood loss must be continuously assessed. Membranes are ruptured at once, regardless of maternal physiologic status. Blood is replaced as quickly as possible, with two to four units minimum needed to maintain maternal stability. In shock the cardiac output is inadequate to provide normal perfusion for the major organs. Intravenous fluids are infused rapidly to keep organs perfused and to prevent irreversible organ damage.

Hypofibrinogenemia occurs because of the consumption of fibrinogen by the retroplacental clot. To correct a critical deficiency of fibrinogen, cryoprecipitate (fibrinogen and factor VIII) is given. Fibrinogen is no longer available for treatment. Coagulation studies are repeated frequently.

Another objective of care is relief from discomfort and anxiety. Analgesics are administered cautiously to prevent further maternal physiologic compromise. Explanations need to be complete but brief. Pain lessens the attention span, and only a small amount of information can be retained at any one time. Thorough explanations can be given later when the mother is physiologically stable.

Delivery of the fetus is accomplished as quickly as possible. Most clients deliver vaginally and within a reasonable length of time. Cesarean section is used for delivery if there is a chance that the fetus may still be alive, if there is little chance that vaginal delivery will follow within four to six hours, or if effective labor does not begin. If delivery is delayed longer, there is an increasing probability of serious maternal renal problems.

MATERNAL COMPLICATIONS

Overall maternal mortality from abruptio placentae is approximately 1 percent. The maternal prognosis depends upon four factors: (1) the amount of blood lost and whether the bleeding is concealed or apparent; (2) the degree of placental separation; (3) the presence of complications; and (4) the interval of time between the abruption and the initiation of treatment.

Hypovolemic Shock

The gravida will often arrive at the hospital in profound shock that is out of proportion to the amount of external vaginal bleeding. Rapid infusion of intravenous fluids and blood replacement as necessary will prevent damage to maternal organs.

Hypofibrinogenemia

Hypofibrinogenemia occurs in 10 percent of gravidas with abruptio placentae. Placental thromboplastic substances escape into the maternal intravascular compartment and deposit fibrin along maternal blood vessel walls, thus depleting the amount of circulating fibrinogen.

Uteroplacental Apoplexy

When hemorrhage is concealed, the red blood cells and serum from the clot may be forced through the myometrium of the uterus, producing a bluish-purple discoloration of the uterus (*Couvelaire uterus*) and loss of contractility of muscle fibers. This loss of contractility interferes with normal postpartum uterine muscle contraction and predisposes to postpartum hemorrhage.

Disseminated Intravascular Coagulation

As a result of myometrial damage and retroplacental clotting, large amounts of thromboplastin are released into the maternal circulation. If this is severe, disseminated intravascular coagulation (DIC) may occur.

Postpartum Infection

Hemorrhage and trauma during labor predispose to postpartum infections. When bleeding is extensive, prophylactic antibiotic therapy may be ordered to decrease the incidence of infection.

Postpartum Hemorrhage

In severe abruptio placentae, uterine contractile efficiency is decreased owing to the extravasation of blood into the uterine muscle.

Renal Failure

Renal failure may occur following ischemia from maternal hypovolemic shock, vascular spasm, or intravascular clotting. Incompatible blood transfusions may also produce renal shutdown. The longer the ischemia persists, the more likely the client is to develop renal problems. Urinary symptoms include oliguria and proteinuria.

Sheehan's Syndrome

Sheehan's syndrome (pituitary necrosis) may result from ischemia (see Chapter 27).

Hepatitis

Hepatitis following blood transfusions may develop in the client with abruptio placentae.

FETAL PROGNOSIS

Overall perinatal mortality following abruptio placentae ranges from 30 to 60 percent, with fetal mortality approaching 100 percent in severe abruption. Mortality results from complications of prematurity or hypoxia. Fetal death in utero is caused by a lowered level of oxygenation that is incompatible with intrauterine survival.

Ruptured Vasa Previa

Vasa previa is associated with velamentous insertion of the umbilical cord. The proximal end of the umbilical cord is attached to the fetal membranes and fetal vessels extend across a membranous bridge to the placenta. When one or more of the fetal vessels cross the internal cervical os, the condition is called *vasa previa*.

A ruptured vasa previa can be difficult to differentiate from abruptio placentae or placenta previa. When a major fetal vessel ruptures and is the source of vaginal bleeding, fetal death is virtually certain. Delivery can rarely be accomplished rapidly enough to salvage the fetus. If the fetal vessel that ruptures is small, the fetus can sometimes be saved if delivery is accomplished quickly.

Ruptured Uterus

Spontaneous or traumatic rupture of the uterus may occur before or during labor, resulting in maternal and/or fetal death.

INCIDENCE

Reported incidence of uterine rupture varies from 1 in 93 to 1 in 8741 pregnancies. The average incidence is approximately 1 in 2000 pregnancies.

TYPES

Uterine rupture may be incomplete or complete. With a complete rupture, all layers of the uterus are involved and there is direct communication between the uterine and abdominal cavities. With an incomplete uterine rupture, the myometrium of the uterus is involved, but the peritoneum remains intact.

SITE OF RUPTURE

During pregnancy, tears most commonly occur in the upper uterine segment. During labor, the thinner lower uterine segment is more likely to rupture.

CAUSES

Causes of uterine rupture are divided into four categories: spontaneous rupture, postcesarean rupture, traumatic rupture, and rupture following other uterine trauma. *Spontaneous rupture of the normal uterus* occurs during labor. These ruptures are most commonly in the lower uterine segment and are often the result of mismanagement of labor. Causes include grand multiparity, cephalopelvic disproportion, abnormal presentations, and improper use of oxytocin. *Postcesarean rupture of the uterus* is the most common cause of ruptured uterus. Previous upper segment scars are more prone to rupture than are lower segment scars. *Traumatic rupture of the uterus* is most often the consequence of operative vaginal deliveries. Causes include version and extraction, difficult forceps deliveries, breech extractions, excessive fundal pressure, and manual dilatation of the cervix. *Rupture of the uterus following other uterine trauma* can occur without warning. Causes include previous myomectomy, cervical lacerations, manual removal of an adherent placenta, endometritis, and hysterotomy.

SYMPTOMS

Symptoms noted with uterine rupture depend upon many factors, including the time of occurrence, the cause of the rupture, the degree of the rupture, the position of the rupture, the amount of bleeding, and whether the fetus is completely or partially expelled from the uterus.

Silent Rupture

With a quiet or silent uterine rupture, the usual signs and symptoms do not occur initially. The nurse may note the presence of maternal tachycardia, pallor, and slight vaginal bleeding. Uterine contractions continue but cervical dilation stops. The silent rupture is most often seen with incomplete rupture of an old cesarean section scar. Symptoms develop over several hours and include abdominal pain, vomiting, faintness, vaginal bleeding, tachycardia, pallor, uterine tenderness, and absence of the fetal heart rate.

Violent Rupture

With a violent rupture, an extremely intense and hard uterine contraction is followed by sharp lower abdominal pain. The client may state that "something gave way." The contractions then stop, the type of pain is altered, and she becomes very apprehensive and restless. The fetus can be palpated abdominally and fetal small parts can be easily identified. Fetal heart tones and fetal movements soon cease. Maternal shock follows.

TABLE 26-9
SAMPLE NURSING CARE PLAN: UTERINE RUPTURE

Mary G., a 32-year-old single gravida 3 para 1 abortion 1 at term is admitted to labor and delivery at 8:00 am in active labor. An initial assessment is done on admission.

Data Base:

32 year old
Grav 3, para 2, abo 1
Single
40 weeks gestation
Prenatal history unremarkable
No known allergies
No medical problems
On no medications, except prenatal vitamins
No prosthesis
Ate last at 10 p.m.
Membranes intact
Pediatrician Dr. H.
Breast feeding
Maternal vital signs: 97.6°F-88-16 B/P 108/74
FHR 148 LLQ
VE at 8 am: 3 cm cervical dilation at −1 station
Presenting part cephalic
Cervix 55% effaced
Dr. R. notified of admission
Routine laboratory tests (CBC, PTT, prothrombin time; UA) done on admission
IV: 1000 ml D5LR started LFA at 8:15 am
Labor progress and parameters within normal limits

10:15 am Labor status: VE 6 cm cervical dilation at 0 station
Cervix 80% effaced
FHR tracing: FHR baseline 130-136 BPM. Average variability noted on external tracing. Occasional accelerations of 15 BPM noted with no other periodic changes. Uterine contractions every 3 minutes, lasting 50 seconds, moderate intensity

11:00 am: Mary c/o severe, stabbing lower abdominal pain. She is restless and diaphoretic. Unable to obtain FHT at this time. Vital signs: 98°F, 144-28, B/P 80/42. Skin cool and clammy. Abdominal palpation reveals tender abdomen, unable to palpate uterine fundus. Fetal small parts identified LRQ. Dr. R. notified

11:05 am: Vital signs: B/P 80/40, P140, R 28, No FHT
Decision to do emergency laporatomy with possible hysterectomy

11:12 am: To surgery

11:16 am: Girl delivered by laporatomy. Apgars 3 and 5. Transferred to neonatal ICU with anesthesiologist and neonatologist in attendance

2:30 pm: Returned to postpartum unit. Report from recovery room: Surgery done: hysterectomy. Vital signs stable. IV of 1000 ml Normal saline infusing at 168 ml.hour. She has received 3 Units packed cells in surgery. Foley catheter draining clear yellow urine. Abdominal dressing dry and intact. Repeat hemoglobin and hematocrit ordered for 6 pm

Nursing Diagnosis	Goals	Nursing Interventions	Rationale	Evaluation
Fluid volume deficit related to internal bleeding secondary to uterine rupture	The client will exhibit minimal effects from fluid volume deficit immediately post-operative	Assess level of consciousness	Uncontrolled bleeding can result in hypovolemia. If the hypo-volemia is severe, blood is shunted to the organs that require the most oxygen, resulting in tissue damage. Blood flow is decreased to the kidney and tissue damage may result. Decreased cerebral blood flow decreases level of consciousness	Sleepy, but oriented to time and place
		Check and record: B/P, P, R q 15 minutes until stable, then q hour times 4, then q 4 hours		P 108, R 24, B/P 100/72 on ad-mission. Remained within normal limits on 15 minute checks
		Take temperature upon arrival in unit and q 4 hours		Temperature 97.6°F
		Assess for hypovolemic shock, if it occurs: Stay with client; Modified Trendelenberg position; Assess vaginal bleeding; Assess abdominal dressings; Frequent vital signs; Notify physician		Vital signs remained within normal limits, no interventions needed. Continue to assess vitals
		Apply antiembolism stockings if ordered		TED hose applied
		Assess lung sounds		Lungs clear bilaterally to auscultation
		Turn, cough, deep breathe, q 2 hours		Position changed Coughing and deep breathing done
		Obtain laboratory work as ordered		Awaiting 6 pm lab work
Potential alteration in nutrition: less than body requirements related to emergency surgery secondary to uterine rupture	The client will remain ade-quately hydrated post-operatively	Maintain NPO status as ordered	Hydration will aid in maintain-ing tissue perfusion	NPO
		Monitor IV infusions Intake and output Assess output hourly Report output under 30 ml/hour to physician		IV of D_5LR ordered at 168 ml/hour. Hung at 3:30 pm after saline infusion completed. Foley output 60 ml/hour
		Assist in administration of blood if ordered	To expand volume and restore clotting factors	Blood on hold awaiting 6 pm laboratory results

TABLE 26-9 (continued)

Nursing Diagnosis	Goals	Nursing Interventions	Rationale	Evaluation
Alteration in comfort: pain related to surgery	The client expresses minor discomfort immediately postoperatively	Assess and evaluate client need for pain medication Incisional pain Vital signs Restlessness Administer Demerol 75 mg IM q 3–4 hours prn as ordered		Pain medication given at 4:30 pm
Knowledge deficit related to emergency surgery and postoperative nursing interventions	The client will verbalize understanding of reason for surgery and postoperative course	Explain reasons for unplanned surgery Answer questions honestly Offer emotional support Encourage questions and verbalizations re: surgery and outcome	Unplanned surgery is a crisis situation Explanations prior to surgery were brief Time needs to be spent offering explanations, answering questions	The reason for the unplanned surgery was explained to Mary. She had many questions, especially concerning the hysterectomy
Alteration in parenting related to compromised neonate	The client will understand and accept the expected neonatal outcome	Offer realistic explanations of neonatal status Keep informed of neonatal status and progress Encourage visits to nursery as soon as possible Take picture of neonate for client to see	Neonatal outcome is guarded. The patient should be told the truth, so she can begin to cope	Nursery nurse spent time with Mary and explained neonate status, etc Mary taken to nursery via cart to see and touch neonate Neonate baptized per Mary's request

Rupture With a Delayed Diagnosis

In this situation, the uterus ruptures but the condition is not diagnosed until the client is in severe hypovolemic shock.

MEDICAL AND NURSING INTERVENTIONS

The vast majority of uterine ruptures can be prevented. During the prenatal period, accurate assessment of the maternal pelvis will avoid potential rupture due to cephalopelvic disporportion. Accurate identification of fetal presentation and position by Leopold's maneuvers and vaginal or rectal examination is important. During labor, careful monitoring of fetal and maternal physiologic status is necessary. Prolonged labor should be avoided. If an oxytocin infusion is used to induce or augment labor, continuous assessment of the mother and fetus are required.

If uterine rupture does occur, prompt recognition of the condition and appropriate interventions will help to reduce maternal and fetal mortality. An immediate laporatomy is performed and the bleeding controlled as quickly as possible. A total hysterectomy is the procedure of choice, although in young women who desire more children, the tear may be repaired if the uterine muscle can be approximated (see Table 26–9 on p. 698 for a sample nursing care plan).

Blood transfusions are needed to replace the blood lost. If only a repair is done, future deliveries will be by scheduled cesarean section to prevent future uterine ruptures.

Explanations are provided for the client and support person before any interventions. If maternal physiologic status is severely compromised, explanations need to be brief with followup explanations after the emergency situation is resolved. Fears and anxieties need to be verbalized, and spiritual support is beneficial.

MATERNAL MORTALITY

The reported maternal death rate ranges from 3 to 40 percent. Main causes of death are shock and blood loss. The maternal prognosis depends upon prompt diagnosis and intervention, the amount of hemorrhage, whether infection results, and the type and site of the rupture.

FETAL MORTALITY

Fetal mortality ranges from 30 to 85 percent. The majority die following placental separation that occurs with the uterine rupture and expulsion of the fetus into the abdominal cavity.

Disseminated Intravascular Coagulation

Disseminated intravascular coagulation (DIC) results in rapid use of blood clotting factors, leading to occlusion of small blood vessels and a predisposition to hemorrhage.

PREDISPOSING FACTORS

The mechanisms of DIC complicate a large number of medical, surgical, and obstetric problems. Obstetric problems that are most commonly associated with DIC are listed in Table 26–10.

TABLE 26–10
OBSTETRICAL PREDISPOSING FACTORS IN DIC

Abruptio placentae
Eclampsia
Retention of a dead fetus
Amniotic fluid embolism
Sepsis
Rapid precipitous labor
Difficult delivery
Oxytocin induction
Retained placenta
Massive maternal hemorrhage

TABLE 26-11
SAMPLE NURSING CARE PLAN: DISSEMINATED INTRAVASCULAR COAGULATION

P.H., a 30-year-old, gravida 5 para 5, delivered a live boy at 7:02 am following oxytocin induction for spontaneous rupture of the membranes. The amniotic fluid was meconium stained. Apgars 7 and 9. Her prenatal history was unremarkable. No known allergies. She was on no medications, with the exception of prenatal vitamins and an iron supplement. No medical problems were present.

Approximately 4 hours following delivery, nursing assessment revealed the following data:

Data Base:

Oozing noted from IM injection site
Diaphoretic
Restless
Slightly confused
B/P 130/74

Pulse 120
Respirations 28
Skin cool and clammy
Dr. V. notified of patient status. Laboratory tests (CBC, PT, PTT, bleeding time) were ordered

Nursing Diagnosis	Goals	Nursing Interventions	Rationale	Evaluation
Fluid volume deficit related to blood loss secondary to clotting deficit	The client survives the disease with minimal or no damage to body organs or tissues	Assess Skin surfaces for: Petechiae Purpura Hematoma Oozing from IM or IV sites Bleeding from mucus membranes GI bleeding Hemoptysis Alterations in level of consciousness	These are typical clinical symptoms of DIC	Oozing noted from IM injection site left hip Epistaxis Small hematoma noted site of delivery room IV Slightly confused

		Monitor vital signs q 15 minutes: Pulse, respirations, B/P Assess skin: Cool Clammy Cyanosis of nailbeds, eyelids Maintain CVP reading at 6–12 mm H_2O Intake and output: Hourly output Check for hematuria Maintain IV as ordered	Fluid volume deficit monitored by assessing parameters at frequent intervals CVP readings measure contractility of heart and adequacy of blood volume Oliguria may indicate inadequate fluid volume	B/P range: 120/74 to 140/92 P—114, regular R—24, slightly shallow Skin cool and clammy, nail beds pink CVP reading remained 7 mm H_2O Output 50 ml/hr
		Assess laboratory tests for results: PT PTT Bleeding time Platelets	Platelets are the reliable index for DIC. Low coagulation factors not reliable, because healthy liver will compensate	Bleeding time 3 minutes PT—130% normal PTT—52 Platelets—75,000 mm^3
		Turn q 2 hours Pad side rails to prevent bruising, hematoma formation Minimize IM or subq injections Apply pressure to oozing sites Minimize B/P cuff readings by maintaining arterial line	Appropriate nursing interventions will decrease incidence of further complications	Turned q 2 hours Padded side rails in place No arterial line in place at this time
Alteration in tissue perfusion related to decreased oxygen exchange and circulation at cellular level	The client will survive the disease with minimal residual effects or sequelae Blood clotting mechanism will return to normal	Administer fluids as ordered Administered blood products as ordered Administer heparin therapy as ordered Monitor for adverse effects: Increased bleeding New purpura, petechiae hematoma PT results	In presence of inadequate tissue perfusion, respirations increase to get rid of excess acid, pulse increases, B/P decreases, perfusion of skin sacrificed to maintain oxygenation to vital organs	IV D5/0.45 NS infusing at 168 ml/hour 1 Unit platelets infused Heparin infusion maintained at 1500 U/hour, via infusion pump No adverse effects noted Will continue to assess

TABLE 26-11 (continued)

Nursing Diagnosis	Goals	Nursing Interventions	Rationale	Evaluation
		Assess: Dyspnea Respiratory distress Poor capillary refill Level of consciousness Cardiac rhythm Lung sounds Respiratory rate Obtain ABGs q 1 hour as ordered		Head of bed elevated 45° Oxygen at 6 L/min ABGs within normal limits Sinus tachycardia noted Lungs clear to auscultation bilaterally
Anxiety related to treatments, environment and risk of death	The client and family will verbalize basic understanding of ordered treatments	Offer explanation of treatments and procedures Minimize extraneous chatter at bedside Use calm approach in dealing with client and family Briefly orient family to intensive care unit	Awareness of treatments and procedures will decrease anxiety	Brief explanation given to client More detailed explanations given to family Family oriented to ICU and policies
Alteration in familiy processes related to critical nature of situation and uncertain prognosis	The family will verbalize understanding of prognosis for the client	Offer explanations at appropriate level of understanding Emotional support Do not give false hope Anticipate grief response	Allow famiily to begin working through grief process	Prognosis discussed with family by physician, reinforced by nurse Verbalized understanding

PATHOPHYSIOLOGY

DIC occurs as a response of the body to a coagulation-producing material entering the circulation. The coagulation-producing material may be decidual tissue, amniotic fluid, or an endotoxin. In response to the stimuli, platelets aggregate and fibrinogen forms. The fibrinogen is converted into fibrin and is deposited into the maternal microcirculation. The adrenal and pituitary glands and the kidneys are especially susceptible to the fibrin deposits.

As the fibrin is deposited, the fibrinolytic system activates to try to clear the blocked circulation, and hemostasis is further compromised. A bleeding defect results that is characterized by prolonged bleeding from small vessels.

LABORATORY VALUES

The bleeding time, partial thromboplastin time, and prothrombin time are prolonged. If the liver is healthy, prolonged coagulation factors are not reliable for diagnosis. Platelet counts are decreased and are a reliable indicator of DIC.

TABLE 26-12
OBSTETRICAL DISORDERS ASSOCIATED WITH DIC AND INTERVENTIONS

- Abruptio placentae
  - Amniotomy to initiate labor and decrease pressure on the retroplacental clot
  - Liberal transfusions
  - Delivery as quickly as possible
- Dead fetus syndrome
  - Coagulation studies
  - Heparin 24 to 48 hours before operative intervention to clear fibrin breakdown products and reestablish homeostasis
- Gram-negative endotoxemia
  - Remove focus of infection
  - Antibiotic administration
  - Blood transfusions
  - Steroids
- Pregnancy-induced hypertension
  - Laboratory studies
  - Prophylactic heparin to reverse thrombocytopenia and fibrin products and increase placental function

MEDICAL AND NURSING INTERVENTIONS (see Table 26-11 on p. 702)

When obstetric patients develop any of the problems that predispose to the development of DIC, assessment for signs that DIC may be developing is an essential component of nursing care. These signs include bleeding from the nose or gums, bleeding from injection sites, tachycardia, restlessness, anxiety, and diaphoresis.

Laboratory tests are assessed for normal or abnormal values. The coagulation profile is usually abnormal. Thrombocytopenia and a decreased hematocrit are suspicious signs that DIC may be developing.

In the obstetric patient, correction of the disorder that caused the DIC to develop will usually correct the defect (see Table 26-12).

Interventions appropriate for treating DIC include: (1) correction of hypovolemia; (2) restoration of reduced levels of coagulation factors and platelets; and (3) clearance of the circulation of FBP produced by fibrinolysis. Vital signs are monitored at frequent intervals. Central venous pressure monitoring may be done with the reading maintained at 6 to 12 mm H_2O. Accurate intake and output are recorded. Oxygen is given via face mask. A lateral or supine position with the right hip elevated will allow adequate oxygenation. Cyanosis, pallor, and cool clammy skin may be observed. Restlessness and confusion are indicative of cerebral hypoxia, so level of consciousness is assessed at frequent intervals. If the client is undelivered, the fetal heart rate and uterine contraction status are assessed.

Administration of blood will help to correct the hypovolemia. If fresh blood is not available, 2 to 3 units of fresh frozen plasma, or 16 to 20 bags of cryoprecipitate or platelets may be given. Appropriate nursing interventions and assessments during administration of any of these products is carried out.

Heparin may be administered intravenously per infusion pump, most commonly in the dosage of 12.5 U per kg per hr after an initial bolus of 5000 units. Heparin is used only when absolutely necessary, since it may increase bleeding if any major part of the vascular system is disrupted.

DYSTOCIA

Dystocia, or difficult labor, may be caused by uterine dysfunction, abnormal presentations and positions, fetopelvic disproportions, or uterine anomalies.

PROLONGED LABOR

Traditionally, any labor that lasted longer than 24 hours was considered a prolonged labor. In obstetrics today, the upper time limit for normal labor is considered 18 hours. Problems should be identified and appropriate interventions implemented long before this time limit is reached.

CAUSES

When no mechanical barrier to the progress of labor is present, the explanation for the prolongation of labor may be obscure. After 12 hours, labors become steadily more dysfunctional. Labor will be less efficient when systemic alterations are present in the gravida. There is an association between dysfunctional labor and maternal dehydration. The woman who approaches labor with excessive fear may be a candidate for dysfunctional labor. Conditions such as intrauterine infections are also associated with dysfunctional labor.

It has been suggested that injudicious use of analgesics, sedatives, and anesthesia may prolong labor although therapeutic doses do not normally reduce uterine contractility.

Other associated factors include postmaturity, overdistention of the uterus, and grand multiparity. Women over 35 years are twice as likely to have dysfunctional labor as are women under 20 years of age (Cohen et al., 1980).

Uterine Dysfunction

Improper functioning of the myometrium when there is no unusual resistance from the presenting part, maternal pelvis, soft tissues, or cervix is implied in dystocia caused by abnormal uterine action. Dystocia due to uterine dysfunction can be identified and managed if the time of the onset of labor is determined, the limits of normal labor are recognized, mechanical dysfunction is ruled out, and the condition of the fetus is known.

THE ONSET OF LABOR

The time of the onset of true labor must be determined. It is often difficult to determine accurately when labor actually begins. The generally accepted definition of the onset of true labor is when the uterine contractions are uncomfortable, are five minutes apart, and there is evidence of cervical dilation.

NORMAL LABOR

Normal labor is almost always associated with a presenting part that fits snugly into the lower uterine segment and is close to the upper cervical rim.

Contractions in a normal labor are characterized by (1) fundal dominance, (2) good intensity at the peak, (3) good relaxation between contractions, and (4) increasing duration. The contractions occur at regular intervals and develop at least 40 mm Hg intrauterine pressure. Between uterine contractions, intrauterine pressure ranges from 6 to 12 mm Hg.

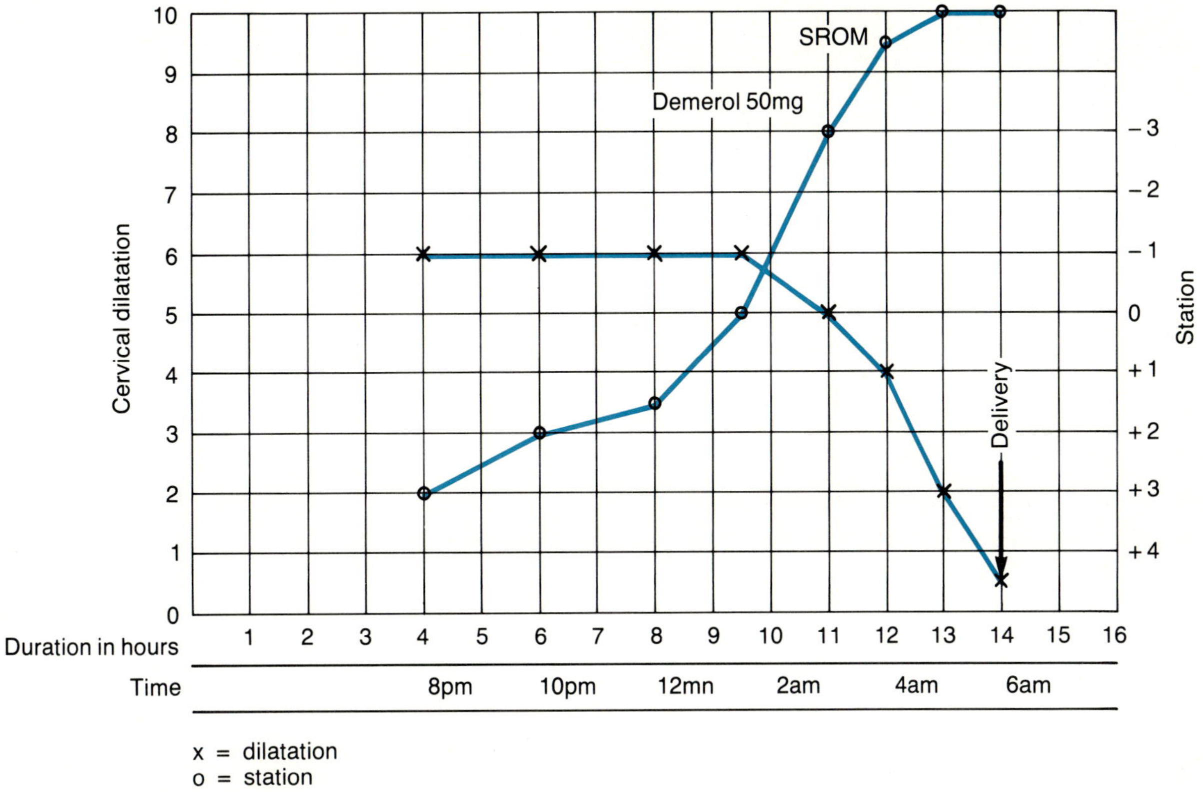

FIGURE 26–3. Normal cervical dilatation curve.

When uterine contractions are effective, the cervix is tight against the presenting part upon vaginal examination. Once labor has begun, it constantly advances, and cervical dilation forms a progressively accelerating curve (see Fig. 26–3).

LABOR GRAPHS

Using a labor graph to plot the progress of cervical dilation will aid in objective assessment of progress and will help to identify dysfunctional labor patterns.

One type of labor graph used to plot labor progress is made by using square-ruled graph paper to plot dilation of the cervix from 0 cm (bottom) to 10 cm (top) on the left ordinate, and stations from −5 (top) to +5 (bottom) on the right ordinate. On the bottom of the graph, the time of the onset of uterine contractions or the beginning of the oxytocin infusion is marked. The client is examined every two hours in the latent phase and every hour in the active phase of labor. The time, degree of dilation (X), and fetal station (O) are graphed (see Fig. 26–4). Interpretation of this graph involves two questions: (1) In what phase is the client? (2) Is labor progressing normally for that phase?

Another graphic analysis of labor, described by Friedman (1978), correlates the duration of labor with the rate of cervical dilation. After graphing the time and the cervical dilation, a sigmoid curve is made when the points of contact are joined (see Fig. 26–5).

The first stage of labor is divided into the latent phase and the active phase. The latent phase is a period of time of some cervical effacement and slow dilation that may last an average of 8 hours in a primigravida and 5 hours in a multipara. The upper limit of normal for a primigravida is 20 hours and for a multipara the upper limit is 14 hours. The active phase begins with the end of the latent

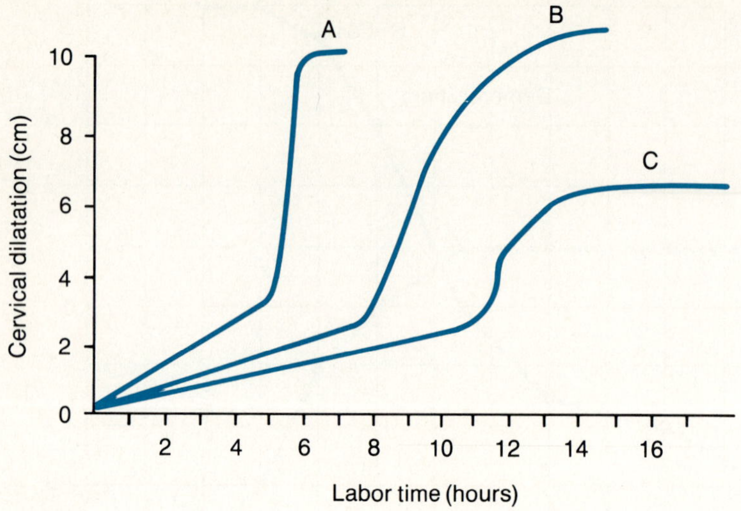

FIGURE 26-4. First stage of labor: A. Multipara. B. Primigravida. C. Secondary arrest of dilatation.

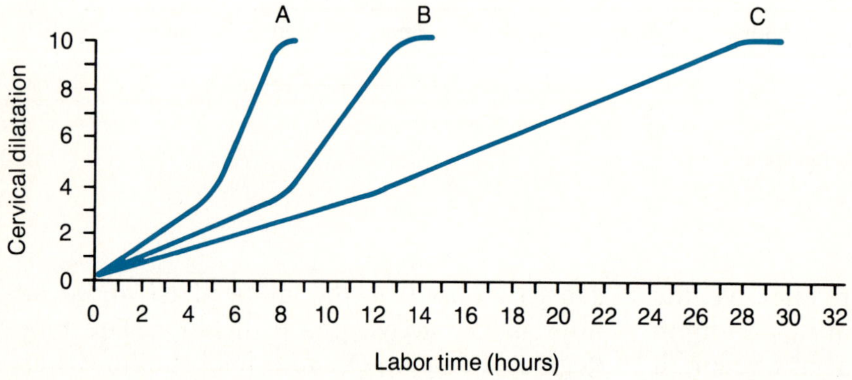

FIGURE 26-5. First stage of labor: A. Multipara. B. Primigravida. C. Primary dysfunction.

phase and ends at complete cervical dilation. The curve on the graph changes from a horizontal slope to a vertical line. The average length of the active phase is 5.8 hours for a primigravida and 2.5 hours for a multipara. The upper limit for the active phase is 12 hours for a primigravida and 6 hours for a multipara. For the first stage of labor primigravidas average 13.3 hours and multiparas average 7.5 hours.

TYPES OF UTERINE DYSFUNCTION

Uterine dysfunction is usually divided into two types: primary and secondary inertia. *Primary uterine inertia*, or hypertonic uterine dysfunction, occurs at the onset of labor. *Secondary uterine inertia*, or hypotonic uterine dysfunction, occurs after the onset of labor; labor starts normally, but then slows significantly or stops altogether.

HYPERTONIC UTERINE DYSFUNCTION

Hypertonic uterine dysfunction, or primary uterine inertia, occurs during the latent phase of labor before active cervical dilation begins.

Characteristics

The uterine contractions are of irregular intensity, ineffectual, uncoordinated, and have no fundal dominance. The contractions are of a poor quality, and the discomfort felt by the patient is out of proportion to the intensity. The uterine muscle is in a state of greater-than-normal tension and does not relax completely between uterine contractions. There is little or no progress in dilation of the cervix or in descent of the presenting part. When the latent phase of labor exceeds 17 to 20 hours in the primigravida, or 11 to 14 hours in the multipara, primary uterine inertia is present.

Causes

Causes include an unripe cervix, abnormal fetal position, fetopelvic disproportion, administration of excessive sedation, unrecognized false labor, uterine overdistention, postmaturity, grand multiparity, and emotional factors.

Maternal Dangers

Maternal dangers in hypertonic uterine dysfunction include exhaustion, dehydration, intrauterine infection, rupture of the uterus, lacerations of the vagina during a difficult delivery, and a negative effect on future childbearing.

Fetal Dangers

Fetal distress may appear during hypertonic uterine dysfunction. Injury to the fetus during a traumatic delivery and possible sepsis are also dangers to the fetus.

Medical and Nursing Interventions

In order to correct the type of uterine contractions present, the pattern must be interrupted. Rest is a primary objective of care. Sedation with morphine and a short-acting barbiturate is given to stop the abnormal contraction pattern (see Table 26–13).

Intravenous fluids are provided to maintain maternal hydration and electrolyte balance. The fetal heart rate and uterine contraction pattern are monitored continuously with the fetal monitor. Maternal vital signs are assessed frequently. External stimuli are decreased, siderails are up, and comfort measures are provided for the mother before administering sedation. Explanations are given to lower anxiety and promote rest.

Normal labor will often begin when the client awakens. Assessment of the onset of normal uterine contractions is important. Oxytocins are not usually given because they will only enhance the abnormal uterine contraction pattern.

HYPOTONIC UTERINE DYSFUNCTION

Hypotonic uterine dysfunction, or secondary uterine inertia, occurs during the active phase of labor.

Active Phase Dysfunction

Active phase dysfunction is present if cervical dilation progresses at less than 1.2 cm per hour in the primigravida or less than 1.5 cm per hour in the multipara (Friedman, 1978).

Characteristics

Uterine contractions that have previously been normal become less frequent, less intense, and of shorter duration. The uterine contractions may become far apart and irregular after 3 to 4 cm cervical dilation. Progress in cervical dilation slows considerably or ceases.

Causes

The specific cause is not known. Associated factors include fetal malposition, fetopelvic disproportion, oversedation, postmaturity, maternal dehydration, maternal exhaustion, grand multiparity, and excessive cervical rigidity (see Fig. 26–6).

TABLE 26-13
SAMPLE NURSING CARE PLAN: HYPERTONIC UTERINE DYSFUNCTION

Diane T., a 24-year-old primigravida at term is admitted to the labor room in early labor at 10:30 pm

Data Base:

24 years old
Married
Gravida 1 para 0
39 weeks gestation
No known allergies
B negative—prenatal antibody titer negative
25 lb weight gain
No medical problems
On no medications except prenatal vitamins
Membranes ruptured at 9 pm—fluid clear, no odor (nitrazine positive on admission)
VE: 1–2 cm cervical dilation
Cervix 50% effaced
Presenting part cephalic at −1 station
Contractions every 4 minutes, lasting 50 seconds, moderate quality
Pediatrician Dr. B.
Breastfeeding
Admission laboratory work done (CBC, PT, PTT, UA), all normal values
Vital signs: 98°F.-88-20 B/P 108/65
Internal fetal monitoring instituted at 10:45 pm according to policy and procedure
IV of d5LR started at 10:40 pm according to physician order
3:00 am labor status: VE 2+ cm cervical dilation
Cervix 60% effaced
Presenting part cephalic at −1 to 0 station
FHR baseline 140–144 BPM, average variability noted, no periodic changes
Uterine contractions q 2 minutes, lasting 80 seconds, good quality
Resting uterine tone 20 mm Hg
Coping poorly with uterine contractions
Utilizing breathing techniques with little success

Nursing Diagnosis	Goals	Nursing Interventions	Rationale	Evaluation
Alteration in the process of labor related to greater than normal tension of uterine muscle secondary to hypertonic uterine dysfunction	The client will deliver without maternal injury, fetal injury, or fetal distress	Identify uterine dysfunction pattern: Plot labor pattern on labor graph Assess uterine contraction pattern for frequency, duration, intensity Client behaviors Progress in cervical dilation FHR pattern Coping ability	Hypertonic uterine dysfunction is characterized by: Uterus in greater than normal state of tension Painful contractions without progress in labor Occurring in latent phase	Progress in labor to this point in time is minimal. Criteria for hypertonic uterine dysfunction pattern is present (see data base)

		Notify physician of labor status Assist with diagnostics Ultrasound Pelvimetry Administer sedation and analgesics as ordered Monitor FHR Monitor uterine contractions Assess hydration status Monitor maternal vital signs	Diagnostics to rule out other causes of lack of labor progress Treatment of hypertonic uterine dysfunction is rest and sedation Labor pattern will often be normal when labor resumes	Dr. B evaluated client status. No ultrasound or pelvimetry ordered Side rails up Voided Clean sheets and gown after partial sponge bath Lights turned down for rest Morphine sulfate gr 1/4 subq as ordered Internal FHR and UC monitoring continued
Knowledge deficit related to alterations in normal labor progress	The client and support person will verbalize understanding of the alteration in labor	Offer explanations re: Cause of lack of labor progress Proposed medical treatment Associated nursing interventions	Explanations will aid in decreasing anxiety and frustration, as well as increase compliance with proposed treatment	The cause of the altered uterine function was explained, along with proposed medical treatment and nursing interventions. They verbalized understanding and agreed with the proposed treatment

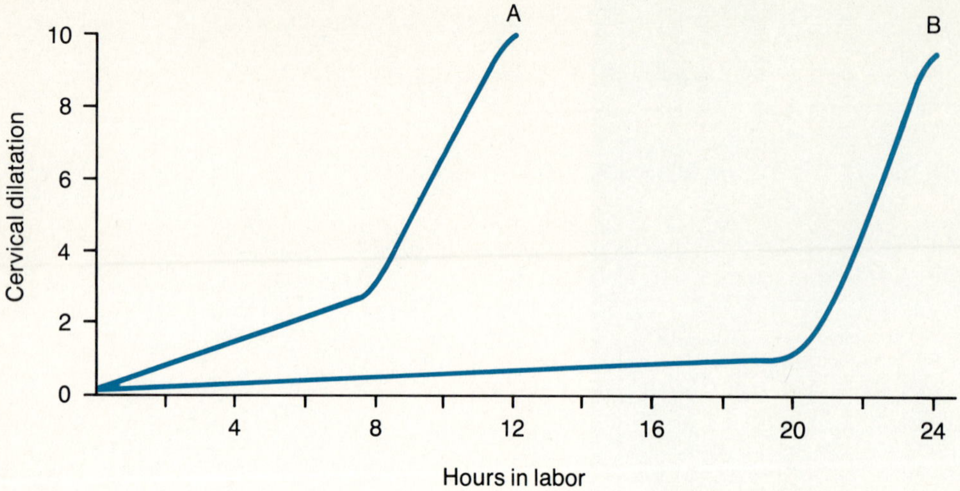

FIGURE 26-6. First stage of labor: A. Normal. B. Prolonged latent phase.

Secondary Arrest Dysfunction

During the active phase of labor, cervical dilation may stop. If there is no change in cervical dilation for two hours when the examination is conducted by the same individual and uterine contractions remain of good quality, secondary arrest of dilation is present (see Fig. 26-6).

Causes

Approximately 50 percent of secondary arrest dysfunction is caused by fetopelvic disproportion (Friedman, 1978). Other causes include malposition of the presenting part, maternal exhaustion, excessive sedation, and inefficient uterine action.

Maternal Dangers

Maternal dangers with hypotonic uterine dysfunction include dehydration, exhaustion, intrauterine infection, increased incidence of postpartum hemorrhage, and mental strain.

Fetal Dangers

When labor is prolonged, the probability of fetal distress is increased. Other dangers include injury from a traumatic, difficult delivery.

Medical and Nursing Interventions

Mechanical factors that may be the cause of the dysfunction are ruled out. A vaginal examination is conducted to ascertain position, station, size of the caput succedaneum (if present), condition of the cervix, and any disproportion. X-ray pelvimetry may be ordered to rule out fetopelvic disproportion or abnormal presentation or position. If the cause of the dysfunction is mechanical and a marked disproportion exists, a cesarean section may be performed.

Explanations and reassurance are given to the client and her partner. Questions and verbalization of fears and concerns are encouraged. Comfort measures (see Chapter 16) are provided by nursing personnel.

If mechanical factors are not the cause of the dysfunction, measures to increase the effectiveness of the uterine contraction pattern are implemented. Maternal hydration status is assessed. If dehydration occurs, rehydration will help to increase the effectiveness of uterine contractions.

The bladder is assessed for distention

that may impede uterine contraction effectiveness and labor progress. Emptying of the distended bladder can aid in cervical dilation and descent of the presenting part. An enema may be ordered to enhance uterine contractions and to prevent mechanical obstruction to descent of the presenting part.

A change in maternal position will aid in increasing uterine contraction effectiveness. A side-lying position is recommended if she is to remain in bed. In this position, uterine contractions are better coordinated and more intense, although they may be less frequent. A position of comfort should be found for the client. If she is allowed out of bed, sitting in a chair or walking may aid in increasing uterine contraction effectiveness (see Table 26–14).

Medical interventions include amniotomy and oxytocin infusion. *Amniotomy* (artificial rupture of the membranes) is performed by the physician to stimulate uterine contractions. The fluid is assessed for color, odor, and amount. Fetal heart tones are continuously monitored for signs of fetal distress. Uterine contractions and progress in cervical dilation are assessed.

For optimal results in labor, a frequency of 22 uterine contractions per hour with an amplitude of 50 to 60 mm Hg intrauterine pressure during contractions is necessary. If needed, an oxytocin infusion for uterine contraction stimulation is begun at 1 mU per minute and the rate increased every 15 to 20 minutes until uterine contractions are 2 to 3 minutes apart, lasting 40 to 60 seconds, and are of good intensity. Oxytocin stimulation is always given piggyback with regulation of the flow rate via an infusion pump. External or internal fetal heart rate and uterine contraction monitoring with a fetal monitor is essential.

In the majority of clients, normal cervical dilation will take place with a normal vaginal delivery as the outcome. If no cervical progress is made, if the gravida's physiologic status becomes unstable, or if fetal distress occurs, a cesarean section is performed.

BANDL'S RING

During normal labor, a physiologic retraction ring forms between the upper and lower uterine segments. In some labors, a specific portion of the myometrium may go into spontaneous spasm as a result of intrauterine manipulations or oxytocin administration and form a pathologic retraction ring. This pathologic retraction ring grips the fetus tightly and prevents fetal descent, causing obstructed labor progress. When fetal obstruction occurs first, followed by a pathologic ring, a condition known as *Bandl's ring* is present. Table 26–15 summarizes the differences between a constriction ring and Bandl's ring.

CERVICAL DYSTOCIA

Cervical dystocia may be primary or secondary. Causes of *primary cervical dystocia* include achalasia of the cervix (inability of a normal cervix to relax and dilate), rigid cervix (abnormal cervical tissue), and conglutination of the external os (sticking together of the external cervical os). *Secondary cervical dystocia* may result from postdelivery scarring, postoperative scarring, and cancer.

If the dystocia is not corrected, the cervix may rupture or detach from the uterus. If the cervix detaches owing to the constant and prolonged pressure during labor, the tissue will come away from the uterus as a ring. The vessels at the site of separation quickly thrombose, so bleeding is not a problem. Management of cervical dystocia may be by manual dilation of the cervix, incisions into the cervix, or cesarean section.

TABLE 26–14
SAMPLE NURSING CARE PLAN: HYPOTONIC UTERINE DYSFUNCTION

Alice, a gravida 4 para 3 at term was admitted at 3:00 pm to the labor room in active labor. Initial nursing assessment was done.

Data Base:

30 years old
Gravida 4, para 3
40 weeks gestation
Prenatal course unremarkable
22 lb weight gain during pregnancy
No known medical problems
On no medications, except prenatal vitamins and iron supplement
Allergic to penicillin, terramycin
O positive
Breastfeeding
Maternal vital signs: Temperature 98.2°F
Pulse 88
Respirations 20
B/P 126/74

Vaginal examination: 4 cm cervical dilation
presenting part cephalic
0 station
Cervix 60% effaced
External fetal monitor applied according to policy and procedure
Uterine contractions: q 4 minutes, lasting 45 seconds, moderate intensity
Labor status at 8:30 pm: VE 5 cm cervical dilation, 0 station
FHR tracing within normal limits
Contractions q 7 minutes, lasting 30 seconds, mild intensity

Nursing Diagnosis	Goals	Nursing Interventions	Rationale	Evaluation
Alteration in the process of labor related to ineffectual uterine contractions	The client will deliver without maternal or fetal problems	Identify dysfunctional labor pattern: Monitor contractions Monitor FHR Assess client behavior Assess cervical progress Use labor graph to plot progress Notify physician of labor pattern Assist with diagnostics to rule out mechanical factors for dysfunction Vaginal examination Ultrasound Pelvimetry	Prolonged labors increase perinatal morbidity & mortality as well as increase maternal complications Hypotonic uterine dysfunction is characterized by: contractions decreasing in frequency duration and intensity Diagnostics done to rule out other causes of dystocia	Uterine contractions becoming more irregular, and less intense FHR remained within normal limits Alice is becoming tired and fatigued with increased irritability noted VE: no progress noted

		Assess hydration status Intake and output Skin turgor Ketonuria		Intake and output assessed Skin turgor good
		Assist with oxytocin infusion (see Table 26–31) Monitor labor status and progress Monitor FHR Monitor contraction pattern Monitor maternal vital signs	Oxytocin is given according to policy and procedure Assess carefully for side effects Assess fetal response to oxytocin infusion	Maintained left lateral position during labor Oxytocin infusion of 1 ml oxytocin added to 1000 ml D_5W started per IVAC infusion pump via piggyback at 1 gtt/min. Infusion rate increased at 15 minute intervals to 4 gtt/min. Uterine contractions q 3 minutes, lasting 50 seconds, good intensity FHR remained within normal limits Maternal vitals stable Spontaneous delivery of live male over intact perineum at 10:22 pm Apgars 8 and 9
Knowledge deficit related to lack of progress in labor secondary to hypotonic uterine contraction pattern	The client and support person will verbalize understanding of abnormal uterine contraction patterns, treatment prescribed and expected labor outcome The client will cope with the stress of labor	Offer explanations at an appropriate level of understanding Stay with client Support and encouragement Assist with relaxation and breathing techniques	Explanations to the client and support person will decrease anxiety and promote cooperation	Explanations given to client and husband Verbalized acceptance of treatment with oxytocin infusion Used breathing and relaxation techniques without difficulty throughout rest of labor

TABLE 26-15
DIFFERENTIATION BETWEEN CONSTRICTION RING AND BANDL'S RING

Constriction Ring	Bandl's Ring
Local ring of hypertonic myometrium	Formed by excessive upper segment retraction
May occur in any part of the uterus	Forms at the junction of upper and lower segments
No uterine thinness or distention below the ring	Uterus below the ring is thin, overdistended
Uterine rupture will not usually occur	Uterus ruptures if ring is uncorrected
Uterus above the ring is relaxed	Uterus above the ring is tense
May occur in any stage of labor	Occurs in the second stage of labor
Position of the ring does not change	Ring will gradually rise in abdomen
Presenting part does not descend	Presenting part becomes jammed in the maternal pelvis
Maternal physiologic status is stable	Maternal physiologic status is not stable
Inefficient uterine action	Uterine action is efficient
Results in obstructed labor	Ring is caused by an obstruction

Abnormal Presentations and Positions

Certain factors cause the fetus to present other than in cephalic presentation or occiput anterior position (see Table 26-16). When malpresentations and malpositions occur, the labor process, the mother, and the fetus are all affected.

TABLE 26-16
FACTORS THAT CONTRIBUTE TO ABNORMAL PRESENTATION AND POSITION

MATERNAL AND UTERINE FACTORS
Contracted pelvis
Pendulous maternal abdomen
Neoplasms
Uterine anomalies
Placental anomalies
History of bony pelvis trauma
FETAL FACTORS
Large fetus
Error in fetal polarity
Abnormal internal rotation
Abnormal fetal attitude
Multiple pregnancy
Fetal anomalies
Polyhydramnios

LABOR EFFECTS

The efficiency of labor is reduced when the presenting part does not enter the pelvis symmetrically. The incidence of fetopelvic disproportion increases and the cervix may dilate slowly and incompletely, the fetal presenting part may fail to descend normally, and labor may be prolonged. Pathologic retraction rings are more common. Premature rupture of the membranes occurs more frequently, and the number of operative deliveries increases.

MATERNAL EFFECTS

Maternal exhaustion occurs with prolonged labor. More stretching of the maternal soft parts and perineum takes place, increasing the incidence of lacerations. Bleeding is increased, both from the lacerations and from uterine atony. Maternal infections are more common, because of premature rupture of the membranes, excessive blood loss, tissue damage, and the increased number of vaginal examinations needed during a lengthy labor. Coping mechanisms of the mother are decreased, and she may complain of increasing discomfort.

FETAL EFFECTS

Excessive molding of the presenting part takes place owing to the imperfect fit into the maternal pelvis. Prolonged labor increases the incidence of anoxia, asphyxia, fetal distress, and intrauterine death. The increased incidence of operative delivery increases the danger of trauma during delivery. Prolapse of the umbilical cord is more common in abnormal position and presentations.

Transverse Arrest

Transverse arrest refers to the arrest of the fetal head in the transverse position, usually in the maternal midpelvis. It is usually caused by uterine inertia or anteroposterior flattening of the maternal pelvis.

The fetal head enters the maternal pelvis at the onset of labor in a transverse position with the sagittal suture lying transversely across the maternal pelvis. In the normal pelvis, anterior rotation of the head will occur and the fetus will deliver with the head in an occiput anterior position.

If the maternal pelvis has a flattened anteroposterior diameter in the midpelvis, the head will tend to travel through the midpelvis in a transverse position. If uterine inertia is present, progress of rotation and descent may stop with the fetal head in the transverse position.

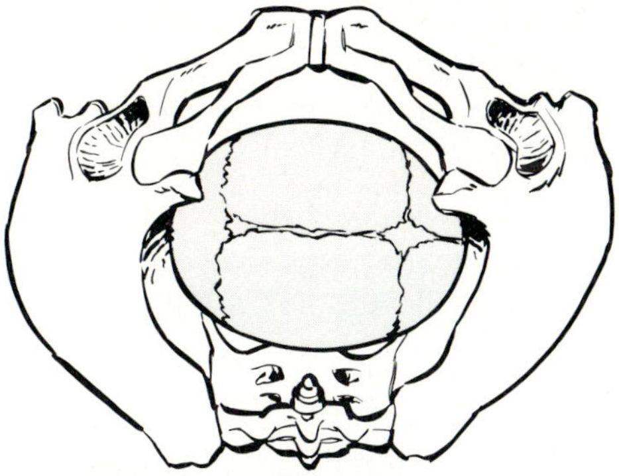

FIGURE 26-7. Transverse arrest of fetal head, vaginal view.

MEDICAL AND NURSING INTERVENTIONS

If the fetal head is in the transverse position, the fetal heart rate is heard loudest in the left lower (LOT) or right lower (ROT) quadrant of the maternal abdomen (see Fig. 26-7). Leopold's maneuvers will reveal the following assessments: (1) vertical lie; (2) the fetal head is at or in the maternal pelvis; (3) the fetal back is felt on the client's left and toward the side (LOT) or on the client's right and toward the side (ROT); (4) fetal small parts are on the right (LOT) or left (ROT); (5) the breech is felt in the uterine fundus; (6) the cephalic prominence can be felt on the right (LOT) or on the left (ROT).

Vaginal examination by the nurse or the physician will yield the following information: (1) the sagittal suture is in the transverse diameter, usually midway between the symphysis pubis and the sacral promontory; (2) the posterior fontanel is toward the client's left at 3 o'clock (LOT) or on the client's right at 9 o'clock (ROT); (3) the bregma is on the right at 9 o'clock (LOT) or on the left at 3 o'clock (ROT).

Maternal position changes can be of some benefit in helping the fetal head to rotate, but medical intervention is usually needed. If the pelvis is normal and the transverse arrest is caused by uterine inertia, oxytocin infusion to augment uterine contractions will often be followed by further descent and anterior rotation with spontaneous or low forceps delivery. If the transverse arrest is caused by a narrowed anteroposterior pelvic diameter, a midforceps rotation and delivery may be performed by the physician. Continuous assessment of maternal vital signs, fetal status, and uterine contractions is essential. The client and her partner need explanations and emotional support.

Occiput Posterior Positions

In an *occiput posterior position,* the occiput and posterior fontanel are in the rear segment of the maternal pelvis.

Occiput posterior positions occur in 15 to 30 percent of all labors. The majority of these rotate anteriorly with no difficulty. They are found more frequently in the android and anthropoid types of pelvis.

MEDICAL AND NURSING INTERVENTIONS

With an occiput posterior position, the fetal heart tones are heard in the right maternal flank (ROP) or left maternal flank (LOP) and may be indistinct owing to the transmission of the heart tones through the fetal scapula.

Assessment of the maternal abdomen will reveal: (1) the lie is vertical with the long axis of the fetus parallel to the long axis of the mother; (2) the fetal head is at or in the maternal pelvis; (3) the fetal back is in the right maternal flank (ROP) or left maternal flank (LOP) and cannot be clearly outlined; (4) fetal small parts can be readily felt on the client's left side (ROP) or right side (LOP); (5) breech is in the uterine fundus; (6) cephalic prominence is on the left (ROP) or right (LOP), but is difficult to feel (see Fig. 26-8).

Vaginal examination will reveal the sagittal suture in the right oblique diameter (ROP) or left oblique diameter (LOP), the posterior fontanel in the right posterior segment of the pelvis (ROP) or left posterior segment of the pelvis (LOP), and the bregma is anterior.

During labor the fetal head can do one of three things: (1) rotate anteriorly, either by long arc rotation of 135 degrees to an OA position, by rotation 90 degrees to an ROA or LOA position, or rotate 45 degrees to an ROT or LOT position; (2) not rotate and remain ROP or LOP; or (3) rotate posteriorly to OP. Spontaneous delivery usually occurs after anterior rotation to OA or posterior rotation to OP.

An arrest in the mechanism of labor may occur high in the maternal pelvis, in the midpelvis (transverse arrest, ROP arrest, LOP arrest, or OP arrest), or at the outlet.

When the occiput posterior position is persistent, the fetal head is shortened in the occipitofrontal diameter and lengthened in the suboccipitobregmatic and mentobregmatic diameters. The resultant caput succedaneum is over the bregma.

Nursing interventions during labor are essentially the same as in an occiput anterior position, with special attention given to fetal monitoring, uterine contraction monitoring, analgesic use, hydration, and comfort measures. Backache is a frequent and persistent accompaniment of occiput posterior positions. Sacral pressure, back rubs, and frequent changes of position may help (see Table 26-17).

When the head is delivered in the posterior position, perineal lacerations are more common. A large episiotomy is usually needed (either RMLE or LMLE) to prevent maternal lacerations.

If there is no progress in the second stage of labor for one hour in the multipara and two hours in the primigravida, operative delivery is considered. The fetal head is rotated to a more favorable position for delivery, either manually by the Pomeroy maneuver or with forceps by the Scanzoni maneuver (a double ap-

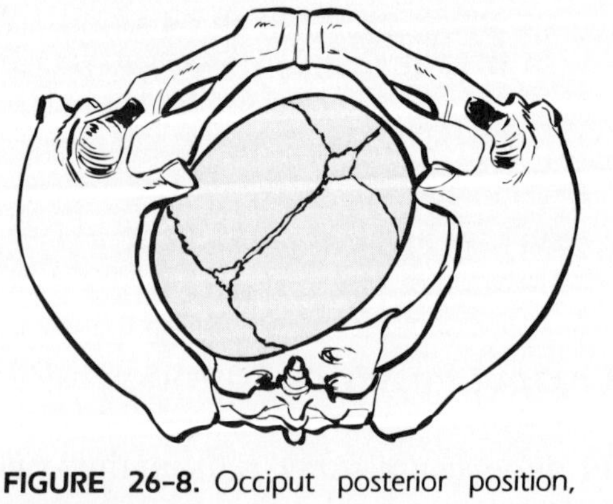

FIGURE 26-8. Occiput posterior position, vaginal view.

plication of forceps: the first application is to rotate the head and the second application is to extract the head) or the Maughan maneuver (one blade is used to rotate the head to transverse; then the other blade is applied to complete the rotation and extraction). When manual or forceps rotations fail, a cesarean delivery may be performed.

Face Presentation

With full extension of the fetal head, the face of the fetus may become the presenting part during labor. In a face presentation, the chin (mentum) is the denominator and the presenting diameter is the suboccipitobregmatic (9.5 cm). The part of the face that presents is the area between the glabella (directly above the root of the nose) and the chin.

The incidence of face presentation varies from once in every 500 to 600 deliveries (Duff, 1981), to once in every 1250 deliveries (Benedetti et al., 1979) and is higher in multiparas. About 70 percent are anterior or transverse, while 30 percent are posterior.

Anything that prevents or delays engagement of the fetal head in flexion can contribute to extension. Causative factors include prematurity, anencephaly, grand multiparity, uterine tumors, cephalopelvic disproportion, placenta previa, premature rupture of the membranes, fetal neck masses, and multiple gestations.

MEDICAL AND NURSING INTERVENTIONS

The fetal heart rate is heard best in the lower quadrant of the maternal abdomen on the same side as the fetal small parts (see Figs. 26-9, 26-10, 26-11).

Abdominal assessment will reveal a vertical lie with the head at the maternal pelvis. The fetal back will be felt on the

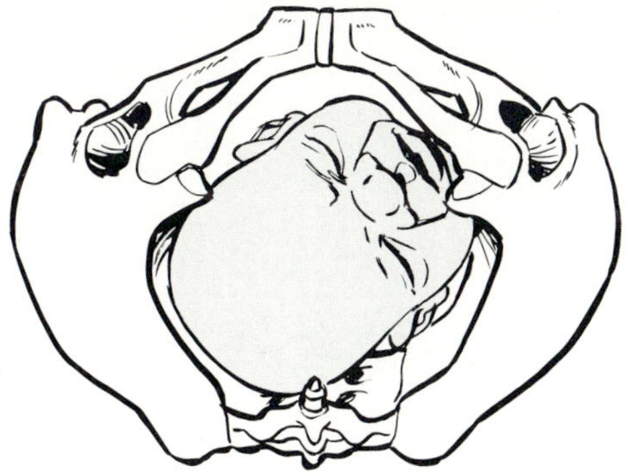

FIGURE 26-9. Face presentation, vaginal view. LMA.

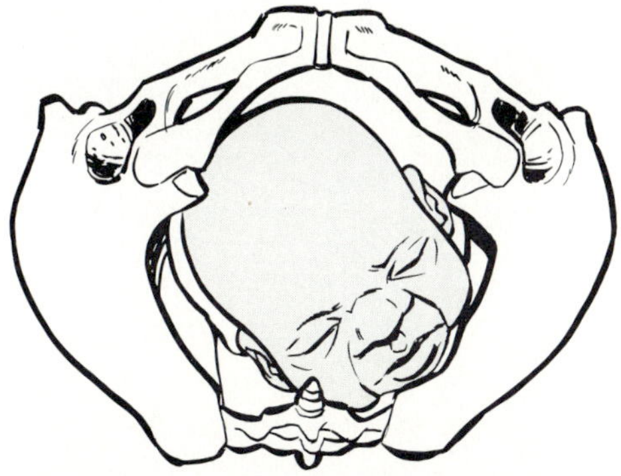

FIGURE 26-10. Face presentation, vaginal view. RMP.

right side of the abdomen (LMA) or on the left side of the abdomen (RMA). The fetal back will be anterior and to the right (LMP) or anterior and to the left (RMP). Fetal small parts may be left and anterior (LMA), right and anterior (RMA), left and posterior (LMP), or right and posterior (RMP). The breech is in the fundus. The cephalic prominence is on the same side as the fetal back.

Vaginal examination will reveal a soft and irregular presenting part and will allow identification of various parts of the face. The long axis of the face is in the oblique diameter of the maternal pelvis. The chin is felt in the left anterior quadrant (LMA), right anterior quadrant (RMA), left posterior quadrant (LMP), or

TABLE 26-17
SAMPLE NURSING CARE PLAN: PERSISTENT OCCIPUT POSTERIOR

Tammy, a gravida 2 para 1 at term gestation was admitted at 6 pm to the labor room in active labor. An initial nursing assessment was done.

Data Base:

Gravida 2 para 1
Age 27
40 weeks gestation
Normal prenatal course
A positive
Allergic to sulfa
No medical problems
On no medications, except prenatal vitamins
Vital signs: 98.2°F, 92, 24 B/P 125/73

Spontaneous rupture of the membranes at 5:00 pm—fluid clear
Uterine contractions started at noon: 5 minutes apart lasting 40 to 50 seconds, moderate intensity
c/o "back labor"
Vaginal examination: Cervix 5 cm dilated
Presenting part cephalic at 0 station
80% effacement of cervix noted
FHT 148. External fetal monitor applied according to policy and procedure

Nursing Diagnosis	Goals	Nursing Interventions	Rationale	Evaluation
Alteration in comfort: pain related to back labor secondary to occiput posterior position	The client delivers without maternal or fetal trauma or complications	Assessment of: Client perception of uterine contractions Fetal presentation Fetal position Cervical dilation Station Maternal vital signs FHR- Leopold's maneuvers	About 10% of deliveries are occiput posterior. These are associated with prolonged labor. Leopold's maneuvers done to aid in determining fetal position FHT may be difficult to hear due to posterior position	Uterine contractions felt in back Presentation cephalic Position ROP VE 5 cm at 0 station Vital signs within normal limits External fetal heart rate tracing in normal limits Leopold's maneuvers: Vertical lie Head in maternal pelvis Fetal back felt on maternal right side Fetal small parts felt on maternal left side Breech in fundus Cephalic prominence felt on left

		Maintain maternal hydration: IV at prescribed rate Intake and output	Maternal exhaustion more common with long labor. OP positions are associated with maternal discomfort	Intake and output noted IV infusing at 8 hour rate
		Promote maternal comfort: Backrub Counterpressure Change position Analgesia		
		Assist in maintaining breathing and relaxation techniques Monitor maternal vitals Monitor FHR and contraction status Monitor labor progress		Using breathing techniques without problem Vital signs stable FHR remained normal 8 pm—VE 6–7 cm at 0 station 10:15 pm—VE 8–9 cm at 0 to +1 station 11:30 pm—VE complete To delivery room Instructed to push with contractions 12:30 am—Fetal head still ROP. Descent minimal. Change of position to no avail. Manual rotation of head by Dr. T. not effective. Midforceps rotation done under saddle block anesthesia Live female delivered at 1:01 am over LML Apgars 8 and 9
Knowledge deficit related to lack of progress in labor with good uterine contractions	The client and support person will verbalize understanding of cause and interventions	Explain lack of labor progress Stay with client and encourage use of breathing and relaxation techniques Answer questions honestly	Maternal exhaustion is more common. Decreased coping is seen with maternal fatigue Knowledge will allay apprehension and promote relaxation and compliance with proposed interventions	Reasons for back labor explained. Verbalized understanding Breathing techniques used

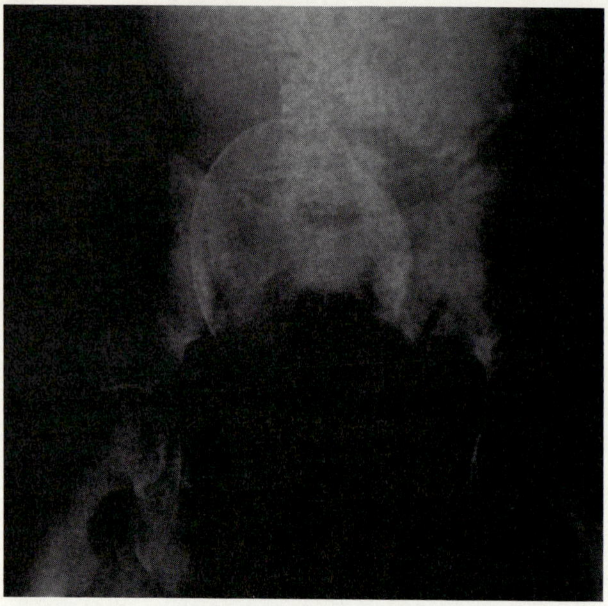

FIGURE 26-11. Pelvimetry report showing a single fetus which appears to be in facial presentation. Prominent hyperextension of the fetal neck is evident.

right posterior quadrant (RMP). Vaginal examinations must be handled gently to avoid injury to the face, especially to the eyes. A flat plate of the abdomen is measured to confirm the position. If the maternal pelvis is normal, anterior face positions are usually allowed to proceed in labor and will often deliver vaginally.

Labor is longer than with occiput anterior presentations because the face is a poor dilator. The face will be badly swollen, bruised, and misshapen at the time of birth. The neonate needs special assessment for laryngeal edema. When the position is mentum posterior, cesarean delivery is usually indicated because the posterior position cannot descend through the maternal pelvic curve for vaginal delivery.

Brow Presentation

When the fetal head is partially extended, the brow may present, with the presenting part the area between the bregma and the orbital ridges. The denominator is the forehead (Fr). The presenting diameter is the verticomental (13.5 cm), which is the longest anteroposterior diameter of the fetal head.

Incidence of brow presentation is from 1 in 1000 deliveries to 1 in 3000 deliveries. The position is often temporary and may convert to an occiput or face position during labor.

Causes include anything that will interfere with engagement of the fetal head in flexion. Cephalopelvic disproportion is the most frequent cause.

MEDICAL AND NURSING INTERVENTIONS

The fetal heart rate is heard best in the left lower (LFrA) or right lower (RFrA) quadrant of the maternal abdomen. Leopold's maneuvers will reveal the following: (1) the fetal head is at the pelvis but is usually not engaged (see Fig. 26-12); (2) the fetal back may be difficult to palpate since it is posterior; (3) fetal small parts are on the opposite side from the back and are anterior; (4) breech is in the fundus; and (5) the cephalic prominence and the back are on the same side.

When the vaginal examination is conducted, the following are noted: (1) the anteroposterior diameter of the head will be felt in the oblique diameter of the

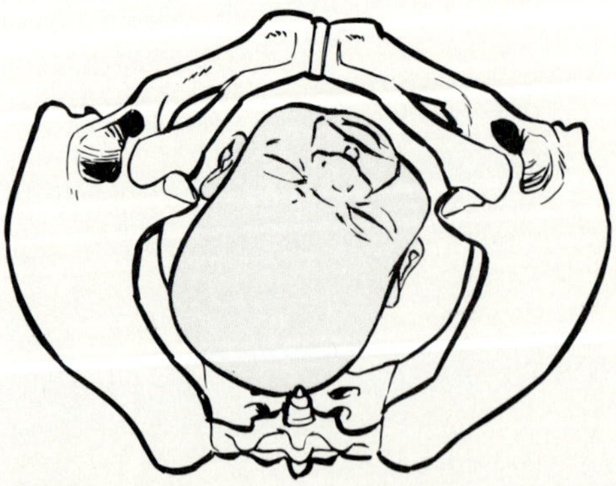

FIGURE 26-12. Brow presentation, vaginal view.

maternal pelvis; (2) the brow presents and can be palpated in the left anterior (LFrA) or right anterior (RFrA) quadrant of the maternal pelvis; (3) the bregma can be palpated easily; (4) the frontal suture can be felt, but the sagittal suture cannot be reached; (5) the supraorbital eye ridges can be felt and will aid in diagnosis.

Unless the fetal head is very small, spontaneous delivery is not possible if the head remains in a brow position. The head may convert spontaneously to a face presentation with further extension, or to an occiput presentation with further flexion.

A cesarean delivery is usually performed if the brow presentation persists, since labor is long and traumatic to the mother. Perineal lacerations are more frequent, owing to the large fetal head diameter that presents at the pelvic outlet. When labor is allowed to progress, excessive molding of the fetal head occurs, causing brain damage and increasing fetal mortality.

Military Attitude

In a *military attitude,* there is neither flexion or extension of the fetal head. The occiput and brow are at the same level in the maternal pelvis. The presenting part is vertex, and the occiput is the denominator.

MEDICAL AND NURSING INTERVENTIONS

Fetal heart tones are heard on the same side as the fetal back (see Fig. 26-13). Abdominal examination reveals: (1) the head is at the pelvic inlet; (2) the back is on one side and the small parts are on the opposite side; (3) the breech is felt in the uterine fundus; (4) there is no marked cephalic prominence on one side or the other, since there is no flexion or extension. On vaginal examination, the sagittal suture is felt in the transverse pelvic diameter. The two fontanels are easy to identify and are at the same level in the maternal pelvis. X-ray pelvimetry can diagnose fetal position and assess the maternal pelvis. Labor is usually longer with median vertex presentations. The majority of the heads will flex and deliver normally.

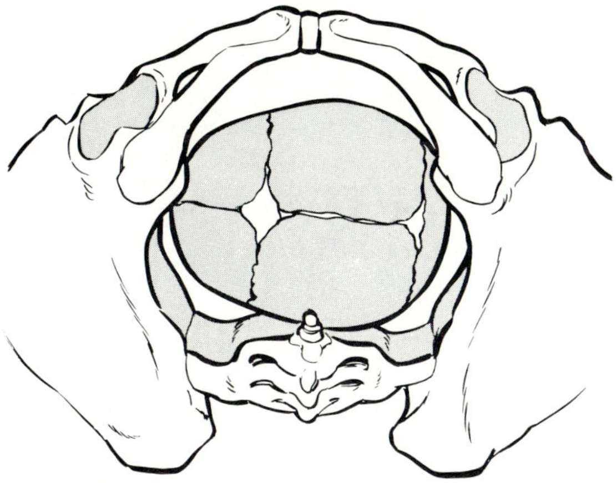

FIGURE 26-13. Military attitude, median vertex presentation.

Breech Presentations

Breech presentation is a longitudinal lie with the breech the presenting part. The fetal pelvis is the leading pole and the denominator is the sacrum. Breech presentations occur in 3 to 4 percent of all deliveries.

ETIOLOGY

Etiologic factors include prematurity, placenta previa, hydrocephalus, grand multiparity, multiple pregnancies, polyhydramnios, congenital uterine anomalies, and tumors of the uterus. Anything that interferes with engagement of the fetal head predisposes to breech presentations. The shape of the uterine cavity that results from placental implantation may in-

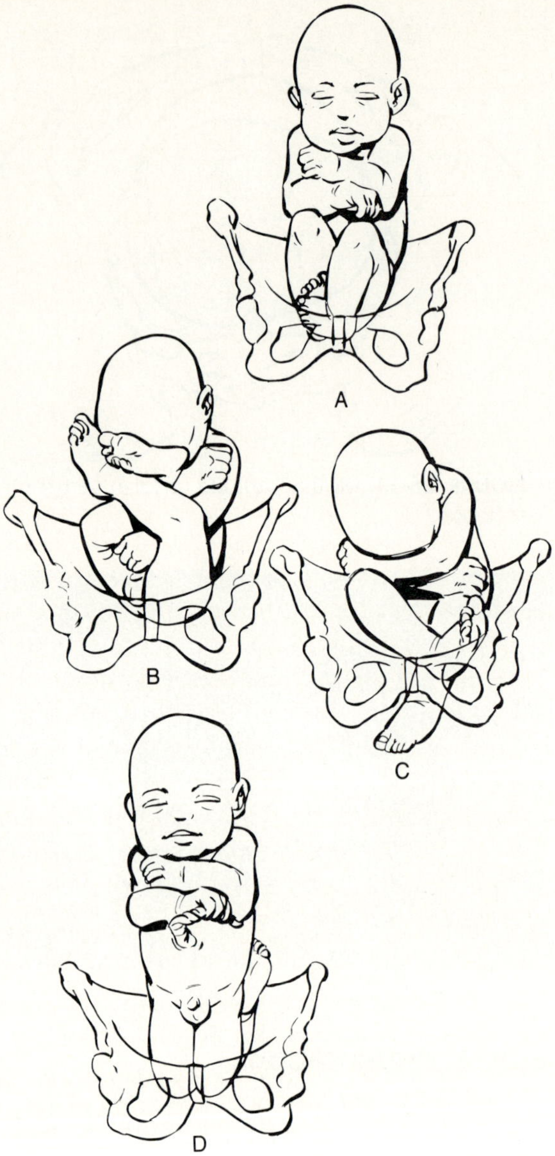

FIGURE 26-14. Types of breech presentations: A. Complete breech. B. Frank breech. C. Footling breech. D. Kneeling breech.

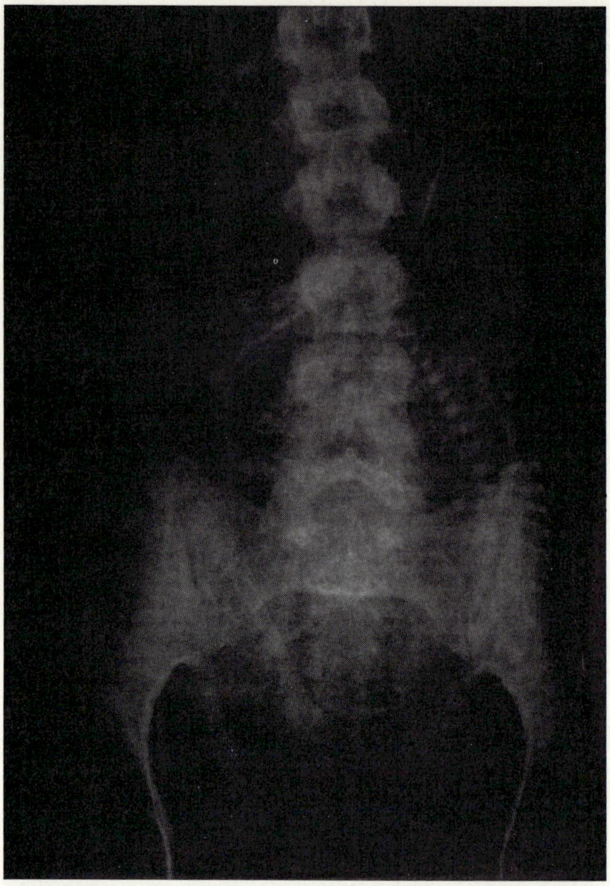

FIGURE 26-15. Abdominal x-ray showing a single floating term fetus in footling breech presentation with the spine directed toward the patient's left.

fluence the occurrence of breech presentations.

There are four types of breech presentations (see Fig. 26-14). The breech may be *complete,* with flexion at the thighs and knees. A *frank* breech has extension at the knees. With a *footling* breech, there is extension at the knees and thighs, with one or both feet the presenting part (see Fig. 26-15). In a *kneeling* breech there is extension at the thighs and flexion at the knees, with one or both knees the presenting part.

MEDICAL AND NURSING INTERVENTIONS

Fetal heart tones are heard loudest at or above the umbilicus on the same side as the back. Leopold's maneuvers usually reveal the following: (1) the fetal head is felt in the uterine fundus; (2) the breech is felt in the maternal pelvis; (3) no cephalic prominence is felt; and (4) fetal small parts can be felt away from the midline. When a vaginal examination is conducted, the presenting part is soft and irregular in a complete breech, the feet and buttocks can be felt in a frank breech presentation, one or both feet can be palpated in a footling breech, or one or both knees may be felt in kneeling breech. A flat plate is done to confirm the presentation. X-ray pelvimetry may be ordered to determine the adequacy of the maternal pelvis and to identify the exact attitude of the fetus and the presence or absence of anomalies.

MATERNAL DANGERS

There is an increased incidence of sepsis, birth canal lacerations, uterine rupture, episiotomy extensions, cesarean deliveries, postpartum hemorrhage, and postpartum infections.

FETAL DANGERS

Breech neonates that are delivered vaginally have three to five times the perinatal mortality than neonates who are delivered in cephalic presentations. Twenty five percent of all breeches are low birth weight. Approximately 6 percent of breech neonates have congenital anomalies.

Injury to the brain and skull occur twice as often as in cephalic presentations. The aftercoming head passes through the pelvis, with excessive compression and decompression taking place. Brain ligaments are stretched suddenly, increasing the risk of intracranial hemorrhage.

Asphyxia occurs more frequently as a result of compression of the umbilical cord between the maternal pelvis and the aftercoming head. Actual cord prolapse is more frequent in frank, footling, and kneeling breech presentations. Aspiration of amniotic fluid and vaginal secretions may occur if the fetus breathes before the head is completely delivered.

The incidence of trauma during vaginal delivery is 12 times higher than in cephalic presentations. Fractures of the humerus, clavicle, and femur may occur, as well as cervical and brachial plexus paralysis. The liver and other abdominal organs may be traumatized if the fetus is not grasped by the hips during delivery of the body.

MANAGEMENT IN THE THIRD TRIMESTER

External Version

Some authorities feel that external version should be attempted at about 32 to 34 weeks gestation with a documented breech presentation. If the obstetrician attempts external version, the procedure is conducted with ultrasound guidance and with no excessive force to avoid abruptio placentae or fetal harm. The fetal loss associated with external version is about the same as with vaginal breech delivery. Therefore, it is generally felt that external version should be avoided, although it is currently being used with success in some perinatal centers.

X-Ray Pelvimetry

X-ray pelvimetry is sometimes indicated in the third trimester for primigravidas and for multiparas with a poor obstetrical history. If the pelvis is small or borderline, an elective cesarean delivery is scheduled. If the pelvis is adequate, a trial of labor is the procedure of choice. Cephalopelvic disproportion is often difficult to assess, owing to x-ray distortion of the fetal head.

METHOD OF DELIVERY

At the onset of labor, a tentative decision is made by the obstetrician as to whether vaginal delivery is feasible or a cesarean delivery is the method of choice. Various protocols have been designed to identify and assess the term breech for possible vaginal delivery. With these protocols, various factors are taken into account: fetal size, type of breech, shape and size of maternal pelvis, position of the fetal head, biparietal diameter of the fetal head, the possible ease of delivery of the fetal shoulders and head, fetal descent during labor, and results of electronic fetal monitoring.

Regardless of the protocol used to determine the safety of vaginal delivery, the final decision is made by the physician. This decision must be made separately for each pregnant woman as she approaches term or goes into labor.

The position of the fetal legs will influence the course and outcome of labor. In a frank breech presentation, the body is splinted by the legs under the chin and may prohibit lateral flexion. Dysfunctional labor is more common in complete breech. The footling breech presents the greatest risk of umbilical cord prolapse.

MEDICAL AND NURSING INTERVENTIONS

Upon admission to the labor room, a complete assessment is conducted, including a review of the prenatal record. The following data should be carefully assessed and recorded: fetal heart tones, location of FHT, gestational age, estimated fetal weight, cervical effacement, type of presentation, station of the presenting part, status of the membranes, and uterine contractions.

Continuous fetal heart rate and uterine contraction monitoring is essential to detect changes that indicate fetal hypoxia. Labor care is as described in Chapter 16. Explanations need to be given that are appropriate to the stage of labor.

A flat plate is obtained to confirm the type of breech, detect flexion or extension of the fetal head, and detect significant congenital malformations that may interfere with normal labor progress.

Vaginal delivery is usually indicated if estimated fetal weight is between 6 and 7 pounds, gestational age is over 36 weeks, the maternal pelvis is adequate, FHR is within the normal range, there is progressive cervical dilation and progressive fetal descent, and adequate anesthesia is available. Vaginal delivery may be spontaneous, assisted, or by extraction. Anesthesia must be available for manipulations that may be needed during delivery. With an assisted breech, once the fetal body is born, a warm dry towel is wrapped around the body to reduce the stimulation of cold air and make it easier to hold the fetal body. Suprapubic pressure will aid in delivery of the fetal head. The hips and bony pelvis are grasped to avoid injury to intra-abdominal organs. An adequate episiotomy is needed and should be performed before the breech crowns.

If there is delay in delivering the fetal head, several measures may be used by the obstetrician to facilitate delivery. In the Wingand-Martin maneuver, the body of the fetus is placed on the arm of the physician, the middle finger of the hand of that arm is placed in the fetal mouth to maintain flexion of the head, and suprapubic pressure is exerted on the head through the maternal abdomen with the other hand. Piper forceps may be used on the aftercoming head to extract it. Breech extraction is the total extraction of the fetus by the obstetrician.

Gravidas in labor with a breech presentation are candidates for cesarean delivery if any of the following criteria are present: frank breech with estimated weight over 2500 gm, hyperextension of the fetal head, elderly primigravida, infertility, insulin-dependent diabetes mellitus, floating presenting part, inadequate pelvis by pelvimetry, or a poor obstetric history.

Transverse Lie

When the long axis of the fetus is at right angles to the long axis of the mother, a transverse lie is present. Frequently, the shoulder is at the brim of the maternal pelvic inlet, giving the transverse lie the name shoulder

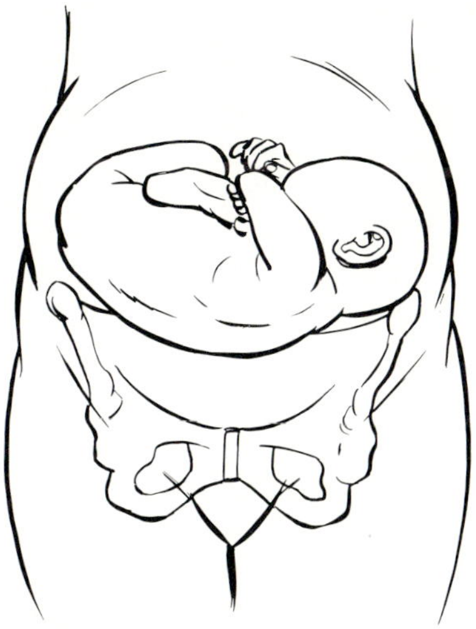

FIGURE 26-16. Transverse lie.

presentation. The fetus may lie directly across the maternal abdomen (see Fig. 26-16) or it may lie obliquely. The denominator is the scapula (Sc).

The incidence of transverse lie is approximately 1 in 500 deliveries. Anything that prevents engagement of either the head or the breech in the maternal pelvis can predispose to a transverse lie. Transverse lie is more common in grand multiparas, the preterm fetus, placenta previa, uterine tumors in the lower uterine segment, contracted maternal pelvis, fetal anomalies, and polyhydramnios.

MEDICAL AND NURSING INTERVENTIONS

The fetal heart rate is best heard below the umbilicus. Abdominal assessment will reveal an asymmetrical abdomen with the long axis of the fetus at a right angle to the long axis of the mother; the uterine fundus lower than expected for the length of gestation; the uterus appears excessively wide; neither fetal pole can be felt in the uterine fundus; the fetal head can be felt in one maternal flank; and the breech in the other flank. When a vaginal examination is done, nothing can be palpated. The bag of waters may extend into the vagina. A flat plate of the maternal abdomen will confirm the diagnosis.

A persistent transverse lie cannot deliver spontaneously. If the membranes rupture, the umbilical cord or arm may prolapse. Internal version may be attempted if complete cervical dilatation has occurred, or on a second twin. A cesarean delivery is usually performed.

Compound Presentations

Compound presentations refer to the prolapse of one or more limbs alongside the head or breech as it enters the maternal pelvis. Occurrence is in approximately 1 of every 500 to 1000 deliveries. Spontaneous conversion frequently occurs. The head may present with one hand and arm (see Fig. 26-17), both hands and arms, one foot, two feet, or an arm and a leg together. The breech may present with a hand or arm prolapsed.

Causes include prematurity, a high presenting part with ruptured membranes, grand multiparity, contracted maternal pelvis, and twins. Diagnosis is made by vaginal examination.

MEDICAL AND NURSING INTERVENTIONS

Because the diameter of the presenting parts combined is larger than the diameter of a single presenting part, mechanical dystocia is more common. If no other complications are present (such as a prolapsed umbilical cord), the labor is allowed to progress. As the cervix completely dilates and the presenting part descends, the arm or leg may rise up out of the maternal pelvis. If there is fetopelvic disproportion caused by the compound presentation, a cesarean delivery is performed.

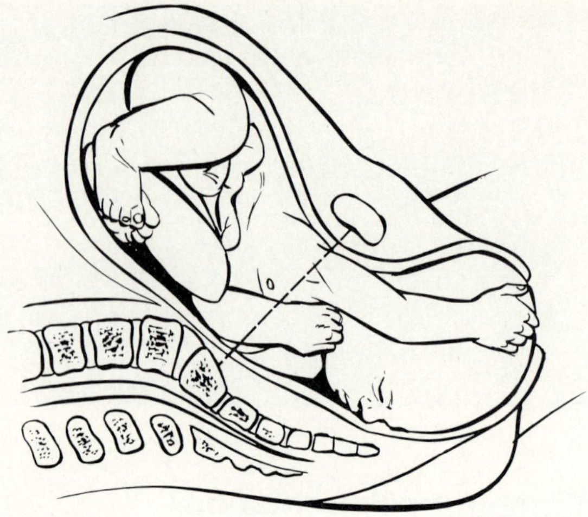

FIGURE 26-17. Compound presentation of head and hand.

Fetopelvic Disproportion

Dystocia may be caused by fetopelvic disproportion. Fetopelvic disproportion refers to the inability of the fetus to pass through the maternal pelvis. With a *relative disproportion,* factors that contribute to the dystocia can sometimes be overcome. In *absolute disproportion,* vaginal delivery is impossible. Problems may be related to the passenger or to the passage.

PASSENGER

Passenger problems include an oversized fetus, abnormal attitude or position of the fetus, moldability of the fetal head, fetal abdominal enlargement, and fetal abnormalities.

Oversized Fetus

The excessively large fetus is defined as one weighing 10 pounds (4545 gm) or more. The excessively large fetus is more common among older Caucasian multiparas and they tend to run in families. Maternal weight gain during pregnancy is often excessive. Mothers with diabetes mellitus and postmaturity are more prone to have oversized neonates. Two thirds of oversized neonates are male. The majority of oversized fetuses are cephalic presentations during labor. Total length of labor is usually not prolonged, but the second stage may last two hours or more. Other problems include:

Maternal problems—The mother is more prone to genital tract lacerations, ruptured uterus, postpartum hemorrhage, and separation of the symphysis pubis.

Fetal problems—Neonatal mortality is increased, and the incidence of injury is higher. Central nervous system problems include fractured skull and intracranial hemorrhage. Peripheral nerve damage including Erb's palsy and brachial plexus palsy may be the result of a traumatic delivery, as may humoral, femoral, and clavicle fractures.

Shoulder Dystocia

Shoulder dystocia is encountered in 2 to 6 per 1000 births and occurs most frequently in the oversized fetus. It results from impaction of the anterior shoulder behind the symphysis pubis and increases morbidity and mortality.

Causes of shoulder dystocia include a short umbilical cord, fetal abdominal enlargement, locked twins, and a uterine constriction ring. Diagnosis is made after the fetal head delivers. The head will recoil back against the maternal perineum and no restitution will take place.

The mother may have extensive vaginal and perineal lacerations following delivery. The fetus may become anoxic and suffer irreparable brain damage. With each uterine contraction large amounts of blood are transferred from the fetal trunk to the head. Venous return from the head is impaired by the angle of the neck. The fetus cannot compensate for the excessive intravascular pressure and anoxia develops accompanied by hemorrhage. If this condition is uncorrected, irreversible brain damage may develop.

Attitude and Position of the Fetus

Even in a borderline maternal pelvis, a fetus with a well-flexed head in an occiput anterior position may deliver normally. The fetus in a face presentation or persistent posterior position may not be able to deliver vaginally even in a normal adequate maternal pelvis.

Moldability

The ability of the fetal head to mold to fit in the maternal pelvis may influence labor. Excessive molding can cause brain damage to the fetus.

Fetal Abdominal Enlargement

The diagnosis of fetal abdominal enlargement is usually made during delivery, after the fetal head is delivered. Fetal mortality is high not only because of trauma to the fetus during delivery but also because the condition that caused the abdominal enlargement may be incompatible with extrauterine life. Generalized edema may occur in neonates of diabetic mothers and erythroblastotic neonates. Fetal ascites is associated with urinary tract anomalies.

Fetal Abnormalities

Congenital fetal abnormalities may cause dystocia. The anencephalic fetus is a poor dilating wedge during labor. The hydrocephalic fetus is associated with dystocia, owing to the large fetal head.

PASSAGE

Passage problems include maternal pelvic size, pelvic shape, congenital or acquired abnormalities of the pelvis, soft tissue abnormalities, and neoplasms.

Maternal Pelvic Size

In terms of dystocia, the important question is the relationship of a given fetus to a given pelvis. The maternal pelvis may be so small that no term fetus can pass through. Reduction in pelvic size may be at the inlet, midplane, outlet, or any combination of the three.

Contraction of the Pelvic Inlet

An inlet contraction is present when the anteroposterior diameter is 10 cm or less and the transverse diameter is 12 cm or less. Fetal effects of a contracted pelvic inlet include failure of engagement, malposition, extreme molding, large caput succedaneum formation, and prolapsed umbilical cord. Labor is often inefficient, with slow cervical dilation and premature rupture of the membranes.

Contraction of the Pelvic Midplane

Midplane contraction is present when the ischial spinous diameter is less than 9.5 cm. Contraction in the midpelvis is a frequent cause of dystocia. Anterior rotation of the occiput may be prevented with a midplane contraction. Extreme molding and caput succedaneum are more common.

Contraction of the Pelvic Outlet

An outlet contraction is present when the distance between the ischial tuberosities is less than 8.0 cm. If the sum of the intertuberous diameter and the posterior sagittal diameter is less than 15 cm, dystocia may result. There is a greater need for forceps deliveries and an increase in maternal perineal lacerations.

Pelvic Shape

The obstetric capacity of the female pelvis is governed by its size and shape. The four types of pelves are discussed in Chapter 13. The gynecoid pelvis offers the best diameters in all three planes for spontaneous vaginal delivery. Occiput posterior positions are common in the android or male-type pelvis, with reduced posterior segments in all three planes. The anthropoid or apelike pelvis has decreased transverse diameters and large anteroposterior diameters, and predisposes to occiput posterior positions at delivery. The platypelloid or flat pelvis has decreased outlet measurements. The highest incidence of cesarean delivery for fetopelvic disproportion is found in this pelvic type.

Many women have mixed types of pelves. A gynecoid pelvis may have an android narrowing at the outlet. Any combination of pelvis in any of the three planes is possible and may contribute to dystocia.

Abnormalities of the Pelvis

Dystocia is also caused by maternal pelves with abnormalities from birth or accident. Kyphosis may complicate delivery, especially when the abnormality is in the thoracic or lumbar region. Scoliosis of the lower spine may interfere with normal labor because of the abnormal curve of the spine.

Soft Tissue Abnormalities

When poor dilatability of the muscles and fascia of the pelvis is present, dystocia is more common, especially in the pelvis with borderline measurements.

Neoplasms

Uterine fibromyomas or ovarian tumors may block the birth canal and present fetal passage during labor.

MEDICAL AND NURSING INTERVENTIONS

When fetopelvic disproportion is suspected, a complete assessment including a history, abdominal palpation, vaginal examination, and x-ray studies is conducted to determine the feasibility of a trial of labor.

Trial of Labor

A trial of labor is a clinical attempt to evaluate fetopelvic disproportion. The gravida is allowed to go into labor under close supervision. The natural forces of labor may overcome a real or suspected disproportion.

The following factors are evaluated carefully during the trial of labor: (1) physiologic status of the mother; (2) psychological status of the mother; (3) fetal well-being; (4) uterine contractions; (5) progress in cervical dilation; (6) descent of the presenting part; (7) molding of the presenting part; and (8) the amount of caput succedaneum.

There are no absolute set time limits for trial of labor. It may last 6 hours or 16 hours. The trial of labor needs to be long enough to make an individual decision on the feasibility of vaginal delivery.

Nursing interventions are the same as in other labors, with an emphasis on psychological support. The anxiety level of the client and her partner will be increased owing to the possibility of cesarean delivery. Unnecessary vaginal or rectal examinations are avoided.

If there is favorable progress of cervical dilation, effacement, and descent of the presenting part with efficient uterine action, labor is usually allowed to continue. If no progress is made with efficient uterine action, a cesarean delivery is recommended.

Uterine Abnormalities

Prolapse of the uterus and uterine abnormalities may predispose to dystocia in the term gravida.

PROLAPSE OF THE UTERUS

In the majority of pregnancies the uterus rises in the abdomen as it enlarges. Occasionally the uterus will descend and protrude downward. Antepartum spontaneous abortions and preterm labor are more common. During labor, cervical dilation may begin outside the vagina. Edema of the cervix may cause cervical dystocia, and cervical lacerations are more frequent. The incidence of puerperal infections is increased. Most clients with a prolapsed uterus have normal vaginal deliveries, but cervical dystocia development could lead to the necessity of a cesarean delivery.

UTERINE ABNORMALITIES

Women with a bicornate uterus are more prone to spontaneous abortions, preterm labor, and premature rupture of the membranes. Breech or transverse lies occur more frequently.

Ineffectual slow labors are common with a double uterus, as is postpartum uterine atony. The cervix of the nonpregnant uterus may interfere with rotation and descent of the fetal presenting part during labor.

Sacculation of the uterus is a functional, transitory pouch that contains all layers of the myometrium. It may occur during pregnancy in the anterior or posterior uterine wall. When anterior sacculation is present, the presenting part can be felt in front of and above the symphysis pubis. Labor and delivery may progress normally or the presenting part may be in the sacculation itself, causing the cervix not to dilate but instead to displace upward as the sac is pushed downward. Posterior sacculation may be seen with a fundus of a retroverted uterus that remains in the pelvis. The anterior wall hypertrophies and the posterior wall forms a sac into which one fetal pole remains. The cervix is above the symphysis pubis and vaginal delivery is impossible.

THREATENED PRETERM LABOR

Preterm delivery accounts for 5 to 12 percent of all births but is associated with 75 to 80 percent of all neonatal deaths that are not caused by congenital malformations. The prevention of preterm labor and delivery is a major challenge to nursing and medicine.

Definition

Preterm labor is defined as labor that occurs between 26 and 37 weeks of pregnancy. Neonates that weight less than 2500 gm (5 pounds, 8 ounces) at birth are classified as low birth weight neonates. The terms premature labor (labor before 37 weeks gestation) and premature neonates (neonates that weight under 2500 gm) are seldom used today because neonatal weight and maturity are not necessarily related to each other or to the length of gestation.

Causes

Preterm labor occurs in a variety of circumstances and situations. Maternal, placental, or fetal factors may be implicated in the preterm labor and delivery. Any of these factors may be purely coincidental or may be found in a significant number of preterm labors. In about one-third of preterm labors, the precipitating factor is premature rupture of the membranes.

Factors that are known to correlate with preterm labor include maternal age, social class, height, weight, prior preterm labors or induced abortions, work situations, smoking, and interruptions in health that may occur in the antepartum period. Specific factors may be divided into low risk (see Table 26–18), medium risk (see Table 26–19), and high risk (see Table 26–20) categories.

Significance of the Problem of Preterm Birth

Preterm labor is one of the more common complications of the third trimester of pregnancy. Delivery of a preterm neonate is a clinical crisis that is often a threat to the life or health of the neonate. The outstanding causes of morbidity and mortality in preterm neonates are respiratory distress syndrome and intracranial hemorrhage. Low birth weight

TABLE 26-18
LOW-RISK FACTORS FOR PRETERM LABOR

Any three of the following factors together equals a high-risk factor

Maternal Factors
- Age: under 16 or over 40 years
- Anemia
- Bacteriuria
- Cholestasis of pregnancy
- Chronic renal disease
- Chronic cardiovascular disease
- Fibroid tumors
- Low socioeconomic factors
- Poor prenatal care
- Repeat first trimester abortions
- Single parent status
- Smoking
- Stature: under 5 feet tall
- Strenuous demanding work
- Weight: under 100 pounds prepregnancy weight

Fetal Factors
- Breech presentations after 30 weeks of gestation

TABLE 26-19
MEDIUM-RISK FACTORS FOR PRETERM LABOR

Any two of the following factors together equals a high-risk factor

Maternal Factors
- Age under 16 years
- Chemical abuse
- Cone biopsy
- Hyperthyroidism
- Narcotic addiction
- One second trimester abortion
- Poorly controlled diabetes mellitus
- Pyelonephritis
- Unexplained vaginal bleeding after 16 weeks gestation
- Uterine anomalies

Placental Factors
- Placenta previa

is an important risk factor for cerebral palsy.

Approximately 7 percent of all neonates born alive in the United States are low birth weight neonates, and most of these are delivered after preterm labors. The incidence of low birth weight neonates is almost twice as high among nonwhites as whites, and is increased six times in multiple gestations.

Medical and Nursing Interventions

Early in the prenatal period, gravidas who have been identified as being at increased risk for preterm labor should be taught the early symptoms of preterm labor, including menstrual-like cramps, rhythmic backache, increase or change in vaginal discharge, intestinal cramping, and rhythmic pelvic pressure.

Normal health measures during pregnancy, including proper nutrition and rest, avoidance of overwork and all excesses, are recommended for all pregnant women, but especially for the gravida who is at increased risk for preterm labor and delivery.

For the gravida who has a prior history of preterm labor and delivery, it is usually recommended that work, travel, and exercise be restricted. A thorough explanation should be provided concerning any proposed restrictions, and understanding and acceptance of these restrictions need to be verbalized by the gravida.

Early diagnosis and treatment of interruptions in health during the antepartum period that may predispose to preterm labor are also important in prevention. Clients with preexisting medical problems such as diabetes mellitus, hyperthyroidism, or cardiac disease should be followed by an internist as well as by the obstetrician. Elective major surgery and extensive dental work are postponed during pregnancy.

After 20 to 24 weeks gestation, weekly visits to the office or clinic are recommended. At these visits, client education concerning the signs and symptoms of preterm labor is reviewed. The cervix is evaluated weekly by vaginal examination to determine dilation, effacement, and consistency. The position and station of the presenting part are evaluated. If excessive uterine activity is reported by the gravida or is noted during the visit, exter-

TABLE 26-20
HIGH-RISK FACTORS FOR PRETERM LABOR

Maternal Factors
Abdominal surgery during pregnancy
Acute systemic bacterial infections
Incompetent cervix
Intrauterine infections
Maternal trauma
Multiple gestation
Pregnancy-induced hypertension
Previous preterm labor
Two or more second trimester abortions
Untreated Cushing's disease
Fetal Factors
Congenital adrenal hyperplasia
Fetal infections
Multiple gestation
Oligohydramnios
Polyhydramnios

nal uterine contraction monitoring may be initiated to evaluate uterine activity. Some physicians advocate modified bed rest.

Diagnosis of Preterm Labor

Numerous tocolytic agents are available to halt preterm labor. These agents are expensive to use, have adverse side effects, and must be administered in parenteral or oral form until preterm labor is no longer a possibility or until it is determined that labor cannot be halted; therefore, before they are instituted, preterm labor must be accurately diagnosed.

The following criteria need to be met before preterm labor is diagnosed: (1) labor occurs between 26 and 37 weeks gestation with an estimated fetal weight between 500 and 2499 grams; (2) regular uterine contractions are occurring at intervals of less than 10 minutes for 30 to 60 minutes; and (3) the uterine contractions are associated with changes in cervical effacement or dilation.

When the gravida first arrives in the labor area, a complete client assessment is done (see Chapter 16). External fetal monitoring is instituted to evaluate fetal and uterine contraction status. At first, the uterine contraction recording may reflect low amplitude, frequent, short, contractions that indicate uterine irritability. If no cervical changes are present, observation for several hours is indicated before the decision to give tocolytic agents is made. Contractions may increase in frequency, duration, and intensity without cervical changes.

Management

When preterm labor is diagnosed, a decision must be made whether to attempt to stop labor or to permit the labor to proceed. Contraindications for inhibition of preterm labor include confirmed fetal death, fetal anomaly incompatible with life, fetal distress, antepartum hemorrhage, PIH, cervical dilation of 4 cm or more, maternal cardiac pathology, maternal insulin-dependent diabetes mellitus, maternal hyperthyroidism, gestational age under 20 weeks, ruptured membranes, chorioamnionitis, or current administration of a betamimetic therapy for a medical condition.

The decision to stop preterm labor is made when the following conditions are present: (1) the fetus is alive, weighs 500 to 2499 grams, and shows no signs of distress; (2) the gestational age is estimated at 26 to 36 weeks; (3) the membranes are intact; (4) no obstetrical or medical complications exist; (5) cervical dilatation is less than 4 cm; (6) uterine contractions are present; and (7) fetal lungs are immature.

Arrest of Preterm Labor

MEDICAL AND NURSING INTERVENTIONS

If the decision is made to attempt to arrest preterm labor, the gravida should remain at bed rest, preferably on her left side. A lateral position will improve uterine blood flow, reduce muscle ischemia, and decrease uterine contraction frequency.

A vaginal examination is done at the beginning of treatment, but is normally not repeated unless it is essential. External fetal heart rate and uterine contraction monitoring is maintained and continuously assessed. An ultrasound is ordered to estimate fetal gestational age and weight, and to rule out gross fetal malformations. An amniocentesis will determine fetal lung maturity.

The client needs to remain well hydrated. Hydration will improve perfusion of all organs, lower ischemia, and may inhibit production of oxytocin.

The psychological status of the client is carefully assessed. She will be anxious not only because of the onset of preterm labor, but also because of the uncertain neonatal outcome. She is encouraged to voice fears and concerns for herself and for her fetus. Thorough explanations are provided to the client and to her partner. They may feel guilt that their actions possibly caused the preterm labor to begin and these feelings need to be dealt with (see Table 26–21).

TOCOLYTIC AGENTS

Most tocolytic agents can suppress uterine contractions and delay delivery for a period of time if administered early in labor. The Food and Drug Administration (FDA) is continuously reconsidering the status of each of these agents. The status of each must be verified before usage for inhibition of labor. Drug classifications that have been used with some success include progesterone derivatives, ethanol, vasodilators, beta-adrenergics, prostaglandin synthetase inhibitors, calcium antagonists, and others (see Table 26–22).

Progesterone Derivatives

Progesterone derivatives may be given to reduce myometrial sensitivity to oxytocin. However, they are not recognized as effective in stopping the progress of preterm labor. In addition, the FDA has recommended that progesterone and progesterone derivatives not be used during pregnancy because of the increased incidence of congenital anomalies.

Ethanol

Ethanol given intravenously in the form of alcohol in dextrose solution acts on the hypothalamus to block the release of oxytocin. Ethanol has been found to postpone delivery for more than 72 hours in selected patients. It is unknown whether the infusion of ethanol to inhibit preterm labor contributes to fetal alcohol syndrome. This unknown, plus the unpleasant side effects associated with its use, has resulted in its being used less frequently to inhibit preterm labor.

Before ethanol administration is begun, contraindications need to be assessed. Ethanol is contraindicated in mothers with epilepsy, urinary tract infections, alcoholism, and diabetes mellitus.

Recommended protocol for ethanol infusion to inhibit preterm labor is:

Intravenous solution: 10% alcohol and 5% dextrose in water

Loading dose: 1.5 ml per kg body weight per hour over 2 hours

Maintenance dose: 0.2 ml per kg body weight per hour for 6 hours or more

Reloading dose: if treatment was discontinued less than 10 hours earlier, new dose is calculated as loading dose times (number of hours divided by 10)

Fetal heart rate and uterine contractions are monitored continuously with external fetal monitoring. Since the patient is NPO, special attention is given to maintaining adequate hydration. An accurate intake and output is kept and documented, and signs of dehydration noted (hypotension, decreased urinary output, poor skin turgor, tachycardia, elevated temperature). Maternal vital signs are assessed frequently.

Explanations are to be provided to the client and her partner. The support person needs to be especially aware of the intoxication that accompanies intravenous ethanol administration in order to understand behaviors that may be exhibited by the client.

When ethanol is infusing, constant attendance by the nurse is essential. An emesis basin and suction should be readily available. Sedation and nausea are common effects, as is inebriation. The client is assessed for alcohol breath, nausea, vomiting, vertigo, ataxia, flushing, disorientation, restlessness, and respiratory depression. Side rails are up. Aspiration is a serious danger, owing to increased gastric secretions. Pneumonia and pulmonary edema have been reported. Blood alcohol levels are drawn and assessed for values. The infusion site is checked frequently for infiltration. Ethanol infusion is given piggyback, with the rate regulated by an infusion pump.

Marked diuresis occurs due to the inhibition of release of the antidiuretic hormone from the neurohypophysis. Hypoglycemia may occur because glyconeogenesis is inhibited.

The fetus is at increased risk of central nervous system depression, so continuous fetal monitoring assessment is important. The fetal cord blood level of alcohol is 20 percent of the maternal plasma level. Neonates born within 12 hours after ethanol administration have lower 1-minute Apgar scores and an increase in respiratory distress syndrome (Zervoudakis et al., 1980). These neonates are at increased risk for central nervous system depression, hypoglycemia, acidosis, and intoxication. At birth, a neutral thermal environment, oxygen, and ventilation are needed, along with fluid and electrolyte replacements.

Beta-Adrenergic Agents

Beta-adrenergic medications stimulate the beta receptors in the sympathetic nervous system. Beta-adrenergic activity includes cardiac acceleration and increased cardiac contractibility, vasodilation of arterioles supplying skeletal muscles, bronchial relaxation, and uterine relaxation.

Beta-mimetic drugs have received extensive trials in the arrest of preterm labor. Those that have met with a degree of success include isoxsuprine hydrochloride (Isuprel), ritodrine hydrochloride (Yutopar), terbutaline sulfate (Brethine), and metaproterenol (Alupent).

Isoxsuprine Hydrochloride

Isoxsuprine hydrochloride (Isuprel) is actually classified as a vasodilator, but is included with the beta-adrenergic drugs because it relaxes the smooth muscle of the uterus by activating the beta-adrenergic receptors. Isoxsuprine hydrochloride is contraindicated in the presence of arterial bleeding, hypotension, and tachycardia.

The following protocol is usually followed when isoxsuprine is used to inhibit preterm labor:

> Loading dose: 500 ml normal saline given by rapid intravenous infusion, followed by isoxsuprine 50 mg diluted in 500 ml normal saline at 1 ml per minute for 45 minutes intravenously
>
> Maintenance dose: 20 mg IM every 6 hours for 24 to 48 hours
>
> When contractions cease, isoxsuprine, 30 to 80 mg orally every three hours. After three or four days, this is reduced to every six hours

Adverse reactions include hypotension, tachycardia, nausea, vomiting, dizziness, abdominal pain, and rash. There is an overall incidence of maternal pulmonary edema of 0.5 percent (Nimrod et al., 1984). If delivery results, the neonate may exhibit a transient tachycardia of 10 to 15 BPM over normal. The FDA has neither approved nor recommended isoxsuprine hydrochloride to inhibit preterm labor.

Ritodrine Hydrochloride

Ritodrine hydrochloride (Yutopar) was approved in 1980 by the FDA for labor inhibition. It acts by stimulation of the beta receptors and inhibition of uterine muscle contractibility. When

TABLE 26–21
SAMPLE NURSING CARE PLAN: THREATENED PRETERM LABOR

C.G. is an 18-year-old gravida 1 para 0 at 29 weeks gestation. Her prenatal course has been uneventful up to this time. Her membranes ruptured spontaneously at 8:00 pm. She states large amount of clear fluid. She arrives at the hospital at 11:30 pm losing a small amount of clear amniotic fluid and complaining of mild, irregular uterine contractions. An initial client assessment is done.

Data Base:

18 years old
Gravida 1 para 0
29 weeks gestation
A positive
Weight gain 13 lb
On no medication, except prenatal vitamins
Denies any allergies
Denies any medical problems
States no trauma, recent intercourse
VE deferred at this time
Nitrazine paper positive for amniotic fluid
External fetal monitor applied according to policy and procedure to evaluate fetal heart tones and uterine contractions
Maternal vital signs: 98.6°F-88-24 B/P 100/75

Nursing Diagnosis	Goals	Nursing Interventions	Rationale	Evaluation
Knowledge deficit related to threatened preterm labor	The client verbalizes understanding of causes and possible treatment of preterm labor	Assess client knowledge of preterm labor Causes Treatment Potential fetal outcome Explain fetal development at this point in gestation Explain reason for hospitalization	Preterm delivery is one of the greatest problems in obstetrics. Preterm deliveries account for the majority of neonatal mortality	C. frightened and anxious Explanations given and understanding verbalized

Anxiety related to probability of preterm delivery	The client experiences minimal anxiety associated with potential preterm labor	Stay with client Reassurance Do not give false hope		
Knowledge deficit related to hospital environment, and nursing procedures	The client verbalizes understanding of interventions proposed	Explain all procedures in appropriate terms Encourage verbalization of concerns Reinforce physician explanations	Explanations will aid in decreasing anxiety and promote cooperation	Speculum and vaginal examination done by Dr. R. Cervix 1 cm dilated, thick PP cephalic Small amount clear fluid observed—nitrazine positive. Fluid specimen on slide for fern test—positive for amniotic fluid
Alterations in comfort related to uterine contractions	The client verbalizes minimal discomfort	Assess client perception of discomfort Assess contraction pattern and FHR status Use nonpharmaceutical measures to relieve discomfort Change position Breathing techniques Relaxation	Accurate assessment of maternal and fetal status needed Analgesia is avoided if preterm labor is present	Uterine contractions q 6 to 8 minutes, lasting 30 seconds, mild FHR within normal limits Breathing techniques explained and demonstrated Using techniques with encouragement Decision made to transfer C. to tertiary perinatal center for delivery Ambulance transport done at 3:30 am with nurse in attendance

TABLE 26–22
NURSING RESPONSIBILITIES IN TOCOLYTIC THERAPY

Identify preterm labor as soon as possible
Position client in left side-lying position to increase uterine blood flow
Thorough client assessment
Electronic fetal monitoring
Assess maternal hydration
Accurate intake and output
Daily weight
Monitor vital signs frequently and according to established protocol
Obtain baseline laboratory tests
Catheterized urinalysis may be ordered to rule out urinary tract infection
EKG may be ordered for baseline cardiac status
Assess lung and bowel sounds
Assess reflexes to determine central nervous system status
Offer support
Give thorough explanations to client and her partner

administered intravenously, it decreases uterine activity and prolongs gestation. After arrest of labor, oral administration helps avoid relapse.

Specific contraindications to administration include antepartum hemorrhage, PIH, chorioamnionitis, cardiac disease, pulmonary hypertension, maternal hyperthyroidism, uncontrolled maternal diabetes mellitus, and bronchial asthma.

Adverse reactions are common and include maternal and fetal tachycardia, hypotension, hyperglycemia, palpitations, arrhythmias, tremors, nausea, vomiting, headache, nervousness, restlessness, anxiety, and chest pain.

When ritodrine hydrochloride is administered intravenously, the client should remain in a left lateral position to reduce hypotension. Maternal hydration status is monitored. A potassium level is ordered before the medication is started. Other laboratory testing is done as ordered.

Explanation must be provided to the client and partner about the procedure and the expected effects. Questions are encouraged.

Recommended protocol for administration of ritodrine hydrochloride is:

Infuse 500 ml of main IV solution rapidly

Piggyback with an infusion pump a solution of 150 mg ritodrine hydrochloride added to 500 ml of IV fluid

Start piggyback infusion at 0.1 mg per minute and increase according to uterine contraction response up to 0.30 or 0.35 mg per minute until uterine contractions stop

Total daily dosage should not exceed 120 mg

Maintain stable infusion of ritodrine hydrochloride for 12 hours after desired result is obtained

Oral ritodrine tablets are started at 10 mg every two hours for 24 hours

30 minutes after first tablet is administered, decrease the ritodrine infusion gradually until the infusion is stopped

After 24 hours of oral ritodrine therapy every two hours, the dosage is decreased to 10 or 20 mg every four to six hours

Maternal blood pressure, pulse, and respirations, and the fetal heart rate are documented every 5 minutes when increasing the dosage of intravenous ritodrine. When the infusion rate is stable, vital signs and fetal heart tones are documented every 15 minutes for a minimum of one hour, then every hour.

Accurate intake and output must be monitored and recorded. External fetal monitoring is used continuously to assess the fetal heart rate and uterine contractions (see Table 26–23).

Specific complications have been documented and must be constantly assessed during ritodrine administration. Hyperglycemia with blood glucose values over 300 mg per 100 ml have been reported in nondiabetic women (Cotton et al., 1981). Urine testing for glucose is done during ritodrine administration. Usually ritodrine is not administered to women who are insulin-dependent diabetics.

Pulmonary edema may result from fluid overload during ritodrine therapy or as a result of accompanying decreased renal excretion of sodium, potassium, and water (Benedetti, 1983). Total fluid intake is usually limited to 2 or 3 liters in 24 hours. Daily weights are measured, and strict intake and

TABLE 26–23
NURSING RESPONSIBILITIES DURING INTRAVENOUS RITODRINE INFUSION

An initial assessment is done
Maintain left lateral position
Intramuscular muscle relaxants may be ordered
  If given before ritodrine is started will decrease anxiety, tremors
Educate client and coach about potential side effects
Obtain laboratory testing as ordered
Institute intravenous fluids as ordered by physician
Administer ritodrine according to protocol via piggyback and infusion pump
Monitor maternal pulse
  Should not exceed 140 BPM for over 10 minutes
Cardiac monitoring is recommended
Assess lung sounds
Monitor FHR and UC with external fetal monitor
Antiembolism stockings may be ordered
  Will help to prevent lower extremity pooling of blood
Avoid fluid overload
Accurate intake and output
Weigh daily
Assess client for potential complications of ritodrine therapy
Encourage verbalization of fears and concerns for self and fetus
Check urine protein and glucose every shift

output measurements are recorded. Chorioamnionitis can increase the incidence of maternal pulmonary edema (Benedetti et al., 1982).

Myocardial ischemia and death have been reported during ritodrine infusion (Benedetti et al., 1983). It is recommended that a baseline electrocardiogram be obtained before ritodrine infusion is started.

Gravidas with a history of migraine headaches have been reported to develop acute cerebral ischemia (Rosene et al., 1982). For this reason, ritodrine must be used with extreme caution in gravidas with a history of migraines.

Decreased serum potassium caused by the movement of potassium from extracellular to intracellular spaces has been documented. Serum lactate can increase due to glycogenolysis and lipolysis. Hemoglobin concentrations may decrease with the expansion of intravascular volume.

When oral ritodrine is given, the client should increase her potassium intake through dietary means. Client teaching emphasizes taking the medication at the prescribed time. Oral dosage is continued until about 37 weeks gestation.

Terbutaline Sulfate

Terbutaline sulfate (Brethine) relaxes smooth muscle of the vascular supply to the skeletal muscles and the uterus, and produces relief of bronchospasm. It is not FDA-approved for labor inhibition at this time.

Contraindications to terbutaline include known hypersensitivity, hypertension, coronary artery disease, and tachycardia. Cautious use is recommended in diabetes mellitus, hyperthyroidism, and cardiac arrhythmias.

Recommended protocol for preterm labor is:

Intravenous infusion of 0.01 mg per minute or 0.25 mg

Increase dosage up to a maximum of 0.025 mg per minute

Maintain dosage necessary to stop uterine contractions for one hour, then gradually decrease to the lowest effective dosage

When uterine contractions cease, given 0.25 mg subcutaneously four times a day or every four hours for three days

Oral dosage for maintenance is 2.5 to 5.0 mg three times a day

Maternal side effects include tachycardia, nervousness, tremors, decreased diastolic and increased systolic blood pressure, lightheadedness, palpitations, nausea, vomiting, and diaphoresis. Nursing responsibilities during terbutaline administration are summarized in Table 26–24.

Metaproterenol Sulfate

Metaproterenol (Alupent), a beta-adrenergic agent, stimulates beta-adrenergic receptors of the sympathetic nervous system and has little or no effect on alpha receptors. The main effect of metaproterenol is relaxation of

TABLE 26-24
NURSING RESPONSIBILITIES DURING TERBUTALINE ADMINISTRATION

An initial assessment is done
Gravida to remain on bedrest in left lateral position
Obtain ordered laboratory testing
Explain potential side effects
Institute intravenous infusion as ordered by the physician
Monitor maternal vital signs
Monitor the FHR and UC with external fetal monitoring
Cardiac monitor
Baseline EKG
Monitor rate and character of maternal pulse
  Pulse rate should not exceed 140 BPM for over 10 minutes
Assess lung sounds
Antiembolism stockings may be ordered to prevent venous pooling
Avoid fluid overload
Strict intake and output
Daily weight
Encourage verbalization of fears and concerns for self and fetus
Permit may be needed (drug not approved by FDA)

smooth muscle of the bronchial tree and the peripheral vasculature which will in turn decrease uterine contractility. This drug may cause central nervous system stimulation and some cardiostimulatory effects that result in tachycardia and hypertension. Metaproterenol has been used investigationally in large dosages to arrest the progress of preterm labor, but has not been approved by the FDA.

Metaproterenol should be used with caution in clients who have hypertension, coronary artery disease, congestive heart failure, hyperthyroidism, or diabetes mellitus, and it is contraindicated in clients with preexisting cardiac arrhythmias associated with tachycardia.

It should not be administered concurrently with other sympatholytic agents owing to the possibility of additive effects. Protocol used for metaproterenol is intravenous infusion at the rate of 10 and 20 μ per minute via infusion pump.

Prostaglandin Synthetase Inhibitors

Prostaglandin synthetase inhibitors such as aspirin, indomethacin (Indocin), naproxen (Naprosyn), and mefenamic acid (Ponstel) are known to be effective in delaying or prolonging labor, but are not approved by the FDA for this purpose. High doses of aspirin during the last three months of pregnancy may prolong pregnancy. These drugs are not recommended for inhibition of preterm labor because significant circulatory effects may be produced in the fetus as well as persistent pulmonary hypertension in the neonatal period.

Calcium Antagonists

Calcium ions are necessary for the activation of the contractile proteins of the myometrium. Two drugs, nifedipine (Procardia) and verapamil (Calan), have been shown to reduce uterine contractibility. When used to arrest preterm labor, doses above the usual range are required, but the preterm labor is usually arrested for 3 to 17 days.

Magnesium Sulfate

Magnesium sulfate acts as a central nervous system depressant and also depresses smooth, skeletal, and cardiac muscle. It is used to inhibit preterm labor in selected clients who cannot receive beta-adrenergic drugs (i.e., diabetes mellitus, cardiovascular disease) or in conjunction with other tocolytics to obtain the desired response.

Magnesium sulfate causes relaxation of the myometrium by suppressing firing of neurons and reducing amplitude of motor and end-plate potentials. It is usually well tolerated by the client, but some side effects include drowsiness, decreased sensory perception, slurred speech, heavy eyelids, flushing, decreased reflexes, decreased gastrointestinal action, and decreased respiratory rate.

Magnesium sulfate crosses the placental barrier and can lead to central nervous system depression in the fetus. The neonate may be lethargic, with reduced muscle tone, decreased sucking reflex, decreased respiratory rate, and

TABLE 26-25
NURSING RESPONSIBILITIES DURING MAGNESIUM SULFATE ADMINISTRATION FOR PRETERM LABOR INHIBITION

Gravida to remain on bed rest in left lateral position
Thorough client assessment is conducted
Obtain ordered laboratory tests
Institute intravenous fluids according to physician orders
Magnesium sulfate is given via piggyback and infusion pump
Vital signs are taken at least every 30 minutes
Note the quality of respirations
Reflexes are checked every 1 to 2 hours
Document increase or decrease in reflexes
Strict intake and output
Urine output should be 30 ml/hour or more
Daily weight
Avoid concurrent use of narcotics
Assess lung sounds
Assess bowel sounds
Antidote of calcium gluconate should be drawn up ready for administration
Monitor FHR and UC with external fetal monitor
Resuscitation equipment must be readily available
Do not leave the client alone

increased serum magnesium levels. These conditions are usually transitory.

Magnesium sulfate is excreted by the kidneys, so urinary output needs to be monitored. The blood level of magnesium sulfate is checked at frequent intervals. Therapeutic levels are usually considered to be 4 to 7 mg per 100 ml. Maternal respiratory depression and arrest can occur when toxic levels are reached (see Table 26-25).

Therapy usually begins with a loading dose after a main intravenous line has been started. Four grams is the usual loading dose for an average size woman. For continuous intravenous administration, a piggyback setup using an infusion pump is employed. The standard solution for maintenance dosage is 20 gm magnesium sulfate mixed in 1000 ml of intravenous solution.

Glucocorticoid Therapy

Glucocorticoids may be prescribed to accelerate fetal lung maturity when preterm labor occurs, thus decreasing the incidence of respiratory disorders in the neonate. The greatest benefits apparently are noted when the pregnancy is at 29 to 32 weeks gestation. Therapy with betamethasone is most effective when delivery is delayed at least two days after treatment is started. Hydrocortisone, 100 mg, is administered as a single injection. If delivery is delayed more than seven days, the treatment is repeated.

Glucocorticoids are contraindicated in severe PIH because of the increased incidence of fetal death associated with the disease process. Cases have been reported of postpartum pulmonary edema when terbutaline sulfate and glucocorticoid combinations are given.

Labor

If delivery of the preterm fetus is elected, or if delivery is unavoidable, every effort must be made to avoid trauma and prevent fetal hypoxia. The preterm fetus has a soft skull, lowered resistance, and tolerates trauma poorly (see Table 26-26). Rapid labors are avoided whenever possible.

A left lateral position is recommended for the gravida, and oxygen is administered throughout labor to promote and maintain adequate maternal-fetal oxygenation. Continuous fetal monitoring is imperative to detect subtle changes that may denote fetal hypoxia. Systemic analgesics are avoided to prevent undue respiratory depression in the neonate. Regional anesthesia or local infiltration of the perineum is used for delivery. If stimulation of uterine contractions becomes necessary, oxytocin stimulation may be used for short periods with the client and fetus under constant surveillance.

Delivery

Vaginal delivery should be slow and gentle to avoid rapid compression and decompression

TABLE 26–26
SAMPLE NURSING CARE PLAN: PRETERM LABOR AND DELIVERY

B.A., a 21-year-old gravida 2 para 1 is 32 weeks gestation. Her pregnancy has been uneventful up to this time. At 2:00 am she awakened with 5-minute contractions. She notified her obstetrician, who told her to come to the hospital. She arrived at the hospital at 3:00 am and was put to bed. An initial assessment was performed.

Date Base:

21 years old
Gravida 2 para 1
32 weeks
A positive
On no medications, except prenatal vitamins
No known allergies
No medical problems
States fell down stairs yesterday
Uterine contractions q 3 minutes, lasting 50 seconds, moderate intensity
Show present
Membranes intact
Vital signs normal
Vaginal examination: 5 cm cervical dilation at +2 station. Bulging membranes. Presenting part cephalic.
Breastfeeding
Labor work done (CBC, PT, PTT, UA), all within normal limits
Dr. A. notified of status
External fetal monitor applied at 3:05 am

Nursing Diagnosis	Goals	Nursing Interventions	Rationale	Evaluation
Potential for injury to fetus related to preterm labor	The fetus will remain well-oxygenated throughout labor and will experience minimal or no trauma during delivery	Monitor FHR with external fetal monitor	Preterm labor and delivery are hazardous for the fetus. The preterm fetus does not have the reserve to combat effects of hypoxia. The preterm infant is more sensitive to maternal analgesia. The left lateral position will improve oxygenation.	FHR remained within normal limits throughout labor and delivery

Alteration in comfort related to uterine contractions secondary to preterm labor	The client will experience minimal discomfort from uterine contractions	Assess uterine contractions: Frequency Duration Intensity Client behavior Assess labor progress Maintain hydration Encourage left lateral position during labor Monitor maternal vital signs Avoid analgesia		Uterine contraction status 3:10 am q 2 min × 50 seconds 3:30 am q 2 min × 60 seconds Vaginal examinations: 3:10 5 cm dilation at +2 station 3:30 10 cm at +3 station Left lateral position maintained throughout labor Oxygen was given per nasal cannula at 3 L/min IV of 1000 ml D_5LR infusing at 128 ml/hour Maternal vital signs remained stable Spontaneous delivery of live boy at 3:38 am over LMLE—Apgars 4 and 6 Neonate to nursery
Knowledge deficit related to preterm labor	The client and coach verbalize understanding of: Causes Potential outcome	Explain: Causes Treatment Expected outcome Stay with patient Offer emotional support	Knowledge will decrease anxiety and fear	Brief explanations given due to advanced labor status. Verbalized understanding
Anxiety related to uncertain fetal outcome	The client verbalizes fears and concerns re: fetal outcome	Work with client to use breathing and relaxation techniques Do not offer false hope or reassurances Encourage questions	Minimal analgesia given to optimize fetal outcome	No analgesics given Breathing techniques utilized throughout labor

of the fetal head. Low forceps and episiotomy are usually used to prevent trauma to the fetal skull during delivery. After delivery, the cord is clamped and cut after 30 to 45 seconds to allow the passage of placental and cord blood in the fetal pulmonary unit.

A cesarean delivery may be performed if fetal distress is present, if there is a breech presentation, or if there is a transverse lie. Many obstetricians consider cesarean delivery less hazardous to the preterm fetus than vaginal delivery.

TABLE 26-27
FACTORS ASSOCIATED WITH PREMATURE RUPTURE OF THE MEMBRANES

Factors
Preterm delivery
Older gravidas
Nonwhites
Multiparous women
Prior instrumentation of the cervix
Cigarette smoking
Incompetent cervix
Low weight gain during pregnancy
Recent coitus
Obesity

Prognosis

Perinatal mortality for the preterm neonate ranges from 25 to 40 percent. Preterm delivery is ideally carried out in a Level III perinatal center to give the neonate the best chance of survival.

PREMATURE RUPTURE OF THE MEMBRANES

Premature rupture of the membranes (PROM) is defined as rupture of the membranes before the onset of uterine contractions. The incidence is about 10 to 12 percent of all deliveries. About 20 percent of these occur before 36 weeks gestation.

Cause

The cause of premature rupture of the membranes is usually not known and often occurs without warning. Predisposing factors are summarized in Table 26-27.

Complications

The major complications following premature rupture of the membranes are the onset of preterm labor and intrauterine infection. At term, spontaneous rupture of the membranes is usually followed by the onset of labor within 24 to 48 hours. When the membranes rupture earlier in pregnancy, the onset of labor may not occur for several days or several weeks.

MATERNAL COMPLICATIONS

The risk to the mother is small compared with that of the fetus. The major maternal complication is ascending intrauterine infection.

FETAL COMPLICATIONS

The major cause of perinatal mortality in PROM is preterm delivery. About 5 percent of neonates born after PROM develop sepsis. The longer the time between rupture of the membranes and the onset of labor, the more likely the fetus is to develop an infection. When membranes are ruptured over 48 hours before delivery, the incidence of infection increases sharply. Infections most commonly noted are infection of the umbilical cord, pneumonia, and septicemia.

During labor that follows PROM, malpresentations and prolapse of the umbilical cord are more common. Fetal prognosis depends upon fetal maturity, presentation, presence of intrauterine infection, and the length of time between rupture of the membranes and delivery of the fetus.

Diagnosis

Diagnosis is obvious if there is a gush of fluid from the vagina followed by continuous drainage of watery fluid. Diagnosis may be more difficult if watery leakage is slight and intermittent.

If diagnosis of rupture of the membranes is doubtful, several tests can be helpful. A sterile speculum examination is conducted by the physician to visually assess the degree of cervical dilation and drainage of amniotic fluid, and to rule out prolapsed cord. If fluid is present, a sterile swab is used to obtain a sample for nitrazine and fern testing (see Chapter 16). If no fluid is seen, the sterile swab should be rubbed over mucosa in the upper posterior vagina, and used for nitrazine and fern testing.

A drop of the liquid obtained can also be mixed with nile blue sulfate, placed on a glass slide, and allowed to dry for 5 minutes. The presence of any orange-staining fetal cells is considered positive for amniotic fluid.

Amniocentesis with ultrasound guidance is sometimes ordered. Five ml of Evans blue dye is injected into the amniotic sac. If the membranes are ruptured, there will be blue staining of a perineal pad within 30 to 40 minutes.

Medical and Nursing Interventions

The management of PROM is determined by the point in gestation at which it occurs. Major considerations in deciding the method of management include the potential for serious fetal or maternal complications. The fetus has an excellent chance of survival if 36 weeks gestation has been reached, and a good chance if 34 weeks is reached. From 24 to 28 weeks gestation, the prognosis ranges from poor to fair, depending on the size and condition of the neonate at birth and neonatal care given after delivery.

The gravida should be admitted to the hospital when the membranes rupture. A complete assessment is conducted, along with an admission vaginal examination to determine cervical dilation and effacement and to rule out prolapse of the umbilical cord. After the initial vaginal examination, no further examinations are needed until active labor begins. An ultrasound is ordered to determine gestational age and locate the placenta.

A conservative approach is employed when the fetus is preterm or the cervix is unfavorable for induction. Fetal lung maturity accelerates when the membranes are ruptured for more than 24 hours and the incidence of respiratory distress is decreased for the neonate. With prolonged PROM (over 24 hours), an elevation in blood corticosteroid levels in the neonate occurs and is thought to accelerate fetal lung maturation.

Maternal and fetal physiologic status are monitored, with special emphasis on assessment for subtle signs of infection or the onset of uterine contractions. Anxiety and feelings of guilt need to be carefully assessed and appropriate interventions instituted.

The use of prophylactic antibiotics in cases of uncomplicated PROM is usually not recommended. Their use does not influence the incidence of amnionitis or sepsis in the neonatal period and the growth of resistant organisms is a major threat to the mother and the neonate. Prophylactic antibiotics given in the absence of complications may lead to neonatal problems. Neonatal effects of antibiotics given to the mother include deafness, dental staining, inhibition of bone growth, anemias, hyperbilirubinemia, and possible damage to the nervous system and kidneys. When prophylactic antibiotics are used, the benefits of usage need to be carefully evaluated against the potential harmful effects to the neonate.

Tocolytics to prevent preterm labor are usually contraindicated with PROM. Glucocorticoids to accelerate fetal lung maturity are used if the gestation is 24 to 34 weeks and if delivery is not expected for at least 24 hours. The gravida is carefully assessed for increased susceptibility to intrauterine infections and postpartum pulmonary edema if glucocorticoids are administered with betamimetic tocolytic agents.

LESS THAN 34 WEEKS GESTATION

If the gestation is 26 to 28 weeks, labor may be induced to prevent maternal ascending infection. After 28 weeks, conservative management can be used with minimal infectious risks to mother or fetus (Varner and Galask, 1981). During the last two months of gestation the fetus gains about 0.5 pound per week. In the absence of complications, in utero existence is considered optimal for the fetus.

The gravida is hospitalized and bed rest is maintained until active leakage of fluid from the vagina ceases. On admission, a complete blood count and urinalysis are ordered. Amniotic fluid is assessed for amount, color, consistency, and odor. Maternal vital signs are assessed frequently, with special attention to maternal temperature and pulse rate. Fetal heart tones are assessed at frequent intervals. Daily white blood cell counts are measured to monitor early signs of infection.

34 to 37 WEEKS

During these weeks, the decision for conservative management or delivery is based on fetal maturity. An ultrasound and amniocentesis are done to assess gestational age and lung maturity. If the fetal lungs are immature, conservative management is indicated. If the fetal lungs are mature (L/S ratio of 2:1), delivery is usually accomplished by induction of labor or cesarean delivery. When the amniocentesis is performed, Gram staining and anaerobic and aerobic cultures are also taken. Bacteria present in any of these cultures indicates the need for prompt delivery to avoid neonatal sepsis. If no infection is present, induction of labor after 16 to 24 hours of documented ruptured membranes is appropriate if the fetal gestational age is 34 weeks or more.

AFTER 37 WEEKS

After 37 weeks gestation, spontaneous rupture of the membranes is usually followed by spontaneous onset of labor within 48 hours. If labor does not begin spontaneously, oxytocin induction is indicated.

Chorioamnionitis

The terms *chorioamnionitis* (inflammation and infection of the amnion and chorion) and *amnionitis* (inflammation and infection of the amnion) are often used interchangeably, although they are not exactly the same. Chorioamnionitis occurs in 0.5 to 1 percent of all pregnancies and in up to 56 percent of pregnancies with PROM (Schreiber & Benedetti, 1980; Guzick & Winn, 1984).

PATHOPHYSIOLOGY

There are three major pathways to intrauterine infection. First, the pathogens can travel an ascending pathway through the cervix. Second, pathogens can travel via the maternal circulation. Third, pathogens can enter the uterus by an iatrogenic source, most commonly as a result of amniocentesis.

DIAGNOSIS

Early diagnosis may be difficult, especially if the membranes are intact. Early signs and symptoms are very subtle. Clinical signs noted may include maternal fever, fetal tachycardia, maternal tachycardia, a foul odor to the amniotic fluid, or uterine tenderness. Laboratory studies are of limited value, since leukocytosis during pregnancy is a normal physiologic occurrence. Endocervical cultures and cultures of amniotic fluid will identify the pathogen.

ANTIBIOTICS

If an infection is diagnosed, antibiotic therapy is begun. The choice of antibiotic depends upon the amount of coverage desired, as well as the potential neonatal effects.

DELIVERY

Delivery is the definitive step to cure the mother and provide optimal therapy for the neonate. Vaginal delivery is preferable for the mother, but for the fetus vaginal delivery must be as atraumatic as possible to be preferable. If vaginal delivery is the procedure of choice, continuous nursing assessments and appropriate interventions are essential (see Chapter 16).

HYDRAMNIOS

Amniotic fluid volume usually increases from early pregnancy until just before term, at which time there is approximately 1000 ml of amniotic fluid.

Oligohydramnios

Oligohydramnios, or an abnormally small amount of amniotic fluid, is associated with several maternal problems and congenital anomalies (Hobbins et al., 1979). Postmaturity, premature rupture of the membranes, intrauterine growth retardation, and low Apgar scores are associated with an excessively small amount of amniotic fluid, as is pregnancy-induced hypertension (Mercer et al., 1984). Fetal anomalies associated with oligohydramnios include agenesis of the ears and genitourinary anomalies, especially renal agenesis.

Polyhydramnios

Amniotic fluid in excess of 1500 to 2000 ml is considered *polyhydramnios* and occurs in 0.4 percent of all pregnancies. Causes of polyhydramnios are varied and include idiopathic causes, diabetes mellitus, congenital anomalies, Rh incompatibility, and multiple gestation. The fetus with a major nervous system anomaly does not drink the usual amount of amniotic fluid, but will usually excrete urine at the normal rate, thus creating an excess of amniotic fluid. With gastrointestinal anomalies proximal to the ileum, there is also a discrepancy between swallowing and urination. Infants of diabetic mothers may have episodes of hyperglycemia in utero that are accompanied by diuresis. Neonatal *micrognathia* (abnormally small jaw) has been reported to play a role in polyhydramnios formation.

DIAGNOSIS

Polyhydramnios is suspected when the uterus is abnormally large for gestational age, fetal heart tones are distant or almost inaudible, and fetal parts are indistinct on abdominal palpation.

An ultrasound is reviewed to confirm polyhydramnios and to detect multiple gestation and obvious congenital anomalies. If a major anomaly is found, the client is informed so that a decision can be made to terminate or to continue the pregnancy. When no major anomalies are found, a comprehensive ultrasound (Stage II scan) is ordered to detect obscure congenital malformations.

MEDICAL AND NURSING INTERVENTIONS

The excess accumulation of amniotic fluid can cause severe maternal distress owing to pressure from the overdistended uterus on the diaphragm and gastrointestinal tract, as well as the decreased venous return from the lower extremities.

In chronic polyhydramnios, accumulation of amniotic fluid is very slow, and maternal distress is usually not as severe as in acute polyhydramnios. With acute polyhydramnios there is a very rapid accumulation of amniotic fluid over the course of a few days or a few weeks. Usually occurring between 21 and 28 weeks of gestation, there is upper abdominal discomfort, dyspnea, and marked edema of the abdomen and vulva.

The gravida is hospitalized and placed on complete bed rest. Amniocentesis may be performed for maternal respiratory distress or marked uterine irritability from overdistention. She is assessed frequently for congestive heart failure. Serial ultrasounds may be ordered to determine the presence of intrauterine growth retardation.

If amniocentesis is ordered to relieve maternal symptoms, withdrawal of fluid should be at a constant rate, about 500 ml per hour. Removal of 1500 to 2000 ml is usually sufficient to relieve symptoms. Reaccumulation of fluid will be rapid and the procedure may need to be repeated every two or three days. Tocolytics are sometimes given to prevent the onset of preterm labor. As the uterus contracts after removal of the amniotic fluid, the diminished intrauterine surface may result in premature separation of the placenta.

PROM may occur, with resultant preterm labor and delivery (Affonso & Danforth, 1981). Prolapse of the umbilical cord is more frequent when the membranes rupture. Cervical dilation patterns are usually normal. During labor and delivery, nursing interventions are the same as discussed in Chapter 16. Specialized care should be available for the neonate at birth. After delivery, assessment for postpartum hemorrhage owing to the previous uterine overdistention is important.

PROLAPSE OF THE UMBILICAL CORD

Prolapse of the umbilical cord is an obstetrical emergency. Although it occurs infrequently, it is associated with a high fetal mortality rate. Umbilical cord prolapse is descent of the cord following rupture of the membranes. The cord may prolapse in one of three positions (see Fig. 26–18): (1) the prolapse may be occult, with the cord beside the presenting part; (2) the umbilical cord may descend into the vagina; or (3) the cord may protrude outside the vagina.

Etiology

An increased risk of prolapsed cord exists whenever the presenting part does not fit snugly into the maternal pelvis. Abnormal presentations, especially transverse lie and breech presentations, are present in the majority of cases. With a preterm fetus, the small presenting part, coupled with the increased incidence of abnormal presentations make the risk of prolapse cord greater. Multiple pregnancy and polyhydramnios also increase the risk of prolapsed cord. An unengaged presenting part predisposes to prolapse of the cord when the membranes rupture. A long cord (80 cm or more) is associated with umbilical cord accidents (Rayburn et al., 1981). When the placenta is located near the cervix, engagement of the presenting part may be prevented. Obstetrical procedures such as amniotomy with an unengaged presenting part and version may cause the umbilical cord to prolapse.

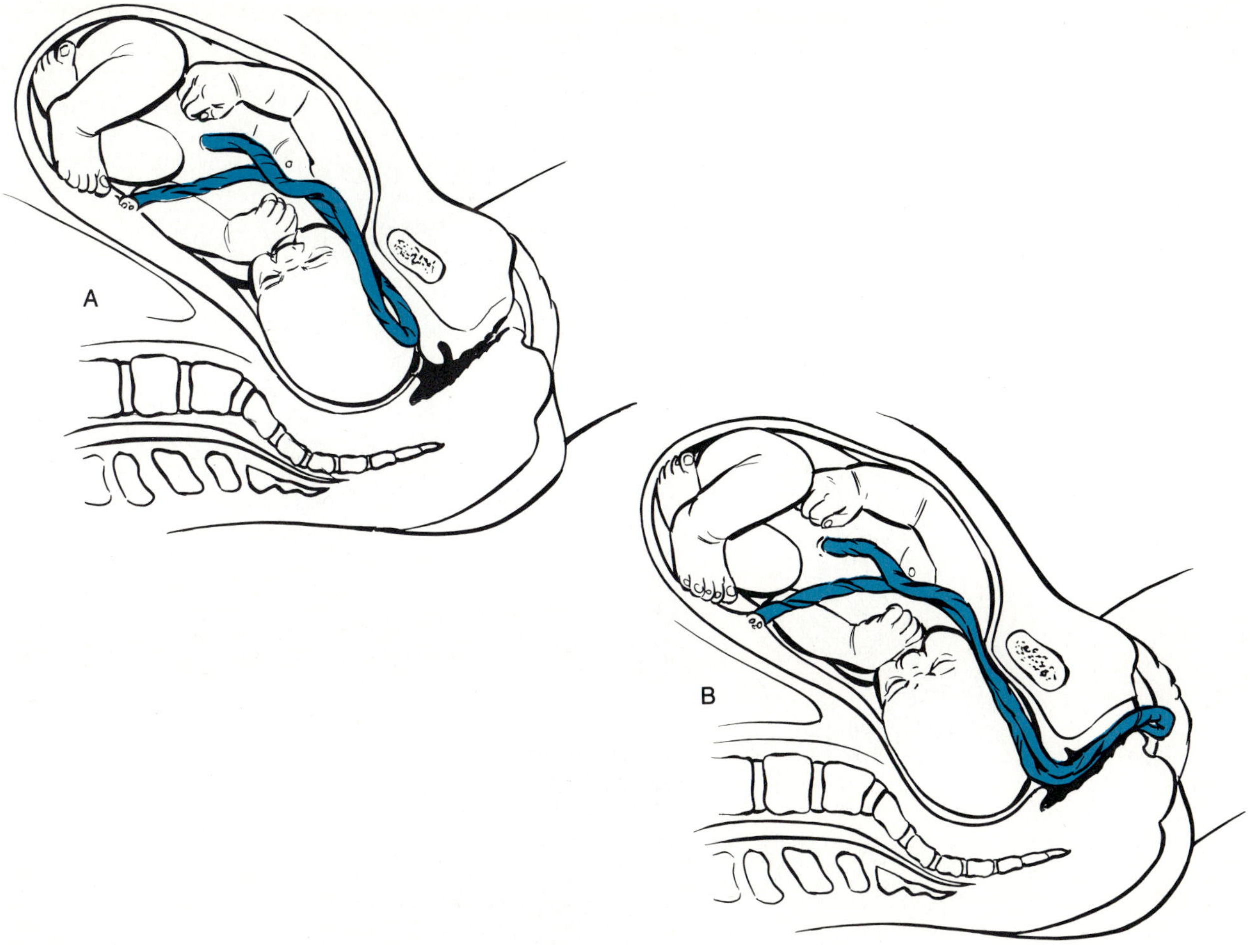

FIGURE 26-18. Prolapsed cord: A. Cord prolapsed at the inlet. B. Cord prolapsed through the introitus.

Prognosis

A prolapsed cord does not affect the progress of labor or the maternal physiologic status. Fetal mortality following prolapsed cord is approximately 35 percent. The longer the interval between diagnosis and delivery and the greater the degree of cord compression, the higher the perinatal mortality. The better the condition of the fetus when diagnosis is made, the greater is the chance of survival. An umbilical cord that strongly pulsates is indicative of a favorable fetal condition. The less traumatic the delivery, the better the fetal prognosis.

Medical and Nursing Interventions

The diagnosis of prolapsed umbilical cord is made by seeing the umbilical cord outside the vulva or feeling the umbilical cord upon vaginal examination. Vaginal examination should be conducted whenever unexplained fetal distress is noted with fetal monitoring and when the membranes rupture (see Table 26–28).

If the fetus is dead, if there are known congenital anomalies incompatible with

TABLE 26-28
SAMPLE NURSING CARE PLAN: PROLAPSED CORD

G.T., a 27-year-old gravida 2 para 1 at term was admitted to labor and delivery in active labor. Initial assessment was completed.

Date Base:

27 years old
Gravida 2 para 1
40 weeks gestation
A positive
No known allergies
No medical problems
On no medications, except prenatal vitamins
27 lb weight gain during pregnancy
Bottle feeding
Maternal vital signs: 99°F-88-20 B/P 100/76
Vaginal examination: 2–3 cm cervical dilation
PP cephalic
−2 to −1 station
BOW intact
Cervix 60% effaced

Uterine contractions q 4 minutes, lasting 40 seconds, moderate intensity
FHR 148 LML
External fetal monitor applied according to policy and procedure
Admission laboratory tests done—within normal limits
2:00 am—PROM occurred—large amount clear fluid noted, no odor.
VE: 3 cm cervical dilation at −1 station
Cervix approximately 85% effaced
Pulsating loop of cord felt on vaginal examination

Nursing Diagnosis	Goals	Nursing Interventions	Rationale	Evaluation
Potential for injury to fetus and mother related to prolapsed umbilical cord	The client will deliver with no maternal or fetal complications	Assess cord for pulsation Continue with fetal monitoring Relieve pressure on cord: Vaginal pressure to elevate PP off cord Knee chest position Modified Trendelenberg position Do not replace cord Oxygen per face mask Notify physician	The shorter the interval between diagnosis and delivery the more favorable the fetal outcome If pressure can be taken off the cord fetal outcome is improved Gravity may help to relieve compression The patient will exhibit decreased ability to cope	When PROM occurred, and loop of umbilical cord identified on vaginal examination, client hips were elevated and vaginal examination maintained to keep pressure off of cord. Dr. R. was notified. Oxygen was given via face mask at 8 L/min. FHR baseline remained normal, with mild variable decelerations noted on fetal monitor tracing
Anxiety related to nursing interventions secondary to cord prolapse	The patient will verbalize fears and concerns	Explanations to client and coach Prepare for delivery by most expeditious route Notify pediatrician and intensive care nursery	Brief but thorough explanations will aid in comprehension	While awaiting arrival of physician, brief explanations were given about cord prolapse and probable method of delivery Dr. R. arrived—decision to do emergency cesarean delivery Preoperative preparation completed To surgery for cesarean delivery—live boy delivered 10 minutes later. Apgars 7 and 8

TABLE 26–29
SAMPLE NURSING CARE PLAN: PRECIPITATE LABOR AND DELIVERY

J.T., a 35-year-old gravida 6 para 5 at term is admitted to labor and delivery in active labor. Initial assessment is completed.

Data Base:

35 years old
Gravida 6 para 5
39 weeks gestation
No known allergies
No medical problems
On no medications, except prenatal vitamins

Uterine contractions q 2 minutes, lasting 60 seconds, intense
Maternal vital signs: 98°F, 96, 24 B/P 140/72
FHT 144 LRQ
Vaginal examination: 8 cm cervical dilation
PP cephalic at +2 station

Nursing Diagnosis	Goals	Nursing Interventions	Rationale	Evaluation
Alteration in the process of labor related to rapid labor and impending delivery	The client and fetus will progress through delivery without injury	Notify physician of labor status Transfer to delivery room Use calm approach Talk to client in calm tones and explain what is happening Open a sterile delivery pack and put sterile drape under buttocks Put on sterile gloves Encourage the client to pant with contractions and gently control progress of head	Labor may progress so rapidly that the nurse will need to deliver A clean environment preferably sterile is needed	J.T. transferred immediately to delivery room Brief explanation given as to labor status A baby boy was delivered over an intact perineum 7 minutes after arrival in the labor unit Apgars were 9 and 9 Maternal and neonatal status stable following spontaneous placental expulsion 1 minute later

	Support the head to prevent rapid expulsion	Rapid expulsion of fetal head should be avoided to prevent intracranial hemorrhage
	Support the perineum	
	Support the head with one hand and wipe the face with the other	
	Palpate for the cord around the neck. If loose, slip over fetal head. If tight, clamp twice and cut between clamps	Immediately after head is delivered, check for nuchal cord If none found, deliver the rest of the fetus
	With next contraction gently help direct anterior shoulder under the symphysis	
	The posterior shoulder will follow	
	Position neonate with head down so that mucus will drain	
	Suction mouth and nose as needed	Suction mouth and nose immediately to clear airway
	Stimulate neonate to cry	
	Dry the neonate	
	Keep neonate and client warm	
	If physician still not present, clamp cord in two places and cut the cord	
	Deliver the placenta if necessary	
	Put the neonate to breast to help in uterine contraction	

extrauterine life, or if the fetus is so immature or preterm that there is no chance of survival, the labor is allowed to proceed.

Interventions to relieve cord compression are instituted immediately upon diagnosis of cord prolapse. A knee-chest or modified Trendelenberg position may aid in decreasing compression on the umbilical cord. The nurse or physician may place sterile gloved fingers into the vagina and push the presenting part of the fetus off the umbilical cord to increase fetal oxygenation. Oxygen is administered via face mask at 7 to 10 L per minute and the fetal heart rate is constantly monitored. *Do not* attempt to replace the umbilical cord into the vagina.

If the cervix is completely dilated (10 cm), vaginal delivery is completed as expeditiously as possible. If cervical dilation is incomplete, cesarean delivery is the treatment of choice to decrease trauma to both mother and fetus.

PRECIPITATE LABOR

A *precipitate labor* is one that totals less than three hours. Predisposing factors include induction of labor, a history of previous rapid labors, grand multiparity, lax unresistant maternal soft tissues, uterine contractions with increased amplitude, and a small fetus in optimal position for labor.

Dangers

Maternal dangers include a possible unattended delivery, birth canal lacerations, and ruptured uterus.

Fetal dangers include impairment of blood flow producing fetal hypoxia, subdural hematoma from tentorial tears owing to the rapid transit through the maternal bony pelvis, and lack of immediate care at delivery.

Nursing Interventions

During antepartal visits to the office or clinic, a complete obstetrical history including the length of previous labors is obtained. The gravida at risk for rapid labors can often be identified early in the antepartal period. These gravidas are instructed on signs and symptoms of labor and when to leave for the hospital or birthing center. Gravidas who have had previous precipitate labors or precipitate deliveries may choose to have an elective induction of labor to prevent a potential unattended delivery with associated increase in neonatal complications.

During labor constant attendance by the nurse is essential. Uterine contractions are continuously assessed and the fetal heart rate is observed for fetal distress. Vaginal examinations are conducted more frequently to determine labor progress.

Psychological support is essential. Gravidas with a history of precipitate labors will be more anxious that they will have the same type of labor again. Coping abilities may be decreased owing to the intensity of uterine contractions and the rapid progress in cervical dilation and descent of the presenting part.

Precipitate labors often result in precipitate deliveries. An unattended delivery can be hazardous for the gravida and for the fetus. If the nurse finds herself in a situation where delivery is imminent, she must be prepared to deliver the fetus herself (see Table 26–29 on p. 752).

PLACENTAL PROBLEMS

Abnormal Configurations

Abnormal configurations of the placenta are influenced by the degree of maternal decidual vascularization and the number and arrange-

TABLE 26–30
ABNORMAL PLACENTAL CONFIGURATIONS

Name	Description	Incidence	Pathogenesis	Nursing Implications
Circumvallate placenta	Chorionic plate is decreased resulting in chorionic villi invading surrounding villi. Fetal membranes fold back on self	1% to 6.5%	1. Inadequate amount of early ovum is converted into the chorion frondosum. Villi invade decidua and grow oblique splitting decidua into two layers 2. Early ovum implants too deeply 3. During early placentation the outer portion of the placenta detaches and rolls inward	May cause bright, moderate painless vaginal bleeding at about 20 weeks gestation Placental insufficiency may result Premature labor Abnormal maternal bleeding following third stage of labor due to improper placental separation Increases incidence of abruptio placentae
Placenta succenturiata	Placenta has one or more accessory lobes attached to the main placenta by 1 artery and 1 vein	0.1 to 0.3%	A group of fetal villi are located a distance from the main part of placenta and do not generate	Postpartum hemorrhage if the accessory lobe is not removed following delivery
Battledore placenta	Umbilical cord is inserted at or near the placental margin All fetal vessels cross the placenta in the same direction (looks like a tennis racket)	5 to 7%	Site of umbilical insertion is determined at implantation by the position of the inner cell mass	Fetal distress Fetal bleeding during labor Contributes to preterm labor

ment of villi that invade the decidua. When the decidua is more highly vascularized in some areas than in others, the resulting villi arrangement may produce an abnormal placental shape (see Table 26–30).

Retained Placenta

The placenta may be retained in the uterus during the third stage of labor, rather than being expelled. When the placenta is not expelled, it is usually because of one of four reasons. On occasion, the placenta may be separated but is not expelled because of ineffective uterine contractions. Second, the placenta may separate normally but is trapped in the upper uterine segment by a uterine constriction ring. Third, the placenta may fail to separate from the uterine wall because of ineffective uterine contractions, an anatomic defect in the uterus, or a decidual abnormality.

In the fourth type of retained placenta, the placenta is abnormally attached to the uterine wall. The uterine decidua is deficient or is entirely absent, and the chorionic villi penetrate the endometrium. The placenta may be completely adherent to the myometrium (*placenta accreta*), the villi may penetrate the myometrium (*placenta increta*), or the villi may reach or penetrate the serosa (*placenta percreta*). When the placenta is totally adherent, gross bleeding begins when attempts are made to remove it. Management may be conservative, in which the placenta is left to absorb, with antibiotics and oxytoxics administered; or radical, with immediate laparotomy and hysterectomy performed.

INDUCTION OF LABOR

Induction of labor is defined as starting labor by artificial methods. The first documented induction of labor was by amniotomy in 1609 by Ambroise Pare. Over the years many methods have been used for induction of labor, including inflatable bags, intranasal oxytocin, and buccal oxytocin. Because these methods have not proved safe for mother and fetus, they have largely been replaced by two methods, amniotomy (artificial rupture of the membranes) and intravenous oxytocin infusion.

Indications

Induction of labor is indicated when certain conditions threaten maternal or fetal well-being, and include PIH, chronic maternal hypertension, prevention of afibrinogenemia when intrauterine fetal death has occurred, antepartum bleeding, to permit treatment of cancer, cyanotic maternal cardiac disease, IUGR, history of rapid labors, premature rupture of the membranes, hypotonic uterine dysfunction (labor augmentation), positive oxytocin challenge test, maternal diabetes mellitus (Classes B-F), Rh isoimmunization, prior intrauterine deaths, and documented postmaturity.

Prerequisites

Prerequisites for induction of labor include a normal cephalopelvic relationship, cervical ripeness, and documented fetal maturity.

A normal cephalopelvic relationship is present when the presentation is cephalic and the head is engaged. A ripe cervix is effaced, centered (anterior), soft, and partially dilated (Lange et al., 1982). An unripe cervix is long, closed, posterior, and firm. Prostaglandins have been used effectively in attaining cervical ripening without uterine contractions (Ulmstem et al., 1982).

Fetal maturity must be documented. At least two clinical criteria must be present and supported by at least one laboratory determination (Committee on Obstetrics, 1981). Clinical criteria include: (1) 39 weeks since last menstrual period; (2) fetal heart tones documented for 20 weeks; and (3) uterine size established by pelvic examination prior to 16 weeks gestation. Laboratory determinations include: (1) 37 weeks have elapsed since positive pregnancy test; (2) ultrasound verification of the fetal biparietal diameter; and (3) amniocentesis verification of fetal lung maturity.

Contraindications

Contraindications to induction of labor include significant cephalopelvic disproportion, patient refusal, fetal distress, unfavorable fetal presentations or positions, unfilled prerequisites, previous classical cesarean delivery, placenta previa, multiple gestations, uterine overdistention by polyhydramnios, and grand multiparity. Inductions should be used with caution in primagravidas, and in women who have had previous uterine surgeries, and a past history of uterine sepsis.

Techniques and Medical and Nursing Interventions

The decision to induce labor by amniotomy, intravenous oxytocin infusion, or a combination of the two rests with the obstetrician. The nurse is the member of the health care team who assists with implementation of the induction.

SURGICAL INDUCTION

Surgical induction or amniotomy is done by the physician, who does a vaginal examination to ascertain presentation, position, station, cervical ripeness, and cervical dilation. With a sterile instrument (uterine dressing forcep, Allis' forcep, amnihook, amniotome), the amniotic sac is punctured, allowing amniotic fluid to escape vaginally.

Appropriate nursing interventions include ascertaining the client's understanding of the procedure. Explanations include: (1) that an amniotomy involves a vaginal examination; (2) that she will feel warm fluid leaking from the vagina and the leakage will continue throughout labor; (3) that uterine contractions will usually begin shortly after the procedure; and (4) reassurance that amniotomy will not harm her or the fetus.

The needed equipment is gathered; sterile instrument, gloves, prep solution or lubricating jelly. The client is positioned on her back with her knees flexed and legs apart, draped to provide privacy.

Prior to the amniotomy, the fetal heart tones are measured (preferably documented with an external fetal monitor). Following amniotomy, continuous assessment of the fetal heart rate and uterine contraction patterns is desirable by external or internal fetal monitoring. If this is not possible, the fetal heart rate may be auscultated and uterine contractions palpated at frequent intervals.

Documentation of the procedure includes the time, who performed the amniotomy, any difficulties noted, the amount, color, and odor of the amniotic fluid, fetal heart rate, and results of the vaginal examination.

MEDICAL INDUCTION

Medical induction by the use of intravenous oxytocin is initiated by the physician, who should remain immediately available throughout the induction (NAACOG, 1979). Certain prerequisites must be met prior to the use of oxytocin for induction. No cephalopelvic disproportion can exist. The cervix must be ripe. An infusion pump must be used for the infusion, along with electronic fetal monitoring equipment. Adequate personnel must be available to monitor maternal-fetal status throughout the induction.

Oxytocin is supplied in 1 ml ampules that contain 10 U. It is rapidly eliminated from or deactivated by the body with a circulatory half-life of 3 to 5 minutes. Uterine effects last 20 to 30 minutes. Oxytocin has some significant cardiovascular and renal effects. The baseline maternal blood pressure initially may decrease slightly in response to oxytocin infusion, with a 30 percent rise being noted after initiation. Cardiac output is increased, with resultant increase in renal blood flow. The average intravenous dose needed to institute uterine contractility ranges from 1 to 10 mU per minute, with the preferred dose the minimum amount needed to maintain normal uterine contractile motility. The majority of women at term will have an adequate labor pattern at 4 to 8 mU per minute (Steer & Beard, 1982; Petrie, 1981). The oxytocin is diluted in an intravenous solution and administered via piggy back with a continuous infusion pump to maintain an exact rate of flow.

Administration

Before initiating an oxytocin infusion for induction of labor, the nurse reviews the client's chart for indications, documentation of fetal maturity, and the obstetrician's order for induction (see Table 26–31). Client education regarding the procedure for induction and the expected results is completed and documented. All equipment needed is assembled: intravenous fluids and tubings, infusion pump, fetal monitor, and blood pressure equipment.

The baseline fetal heart rate and uterine

TABLE 26-31
NURSING RESPONSIBILITIES IN INDUCTION BY OXYTOCIN INFUSION

Complete initial client assessment
Evaluate and document cervical status, station, presenting part, membrane status, and indications for induction
Explain procedure to the client and her coach
Apply fetal monitor and obtain 20-minute baseline strip
Maintain client in left lateral position or position of comfort
Ensure adequate hydration status (125 ml/hour)
Initiate main intravenous line
Set up oxytocin infusion according to the physician's order. Rotate the intravenous solution to ensure adequate mixing
Piggyback oxytocin infusion to main intravenous line via infusion pump at the port nearest the IV insertion site and commence infusion at a beginning rate of 0.5 to 1 mU/min or at the rate ordered by the physician
Remain with the client continuously for at least the first 20 minutes, minimum, to evaluate uterine response, labor pattern, and fetal heart rate response
Advance oxytocin infusion rate in 1 to 2 mU/min increments every 15 to 20 minutes according to uterine response until the uterine contraction pattern is every 2 to 3 minutes, with a duration of 50 to 60 seconds
Record B/P with each increase in oxytocin rate
Increment dosage of oxytocin above 20 mU/min should not exceed 4 mU/min for 20 minutes. Do not double oxytocin after 4 mU/min as it increases the risk of uterine hyperstimulation and may decrease the frequency of uterine contractions
Document on the fetal monitor strip and the client's chart:
- Nurse's full name on the strip at the beginning of the shift
- Initial the strip thereafter
- Client name, hospital number, date, time, indication for monitoring, and whether induction or augmentation
- Maternal vital signs
- Hourly documentation of assessment of fetal heart rate for baseline, variability, periodic changes
- Oxytocin dosage changes
- Hourly documentation of uterine contraction pattern for frequency, duration, and intensity
- All procedures, vaginal examinations, medications, position changes, etc.
- Any interventions done pertinent to uterine contraction pattern or fetal heart rate

activity status is determined for a minimum of 20 minutes prior to starting the oxytocin infusion. Maternal physiologic parameters are obtained.

The primary intravenous fluid is started while obtaining a 20-minute fetal heart rate and uterine activity baseline. The piggyback oxytocin infusion is prepared. Normally the oxytocin infusion contains 10 mU oxytocin per ml solution (0.5 ml in 500 ml intravenous solution or 1 ml in 1000 ml intravenous solution).

The physician must be present when the oxytocin infusion is started, usually at the rate of 1 to 2 mU per minute. After initiation of the oxytocin infusion via infusion pump, the physician must be immediately available. The nurse maintains the induction by assessing and recording the fetal heart rate and uterine activity every 10 to 15 minutes. The dosage level of oxytocin is increased according to assessment of uterine activity (see Table 26-32). The fetal heart rate in relation to

TABLE 26-32
OXYTOCIN FLOW RATES AND DOSAGES WITH CONVERSION TABLE

mU (chamber size 15 gts/min)	Flow rate
IVAC infusion (gtts/min)	
0.6	1 gtt
1.2	2 gtt
2.4	4 gtt
3.6	6 gtt
4.8	8 gtt
6.0	10 gtt
7.2	12 gtt
8.4	14 gtt
9.6	16 gtt
10.8	18 gtt
12.0	20 gtt
13.2	22 gtt
IMED infusion	
0.5	3 ml/hr
1.0	6 ml/hr
2.0	12 ml/hr
3.0	
4.0	24 ml/hr
5.0	
6.0	36 ml/hr
7.0	
8.0	48 ml/hr
9.0	
10.0	60 ml/hr
11.0	

uterine activity is assessed and documented. Maternal vital signs are assessed at frequent intervals.

Dosage is stabilized with uterine activity maintained at 2- to 3-minute uterine contractions of 50 to 60 seconds duration, with an intensity of approximately 50 mm Hg intrauterine pressure (if direct intrauterine monitoring of uterine contractions is used).

Complications

Induction of labor carries with it the risk of certain complications, including prolapse of the umbilical cord, uterine hyperstimulation, tetanic uterine contractions, fetal distress, chorioamnionitis, water intoxication, and hyperbilirubinemia in the neonate.

Prolapsed Umbilical Cord

Prolapse of the umbilical cord may occur if an amniotomy is done when the presenting part is not engaged or if the fetus is in other than a cephalic presentation. Nursing interventions include assessing for the presence of a prolapsed umbilical cord (see Table 26-28).

Uterine Hyperstimulation

The increase in uterine contractility that occurs with oxytocin administration is dose-related. Any dosage above the threshold level increases the amplitude and frequency of uterine contractions. The threshold varies with each patient.

When uterine hyperstimulation occurs, the oxytocin dosage is decreased by two increments and the uterine activity is constantly observed for 20 minutes (NAACOG, 1979). Hyperstimulation occurs when uterine contractions are more often than every 2 minutes or when the baseline uterine tone increases to over 15 to 30 mm Hg pressure as observed with an internal pressure catheter. If normal baseline tone and uterine contractions are not established and maintained, it may be necessary to discontinue the oxytocin infusion. When normal uterine tone and activity have been reestablished, stimulation of uterine activity may be resumed.

Tetanic Contractions

A *tetanic uterine contraction* is a sustained contraction with no relaxation of the uterine muscle. The contracting uterus needs more oxygen than is available, resulting in hypoxia and lactic acidosis. If this is prolonged, the deficiency in oxygen may lead to nonrelaxation of the uterus (uterine tetany) with uteroplacental insufficiency and resultant fetal distress.

When tetanic contractions occur, assessments include those for abruptio placentae (see Table 26–8) and uterine rupture (see Table 26–9). Immediate discontinuation of the oxytocin infusion and notification of the physician are appropriate nursing interventions. Maternal vital signs are assessed for signs of shock, the fetal heart rate is assessed for signs of distress, and uterine contraction activity is assessed for return to normal baseline and contraction patterns.

Fetal Distress

Immediate discontinuation of the oxytocin infusion and notification of the physician are appropriate when fetal distress is noted. The client is maintained on her left side with oxygen by face mask if the distress pattern is caused by inadequate placental perfusion. If the distress is caused by cord compression, the maternal position is changed (see Table 16–13).

Chorioamnionitis

Chorioamnionitis may occur after the membranes are ruptured. Maternal vital signs, especially the temperature and pulse are assessed for elevations. The fetal heart rate baseline is assessed for tachycardia (over 160 BPM), which may occur up to 24 hours before the maternal temperature becomes elevated. The odor of the amniotic fluid is assessed.

Water Intoxication

Oxytocin has an antidiuretic effect through its action on the distal convoluted tubules and collecting ducts. It causes increased water reabsorption from the glomerular filtrate. The combination of oxytocin in association with large amounts of electrolyte-free glucose in water can lead to retention of fluid, low serum chloride levels, and progressive oliguria. Water intoxication can be avoided by monitoring the amount of water and oxytocin administered to the client and accurately monitoring intake and output. An electrolyte solution and increased concentrations of oxytocin are used to limit the fluid volume infused when oxytocin dosages are over 20 mU per minute.

Hyperbilirubinemia in the Neonate

When the fetus has substantial exposure to oxytocin infusions, there is an increase in plasma bilirubin at birth. There have been several reasons proposed for this increase in bilirubin: oxytocin may interfere with hepatic maturation, increase bilirubin production, decrease the conjugation and excretion of bilirubin, and alter the red blood cells, making them more likely to be removed from the circulation.

Monitoring the amounts of oxytocin administered during induction or augmentation of labor will help to avoid this problem. Notification of the special care nursery when intravenous oxytocin is administered will alert them to the possibility of significant jaundice in the neonate.

UTERINE INVERSION

In uterine inversion, the top of the endometrial cavity protrudes through the cervix into the vagina and may even protrude outside the introitus. Inversion may be partial or complete.

The reported incidence of uterine inversion ranges from 1 in 100,000 to 1 in 500,000 deliveries. Causes include multiparity with lax abdominal muscles and walls, and faulty management of the third stage of labor with excessive fundal pressure (Crede's maneuver), or traction on the umbilical cord before placental separation. Some inversions are spontaneous. More than half the reported cases have occurred in primiparas.

Diagnosis

Acute uterine inversion is diagnosed when an unusual hard mass is felt in the vagina or is seen protruding from the vaginal introitus. Shock out of proportion to blood loss is usually seen, probably caused by the tension on the nerves of the broad ligament and irritation of the peritoneum. The fundus of the uterus is not felt on abdominal palpation.

Medical and Nursing Interventions

Immediate replacement of the uterus by the physician is the procedure of choice when diagnosis is made. Blood is drawn for type and crossmatched, and maternal vital signs are monitored. A second intravenous line is established to help maintain fluid volume. The uterus is replaced under anesthesia to its original position. If manual replacement is not possible, immediate surgery may be required. Antibiotics are given prophylactically to prevent postpartum or postoperative infections.

VERSION AND EXTRACTION

Version is a procedure in which the fetus is turned in utero for the purpose of changing fetal presentation. With a *cephalic version*, the resulting presentation is cephalic. *Podalic version* results in a breech presentation. Extraction is the immediate forceful delivery of the fetus.

External Version

External version is version in which all manipulations are done externally through the maternal abdominal wall.

PREREQUISITES

Before external version is attempted by the physician, certain prerequisites must be met: the pregnancy must be single, the fetal position must be accurately identified, no cephalopelvic disproportion can exist, the fetus must be freely moveable, the membranes must be intact, uterine relaxation is necessary, and the maternal abdominal wall must be lax and thin. External version is ideally carried out with the aid of ultrasonography.

CONTRAINDICATIONS

Contraindications to external version include deep engagement of a breech presentation, congenital anomalies, fetal death, multiple pregnancy, premature rupture of the membranes, antepartum bleeding, and previous uterine surgeries.

NURSING INTERVENTIONS

Before the physician initiates external version, the procedure is explained thoroughly to the client. For an external version to be successful, client cooperation is essential. Maternal vital signs and fetal heart tones are obtained before external version. The bladder is emptied, the client lies flat on her back with a pillow under her head, the abdomen is uncovered, and the knees are flexed.

During external version, premature separation of the placenta may occur. The uteroplacental circulation may be interfered with during the fetal manipulations. Preterm labor may follow fetal manipulations.

Following external version, fetal position is documented. Maternal vital signs and fetal heart tones are taken and documented.

MEDICAL AND NURSING INTERVENTIONS

Fetal heart rate is monitored throughout the procedure. The client's bladder and rectum are emptied. An intravenous infusion is started, blood is available, and maternal vital signs are monitored. The client is placed in a lithotomy position and anesthetized. During the version, maternal and fetal physiological status are constantly monitored.

Internal Version

With *internal version,* turning of the fetus is accomplished with the fingers or hand inside the uterus. The feet are grasped, and the fetus is turned to a footling breech presentation.

INDICATIONS

Internal version is done when immediate rapid delivery is essential, e.g., prolapsed umbilical cord, compound presentation with an arm prolapsed below the fetal head, second twin when descent does not occur within 30 minutes of delivery of the first twin, or transverse lie. It is done in the delivery room with adequate anesthesia.

DANGERS

Maternal dangers from internal version include rupture of the uterus, cervical lacerations, abruptio placentae, or postmanipulative infection. Dangers to the fetus include intrauterine asphyxia, anesthesia narcosis, intracranial hemorrhage, and trauma.

PREREQUISITES

Before internal version is attempted by the obstetrician, accurate diagnosis of fetal position is essential. The fetus must be alive. No cephalopelvic disproportion can exist, and the cervix must be completely dilated.

OPERATIVE DELIVERIES

Forceps Deliveries

Obstetric forceps were invented by Peter Chamberlin in the early 1700s to extract the fetal head during labor. The obstetric forceps consist of two crossing blades that fit over the fetal head. There are many different types of forceps (see Figs. 26–19 and 26–20), some for general duty and others for specialized functions.

USES

Obstetrical forceps are used either for traction or rotation of the fetal head during delivery.

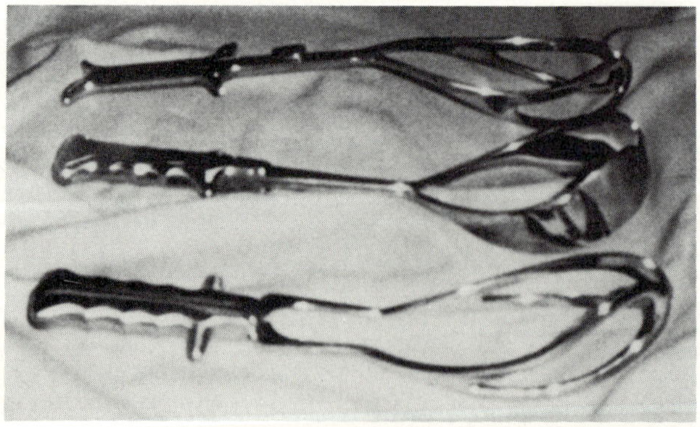

FIGURE 26–19. Types of obstetrical forceps: Simpson forceps. Tucker-McLean forceps. Kielland forceps.

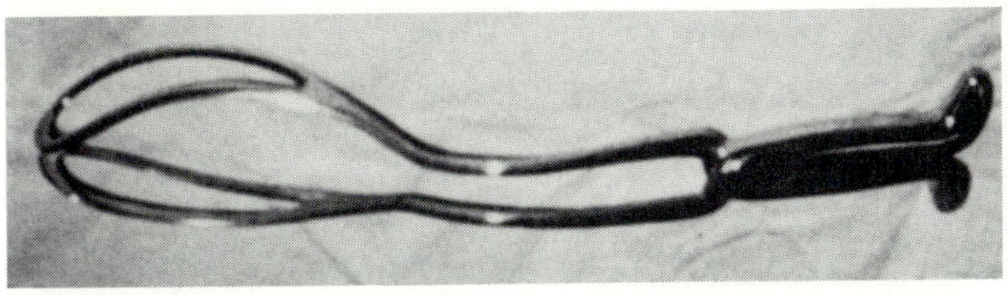

FIGURE 26-20. Piper forceps.

TYPES OF FORCEPS DELIVERIES

Low or Outlet Forceps

Low forceps are applied after the fetal head has reached the perineal floor and the sagittal suture of the fetal head is in the anteroposterior diameter of the pelvic outlet.

Midforceps

With midforceps the forceps are applied before the criteria for low forceps are met but after engagement has taken place. The biparietal diameter of the fetal skull has passed through the maternal pelvic inlet. Any forceps delivery that requires artificial rotation of the fetal head, regardless of the station of the head, is designated a "midforceps rotation."

High Forceps

High forceps are applied to the fetal head before it is engaged in the maternal pelvis. They are seldom, if ever, used in obstetrics today.

INDICATIONS

A forceps delivery is justified if the risk to the mother and to the fetus is less than the risk of waiting for spontaneous delivery to occur. Maternal exhaustion is noted by dehydration, concentrated urine, and elevated temperature and pulse. When maternal exhaustion occurs, uterine dysfunction may follow, and a forceps delivery will shorten the second stage of labor. When maternal disease (pregnancy-induced hypertension, cardiac disease, pulmonary disease) is present, it may be desirable to shorten the second stage of labor and avoid prolonged bearing-down efforts.

Fetal distress indicates the need for immediate delivery. If the prerequisites are met, low or outlet forceps will expedite delivery of the fetus and increase the chance for extrauterine survival.

When failure of descent or failure of internal rotation of the fetal head during the second stage of labor occurs, forceps delivery is indicated.

Elective forceps are used to prevent fetal distress and reduce injury and discomfort to the mother. The rationale for elective forceps delivery includes reducing the incidence of pelvic and perineal relaxations, avoiding painful hemorrhoids that occur following prolonged bearing-down, and preventing trauma to the fetal head from prolonged perineal pressure.

PREREQUISITES

Before forceps are applied by the physician, certain prerequisites must be met. The vertex must be presenting and be at no higher than a 0 station. Complete cervical dilation and ruptured membranes are needed. There should be no evidence of cephalopelvic disproportion, and no bony or soft tissue obstruction. The physician must be able to accurately diagnose fetal position and station. The maternal bladder and bowel must be empty. Aseptic conditions must be maintained. Adequate anesthesia must be available.

CONTRAINDICATIONS

Contraindications to use of obstetrical forceps include absence of indications for use, incomplete cervical dilation, marked cephalopelvic disproportion, fetal head not engaged, and lack of expertise by the physician.

HAZARDS

Even in the hands of an experienced physician, obstetrical forceps are not without hazards. Maternal hazards include lacerations of the cervix and vagina, ruptured uterus, injury to the bladder and rectum, and fracture of the coccyx. Fetal hazards include cephalhematoma, intracranial hemorrhage, skull fracture, brachial plexus palsy, facial paralysis, and cord compression.

MIDFORCEPS DELIVERY

Midforceps delivery may be indicated in malpositions of the fetal head such as persistent occiput posterior positions, transverse arrest, uterine inertia occurring during the second stage of labor, and life-threatening maternal or fetal conditions. In any circumstances where midforceps are used, the decision is made by the physician according to the circumstances of that particular moment.

NURSING INTERVENTIONS

Accurate and careful assessment of maternal vital signs and the fetal heart rate is necessary. Explanation by the physician may need to be reinforced by the nurse.

Postpartum, maternal vital signs are monitored for signs of hypovolemic shock caused by excessive bleeding. Uterine firmness is assessed to prevent uterine atony and hemorrhage.

The neonate is assessed for any indication of injury—brachial plexus palsy, facial palsy, skull fracture, bruising, or forcep marks.

VACUUM EXTRACTOR

Popular in Europe, the vacuum extractor is used as an alternative to forcep vaginal deliveries. It consists of a metal suction cup which is fixed to the fetal scalp with a negative pressure of 0.7 to 0.8 kg. The fetal scalp is drawn into the cup, creating an artificial caput succedaneum.

Indications are the same as for forceps, with the exception that it cannot be used for face presentations or on the aftercoming head in breech presentations. The vacuum extractor can be applied at any time after 5 cm cervical dilation.

Maternal complications include vaginal or cervical lacerations caused when maternal tissue is caught between the cup and the fetal head. Fetal problems include artificially induced caput succedaneum, minor scalp abrasions, and cephalhematoma.

Cesarean Delivery

Cesarean delivery is the delivery of the fetus through an incision made in the maternal abdominal wall and the uterus. The first professional cesarean delivery in the United States was done in 1827.

INCIDENCE

The reported incidence of cesarean delivery varies from 10 to 30 percent of all deliveries. Over the last decade, the incidence of cesarean births has increased dramatically. Many factors have influenced these increases. Cesarean births are much safer for the mother and fetus today than in the past. Low birth weight neonates are delivered more often by cesarean delivery to reduce the trauma associated with a vaginal delivery. Primigravidas are more likely to have a primary cesarean delivery than are multigravidas. The trend toward regionalization and delivering high-risk mothers and neonates in tertiary perinatal centers has also increased the incidence of cesarean delivery.

INDICATIONS

Indications for cesarean delivery can be absolute or relative. A condition that makes vaginal delivery impossible is an *absolute indication.* With a *relative indication,* vaginal delivery may be possible, but cesarean delivery is felt to be safer for the mother or the fetus.

Four diagnostic categories account for 80 percent of all cesarean deliveries: repeat cesarean delivery, dystocia, breech presentations, and fetal distress (Shearer, 1981). Indications are summarized in Table 26–33.

Repeat cesarean deliveries are done when the gravida has a history of a cesarean delivery with the last or previous pregnancies. There are two schools of thought concerning repeat cesarean deliveries. One school maintains that if a previous cesarean delivery was done for other than disproportion and if there are no contraindications to labor and vaginal delivery with this pregnancy, a trial labor may be allowed. The other school maintains that once a cesarean, always a cesarean.

TABLE 26–33
INDICATIONS FOR CESAREAN DELIVERY

- Repeat cesarean delivery
- Dystocia
  - Fetopelvic disproportion
  - Malpositions
  - Soft tissue dystocia
  - Failed forceps deliveries
  - Neoplasms
  - Malpresentations
  - Congenital uterine anomalies
  - Lack of progress in labor
- Breech presentations
- Fetal distress
- Other indications
  - Previous uterine surgeries
    - Myomectomy
    - Hysterotomy
    - Cervical suturing
  - Maternal pathophysiology
    - PIH
    - Cardiac disease
    - Diabetes mellitus
    - Chronic kidney disease
  - Maternal hemorrhage
    - Placenta previa
    - Abruptio placentae
  - Previous fetal death or damage
  - Progressive Rh incompatibility
  - Elderly primigravida
  - Postmaturity
  - Previous vaginal repair
  - Active genital herpes

TYPES OF CESAREAN DELIVERIES

There are four basic types of cesarean deliveries: lower segment, classical, extraperitoneal, and cesarean hysterectomy.

Lower Segment Cesarean Delivery

Lower segment cesarean delivery can have either a vertical or a horizontal abdominal incision (see Figure 26–21). It permits safe abdominal delivery even when uterine infection is present. The uterine incision is made through the lower uterine segment, which minimizes blood loss. The resultant uterine scar is stronger.

Classical Cesarean Delivery

In a classical cesarean delivery a vertical incision is made into the maternal abdomen and the wall of the body of the uterus (see Figure 26–21). This incision is useful when the fetus is transverse or when adhesions are present in the lower uterine segment or the bladder area. There is more maternal blood loss than with a lower uterine segment incision and there is a higher incidence of uterine rupture with subsequent pregnancies.

Extraperitoneal Cesarean Delivery

This procedure was designed to allow access to the lower uterine segment by lateral displacement of the bladder and peritoneal fold. The technique is relatively difficult and often results in accidental entry into the peritoneal cavity and injury to the maternal bladder. It is used in grossly infected cases to prevent peritonitis and is seldom done today.

Cesarean Hysterectomy

In this procedure, a cesarean section is done followed by a hysterectomy. Indications include uncontrolled maternal hemorrhage, placenta accreta, unrepairable rupture of the uterus, and cancer of the cervix or ovary.

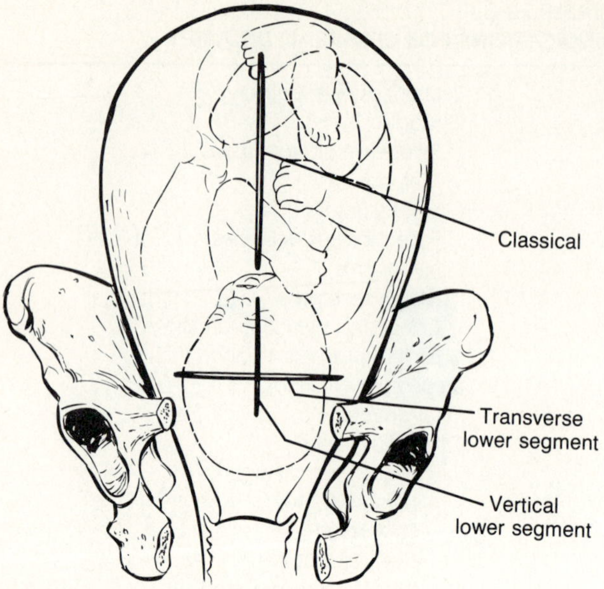

FIGURE 26-21. Types of cesarean delivery.

MATERNAL COMPLICATIONS

Infections of varying types, including intrauterine abscesses, respiratory and urinary tract infections, wound abscesses, and generalized sepsis are still the major postoperative problems. Hemorrhage, adhesions, fistulas, sinuses, wound dehiscence, subsequent uterine rupture, injury to adjacent structures, blood transfusion complications, thromboembolism, aspiration pneumonia, and anesthesia complications have all been reported in the literature.

FETAL COMPLICATIONS

Many fetal complications following cesarean delivery are the result of maternal obstetrical complications. Maternal conditions such as PIH, hypertension, Rh isoimmunization, and placenta previa require delivery before fetal maturity, thus increasing the incidence of respiratory distress in the neonate. Small-for-gestational-age and large-for-gestational-age neonates are also the result of existing maternal complications. The effect of maternal drug administration may be seen in the neonate. Maternal hypertension can result in fetal hypoxia and neonatal acidosis.

NURSING INTERVENTIONS

Emotional preparation for women who are to have a cesarean delivery is of vital importance. The woman who is to have an elective cesarean delivery has ample time for psychological preparation. She may have disturbing memories of her previous cesarean birth and her postoperative period, which must be worked through before this cesarean. Her partner also needs to be prepared emotionally for this experience.

Women who are having an unplanned cesarean are emotionally unprepared for the surgery. They are often tired and discouraged from labor, and worried about themselves and the fetus. Preoperative preparations are often done quickly and without thorough explanations. Anxiety levels are high, so listening is selective. Explanations, even though brief, must be offered to the client and to her partner. Time needs to be spent during the postoperative period with both parents to reconstruct the events leading to the cesarean, and to aid them in working through the grieving process since their attempt at vaginal delivery was unsuccessful.

Emotional care is an important aspect of nursing interventions for either planned or unplanned cesarean delivery, in addition to the usual preoperative and postoperative nursing interventions. A nursing care plan for a gravida having an unplanned cesarean delivery can be found in Table 26-34.

PERINEAL AND CERVICAL INJURIES

Perineal Lacerations

CAUSES

Causes of perineal lacerations that occur during delivery include rapid and sudden expul-

TABLE 26–34
SAMPLE NURSING CARE PLAN: UNPLANNED CESAREAN DELIVERY

A.B., a 24-year-old, gravida 1 para 0 at term was admitted in active labor at noon. On admission, she was 3 cm cervical dilation at −1 station. The presenting part was cephalic. FHR were within normal limits via external fetal monitoring. Uterine contractions were 3 minutes apart, lasting 50 seconds, and of good intensity. After 4 more hours of good uterine contractions, she had not changed in terms of cervical dilation or station. FHR baseline remained 140 to 150 BPM, variability was decreased, and late deceleration patterns were noted. Nursing interventions were not effective in relieving the fetal heart rate deceleration pattern. Dr. F. did a fetal scalp pH, which showed pH of 7.17. A decision was made to do an emergency cesarean delivery.

Nursing Diagnosis	Goals	Nursing Interventions	Rationale	Evaluation
Knowledge deficit related to cesarean delivery	The client and coach verbalize understanding of and reason for cesarean delivery	Assess client knowledge regarding cesarean Discuss need for cesarean Briefly explain: Preoperative preparation Consent Laboratory tests Abdominal prep Foley catheter Types of anesthesia	Knowledge will decrease anxiety and aid in preoperative preparation	Reason for cesarean explained—verbalized understanding
Anxiety related to uncertain fetal outcome secondary to documented fetal distress in labor	The client has the opportunity to verbalize fears and concerns for the fetus	Assess client understanding of present fetal status and expected outcome	Client needs to know current status and expected outcomes to begin psychological acceptance	A. crying over possible poor fetal outcome Minister gave added support during preoperative preparations
Alteration in self-concept related to interrupted labor and delivery plans	The client verbalizes understanding of alteration in planned delivery	Identify behaviors that may signify guilt feelings Encourage ventilation of fears and concerns Offer reassurance Be nonjudgmental	Client needs to understand there is no guilt	No problem at this time

sion of the presenting part during delivery, a large fetus, difficult midforceps delivery, difficult breech extractions, pelvic outlet contractions, and friable maternal tissues.

CLASSIFICATION

Perineal lacerations may be classified into four degrees:

First degree. Involves vaginal mucosa, fourchette, and perineal skin.

Second degree. Involves vaginal mucosa, fourchette, perineal skin, and perineal muscle.

Third degree. Involves vaginal mucosa, fourchette, perineal skin, perineal muscle, and the rectal sphincter.

Fourth degree. Involves vaginal mucosa, fourchette, perineal skin, perineal muscle, rectal sphincter, and the anterior rectal wall.

Vulvar and Anterior Vaginal Wall Lacerations

These lacerations may be located in the tissue on either side of the urethra, labia minora, lateral vaginal wall, clitoris, urethra, and bladder. Upper vaginal wall lacerations are more common with operative vaginal deliveries and bleed profusely.

Cervical Lacerations

SUPERFICIAL CERVICAL LACERATIONS

Superficial lacerations of the cervix occur during almost every labor as the cervix effaces and dilates. These small surface lacerations heal spontaneously and require no treatment or suturing.

DEEP CERVICAL LACERATIONS

Deep lacerations occur during precipitate labors, with a rigid or scarred cervix, during forceful delivery of the fetus through an incompletely dilated cervix, breech extractions, and delivery of a large fetus.

Deep cervical lacerations are diagnosed when the cervix is inspected following delivery. The cervix is grasped with ring forceps so that the total cervix can be visualized. Careful repair of deep lacerations is important to control postpartum bleeding and to prevent excessive scarring and erosions.

CERVICAL INCISIONS

When immediate vaginal delivery is required and the cervix is incompletely dilated, Duhrssen's cervical incisions may be used to facilitate delivery of the fetus. These incisions are made at 2, 6, and 10 o'clock, which creates the equivalent of complete cervical dilation and allows the fetus to deliver vaginally.

ANNULAR CERVICAL DETACHMENT

During a prolonged labor, the anterior lip of the cervix may become compressed between the fetal head and the maternal symphysis pubis. This compression leads to poor circulation in the cervix, anoxia of the cervical tissue, and eventual necrosis. A tear starts at the junction of the vagina and the cervix, and continues with detachment taking place at 4 to 5 cm cervical dilation. Annular detachment occurs with true cervical dystocia. Since the vessels are thrombosed before detachment occurs, bleeding is not a problem and no treatment is usually needed.

AMNIOTIC FLUID EMBOLISM

Amniotic fluid embolism is a rare complication of labor that occurs in 1 in 8,000 to 1 in 80,000 live births. A small amount of amniotic fluid is infused into the maternal circulation, causing respiratory distress, cardiovascular collapse, and possible maternal death. Maternal mortality approaches 86 percent.

RISK FACTORS

Predisposing factors associated with the occurrence of amniotic fluid embolism include difficult rapid labor, oxytocin infusion, large fetus, intrauterine fetal demise, meconium-stained amniotic fluid, multiparity, advanced maternal age, cervical tears, abruptio placentae, ruptured uterus, cesarean delivery, presence of IUD throughout pregnancy, and intra-amniotic injection of hypertonic saline for midtrimester abortion.

SYMPTOMS

Amniotic fluid embolism seldom occurs in the absence of labor (Sterner et al., 1984). The onset of symptoms may occur during labor, delivery, or in the early puerperium. The client suddenly develops acute respiratory distress and shock. She has chest pain, dyspnea, tachycardia, and cyanosis. She may convulse and become comatose. Pulmonary edema with pink frothy sputum, afibrinogenemia, and uterine relaxation with hemorrhage also occur.

PATHOPHYSIOLOGY

The two major infusion sites of entry are the endocervical veins and the uteroplacental area. The exact mechanism of entry is not known, but it is postulated that amniotic fluid that contains fetal debris, such as squamous cells, lanugo, and fat, enters the maternal circulation (Kitzmiller, 1982). Once in the maternal venous system, the fluid returns through the right heart and becomes lodged in the pulmonary vasculature. The lungs become edematous, with hemorrhage of the alveoli, and emboli formation. The right side of the heart is often dilated and may contain amniotic fluid. Pulmonary hypertension occurs as a result of fetal debris and vasopasm.

MORTALITY

Maternal mortality is high, with the majority of deaths resulting directly from the embolism. Fetal mortality is high if the embolism occurs during labor and delivery.

MEDICAL AND NURSING GOALS

If the mother is undelivered, delivery is accomplished as rapidly as possible. The high-risk nursery is alerted to the possibility of a compromised neonate.

Medical and nursing goals in treatment of the mother include life support, reduction of pulmonary hypertension, increasing tissue perfusion, relief of bronchospasm, supportive care, and replacement of coagulation factors.

In spite of the many complications that may affect the mother and fetus during labor and delivery, intelligent and accurate nursing assessments and interventions will continue to decrease mortality during this period.

BIBLIOGRAPHY

Affonso, D.D. & Stichler, J.F. Cesarean section birth. Women's reactions. *American Journal of Nursing,* 1980, **80,** 468.

Barden, T.P., Peter, J.B. & Merkatz, I.R. Ritodrine hydrochloride: A betamimetic agent for use in preterm labor. Part I. *American Journal of Obstetrics & Gynecology,* 1980, **56,** 1.

Benedetti, T.J. Maternal complications of parenteral β-sympathomimetic therapy for premature labor. *American Journal of Obstetrics & Gynecology,* 1983, **145,** 1.

———, Hargrove, J. & Rosene, K.A. Maternal pulmonary edema during premature labor inhibition. *Obstetrics & Gynecology,* 1982, **59**(suppl), 33.

Berkowitz, G.S. An epidemiologic study of preterm delivery. *American Journal of Epidemiology,* 1981, **112,** 1092.

Blanco, J.D. & Gibbs, R.S. Infections following classical cesarean section. *Obstetrics & Gynecology,* 1980, **55,** 167.

Brown, S.M. & Tijani, N.A. Terbutaline sulfate in the prevention of recurrence of premature labor. *Obstetrics & Gynecology,* 1981, **57,** 22.

Burchell, H.J., et al. Uterine contraction patterns in abruptio placenta. *South African Medical Journal,* 1985, **67,** 48-50.

Cohen, W.R., et al. Risk of labor abnormalities with advancing maternal age. *Obstetrics & Gynecology,* 1980, **55,** 414.

Committee on Obstetrics. Maternal and fetal medicine. Assessment of fetal maturity. American College of Obstetrics & Gynecology, 1981.

Cotton, D.B., et al. The effects of terbutaline on acidbase serum electrolytes and glucose homeostasis during management of preterm labor. *American Journal of Obstetrics & Gynecology,* 1981, **141,** 617.

Creasy, R.K., et al. Oral ritodrine maintenance in the treatment of preterm labor. *American Journal of Obstetrics & Gynecology,* 1980, **137,** 212.

Duff, P. Diagnosis and management of face presentation. *Obstetrics & Gynecology,* 1981, **57,** 105.

External cephalic version used for 'breeches.' *Clinical Aspects of High Risk Pregnancy,* 1984, **2,** 7.

Flood, B. & Naeye, R.L. Factors that predispose to premature rupture of the fetal membranes. *Journal of Obstetric, Gynecological & Neonatal Nursing,* 1984, **13,** 119.

Friedman, E.A. *Labor, evaluation and management.* New York: Appleton-Century-Crofts, 1978.

Gibbs, R.S., et al. Management of acute chorioamnionitis. *American Journal of Obstetrics & Gynecology,* 1980, **136,** 709.

Gold W.R. & Levine, A.M. Pinpointing a major source of OB malpractice claims. *Contemporary Obstetrics & Gynecology,* 1982, **20,** 214.

Guzick, D.S. & Winn, K. Chorioamnionitis links to 25% of premature births. *Clinical Aspects of High Risk Pregnancy,* 1984, **2,** 1.

Harris, B.A. Dealing with a difficult delivery. *Emergency Medicine,* 1984, **16,** 24.

Jagani, N., Schulman, H., et al. Role of the cervix in the induction of labor. *Obstetrics & Gynecology,* 1982, **59,** 21.

Katz, M., et al. Cardiovascular complications associated with terbutaline treatment for preterm labor. *American Journal of Obstetrics & Gynecology,* 1981, **139,** 605.

Kitzmiller, J.L. & Lucas, W.E. Studies on a model of amniotic fluid embolism. *Obstetrics & Gynecology,* 1982, **39,** 626.

Lange, A.P., et al. Prelabor evaluation of inducibility. *Obstetrics & Gynecology,* 1982, **60,** 137.

Liggins, G.C. New concepts of what triggers labor. *Contemporary Obstetrics & Gynecology,* 1982, **19,** 131.

Marshall, C. The art of induction/augmentation of labor. *Journal of Obstetric, Gynecological & Neonatal Nursing,* 1985, **14,** 22-27.

Mercer, L.J., et al. A survey of pregnancies complicated by decreased amniotic fluid. *American Journal of Obstetrics & Gynecology,* 1984, **149,** 355.

NAACOG. Induction of labor. *NAACOG Technical Bulletin No. 4,* 1979.

NAACOG. Preterm labor and tocolytics. *OGN Nursing Practice Resource #10,* 1984.

Nimrod, C., et al. Pulmonary edema associated with isoxsuprine therapy. *American Journal of Obstetrics & Gynecology,* 1984, **148,** 625.

Ouelette, S.M. Some success with terbutaline for inhibition of preterm labor. *Hospital Forum,* 1981, **16,** 1179.

Petrie, R.H. The pharmacology and use of oxytocin. *Clinics in Perinatology,* 1981, **8,** 35.

Phillipsen, T., et al. Pulmonary edema following ritodrine-saline infusion in premature labor. *Obstetrics & Gynecology,* 1981, **58,** 304.

Rayburn, W.F., et al. Umbilical cord length and intrapartum complications. *Obstetrics & Gynecology,* 1981, **57,** 450.

Read, J.A., et al. Randomized trial of ambulation versus oxytocin for labor enhancement. A preliminary report. *American Journal of Obstetrics & Gynecology,* 1981, **139,** 669.

Rosene, K.A., et al. Cerebral ischemia associated with parenteral terbutaline use in pregnant migraine patients. *American Journal of Obstetrics & Gynecology,* 1981, **143,** 405.

Schreiber, J. & Benedetti, T. Conservative management of preterm premature rupture of the fetal membranes in a low socioeconomic population. *American Journal of Obstetrics & Gynecology,* 1980, **136,** 92.

Shearer, E. NIH consensus development task force on cesarean childbirth. The process and the result. *Birth & Family Journal,* 1981, **8,** 24.

Shortridge, L.A. Using ritodrine hydrochloride to inhibit preterm labor. *MCN,* 1983, **8,** 58-61.

Smith, J.J., et al. Placenta previa reappraisal and new therapeutic classification (HALO). *New York State Journal of Medicine,* 1982, **82,** 1037.

Spisso, K.R., et al. The use of magnesium sulfate as the primary tocolytic agent to prevent premature delivery. *American Journal of Obstetrics & Gynecology,* 1982, **142,** 840-845.

Steer, P.J. & Beard, R.S. Bettering control of oxytocin infusions. *Contemporary Obstetrics & Gynecology,* 1982, **19,** 117.

Sterner, S., Campbell, B. & Davies, S. Amniotic fluid embolism. *Annals of Emergency Medicine,* 1984, **13,** 343.

Stewart, P., Kennedy, J.H., et al. Spontaneous labor. When should the membranes be ruptured? *British Journal of Obstetrics & Gynecology,* 1982, **89,** 30.

Taenaka, N, Shimada, Y, Kawhi, M., et al. Survival from DIC following amniotic fluid embolism. *Anaesthesia,* 1981, **35,** 389-393.

Takahashi, K., Diamond, F., et al. Uterine contractility and oxytocin sensitivity in preterm, term, and postterm pregnancy. *American Journal of Obstetrics & Gynecology,* 1980, **136,** 774.

Ulmsten, U., Wingerupt, L., et al. Intracervical application

of prostaglandin gel for induction of term labor. *Obstetrics & Gynecology,* 1983, **59,** 336.
Varner, M.W. & Gakasjm R.P. Conservative management of premature rupture of the membranes. American Journal of *Obstetrics & Gynecology,* 1981, **140,** 39.
Watson, P., Besch, N. & Bowes, W.A., Jr. Management of acute and subacute puerperal inversion of the uterus. *Obstetrics & Gynecology,* 1980, **55,** 12.
Ying, Y.K. & Tejani, N.A. Angina pectoris as a complication of ritodrine hydrochloride therapy in premature labor. *Obstetrics & Gynecology,* 1982, **60,** 385.
Zervoudakis, I., Krauss, A. & Fuchs, F. Infants of mothers treated with ethanol for premature labor. *American Journal of Obstetrics & Gynecology,* 1980, **137,** 713.

chapter 27

COMPLICATIONS DURING THE PUERPERIUM

OBJECTIVES

Upon completion of this chapter, the reader will be able to:

1. Define postpartum hemorrhage.
2. State the three causes of postpartum hemorrhage; identify symptoms of each; discuss appropriate nursing interventions.
3. Discuss the types of puerperal infection; identify appropriate nursing interventions.
4. Given a client with a venous thrombosis, identify predisposing factors, symptoms, and nursing interventions.
5. Differentiate between engorgement and mastitis.
6. Discuss prevention, causes, and treatment of postpartum urinary tract infections.
7. Identify signs, symptoms, and behavioral changes that occur with postpartum psychosis.

KEY TERMS

Endometritis
Hematoma
Mastitis
Parametritis
Postpartum hemorrhage
Retained placenta
Subinvolution
Uterine atony
Uterine inversion

The more common complications during the puerperium include postpartum hemorrhage, infections, and thrombophlebitis. Many less common complications may occur, including postpartum psychosis, renal failure, postpartum vulvar edema, Chiari Frommel syndrome, and adult respiratory distress syndrome.

POSTPARTUM HEMORRHAGE

Postpartum hemorrhage is most often defined as blood loss in excess of 500 ml following delivery. Hemorrhage during the puerperium accounts for about one-fourth of deaths from obstetrical hemorrhage.

Most commonly, postpartum hemorrhage occurs within the first hour after delivery (fourth stage of labor) but may occur two or more weeks after delivery. Although uterine atony, lacerations of the reproductive tract, and retained placenta are the most common causes, other causes are of equal importance (see Table 27–1).

Predisposing Risk Factors

In the majority of cases, postpartum hemorrhage can be predicted before it occurs. Many predisposing factors can be identified as high-risk factors for postpartum hemorrhage (see Table 27–2).

TABLE 27–1
CAUSES OF POSTPARTUM HEMORRHAGE

Early Hemorrhage
- Uterine atony
- Lacerations of the vagina, cervix, perineum, or lower uterine segment
- Retained placenta
- Uterine inversion
- Blood dyscrasias

Late Hemorrhage
- Retained placental fragments or membranes
- Subinvolution of the uterus
- Hematoma

PREVENTION OF HEMORRHAGE

Specific nursing assessments and interventions will often prevent the occurrence of early postpartum hemorrhage. Assessing for predisposing risk factors during the initial patient assessment (see Table 16–1) and from the prenatal record will identify the potential hemorrhage patient.

Following delivery, the uterine fundus must be checked frequently and massaged as necessary to keep it well contracted and to expel clots. Frequent assessment of maternal vital signs will identify impending hypovolemic shock. Careful and accurate assessment of intake and output during labor will prevent hypovolemia and aid in prevention of hemorrhage after delivery. Administration of the correct oxytocic medications in the prescribed dosage at the ordered time will decrease the

TABLE 27–2
PREDISPOSING RISK FACTORS FOR POSTPARTUM HEMORRHAGE

- History of previous hemorrhage
- Grand multiparity
- Uterine fibroids
- Idiopathic thrombocytopenia purpura
- Chronic anemia
- Abruptio placentae
- Placenta previa
- Uterine overdistention from multiple pregnancy, polyhydramnios, fetus over 4500 grams, etc.
- Prolonged labor
- Precipitate labor
- Traumatic labor and/or delivery
- Chorioamnionitis
- Cesarean delivery
- General anesthesia
- Induction of labor
- Coagulation defects
- Pregnancy-induced hypertension
- Dystocia
- Administration of tocolytic medications

occurrence of bleeding. Reevaluation of the client status before leaving the delivery or birthing room in terms of bleeding and potential for bleeding will aid in planning the type of nursing interventions needed during the fourth stage of labor.

Symptoms

The symptoms observed in postpartum hemorrhage depend upon the maternal blood volume and degree of anemia (if any) before delivery. Bleeding from uterine atony can be differentiated from bleeding caused by lacerations in the uterus. Bleeding caused by lacerations is bright red and occurs despite a firm, well-contracted uterine fundus, whereas bleeding from uterine atony is usually darker and has clots with a boggy, noncontracted uterine fundus.

Moderate maternal blood loss may not be reflected by severe hypotension or tachycardia. There may be no sudden massive hemorrhage but rather a steady vaginal bleeding that is moderate in amount but persists until serious hypovolemia occurs.

Medical and Nursing Interventions

GENERAL PRINCIPLES

Fresh blood products and plasma expanders are available for identified high-risk clients, since stored blood has decreased factors V, VIII, and platelets, causing increased oxygen affinity and less release to peripheral tissues. Stored blood also has an increased potassium and ammonia content.

An intravenous line with a large bore needle is kept open until the mother is stable. Hemoglobin, hematocrit, and coagulation factors are obtained and assessed. Oxytocin is administered after delivery to contract the uterus and keep it well contracted.

With massive hemorrhage the goal is to maintain the maternal hematocrit at 30 percent or more and the urinary output at 30–60 ml per hour. Arterial blood gases are measured at the onset of bleeding and after every 5 units of packed cells are administered. Platelet counts are made with every 6 to 8 units transfused. The client is given 100 percent oxygen by mask and antibiotics to prevent puerperal infections. Nursing responsibilities in postpartum hemorrhage are identified in Table 27-3.

On occasion, therapeutic measures are ineffective in reversing hemorrhage. Surgery may be indicated to control hemorrhage, including uterine vessel ligation, hypogastric artery ligation, and hysterectomy.

UTERINE ATONY

Uterine atony, the most common cause of postpartum hemorrhage, is the inability of the myometrium to contract and con-

TABLE 27-3
NURSING RESPONSIBILITIES IN POSTPARTUM HEMORRHAGE

Identify clients at increased risk for hemorrhage
Accurate assessments and observations
Uterine massage
Monitor vaginal bleeding
Perineal pad count
Monitor maternal vital signs
Administer oxygen via face mask
Intake and output
Monitor intravenous infusions
Administer oxytocins as ordered
Assist in administration of blood transfusions if ordered
Keep the physician informed of client's status
Assess level of consciousness
Give explanations to the client and support person
Obtain laboratory tests as ordered
Prepare for surgery if necessary
Provide support

strict the blood vessels within the muscle fibers, resulting in open sinuses at the site of placental separation.

Medical interventions include fundal massage and oxytocin administration. If the uterus does not respond to massage, the uterine cavity is reexamined. Intrauterine packing may be used to help slow blood loss if bleeding cannot be stopped while operative preparations are being made.

Nursing interventions include massaging the uterus until it is firm, taking care not to overmassage to the point of uterine relaxation. Intravenous fluids are started or maintained to increase fluid and blood volume. Oxytocin is given as ordered by the physician, usually mixed in an intravenous solution and given at a rate to contract the uterine muscle and keep it contracted. Maternal vital signs are assessed at frequent intervals. Explanations are provided to the client and support person, and emotional support is provided.

LACERATIONS OF THE VAGINA, CERVIX, PERINEUM OR LOWER UTERINE SEGMENT

Unrepaired tears, especially those deep in the vagina, cervix, or lower uterine segment, can result in profuse vaginal bleeding.

Medical preventative interventions include inspecting the vagina, cervix, and lower uterine segment after delivery and repairing lacerations that have occurred. Hemostasis is maintained by beginning the repair at the uppermost level of the tear. If hemorrhage occurs after the client has left the delivery room, she should be returned for reexamination and repair of any additional lacerations.

Nursing interventions include frequent recovery room (fourth stage of labor) assessments of vital signs, fundus, and lochia. If vaginal bleeding persists and the uterine fundus is firm, the physician is notified. Explanations of the need for return to the delivery room are given at an appropriate level of understanding. An operative permit is signed for examination under anesthesia before the client is returned to the delivery room.

RETAINED PLACENTA

Any piece of the placenta that remains in the uterus following completion of the third stage of labor interferes with vascular constriction and creates increased bleeding problems.

The placenta is expelled only after placental separation takes place. If there is incomplete separation of the placenta and increased vaginal bleeding, the placenta is removed manually. Following either placental expulsion or manual removal of the placenta, the placenta is carefully inspected to determine cotyledon absence or the presence of an accessory lobe. After placental removal, the physician will examine the uterine cavity for placental tissue.

UTERINE INVERSION

If uterine inversion occurs and the uterus turns out during the third stage of labor, shock out of proportion to external blood loss quickly follows. Prompt diagnosis and immediate replacement of the uterus are the mainstays of management.

Nursing interventions include monitoring of maternal vital signs, and providing support and explanations to the client and her partner.

BLOOD DYSCRASIAS

Any of the blood dyscrasias can affect the pregnant or newly delivered client and cause postpartum hemorrhage. Afibrinogenemia may follow abruptio placentae, prolonged retention of a dead fetus, and amniotic fluid embolism. Reduction in fibrinogen levels leads to interference with blood clotting mechanisms.

Nursing interventions include assessing for risk factors that predispose to defects in blood coagulation and frequent assessments of maternal parameters.

Delayed Hemorrhage

Delayed hemorrhage is caused by retained placenta fragments or membranes, subinvolution of the uterus, and hematoma formation.

RETAINED PLACENTAL FRAGMENTS OR MEMBRANES

When placental fragments or fetal membranes are retained for a week or more, necrosis occurs and a placental polyp develops. A dilation and curettage is completed to remove the polyp and prophylactic antibiotics are given.

SUBINVOLUTION OF THE UTERUS

Delayed return of the puerperal uterus to normal size and function is called *subinvolution.* Causes include retained placental fragments, uterine fibroids, and endometritis. A large flabby uterus, prolonged lochial flow or profuse vaginal bleeding, and backaches are frequent symptoms.

Treatment is aimed at correcting the cause. Ergonovine (Ergotrate) or methylergonovine (Methergine) are administered to hasten involution and contract the uterus. Dilation and curettage may be needed to remove the uterine contents. Antibiotics are prescribed to correct endometritis and other pelvic infections.

HEMATOMAS

When blood escapes from an injured blood vessel into the connective tissue of the external genitalia or beneath the vaginal mucosa, a hematoma forms. Most hematomas are small and located under the skin of the perineum (vulvar hematomas). If the vessels under the vaginal mucosa rupture, large amounts of blood can collect in the submucosal tissues as a vaginal hematoma. Occasionally, the hematoma may extend upward into the broad ligament.

Large vulvar hematomas cause severe perineal pain and are characterized by the appearance of a tense, sensitive mass of varying size covered by discolored skin. It is often seen on the side opposite the episiotomy. The client may be unable to void.

Assessment of the perineum will identify a swollen mass that is firm and quite tender to touch. It soon becomes discolored. Vaginal hematomas may be difficult to see, but client complaints of severe perineal pain and rectal pressure will aid in diagnosis. When the hematoma is small, no specific medical treatment may be needed. If the hematoma contains a large amount of blood, shock symptoms are noted. Accurate nursing observations and assessments, along with ice packs, analgesic medications, and good perineal hygiene, may be all that is required. The client may be given antibiotics prophylactically. Large hematomas that are enlarging require evacuation. The client is returned to the delivery room or is taken to the operating room, adequate anesthesia is administered, the hematoma is opened, blood clots are evacuated, and the bleeders are ligated. A pack may be placed in the opened hematoma by the physician and left in place for 24 hours, or the area may be resutured. Antibiotics are administered prophylactically and the client is assessed frequently for fresh bleeding, new hematoma formation, and infection.

PATIENT TEACHING

With the current emphasis on early discharge, the new mother may be discharged home with her newborn within several hours after delivery. Nursing interventions focus on client teaching. Normal uterine involution and lochial progression are identified. Signs and symptoms that should be reported immediately to the physician are stressed and include: excessive bleeding, bright red bleeding, a boggy fundus that will not firm with massage, abnormal clotting, elevations in temperature, foul-smelling lochia, and unusual pelvic discomfort.

Complications

SHEEHAN'S SYNDROME

About 15 percent of women who survive severe hypovolemic shock associated with postpartum hemorrhage develop *Sheehan's syndrome* (anterior pituitary necrosis). Infarction of all or a portion of the anterior pituitary gland leads to a decrease in or a total loss of thyroid, adrenal, and ovarian function.

Endocrine gland hypofunction in Sheehan's syndrome is characterized by failure of lactation, decreases in breast size, loss of pubic and axillary hair, genital atrophy, myxedema, amenorrhea, apathy, and fatigue.

Medical treatment includes long-term hormone replacement therapy with thyroid hormone, estrogens, and cortisone and a high-protein high-carbohydrate diet. Associated nursing interventions include client teaching (medications and diet) and emotional support.

The long-term effects of Sheehan's syndrome are infertility, decreased resistance to infection, and premature aging. Prognosis depends upon the amount of supplemental therapy required and the degree of function that remains in the anterior pituitary gland.

INFECTIONS

Infections following delivery are of three main types: puerperal, mastitis, or urinary tract. Puerperal infections are infections of the reproductive system organs after delivery and include endometritis, parametritis, and localized perineal infections.

The diagnosis of infection is based on the accepted standard for puerperal morbidity: a temperature of 100.4°F (38°C) or higher on two successive postpartum days, not including the first 24 hours after delivery. The temperature is taken by mouth at least four times a day.

Puerperal Infections

PREDISPOSING FACTORS

The greatest likelihood of puerperal infections occurs after prolonged rupture of the membranes, prolonged labor with frequent vaginal examinations, intrauterine manipulations for fetal delivery and placental expulsion, and cesarean delivery.

Other factors have also been implicated during the antepartum and intrapartum periods. Predisposing antepartum factors include anemia, low socioeconomic status, poor nutrition, and sexual intercourse after the membranes have ruptured.

Intrapartally, three factors are considered important in increasing the risk of puerperal infection. First, bacterial contamination of the uterus may occur during examinations or operative manipulations. Although sterile gloves are worn, bacteria already present on the vulva and in the vagina may be carried into the uterine cavity. Sterile gloves or instruments may become contaminated by pathogens as the result of droplet infection. This is the basis for wearing caps and masks in the delivery or birthing room as well as for the exclusion of all persons with upper respiratory infections during labor and delivery. Second, excessive blood loss during labor and delivery predisposes to puerperal infection owing to decreased resistance to pathogens. Third, trauma associated with lacerations and operative deliveries provides portals of entry and an excellent culture medium for pathogenic bacteria.

CAUSE

Sources of reproductive tract infections are endogenous or exogenous. Bacteria in the normal vaginal flora often become virulent when trauma to tissues occurs. Pathogens may be introduced via transmission from personnel, breaks in aseptic technique, or contamination from other sources. Common causative organisms include streptococci, E. coli, Staphylococcus albus, hemolytic Staphylococcus aureus, Clostridium perfringens, and Neisseria gonorrhoeae.

PATHOLOGY

When the third stage of labor is completed, the placental attachment site is raw, elevated, and dark red. The surface is nodular, owing to the numerous veins, and offers an excellent portal of entry for microorganisms. Uterine decidua is very thin (2 mm) and has many small openings that offer a portal for pathogens. In addition, small cervical, vaginal, and perineal lacerations, as well as the episiotomy site provide entry ports for pathogens. The resultant inflammation and infection can remain localized or can extend via blood or lymph vessels to other tissues.

PREVENTION

Many puerperal infections can be prevented through appropriate medical and nursing interventions. Prompt treatment of anemia during the antepartal period, good nutrition, avoidance of coitus in late pregnancy or when the membranes are ruptured, strict aseptic technique throughout the labor process, sterile perineal pads, and separation of infected and noninfected patients all will help in preventing puerperal infections, as will client teaching about peri care and proper handwashing.

ENDOMETRITIS

Endometritis, or infection of the endometrium of the uterus, is a common puerperal infection. Early postpartum endometritis occurs within 48 hours of delivery and is usually caused by both aerobic and anaerobic bacteria. Late postpartum endometritis is caused by bacteria including C. trachomatis.

TABLE 27-4
SYMPTOMS OF POSTPARTUM ENDOMETRITIS

Early
Mild temperature elevation
Late
Chills
Temperature elevation (saw-tooth pattern of elevation up to 103 to 104°F)
Tachycardia
Malaise
Loss of appetite
Headache
Backache
Generalized discomfort
Severe afterpains
Large tender uterus
Copious or decreased dark brown, foul-smelling lochia
Leukocytosis

Following vaginal delivery, the reported incidence ranges from 0.9 to 3.0 percent, with 10 to 50 percent incidence reported following cesarean delivery. Inflammatory changes occur in the superficial endometrial layers, with leukocyte infiltration into the myometrium.

Symptoms

Early postpartum endometritis may present with only a low-grade temperature. Endometritis that occurs 48 to 72 hours after delivery will have more pronounced symptoms (see Table 27-4).

Medical and Nursing Interventions

Prevention of endometritis by identification of clients at risk and control or elimination of predisposing factors is important. Other diseases are ruled out before the diagnosis is made, including urinary tract infections, mastitis, appendicitis, viral diseases, and septic pelvic thrombophlebitis.

Treatment depends on the severity of symptoms. Antibiotics are prescribed after blood cultures and lochial cultures are obtained. Supportive therapy of fluids and electrolytes is instituted and good nutritional status is maintained.

Maternal vital signs are monitored every four hours and as needed. General reactions of the client to infection such as malaise and diaphoresis are observed, assessed, and documented. Intake and output are recorded to maintain adequate hydration. Isolation is usually ordered, so explanations regarding isolation and separation from the neonate are provided. Every effort is made to maintain contact between the client and her neonate. Frequent reports of neonatal progress and bringing the baby to the door of the room so she can see him are two ways contact can be maintained.

Ergonovine (Ergotrate) or another oxytocic may be ordered to increase uterine tone. A mid-Fowler's position in bed is encouraged to promote gravity flow of drainage.

PARAMETRITIS

Parametritis, or pelvic cellulitis, is puerperal infection that has spread beyond the endometrium into the surrounding pelvic structures including the broad ligament. Pelvic cellulitis is often unilateral, with the infection limited to the base of the broad ligament, but it may be bilateral and extend to the pelvic walls and umbilicus.

Symptoms

Symptoms noted include a prolonged high temperature, chills, elevated leukocyte count, and positive blood and urine cultures. Pain and tenderness are noted on one or both sides of the abdomen.

As the process advances, the uterus may become fixed by the exudate and a mass may develop in the broad ligament. In the majority of cases, absorption of the exudate occurs, but it may take several weeks.

Medical and Nursing Interventions

Antibiotics must be used to treat the infection. Nursing assessments include possible abscess formation. If an abscess forms, surgical drainage is necessary.

EPISIOTOMY INFECTION

Local pain and dysuria, with or without urinary retention, are the usual symptoms of a simple episiotomy infection. The skin and underlying soft tissue of the posterior portion of the vulva are most commonly involved. Staphylococcus or enteric gram-negative bacteria are the usual pathogens.

Management of these localized infections includes emotional support. Removal of the sutures will enhance drainage. Analgesics and Sitz baths will help to relieve perineal pain. Antibiotics are usually prescribed during the acute phase of the infection.

Mastitis

Mastitis, infection of the breast, occurs in about 1 percent of puerperal women. The source of the infection may be the hands of the client, personnel caring for her, the neonate, or it may be blood-borne.

PREVENTION

The best preventative measures are good breast hygiene, aseptic technique, and checking the nipples for cracks, which are portals of entry for pathogens.

SYMPTOMS

The symptoms include:

Marked breast engorgement
Chills
Elevated temperature
Tachycardia
Malaise
Acute breast pain
Breast tenderness

Physical assessment reveals erythema over the infected breast or breast segment, axillary lymph gland enlargement, and marked tenderness to palpation.

MEDICAL AND NURSING INTERVENTIONS

Cultures of breast milk and other nipple drainage are taken and appropriate antibiotic therapy initiated. Breastfeeding may be discontinued during antibiotic administration, depending on the antibiotic ordered. Application of heat or cold (depending on the stage of infection) is recommended. A support bra should be worn at all times. Personal hygiene is reviewed and stressed. Small side pillows for extra breast support when lying down may help decrease discomfort. If an abscess develops, incision and drainage are performed.

Urinary Tract Infections

Postpartum urinary tract infections are usually caused by E. coli. Several factors predispose to their development: increased bladder capacity, decreased bladder tone, decreased perception of the need to urinate, and insufficient emptying of the bladder.

SYMPTOMS

Symptoms noted with puerperal urinary tract infections vary with the location of the infection. Lower urinary tract infections are characterized by frequent small voidings or an inability to urinate, dysuria, hematuria, bacteriuria, and pus cells in the urine. Symptoms of upper urinary tract infections include chills, elevated temperature, tenderness over one or both kidneys, malaise, nausea, and vomiting.

MEDICAL AND NURSING INTERVENTIONS

A catheterized or clean catch urine specimen is obtained and sent to the laboratory for urinalysis, culture, and sensitivity. Oral fluids are encouraged. Antibiotic therapy is prescribed for seven to ten days. Assessment for increase or decrease in symptoms is important. The importance of taking all of the medication prescribed is stressed to the client. Maternal vital signs are monitored for changes.

THROMBOPHLEBITIS

Thrombophlebitis occurs in fewer than 1 percent of puerperal patients and is divided into three different types: superficial, femoral, and pelvic thrombophlebitis.

SUPERFICIAL THROMBOPHLEBITIS

Superficial thrombophlebitis usually involves the superficial saphenous veins and is characterized by tenderness along the vein with increased skin temperature in the involved region. Little edema or redness is noted. Treatment is with analgesics, elastic leg support, and rest with the leg elevated. Anticoagulants are not administered.

FEMORAL THROMBOPHLEBITIS

Thrombophlebitis involving the femoral vein is characterized by fever, pain, and swelling in the affected leg. Other symptoms include tachycardia, positive Homan's sign (calf pain on dorsiflexion of the foot), mottling, and leukocytosis.

Treatment includes bed rest with elevation of the affected leg. A foot cradle or sheet spreader is used to keep the bed covers off the leg. Analgesics are prescribed as necessary for discomfort. Intravenous heparin is administered. If the temperature is elevated, antibiotics are given.

PELVIC THROMBOPHLEBITIS

Characteristic symptoms of pelvic thrombophlebitis are severe chills and high temperature. Following the chills, there is a precipitous fall in temperature. Anaerobic streptococcus is the usual causative organism. Antibiotics and heparin are the treatments of choice.

OTHER COMPLICATIONS

Postpartum Neurosis

Approximately 1 to 3 percent of delivered patients develop a postpartum neurosis that is nonpsychotic in nature. There are almost no precipitating factors, although it has been proposed that hormonal factors or folic acid deficiency may contribute to its occurrence.

Pregnancy-associated factors that may help to identify patients at risk for postpartum neurosis include (Braverman and Rout, 1978):

- Feeling unloved or rejected by the husband
- Undesired pregnancy
- Past history of postpartum depression
- Single status
- Marital turmoil
- Unplanned pregnancy

Depression varies from mild and temporary to severe and lengthy and is the most common symptom observed. Neurasthenia, with complaints of extreme fatigue, sleeplessness, emotional lability, and irritability, may last from a month to a year. Sexual difficulties, psychosomatic complaints and phobias that include a fear of infanticide and insanity are common. If postpartum neurosis develops, the client should not be left alone, since mood changes occur rapidly and she may be unable to care for herself or her baby.

Postpartum Psychosis

Symptoms of postpartum psychosis usually appear about the third day after delivery. Early symptoms include insomnia, restlessness, exhaustion, depression, irritability, and mood swings. As the psychosis worsens, the client becomes suspicious, confused, and incoherent, makes irrational statements, expresses excessive concern over trivia, and may refuse to eat.

The cause is unknown, but possible precipitating factors have been identified. The birth experience, personality traits, environmental factors, psychological adaptation to pregnancy, hormone withdrawal following delivery, and fear of the maternal role have all been implicated as possible factors in the development of puerperal psychosis.

Other Complications

CHIARI-FROMMEL SYNDROME

Chiari-Frommel syndrome is a rare puerperal complication characterized by prolonged galactorrhea that is not associated with breastfeeding.

Symptoms include profuse leaking of fluid from the breasts, headaches, hearing loss, visual loss, and genital atrophy, possibly caused by a pituitary tumor or prolonged phenothiazine treatment. There is no effective treatment. Clomiphene citrate (Clomid) may induce ovulation, and bromocryptine (Parlodel) will aid in suppressing lactation.

ACUTE RENAL FAILURE

Acute renal failure in the puerperium occurs as a sequel to uterine hemorrhage, septic abortion, or eclampsia.

POSTPARTUM VULVAR EDEMA

Postpartum vulvar edema usually begins two to three days after delivery. The client develops unilateral vulvar and perineal edema with induration that spreads to the opposite side and inner pelvis within two to three days. Fever and marked leukocytosis are present. On about the fourth of fifth postpartum day, vascular collapse may occur. The cause is unknown, but the edema may respond to antibiotic therapy. Nursing assessment of physiologic and psychological status is important.

Knowledge of the normal puerperal changes that occur will aid in identifying deviations that may signify development of complications. The nurse, working in conjunction with the client and physician, can assist in recovery with appropriate assessments and interventions.

BIBLIOGRAPHY

Ballinger, C.B. Emotional disturbance during pregnancy and following delivery. *Journal of Psychosomatic Research,* 1982, **26,** 629–634.

Bowes, W.A., Jr. (Ed.). The puerperium. *Clinics in Obstetrics & Gynecology,* 1980, **23,** 971.

Braverman, J. & Roux, J.F. Screening for the patient at risk for postpartum depression. *Obstetrics & Gynecology,* 1978, **52,** 731–736.

Easterling, W.E., Jr. & Herbert, W.N.P. The puerperium. In D.N. Danforth (Ed.). *Obstetrics and gynecology* (4th ed.). Philadelphia: Harper & Row, 1982.

Eschenbach, D.A. New concepts of obstetric and gynecologic infection. *Archives of Internal Medicine,* 1982, **142,** 2039–2044.

Pass, M.A., Gray, B.M. & Dillon, H.C., Jr. Puerperal and perinatal infections with group B streptococci. *American Journal of Obstetrics & Gynecology,* 1982, **143,** 147.

chapter 28

THE PREGNANT ADOLESCENT

OBJECTIVES

Upon completion of this chapter, the reader will be able to:

1. Discuss the ramifications of adolescent pregnancy.
2. Identify the factors that may account for the increase in adolescent pregnancy.
3. Discuss the role of sex education in prevention of adolescent pregnancy.
4. Identify contraceptive methods appropriate for the adolescent.
5. Identify complications of pregnancy that are more frequent in the adolescent.
6. Identify appropriate nursing interventions for the adolescent parent in the antepartum, intrapartum, and postpartum periods.
7. Discuss involvement of the adolescent father during pregnancy.
8. Identify resources that are available for adolescent parents.

KEY TERMS

Adolescence
Adolescent
Psychological development
Puberty

Adolescent pregnancy is a socioeconomic problem with specific implications for medicine and nursing. Each year more than 1 million American teenagers become pregnant, with 80 percent of these unmarried. There are more than 500,000 infants born each year to women under 20 years of age (U.S. Department of Public Health, 1985). Many of these (over 30,000) are born to teenagers under the age of 15. If this present trend continues, 40 percent of today's 14-year-old girls will be pregnant at least once before the age of 20.

Adolescent pregnancy imposes hardships on all generations of the family, regardless of the family structure in which it occurs. The young mother with small children is more likely to live below the poverty level. More than half do not complete high school, earn less money, and are more likely to be on welfare.

In the last ten years there has been a decline in the overall number of pregnancies in women between the ages of 16 and 19 years, with an increase in pregnancies under the age of 15. Pregnancy rates have remained fairly constant among minority girls under 15 years of age, with the increase occurring in white middle-class females. Nearly half of black females in the United States have been pregnant at least once by age 20. Among black females, the pregnancy rate is almost twice that among white females.

Although black adolescents have a higher overall pregnancy rate than whites, white adolescents far surpass their peers in other countries in rates of pregnancy. According to the Alan Guttmacher Institute, the United States leads all developed nations in pregnancy rates among girls aged 15 through 19, although they are not more sexually active than their counterparts.

The issue of adolescent pregnancy affects many facets of society. The economic impact of interrupted education and low-paying jobs has far-reaching implications for our society. The social issues of abortion rights, adolescent access to contraceptives, sex education in our school systems, welfare programs, and family structures are affected by pregnancy among adolescents.

In the last 30 years, societal mores and attitudes have changed dramatically. Thirty years ago, there were many teenage pregnancies, but the majority occurred among married teenagers. Early marriages were often the solution to an unwed teenager's pregnancy. Abortion was not a legal option for the pregnant teenager. Other pregnant teens moved away during their pregnancies, had their babies, gave them up for adoption, and returned home. Few kept their babies and maintained unmarried status.

Today legal abortion is an option used by about 45 percent of pregnant teenagers as the solution to pregnancy. For those teenagers who elect to carry their pregnancies, about 75 percent are illegitimate. Of illegitimate infants, only about 5 percent are given up for adoption.

INCREASES IN ADOLESCENT PREGNANCY

The adolescent in our urban society faces many tasks in the maturational process. Our culture dictates that even the mature adolescent remain partially dependent. Society expects the adolescent to accomplish separation from parents, determination of a sexual role, development of a value system, and selection of a vocation. At the same time as it expects these maturational tasks to be accomplished, society places constraints on adolescents that inhibit accomplishment of these tasks.

Physical Changes at Puberty

The growth spurt of the adolescent is the second major period of accelerated growth in the human. The first growth spurt starts at birth and lasts until about two-and-a-half years of age. During this growth spurt the infant doubles, triples, and quadruples his birth weight. Following this growth spurt, childhood is a quiescent period of growth. When the child reaches preadolescence, there is another sudden increase in the rate of growth that initiates pubertal changes.

The adolescent growth spurt involves all muscular and skeletal dimensions of the body. In most boys, puberty begins between the ages of 13 and 15, with growth continuing until approximately 21 years of age. In girls, pubertal changes start between 10 and 13 years of age, and growth ends at approximately age 18.

The sequence of events during adolescence is fairly predictable, although there is large variation from individual to individual. About one year before the onset of the height spurt, the child will show a marked increase in fat deposition, lasting for about two years, then diminishing as the skeletal growth rate and muscle mass increase. Girls deposit more subcutaneous fat than boys and lose it at a slower rate.

The maturational changes in the reproductive system are related to the rapid growth of the musculoskeletal system. Reproductive system changes are usually poorly understood and often ignored by health professionals who work with adolescents. Boys are often hesitant to talk to the nurse about reproductive development, while girls are apt to talk more freely with the nurse about sex and sexual development.

PUBERTAL DEVELOPMENT IN BOYS

Male pubertal development takes place over approximately a four-year period. The following progressive changes take place: (1) increase in the size of the testes and reddening of the scrotum; (2) the appearance of lightly pigmented hair at the base of the penis coinciding with the onset of the overall growth spurt; (3) increase in the length and width of the penis; (4) appearance of circumanal, perineal, and axillary hair; (5) pubic hair becomes adult in amount and type; (6) appearance of facial hair; and (7) deepening of the voice.

PUBERTAL DEVELOPMENT IN GIRLS

In girls, breast development usually is the first sign of puberty. Breast development occurs in stages: (1) preadolescent elevation of papilla; (2) breast bud stage with elevation of the breast and papilla as a small mound; (3) enlargement and elevation of breast and areola without separation of the contours; (4) projection of the areola and papilla to form a mound above the level of the breast; and (5) maturity, with projection of papilla and recession of the areola into the breast contour. A frequent complaint of adolescent girls is tenderness during the breast bud stage. This concern is frequently communicated to the nurse and should serve as a signal for health education.

Growth and development of the uterus and vagina begin at about the same time as the breast bud appears. The vaginal pH becomes acid, and the epithelial layers become gray, mucoid, and thickened from estrogen effects. During this period the adolescent may notice a slight vaginal discharge.

Pubic hair first appears on the labia, then the mons veneris. Within approximately two years, the pubic hair takes on the adult triangular configuration. Menarche most commonly appears between the ages of 10 and 13 years, after the spurt in height has occurred. Linear growth occurs following menarche but at a slower rate.

PSYCHOLOGICAL DEVELOPMENT IN ADOLESCENTS

The adolescent period is one of extreme mood swings, and is called by some psychologists the second negative phase. The adolescent is subject to frequent mood changes, at one moment depressed, the next happy. He or she is frequently rebellious and "touchy," yet still demanding and dependent. The adolescent tests and struggles as he struggles for independence in the process of establishment as an adult.

This period of growth is one of adjustment to new feelings, impulses, and stress. Needs of the adolescent are many. Endocrine changes concurrent with adolescence produce many tensions. Temper outbursts and unreasonable behavior are frequent occurrences.

Establishment of Independence

Major causes of difficulties in adjustment during adolescence occur as the teenager tries to establish independence and assume a role as an adult. The adolescent years are anxious years. Behaviors that are seen as rebellious result from attempts to show parents that he is no longer a child and is capable of making independent decisions.

Relationships With Siblings

Poor sibling relationships commonly occur during the adolescent years. It is not unusual for teenagers to have frequent disagreements, to become critical and derogatory toward one another, and to be embarrassed over public behavior of their brothers and sisters. This is normal during adolescence and reflects a concern and awareness of self-image.

Peer Groups

Peer group support is very important to the adolescent. The adolescent lacks self-confidence, and the peer group functions to provide support and security at a time of life when insecurity seems insurmountable for the teen.

Sexual Activity

American adolescents are more sexually active than they used to be. During the 1970s, sexual intercourse among unmarried teenagers increased by two-thirds. In 1982, 1 of 5 15-year-old girls admitted to having had intercourse, as did one-third of 16-year-olds and 43 percent of 17-year-olds (Zelnick & Young, 1982).

Why this dramatic increase? The average age of menarche has dropped to 12.5 years for whites and 11.8 years for blacks. There are heavy sexual messages in all media that bombard the senses with the insinuation that sophistication is equated with sexual activity. Peer mores are established through a comparison and testing of the standards of morality, deriving a set of flexible standards for the adolescent.

Adolescents try to achieve a balance between impulse and control. They need to learn to assume responsibility for sexual expression. Society can help them assume responsibility by increasing involvement in two areas: sex education and contraceptive information.

SEX EDUCATION FOR THE ADOLESCENT

Adolescent feelings and attitudes about sex often reflect those of their parents. If questions about sex are handled with hesitancy and uneasiness in the home situation, the adolescent soon gets the impression that these matters are not to be discussed at home, and looks elsewhere for information. Many parents are so uncomfortable with sexual discussions that they prefer information to be obtained from outside the home environment. Parents may feel that giving sexual information will lead to acting out sexual scenes by the adolescent.

When the parents fail to give accurate information about sexual changes or sexual feelings to the adolescent, the responsibility is often shifted to the schools.

Sexual information needed by the adolescent depends, in part, on the amount and type of information already provided in the home. Often information given is not at a level appropriate to the adolescent's understanding.

The child will also only assimilate information that he is ready to accept.

Nursing Interventions

Sexual information should be presented by a qualified person in order to ensure accurate dissemination and factual information at a level of understanding appropriate to the stage of development. Early adolescents are concerned with physical and emotional changes that are occurring. A basic knowledge of anatomy and physiology is appropriate teaching for the early adolescent. Older adolescents are more concerned with sex, sexual changes, and how to behave in certain situations. A comfortable atmosphere that is conducive to questions and discussion is needed. The adolescent is encouraged to verbalize individual concerns. All discussions and questions are treated in a nonjudgmental manner. It is important for the nurse to demonstrate that restraint in handling impulses is possible, while at the same time demonstrating to the adolescent an appreciation of how difficult it is for young people to go through adolescence and handle these feelings and desires. Sexual information should not be accompanied by moralistic warnings. These warnings will only increase curiosity, anxiety, and guilt.

Discussions should include subjects that are particularly anxiety-producing in the adolescent: sexual function, masturbation, venereal disease, nocturnal emissions, and sexual relationships. The timing of these discussions is ideally when the subjects are brought up by the adolescent.

Visual aids such as plastic models and charts are useful when discussing sexual development with adolescents. Allowing the adolescent to talk about "other kids" or what his friends think is a useful approach in dealing with sexual topics. Questions are encouraged to identify what information is needed, rather than presenting information totally in a specific format.

Written material is useful to supplement information, but should not be used to the exclusion of visual aids and discussions. It is often difficult for the adolescent to verbalize a specific question, and written information may provide the information the adolescent seeks.

The end result of sexual education for the adolescent is the impression that there are responsible adults who understand the teenager's feelings and who wish to be helpful during the striving toward adulthood.

CONTRACEPTION

Approximately 62 percent of teenage pregnancies are associated with no birth control usage. Inconsistent use accounts for 30 percent of pregnancy in adolescents. With some adolescents, inadequate or inaccurate information seems to be the major cause of unwanted pregnancies. In other adolescents, the knowledge is adequate, but motivation for consistent usage is lacking. Despite the increasing availability of contraception education to the public, there are many misconceptions and much misinformation.

Teenagers usually do not identify either schools or health professionals as sources of contraceptive information, but rely on the peer groups as sources of information. The majority of teenage girls know where to obtain family planning information and supplies but do not use them. One factor that is identified in contraceptive use is client instruction. In order to use a contraceptive method successfully, a thorough knowledge of the method chosen is required.

Choosing a method of contraception for the

adolescent creates another dilemma. Many of the available birth control methods are not appropriate or reliable for the adolescent, because of either physical effects or psychological readiness to use the selected form of contraception.

Oral contraceptives are less popular today. Side effects may prohibit their selection and use of hormones when sexual activity is sporadic make them a less than desirable contraceptive form for the adolescent. Intrauterine devices are becoming less acceptable (and less available), owing to the documented increases in pelvic inflammatory disease and ectopic pregnancy. Diaphragm use may not be acceptable to the adolescent, as it is contrary to spontaneity in sexual activity. In addition, many adolescents are squeamish about touching their genitals.

According to Planned Parenthood, the most practical and realistic birth control method for teenagers is the condom and foam (Morgan and Barden, 1985.) Even though they are slightly less effective than some other methods, they are inexpensive, readily available, and the condom offers protection against venereal disease.

Nursing Interventions

Counseling to both sexes includes understanding contraceptive use. Feelings need to be explored to gain reassurance in decision making. The adolescent needs to know how to share responsibility in contraceptive use.

Scientific knowledge of reproductive physiology is presented at an appropriate knowledge level to aid in selection of a contraceptive method and sharing of responsibility. A nonjudgmental approach used in a nonthreatening environment will generate the best results for the adolescent who is sexually active.

ADOLESCENT PREGNANCY

During adolescence, individual identity is established. Relationships with parents are altered as peer relationships are identified and established. The adolescent feels dependent and independent at the same time, and frequent alterations and swings in behavior are common. Risk-taking behaviors are common and may be initiated without identifying long-term consequences.

Psychological Traits

What psychological traits characterize the pregnant adolescent? Many studies have attempted to identify psychological differences in teens who get pregnant. The pregnant teen has been characterized as a neurotic lonely girl whose emotional needs have not been met in the home and who seeks emotional stability outside of the home. Unwed mothers and fathers tend to come from homes dominated by one parent, usually the mother, and the girl may purposely become pregnant to punish the parent. Premature sexual expression and activities are characterized as caused by a lack of parental supervision and discipline that creates defective ego control in the presence of sexual drive. Some studies have identified teenage pregnancy following the loss of a significant other in the family situation.

Despite these studies identifying certain personality traits apparent in some pregnant adolescents, it is generally agreed that there is no identifiable psychological "type" who becomes pregnant.

Out-of-wedlock pregnancy is identified as the beginning of a cycle that includes a failure to continue education, a dependency on a state welfare system, prohibition of stable family relationships, and continuation of the cycle of illegitimacy.

Risks in Adolescent Pregnancy

Certain tasks are faced by the pregnant adolescent: (1) confirmation of the pregnancy; (2) acceptance or denial of the fact of pregnancy; (3) involvement of the family unit; (4) the decision of whether to marry or not to marry; and (5) the question of termination or continuation of pregnancy. If the pregnancy is continued, the question of adoption or retention of the child must be faced.

HEALTH RISKS

The pregnant adolescent is vulnerable to unique problems of pregnancy that are created by her own physical and emotional immaturity. The death rate from pregnancy complications is much higher in girls under age 15. Pregnancy-induced hypertension is more common among adolescents, most probably influenced by undernutrition and inadequate prenatal care. Preterm or prolonged labor is also more frequent in the adolescent.

The need for early and continuous medical care and supervision during pregnancy is often not understood. Delay in going to a clinic or physician for prenatal care may be caused by shame, fear of parental reaction, or ignorance of the fact of pregnancy. Inadequate prenatal care often compounds the problem of adolescent pregnancy by poor eating habits, smoking, or substance abuse.

The fetus in an adolescent pregnancy is also at increased risk. Low birth weight is more common in neonates of adolescents, and may suffer from immature organ systems, difficulty in maintaining a neutral thermal environment, mental retardation, congenital malformations, and an increased risk of death during infancy.

PSYCHOLOGICAL RISKS

The adolescent mother and her infant also suffer risks from social and economic factors. Two of three pregnant girls drop out of school when pregnant and do not return. Lack of job skills may force them into low-paying dead-end jobs. The rate of attempted suicide and child abuse is high among these families.

Needs

The way in which the needs of the unwed expectant mother are met will be the result of the interaction of identification of needs, resources available, and her personal desires. Certain specific needs of the unwed adolescent have been identified: (1) early diagnosis and continued health supervision of pregnancy; (2) plans for pregnancy, delivery, the newborn, and the future; (3) awareness of resources available; (4) knowledge about sexual functioning; (5) child care instruction and support in child care during early infancy; (6) support for reproductive decisions she makes, whether to terminate pregnancy, continue pregnancy and keep the baby, or continue the pregnancy and give the infant up for adoption; and (7) continuation of the adolescent maturational process that has been interrupted by pregnancy.

Antepartum Period

Coping ability of the adolescent during the antepartum or prenatal period depends on certain factors: stage of development, stage of adolescence, value system, relationship with parents, culture, relationship with boyfriend, physical condition, and resources available.

When pregnancy is confirmed, the young mother's first reaction will vary from anger, tears, fear, or even complete apathy. She needs a chance to react in her own individual way and needs to be encouraged to express her feelings.

Following the initial shock phase when pregnancy is confirmed, she will begin to understand that she has important choices to make that will affect her future and that of her unborn child. Once pregnancy is confirmed in the adolescent, her choices include continuation of the pregnancy and keeping the baby, continuation of the pregnancy and giving the baby up for adoption, or termination of pregnancy.

As she begins to work through her choices, resources need to be identified to aid her in making her decisions.

NURSING INTERVENTIONS

The nurse who is knowledgeable about adolescent decision-making abilities can aid the adolescent in making the decision that is best for her particular situation. Information is presented in a factual manner at an appropriate level of understanding to the adolescent and her support person (preferably a parent) to aid her in accepting the fact of pregnancy and making the reproductive decision necessary.

The adolescent may be afraid to openly discuss pregnancy or pregnancy alternatives with either her family or the nurse. She may be afraid of judgment on the part of her parents and the nurse.

The perception of the significance of pregnancy will vary greatly from adolescent to adolescent, depending at least in part on the level of maturation when the pregnancy is diagnosed. Other factors include her level of ambivalence, her future goals, the meanings she associates with pregnancy, and her sexual partner's attitudes about the pregnancy.

Working with an adolescent during pregnancy can be difficult for the nurse. Adolescent reactions to situations are often unpredictable, and the nurse may have difficulty in coping with the expressed or unexpressed reactions. The nurse must be aware that the adolescent is basing her decisions on a different developmental level. When this level is identified, it will be easier for the nurse to aid the adolescent.

TERMINATION OF PREGNANCY

If the adolescent is contemplating termination of pregnancy, the problems become complex. The complexity stems from many sources, which may be conflicting. The adolescent may want to please her parents and her sexual partner, affirm her own values and ethics, balance her career and motherhood goals, complete her education, and enjoy the adult status provided by motherhood (Brown, 1983).

Nursing Interventions

The nurse plays an important role in the decision made by the adolescent. Open, frank, and nonjudgmental characteristics are needed by the nurse in dealing with the pregnant adolescent who is contemplating termination of pregnancy. The abortion procedure used is determined by the length of pregnancy and must be explained fully to the girl. While this information is factual, other factors need to be resolved if pregnancy termination is decided, especially arrangement of transportation and finances. If the pregnancy is to be kept a secret, arranging for time off from school may be a problem that must be resolved.

Another important factor is the girl's relationship with her parents. Parental reactions may demand that the girl terminate the relationship with her partner, refrain from further sexual activities, initiate contraception, and impose a curfew. These demands will place considerable stress on the girl.

Moral issues and religious affiliations may also compound a decision to terminate a pregnancy. These young girls are caught between their desire to terminate the pregnancy and opposition to abortion for moral or religious reasons. Referral to clergy may be of benefit.

Different cultures have different attitudes toward abortion. The pregnant adolescent will in part base her pregnancy decision on the standards dictated by her cultural or ethnic backgrounds.

Before nurses can counsel adolescents who are facing decisions about pregnancy termination, they must be aware of their own feelings and attitudes about pregnancy, adolescents, and abortion. If the nurse is not comfortable with these issues, she should refer the girl to another health professional who can assist in decision making.

The irreversibility of abortion may be a relief for some adolescents. For others, it may lead to intense feelings of guilt. With nursing guidance and teaching, the majority of adolescents will make the decision that is best for them at this point in their life, cope as well as possible, accept the finality of the abortion, and continue their lives.

CONTINUATION OF PREGNANCY

If the decision is made to continue with the pregnancy, the continuation of prenatal care is paramount. Prenatal visits by the adolescent may be decreased because of pregnancy denial, ignorance, a casual attitude, nonavailability of services, or inappropriate methods of service delivery.

One way of providing continuation of prenatal care for the adolescent is through childbirth preparation classes geared to her particular level of development. Adolescents often hold a highly fantasized view of pregnancy and parenthood. Childbirth preparation classes will help them to prepare not only for pregnancy and labor and delivery, but will help prepare them for realistic parenting. The atmosphere of these classes should be informal but informative. Questions are encouraged and group discussions allow the pregnant teen to realize that she is not alone in her questions and concerns. Teens are encouraged to bring along a support person who will become a labor coach during labor and delivery. The importance of the support person is emphasized, not only for the support that will be provided to the girl, but as an aid in resolution of some of the family conflicts that have arisen because of the pregnancy.

Teaching topics are arranged according to the phase of pregnancy, and include nutrition, fetal development, labor and delivery, infant care, the importance of well-baby checkups following delivery, parenting skills, and contraception. Role playing is one useful means of imparting information during these classes.

Nutrition for the Pregnant Adolescent

When adolescence and pregnancy are superimposed on each other, proper nutrition is of utmost importance. Proper nutrition can prevent or modify some of the common hazards faced by the pregnant teen and her growing fetus.

Energy or calorie intake must be sufficient to allow tissue development in the girl and her developing fetus, protein synthesis, and to meet the increasing energy demands of pregnancy. When calorie intake is limited, dietary protein consumed will be used for energy and not for synthesis of new tissues. At least 300 extra calories a day are needed. One way of identifying adequate calorie intake is monitoring the pattern of weight gain during pregnancy. Specific nutritional needs of the pregnant adolescent during pregnancy are discussed in Chapter 11.

INVOLVING THE ADOLESCENT FATHER

Tradition identifies the adolescent father as the irresponsible, promiscuous villain victimizing the adolescent female. In actuality, that is not generally true. Many of these young men would like to marry their partners and give whatever financial, social, and psychological support they can. They are anxious to participate in the parenting of their children but need help and support to assume a responsible role.

Adolescent fathers often come from backgrounds similar to the pregnant girl. Their income is low and they have not completed their education. If they drop out of school to work and provide financial support, they head straight for low-paying jobs.

It is often difficult for health care personnel to reach and work with young fathers. There are few programs organized to help teenage fathers. Many prenatal clinics do not include the father in their plans.

The adolescent father-to-be has many conflicts to resolve. His idea of what a father is supposed to do may be minimal or nonexistent. He may come from a home with minimal or absent paternal contact, giving him no role model to imitate.

Even when he desires to provide financial support, there is considerable stress and concern. His low-paying job may not even provide necessities, and this may be seen as a threat to his masculinity. If he remains committed throughout pregnancy, he will lose peer relationships that are needed for his further maturation. The girl's family may be angry with him, and his family may be disappointed and angry. His relationship with the girl will change dramatically. He will have to deal with body image and psychological changes normal during pregnancy without the appropriate knowledge to aid in coping.

Nursing Interventions

Nursing interventions include education and guidance for the adolescent father. He should be given an opportunity to feel a part of the pregnancy. Participation in childbirth preparation classes and parenting programs is invaluable. A nonthreatening environment with a nonjudgmental approach, and education at an appropriate level for understanding will provide him the means for involvement during pregnancy.

Intrapartum Period

There is no one single predictable response of a gravida in labor. Each client brings to labor her total self, which includes physical characteristics, psychological makeup, cultural identity, and ethnic background. Among adolescents in labor, there are also no absolute predictable responses.

Certain responses are more prevalent in the adolescent. She may have difficulty separating pain from outcome and view the discomforts of labor as an ordeal or punishment. A lowered pain threshold is coupled with lack of knowledge and anxiety, creating a stressful situation, at best, and a crisis situation, at worst. Regression to childish behavior is not uncommon.

Her modesty may lead to embarrassment about being exposed. Obtaining cooperation is often difficult, owing to anxiety, feelings of helplessness, and loss of control over the situation.

NURSING INTERVENTIONS

The focus of nursing interventions during labor is to help the adolescent to attain and maintain a sense of control. A nonjudgmental approach that is firm without being authoritative will give direction to the behavior of the adolescent during labor.

If no support person is present, the nurse is both a coach and a support person in addition to her other duties. If a support person is present, the nurse should encourage the supportive coaching role without interfering with established relationships. The parent and boyfriend may both be present and competing for the girl's attention, requiring diplomacy in handling the situation.

Explanations are provided honestly at an appropriate level of understanding. Do not talk down to the teenager; they are adolescents who need help in coping with the situation.

Postpartum Period

Adolescents tend to have a lower pain threshold and will often complain about physical discomforts during the early puerperium. Behaviors may be regressive, and the adolescent may refuse to assist in or perform self-care.

NURSING INTERVENTIONS

The nurse should set limits for the adolescent who displays regressive or demanding behaviors. Assessment of needs is important. Teaching is begun when the adolescent is open and receptive to instruction. The first few days postpartum, the young mother will be enjoying the flood of attention from family and friends. When she displays an interest in or a willingness to learn about self-care or infant care, information is provided at an appropriate level. Health education needs of adolescent mothers are many, and include self-care needs, the infant's medical needs, contraceptive information, and parenting skills.

FOLLOWUP ASSESSMENTS

Having an infant during adolescence has been associated with child abuse and poor parenting skills. A lack of readiness for parenting has been documented in the adolescent (Jones et al., 1980), and these mothers have difficulty in responding to their infant's needs (Mercer, 1980). The adolescent appears more insecure in the maternal role and usually relies on her mother for medical advice. Expectations for her infant are often unrealistic. Followup needs for the adolescent are identified by the health professional.

Resources

Home visits for continued assessment and teaching are invaluable for the adolescent. Nurses making home visits will need to be familiar with resources available in the community, and proficient at making assessments of current performance and ongoing needs. Followup visits should aid in minimizing the stresses of daily maintenance as well as assist in involvement with available services that offer positive alternatives and benefits to the adolescent parent.

Available followup services that should be provided include ongoing medical care for the mother and child. A supplemental food program specifically designed to meet the needs of pregnant and postpartum women and children is Women and Infant Care (WIC). This program offers nutritional education for these clients and provides supplemental high-protein foods beginning in the prenatal period, and lasting six months postpartum for bottle feeding mothers and one year postpartum for breastfeeding mothers, and up to age five for the child. A major advantage of this program is that proof of ongoing medical supervision is required to be eligible for the benefits.

The nurse needs to refer the mother for available financial aid. Transportation services may need to be arranged for obtaining needed services such as clinic or physician appointments.

Parenting services such as parent training classes, child care classes, and telephone hot lines should be accessible to the adolescent parent. Child care services for infants and preschool children are available in most communities.

Career counseling that will aid in planning

for the future should be made available. Interests and career options are explored with adolescent parents to help them pursue individual goals.

Caring for the pregnant adolescent is a major nursing challenge. Meeting the needs of adolescent parents is a time-consuming, demanding, often frustrating, but at the same time, highly rewarding role for the nurse. In modern society, an important segment is still receiving less than optimal care and services. We must focus on meeting the needs of this segment of our population to ensure the continued growth of our society.

BIBLIOGRAPHY

Abrams, B. Helping pregnant teenagers eat right. *Nursing 81,* 1981, **11,** 46.

Admire, G. & Byers, L. Counseling the pregnant teenager. *Nursing 81,* 1981, **11,** 62.

Baldwin, W. Adolescent pregnancy and childbearing—an overview. *Seminars in Perinatology,* 1981, **5,** 1-8.

Bartel, C.H. Old enough to get pregnant . . . too young to have babies. *Nursing 81,* 1981, **11,** 44.

Bierman, B. & Street, R. Adolescent girls as mothers. Problems in parenting. In I. Stuart & C. Wells (Eds.). *Pregnancy in adolescence. Needs, problems and management.* New York: Van Nostrand, 1982:407–425.

Brown, M.A. Adolescents and abortion. A theoretical framework for decision making. *Journal of Obstetric, Gynecological & Neonatal Nursing,* 1983, **12,** 241.

Burbach, C.A. Contraception and adolescent pregnancy. *Journal of Obstetric, Gynecological & Neonatal Nursing,* 1980, **9,** 319.

Copeland, D. Unwed adolescent primigravidas identify subject matter for prenatal classes. *Journal of Obstetric, Gynecological & Neonatal Nursing,* 1979, **8,** 248.

Daniels, M.B. A clinic for pregnant teens. *American Journal of Nursing,* 1983, **83,** 68.

Howard, J.S. & Sater, J. Adolescent mothers. Self-perceived health education needs. *Journal of Obstetric, Gynecologic, & Neonatal Nursing,* 1985, **14,** 399.

Jones, F.A., et al. Maternal responsiveness of primiparous mothers during the postpartum period. Age differences. *Pediatrics,* 1980, **65,** 579.

Mercer, R. Assessing and counseling teenage mothers during the perinatal period. *Nursing Clinics of North America,* 1983, **18,** 293.

———. A theoretical framework for studying factors that impact on the maternal role. *Nursing Research,* 1981, **30,** 73.

———. Teenage motherhood. The first year. Part I. The teenage mother's views and responses. Part 2. How their infants fared. *Journal of Obstetric, Gynecologic & Neonatal Nursing,* 1980, **9,** 16.

Morgan, B.S. & Barden, M.E. Unwed and pregnant. Nurse's attitudes towards unmarried mothers. *MCN,* 1985, **10,** 114.

Panzarine, S. & Elster, A. Prospective adolescent fathers. Stresses during pregnancy and implications for nursing intervention. *Journal of Psychosocial Nursing,* 1982, **20,** 21-24.

———, et al. A systems approach to adolescent pregnancy. *Journal of Obstetric, Gynecologic & Neonatal Nursing,* 1981, **10,** 287.

Peterson, C., et al. Psychiatric aspects of adolescent pregnancy. *Psychosomatics,* 1982, **23,** 723.

Ray, D.V. & Estok, P.J. Infant feeding choice and the adolescent mother. *Journal of Obstetric, Gynecological & Neonatal Nursing,* 1984, **13,** 115.

Ryan, G. & Schneider, J. Teenage obstetrical complications. *Clinics in Obstetrics & Gynecology,* 1980, **21,** 1191.

Sewall, K.S. Peer group reality therapy for the pregnant adolescent. *MCN,* 1983, **8,** 67.

U.S. Bureau of the Census. *Statistical abstracts of the United States* (103rd ed.). Washington, D.C.: U.S. Government Printing Office, 1982.

U.S. Department of Public Health. Women's Health. Report of the Public Health Service Task Force on Women's Health Issues. *Public Health Reports,* 1985, **100,** 74-106.

Yoos, L. Developmental issues and the choice of feeding method of adolescent mothers. *Journal of Obstetric, Gynecologic & Neonatal Nursing,* 1985, **14,** 68.

Zelnick, M. Second pregnancies in premaritally pregnant teenagers. *Family Planning Perspective,* 1980, **12,** 69.

——— & Young, K. Sex education and its association with teenage sexual activity, pregnancy, and contraceptive use. *Family Planning Perspective,* 1982, **14,** 117.

UNIT VII

ASSESSMENT AND MANAGEMENT OF NEONATAL DISORDERS

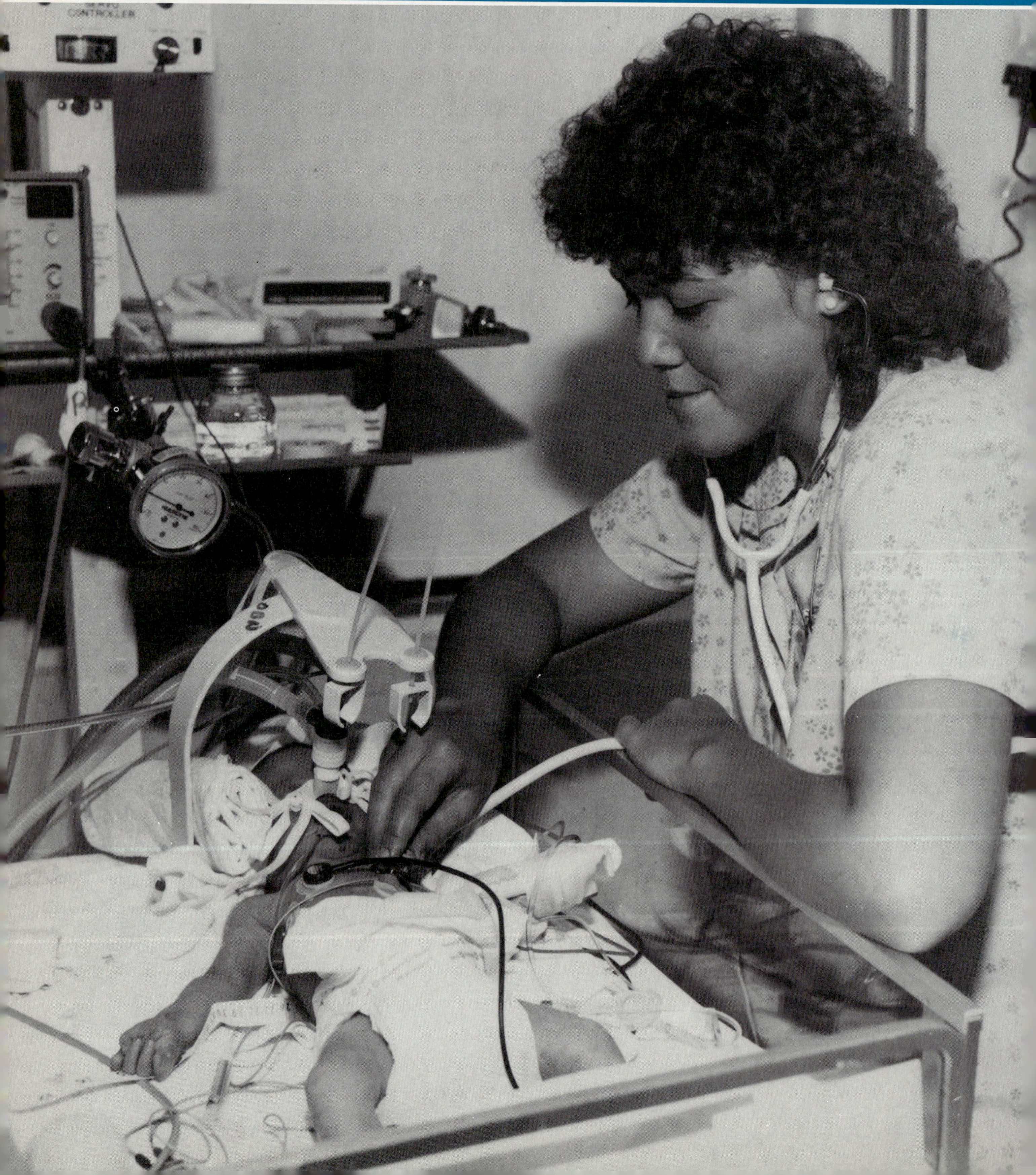
CONTROLLER

UNIT VII

ASSESSMENT AND MANAGEMENT OF NEONATAL DISORDERS

UNIT VII

ASSESSMENT AND MANAGEMENT OF NEONATAL DISORDERS

chapter 29

HIGH-RISK NEONATAL CARE

OBJECTIVES

After completing this chapter, the reader will be able to:

1. Describe physiologic parameters used to identify the high-risk neonate.
2. Explain the physiologic mechanisms involved in asphyxia of the neonate, identify resulting symptomatology, and describe appropriate nursing interventions.
3. Discuss neonatal hypoglycemia, noting nursing assessments, factors that place the neonate at risk for the development of hypoglycemia, and nursing responsibilities.
4. Describe the categories of neonates at risk for the development of cold stress, explain the resulting consequences, and discuss preventive nursing measures.
5. Describe nursing assessments used to identify the neonate with respiratory disorders.
6. Differentiate transient tachypnea from respiratory distress syndrome.
7. Identify the parameters used in blood gas analysis of the neonate and state the normal ranges.
8. Explain the mechanisms of meconium aspiration and discuss preventive measures and nursing interventions.
9. Explain the pathophysiology of respiratory distress syndrome (hyaline membrane disease), clinical manifestations, and medical and nursing interventions.
10. State the causes of pulmonary air leaks and describe related clinical manifestations.
11. Describe and discuss nursing interventions used to promote the physiologic welfare of the compromised neonate.
12. Discuss nursing responsibilities involved when providing alternative feeding methods for the compromised neonate.
13. Give examples of nurturing activities included in the care of the ill neonate.
14. Cite methods used to involve the parents in the care of the ill neonate.

KEY TERMS

Acidosis
Air leaks
Alkalosis
Arterial blood gases
Asphyxia
Chest physiotherapy
Chest retractions
Chin tug
Cyanosis
Gavage feeding
Grunting
Hypocalcemia
Hypoglycemia
Hypothermia
Hypovolemia
L/S ratio
Meconium aspiration
Nasal flaring
Perinatal period
Respiratory distress syndrome
Transcutaneous O_2 monitoring
Transient tachypnea (Type 2 respiratory distress syndrome)

The neonate at birth represents the culmination of genetic, antepartal, and intrapartal factors which affect its immediate and future well-being. In the best of circumstances, this neonate should represent the acme of perfection at birth. Unfortunately, this grandiose goal is not achievable in each and every pregnancy and birth. Many neonates, when born, have already experienced in utero insults and birth trauma, which severely jeopardize their future welfare. Their survival, and perhaps their quality of life is entrusted to the knowledge, skill and expertise of the health care team responsible for their care.

PERINATAL CARE

In an effort to prevent such precarious neonatal circumstances, family-centered maternity care has directed attention to the high-risk pregnancy, which may result in health problems in both the mother and fetus. Centers formerly active in neonatal intensive care have expanded to become perinatal centers, which promote the welfare of the high-risk childbearing family during the perinatal period. This period begins during the 20th week of gestation and continues through the 28th day of postnatal existence.

In 1978, federal involvement in maternity care centered on the provision of intensive care facilities for high-risk perinatal clients. Regionalized centers were developed for three levels of high-risk perinatal clients. Level I hospitals provide care to the normal, uncomplicated gravida and neonate. Care at Level II focuses on the client with more complex needs associated with high-risk factors. These secondary care centers are capable of providing initial care for the severely augmented pregnancy or compromised neonate, but transfer of the client to a Level III nursery is often necessary. Level III, or tertiary, centers provide the most sophisticated type of care, employing comprehensive medical and nursing modalities, technology, and equipment. They are usually affiliated with large medical schools and institutions located in well-populated areas. Part of their responsibility as Level III centers is to serve as consultants to the network of centers within a specified region.

This provision for regionalized care makes it possible for most high-risk perinatal clients (maternal and neonatal) in any geographic area, to receive the benefits of the most sophisticated maternity care. They also provide more economical delivery of maternity care to large numbers of people.

Nurses involved in the practice of high-risk perinatal nursing must have developed knowledge and skills inherent in assessment, planning, intervention, and evaluation of perinatal clients. Table 29–1 presents a statement set forth by the American Nurses' Association Council of High-Risk Perinatal Nurses defining the scope of practice of high-risk perinatal nursing.

Implications for and circumstances warranting the initiation of care for the maternal-fetal unit during the antepartal and intrapartal period have been discussed in Unit VI. The high-risk neonate, however, is a distinct entity at the time of birth and requires specialized care.

HIGH-RISK NEONATAL NURSING

Delivery of nursing care in the neonatal unit is based on developed practice guidelines that include the cognitive and technical skills necessary for implementation of the nursing process. Assessment skills enable the neonatal nurse to differentiate characteristics of the high-risk neonate from those exhibited by the normal neonate. She is then, in collaboration with other members of the health care team, able to plan and initiate therapeutic regimens necessary for the care of the high-risk neonate.

TABLE 29-1
SCOPE OF HIGH-RISK PERINATAL NURSING PRACTICE

High-risk perinatal nursing practice includes, but is not limited to the following:

1. **Assessment.** Assessing the psychosocial and physiological status of the high-risk childbearing family by differentiating levels of perinatal risk; by initiating and utilizing multiple sources and assessment tools for data collection, such as histories, physical examinations, and appropriate laboratory data; and by interpreting data that leads to nursing diagnoses.
2. **Plan of care.** Establishing an appropriate plan of intervention with the high-risk perinatal family based on nursing diagnoses by collaborating with the family and other health care providers; by differentiating immediate and long-term health care goals with the family; and by determining and coordinating the plan of action to meet these identified goals.
3. **Intervention.** Implementing the interventions with the high-risk perinatal family that are based on the plan of care including initiating technical procedures and therapeutic regimes; maintaining a therapeutic environment; intervening in life-threatening situations; teaching, counseling, and facilitating family development; preventing further complications; and promoting optimum health development of the high risk perinatal family.
4. **Evaluation.** Evaluating the plan of care of the high-risk perinatal familiy by evaluating the interventions; evaluating the effects of the interventions on the family; evaluating the family's progress toward the identified goals; and initiating changes in the plan of care based on new data and resources and on the environment.

Excerpt from the American Nurses' Association. A statement on the Scope of High-Risk Perinatal Nursing Practice. 1980. Reprinted with permission of the American Nurses' Association.

The nurse involved with the care of the critically ill neonate requires specialized knowledge and skills achieved through advanced education, experience, and continuing education in neonatal nursing.

The intensive care unit has the equipment necessary to resuscitate and maintain respiration and cardiac functions of the high-risk neonate. Provisions for maintenance of thermoregulation such as radiant warmers or Isolettes are required. One-to-one nursing care must be provided when the critical neonate requires it.

THE HIGH RISK NEONATE

Identification of Risk Factors

Classification of a neonate as high-risk may be the result of antepartal, intrapartal, or neonatal risk factors. Factors that may contribute to the birth of a high-risk neonate have been discussed previously (see Table 22-1 and Tables 24-1 and 24-2). When any of these factors appear in an antepartal history or are present in a gravida during the intrapartal period, they should be made known to the nursing personnel in the neonatal unit in preparation for the supportive and therapeutic care that may be required by the neonate. Immediate care of the high-risk neonate begins in the delivery room and is further complimented by continued intensive care in the neonatal nursery. Parameters that are essential in either area for the identification of the high-risk infant are:

APGAR SCORING

7–10	Low risk resuscitation unnecessary, insure patent airway
4–6	Moderate risk. May need assistance in establishing respirations
1–3	High-risk. Resuscitation measures needed immediately

The 1-minute Apgar score indicates the need for immediate resuscitation measures, while the 5-minute Apgar, when low, indicates in utero asphyxia. The 5-minute score appears to give the best indication of future neurologic outcomes. Continued evaluation is needed when resuscitative measures are employed. The basics of neonatal resuscitation are found in Chapter 16.

ASSESSMENT OF ALL PHYSICAL AND NEUROLOGIC PARAMETERS

Table 22-4 provides a tool for the assessment of neonatal risk factors. Any neonate whose general appearance indicates compromise should receive immediate supportive care; the physical examination is delayed until these measures have been instituted.

DETERMINATION OF GESTATIONAL AGE

A generalized assessment of gestational age immediately after birth will serve as a basis for initial nursing interventions. The complete gestational age assessment is made when the neonate is stable or when all necessary resuscitative measures have been undertaken. Figures 22-24 to 22-27 describe gestational age assessment criteria.

THE COMPROMISED NEONATE

The period immediately following birth has the highest rate of perinatal and neonatal mortality. The neonate who is experiencing cardiac or respiratory problems will have difficulties adapting to an extrauterine environment, and unless immediate resuscitative measures are begun, physiologic and neurologic damage or death may occur. Fundamental to the assessment of the compromised neonate is an understanding of the physiologic alterations that require immediate intervention. Alterations of cardiorespiratory functioning are frequently related to asphyxia, birth trauma, intrapartal hemorrhage, fetal sepsis, fetal anomalies, abnormalities of the central nervous system, gestational age, and medications administered to the mother during labor and delivery.

Asphyxia

All neonates at birth are slightly asphyxiated from carbon dioxide accumulations in the blood which stimulate carotid and aortic chemoreceptors to transmit impulses to the medulla oblongata of the brain and thus, initiate respirations. At this time, the average PCO_2 is 58 mm Hg, PO_2 is 20 to 30, and pH of the blood is about 7.28. Within 15 seconds after birth the normal neonate will take his first breath. Any delay in respirations over 30 seconds is considered abnormal, except in preterm neonates, whose immature central nervous systems impair stimulation of respiratory efforts.

The fetus may experience asphyxia in utero owing to maternal hypoxemia, placental abnormalities, insufficient placental perfusion, cord compression, or abnormalities of fetal circulation. Fetal heart rate patterns have usually provided some indication of compromised fetal status by decreased variability, a brief period of tachycardia followed by bradycardia, and variable or late decelerations. At birth, these neonates are often severely depressed, acidotic, apneic, and, if mature, may have meconium-stained amniotic fluid. Asphyxia resulting from fetal or neonatal events requires resuscitative measures (see Chapter 16).

Asphyxiating events, occurring either in utero or following birth, result in increasing CO_2 levels, with respiratory acidosis, inadequate oxygenation of tissue cells, and tissue hypoxia. In the absence of oxygen, anaerobic glycolysis replaces aerobic metabolism, which causes increased production of lactic acid, decreased blood pH, and metabolic acidosis. In an effort to protect vital organs from the respiratory and metabolic acidosis, vasoconstriction occurs in the less vital organs and blood circulation is increased to the vital organs. If hypoxia (decreased PO_2) is allowed to continue, the blood supply to the vital organs also diminishes, and physiologic insults extend to the cardiac system, brain, kidney, and liver.

Clinical symptoms will depend on the cause of asphyxia, the onset (whether in utero or neonatal), the duration, severity, organ response to hypoxia, circulation, gestational age, treatment, and response. Following resuscitative measures, and contingent upon the condition of the neonate in the delivery room, he is transferred to the special care nursery, intensive care nursery, or tertiary neonatal center.

Apart from the assessments performed on a normal neonate, special emphasis is placed on frequent or continual assessment of respiratory, cardiac, temperature, and neurologic status. All assessments are performed in the least stressful manner for the neonate. The extent of examinations and procedures depends on the condition of the neonate.

The neonate who has mild asphyxia will generally continue to improve within the first 24 hours with supportive care and anticipatory management. When a more severe degree of asphyxia has occurred, physiologic deterioration within the first 24 to 48 hours results in stupor, coma, or death.

The neonate with asphyxia is prone to hypothermia. If he is allowed to deteriorate to cold stress, the outcome is considerably reduced.

Resulting sequelae and symptoms of neonatal asphyxia during the first three days following birth are found in Table 29–2.

Treatment modalities for neonatal asphyxia are concerned with the prevention of neurologic damage and the maintenance of physiologic homeostasis. Careful monitoring of fluid and electrolyte balance is important to prevent increased pulmonary or cerebral edema and to protect renal function. Monitoring of respiratory status and blood gases is essential to prevent hypoxia and acidosis. Since glycogen stores may be depleted easily during asphyxia it is important to carefully monitor blood sugar levels. Of primary concern is the avoidence of hypothermia, which increases glucose use. Careful attention is given to cardiac status, with emphasis on assessments for symptoms of increased venous pressure, congestive heart failure, cardiogenic shock, and right-to-left shunting of the blood through the ductus arteriosus. Assessment of the gastrointestinal system includes abdominal distention, vomiting, and blood in the stools, which may indicate necrotizing entercolitis (see Chapter 31 for a complete discussion). Hyperbilirubinemia may also be noted, owing to hepatic damage and interventions may be necessary. Assessment of neurologic status is ongoing with attention to subtle deviations indicative of seizure activities such as blinking and abnormal pupillary responses.

Hypoglycemia

Hypoglycemia may be defined as a glucose level below 40 mg per 100 ml, with a Dextrostix evaluation and 30 mg per 100 ml or less when whole blood is used. Specific diagnostic criteria for the full-term neonate require two blood glucose levels of 30 mg per 100 ml or below during the first three days following birth and 40 mg per 100 ml from then on.

INCIDENCE

All neonates have a precepitous drop in blood glucose levels immediately following birth. However, most neonates are able to stabilize at a normal level (40 to 80 mg per 100 ml) within a few hours. Neonates who have been stressed may have difficulty maintaining glucose levels and develop pathology associated with hypoglycemia. Identification of high-risk factors for hypoglycemia include:

Gestational age classification

SGA. Occurs in 20 to 40 percent of SGA neonates because of low glycogen stores and alterations in glycogenolysis and glyconeogenesis.

Preterm. 40 to 50 percent of preterms will have low blood sugar levels, due to inadequate storage of glycogen, altered glyconeogenesis, and hypothermia.

Asphyxia. Due to rapid depletion of glycogen stores involved in stressed metabolic processes.

Neonates of Diabetic Mothers. High maternal glucose levels stimulate fetal production of insulin at increased levels. When maternal supply is eliminated following birth, insulin production remains high in relation to the amount of blood glucose, causing hypoglycemia. Some 45 to 50 percent of these

TABLE 29-2
SEQUELAE AND SYMPTOMS OF NEONATAL ASPHYXIA

Sequelae	Symptomatology*
CARDIOVASCULAR SYSTEM	
Cardiac myopathy	
Increased venous pressure	Premature at risk for intraventricular hemorrhage
Cardiogenic shock	Hypotension
Right-to-left shunt	Return to fetal circulatory pattern
Tricuspid insufficiency	Heart murmur
	Cardiomegaly
Cor Pulmonale	Persistent hypertension
Congestive heart failure	Lethargy
	Tachycardia
	Central cyanosis
PULMONARY SYSTEM	
Increased pulmonary pressure	
Delayed absorption of lung fluid	
Pulmonary edema	Hypoxemia
	Hypercarbia
Reduced pulmonary surfactant	
Respiratory distress syndrome	Tachypnea
	Nasal flaring
	Apnea
	Periodic breathing
	Retractions
	Grunting
RENAL SYSTEM	
Renal ischemia	Oliguria
Tubular necrosis	Anuria
Glomerular filtration reduced	Electrolyte imbalances
	Hypocalcemia (after 24 hours)
	Hyponatremia (after 12 hours)
	Hyperkalemia
Renal failure	
GASTROINTESTINAL SYSTEM	
GI bleeding	Blood in stools
Malabsorption of nutrients	
Necrotizing enterocolitis	Abdominal distention
	Vomiting
Hepatic cellular damage	Hyperbilirubinemia
CENTRAL NERVOUS SYSTEM	
Cerebral edema	
Intracranial hemorrhage	Bulging tense fontanels
	Altered consciousness
Increased intracranial pressure	Multifocal seizures
	Lip-smacking
	Cycling movements of arms & legs
	Blinking

TABLE 29-2 (continued)

Sequelae	Symptomatology*
CENTRAL NERVOUS SYSTEM (continued)	
	Hypotonia or hypertonia
	Alert staring expression to eyes (after 12 hours)
Cerebral palsy	Absent reflexes
	Poor suck and swallowing reflexes
Ataxia	Moro reflex diminished or absent
Mental retardation	Lethargy
	Vomiting/inadequate suck
Seizures	Seizuring most frequently seen after 12 to 36 hours
Hydrocephalus	Wide-separated sutures
	Bulging fontanels
	Stupor/coma
METABOLIC CONSEQUENCES	
Hypoglycemia	Decreased blood glucose
	Jitteriness
Hypothermia	Temperature instability
Decreased ATP	Altered electrolytes
Altered arterial blood gases	High $PaCO_2$
	Low PaO_2
	Decreased pH
	Low blood HCO_3
SEPSIS	
	Anemia
	Apnea
	Irritability
	Hypo or hyperthermia
	Petechiae

*These symptoms may also indicate other disorders and should be viewed in that context.

infants become hypoglycemic within the first 8 hours.

Rh hemolytic disorders. Hyperplasia of the fetal islet cells of the erythroblastotic neonate (see Chapter 31) will cause hyperinsulinism and low blood sugar.

Hypothermia. Supplies of glycogen are rapidly used to produce heat, and neonates who have cold stress will readily become hypoglycemic.

Polycythemia. Hyperviscosity of the blood causes complications such as respiratory distress, hyperbilirubinemia, and congestive heart failure, all of which intensify hypoglycemia.

Other Disorders. Adrenal insufficiency, tumors, galactosemia (disorder of galactose metabolism), congenital heart disease, shock, sepsis, and maternal drugs.

CLINICAL MANIFESTATIONS

Clinical manifestations of hypoglycemia are, for the most part, related to dysfunction of the central nervous system and are exhibited in alterations of the respiratory system, systemic alterations, and overt central nervous system symptoms. Neonates exhibiting any of the following symptoms should be closely observed for hypoglycemia:

- Apathy
- Jitteriness
- Tremors
- Hypotonia
- Irritability
- Eye rolling
- High-pitched or weak cry
- Poor feeding
- Tachypnea
- Apnea
- Pallor
- Cyanosis
- Vomiting
- Seizures
- Sweating

The hypoglycemic neonate may be asymptomatic or symptoms may be episodic, developing over a period of time from a few hours after birth to a week or ten days. Causative factors must also be differentiated, since the same symptoms may occur in other neonatal complications, such as central nervous system disorders, sepsis, metabolic disorders, and respiratory disorders.

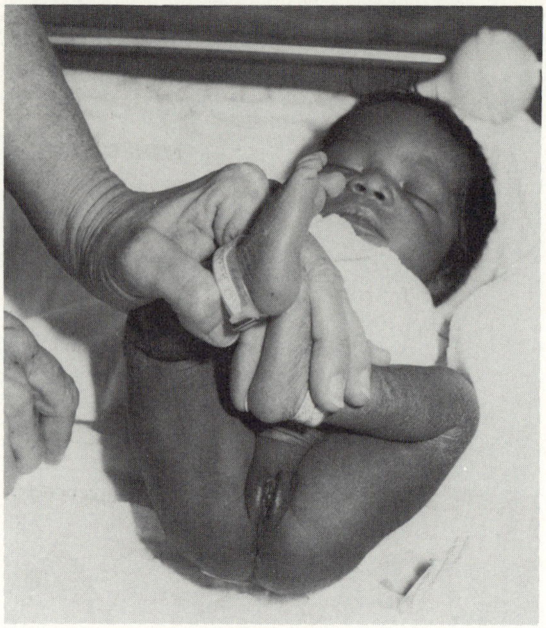

FIGURE 29-1. Site of heel stick puncture on right heel of preterm neonate. Also note the prominent clitoris and wide-spread labia majora.

DIAGNOSIS

All neonates admitted to the nursery should have glucose determinations assessed within one hour following birth. When Dextrostix tests are performed, a sample of blood is obtained from a stick in the lateral aspect of the heel (Fig. 29-1). Levels found to be 40 mg per 100 ml or less are indicative of hypoglycemia, and further assessment and interventions are necessary. Specimens may also be obtained from direct analysis of whole blood or plasma. Normal plasma levels (35 mg per 100 ml) are somewhat higher than whole blood levels (30 mg per 100 ml). When the neonate is 72 hours old, plasma glucose levels should be 45 mg per 100 ml or better. Lower levels of blood glucose are found in preterm and SGA neonates with plasma levels of 25 mg per 100 ml and whole blood levels of 20 mg per 100 ml.

MEDICAL AND NURSING INTERVENTIONS

Therapeutic interventions for hypoglycemia consist of administration of glucose by oral and/or intravenous administration with an infusion pump. Oral glucose may be given in feedings of 5 or 10 percent dextrose in water or formula, followed by glucose determinations. Symptomatic and low birth weight neonates will generally require IV administration of 6 to 8 mg per kg per minute of 10 percent glucose. Infusion pumps are necessary to insure a steady rate of administration, thereby decreasing fluctuations in neonatal insulin response. Glucose levels are monitored every 15 minutes to determine if an increase or decrease in infusion rate or concentration is needed. The blood glucose should be maintained at 30 to 40 mg 100 ml. When the glucose level is stabilized, the rate is slowly tapered, decreasing about 2 gm per kg per minute if consistent with stabilization. It is essential that IV infusions of glucose not be abruptly discontinued, as reactive hypoglycemia may occur (Avery, 1981). Continued monitoring of glucose levels is necessary every 4 hours for the next 24

TABLE 29-3
NURSING RESPONSIBILITIES IN NEONATAL HYPOGLYCEMIA

IDENTIFICATION OF NEONATES AT RISK FOR HYPOGLYCEMIA

Assessment of antepartal, intrapartal, and neonatal risk factors

ASSESSMENT OF ALL NEONATES FOR HYPOGLYCEMIA

Dextrostix or blood glucose level determination on all neonates within one hour of birth
Observe all neonates for symptoms of hypoglycemia
Report any abnormal glucose levels or symptoms to physician

MONITORING OF GLUCOSE LEVELS OF ALL NEONATES AT-RISK FOR HYPOGLYCEMIA

Monitor:
- LGA neonate—every hour for 8 hours following birth, then as needed
- Preterm AGA neonate—every 4 hours for 1st 24 hours, then as needed
- SGA neonate—every 4 hours for 1st 24 hours, then every 8 hours for next 72 hours
- Any neonate exhibiting symptoms every hour

ADMINISTERING AND MONITORING TREATMENT OF HYPOGLYCEMIC NEONATE

Initiate small frequent feedings to maintain stable glucose levels and provide caloric intake
Give supplementary oral glucose feedings when indicated.
Administer and monitor IV glucose infusion as ordered
- Use infusion pump to provide constant infusion rate
- Administer infusion in peripheral vein of upper extremity to avoid varicosities of lower extremities
- Monitor IV site carefully for infiltration that causes tissue necrosis, especially in the preterm neonate

EVALUATION OF THERAPEUTIC INTERVENTIONS

Monitor glucose levels every 15 minutes until stable
When levels have stabilized, decrease glucose rate in indicated decrements
Evaluate every hour during rate decrease
When glucose infusions completed, evaluate every four hours for the next 24 hours

PREVENTION OF NEUROLOGIC IMPAIRMENT

Elimination of environmental factors promoting hypothermia
Prompt treatment of all hypoglycemic neonates
Continued and careful observation of all neonates following treatment for hypoglycemia

hours. The output and specific gravity of the urine are monitored to prevent dehydration from hyperglycemic osmotic diuresis.

Three other medications may be used to promote elevation of blood glucose levels. Glucagon and epinephrine stimulate the release of liver glycogen for conversion to glucose (Avery, 1981). However, SGA neonates with insufficient glycogen stores may not have a significant therapeutic response. Likewise, epinephrine has an anti-insulin action that may be beneficial, but because of its potential to promote lactic acidosis, it must be used with caution. Promotion of gluconeogenesis may be enhanced by the use of steroids. These medications are used only in the more severe, intractable cases of hypoglycemia.

Nursing interventions and responsibilities are centered on six main goals (see Table 29–3). These goals include:

- Identification of neonates at risk for hypoglycemia
- Assessment of all neonates for hypoglycemia
- Monitoring of glucose levels of all neonates at risk
- Administering and monitoring treatment of hypoglycemic neonates
- Evaluation of therapeutic interventions
- Prevention of neurologic impairment

Hypothermia (Cold Stress)

A neutral thermal environment is vital for normal extrauterine adaptations following birth. Aspects of neonatal thermal regulation discussed in Chapter 21 are also applicable to the high-risk neonate.

Several categories of neonates are more susceptible to the effects of hypothermia than are others including:

Preterm neonates. Because they have less subcutaneous tissue and brown fat, increased ratio of body surface to mass, decreased flexion of the extremities and immaturity of the central nervous system.

SGA neonates. Because they have less subcutaneous tissue and brown fat and increased ratio of body surface to mass.

Hypoxic neonates. Because they have insufficient amounts of oxygen and rapid depletion of glycogen stores.

Neonate with CNS depression. Hinders the release of norepinephrine from sympathetic nerve endings.

Depressed neonate. Neonates who were depressed in utero by analgesics or anesthetics given to the mother.

Hypoglycemic neonates. Because they have inadequate glucose to meet caloric needs for metabolism.

When a neonate is chilled, oxygen consumption is increased in order to facilitate metabolism of available glucose. Following the increase in metabolism, if the neonate is still cold, his sympathetic nerve endings are stimulated to release norepinephrine, which in turn stimulates the metabolism of brown fat. Effects of norepinephrine are subsequently reflected in an increase in pulmonary vascular resistance, which inhibits pulmonary blood flow and reduces blood oxygenation. If the mechanisms for heat production are not intact or if heat loss is allowed to continue, oxygen consumption and brown fat metabolism are further increased. Fatty acids begin to accumulate from increased brown fat metabolism. Eventually, delivery of oxygen to the tissues is insufficient, and anaerobic metabolism replaces aerobic metabolism, which changes the end product of glucose metabolism to lactic acid instead of CO_2 and water. The combined effects of lactic acid from anaerobic metabolism and fatty acids produced by increased metabolism of brown fat cause a drop in the pH of the blood and the development of metabolic acidosis (see Fig. 29–2).

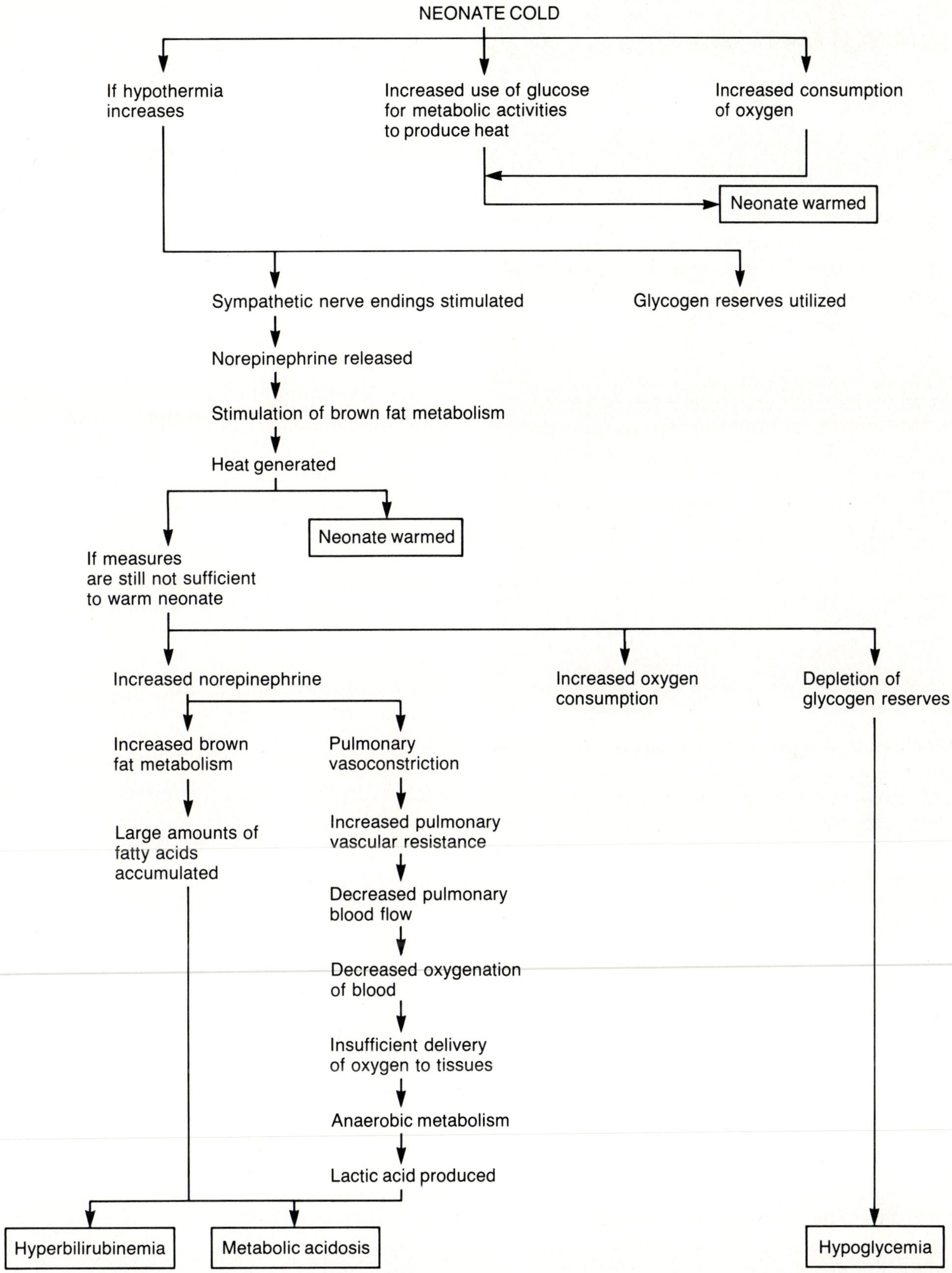

FIGURE 29-2. Mechanism of neonatal cold stress.

NURSING RESPONSIBILITIES

Careful monitoring of the neonate's temperature is important. Observable symptoms of cold stress may not be apparent until there is a profound decrease in core temperature. Axillary temperature evaluations or heat probes are employed, since skin temperature will drop before core temperature. When hypothermia occurs, placement of the thermometer in the axillary region, with its supply of brown fat, may give a false indication of the temperature owing to the highly vascular nature of brown fat tissue and the consequent increased circulation to those areas. Symptoms that alert the nurse to developing hypothermia are:

- Shallow, irregular respirations, retractions
- Diminished reflexes
- Bradycardia
- Oliguria
- Lethargy
- Subnormal temperature

Nursing responsibilities focus on the prevention of hypothermia, as mentioned in Chapter 21. However, the neonate who is suspected of hypothermia should be warmed slowly, have blood glucose levels assessed and arterial blood gas determinations made. The hypothermic neonate becomes at risk for the development of hypoglycemia, hyperbilirubinemia, right to left shunts, and intracranial hemorrhage, depending on the severity and the gestational age of the neonate.

Hypocalcemia

Hypocalcemia is present when serum calcium levels are 7.0 mg per 100 ml or less. Neonates considered at risk for hypocalcemia are:

- Neonates who experienced asphyxia
- Neonates of diabetic mothers who are insulin-dependent
- Preterm neonates and SGA neonates
- Neonates whose mothers have hypoparathyroidism
- Neonates who were delivered after a prolonged or difficult labor or with placenta previa
- Neonates who have received sodium bicarbonate for treatment of metabolic acidosis
- Neonates who have received citrated blood during exchange transfusions
- Neonates receiving whole cow's milk for feedings
- Neonates of mothers who were medicated antepartally with magnesium sulfate

The development of hypocalcemia is related to in utero events. During the last trimester of pregnancy an increased maternal supply of calcium to the fetus provides a ready supply at birth. The neonate born prematurely does not have the opportunity to develop these calcium stores and may, therefore, have a calcium deficit at birth. This problem may be further intensified by the hypoparathyroidism characteristic of preterm neonates.

Disorders of vitamin D metabolism, increased phosphorus production, increased calcitonian produced by the thyroid gland, and hypomagnesemia appear to affect calcium production in the neonate. Several disorders, such as hypoglycemia, maternal hypothyroidism, and neonatal asphyxia, alter these factors and contribute to the development of hypocalcemia.

Hypocalcemia is also encountered in neonates who consume cow's milk that has a high level of phosphates, which is incompatible with proper functioning of the parathyroid gland. Symptoms of hypocalcemia are not apparent in these neonates until about one week after birth.

When hypocalcemia is attributed to factors other than cow's milk feedings, symptoms may be exhibited within the first 48 hours following birth. The following symptoms may be indicative of hypocalcemia:

- Jitteriness
- High-pitched cry
- Apnea

Chvostek's sign (facial muscle spasms elicited by a tap to facial nerves)
Irritability
Hypotonia
Carpopedal spasms
Abdominal distention
Vomiting
Tetany
Seizures

Treatment of hypocalcemia consists of oral or IV administration of calcium therapy, which is generally in the form of calcium salts such as calcium gluconate and calcium lactate. Calcium chloride is irritative to the gastric system, causing vomiting and frequent bowel movement and contributing to the development of necrotizing enterocolitis; it is, therefore, not recommended.

An initial IV bolus of 10 percent calcium gluconate may be administered at a rate of 1 to 2 ml per kg body weight over a 10-minute period for acute hypocalcemia. Careful administration is critical, since rapid infusions may precipitate bradycardia, dangerous arrhythmias, and circulatory failure. Constant monitoring of cardiac status is necessary when IV infusions are employed. Separate lines for IV infusions are used, owing to the incompatibility of calcium with drugs such as sodium bicarbonate, which forms a precipitate when mixed in the same IV line. Calcium is not administered IM, as it is a tissue irritant and may cause tissue necrosis. For this same reason, when calcium is administered IV, measures are taken to prevent leakage into the tissues.

If the neonate is asymptomatic and calcium levels are low, treatment consists of calcium in divided doses until calcium levels have returned to normal and are stabilized.

RESPIRATORY DISORDERS

Assessments

Establishment of effective respiratory functioning and concomitant respiratory efforts are crucial to the survival of the neonate. Astute nursing assessments of the neonate's respiratory status are necessary to detect any subtle change in respiratory function or the presence of respiratory insufficiency. These assessments include:

Observation of breathing movements and respiratory efforts
Auscultation of breath sounds
Determination of respiratory rate and rhythm
Observation of skin color

CHEST RETRACTIONS

Breathing efforts of the normal neonate are primarily diaphragmatic, observed as a rise and fall of the abdomen with each respiration. When breathing becomes difficult, there may be inward drawing of the chest wall with each inspiration, visible at either the level of the sternum (*xiphoid retractions*), between the ribs (*intercostal retractions*), below the inferior costal margins (*subcostal retractions*), or above the clavicles (*supraclavicular retractions*).

As the respiratory efforts increase, retractions become more pronounced and interfere with lung expansion. Characteristic breathing patterns occur with inspiration lags or "see-saw" respirations. In an effort to determine the severity of respiratory insult, the Silverman-Andersen index may be used to grade respiratory status according to chest movements, retractions (xiphoid and intercostal), flaring of the nares, and expiratory grunt (see Fig. 29-3).

NASAL FLARING

In an effort to inhale more air, the neonate will attempt to increase the size of the nasal passages by flaring the nostrils and decreasing the resistance of the nasal air passages. The effectiveness of this mechanism is limited, and its presence indicates decreasing respiratory status.

CHIN TUG

Chin tug may also be observed in neonates with respiratory distress. The increased respira-

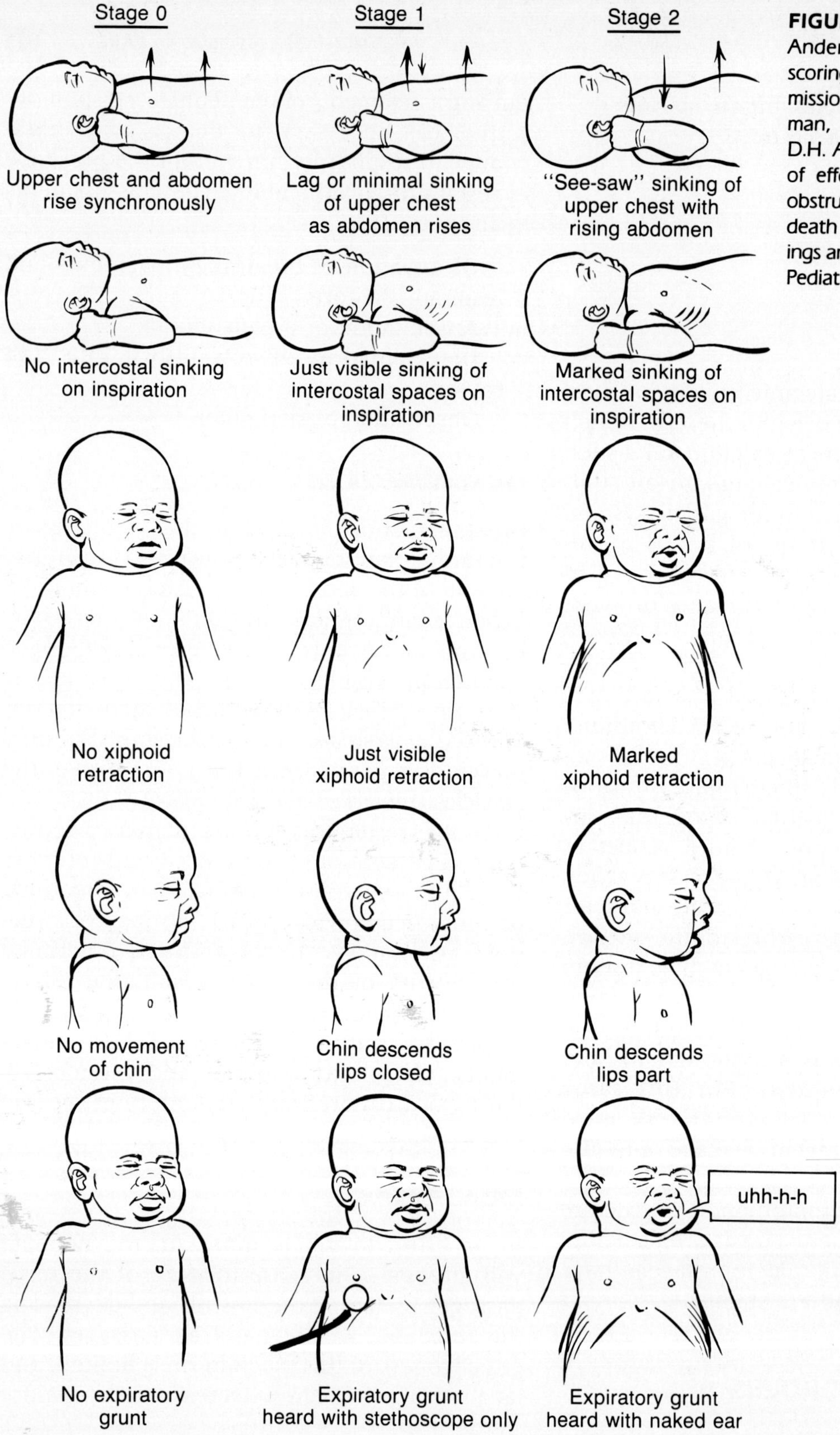

FIGURE 29-3. Silverman-Andersen index retraction scoring. Reprinted with permission. Adapted from Silverman, W.A. and Andersen, D.H. A controlled clinical trial of effects of water mist on obstructive respiratory signs, death rate and necropsy findings among premature infants. Pediatrics, **17** (1), 1956: 1-9.

Retraction scoring. Four inspiratory criteria: (1) movement of upper chest and abdomen; (2) intercostal movement; (3) xiphoid movement; (4) chin movement, and 1 expiratory criterion; (5) presence or absence of grunting were arbitrarily graded into 3 stages (0, 1 and 2). The "retraction score" was computed by adding the values (0,1 and 2) assigned to each criterion at the time of a single observation. Thus, a "retraction score" of zero indicated no retractions and a score of 10 indicated maximal retractions.

tory effort causes a downward pull on the chin, as if it were being tugged. The mouth may or may not fall open, but as severity increases, the lips are parted.

GRUNTING

Another compensatory mechanism used by the neonate in respiratory distress is grunting. Grunting is the sound heard when expirations occur against a partially occluded glottis. The effect of this modified Valsalva maneuver is to increase lung volume, prolong expirations, and thereby improve gas exchange in the lungs. Grunting may be heard with a stethoscope or as an audible grunt. The presence of grunting is an indicator of respiratory difficulties and should be reported to the physician when it is first detected.

BREATH SOUNDS

Breath sounds are auscultated in every neonate on admission to the nursery and whenever respiratory distress is suspected or present. The bilateral anterior and posterior aspects of the chest are auscultated and contrasted, noting the presence and location of rales, rhonchi, and diminished breath sounds. During the transitional period, lung sounds in certain areas of the chest may be absent, owing to the presence of unabsorbed fetal lung fluid, but it may also suggest atelectasis or pneumothorax. Accuracy of the location of abnormal breath sounds is dubious because of the small size of the lungs, which readily transmit sounds through the entire lung field. Rales may be heard in the alveoli and the terminal bronchioles and are distinguished as interruptive discrete crackling sounds during inspiration. Rhonchi are heard in the large bronchioles and produce a continuous, coarse sound during both inspiration and expiration. Wheezing, stridor (crowing sound), and prolonged expirations also suggest obstruction in the air passages. Any abnormal or absent chest sounds should be noted, location distinguished, and the physician notified.

RESPIRATORY RATE AND RHYTHM

During the transitional period of neonatal adaptation, fluctuations in respiratory rate and rhythm occur. Respiratory rate may range between 60 and 90 breaths per minute, with periods of irregularity and tachypnea. However, within 12 hours after birth, including the transitional period, the respiratory rate should be between 30 to 60 breaths per minute and regular.

TRANSIENT TACHYPNEA (TYPE 2 RESPIRATORY DISTRESS SYNDROME)

Tachypnea may be transient as a response to delayed absorption of lung fluid or as an indicator of respiratory distress. Transient tachypnea is frequently found in preterm neonates and those delivered by cesarean delivery, because of their inability to clear the fluid from the lungs by chest compression during the birthing process. The respiratory rate is generally more than 80 breaths per minute and some slight retractions may be noted. The exchange of gases is usually within a normal range (P_aO_2 50 to 80 mm Hg, P_aCO_2 33 to 45 mm Hg, and pH 7.35 to 7.45), although mild hypoxia and hypercapnia may be present.

Transient tachypnea is treated by careful observation and respiratory assessments every 15 minutes until improvement occurs. It may be necessary to institute oxygen therapy to prevent hypoxemia and persistent fetal circulation. During periods of tachypnea, the neonate does not receive any oral feedings, and intake and output are carefully monitored. X-rays of the chest frequently reveal fluid in the pleural spaces of the lungs, increased lung volume, and vascularity. Tachypnea may also be an indication of pneumonia and respiratory distress syndrome, especially in the preterm neonate.

APNEA

Apnea that last 20 seconds or longer or that is associated with bradycardia, cyanosis, or pallor is considered abnormal and indicative of complications. It must be differentiated from periodic breathing, which is the cessation of respirations for 5 to 10 seconds followed by an increased rate of 50 to 60 per minute for 10 to 15 seonds. Periodic breathing is considered normal and is not associated with bradycardia or cyanosis. It often occurs during periods of REM sleep but is usually not observed in the first few days of life. Preterm neonates will demonstrate periodic breathing. Apnea, however, is a symptom for which the cause must be determined. Apnea is often seen in the preterm neonate and will be discussed in Chapter 30.

CYANOSIS

Acrocyanosis of the hands and feet, and circumoral cyanosis of the area surrounding the mouth, are considered normal following birth. These manifestations of peripheral cyanosis are a result of the immaturity of the peripheral circulation, vasomotor instability, and hypothermia. Neonates who have encountered venous stasis of an extremity in utero such as a footling breech or a nuchal cord often has a noticeable cyanotic foot or face. In all of these instances, the cyanosis improves with the establishment of adequate peripheral circulation and temperature stabilization. When neonatal sepsis or hypovolemia is present, peripheral cyanosis may be noted and is considered pathologic.

Certain characteristics help the nurse to distinguish peripheral physiologic cyanosis from the pathologic type. For instance, when an extremity appears to be cyanotic, it may be warmed by the application of a moist heat pack for a short interval. If the color returns, the most likely cause is lowered temperature or vasoconstriction. Assessing the neonate's temperature confirms hypothermia. Placing him under a heat lamp will also improve the color. Hypothermic neonates often display a mottled appearance, which is also helpful in when assessing the cyanosis related to hypothermia. If neither the heat lamp nor application of heat packs improves the color, pathology may be suspected.

Central cyanosis always demands immediate treatment and is considered a serious symptom. It may be differentiated from peripheral cyanosis by the cyanotic appearance of the mucous membranes and tongue as well as the nail beds and extremities. The main causes of central cyanosis are respiratory or cardiac factors, although metabolic, hematologic and central nervous system disorders may be implicated. Table 29–4 provides examples of cyanotic disorders related to these systems.

Insight into the cause of central cyanosis presents a more complex problem. For the most part, the largest percentage of central cyanosis is caused by respiratory or cardiac disorders, and differentiating characteristics are assessed. The neonate displaying cyanosis from respiratory dysfunction will have little change in the degree of cyanosis while crying, but cyanosis associated with cardiac problems is intensified during crying episodes. Suctioning the neonate who appears to have mucus problems will relieve cyanosis if a mucus obstruction is impairing air flow; however, suctioning the neonate with cardiac problems increases stress and consequently the degree of cyanosis. For this reason, neonates with cardiac problems also become more cyanotic when bottle- or breastfeeding. The neonate with cardiac problems also exhibits tachypnea, much the same as the neonate with respiratory disorders, but tachypnea of cardiac origin is usually not associated with labored respirations or retractions.

Initiating oxygen therapy does not appreciably increase the P_aO_2 or alter cyanosis of the neonate with cardiac problems. On the other hand, the neonate with respiratory problems will usually, with the initiation of oxygen therapy or an increase in concentration, reflect a change in the P_aO_2 level.

Assessment of cardiac status is necessary to direct attention to the presence of heart murmurs, altered rates and rhythms, displacement of the PMI, and evaluation of pulses. When indicated, electrocardiograms and echocardio-

TABLE 29-4
EXAMPLES OF DISORDERS CAUSING CENTRAL CYANOSIS*

RESPIRATORY DISORDERS

Respiratory distress syndrome
Obstruction of the respiratory tract (mucus, bilateral choanal atresia, etc.)
Meconium or amniotic fluid aspiration
Pneumonia
Diaphragmatic hernia
Pneumothorax

CARDIAC DISORDERS

Persistent fetal circulation
Cyanotic congenital heart lesions
(Transposition of the great vessels, pulmonary stenosis, truncus arteriosus, tricuspid atresia, anomalous venous return, tetralogy of Fallot, etc.)
Congestive heart failure

CENTRAL NERVOUS SYSTEM DISORDERS

Asphyxia
Intracranial hemorrhage
Cerebral edema

METABOLIC DISORDERS

Hypoglycemia

HEMATOLOGIC DISORDERS

Methemoglobinemia
(genetic disorder causing decreased oxygen carrying capacity of the blood)

*This list is not intended to be a complete list of cyanotic disorders but serves as an example of causative factors.

grams are employed. Chest x-rays and determination of arterial blood gases and hematologic values are also important diagnostic tools.

Cyanosis is not a reliable indicator of oxygenation. Central cyanosis, as previously stated, is always considered a serious symptom; however, neonates may become severely hypoxic before cyanosis is detected. Detection of cyanosis is affected by the hemoglobin level, jaundice, gestational age, lighting used for observation, and opinions of the observer.

ARTERIAL BLOOD GASES

Fundamental to the assessment of respiratory homeostasis of the compromised neonate is the determination of arterial blood gases. These measurements indicate the adequacy of oxygenation and the ability of the body to maintain a normal acid-base equilibrium.

The acid-base determination is measured by evaluating the pH of the blood. When the pH of the blood is lowered, a corresponding acidosis (increased hydrogen ions) is likely and, conversely, when the pH is elevated, the increase in base components causes an alkalosis (decreased H ions). In order for the pH of the blood to remain within a normal range (7.35 to 7.45), the interaction of respiratory and metabolic processes must exist.

Metabolic cell activities release acids, some of which (volatile, carbolic acid) are converted to CO_2, and some of which must be buffered (nonvolatile lactic, sulfuric and phosphoric acids). The respiratory system serves as the channel for elimination of CO_2, while the kidney eliminates the blood-buffered nonvolatile acids. Buffering refers to the mechanism that monitors and minimizes the effects of changes in H ion concentration by releasing or usurping H ions when there is a deficit or excess in the blood. The buffers of the blood are: hemoglobin, acid and alkaline phosphates, proteins, and the primary buffer system, bicarbonate/carbonic acid. Nonvolatile acids are dependent on the bicarbonate/carbonic system, which exists in a ratio of 20:1. When homeostasis is present, both the respiratory and metabolic pathways function cooperatively to provide a normal pH.

Disturbances of respiratory or metabolic activities may cause an alteration in the conversion and elimination of acids that potentiates development of either acidosis or alkalosis. To differentiate causation, a distinction is made between the characteristics of respiratory acidosis, respiratory alkalosis, metabolic acidosis, and metabolic alkalosis:

Respiratory acidosis. A disturbance in gas exchange caused by inadequate ventilation, which promotes retention of CO_2. Consequently, the $PaCO_2$ is elevated and the pH of the blood is decreased.

Respiratory alkalosis. A decreased level of acid in the blood caused by conditions that lower the $PaCO_2$, such as, hyperventilation. The pH rises and respiratory alkalosis develops.

Metabolic acidosis. Condition which impairs the excretion of acids through the kidneys or promotes increased production of acids in the body, such as anaerobic metabolism and/or conditions that allow increased loss of base components. This results in a base deficit with a decrease in HCO_3^- and pH.

Metabolic alkalosis. Base components (bicarbonate ions) are increased beyond normal (20 to 25 mEq/L), resulting in a base excess and elevated pH of the blood.

If any of the above conditions arise, the body will employ compensatory mechanisms to reestablish the normal range of pH. These mechanisms serve as temporary measures until the original or contributing cause of the disturbed acid-base balance can be remedied. Therefore, when assessing arterial blood gases, compensatory mechanisms may reflect a normal pH while the bicarbonate or CO_2 levels, in their effort to compensate for the imbalance, will show varying degrees of alterations. Careful attention must be paid to assessment of all factors of blood gas analysis in relation to the *existing* condition. The aim of treatment is to correct the condition rather than supporting compensatory mechanisms. For instance, respiratory acidosis related to impaired ventilation is best treated by improving ventilation rather than striving to increase bicarbonate retention (Merenstein & Gardner, 1985).

The $PaCO_2$ of the blood denotes the partial pressure (force exerted by gas as it moves from one state to another or intercompartmentally) of carbon dioxide and is an indication of the effectiveness of ventilation and respiratory parameters of acid-base balance. $PaCO_2$ values are inversely related to ventilation. When hyperventilation occurs, the $PaCO_2$ decreases, but it rises in the presence of hypoventilation. If $PaCO_2$ is increased above the normal level (33 to 45 mm Hg) and the pH of the blood is decreased, respiratory acidosis may be suspected.

Base excess is an indicator of the amount of bicarbonate buffers in the blood. It is calculated rather than measured and is derived from the use of a nomogram (Siggard-Anderson) when hemoglobin, pH, $PaCO_2$, and/or plasma bicarbonate levels are known. The values are expressed in either negative (deficit of base) or positive values (excess of base). A metabolic alkalosis is indicated by a plus value above the normal range, and a metabolic acidosis is exhibited by a negative value below the normal range which is +4 to −4 mEq/L.

The bicarbonate level provides an indication of the metabolic parameter of acid-base balance. An increase in the bicarbonate levels (HCO_3) over normal (20 to 25 mEq/L) will give rise to alkalosis, while a decrease in HCO_3

indicates an excess of acid or lack of base and consequently acidosis and decreased pH.

Oxygenation of the blood refers to the amount of hemoglobin that is in combination with oxygen. Combination occurs when oxygen binds to hemoglobin and in this form is made available to the tissues. Measurements of indirect oxygen levels may be made by arterial blood gas assessments and are referred to as the PaO_2 levels. In the normal neonate the range of PaO_2 is between 50 and 80 mm Hg. Pa refers to the partial pressure of oxygen in the blood.

Many factors will alter the PaO_2 of the neonate's blood, and in so doing will affect the amount of oxygen available to the tissues. Alterations in hemoglobin levels (anemia), inadequacies of cardiac function (failure of heart to pump blood to tissues), and insufficient oxygenation (asphyxia) contribute directly to hypoxia of the tissues. PaO_2 can measure the oxygen content of the blood but it cannot measure the extent of tissue hypoxia. It does, however, measure the amount of oxygen within the arterial blood available for tissue oxygenation.

Oxygen saturation indicates the amount of oxygen in the hemoglobin. The greater the percentage of saturation the more oxygen that is available for tissue oxygenation. Oxygen saturation is affected by the affinity of hemoglobin for oxygen, or in other words, the ability of hemoglobin to take up oxygen. An increasing affinity of hemoglobin allows more oxygen to be combined with hemoglobin but prevents less from being released to the tissues. Neonatal cold stress, alkalosis, and characteristics of fetal hemoglobin increase the affinity of hemoglobin for oxygen, but at the same time less is released to the tissues.

PaO_2 levels also affect oxygen saturation, in that the lower the PaO_2 level, the lower the percentage of saturation. The normal oxygen saturation level is 95 to 98 percent and any level below 70 percent is incompatible with tissue oxygenation. Cyanosis becomes noticeable when oxygen saturation is approximately 75 to 80 percent and is associated with a PaO_2 level of 42 to 52 mm Hg in the adult and 32 to 41 mm Hg in the neonate (Korones, 1981). Therefore, the neonate who is cyanotic will be less oxygenated than the adult with cyanosis.

When assessing blood gases, the pH serves as the initial indicator of acid-base imbalance. Assessment of CO_2 levels may then be evaluated for the presence of a respiratory problem. If the CO_2 level is not altered, assessment of the HCO_3 level is necessary for assessment of metabolic acidosis.

Effective compensatory mechanisms will alter the indices of uncompensated acidosis or alkalosis. Therefore, when assessments are made, indications of shifting $PaCO_2$ levels and/or bicarbonate levels opposite what is expected in relationship to the pH level may indicate partial compensation.

Normal ranges of arterial blood gas analysis of the neonate may be found in Table 29–5.

TABLE 29–5
NORMAL RANGE OF ARTERIAL BLOOD GAS ANALYSIS OF THE NEONATE

pH	7.35–7.45
$PaCO_2$	35–45 mmHg
HCO_3	20–25 mEg/L
PaO_2	50–80 mmHg
Base excess	−4 to +4 mEq/L
O_2 saturation	95–98%

Meconium Aspiration

Episodes of intrauterine hypoxia may cause relaxation of the anal sphincter, which permits the passage of meconium into the amniotic fluid. With severe hypoxia, the fetus gasps in utero and aspirates the meconium-stained amniotic fluid. In most instances, however, the meconium is aspirated at birth, when the neonate takes his first breath. Aspirated meconium particles obstruct the air passages, precipitating atelectasis, emphysema, pneumomediastinum, pneumothorax, and the development of infection or a chemical (meconium irritant) pneumonitis.

INCIDENCE

Meconium aspiration occurs in approximately 10 percent of all deliveries and 20 percent of deliveries with meconium-stained amniotic fluid. Predisposing factors are related to in utero hypoxia, breech deliveries, postterm neonates, and traumatic deliveries.

PREVENTION

Prevention of meconium aspiration begins with diagnosis of fetal events precipitating fetal hypoxia. Careful fetal monitoring and assessments of fetal distress are necessary to prevent or detect fetal hypoxic insults.

Any neonate who is born with meconium-stained amniotic fluid or meconium-stained vernix caseosa, fingernails, or umbilical cord is considered a candidate for meconium aspiration. Prompt suctioning should be undertaken when the head is first delivered and before the neonate takes a breath. A bulb syringe or DeLee suction trap may be used to remove mucus from the oropharynx immediately upon delivery of the head. The DeLee suction trap (see Fig. 29-4) allows placement of a catheter into the oropharynx to facilitate more effective suctioning. The catheter is attached to the mucus trap, and the mouth of the trap is placed into the nurse's mouth. Mucus is removed when the nurse sucks on the mouthpiece and creates suction that draws the mucus into the trap. If meconium has been aspirated, it may be necessary to visualize the cords by laryngoscopy and if meconium is present to utilize endotracheal suctioning.

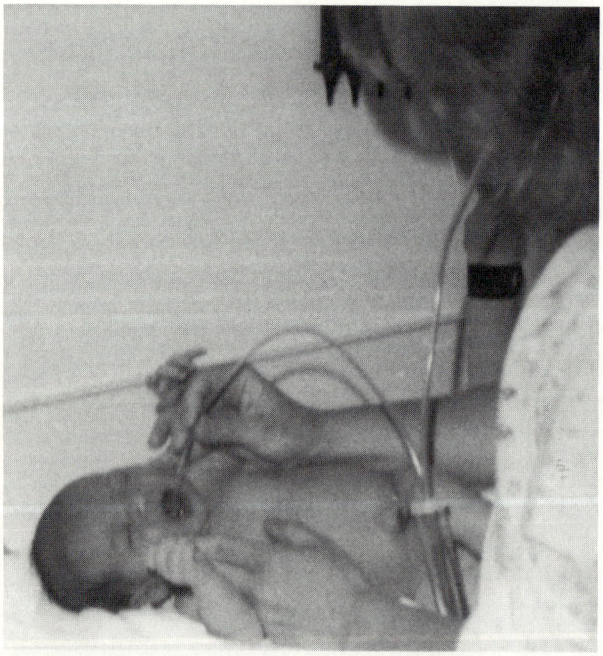

FIGURE 29-4. Nurse using DeLee suction trap.

MEDICAL AND NURSING INTERVENTIONS

Level of intervention depends on the severity of the aspiration. Assessments of respiratory parameters are necessary following meconium aspiration and are conducted at frequent intervals. Signs of respiratory distress may be manifested by rapid, shallow respirations, rales and rhonchi, prolonged expirations, retractions, and barreling of the chest.

X-ray examinations are necessary to detect infiltrates and a developing pneumomediastinum or pneumothorax. Complications such as right to left shunting, acidosis, cardiomyopathy, and asphyxia are also possible. Nursing goals are directed toward careful monitoring of respiratory status, arterial blood gases, intake and output, vital signs, thermoregulation, and hydration. Without complications, recovery occurs in about 48 hours.

Respiratory Distress Syndrome (Hyaline Membrane Disease)

Respiratory distress syndrome (RDS), or hyaline membrane disease, as it is often called, is a severe respiratory disorder associated with deficiencies of pulmonary surfactant, generally caused by the immaturity of the lung. It is characterized by deficient production of the phospholipid lecithin and an alteration in the production of phosphatidyl glycerol(PG). Normally, if the neonatal lungs are mature, the phospholipids lecithin and sphingomyelin are present in surfactant in a ratio of 2:1. When lecithin and sphingomyelin are present in this ratio, surfactant is capable of providing alveolar stability. Without surfactant, surface tension of the alveoli increases, functional residual capacity is not established or maintained, and the alveoli collapse upon expiration.

RDS is also associated with birth asphyxia, which may lower the pH of the blood (below 7.25) and destroy the Type II epithelial alveolar cells responsible for the production of surfactant.

Failure to produce surfactant in utero and failure to maintain production after birth are of equal importance in the development of RDS.

INCIDENCE

Approximately 30 percent of all neonatal deaths may be attributed to RDS, with a 35 percent increase in preterm neonates. It is more common among white male neonates than black or female neonates. Although prematurity correlates closely with the development of RDS, other factors such as perinatal asphyxia, maternal diabetes, maternal hemorrhage, cold stress, hypoglycemia, and cesarean delivery are also considered predisposing or contributing factors.

PATHOPHYSIOLOGY

When insufficient surfactant production prevents the development of functional residual capacity and allows increased alveoli surface tension, the alveoli will collapse after each expiration, and a diffuse atelectasis results. Interference with gas exchange occurs owing to unequal and reduced alveolar ventilation, followed by the development of hypoxia and hypercapnia. The resulting inadequate tissue oxygenation promotes anaerobic metabolism and metabolic acidosis, while insufficient ventilation contributes to the retention of CO_2 and the development of respiratory acidosis.

The cycle is intensified as acidosis and inadequate ventilation advances, causing pulmonary arteriolar vasoconstriction, pulmonary hypoperfusion, increased vascular resistance, and shunting of blood through the foramen ovale and ductus arteriosus (right-to-left shunt) (see Fig. 29–5). All these factors serve to increase hypoxia and further curtail the development of surfactant. Eventually, the alveoli breakdown and there is effusion of fibrin and cellular products into the air spaces, producing the characteristic hyaline membrane appearance of the lungs.

CLINICAL MANIFESTATIONS

In the first few minutes following birth, the neonate will often appear normal and receive satisfactory Apgar scores. Within the first two hours after birth, however, the neonate uses up surfactant reserves and may begin to develop symptoms indicative of respiratory distress such as:

Initial symptoms	Tachypnea > 60 Expiratory grunt Intercostal retractions
As condition progresses symptoms of	Nasal flaring Cyanosis Apnea Seesaw respirations Chin tug Pallor—ashen color Edema—pitting edema in extremities Hypotonia Oliguria

In the early stages, auscultation of lung sounds are normal, but as the disorder

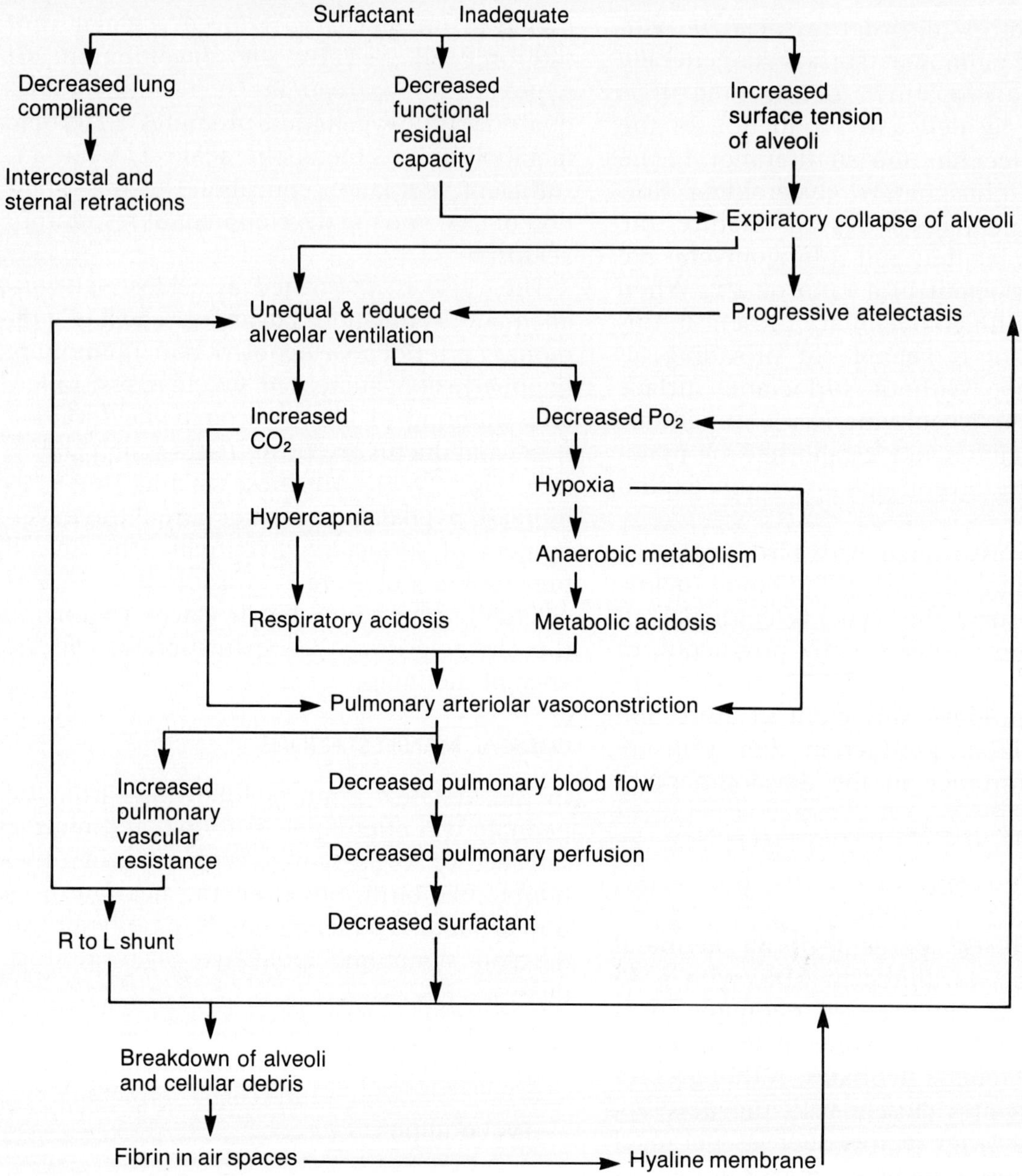

FIGURE 29-5. Mechanism of respiratory distress syndrome.

progresses lung sounds may be diminished, absent, or heard as coarse, sandpaperlike sounds. Lung compliance (elasticity) is reduced and the neonate appears to struggle for each breath. Analysis of arterial blood gases may reveal a decreased pH (7.20 to 7.30), PaO_2 of 40 mm Hg or less, a rise in the $PaCO_2$ (over 60 mm Hg), and alterations in base deficit and bicarbonate, thus reflecting both a metabolic and respiratory acidosis. Hypoxia also interferes with heat production, and hypothermia may quickly ensue.

The severity of symptoms increases during the first 72 hours and then appears to peak, with improvement following over the course of a few days to two weeks. Neonates who have more severe distress may digress to a level incompatible with life within the first 72 hours. Complications that may arise include: patent ductus arteriosus, pneumothorax, disseminated intravascular coagulation (DIC), intracranial hemorrhage, sepsis, bronchopulmonary dysplasia, pulmonary infections, retrolental fibroplasia, neurologic impairment, respiratory and circulatory failure and death.

DIAGNOSIS

Diagnosis is based on the perinatal history, birthing events, gestational age, clinical symptoms, x-ray findings, blood gas analysis, and biochemical and electrolyte evaluations. Typical x-ray findings reveal a *reticulogranular* (ground-glass) pattern with diffuse atelectasis. With progression of the disorder, air bronchograms or "white-out" areas may be seen on x-ray visualization. Samples from gastric aspiration or amniotic fluid may be obtained to measure the L/S ratio and PG levels for evaluation of lung maturity.

MEDICAL AND NURSING INTERVENTIONS

Foremost in considerations related to RDS is the prevention of delivery of neonates with immature L/S ratios. When elective cesarean deliveries or inductions are anticipated, amniocentesis for determination of L/S ratio and complete lung profiles are indicated.

Supportive measures are the key elements in the treatment of respiratory distress syndrome. Since RDS represents a surfactant deficiency state, time offers the opportunity for maturing of the lungs, establishment of the L/S ratio, and resolution of the associated manifestations. Fortunately, with proper supportive measures, resolution usually takes place within the 72 to 86 hours following the onset of symptoms. During the acute phase of the disorder a focus is placed on prevention or correction of acidosis and hypovolemia, thermoregulation to minimize oxygen consumption and inhibit vasoconstriction, assisting ventilation, nutritional support, and psychological support of the parents.

Ventilation

Essential to supportive care is the provision of effective ventilation, which facilitates correction of respiratory acidosis. At the onset of ventilation difficulties, the neonate will attempt to lower the $PaCO_2$ by crying and hyperventilating. When he becomes fatigued, these measures are inadequate and supplemental oxygen or assisted ventilation is necessary.

An Oxyhood (see Fig. 29–6) may be employed to administer warmed, humidified oxygen to the neonate as long as the blood gas parameters remain within a normal range with oxygen concentrations less than 40 percent. An Isolette (see Fig. 29–7) may be used with oxygen supplied within the unit; however, it is difficult to maintain an oxygen concentration when the side portholes are opened to provide care to the neonate, therefore, use of the Isolette is not recommended in these circumstances.

If respiratory status continues to deteriorate, oxygen concentrations of 50 to 60 percent are needed to maintain the PaO_2 at 50 mm Hg, and $PaCO_2$ levels increase to 40 to 45 mm Hg, the use of continuous positive airway pressure (CPAP) may be necessary to provide a constant pressure within the lungs and prevent the alveoli from collapsing. Mechanical ventilation is considered when $PaCO_2$ levels rise beyond 55 to 60 mm Hg, PaO_2 has fallen below 50 mm Hg with 100 percent oxygen, the pH drops (below 7.25), severe retractions, apnea, bradycardia, and grunting are present, and the respiratory rate increases over 80 per minute.

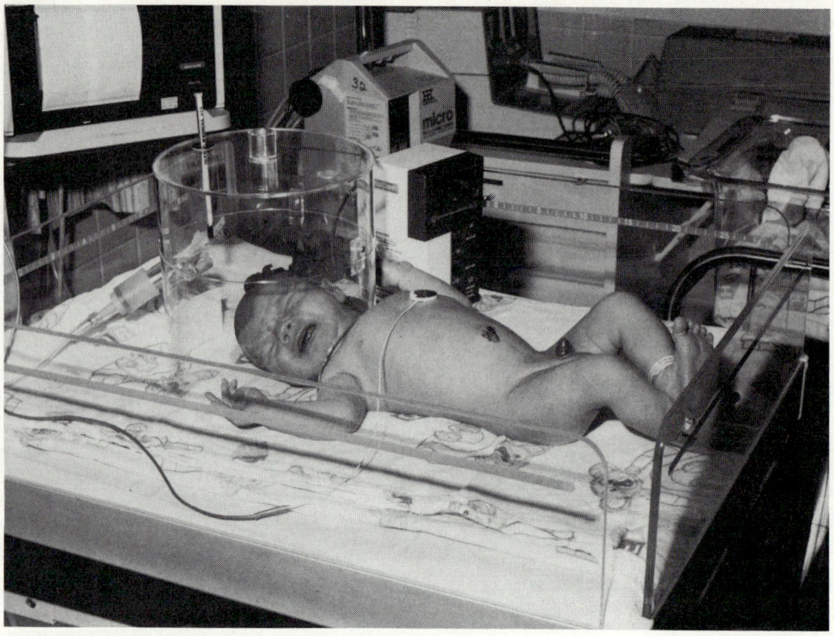

FIGURE 29-6. Oxyhood.

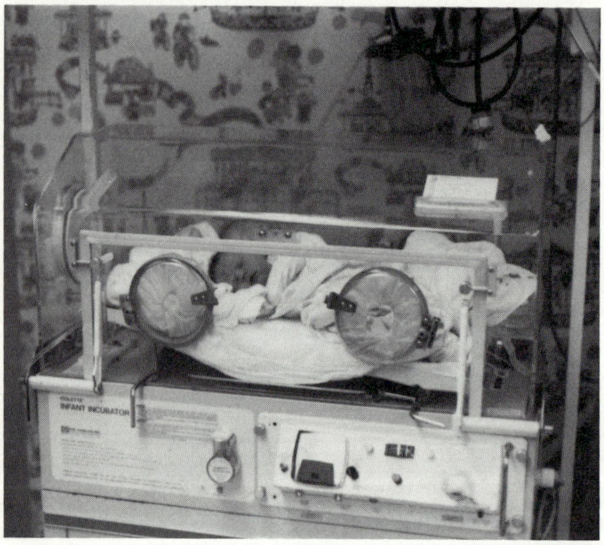

FIGURE 29-7. Isolette.

Improvement will be indicated by a rising PaO_2 and normal $PaCO_2$. When PaO_2 reaches 60 mm Hg, concentrations of oxygen are reduced in narrow (5 percent) decrements followed by measurements of PaO_2.

Signs of intolerance indicate a need to again increase concentration. If the neonate remains stable, however, the process is continued until he may be maintained on room air only.

Acidosis

Correction of acidosis with an alkaline solution such as sodium bicarbonate, is only cautiously used when the acidosis is determined to be metabolic in origin, as assessed by blood gas analysis and an ineffective response to oxygen. Base deficit, in this instance, is usually found to be 10 to 12 mEq/L. Sodium bicarbonate is not administered if ventilation is inadequate or in the presence of true respiratory acidosis. Sodium bicarbonate will release CO_2 as it breaks down, which will only compound the problem if the additional CO_2 can not be eliminated because of inadequate ventilation. If sodium bicarbonate is used, it is diluted in a ratio of 1:1 with sterile water before administration to avoid damage to the blood vessels. It is given slowly to decrease the effects of increased osmolarity, which could alter intravascular and extracellular fluid compartments, possibly contributing to capillary rupture and the development of intracranial hemorrhage. In instances where both respiratory and metabolic acidosis exist, attention is directed to correction of ventilation before sodium bicarbonate is used. When used, careful observations of respiratory status are made, arterial blood gases are assessed, and signs of intracranial hemorrhage, hypernatremia and pulmonary edema are carefully noted.

Hypovolemia

Assessments for hypovolemia are necessary in RDS to insure maintenance of hematocrit levels between 45 and 60 percent. Measurements of B/P and hematocrit levels are monitored at frequent intervals to denote hypotension and related hypovolemia. Hypovolemia associated with RDS may be caused by low serum albumin levels or vasodilitation that occurs as acidosis is corrected (Avery, 1981). Therefore, it is important for the nurse to carefully monitor the B/P, as the parameters of arterial blood gases improve. Prudent management and accurate recordings of the amount of blood removed for blood sampling is important to avoid circulatory stress and to determine levels of replacement with plasma, blood, or albumin.

Nutrition and Hydration

The goals of nutritional management for the neonate with RDS are to: (1) maintain adequate hydration, (2) provide adequate caloric intake necessary to meet the demands of increased metabolic activities interfaced with depletion of glycogen stores, and (3) prevent electrolyte imbalances.

Initially, IV glucose may be administered to prevent dehydration and hypoglycemia. Careful monitoring of the infusion rate is important to prevent fluid overload, congestive heart failure, hyperglycemia, and electrolyte losses. Gavage feedings may be given if adequate gastrointestinal functioning is present. Increased energy demands required with nipple feeding may prohibit bottle feedings until the respiratory distress is minimized and the respiratory rate is not more than 60 per minute. The neonate who remains severely depressed may require total parenteral nutrition. Fluid requirements may be met by utilizing the following schedule.

1st 24 hours	60–80 ml/kg/24 hours
2nd 24 hours	80–100 ml/kg/24 hours
3rd 24 hours	100–120 ml/kg/24 hours
4th 24 hours	120–150 ml/kg/24 hours

Increasing to 150 ml/kg/24 hours

Fluid requirement allowances are made for insensible and sensible water loss and may be more restricted for the low birth weight neonate or one with cardiac problems. Caloric intake requires 120 kcal per kg per 24 hours. Hydration will provide information for determination of fluid and caloric needs. Symptoms of dehydration are observed as:

Poor skin turgor

Sunken eyeballs

Elevated hematocrit (45 to 60 percent normal range)

Increased specific gravity of the urine (1.008 to 1.012 normal range)

Elevated serum Na^+ (136 to 143 mEq/L normal range)

TABLE 29-6
NURSING RESPONSIBILITIES INVOLVED IN CARE OF THE NEONATE WITH RESPIRATORY DISTRESS SYNDROME

INITIAL ASSESSMENT

Perform Apgar assessment on all neonates at 1 & 5 minutes following birth
Assess respiratory status of neonates on admission to nursery
Assess vital signs, B/P, and auscultate heart & lung sounds

IDENTIFY NEONATES AT RISK FOR DEVELOPMENT OF RDS

Perform gestational age assessment
Carefully observe neonates who have experienced asphyxia following birth
Review perinatal history and neonatal history with attention to maternal diabetes, maternal hemorrhage, fetal distress, maternal sedation, birth trauma, sepsis

PROVIDE RESPIRATORY SUPPORT

Maintain oxygenation to meet metabolic requirements
Administer oxygen as ordered according to FiO_2 with hourly measurements of concentration and maintenance of arterial PO_2 between 50 and 80 mm Hg
Use transcutaneous monitor for PO_2 measurements, calibrate as indicated, and change sensor location every two hours
Calibrate oxygen analyzer every eight hours
Analyze oxygen every two hours and prior to blood gas evaluations
Provide warm, humidified oxygen by Oxyhood or Isolette
If using oxyhood change hood and humidifier every 24 hours, with Isolette change oxygen tubing and humidification source every 24 hours
Use only sterile distilled H_2O in humidifiers
Monitor respiratory efforts, noting signs of increasing respiratory distress: tachypnea, grunting, retractions, nasal flaring, apnea, see-saw respirations, chin tug, pallor, cyanosis
Assess neonatal physiologic response, noting hypotonia, oliguria, lethargy, bradycardia, edema, abdominal distention, irritability, unresponsiveness, poor skin turgor
Assess heart and lungs sounds hourly at rest or as indicated by condition, noting lung rales or rhonchi, location or absence of breath sounds, characteristics of inspiratory and expiratory breath sounds over all aspects of lung field; heart rate and rhythm, location of PMI, murmurs
Assess vital signs and B/P every 30 minutes until stable and then every one to two hours
  Utilize cardiac and respiratory monitors as needed
  Assess for location and quality of all pulses & capillary refill
Suction prn
Provide postural drainage and percussion as ordered
Assess need for assisted ventilation, noting:
  (1) inability of neonate to maintain PaO_2 at 50 mm Hg in oxygen concentrations of 50 to 60 percent
  (2) $PaCO_2$ levels >45 mm Hg
  (3) pH level below 7.25
Have emergency medications and equipment (suction, bagging) immediately available
Employ CPAP or PEEP as ordered by the physician
  Administer ventilator care to neonate as outlined in neonatal intensive care standards and procedures

MAINTAIN NEUTRAL THERMAL ENVIRONMENT

Utilize radiant warmer or Isolette to maintain axillary temperature at 36.6° to 37°C (98° to 98.6°F)
Assess temperature every 30 minutes until stable
Assess physiologic status for indications of hypothermia
Monitor oxygen temperature

TABLE 29-6 (continued)

ASSESS LABORATORY PARAMETERS OF NEONATE

Monitor arterial blood gas levels (see Figure 29-5 for normal values)
- Obtain samples only when neonate is resting and not during crying episodes which alters values
- Assess every two to three hours according to condition and following increase or decrease in oxygen concentrations

Determine blood glucose levels
- Report
  - Dextrostix below 40 mg per 100 ml
  - Whole blood levels 30 mg per 100 ml or below and above 130 mg per 100 ml

Monitor total serum bilirubin levels (normal level is 5-12 mg per 100 ml)
- Observe for jaundice
- Provide phototherapy when indicated and as ordered by physician

Monitor hematocrit levels as needed (normal levels, 45-60%)
Assess electrolytes and serum protein
Record time and amount of blood obtained for samples

PROVIDE ENVIRONMENT CONDUCIVE TO HOMEOSTASIS

Minimize environmental stimuli
Handle as little as possible but change position every two hours
Elevate head slightly, avoid hyperextension
Organize and plan management to minimize stress
Maintain aseptic technique or when indicated sterile technique
Assess for signs and symptoms of infection

MANAGE AND MONITOR FLUID AND NUTRITIONAL SUPPORT

Provide nutritional intake with attention to caloric needs, electrolyte balance, hydration, and glucose levels
If IV administered, maintain infusion rate by use of infusion pump; change IV tubing every 24 hours
Observe vital signs for indications of circulatory overload
Monitor IV sites for infiltration and infection
Monitor intake and output
- Record all stools and characteristics (color, consistency, and amount)
- Measure urine output, specific gravity, glucose, and pH

Weigh neonate daily
- Record and report unexpected increments or decrements in weight

Assess for symptoms of dehydration
If gavage feeding, administer slowly to avoid stressing neonate
- Calculate return residual following insertion of catheter
- Position on right side following feedings

Assess ability to nipple feed, sucking and swallowing reflex, energy expenditure during feeding

ADMINISTER MEDICATIONS AS ORDERED

Accurately record medication, doşe, time, and route of administration
Assess and evaluate therapeutic and adverse effects of all medications given

NOTIFY PHYSICIAN IMMEDIATELY IF CONDITION OF NEONATE DETERIORATES

PROVIDE PARENTERAL SUPPORT

In conjunction with physician, provide parents with explanations of disorder, treatment, and prognosis
Allow parents opportunity to ask questions
Provide opportunity for parents to see and touch neonate
Include parents whenever possible in care of neonate

TABLE 29-7
SAMPLE NURSING CARE PLAN: RESPIRATORY DISTRESS SYNDROME

Neonate boy H is 2 hours old. He was delivered by cesarean section, owing to a late deceleration fetal heart rate pattern exhibited during the active phase of labor. Apgar scores at 1 minute were 6, and 8 at 5 minutes. Gestational age examination and correlation with maternal due date indicated Baby G to be 37 weeks gestational age. He weighed 2700 gm at birth. This is the first baby for Glenn and Ann H.

Data Base:

Admission assessment at 8:30 am revealed the following data:
Maternal prenatal history negative
Intrapartal history indicates late deceleration fetal heart rate pattern
Delivered by C-section at 8:20 am
Weight 2700 gm
Length 48.3 cm
Gestational age 37 weeks
Respirations 48, regular, no increased respiratory effort acrocyanosis of hands and feet; bilateral lung sounds present and clear no rales and rhonchi
Apical pulse 120
B/P 68/42
Temperature 36°C rectally
Heart sounds clear and with no murmurs, PMI at 4th intercostal space in midclavicular line
Active motion present, crying
Umbilical cord clamped with 2 arteries, 1 vein, no bleeding
Head circumference 34 cm
Chest circumference 32 cm

Dextrostix 60 mg/100 ml at 9:00 am
Head to toe examination within normal limits
Placed in Isolette for observations following C-section
Maintained on cardiac, respiratory and temperature monitors
At 9:00 am nursing assessments note the following changes in physiologic status of the neonate:
Tachypnea, respiratory rate of 72 breaths/min
S1 intercostal retractions
Grunting assessed with stethoscope
Placement of transcutaneous monitor reveals PaO_2 of 48 mm Hg
Apical pulse rate, 150
The physician is notified and arterial blood gas analysis, hematocrit, and glucose levels are ordered. An order is also given for the administration of oxygen per oxyhood at FiO_2 of 30 percent and radiant warmer to be used.
Arterial blood gas analysis at 9:15 am reveals:
pH 7.28 — O_2 sat 90%
$PaCO_2$ 52 mm Hg — Bicarbonate 24 mEq/L
PaO_2 45 mm Hg — Hematocrit 50%

Nursing Diagnosis	Goals	Nursing Interventions	Rationale	Evaluation
Ineffective breathing pattern related to inadequate ventilation	The neonate will exhibit absence of altered breathing pattern	Slightly elevate neonate's head—avoid hyperextension Change neonate's position every 2 hr	Provides unrestricted air passages for maximum air intake Prevent stasis of lung fluids	Head of bed slightly elevated—air passages unrestricted
		Provide oxygen-enriched environment consistent with arterial blood gas	Provides constant supply of oxygen for respiratory and metabolic use	9:15 am—In Oxyhood with FiO_2 of 30% $tcPO_2$ 9:15 50 mm Hg

		Maintain $tcPO_2$ at 50–80 mm Hg in oxygen concentrations less than 40%	Concentrations of oxygen which increase $PaO_2 > 100$ mm Hg are hyperoxic with toxic effects on eyes and lungs	9:30 50 mm Hg 9:45 54 mm Hg 10:00 56 mm Hg 10:15 58 mm Hg
		Warm and humidify all oxygen used	Cool oxygen directly to the face will stimulate hypothermic response in neonate	Nebulizer providing humidified, warmed O_2 at ambient air temp as monitored by hood thermometer
	The neonate will maintain effective ventilation as demonstrated by relief of respiratory distress symptoms	Monitor respiratory and cardiac status	Provides indication of respiratory or circulatory failure	Neonate remains on monitors Respirations and apical pulse: 9:15 am 68 140 9:30 am 72 136 9:45 am 62 136 10:00 am 60 124 10:15 am 64 120
		Auscultate lungs sounds q hr	Provides indication of absence of lung sounds which may denote complications such as atelectasis or pneumothorax	9:00 bilateral breath sounds, clear to auscultation 10:00 bilateral breath sounds slightly diminished
		Assess for symptoms of decreasing respiratory status Apnea Chin tug Nasal flaring Grunting Retractions		Color pink, slight intercostal retractions
Potential for tissue hypoxia related to impaired oxygenation	Neonate will meet increased oxygen and glucose demands needed for accelerated respiratory and metabolic use	Maintain neutral thermal environment	Decreases oxygen consumption utilized to generate heat	Radiant warmer with heat probe used to stabilize temperature at 37.6°C
		Assess for indications of vasoconstriction	Pallor, transient elevation in B/P, and poor capillary filling may indicate acidosis and decreased oxygenation of tissues	9:15 am color pink B/P 68/42 9:45 am color pink B/P 62/36
		Minimize neonatal stress by efficient management and administration of care Limit environmental stimuli	Stress increases neonatal oxygen & glucose consumption	Periods of uninterrupted rest provided for neonate
		Monitor arterial blood gases as ordered (q 2 hr)	Indicates development or correction of respiratory or metabolic acidosis	10:00 am pH 7.30 $PaCO_2$ 50 mm Hg PaO_2 54 mm Hg

TABLE 29-7 (continued)

Nursing Diagnosis	Goals	Nursing Interventions	Rationale	Evaluation
		Monitor blood glucose levels & assess for symptoms of hypoglycemia Jitterness Apathy Tachypnea Irritability Tremors Hypotonia Vomiting	Increased metabolic and respiratory efforts reduce glycogen stores Decreased gestational age alters development of brown fat	O_2 Sat 92% Bicarbonate 25 mEq/L Dextrostix—60 mg/100 ml at 10:00 am
	Maintain fluid & electrolyte balance necessary for physiologic needs	Maintain fluid electrolytes, glucose, and medications in prescribed regimen	Dehydration alters intra and extracellular fluids thereby reducing blood volume and physiologic homeostasis Rapid dehydration may occur in low birth weight neonates	Skin turgor good IV infusing at prescribed rate
		Monitor weight q 12 hr	Rapid loss or gain may indicate dehydration or fluid retention respectively	Admission weight 2700 gm
		Maintain caloric needs by administration of feedings as tolerated	Gavage or parenteral feedings used when necessary to lessen expenditures of energy by neonate	
		Measure and record intake and output	Provides indication of hydration	
		Measure specific gravity of urine	Diuresis will coexist with improvement of RDS Specific gravity increased when dehydrated	9:30 am voided 30 ml, specific gravity, 1.008

Potential alterations in safety related to potential for sepsis	Demonstrate absence of alterations in homeostasis due to infection	Maintain aseptic technique when giving care to the neonate	Reduces risk of nosocomial infection	
		Change humidifiers, tubing, and IV tubing every 24 hr	Humid environment provides opportunity for bacterial growth	Scheduled for humidifier & tubing replacement established q 24 hours
		Assess for indications of sepsis Administer antibiotics as ordered	Cord stump site at increased risk for infection	
Potential for alterations in parenting related to impaired parent-neonate bonding	Begin attachment and bonding with parents	Explain all medical & nursing interventions to parents	Relieves anxiety about equipment & complexities of treatment	Explanation of neonate's status and rationale given. Parents asked questions & verbalized concerns
		Provide opportunity for parents to touch & if possible, hold neonate	Promotes bonding	Parents at neonates bedside, touched & stroked neonate
		Encourage parents to ask questions and verbalize feelings	Relives guilt feelings	
		Answer all questions when asked	Provides reassurance	
		Ask parents for picture of themselves to place within neonate's view	Enables parents to conceptualize their parenting role	Discussed articles to place in crib, parents will bring photo
		Provide picture of neonate for parents	Promotes identification with neonate	Snapshot of neonate taken & given to parents
		Encourage visits to the nursery or telephone calls	Relieves anxieties as they arise	

Elevated serum protein (4.8 to 7.4 gm per 100 ml normal range)

Decreased urinary output (150 to 250 ml per 24 hours) 30 ml per kg per 24 hours normal range)

Weight loss greater than 5% of total body weight over a 24 hour period

Parental Support

Efforts are made to provide the parents with an explanation of the disorder, its manifestations, treatment and supportive measures taken. They are encouraged to touch the neonate and if possible hold him. Honest explanations create trust and all discussions and explanations are presented with that consideration as a priority; however, emphasis is placed on the positive aspects without giving false hope or unrealistic assessment. (Supportive nursing measures for parents of ill neonates are discussed in Chapter 32.)

Table 29-6 provides a review of nursing responsibilities for the neonate with respiratory distress syndrome, and Table 29-7 provides a sample nursing care plan.

Air Leaks

Air leaks from the alveoli of the lungs result in air movement along perivascular and peribronchial lymphatic sheaths, with accumulations in the mediastinum, plural spaces, and other compartments of the chest. Accumulations may be encountered in any of the following compartments:

Pneumomediastinum. Collections of air within the mediastinum produce x-ray visualization of an elevated thymus and occasionally a "halo" effect encircling the heart. Air accumulations bordering the heart decrease heart sounds. Treatment may include administrations of 100 percent, oxygen although spontaneous resolution is the usual prognosis.

Pneumothorax. Air accumulates in the pleural cavity, producing an abrupt alteration in respiratory status. Decreased breath sounds, hyperresonance of the chest, irritability, and a shifted PMI are characteristic diagnostic features found in combination with x-ray confirmation of air in the pleural spaces.

Pneumopericardium. This complication results after involvement of one of the previously mentioned air leaks and results in accumulation of air in the pericardium of the heart. Blood pressure drops dramatically within a few moments following the air leak. Air in the pericardial area creates a cardiac tamponade, restricting the heart muscle and reducing cardiac filling. Symptoms of decreasing pulse pressure, absence of heart sound, and bradycardia ensue. Death follows rapidly unless air is immediately removed from the pericardium by needle aspiration.

Pneumoperitoneum. Air that migrates from a pneumomediastinum into the peritoneal cavity produces a pneumoperitoneum. Differentiation of this condition from intestinal perforation is critically important, as intestinal perforations require immediate surgery whereas pneumoperitoneum is usually benign and does not require treatment.

ETIOLOGY

Obstructions to ventilation (blood, mucus, meconium), noncompliance of the lungs (RDS, pneumonia, hypoplastic lungs), and excessive pressure in the lungs (first breath, positive pressure ventilation) are associated with air leaks. Any force that encourages overdistention of the alveoli is considered a risk factor. Vigorous resuscitation measures, such as bagging with bag and mask or endotracheal intubation, also have positive correlation with air leaks, owing to increased pressure within the alveoli.

CLINICAL MANIFESTATIONS

Symptoms that alert the nurse to the possibility of air leaks include:

- Restlessness of the neonate
- Tachypnea
- Grunting
- Shifted PMI
- Retractions
- Bradycardia or tachycardia
- Sudden drop in B/P
- Narrow pulse pressure
- Decreased or shifted breath sounds (either bilateral or unilateral)
- Increasing oxygen requirements
- Pronounced cyanosis
- Asymmetrical chest
- Abdominal distention
- Downward displacement of the liver or spleen
- Hyperresonance of chest
- Lethargy
- If on assisted ventilation, a sudden change in inspiratory pressure requirements

Depending on the type of air leak, symptoms may vary from minimal, with benign effects, to severe, with rapid deterioration and death. Early symptoms of a pneumothorax may only consist of restlessness and tachypnea, but as the process continues, the PMI shifts and becomes an important diagnostic feature. Likewise, the very sudden drop in B/P, narrowing pulse pressure, and rapidly deteriorating respiratory and cardiac status are critical diagnostic aids associated with pneumopericardium.

MEDICAL AND NURSING INTERVENTIONS

Observations for indications of air leaks are made on all preterm neonates, neonates resuscitated at birth, those with RDS, and those using mechanical ventilation, especially when high ventilator pressures are used. When symptoms suggesting air leaks occur, the physician is immediately notified and provision for arterial blood gases, transillumination of the chest, and chest x-ray may be anticipated. The head of the bed is slightly elevated to relieve pressure. Oxygen concentrations of 100 percent may be ordered to facilitate removal of nitrogen from the pleural spaces. Nitrogen is normally absorbed slowly, but when high concentrations of O_2 are administered, nitrogen is readily "washed out" (reduced partial pressure) of the blood. This raises the nitrogen gradient and facilitates the transfer of nitrogen from the pleural spaces to the blood, enhancing the resolution of the pneumothorax (Oellrich, 1985). If the condition is critical, emergency treatment may involve needle aspiration of the chest or insertion of chest tubes to remove air from the pleural spaces and restore negative pressures to the lung.

Chest tubes are placed, using sterile technique under local anesthesia. They are sutured in place, covered with vaseline gauze, and every effort is made to insure an air-tight insertion site. Two rubber-tipped hemostats and another vaseline gauze square are taped to the bedside in case of a break in the system or dislodgement of the tube. Care of the neonate with chest tubes is reviewed in Table 29–8.

NURSING INTERVENTIONS FOR THE COMPROMISED NEONATE

Maintaining Ventilation

AIRWAY CLEARANCE

The necessity of maintaining a clear passage for air exchange is emphasized from the onset of birth, through the transitional period, and during normal newborn adaptations. For most neonates,

TABLE 29-8
NURSING RESPONSIBILITIES OF THE NEONATE WITH CHEST TUBES

Frequent auscultations of the chest (q 1 hr) to denote PMI shifts and evaluate breath sounds
If water seal drainage is used, observe placement of bottles below chest level to prevent water from entering pleural space
Secure and stabilize bottles and all connections
Note and record the characteristics and amount of any drainage in the tube or bottle
Remember, it is a pressure closed system, so never open or empty bottles
Check tubing for kinks or obstruction
Note fluctuations in water level of the tube in the bottle which indicates inspiration and expiration
Position neonate as ordered
Note bubbling in bottle, which indicates air removal (if it is continuous check for air leaks in tubing)
Monitor respiratory status, vital signs (q 30 minutes and blood gases as ordered)
Do not weigh neonate unless specifically ordered and, if so, handle with caution to avoid dislodgement of the tube
If tubing becomes dislodged, cover the opening with a vaseline gauze strip—hold securely over opening—do not leave neonate and send someone to notify physician immediately
Notify physician of any deterioration of status

removal of mucus from the mouth and nasal areas when necessary is all that is required.

Neonates with meconium aspiration or accumulated secretions may require suctioning with a DeLee mucus trap, as previously discussed, or by oronasopharyngeal suctioning with negative pressure supplied by a wall suction apparatus. In this instance, a sterile catheter is obtained and attached to the connecting tube of the wall suction. The tip of the catheter is moistened with sterile water and the wall suctioning is turned on with a pressure setting of 60 to 80 mm Hg. With the finger placed over the suction control or the catheter pinched, the tube is inserted into the oral pharyngeal cavity. Suctioning is begun as the finger is removed from the suction control. The catheter is rotated as it is removed in order to prevent sustained pressure on the mucus membranes. It is then rinsed in sterile water and the same procedure is used to suction the nares. Suctioning periods are not extended for intervals longer than 5 seconds, since oxygen removal also occurs with suctioning. The nurse continually observes for indications of vagal stimulation and related cardiac arrythmias as the suctioning is performed. If arrythmias or respiratory distress are noted, 100 percent oxygen may be administered for a short interval. Suction tubes must never be forced through the airway; if resistance is met, the catheter is removed and the physician is notified.

POSITIONING

Neonates with respiratory problems are positioned with the head of the bed slightly elevated (30 to 40 degrees) and a small rolled towel placed just behind the shoulders. This position increases expansion of the thorax, decreases pressure on the diaphragm, and extends the trachea, facilitating movement of air through the air passages. Hyperextension is avoided, as it emphasizes proximation of the vocal cords, narrowing of the glottis, and restriction of air flow.

To ensure drainage of the lung segments, the neonate's position is changed at least every two hours. His arms are placed at the side to avoid the extra weight of the appendages on the chest or abdomen.

Oxygen Therapy

Supplementary oxygen provides an important adjunct for maintenance of ventilation and oxygenation of the compromised neonate. Although beneficial results may be achieved with oxygen therapy, oxygen is not without adverse effects. Therefore, it must be considered as a medication and its use must follow the same guidelines as the administration of any medication.

Oxygen administered to the neonate requires a physician order, stating the method of delivery, dosage, and provisions for monitoring concentrations according to blood gas analysis or transcutaneous PO_2 monitoring. The dosage of oxygen is indicated by the fraction of inspired air (FiO_2) and not by liters per minute. For instance, FiO_2 of 0.30 would indicate a 30 percent concentration of oxygen. To further substantiate the dosage of oxygen, measurements of arterial O_2 levels and pH are needed during oxygen therapy. PaO_2 is considered within a normal range between 50 to 80 mm Hg. There is no specific concentration of oxygen that will always result in this desired PaO_2 level. In other words, the oxygen concentration (FiO_2) is individualized according to the PaO_2 and pH of each neonate. When a neonate experiences severe respiratory distress, maintaining PaO_2 levels within a normal range may necessitate oxygen concentrations of 60 to 80 percent. As the condition improves, concentrations required to maintain the normal range of PaO_2 may fall to 40 percent.

Oxygen concentrations resulting in a PaO_2 over 100 mm Hg (hyperoxia) have been implicated in the development of retrolental fibroplasia (retinal damage; see Chapter 30). Adverse effects have also been suspected in the kidneys and red blood cells. It must be noted that the potential for damage is not indicated by the oxygen concentration but by the effects that particular concentration has on the PaO_2 of the blood.

The effect of oxygen therapy is not measured by the presence or lack of cyanosis. Neonates who are severely hypoxic may not demonstrate cyanosis, while those with PaO_2 within a normal range may have some degree of cyanosis.

During oxygen administration, oxygen analyzers are used to measure the concentration of oxygen supplied to the neonate. Oxygen is mixed with compressed air in a mixing chamber to arrive at the designated concentration. Analysis of concentration is performed every two hours and before arterial blood gases are drawn. To insure accuracy of the analyzer it should be calibrated every eight hours.

All oxygen is warmed and humidified (30 to 40 percent) before administering to the neonate. Cold oxygen is never blown over the neonate's face, as it will stimulate a hypothermic reaction and apnea. Oxygen delivered without humidity is drying and irritating to the mucous membranes.

When the condition of the neonate deems it appropriate to reduce oxygen concentrations, it is gradually decreased with decrements of 5 percent every three to four hours until concentrations reach 35 to 40 percent. Reductions of 2 percent are then made every one to two hours until the neonate is receiving room air only (21 percent oxygen). Neonates who have received oxygen therapy for short intervals may have oxygen concentrations reduced more quickly.

In emergency situations, the nurses may administer oxygen without an order until the physician is notified and treatment is instituted. If the nurse's assessment indicates an immediate need for oxygen, it is administered at concentrations below 40 percent with transcutaneous O_2 monitoring and pending further orders from the physician. If bagging of the neonate is necessary, 100 percent oxygen concentration may be used.

TRANSCUTANEOUS O_2 MONITORING

Continuous measurements of PaO_2 levels may be determined by noninvasive transcutaneous O_2 monitoring. A heated skin electrode (44°C) is placed on the skin, and as the area is warmed vasodilatation occurs. The PaO_2 level is measured by detecting the amount of O_2 diffusing through the skin. The electrode must be placed in an area free from bony protuberances, with good circulation. The area is cleansed with alcohol to remove skin oils. The skin area beneath the electrode will become red, which is considered a normal reaction. If the electrode is left in the same place for an extended period of time, however, tissue trauma can result. To prevent this, the electrode site is changed every two hours.

Transcutaneous O_2 monitoring furnishes a continuous assessment of $P_{Tc}O_2$ levels and provides an indication of developing trends in respiratory status. The stress of diagnostic and therapeutic procedures may also be assessed. When the nurse observes the $P_{Tc}O_2$ level dropping while she is giving care to the neonate, she may find it necessary to interrupt the procedure or to delay further manipulations until $P_{Tc}O_2$ levels rise and the neonate is able to tolerate the stress of care. Studies have documented variations in $P_{Tc}O_2$ levels caused by crying, positioning, and suctioning; thus, care for each neonate is guided by the effects of procedures or manipulations on the transcutaneous PO_2 level.

An additional diagnostic advantage is realized when $P_{Tc}O_2$ monitors are used to identify shunting through the ductus arteriosus. Electrodes are placed in the upper part of the right chest and on the abdomen. If the transcutaneous PO_2 is measured higher by the right chest electrode than by the electrode on the abdomen, a right to left shunt may be suspected.

The $P_{Tc}O_2$ monitored levels correlate well with arterial blood measurement of PO_2; however, caution must be used when assessments are made. If $P_{Tc}O_2$ levels are within a normal range and clinical symptoms indicate decreasing respiratory status, malfunction of the monitor is suspected. Monitors appear to be sensitive to atmospheric weather changes and are also affected by long-term use in one neonate. Neonates with extreme hypotension (shock) and poor capillary perfusion are not accurately monitored by transcutaneous PO_2 levels because of decreased circulation. It is essential to establish a baseline correlation between arterial PO_2 levels and transcutaneous PO_2 levels to differentiate between alterations in PO_2 levels due to circulatory impairment from those of respiratory inadequacy.

Transcutaneous PCO_2 monitors are used for sampling PCO_2 levels and function, basically on the same principle as transcutaneous PO_2 monitors. They are beneficial when evaluating the effectiveness of ventilation therapy and in monitoring PCO_2 levels.

Administration of Oxygen

ISOLETTE

Neonates cared for in Isolette incubators may be provided with humidity, controlled temperature, oxygen, and an isolated environment. The temperature of the Isolette is closely monitored to maintain the neonate's temperature in a range of 97.9°F (36.6°C) and 98.6°F (37.0°C). All oxygen directed to the Isolette is warmed and humidified. Controlled concentrations of oxygen are difficult to maintain in the Isolette because of frequent porthole opening when caring for the neonate.

OXYHOOD

Oxyhoods are plexiglass chambers placed directly over the neonate's head to provide an oxygen-enriched environment. They are designed for increased concentrations of oxygen and are available in different sizes corresponding to the weight of the neonate. Small hoods are indicated for neonates under 2.5 pounds, medium for neonates between 2.5 pounds and 8 pounds, and large for neonates over 8 pounds. The top of the hood may be removed during care without significantly altering oxygen concentrations, since oxygen is heavier than air. Small openings in the sides of the hood and a neck opening allow expired CO_2 to be removed from the chamber; these openings should never be blocked. Temperature probes and oxygen analyzers are used within the hood to insure correct temperature and O_2 concentrations. An adequate flow of approximately 10 to 15 liters of oxygen and compressed air is needed to wash out CO_2 levels when using an oxyhood.

As with all devices for oxygen administration, oxygen should be warmed and humidified before administration to the neonate. Transcutaneous oxygen monitoring and arterial blood gas analysis are used to monitor PaO_2 levels.

ASSISTED VENTILATION

When ventilation of the neonate is impaired, auxiliary methods of enhancing ventilation of the lungs may be employed. Methods used to assist ventilation of the lungs are bag and mask, CPAP (continuous positive airway pressure), and mechanical ventilation with PEEP (positive end expiration pressure).

Bag and Mask

"Bagging" a neonate refers to the use of a bag and mask device, which provides ventilation to the neonate needing immediate resuscitation. Two main types of devices are used to provide bag and mask resuscitation: (1) the anesthesia bag and (2) the self-inflating bag (see Fig. 29–8).

The anesthesia bag and mask provides 100 percent concentration of oxygen to the neonate from an external source of oxygen. They are capable of providing positive end pressures when needed. The self-inflating bag uses room air and is not dependent on an external oxygen source. Self-inflating bags are not capable of delivering precise concentrations of oxygen and can not be employed to provide positive end pressures.

Before ventilation is initiated the oropharyngeal cavity is suctioned if possible to remove mucus and clear the air passages. The neonate's head is placed in a slight "sniffing" position and the proper

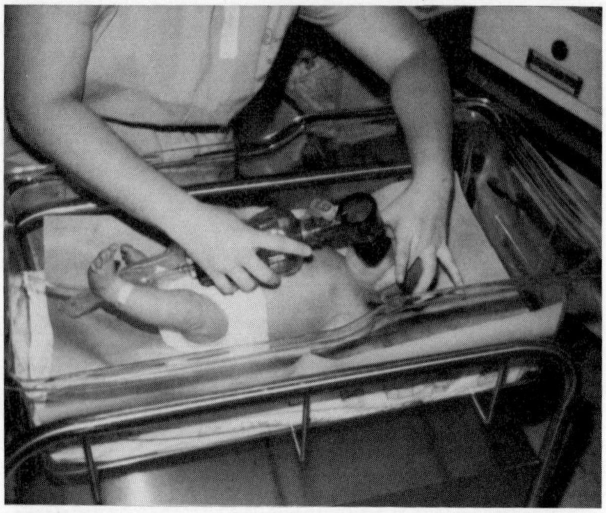

FIGURE 29-8. Bag and mask.

sized face mask is placed over the nose and mouth to create a seal. Ventilation is begun as described in Chapter 16, with pressures less than 30 cm H_2O at a rate of 30 to 50 per minute using a manometer. Assessment of the adequacy of ventilation may be made by observing the rise of the chest and auscultation of equal breath sounds.

When the chest wall rises, the pressure is reduced to 15 to 20 cm H_2O administered 20 to 30 times per minute. Overbagging is avoided, as the rapid decrease in CO_2 may cause apnea. Assessments are made to determine the presence of a distended abdomen, created as air is inadvertantly introduced into the stomach. In this instance, or if bagging is continued beyond 5 to 7 minutes, a nasogastric tube is inserted to relieve abdominal distention that could further impair respiratory efforts. Bagging is discontinued when respirations are established; if improvement does not occur, endotracheal intubation may be necessary.

Apart from resuscitation at birth, bag and mask therapy may be employed when neonates experience periods of apnea, when mechanical ventilation is interrupted, when providing intermittent positive pressure for short intervals, and following suctioning to prevent hypoxemia.

CPAP

CPAP ventilation provides a means of increasing functional residual capacity by maintaining continuous positive airway pressure. The end result is the reduction of CO_2 levels, improvement of oxygenation, and a decreased incidence of atelectasis and right to left shunting. It is provided by nasopharyngeal tubes, endotracheal tubes, or nasal prongs.

During CPAP administration, warmed humidified air and oxygen mixtures are delivered during spontaneous respirations. The mixture is contained within the lungs under prescribed amounts of pressure. A pressure release valve is included with most devices in order to prevent unsafe levels of pressure; however, some type of seal is required to prevent loss of pressure. An orogastric tube is used to prevent abdominal distention.

Indications for CPAP vary with symptomatology, but a PaO_2 of less than 50 mm Hg in 60 percent oxygen concentration for an extended time and continued periods of apnea often necessitate the use of CPAP.

PEEP

PEEP is end-expiratory pressure provided by a mechanical ventilator. The air supplied to the lungs by the ventilator is sustained at a given pressure during expiration, to increase functional residual capacity of the lungs. The pressure prevents the lungs from collapsing and extends the period for diffusion of inspired air. Mechanical ventilation is indicated by apnea, when PO_2 levels are below 50 mm Hg with oxygen concentrations of 100 percent, when respiratory acidosis is present with a pH of less than 7.25, and when CO_2 levels are over 55 to 60 mm Hg.

Nursing assessments, responsibilities, and interventions for the neonate receiving assisted ventilation require advanced knowledge and clinical practice in neonatal intensive care nursing.

Physiotherapy of the Chest

Chest physiotherapy is performed to relieve congestion in the lungs by loosening and draining secretions from the respiratory tract. Three basic principles are involved in chest physiotherapy: positioning, percussion, and vibration of the chest.

Positioning of the neonate enables gravity to aid in the removal of secretions by draining the smaller bronchi into the larger bronchi and trachea, where they can be coughed up or suctioned. Various positions are used to insure drainage of all lung segments. Chest physiotherapy may be performed by the nurse with the neonate in the crib (Isolette, radiant warmer, etc.) or while holding him in her lap.

With the neonate in the selected position, the nurse percusses the chest wall to loosen secretions and facilitate their removal. Percussion is performed in the adult using cupped hands; however, with a small neonate the cupped hands of the adult are too large to create the suction needed on the small chest. Various devices have been adapted to achieve the cupping action for the small chest, including bottle nipples, small padded medicine cups, or face masks (bag and mask type). The cupping action is vigorous but not forceful. Cupping is performed with each position change and covers the entire area pertinent to that position. Percussion in each area of the chest is performed for 1 to 3 minutes with a total of 15 to 20 minutes for the complete procedure.

The third step in chest physiotherapy involves vibrating the chest area following each episode of cupping and before changing to another position. Vibrating the chest allows the loosened secretions to move forward toward the trachea. To be most effective, vibrations are performed on expiration in coordination with expiratory airflow. A padded electric toothbrush is frequently used to perform the vibrating function.

Following each episode of percussion and vibration, secretions are removed by suctioning the oronasopharyngeal cavity. The neonate is assessed for tolerance of the procedure and if stressed, percussion and vibration of other chest areas is temporarily delayed. Chest physiotherapy should not be performed until 30 minutes prior to or after feedings to prevent regurgitation. Small and preterm neonates are not positioned with the head down, as there is an increased risk of intraventricular hemorrhage. Figure 29–9 designates positions and percussion areas for chest physiotherapy.

Blood Sampling and Intravascular Techniques

Blood sampling necessary for evaluation of respiratory and physiologic parameters is obtained from heel sticks, venipuncture, arterial punctures, or umbilical artery catheter.

CAPILLARY SAMPLING (HEEL STICKS)

Heel stick sampling may be used to obtain glucose levels and to test for galactosemia and phenylketonuria, but they

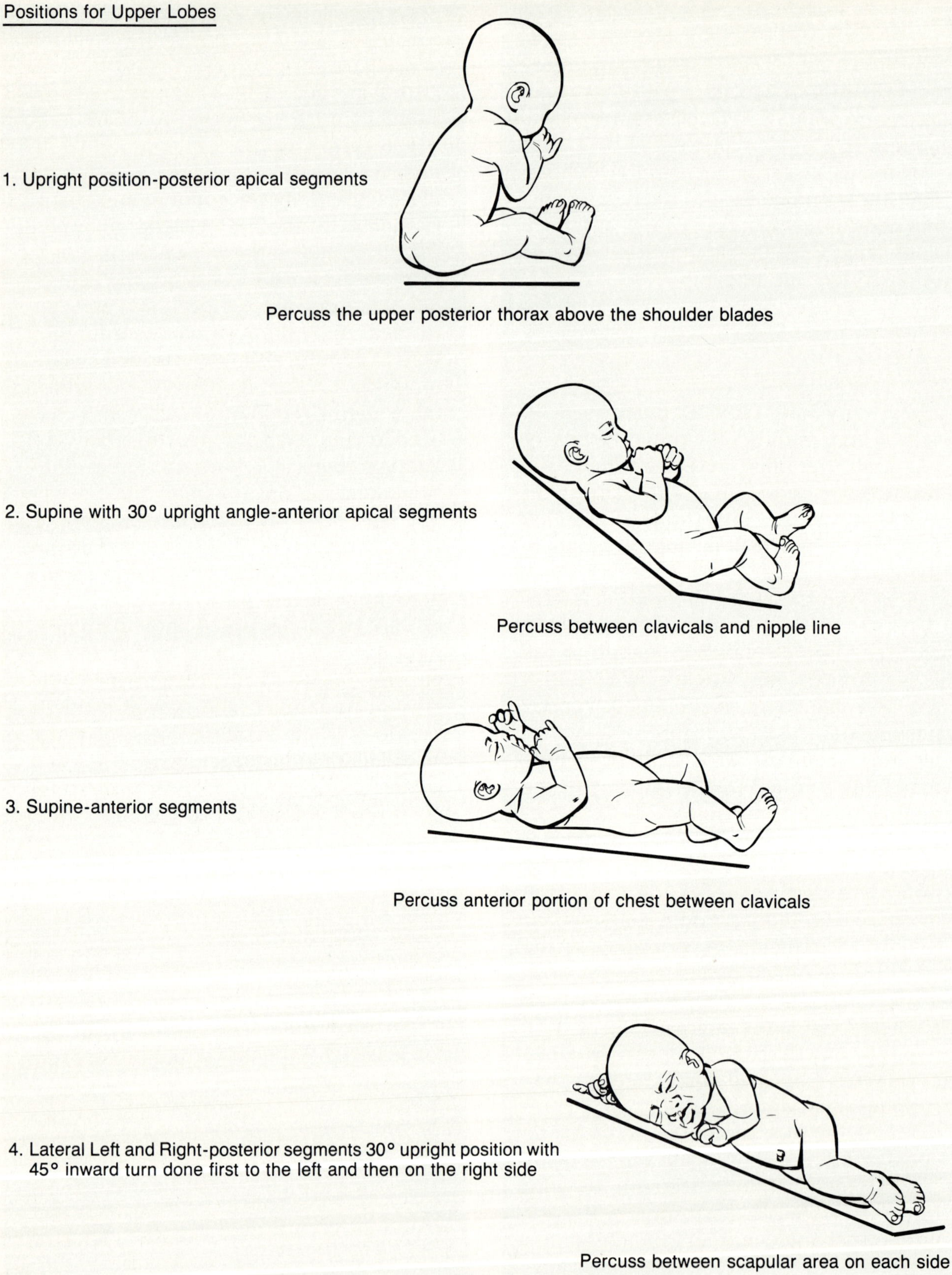

FIGURE 29-9. Positioning and percussion involved in chest physiotherapy of the neonate.

Positions For Middle Lobes

1. Supine-Tilt head downward 15° and rotate body 45° to the left
   Tilt head downward 15° and rotate body 45° to the right

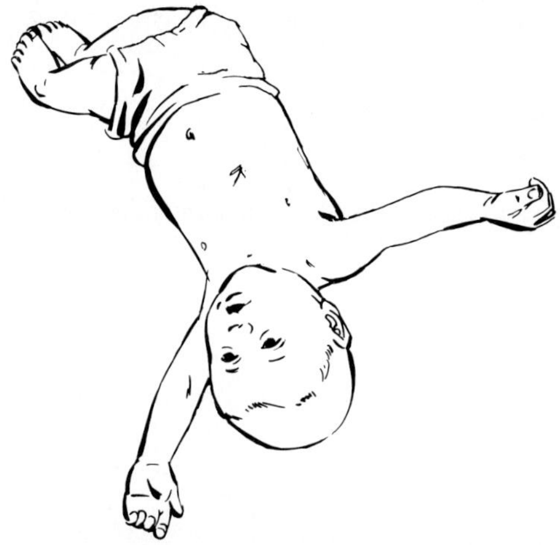

Percuss side and chest areas level with the nipples on each side.

Positions For Lower Lobes

1. Prone-superior segments of lower lobes

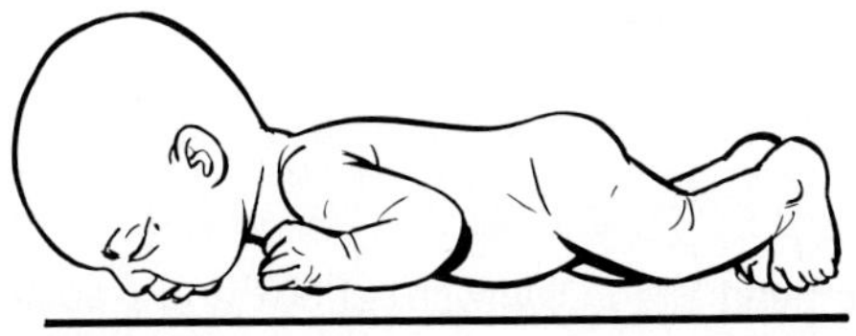

Percuss back level with lower rib cage

2. Supine with head tilted downward at 30° angle-anterior basal segments

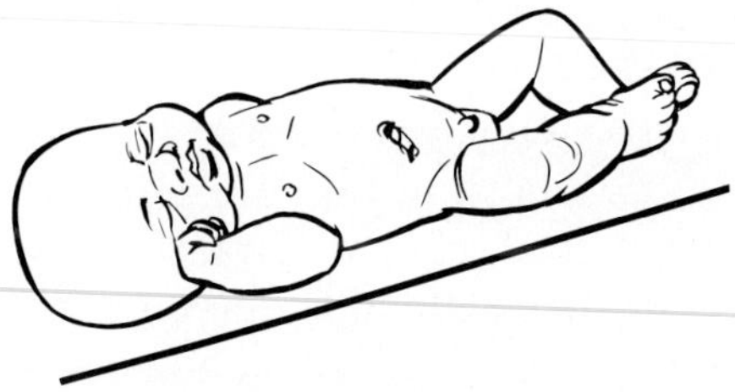

Percuss anterior chest level with lower rib cage

FIGURE 29-9. (continued)

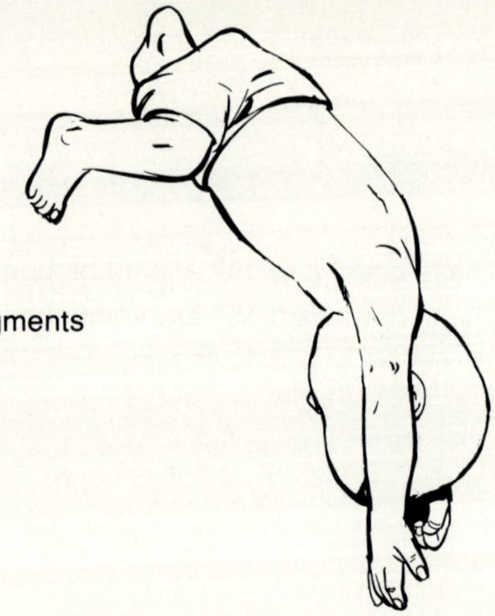

3. Left and Right side with head tilted downward 30°-lateral basal segments

Percuss each side level with lower rib cage

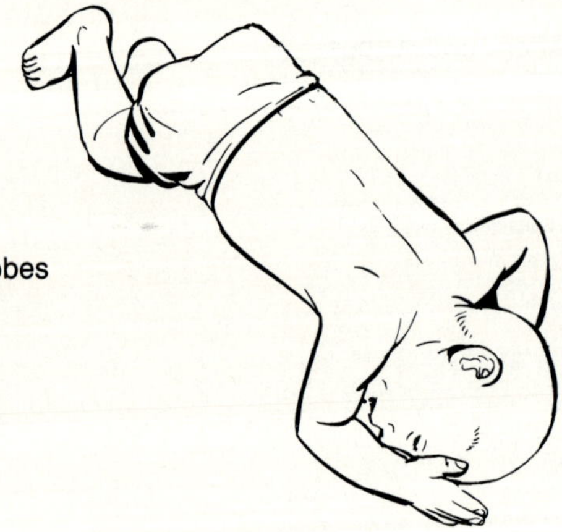

4. Prone with head tilted downward at 30° angle-posterior lower lobes

Percuss back level with lower rib cage

FIGURE 29-9. (continued)

are not considered a reliable or accurate method of assessing blood gases. When capillary blood is obtained in this method, the heel of the neonate is warmed to increase circulation to the area. Following cleansing of the site and performance of the heel stick, the first drop of blood is discarded and the sample is then collected. The blood should flow without pinching or squeezing the site, since such a maneuver will increase the serum content of the sample and consequently invalidate it. Heel stick values are altered when the circulation is poor or when the neonate is hypothermic. Values from heel stick samples will provide pH and PCO_2 levels but are not considered accurate for PO_2 or hemoglobin and hematocrit levels.

ARTERIAL SAMPLING

Arterial blood sampling is obtained from arterial puncture of the radial or temporal artery or by umbilical artery catheterization. Arterial punctures are indicated when frequent sampling is not necessary. They are used to provide accurate assessments of all components of blood gas analysis. After the puncture has been completed and the sample obtained, pressure is applied to the puncture site for 5 to 10 minutes to prevent hemorrhage. Careful nursing assessments are made of the puncture site following each puncture to detect hemorrhage or a developing hematoma.

Umbilical Artery Catheterization

When blood gas analysis from arterial sampling is needed, umbilical artery catheterization may be the method of choice. Catheterization is performed by a physician, using sterile technique and with cardiac monitors in place. The catheter is inserted through the umbilical artery into the aorta and placed at the level of the third to fourth lumbar vertebra. Placement of the catheter is confirmed by x-ray visualization. Vascular complications may follow catheterization, and nursing observations are necessary to avoid traumatic results. Complications associated with umbilical artery catheterization include:

Arteriospasms: Note blanching or cyanosis of feet or toes.

Development of thrombi and emboli: Note absence of peripheral pulses and changes in B/P.

Infection: Observe site for redness, drainage, or odor.

Hemorrhage from the site: Assess for bleeding.

Bowel infarction: Observe for abdominal distention and vomiting.

All samples used for blood gas analysis should be labeled, stating the O_2 concentration and flow rate of the oxygen delivered to the neonate, method of oxygen delivery (hood, mask, Isolette, ventilator [CPAP, PEEP], and settings), B/P, respiratory rate, temperature, apical pulse, and transcutaneous PO_2. The amount of blood withdrawn for each sample and the time are also recorded.

Umbilical Vein Catheter

Catheterization of the umbilical vein is indicated for measurement of central venous pressure and exchange transfusion. The catheter is placed through the umbilical vein into the inferior vena cava. Confirmation of the placement site is visualized by x-ray. Umbilical vein catheterization is used infrequently due to the increased incidence of infection.

Care of umbilical lines requires advanced skill and knowledge and is an important component of neonatal intensive nursing care content.

PERIPHERAL INTRAVENOUS LINE

Scalp veins and veins in the distal portion of the arm are used for intravenous administration of glucose, fluids, electrolytes, medications, and blood products. The antecubital fossa site is not satisfactory, since neonatal arm movements increase the risk of infiltration. Lower extremities are also not recommended owing to the increased incidence of phlebitis associated with their use.

The use of Buretol chambers, infusion pumps, and pediatric filters is recommended as a means of control for IV therapy. Chambers are regulated to contain no more than one hour volume, and careful observation of infusions are necessary. Protocol for IV administration includes:

Immobilization of site area—do not obscure from view.

Check infusion site for:
Infiltration—hard, cold edematous area
Infection—redness, edema
Restrain neonate as necessary—do not allow restraints to remain in same location for more than two hours
Observe for fluid overload—dyspnea, cyanosis, rales, cardiac arrhythmias
Observe for dehydration—sunken eyeballs, decreased urinary output, poor skin turgor, elevated hematocrit, increased specific gravity, weight loss, elevated temperature, depressed fontanels
Measure all intake and output
Weigh diapers
Determine specific gravity
Observe for signs of electrolyte imbalance
Sodium—irritability, lethargy, depression, CNS change
Calcium—jittery, GI upsets, apnea, twitching seizures
Potassium—weakness, abdominal distention, hypotonia, cardiac irritability
Magnesium—apnea, hypertonia, twitching, seizures
Weigh neonate q 24 hours
Change IV tubing q 24 hours
Change IV site q 24 to 48 hours (intracatheters are changed every 72 hours)
Monitor vital signs and B/P—during administration of blood and blood products, monitor q 15 minutes

BLOOD PRESSURE ASSESSMENT

Blood pressure in the neonate is assessed by external or internal techniques. The most widely used external technique is provided by Doppler assessment, which uses ultrasound monitoring. Systolic and diastolic pressure readings are displayed digitally and may also be heard with the stethoscope placed over the brachial artery. Some models provide heart rate and mean pressure readings. Correct cuff size should be used measuring the width of the cuff to be 40 percent of the circumference of the midpoint of the arm or leg. In general, the cuff size is about 1 to 2 inches wide and 3 inches long.

Using the palpation method and stethoscope will only provide the systolic measurement, and hence, is not considered an accurate assessment of neonatal blood pressure.

If the neonate has an arterial catheter in place, blood pressure can be measured using the intra-arterial B/P monitor. This internal method of blood pressure measurement is accurate and provides continuous assessment. It is an invasive procedure, however, and is usually not used unless arterial catheterization has already been instituted. Likewise, a catheter inserted into the umbilical vein may be used for measurements of central venous pressure.

Blood pressure measurements will vary with gestational age and weight. In general, the normal range is a systolic reading of 50 to 80 and diastolic of 30 to 40 for the full-term neonate, and 45 to 65 systolic with 25 to 35 diastolic readings in neonates 1000 to 2500 gm. Careful measurement of B/P is essential when caring for the ill neonate. For instance, hypotension may indicate the increasing severity of respiratory distress syndrome, developing pneumopericardium, and shunting through the ductus arteriosus. Coarctation of the aorta may be indicated when the systolic blood pressure is higher in the upper extremities than in the lower extremities.

Feeding the Compromised Neonate

The method chosen to feed the ill neonate will depend on his ability to suck and swallow, adequacy of gastrointestinal functions, the degree of stress placed on the neonate by the feeding method, gestational age, and nutritional needs. Early feedings are important to maintain glucose levels, to prevent dehydration, to establish gastrointestinal functioning, to promote vitamin K synthesis, to eliminate bilirubin, and to develop the suck and swallow reflex.

The first oral feeding (2 to 4 ml of sterile water) is initiated within the first hour of birth if the neonate is able to tolerate it; if not, IV administration of glucose may be ordered by the physician to prevent depletion of glycogen stores and consequent sequelae. Oral feedings are not attempted if the neonate shows indications of respiratory complication, complications of asphyxia or symptoms of shock (decreased B/P, cold clammy skin, diaphoresis), or both.

Breastfeeding may be initiated if the neonate is capable of sucking and his condition permits it. When possible, the mother feeds the neonate in the special care nursery where his feeding response and condition may be observed by the nurse. If it is not possible for the mother to nurse the neonate because of his condition, her breast may be pumped and the milk fed to the neonate in the manner consistent with his condition. Milk from the preterm mother is higher in protein, total energy, and lipids, and is somewhat lower in trace elements. If the preterm neonate is fed only breast milk, he may require additional supplements of vitamin D and calcium (Avery & Taeusch, 1984).

Formula feeding begins after it has been determined that the sterile water feeding was tolerated. Determination of the type and amount of feeding will depend on the weight, condition, and nutritional needs of the neonate (see Chapter 23). The aim of nutritional support of the ill neonate is to supply him with adequate calories and nutrients to foster growth without stressing the gastrointestinal system or metabolic activities. In general, fluid and caloric requirements are generally considered to be:

Fluid

Full term: 150 to 200 ml per kg of body weight/24 hours

Low birth weight: 60 to 150 ml per kg of body weight/24 hours

Insensible water loss will affect fluid requirements. The neonate receiving phototherapy or under a radiant warmer will have increased fluid loss and therefore increased fluid needs.

Calories

Full term: 110 to 120 kcal per kg of body weight/24 hours

Low birth weight: 149 kcal per kg of body weight/24 hours

During the first oral feedings the nurse assesses the following neonatal responses:

Gag reflex, sucking and swallowing reflexes

Bubbling response

Choking during feedings

Presence of excessive amounts of mucus

Presence of cyanosis during feeding

Total time duration of feeding

Total amount taken

Upon completion of the feeding, the neonate is placed on his right side, with the head of the bed elevated to facilitate emptying of the stomach and prevent regurgitation. Assessments are then made of the neonate's ability to tolerate the feeding. The following factors are observed:

Mobility of the intestinal tract

Bowel sounds should be heard with a stethoscope

Observe for abdominal distention, loops of bowel visible under the abdominal skin, regurgitation, vomiting (note amount, characteristics and if projectile), and pain (evidenced by crying and legs drawn up)

Note the characteristics of stools—meconium, diarrhea, acholic (light colored stool due to absence of bile in intestines), blood in stools, mucus, amount of stool, and consistency, and test for presence of glucose, which indicates the neonate's ability to handle glucose

Assess amount and characteristics of urinary output

GAVAGE FEEDING

If oral feedings are not compatible with the condition of the neonate or if he tires too easily during feedings, intermittent gavage feedings may be ordered. Gavage feeding involves the insertion of a catheter-type tube through the mouth or nose into the stomach for the purpose of giving nourishment (see Fig. 29–10 for intermittent gavage feeding procedure). Oral placement is preferred, since the neonate breathes through his nose until about 3 months of age and placement of the tube in the nose may interfere with breathing. However, there is an increased incidence of vagal stimulation and gagging when an oral tube is passed. Nasogastric insertion is employed when the need for frequent feedings makes it desirable to leave the tube in place, avoiding the stress and trauma of reinsertion for each feeding. If the tube is left in place, confirmation of the insertion site as outlined on Figure 29–10 is necessary before each feeding. At the completion of the feeding, 1 to 2 ml of sterile water is injected through the tube to clear it in preparation for the next feeding. Indwelling tubes are changed every 48 to 72 hours.

Continuous gavage feedings may be indicated when the neonate is not able to tolerate the volume of feeding given by intermittent gavage feedings. In this instance, the tube is placed and an infusion pump is used to supply formula at a rate of 1 to 2 ml per hour and increased as tolerated. Gastric residuals must be checked frequently and the neonate is observed for abdominal distention, regurgitation, and dislodgement of the tube.

TRANSPYLORIC FEEDING METHODS

Transpyloric feeding techniques are continuous nasoduodenal and nasojejunal methods. Both of these techniques involve passing the feeding tube beyond the stomach into the duodenum or jejunum. Before the tube is inserted, measurements are made from the bridge of the nose to the xiphoid process plus 2 cm for the nasojejunal technique. With the neonate on the right side, the tube is slowly passed through the nose and stomach and into the desired area of the small intestine. Placement of the tube is a lengthy procedure, and gastric aspirates are checked as the tube is passing. If the pH is below 5, the tube is thought to be in the stomach and if the pH is 5 to 7, it is located in the intestine. X-rays are then taken to confirm tube placement.

Transpyloric techniques are not routinely used but may benefit the neonate

FIGURE 29-10. Procedure for intermittent gavage feedings.

Purpose:

To provide nourishment for the neonate who is unable to nurse or nipple feed due to physiologic status.

Procedure:

1. Assemble equipment:
   Gavage tube—#5 to 8 FR catheter
   Syringe—20 ml
   Stethoscope
   Sterile H_2O
   Prescribed formula
   Tape
2. Wash hands before beginning procedure.
3. Restrain neonate as needed.
4. Using gavage tube, measure from the ear to the tip of the nose and then to the xiphoid process.
5. Mark the distance on the tube with tape.
6. Moisten the tip of the tube with sterile water.
7. Insert the moistened tube into the mouth of the neonate and as he swallows, pass the tube into the stomach stopping at the tape. Remove immediately if the neonate begins to struggle to breathe, coughs, or becomes cyanotic.
8. Verify placement of the tube.
   8.1 Aspirate gastric contents with syringe and note the characteristics and amounts of gastric residual. Return residual to stomach if not otherwise ordered.
   8.2 Carefully inject 1 to 2 ml of air into the tube and immediately listen with the stethoscope for the entrance of the air into the stomach.
   8.3 Place the free end of the tube into sterile H_2O and observe for bubbling of the water with each respiration. If bubbling is present and does not cease, withdraw the tube immediately. (This method is considered the least acceptable since air may be in the stomach causing bubbling to occur even when the tube has been properly placed.)
9. After placement of the tube has been confirmed, pour the formula into the syringe and while holding it about 4 to 6 inches above the head, allow the formula to flow by gravity. A little pressure on the syringe may be needed to initiate the flow, however do not continue to force the formula into the stomach. The formula should flow smoothly and steadily at a rate compatible with a normal feeding. Control of the rate of flow is obtained by raising or lowering the height of the syringe.
10. Offer neonate pacifier to suck on as the feeding is given.
11. During feeding, observe the neonate for respiratory distress, bradycardia, gagging, and regurgitation. If noted, immediately pinch off tube and remove.
12. After the entire feeding has been given, pinch off the tube to avoid aspirations of formula droplets into the pharynx and smoothly and quickly remove the tube. If the tube is to be left in place, rinse with 1 to 2 ml of sterile H_2O. Do not block or place stopper in the end of the tube as this encourages regurgitation of gastric contents into the esophagus.
13. Remove the restraints and bubble neonate. Hold, stroke, or rock neonate while bubbling.
14. Elevate the head of the bed and place neonate on his/her right side.
15. Record time of feeding, type of formula, amount of residual amount of formula taken, and the neonate's response to the feeding. Amount used for rinsing tube must also be recorded if tube is left in place.

who has delayed gastric emptying and pooling of gastric contents. These neonates are prone to regurgitation and when transpyloric feedings are begun, this risk is eliminated and weight gain is enhanced. Other benefits derived include: decreased incidence of vagal stimulation and associated bradycardia when passing gavage tube, decreased risk of aspiration, and less stress on the neonates when frequent passing of gavage tubes are eliminated.

Small amounts of formula are administered at the onset of treatment and gradually increased at subsequent feedings as tolerated. Some physicians prefer to give 5 percent glucose for the initial feeding and then, if tolerated, half-strength formula followed by full strength.

Transpyloric feedings may be beneficial to the ill neonate, but complications are associated with their use. The most frequently observed include perforations of the intestine, necrotizing enterocolitis (see Chapter 31), and infection.

Nursing responsibilities for the neonate receiving transpyloric feedings include: assessing for abdominal distention determined by measurement of the abdomen every three hours, monitoring infusion rate and fluid levels hourly (not more than three hours within the set at a time), determining residuals every three hours, monitoring stools and prevention of infections by changing external setup every eight hours. A nasogastric tube is inserted for back-flow and residual checks; nasojejunal tubes are not aspirated.

TOTAL PARENTERAL NUTRITION

Total parenteral nutrition (TPN) is a method of providing nutritional support for the neonate by means of intravenous infusions of amino acids, glucose, trace elements, essential fatty acids, minerals, vitamins, and electrolytes. A concentrated solution is prepared to meet the specific caloric, fluid, electrolyte, and nutritional needs of the individual neonate.

Indications for use, as defined by Iffy and Charles (1984), are:

- Neonates with congenital gastrointestinal anomalies
- Neonates with necrotizing enterocolitis
- Intractable diarrhea
- Malabsorption syndrome
- Low birth weight neonates with poor sucking or gastrointestinal functioning
- Neonates with respiratory distress and cardiorespiratory disorders

The solution is administered via peripheral or central venous line. Central venous insertion is performed with sterile surgical technique and involves passing the catheter through the jugular or subclavian veins into the superior vena cava with placement at the entrance of the right atrium.

Solutions with concentrations of glucose over 10 percent are not administered through peripheral veins, owing to the irritative properties of high concentrations of glucose which increases the risk of phlebitis.

Since fat emulsions (intralipids) provide a more concentrated source of calories, they may also be needed to provide nutrition for the neonate. However, intralipids may not be mixed with glucose solutions. This necessitates piggybacking the intralipid through a Y-connection located below the filter (to prevent clumping) and as close to the insertion site as possible.

At the onset of total parenteral nutrition, low concentrations of glucose and amino acids are given. Gradually, over a period of several days, the strength and concentration of the solution is increased until full nutritional needs are met. The infusions are administered by an infusion pump, calibrated microdrip chamber, and an in-line millipore filter. TPN lines may not be used for the administration of medications or blood.

Complications of TPN include sepsis (Candida, Staphylococcus), phlebitis, thromboemboli, hyperglycemia or hypoglycemia, dehydration (owing to the higher concentrations of glucose), and dislodgement of the tube.

Nursing responsibilities involve monitoring flow rates and pump infusion settings, evaluation of urine for glucose, specific gravity, and protein, Dextrostix evaluations, monitoring for indications of sepsis, maintaining aseptic environment to prevent infection, changing tubing, filters, and chambers every 24 hours, observations for infiltration and tissue deterioration, provisions for oral hygiene for the neonate, and assessments of intolerance to hyperalimentation solution.

Nurturing the Ill Neonate

As techniques for providing care to the ill neonate continually advance, the nurse becomes enmeshed in a very technical environment that demands attention to the intricacies, mechanics, and operations of highly specialized equipment. The benefits for the neonate from this environment cannot be denied, but while attention is focused on the physiologic aspects of care for the ill neonate, the psychological and development aspects are often overlooked. It may be difficult for the nurse to imagine how she can provide a loving, caring atmosphere for the neonate who is "hooked up" to a plethora of tubes, electrodes, and monitors. Yet, the nurturing aspect of neonatal care is just as important as provision for physical care.

One of the first considerations the nurse makes is the manner in which she can provide care that will promote the psychological welfare of the neonate. Attention to methods of interacting with the neonate often provides guidelines for care. For instance, when the neonate is in the light sleep state, are intrusive disturbances such as positional changes made when unnecessary, or does the nurse wait until the neonate is in a more alert state? Other often overlooked nurturing activities are stroking, fondling, and simply talking to the neonate in a soothing voice. Even gravely ill neonates will benefit from these caregiving gestures if they are provided in a gentle, reassuring manner. Neonates need loving attention throughout the entire 24-hour period and not just when parents are available to provide it.

Bright lights, equipment noises, and loud voices are not soothing to any neonate, much less those who are stressed by illness. Without a doubt, many of these stressors cannot be reduced. Yet, gentle reassurance as the neonate attempts to adapt to his environment is important. As discussed earlier, from the first moments following birth, the neonate begins to interact with his environment by giving behavioral cues that indicate his needs. This task is monumental for the neonate who is physically stressed. Can you imagine trying to interact with your environment with a covering over your eyes, a tube in your mouth and perhaps one in your nose, and your arms restrained as a needle is stuck into you? How responsive or comforting is an environment filled with invasive procedures, discomfort, and mechanical barriers?

The astute, caring nurse is attentive to all behavioral clues the neonate may attempt to convey, even a facial grimace and most certainly a cry. Attention is given to the neonate's attempt to habitate and efforts toward self-quieting. To illustrate, feedings are given when the neonate is in a more responsive state, eliminating the need to wake him when he has been successful in his efforts to habitate. In the same light, the neonate who is awake and crying is attempting to convey a need, and to ignore that cue does not promote the neonate's efforts to interact with his environment. The manner in which the nurse responds to the cue is also important. To simply place a pacifier in the neonate's mouth is generally not acceptable, when rocking, stroking, or fondling would provide the nurturing so important to his development.

In order to foster development of the neonate, therapeutic stimulation is included in the provision of care. Stimulation may be provided by auditory, tactile, and visual methods. A holistic approach to neonatal care involves the use of stimuli in a manner that will facilitate his development. Stimulation begins with gentle reassuring motions provided by the caregiver. The neonate cannot attend to purposeful developmental stimuli until he has experienced comforting interactions with his caregiver. In the intensive care setting, he is constantly bombarded with intrusive stimuli and to initiate developmental stimuli before he has experienced comforting and trust only increases stress.

Therapeutic auditory stimuli are provided by the soft, soothing voice of the caregiver or parents to pacify and interact with the neonate. Talking with the neonate while giving care and playing soft music by his bedside are realistic methods of providing auditory stimuli. Parents may also be encouraged to make tape recordings of their voices to be played frequently to the neonate.

Therapeutic tactile stimulation can be provided by stroking, cuddling, and fondling activities, employed not only when giving care to the neonate but also as a soothing gesture when he is reacting to a stressor. Gentle stimulation provided by passive movement of the arms and legs or positional changes also provides tactile development.

Intense visual stimulation such as bright lights directly in the eyes will hinder neonatal response to therapeutic visual stimulation and should be avoided when possible. Visual stimulation that fosters development may be provided in a variety of ways. One of the most important is eye-to-eye contact. If possible, this should be done with the neonate in an en face (directly facing) position during a period of alertness. As the condition of the neonate improves, bright patterned objects may be placed within his sight to provide visual stimulation.

Overstimulation or inappropriate stimulation may be as traumatic as lack of stimulation. By observing behavior and behavioral cues, the nurse is able to determine the effect of stimulation on the neonate during different levels of responsiveness. Overloading the neonate with stimuli increase the neonate's stress and results in alterations in physiologic as well as psychological adaptations. The nurse must appropriately respond to the levels of stress experienced by the neonate and organize and manage care accordingly. This information is communicated to all nurses providing care for the neonate as a basis for the development of nursing diagnosis and subsequent nursing care plans. Nursing orders must be written that outline specific details of nursing intervention adapted to the care of the neonate based on his individual response.

Information regarding behavioral response of the ill neonate must also be communicated to the parents. As they become involved in his care, their knowledge of his behavioral responses will enable them to provide nurturing consistent with his developmental needs. They, too, become involved in the development of the nursing care plan for their infant. In her discussions with parents, the nurse emphasizes the characteristics of the neonate that will help them to identify with their baby as an individual and not as a diagnosis. For instance, the nurse may point out the ways in which the neonate likes to be held, the conditions he finds stressful, the manner in which he expresses specific needs, his efforts at adaptation, and the activities which appear to most readily soothe him. These behavioral aspects are just as important as the reports given to the parents regarding their infant's physiologic status. In fact, they are indicators of the neonate's progress and will often be the areas that parents will ask about when speaking with the nurse. Knowing that they can directly and beneficially contribute to the care of the ill neonate helps parents to adapt to their own stress and will help them focus on their relationship with the baby instead of his mechanical support systems.

The needs of parents with ill neonates are complex and individualized (for a complete discussion, see Chapter 32).

There is no way that we can insure the perfect physiologic, psychological, or developmental environment for the ill neonate; however, as nurses, we can promote nursing measures that have positive consequences rather than negative effects. We must take the hand of the neonate and provide him with loving support and exemplary nursing care as he progresses through these very critical moments of life.

BIBLIOGRAPHY

Avery, G. *Neonatology* (2nd ed.). Philadelphia: Lippincott, 1981.

Avery, M. E. & Taeusch, H. *Schaffers' diseases of the newborn* (5th ed.). Philadelphia: Saunders, 1984.

Bellag, L. The expanded nursing role in the neonatal intensive care unit. *Clinical Perinatology,* 1980, **7,** 159.

Blackburn, S. The neonatal ICU: a high-risk environment. *American Journal of Nursing,* 1982, **82,** 1708-1712.

Braithwaite, S. Caring for special babies: the ethics of neonatology—part 1. *Nursing Times,* 1984, **80,** Jan. 25-31, 24.

Burgess, W. & Chernick, V. *Respiratory therapy in newborn infants and children.* New York: Thieme-Stratton, 1982.

Cagan, J. Evaluation of a discharge planning tool for use with high-risk infants. *Journal of Obstetric, Gynecological & Neonatal Nursing,* 1983, **12,** 275-281.

Coen, R., McCutchen, C., Wermer, D., et al. Continuous EEG monitoring of the asphyxiated infant. *Clinical Research,* 1981, **29,** 133.

Cohen, M. A. Trancutaneous oxygen monitoring for sick neonates. *MCN,* 1984, **9,** 324.

Dingle, R., Grady, M. & Lee, J. et al. Continuous transcutaneous O_2 monitoring in the neonate. *American Journal of Nursing,* 1980, **80,** 890.

Field, T. & Sostek, A. *Infants born at risk: Physiological, perceptual and cognitive processes.* New York: Grune & Stratton, 1983.

Fuchs, P.: Understanding continuous mechanical ventilation. *Nursing 79,* 1979, **9,** 26-33.

Gist, K. & Coen, R. Assessment techniques used in high-risk newborn follow-up programs: a review. *Perinatology/Neonatology,* 1981, **5,** 31.

Gorski, P. A. Behavioral and environmental care: new frontiers in neonatal nursing. *Neonatal Network,* 1985, **3,** 8-11.

Hansen, F.: Nursing care in the neonatal intensive care unit. *Journal of Obstetric, Gynecological & Neonatal Nursing,* 1982 **11,** 17-20.

Hodson, W. & Truog, W. *Critical care of the newborn.* Philadelphia: Saunders, 1983.

Iffy, L. & Charles D. *Operative perinatology.* New York Macmillan 1984.

Jones, M. Respiratory distress syndrome and the induction of fetal lung maturity by the use of glucocorticoids. *Journal of Obstetric, Gynecological & Neonatal Nursing,* 1977, **6,** 21-28.

Koch, J. Code pink: a system for neonatal resuscitation. *JOGN, Journal of Obstetric, Gynecological & Neonatal Nursing,* 1978, **7,** 49-53.

Korones, S. *High-risk newborn infants.* St. Louis: Mosby, 1981.

Levine, M. P., Carey, W. B., Crocker, A. C. & Gross, R.T.: *Developmental behavioral pediatrics.* Philadelphia: Saunders, 1983.

Martin, T. & Burnett, P. Development of a neonatal intensive orientation program. *Journal of Obstetric, Gynecological & Neonatal Nursing,* 1982, **11,** 175-179.

Merenstein, G. & Gardner, S. *Handbook of neonatal intensive care.* St. Louis: Mosby, 1985.

NAACOG. *Standards for obstetrical, gynecologic, and neonatal nursing* (3rd ed.) Washington D.C.: NAACOG, 1986.

Nelson, K. & Ellenberg, J. APGAR Scores as predictors of chronic neurologic disability. *Pediatrics,* 1981, **68:**36.

Noga, K. High-risk infants: the need for nursing followup. *Journal of Obstetric, Gynecological & Neonatal Nursing,* 1982, **11,** 112-115.

Nugent, J. Acute respiratory care of the newborn. *Journal of Obstetric, Gynecological & Neonatal Nursing,* 1983, **12,** 31s-44s.

Oellrich, R. Pneumothorax, chest tubes and the neonate. *MCN,* 1985, **10,** 29-35.

Patteson, D. & Raff, B. Neonatal respiratory depression. March of Dimes Birth Defects Foundation. Series 1-Module 5. 1982.

Perelman, R. & Farrell, P. Analysis of causes of neonatal death in the United States with specific emphasis on fetal hyaline membrane disease. *Pediatrics,* 1982, **70,** 570.

Perry, R. *Perinatal nursing practice.* St. Louis: Mosby, 1981.

Reid, T. Newborn cyanosis. *American Journal of Nursing,* 1982 **82,** 1230-1234.

Shogan, M. Intensively caring . . . neonatal nursing. *Critical Care Nurse,* 1984, **4,** 32.

Wennberg, R. & Goetzman, B. *Neonatal intensive care manual.* Chicago: Year Book, 1985.

chapter 30

DISORDERS OF GESTATIONAL AGE AND BIRTH WEIGHT

OBJECTIVES

Upon completion of this chapter, the reader will be able to:

1. Describe physiologic characteristics associated with prematurity and explain their effects on the extrauterine adaptation of the preterm neonate.
2. Differentiate between apnea of prematurity and periodic breathing and identify nursing responsibilities involved in the care of the preterm neonate with apnea.
3. Explain the association of oxygen therapy with the development of retrolental fibroplasia and bronchopulmonary dysplasia.
4. Discuss patent ductus arteriosus and its significance on preterm extrauterine adaptations.
5. Discuss nursing assessments, interventions, and management necessary to meet the needs of the preterm neonate.
6. Discuss nursing measures used to promote growth and development of the preterm neonate and to foster parental relationships.
7. Identify intrauterine growth retardation factors associated with small-for-gestational-age neonates.
8. Describe the characteristics of the small-for-gestational-age neonate and discuss the special needs of neonates in this classification.
9. Distinguish factors related to the birth of a large-for-gestational age neonate.
10. Examine the needs of the infant of a diabetic mother (IDM) neonate and identify appropriate nursing responsibilities involved in his care.
11. Discuss postmaturity, its effects on the neonate, and related nursing interventions.

KEY TERMS

Apnea
Appropriate-for-gestational age
Bronchopulmonary dysplasia
Full-term neonate
Infant of diabetic mother (IDM)
Intrauterine growth retardation
Large-for-gestational-age
Patent ductus arteriosus
Periodic breathing
Postterm neonate
Preterm neonate
  Extremely preterm
  Moderately preterm
  Borderline preterm
Retrolental fibroplasia
Small-for-gestational-age

Gestational age can significantly influence neonatal morbidity and mortality and must be considered an important influencing factor of neonatal welfare. Gestational age factors are not considered disorders or diseases, but alterations that necessitate supportive medical and nursing management. In previous years, gestational age was viewed only in terms of the preterm neonate. Yet, many neonates considered full-term or postterm experienced problems, too. The problems of these compromised neonates offered a convincing argument for the development of a system that assessed all neonates in light of their gestational age. Classifications were developed that provide a frame of reference for the management of neonates based on their individual characteristics as related to their gestational age. Although classification of gestational age has been discussed in Chapter 22, a review of the categories is as follows:

Preterm	Gestation of 37 weeks or less Characteristics classified according to SGA (small for gestational age), AGA (appropriate for gestational age), and LGA (large for gestational age)
Full-term	Gestation of 38 to 41 weeks Characteristic classified according to SGA, AGA, LGA
Postterm	Gestation of 42 weeks or more Characteristics classified according to SGA, AGA, LGA

Knowledge gleaned from the application of this classification system in newborn nurseries has provided insight into the care of neonates with special gestational age-related problems. It is now known that even though the highest mortality rate is seen in small-for-gestational-age preterm neonates, there may also be problems related to the gestational age of the full-term neonate and the postterm neonate. Each grouping has specific problems related to the characteristics inherent in the classification.

Estimation of gestational age is done prenatally by assessing:

Maternal menstrual history
Fundal height measurements
First occurrence of quickening
Ultrasound examinations
Analysis of amniotic fluid components

Information obtained from the maternal history is then correlated with the Apgar scores of the neonate at birth and the postnatal assessment.

Following birth, the Dubowitz or Ballard gestational age assessment (see Figs. 22–24, 22–25, and 22–27) are incorporated into the neonatal physical examination, preferably within the first 24 hours. Gestational age is determined and, along with the individual characteristics and problems of the neonate, used to develop a plan of care incorporating:

Continued assessment and evaluation of the physiologic, and neurologic parameters and laboratory data of the neonate

Modification of the environment to facilitate neonatal adaptation (temperature, oxygen, avoiding unnecessary stimuli, provision for quiet, uninterrupted rest, protection from infection, etc.)

Provision for fluid and nutritional needs to meet the metabolic and growth requirements of the neonate

Provision of care attending to the physical, developmental, and nurturing needs of the neonate

Provision for bonding with parents and inclusion of them in planning and care giving

THE PRETERM NEONATE

INCIDENCE

The incidence of preterm births is approximately 6 to 7 percent of all births. Survival of the preterm neonate appears to have a strong correlation with neonatal weight, suggesting a survival rate approaching 100 percent with neonatal weight over 1500 gm, 85 percent survival in the weight range of 1000 to 1500 gm, and 60 percent survival in the very low birth weight neonates of 750 to 1000 gm. Neonates in the very low birth weight category frequently (16 percent) have an increased incidence of cerebral palsy, visual and auditory problems, lung disorders, gastrointestinal problems, infection, mental retardation, hydrocephalus, and failure-to-thrive, which may require long-term hospitalization and costly expense to the family. In spite of these complications, improvements in care, the development of neonatal intensive care facilities, and the availability of more resources has dramatically reduced the mortality rate of preterm neonates.

CLASSIFICATION OF PREMATURITY

The degree of prematurity will significantly influence the characteristics and subsequent care of the preterm neonate. The word prematurity, in this case, denotes immature physiologic and neurologic development, impairing adaptation to extrauterine life. The better prepared the neonate is to meet the challenges of birth and extrauterine existence, the more apt he is to survive.

Classification of preterm neonates has been defined by Usher (Avery, 1981) as:

Extremely premature 24–30 weeks
Moderately premature 31–36 weeks
Borderline premature 37–38 weeks

The intensity of care will be, for the most part, influenced by the degree of prematurity and birth weight. Extremely premature neonates of very low birth weight and moderately premature neonates customarily require more sophisticated technology, and medical and nursing expertise, while the borderline premature may only require careful observation and supportive care as necessary. These classifications are used only as guidelines and can not be indiscriminately cited as the basis for neonatal care.

CHARACTERISTICS OF THE PRETERM NEONATE

The preterm neonate displays characteristics consistent with the degree of immaturity of organ systems and development. Certain characteristics may be observed in preterm neonates in different degrees, depending on gestational age.

One of the most observable characteristics is the lack of subcutaneous fat. Fat deposits are not present until the later weeks of pregnancy and their absence is noted in almost all levels of prematurity (see Fig. 30–1). The lack of subcutaneous fat imparts a scrawny look to the neonate. The skin may appear wrinkled and, in the areas of the abdomen and head, almost transparent, especially in the extremely

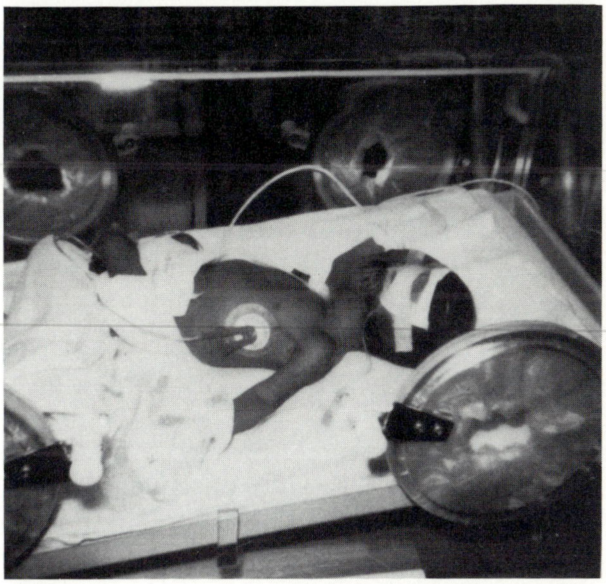

FIGURE 30–1. Preterm neonate of 37 weeks gestation. Note lack of fat deposits and somewhat scrawny appearance of neonate.

preterm neonate. Edema is often noted in the hands and feet, giving the skin a shiny appearance. Abundant amounts of lanugo can be found on the shoulders, back, and forehead except in the case of the extremely preterm neonate, who has very little. Borderline prematures may have some vernix caseosa present, but other categories of preterm neonates display little.

General inspection of the neonate reveals the head to be disproportionately large in relation to the trunk. The head bones may be pliable, feel soft, with some overlapping of the suture lines. The hair of the preterm neonate is fuzzy and wooly, with sparse distribution in the very small premature. Long, thin extremities appear to hang limply at the side of the small preterm neonate with thin, fragile fingernails and toenails. Attempts to elicit a grasp reflex may produce minimal results. Ear cartilage is soft with little recoil and the ears appear delicate and close to the head, again, depending on the degree of prematurity.

Plantar creases on the soles of the feet cover the anterior two thirds of the foot of the borderline premature, but only the anterior transverse creases are present on the neonate of 36 weeks. Breast tissue is barely noted in the extremely preterm neonate, but some budding may be seen in the borderline premature. The female genitalia reveal a prominent clitoris with poorly developed labia majora. The scrotum of the male is minimally rugated and the testes may be undescended.

A description of neurologic assessment using the Dubowitz or Ballard maturity rating and classification is found in Chapter 22.

PHYSIOLOGIC CHARACTERISTICS

Immaturity of the preterm may be noted in many organ systems, and consequently their related functions are altered. The physiologic alterations listed on pages 857–858 must be considered when planning care for the neonate.

COMPLICATIONS OF PREMATURITY

As evidenced by the previous discussion, the preterm neonate is at risk for development of complications simply because of the immaturity of his physiologic development. Complications such as hypoglycemia, hypothermia, hyperbilirubinemia, anemia, poor nutrition, fluid and electrolyte imbalance, and infection are all inherent in the immature response to extrauterine existence. The preterm neonate is also at risk for development of several specific complications that further jeopardize his existence.

Respiratory Distress Syndrome

This disorder is not limited to the preterm neonate but is found frequently as a complication of prematurity. Its manifestations and medical and nursing interventions have been discussed in Chapter 29. Since the incidence of this disorder is greatly increased in the preterm neonate, the nurse must be observant for any evidence of clinical symptoms.

Apnea

Apnea is defined as the cessation of breathing for more than 20 seconds and is generally associated with bradycardia, pallor, or cyanosis. Periodic breathing, which is the cessation of respiration for 5 to 10 seconds followed by an increased rate for 10 to 15 seconds, is considered normal in preterm neonates. Mistakenly identifying apnea for periodic breathing can have devastating, if not fatal, effects on the neonate. Apnea is not uncommon, occurring in as many as 80 percent (Vestal & McKenzie, 1983) of neonates with a birth weight less than 1000 gm. All neonates less than 34 weeks gestation should be monitored for apneic episodes.

Apnea is not considered a disorder in itself but is an indication of altered physiology,

RESPIRATORY SYSTEM

Immaturity of respiratory response at birth delaying the onset of respirations
Reduced lung compliance which inhibits the ability of the lung to take in air
Increased incidence of asphyxia often necessitating the use of resuscitative measures
Reduced production of mature surfactant which reduces functional residual capacity, increases alveolar surface tension and allows the alveoli to collapse, promoting the onset of respiratory distress syndrome
Characteristic periodic breathing and periods of apnea which encourages CO_2 retention and hypoxia

CARDIOVASCULAR SYSTEM

(Review Figure 21-1 for normal circulatory adaptations at birth)
Prone to development of persistent fetal circulation due to a combination of the following factors:
- Increased pulmonary resistance from effects of hypoxia, which prohibits dilation of pulmonary blood vessels and decreases pulmonary blood flow
- Lack of an effective constrictive response of the ductus arteriosus to oxygen, promoting a patent ductus arteriosus
- Effects of response to treatment for respiratory distress syndrome (see discussion on patent ductus arteriosus)

HEMATOLOGIC SYSTEM

Increased fragility of capillaries, abnormal platelets, and coagulation function promoting the incidence of hemorrhage
Increased incidence of intraventricular hemorrhage
Increased affinity of hemoglobin for oxygen
Prone to anemia due to exaggerated physiologic anemia of the newborn, vitamin E deficiencies, less circulating iron, and declining hemoglobin levels

GASTROINTESTINAL SYSTEM

Immaturity of digestive system noted by reduced production of gastric enzymes and acids inhibiting the ability of the neonate to digest and absorb nutrients
- Poor digestion of fats due to decreased amount of bile salts and lipases
- Inadequate production of liver enzymes needed for synthesis of some amino acids

Poorly developed suck and swallow reflex which deters feeding
Fatigue during feedings
Need for increased amounts of calories but a small stomach capacity
Frequent incidence of regurgitation due to immaturity of cardiac and pyloric sphincter response
Increased insensible water loss
Frequent inability to tolerate feedings due to immaturity of gastrointestinal functioning, resulting in diarrhea or constipation
Impaired synthesis of vitamin K due to decreased intestinal functioning
Increased incidence of necrotizing enterocolitis, resulting from hypoxic insults

HEPATIC SYSTEM

Tendency to hyperbilirubinemia due to:
- Low serum albumin levels necessary for transportation of unconjugated bilirubin to liver for conjugation
- Decreased amounts of Y protein in liver needed for storage of bilirubin for conjugation
- Increased amounts of heme from breakdown of RBCs

HEPATIC SYSTEM (continued)

Presence of acidosis, which diminishes the attraction of bilirubin to albumin
Increased production of free fatty acids related to hypoglycemia. Fatty acids must also bind with albumin and are therefore in competition for a binding site with bilirubin

RENAL SYSTEM

Reduced glomerular filtration, tubular reabsorption, and plasma blood flow, resulting in the potential for edema, dehydration, decreased renal threshold for bicarbonate-altering buffering capacity, glycosuria, and altered drug excretion.
Decreased ability to accommodate solute and water loads

CENTRAL NERVOUS SYSTEM

Immature neurologic development
Poor or absent reflexes
More susceptible to adverse effects of unconjugated bilirubin
Immaturity of respiratory center

METABOLIC ACTIVITIES

Temperature instability
Tendency to hypothermia due to:
- Reduced glycogen stores
- Reduced brown fat deposits
- Minimal ability or inability to assume attitude of flexion to conserve heat
- Large surface area in relation to body weight
- Reduced subcutaneous fat promoting heat loss by conduction, radiation, and convection
- Impaired ability to use shivering mechanism for heat production

Tendency to hypoglycemia due to reduced glycogen stores, rapid utilization of glucose supplies to produce warmth, and immaturity of enzyme system needed for carbohydrate metabolism

IMMUNE SYSTEM

Increased susceptibility to infections due to decreased antibody levels
Inadequacy of cellular defense mechanism

which may result in hypoxia and deterioration of physiologic status. Periods of apnea are often associated with hypothermia, hypoglycemia, hypocalcemia, sepsis, respiratory distress syndrome, intracranial hemorrhage, patent ductus arteriosus, metabolic disorders, immaturity of the respiratory system, hypocalcemia, anemia, and central nervous system disorders.

The apnea of prematurity commonly is not seen until 24 hours following birth. During an apneic episode, respirations cease for a period of 20 seconds or more, the heart rate slows, and the neonate may appear pale, cyanotic, or dusky. Stimulation is immediately necessary to interrupt the apnea; it may be provided by stroking the infant, changing his position, or manipulating the crib. In most instances the neonate will resume breathing; however, periods of apnea may be expected to continue. When stimulation does not interrupt the apneic episode, resuscitative measures are in order. The nurse may find it necessary to administer bag and mask ventilation until breathing resumes. If the apnea increases in severity or frequency, CPAP ventilation may be indicated.

Two drugs have been used in the treatment

of apnea, caffeine and theophylline. Their action, although not clearly understood, appears to result in an increase in the level of cyclic AMP, increasing CO_2 sensitivity and respirations. Following the initial dose, evaluation of serum theophylline levels is necessary to determine and maintain therapeutic doses and to prevent toxic levels. Adverse effects from theophylline therapy include: stimulation of the myocardium, tachycardia ($>$ 200), gastrointestinal bleeding, abdominal distention and vomiting, stimulation of the central nervous system, and seizures.

NURSING RESPONSIBILITIES

Nursing responsibilities involve careful monitoring of all preterm neonates for evidence of apneic spells. Apnea monitors that will sound an alarm when a period of apnea occurs may be used. The episode can then be interrupted. Documentation of the time, duration, and frequency of apneic periods, the characteristics of the neonate during the episode (bradycardia, cyanosis, etc.), and the response to treatment is necessary to serve as a basis for diagnosis and subsequent treatment. Apneic neonates should never be left unattended in the nursery, even though the apnea alarm is set. Laboratory assessments are necessary to determine blood gases, hemoglobin, and hematocrit levels.

Explanations are provided to the parents to help them understand the need for monitoring the neonate in the nursery and the interventions used to correct apneic episodes. Parents are often concerned about the relationship of apnea and the future development of sudden infant death syndrome (SIDS). The cause of SIDS is not known at this time and no relationship has been established between preterm neonatal birth apnea and SIDS. It is known, however, that SIDS is three times more common in preterm neonates. The value of using sleep monitors in the home is questionable, but in some instances may be indicated. Parents of apneic preterm infants should be taught stimulation methods and mouth-to-mouth resuscitation of infants.

Retrolental Fibroplasia

In the presence of high concentrations of oxygen, with elevated PO_2 levels, the vessels of the immature retina constrict, resulting in degenerative vascular changes of the retina and the formation of scar tissue. Later, as the scar tissue contracts, the retina detaches, a membrane forms over the lens, and subsequent blindness ensues.

The disorder appears to be limited to preterm neonates who have been exposed to high concentrations of oxygen, although there have been some reported cases in preterm neonates not exposed to high oxygen concentrations. Prevention of hyperoxemia is the most direct approach to avoiding retrolental fibroplasia. Careful monitoring of blood gases and oxygen concentrations is essential when preterm neonates are receiving oxygen therapy. Whenever the preterm neonate receives high oxygen concentration, such as bagging with 100 percent oxygen, the risk of developing retrolental fibroplasia is incurred.

Periodic eye examinations following administration of high concentrations of oxygen or during oxygen therapy may reveal preliminary retinal changes and require a change in oxygen management. Eye examinations are also performed by the physician before the baby is discharged and during the first 6 months of life.

Better management of oxygen administered to the preterm neonate has decreased the incidence of retrolental fibroplasia. Nursing responsibility requires an understanding of the cause and effect relationship of oxygen and retrolental fibroplasia and the ability to prudently administer and monitor oxygen therapy.

Bronchopulmonary Dysplasia

Bronchopulmonary dysplasia is a condition of the immature lung characterized by damage to the epithelial linings of the alveoli and bronchi, with fibrosis and the formation of cystic air lesions, causing pulmonary insufficiency. It is commonly associated with neonates who had respiratory distress syndrome (hyaline membrane disease) and were treated with mechanical ventilation.

RISK FACTORS

Risk factors associated with the development of bronchopulmonary dysplasia are increased by prematurity, patent ductus arteriosus, high concentrations of oxygen ($>$ 60 percent), positive pressure ventilation, and endotracheal intubation. No one factor can be cited as the direct cause, and a combination of these factors most likely contributes to the onset of the disorder.

CLINICAL COURSE AND SYMPTOMATOLOGY

The neonate with bronchopulmonary dysplasia exhibits tachypnea, dyspnea, hypoxemia, apnea, and increasing oxygen dependency, generally following respiratory distress syndrome and after several days of treatment with positive pressure ventilation.

X-ray findings reveal typical diagnostic changes indicating damage, repair, and the formation of cystic lesions incurred through four distinct stages. As the disorder progresses, obstruction, hyperinflation, and emphysema of the lungs occur, potentiating the development of air leaks, pulmonary hypertension, and right heart failure.

MEDICAL AND NURSING MANAGEMENT

Supportive management is the primary focus of treatment. Nursing responsibilities involve careful assessment of respiratory parameters with attention to observations for indications of pulmonary edema such as rales and wheezes. Oxygen monitoring is essential as efforts are made to maintain the PaO_2 over 60 mm Hg. If pulmonary congestion is noted, fluids may be restricted and the use of diuretics employed. Calorie intake is increased to hasten repair of the lung tissue and to foster continued lung development. Recovery is slow and variable, in some instances taking several years to resolve completely. Residual pulmonary dysfunction may continue to occur during childhood.

Patent Ductus Arteriosus

In the normal full-term neonate following birth a gradual decrease in pulmonary pressure and an increase in systemic pressure coupled with the constrictive response of the muscle cells of the ductus arteriosus to oxygen, initiates the closure of the ductus arteriosus in the first day of life and establishes pulmonary circulation. Meanwhile, the increased left atrial pressure and decreased right atrial pressure caused by elimination of the placenta, facilitates the closure of the foramen ovale (see Fig. 21–1). Normal neonatal circulation can then occur.

Interference in any of the mechanisms involved in closure of these fetal shunts can result in a continuation or return to fetal circulation. Preterm infants are at risk for failure of the shunts to close owing to several factors: (1) the muscle cells of the ductus arteriosus are not as well developed and therefore the constrictive response is altered; (2) hypoxia or asphyxia of preterm neonates alters the amount of oxygen delivered to facilitate closure, and (3) the frequency with which preterm neonates encounter respiratory distress syndrome.

In respiratory distress syndrome, the pulmonary vascular resistence remains high owing to pulmonary arteriolar vasoconstriction, and a right-to-left (pulmonary artery to aorta) shunt of the blood through the ductus arteriosus occurs, resulting in unoxygenated blood in the systemic circulation. With improvement of respiratory distress syndrome, pulmonary vascular resistence may rapidly decrease and the blood is then shunted from left-to-right (aorta to pulmonary artery) (see Fig. 30–2), resulting in a patent ductus arteriosus, with increased amounts of blood going back into the pulmonary circulation. In normal circulation, oxygenated blood from the lungs returns to the left atrium and is directed to the left ventricle, where it is pumped out to the systemic circulation via the aorta. It becomes evident that a left-to-right shunt from the aorta to the pulmonary artery creates a vicious circle, placing great demands on the pumping action of the left ventricle.

Preterm neonates may fall victim to a left-to-right shunt even in the absence of respiratory distress syndrome. As previously mentioned, their ductal constrictive response to oxygen is lessened and at birth the drop in pulmonary resistence is rapid, which eliminates the pressure changes needed for closure of the ductus arteriosus.

Effects of patent ductus arteriosus depend on the amount of closure of the ductus. If the opening is small, the effects are minimal. When the opening is large, however, the effects increase in magnitude as the left ventricle struggles to accommodate the large blood volume, and heart failure may ensue.

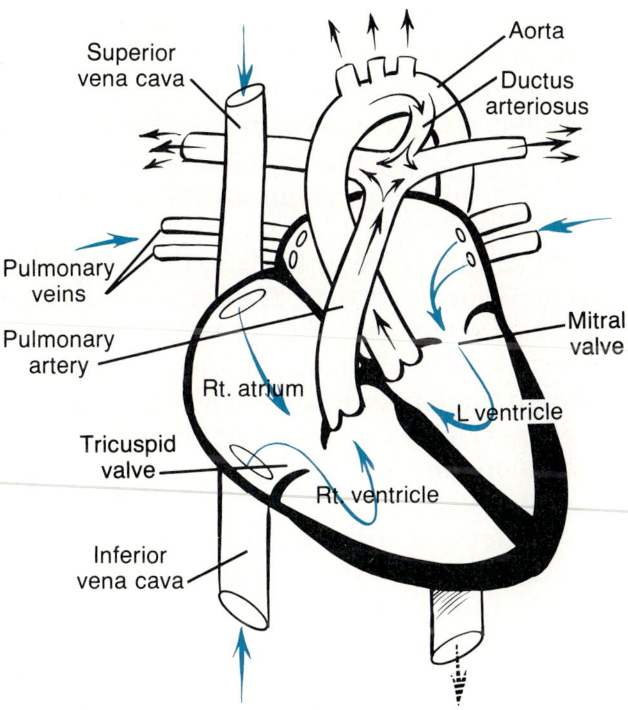

FIGURE 30–2. Patent ductus arteriosus. Dark line represents the flow of the blood through the heart and lungs with shunting of the blood from the left to the right (aorta to pulmonary artery) via the ductus arteriosus. This results in an increased blood supply to the pulmonary circulation and stresses the left ventricle as well as decreasing the blood to the systemic circulation.

CLINICAL SYMPTOMS

Clinical symptoms may reveal a heart murmur heard at the mid to upper left sternal border, bounding pulses, widening pulse pressure, enlarged heart, and symptoms of congestive heart failure (tachycardia, tachypnea, dyspnea, and respiratory rales). If the opening is small, the neonate may not exhibit any symptoms but is susceptible to respiratory infections. X-ray examinations and echocardiograms may be helpful in establishing a diagnosis when left ventricular hypertrophy is revealed in infants with a large ductus, but they are seldom diagnostic for a small ductus.

MEDICAL AND NURSING INTERVENTIONS

Studies have indicated that prostaglandins may affect the patency of the ductus arteriosus. Therefore, the use of prostaglandin inhibitors such as indomethacin may be helpful in effecting closure. This relatively new method of treatment has had some success, although its effects are not as pronounced in the very low birth weight neonate. Surgical treatment involves ligation of the ductus and is usually completed in the first year of life unless complications require earlier closure.

Nursing responsibilities require assessments for developing symptoms consistent with a patent ductus arteriosus and discriminatory monitoring of respiratory, cardiac, and laboratory parameters.

Associated Complication of Prematurity

In addition to the problems already mentioned, the preterm neonate is at risk for the development of complications such as asphyxia, hypoglycemia, hypocalcemia, and hypothermia. Other complicating factors and disorders, including hyperbilirubinemia, necrotizing enterocolitis, sepsis, anemia and intraventricular hemorrhage, are discussed in Chapter 31.

CARE OF THE PRETERM NEONATE

Thermoregulation

Because the preterm neonate is at risk for development of hypothermia, immediate measures are taken following birth to prevent heat loss and to maintain neonatal temperature in a neutral thermal range. Protective measures include quickly drying the neonate, placing a covering on his head, and placing him under a radiant warmer. If his condition permits, he may be wrapped in prewarmed blankets and placed in the warmth of his mother's arms.

After he is admitted to the nursery, the same principles of thermoregulation are continued, using a radiant warmer, Isolette or incubator. Any factors that would place him at risk for development of hypothermia are assessed, evaluated, prevented, or corrected. Even when preterm neonatal temperatures appear to be stabilized, the infant may not be able to maintain that temperature without large expenditures of energy. Therefore, the protective thermal environment of the Isolette or incubator may still be necessary, even after the temperature has stabilized.

Insensible water loss is increased in preterm infants and may be further intensified by the use of radiant warmers and Isolettes. The nurse must assess the neonate for any signs of dehydration and maintain accurate intake and output records.

Nutrition and Fluid Requirements

Gestational age, birth weight, respiratory and cardiac status, and glucose levels serve as the basis for determination of nutritional requirements and feeding methods for the preterm neonate. If the sucking, swallowing, and gag reflexes are poorly developed or absent, or if expenditures of energy are considered too great during oral feedings, gavage or transpyloric feedings are indicated. When the immaturity of the neonate's gastrointestinal system interferes with nutrition, total parenteral nutrition (TPN) may be employed. Neonates of less than 32 weeks gestation generally require gavage or TPN feedings. Methods of feeding are determined according to the criteria discussed in Chapter 29.

Initial oral feedings begin with 1 to 2 ml of sterile water and may proceed to 5 percent glucose water, formula, or breastfeeding, as tolerated. The neonate may be placed on a two- to three-hour feeding schedule; however, feeding schedules vary according to neonatal condition and the policy of the individual hospital.

Mothers of preterm neonates are encouraged to breastfeed their infants if they desire, even though nursing may not be immediately possible because of the neonate's condition. The breast can be pumped and the breast milk fed to the neonate by another method until he is strong enough to nurse. Providing breast milk to their infants helps mothers to identify with them and fosters mother-infant relationships.

Formula-fed preterm neonates have different

nutritional requirements than full-term neonates and, consequently, will need special formulas to meet these requirements. Immaturity of the digestive system inhibits the digestion of fats owing to insufficient amounts of lipases and, therefore, special allowances are made for the inclusion of medium-chain triglycerides, which do not require lipases or bile salts for breakdown. The preterm neonate is unable to digest carbohydrates in the form of lactase, necessitating carbohydrate substitutions in the form of polycose which decreases the solute load while providing adequate caloric intake. Special preterm formulas also contain a higher proportion of protein in the form of whey than in the form of casein (60:40 ratio), which renders it more digestible. Certain amino acids, are not synthesized by the preterm neonate because of the lack of specific liver enzymes, and these amino acids must be accommodated in preterm formulas. In general, the preterm neonate needs more calories and protein, with attention to electrolyte balance, osmolality, and solute load.

The low birth weight preterm neonate will, on an average, require 149 kcal per kg body weight per day. This requirement will vary with the needs and weight of the individual neonate and may range from 120 kcal per kg to 160 kcal per kg. Nutritional supplements may be needed in the form of vitamins, with a special emphasis of vitamin E. Preterm neonates are born with a deficiency of vitamin E and demonstrate an inability to absorb adequate amounts from food sources. Vitamin E is needed for red blood cell integrity, which prevents hemolysis of red blood cells and the development of hemolytic anemia.

At birth, preterm neonates are also deficient in iron and may need iron supplements. Iron, however, interferes with absorption of vitamin E, and this factor must be considered when determining the need for iron supplements. Iron supplements may be delayed until the third month of life to avoid interference with vitamin E absorption. The need for multiple vitamins, including vitamins A, B, C, and D, is also assessed.

Following feedings, the nurse observes the infant for regurgitation, abdominal distention, and vomiting. If gavage feedings are used, residuals are always checked and recorded before each feeding. The neonate may be positioned on his right side with the head of the bed elevated.

Preterm neonates have increased insensible water loss, necessitating careful assessment and management of fluid and electrolyte balance. Fluid requirements range from 80 to 200 ml per kg of body weight per day. Efforts to compensate for fluid loss on the first day generally require IV administration of 5 or 10 percent glucose at a volume of 80 to 100 ml per kg of body weight. Initial administration of 10 percent glucose may be needed to prevent hypoglycemia associated with preterm immaturity of enzyme systems, rapid utilization of available glucose, deficiency of glycogen and brown fat, and increased levels of thermal stress. On the second day, fluid volume is increased by 20 to 40 ml, with the addition of 2 to 3 mEq per kg per day of sodium chloride. Thereafter, potassium and calcium are added when urine output is adequate and fluid volume is increased to 140 to 200 ml per kg per day.

NURSING RESPONSIBILITIES

Nursing responsibilities require careful monitoring of fluid intake and output, with management focusing on the prevention of dehydration and fluid overload. Principles of fluid management require:

- Daily weight of the neonate—no losses greater than 5 percent of total body weight per day
- Monitoring intake and output
- Assessments for clinical symptoms of dehydration (sunken eyeballs, depressed fontanels, poor skin turgor), fluid retention (edema, abnormal weight gain, rales, pulmonary congestion, increasing respiratory requirements)

Monitoring laboratory values with attention to elevated hematocrit, serum electrolytes, serum calcium, and pH

Monitoring glucose levels with Dextrostix or blood glucose levels every 30 minutes until stable. Observe for both hypoglycemia and hyperglycemia. Preterm infants can quickly become hyperglycemic when receiving 10 percent glucose infusions

Attention to increased insensible water loss of neonates undergoing phototherapy for jaundice or those using radiant warmers. Consider provisions for plexiglass heat shields or plastic wraps for the neonate to decrease insensible water loss

Promoting Growth and Development

The nurse is responsible for assessing all the physiologic parameters of the preterm neonate that provide insight into his immediate needs as well as those associated with successful adaptation and growth. Continued assessments and evaluations of respiratory, cardiac, gastrointestinal, renal, and neurologic status provide the basis for determination and implementation of short-term and long-term health care goals. Nursing care requires the use of cognitive and technical skills to recognize and respond appropriately to interruptions in the physiologic status of the preterm neonate. Emphasis is placed on provision of restorative care, which will enable the preterm neonate to recover from the physical insult of preterm birth and to advance to a physiologic level where growth and development occur.

Fundamental to the provision of nursing care that facilitates growth and development, is the need for an environment that protects the vulnerable preterm neonate. The altered immune system of the preterm neonate places him at risk for infection. During the last trimester of pregnancy, immunoglobulin IgG crosses the placenta in increasing amounts. Because of his gestational age, the preterm neonate does not receive the full benefits of these antibodies and consequently will have decreased immunity at birth. Skin barriers against infection are also lessened because of fragility and permeability of the immature skin. For these reasons, strict aseptic technique is required when caring for the preterm neonate, and the use of sterile linen is often recommended. Careful handling of the neonate aids in the prevention of skin breakdowns, as will attention to the placement of tape, restraints, monitors, and tubes. IV sites and umbilical cords are areas frequently associated with infection and should be carefully monitored for inflammation, swelling, and discharge. The nurse is also alert for symptoms of systemic infections such as lethargy, apnea, acidosis, temperature instability, hypotension, and abdominal distention. All procedures or invasive techniques must be performed with consideration for the possibility of infection and the necessary precautions taken.

Handling and manipulation of the preterm neonate should be kept at a minimum to prevent stress. Management of his care is planned to prevent unnecessary intrusive procedures and to protect from disruptive environmental stimuli. Therapeutic stimulation involves reassuring stroking, soft vocal communication, and eye-to-eye contact. The addition of other types of stimuli is based on the neonate's condition and his behavioral responses. Assessments are conducted to detect any adverse response to stimuli exhibited by increased heart or respiratory rate (or both), decreased transcutaneous PO_2 levels, skin color changes, abnormal reflex responses, disorganized movements, and regurgitation. On the other hand, alert responses by the neonate to voice or tactile stimulation may indicate readiness for increased therapeutic developmental activities. These may include such simple activities as eliciting the grasp reflex or gentle rocking.

Included in the developmental needs of the

neonate is the formation of parental relationships. Fostering parental relationships with the preterm neonate includes early opportunities for the parent-infant bonding. If the preterm neonate cannot leave the confines of the special care nursery, the parents are brought to his bedside as soon as possible following birth. As with any compromised neonate, parents are encouraged to stroke and talk to him and participate, when possible, in caregiving activities.

Efforts are made to coordinate information given to the parents by all members of the health care team so they receive consistent, nonconflicting data about their infant. The nurse must be prepared to accept the response of the parents in a nonjudgmental and understanding manner. Reactions to the birth of a preterm neonate may vary from feelings of inadequacy over inability to carry the pregnancy to term, guilt because of some action that they feel precipitated the premature delivery, disappointment with the unfinished appearance of their baby, fear they will harm him if they touch him, reluctancy to become attached to him for fear he will die, and fear that he may live and they will be incapable of meeting his special needs.

To further complicate the situation, the acquaintance process of the preterm infant with the parents is influenced by neonatal behavioral response. The inconsistency and unpredictable nature of preterm responses confuses parents. The socially reinforcing responses such as alertness and consolability are often not demonstrated by the preterm neonate, which in turn diminishes parental confidence in their parenting ability. Feelings of closeness and desires to cuddle the baby are altered by the presence of equipment and the neonate's fragile appearance. Parents simply often do not know how to relate to this child who is so different from their original expectations.

The nurse can enhance the parent-infant relationship by providing parents with insights into the behavior of their baby. Following an assessment of the interaction of the parents with the baby, the nurse plans interventions needed to help the parents. These interventions include involving the parents in the care of the infant, providing time for the parents to be alone with the baby, listening attentively and answering all questions they may have, providing support without giving false hope, helping them to plan home care of the baby, and acquainting them with community resources available. Nursing interventions are individualized to the need of the parents and the baby. Although these suggestions are important considerations, they must not be considered all-inclusive.

Following discharge of the baby from the hospital, continued followup services are important to insure continued developmental and physical management and to facilitate positive parenting. The followup program is explained to the parents before their baby is taken home, providing them with a feeling of continued support from the health care team that has been involved in their infant's care. They are reassured that supportive services are available to them and that the concerns and support of the health care team does not end when the baby is taken home.

SMALL-FOR-GESTATIONAL-AGE NEONATE

The most commonly accepted definition of the small-for-gestational-age (SGA) neonate is any neonate whose birth weight falls below the tenth percentile for his given gestational age (see Fig. 22–22). These neonates may be preterm, full-term, or postterm, but the defining characteristic specifies that they are small for their designated gestational age. The diagnosis of SGA is made on the basis of evaluations using gestational age assessments for the neonate as compared with birth weight.

SGA occurs in about 3 percent of all births and carries an increased risk of neonatal mortality.

The underlying cause of SGA neonates is an interruption in the normal pattern of in utero growth. Factors that may contribute to alterations are of fetal, placental or maternal origin (see Table 30–1). Poor maternal nutrition has not been clearly established as a specific causative factor of SGA, although it may contribute to some of the other known factors. Many maternal factors can be altered or prevented by the client and must be considered a responsibility of the nurse in prenatal management of the client.

Characteristics associated with intrauterine growth retardation are related to the onset, length, duration, and severity of the in utero growth interference. When neonates have experienced chronic growth retardation with onset in the early developmental period, their weight, length, weight-length ratio, and head circumference measurement will be less or smaller than normal but will be in proportion. This neonate is small, but he does not appear to be wasted or out of proportion, only small.

Neonates who encounter growth retardation factors in the last weeks or days of in utero gestation, such as placental insufficiency, will appear scrawny and out of proportion. Length and head circumference are in the normal range but there is a noticeable absence of subcutaneous fat and muscle mass. Their hair is sparse and the skin appears dry, scaley, and wrinkled.

Neurologic functioning is not generally affected in either of the categories of small-for-gestational-age neonates unless other related problems exist. The neonate will usually appear alert and responsive, with normal reflexes. He has a developed sucking and swallowing reflex and usually can be formula- or breastfed without difficulty.

Although the external characteristics of the small-for-gestational-age neonate often alert the nurse to the identification of these neonates, not all SGA neonates are so readily apparent (see Fig. 30–3). It is important to perform a gestational age assessment on every newborn. For instance, the neonate who is term but small-for-gestational-age may have the same weight and scrawny look as a neonate who is preterm and appropriate for gestational age. Both neonates have the same weight but their appearance and weight are related to different causes and their specific needs can be vastly different.

The SGA neonate will generally not have problems associated with immaturity such as respiratory distress syndrome, patent ductus

TABLE 30–1
INTRAUTERINE GROWTH RETARDATION FACTORS ASSOCIATED WITH SMALL-FOR-GESTATIONAL-AGE NEONATES

Fetal Factors	Placental Factors	Maternal Factors
Genetic factors	Placental infarcts	Smoking
Chromosomal abnormalities	Partial abruptio placentae	Alcohol consumption
Congenital infections (rubella, cytomegalovirus, toxoplasmosis)	Placenta previa	Narcotic use
Metabolic disorders (galactosemia, etc.)	Abnormal cord insertions	Pregnancy induced hypertension
Congenital malformations	Single umbilical artery	Chronic renal disease
Multiple gestations twins, etc.)	Placental insufficiency	Diabetes (Class D-E-F)
	Small placenta	Residing at high altitudes
		Hypertensive cardiovascular disease
		Grand multiparity
		Low socioeconomic class
		Young teenage pregnancy
		Sickle cell anemia
		X-rays

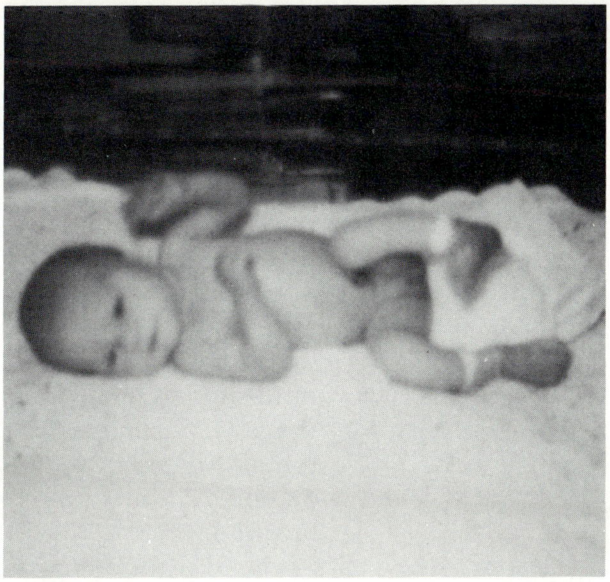

FIGURE 30-3. Postterm, small-for-gestational-age neonate.

arteriosus, and apnea, but will have complications related to growth-retarding stress disorders or abnormalities. Because of their in utero stress, they are prone to birth asphyxia with associated sequelae, hypocalcemia, and meconium aspiration. Reduced subcutaneous fat and depleted brown fat deposits place them at risk for neonatal cold stress, metabolic acidosis, and hyperbilirubinemia. In their efforts to produce heat, metabolic activities are increased, depleting available glucose and glycogen stores, also placing them at risk for hypoglycemia. Oxygen deprivation in utero stimulates the production of red blood cells, which increases hemoglobin and hematocrit levels and favors the development of polycythemia (hematocrit level above 65 percent).

The ultimate effects of growth retardation associated with small-for-gestational-age neonates depends on the cause, degree of utero insult, and any resulting complications. During childhood, as a rule, these children are smaller in stature but within normal ranges. It is important to ascertain the causation of SGA so that appropriate medical and nursing management may be instituted and further complicating factors avoided.

Nursing interventions will focus on the following:

Identification of neonates at risk for SGA

Gestational age assessment to identify the SGA neonate

Implementation of nursing measures to prevent hypoglycemia and hypothermia

Assessments for complications with emphasis on:

Complications of asphyxia and meconium aspiration

Hypoglycemia, hypocalcemia, and hypothermia

Hyperbilirubinemia, polycythemia, and cerebral edema

Assessments of respiratory and cardiac status for indications of respiratory distress

Evaluation of physical and neurologic status to aid in identification of causes of SGA

Provisions for caloric and fluid requirements.

Administer glucose orally or IV within the first hour of life and provide adequate nutrition to meet metabolic needs

Assess and evaluate laboratory parameters

Do Dextrostix evaluation of neonate on admission to the nursery and every 2 to 4 hours

Assess hemoglobin and hematocrit levels—report hematocrit over 65 percent

Provide environment consistent with the prevention of infection, stress, and fatigue

Promote parent-infant bonding

LARGE-FOR GESTATIONAL-AGE NEONATE

Large for gestational age neonates (LGA) are those whose birth weight places them above the 90th percentile of normal for their gestational age. LGA neonates may be preterm, full-term, or postterm.

Neonates of diabetic mothers are often large-for-gestational-age at birth (see Fig. 30–4). Elevated maternal glucose levels provide the growing fetus with an abundant supply of glucose, increasing his stores of fat and consequently his weight and size. At the same time, the increase in glucose stimulates the fetal pancreas to increase the production of fetal insulin, since maternal insulin does not cross the placenta. At birth the rich supply of maternal glucose is eliminated, while levels of fetal insulin remain high. The neonate rapidly uses his supply of glucose and glycogen stores to support metabolic activities, and this coupled with the hyperinsulinism increases the risk of hypoglycemia.

The infant of the diabetic mother (IDM) appears fat and enlarged, with characteristic cushingoid facial and neck features and an overall ruddiness. *Macrosomia* (enlargement) is displayed in the organs, as well, with enlargement of the liver, spleen, and heart. The neonate may appear edematous owing to his puffy appearance, but in reality these neonates have decreased extracellular fluid and total body water. They often are initially lethargic but may develop symptoms of irritability, jitteriness, and tremors associated with complications as seen in the following conditions:

Hypoglycemia	Related to hyperinsulinism following birth
Hypocalcemia	Associated with prematurity and hyperphosphatemia or asphyxia
Polycythemia	Complicating factor of decreased extracellular fluid
Hyperbilirubinemia	Associated with premature delivery of IDM neonate. May be influenced by decreased extracellular fluid and birth trauma hemorrhage (cephalhematoma). Noted between 48 and 72 hours following birth
Respiratory distress syndrome	Associated with premature delivery
Congenital anomalies	

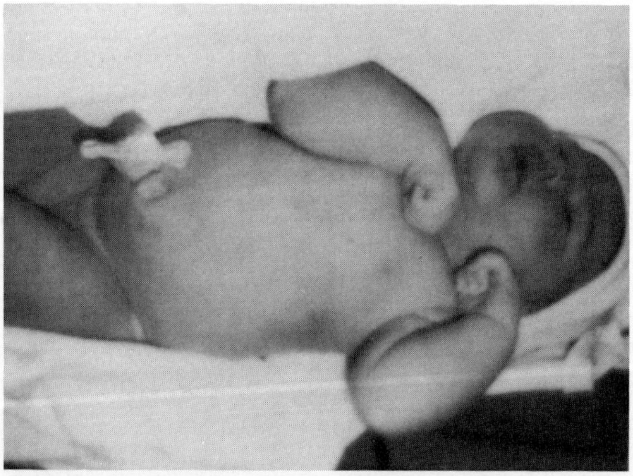

FIGURE 30–4. IDM Neonate. Infant of diabetic mother. Note large-for-gestational-age characteristics of neonate.

Table 30–2 provides a sample nursing care plan for the large-for-gestational-age neonate.

Although LGA neonates are frequently babies of diabetic mothers, other factors may be responsible for increased size. Genetic predisposition may be the reason for a neonate's large size, especially if both parents are large. Accelerated growth is also seen in neonates with erythroblastosis (see Chapter 31), transposition of the great vessel (see Chapter 31), and Beckwith's syndrome (hereditary disorder with accompanying gigantism, omphalocele, and enlargement of the tongue). Commonly, second and third pregnancies will produce larger neonates than first pregnancies. Male neonates are, for the most part, larger than females but are not necessarily larger-for-gestational-age.

LGA neonates, as well as IDM neonates, are prone to the following complications:

Birth injuries	Fractures of the clavicle Facial nerve paralysis Erb's paralysis Diaphragmatic paralysis
Cephalhematoma	

Ecchymosis
Increased intracranial pressure

Large-for-gestational-age neonates may, because of their large size, appear to be well on their way to successful extrauterine adaptation. This is, in fact, not true, for these neonates may be as severely jeopardized as the premature or SGA neonate. They require careful observation, assessment, and care following birth. Nursing responsibilities involved in the care of the LGA neonate include:

Assessment of gestational age related to birth weight
Identification of factors causing LGA neonate
Assessment for associated complications (see previous discussion)
Careful monitoring of temperature and respiratory and cardiac status
Frequent glucose determinations and laboratory assessments with attention to calcium levels, bilirubin levels, hemoglobin and hematocrit, and acid-base balance
Provision for glucose, fluid, and caloric intake in a manner consistent with condition of neonate
Prevention of infection

THE POSTTERM NEONATE

Neonates delivered after 42 weeks gestation are classified as postterm. The mechanisms responsible for postmaturity are at this time unknown, although etiology has been associated with anencephaly and trisomy 18, as well as first-time mothers over 35 years of age. The incidence is between 5 and 10 percent, with a 7 to 8 percent mortality.

Characteristics displayed by the postmature neonate are contingent upon placental functioning and related placental insufficiency. When placental insufficiency coexists with postmaturity, the resulting symptoms have been collectively called the postmaturity syndrome. In the less severe manifestations of postmaturity (stage 1) the skin of the neonate appears pale, cracked, very dry, peeling, and wrinkled with a noticeable absence of vernix caseosa. The fingernails and hair are long, but no lanugo is noted. The neonate is thin, appears dehydrated, and has little subcutaneous fat. His measurements are in proportion, although he looks like he has lost weight. In spite of his alert expression, he often looks worried and distressed.

If the placental insufficiency has been more severe (stage 2) and a degree of fetal distress has been present, there may be meconium staining of the amniotic fluid, fingernails, and umbilical cord. With increased stress duration (stage 3), the staining takes on a yellow appearance and the skin has a yellowish discoloration.

Complications are not caused by the fact that the neonate was postmature but by the degree of inadequate placental functioning that accompanied the postmaturity. Neonates who experienced minor placental changes in utero may have few symptoms other than long fingernails, dry peeling skin, and little vernix caseosa. Those with a more severe degree of placental insufficiency, may have more severe complications, including asphyxia, meconium aspiration, hypoglycemia, polycythemia, cold stress, metabolic problems, and congenital anomalies.

When a pregnancy has gone beyond term and is considered postterm, careful evaluations of fetal status are necessary. Tests are done to determine fetal welfare (see Chapter 24). If it is determined that the welfare of the fetus is in jeopardy, induction of labor or delivery by cesarean section is advised.

Nursing responsibilities following delivery may involve nursing management of the neonate suffering from birth asphyxia, meconium aspiration, and related problems. Supportive measures include assessment and maintenance of respiratory and cardiac status, provision for adequate and stable thermoregulation, prevention of hypoglycemia with adequate nutrition

TABLE 30–2
SAMPLE NURSING CARE PLAN: LARGE-FOR-GESTATIONAL-AGE IDM NEONATE

Baby boy Z was born on February 14 at 11:00 pm following a spontaneous LOA delivery. He is the first child of Donna Z., a client with diabetes mellitus diagnosed five years ago. At birth, boy Z had Apgar scores of 8 at 1 minute and 9 at 5 minutes. Physical assessments on admission to the nursery were within the normal range; however, using gestational age assessments criteria, baby boy Z is assessed as large-for-gestational-age.

Data Base:

The following data was revealed:

Weight 4250 gm	Respiratory rate 42
Length 48 cm	Apical pulse 128
Temperature 37.0°C, taken rectally	Dextrostix glucose evaluation 45/mg/100 ml

Nursing Diagnosis	Goals	Nursing Interventions	Rationale	Evaluation
Potential for alterations in nutrition: less than body requirements secondary to potential for hypoglycemia	The neonate will remain asymptomatic for hypoglycemia	Following initial admission evaluation of Dextrostix glucose level or laboratory evaluation schedule repeat assessments of blood sugar as follows: Assess every 30 minutes for 3 hours and then if stable 1 per hour for next 4 hours followed by 1 every 8 hours	Frequent evaluations of glucose levels provide indication of decreasing blood glucose and the development of hypoglycemia	Glucose evaluations performed as planned: Blood glucose levels remained above 45 mg/ml at each assessment (refer to neonate's chart for values and assessment times)
		Notify physician of Dextrostix level below 45 mg/100 ml or as indicated on laboratory assessment	Provides assessment for necessity of glucose oral or IV therapy to maintain glucose level within the normal range	
		Observe neonate for clinical symptomatology of hypoglycemia. Note: Lethargy Irritability Hypotonia Tremors Poor feeding Respiratory distress	Symptoms may indicate developing hypoglycemia and should be evaluated Brain damage may be consequence of untreated hypoglycemia	Hourly assessments of neonate with emphasis on symptoms of hypoglycemia No symptoms noted during six-hour evaluation period

		Pallor Apnea High-pitched cry Vomiting		
		Assess for complications associated with IDM neonate Hyperbilirubinemia Polycythemia Birth injuries		
		Assess neonate's ability to oral feed and tolerance of feedings. Give 2 ml of sterile water in first hour following birth and assess sucking and swallowing capabilities If sterile water tolerated and neonate able to feed, provide glucose water, formula or breast feeding within first hour following birth	Poor sucking and swallowing reflex or choking indicates necessity of using alternate feeding method such as gavage or IV Early feedings necessary to prevent precipitous drop in glucose levels from effects of hyperinsulinism	2 ml of sterile water taken at 11:30 pm—tolerated well Sucking and swallowing reflex well developed, no choking while feeding 15 ml of formula taken @ 12:00 am and 3:00 am on 2/15 Formula feedings tolerated well
		Avoid fatiguing neonate during feedings	Energy expenditures increase metabolic activities and use of glucose supplies	No distress noted during feedings Rest period provided immediately following each feeding
Potential for activity intolerance secondary to unstable glucose levels	The neonate will experience a limited amount of physiologic stress associated with care	Assess and monitor levels of physiologic stress neonate encounters when: Feeding Eliminating Diapering Assessing vitals Crying Laboratory assessments Physical examinations	Monitoring of cardiac and respiratory parameters will aid in identifying stress intolerance during care	Respiratory and cardiac parameters remain within normal range during care giving activities (Refer to neonate's chart for values)
		Plan nursing interventions and care to provide rest periods interspaced with care activities	Eliminates frequent or sustained periods of stress Allows recuperative period from stressful activities	All care planned and given with regard for intensity of stress on neonate and periods of rest provided following any care given

TABLE 30–2 (continued)

Nursing Diagnosis	Goals	Nursing Interventions	Rationale	Evaluation
		Control environmental stimuli to prevent unnecessary stress Avoid loud noises Provide comfort measures when neonate is crying Avoid use of developmental stimuli until neonate is stable	Unnecessary stimuli will have the potential to fatigue neonate	Neonate placed in quiet area of the nursery away from the alarms of monitored neonates
Potential for alteration in tissue perfusion related to increased risk for hypothermia	The neonate will exhibit temperatures within a neutral thermal range	Following admission assess temperature Every hour for 2 hours Every 4 hours for first 24 hours Monitor with temperature probe if needed	Temperature evaluations provide indication of impending hypothermia which decreases tissue oxygenation	Temperature probe used to monitor temperature Neonate's temperature remained within normal limits during six-hour evaluation period (see chart for levels and assessment times)
		Utilize measures to support neutral thermal range Warm blankets Head covering Radiant warmer Isolette, incubators	Neutral thermal range will help prevent increased oxygen consumption, depletion of glucose sources, and physiologic stress during increased metabolism involved in heat production	
	The neonate will experience minimal heat loss	Avoid environmental factors which will encourage heat loss through: Conduction Convection Radiation Evaporation		Neonate in Isolette with controlled temperature maintaining axillary temperature at 37.0°C (98.6°F)

and frequent monitoring, and sufficient caloric intake to meet growth demands.

Consideration must also be given to the effect of the late birth on the parents. When a pregnancy is postterm, parental concern over the welfare of the neonate is intensified. The pregnant woman is not only uncomfortable because of her increased size, but she is also worried about her baby. The necessity of diagnostic tests and possible cesarean delivery increases the anxieties shared by the parents, and when the neonate finally does arrive they may be filled with myriad emotions. Their first reaction is relief that the pregnancy is terminated and that the baby is healthy. However, the appearance of the baby may come as a surprise and they may again become concerned over his welfare, especially if his condition is in any way compromised.

Supportive nursing interventions focus on helping parents to resolve guilt feelings or resentments associated with the inability to terminate the pregnancy before the welfare of the infant was jeopardized. Their concerns over the appearance of the baby must also be addressed as they are reassured of his future growth and development.

BIBLIOGRAPHY

Affonso, D. & Harris, T. Postterm pregnancy: Implications for mother and infant, challenge for the nurse. *Journal of Obstetric, Gynecologic & Neonatal Nursing,* 1980, **9,** 139-145.

Baumgart, S. Radiant energy and insensible water loss in the premature infant nursed under a radiant warmer. *Clinical Perinatology,* 1982, **9,** 483-503.

Boggs, K. & Rau, P. Breastfeeding the premature infant. *American Journal of Nursing,* 1983, **83,** 1436-1439.

Bowes, W. Delivery of the very low birth weight infant. *Clinical Perinatology,* 1981, **8,** 183-195.

Bragdon, D. A basis for the nursing management of feeding the premature infant. *Journal of Obstetric, Gynecologic & Neonatal Nursing,* 1983, **12,** 51s-57s.

Cagan, J. & Meier, P. Evaluation of a discharge planning tool for use with families of high-risk infants. *Journal of Obstetric, Gynecologic & Neonatal Nursing,* 1983, **12,** 275-281.

Carey, B. Intraventricular hemorrhage in the preterm infant. *Journal of Obstetric, Gynecological & Neonatal Nursing,* 1983, **12,** 60s-69s.

Cohen, R. S., Stevenson, D. K., Malachowski, N., et al. Favorable results of neonatal intensive care for very low birth weight infants. *Pediatrics,* 1982, **69,** 621-625.

Cole, J. & Frappier, P. Infant stimulation reassessed: A new approach to providing care for the preterm infant. *Journal of Obstetric, Gynecological & Neonatal Nursing,* 1985, **14,** 471-477.

D'Apolito, K. The neonate's response to pain. Part 2. *MCN,* 1984, **9,** 256-257.

DiMaggio, G. & Sheetz, A. The concerns of mothers caring for an infant on an apnea monitor. *MCN,* 1983, **8,** 294-297.

Donlen, J. & Lynch, P. Teenage mother . . . high-risk baby. *Nursing 81,* 1981, **11,** 51-56.

Escalona, S. Babies at double hazard: early development of infants at biologic and social risk. *Pediatrics,* 1982, **70,** 670-676.

Favorito, J., Pernice, J. & Ruggiero, P. Apnea monitoring to prevent SIDS. *American Journal of Nursing,* 1979, **79,** 101-104.

Ferguson, C. Care of the infant with sclerema neonatorum. *Journal of Obstetric, Gynecological & Neonatal Nursing,* 1983, **12,** 391-394.

Fitzharding, P. Current outcome: ICU populations, neonatal neurological assessment and outcome. Report of the 77th Ross Conference in Pediatric Research, Columbus, OH: Ross Laboratories, 1980.

Fore, C. & Holmes, S. A care-by-parent unit revisited. *MCN* 1983, **8,** 408-410.

Iyer, P. My baby was premature. *Journal of Obstetric, Gynecological & Neonatal Nursing,* 1981, **10,** 304-307.

Korones, S. *High-risk newborn infants.* (3rd ed.). St. Louis: Mosby, 1981.

Kuller, J., Lund, C & Tobin, C. Improved skin care for premature infants. *MCN* 1983, **8,** 200-203.

Lazzara, A., Ahmann, P., Dykes, F, Brann A. & Schwartz, J. Clinical predictability of intraventricular hemorrhage in preterm infants. *Pediatrics* 1980, **65,** 30-39.

Lemons, J. Neonatal glucose metabolism and the infant of the diabetic mother. *Critical Care Quarterly,* 1981, **4,** 59-69.

McCormick, A. Special considerations in the nursing care of the very low birth weight infant. *Journal of Obstetric, Gynecological & Neonatal Nursing,* 1984, **13,** 357-363.

McGovern, M. Caring for special babies: Separation of the baby from the parents. Part 2. *Nursing Times,* 1984, **80,** 28-30.

Miles, M. Assessing parental stress in intensive care units. *MCN* 1983, **8,** 354–359.

Myers, T., Milsap, R., Krauss, A., Auld, P. & Reidenberg, M. Low dose theophylline therapy in idiopathic apnea of prematurity. *Journal of Pediatrics,* 1980, **96,** 99.

Roncoli, M. & Brooten, D. Low-birthweight infants: Balancing the scales of care. *Nursing and Health Care,* 1985, **6,** 199-201.

Saucier, P.: Persistent fetal circulation. *Journal of Obstetric, Gynecological & Neonatal Nursing,* 1980, **9,** 50-53.

Trotter, C. Perinatal factors and the developmental outcome of preterm infants. *Journal of Obstetric, Gynecological & Neonatal Nursing,* 1982, **11,** 83-89.

Usher, R. The special problems of premature infants. In G. Avery. *Neonatology* (2nd ed.). Philadelphia: Lippincott, 1981.

Vestal, K. & McKenzie, C. *High risk perinatal nursing.* Philadelphia: Saunders, 1983.

chapter 31

DEVELOPMENTAL AND ENVIRONMENTAL DISORDERS

OBJECTIVES

Upon completion of this chapter, the reader will be able to:

1. Describe the clinical manifestations of physiologic jaundice and explain related physiology.
2. Describe nursing assessments used to differentiate pathologic from physiologic jaundice.
3. Discuss nursing interventions used when caring for the neonate with jaundice.
4. Discuss the pathophysiology of neonatal hemolytic disease.
5. Describe nursing interventions used in the management of the neonate with necrotizing enterocolitis.
6. Describe the clinical manifestations of polycythemia
7. List four ways in which neonates may be exposed to pathogenic organisms.
8. Relate symptomatology that may be indicative of neonatal infection.
9. Describe the clinical manifestation of neonatal alcohol and drug dependency.
10. Identify the nursing responsibilities involved in caring for the neonate with intracranial hemorrhage.
11. Briefly discuss the nursing management of the neonate with Erb-Duchenne, diaphragmatic, and facial paralysis.
12. Contrast the two main classifications of congenital heart disease and cite examples of each.
13. Describe nursing assessments used in the management of neonatal cardiac anomalies.
14. Describe clinical manifestations and nursing assessments of neonates having selected congenital anomalies.

KEY TERMS

Anemia
Birth anomalies
Birth injuries
Congenital heart anomalies
Fetal alcohol syndrome
Hemolytic disease
Hydrops fetalis
Hyperbilirubinemia
Kernicterus
Necrotizing enterocolitis
Neonatal drug exposure
Neonatal sepsis
Polycythemia
Serum bilirubin levels

One of the foremost considerations involved in the management of the high-risk neonate is an understanding of factors encountered in the intrauterine environment that influence extrauterine adaptations. Not every adverse factor of a neonate's intrauterine environment can be known or its influence fully appreciated. Yet, knowledge gained from medical and nursing science has given us insight into some of the complications a neonate may encounter from the effects of his fetal environment and his development within that environment. Our task, as nurses, is to understand the neonate entrusted to our care as he was before birth and as he is now. Thus, in collaboration with other members of the health team, we are able to manage the neonate's care with insight into individual needs and to plan realistic goals and interventions consistent with those needs.

NEONATAL HYPERBILIRUBINEMIA

Bilirubin is derived from the breakdown of red blood cells (see Chapter 21). In order for bilirubin to be eliminated from the body, it must be transported to the liver via serum albumin for conjugation, becoming water-soluble before excretion.

When any alteration exists in the mechanisms or processes necessary for conjugation or elimination of bilirubin from the body, the free, unconjugated bilirubin may be deposited in skin, kidney, cardiac, or brain tissue. If accumulations in the blood and organs reach toxic levels, pathologic effects may jeopardize the life of the neonate.

CAUSATIVE FACTORS

Factors that favor development of hyperbilirubinemia may be of a relatively benign nature or may be associated with more serious complications. *Physiologic hyperbilirubinemia* is usually related to (1) immaturity of the hepatic conjugating system; (2) alterations in excretion of bilirubin; (3) alterations in the production of glucuronyl transferase; and (4) large volumes of RBCs present for breakdown, as seen in cephalhematoma or bruising. In these instances, the severity of the disease is usually minimal and improvement occurs without treatment or with the use of phototherapy.

Hyperbilirubinemia may, in addition, be found in neonates who are breastfed, or who exhibit neonatal complications such as asphyxia, hypoglycemia, hypothermia, polycythemia, acidosis, biliary obstructions, sickle cell anemia, and sepsis.

The most common cause of *pathologic* hyperbilirubinemia is associated with Rh and ABO neonatal blood incompatibilities. When bilirubin accumulations rise to toxic levels, unconjugated bilirubin is deposited in the basal ganglia of the brain, resulting in a condition called *kernicterus.* The ensuing neurologic damage presents symptoms of lethargy, hypotonia, high-pitched cry, diminished or absent Moro and sucking reflex, and vomiting. As the condition progresses, advanced neurologic damage results is hyperirritability, hypertonia, seizures, and opisthotonos. Permanent neurologic damage may occur with the development of cerebral palsy, seizure disorders, deafness, motor dysfunctions, maladaptive behavior, mental retardation, and death.

It is possible for kernicterus to develop at low levels of bilirubin (10 mg per 100 ml) in the preterm neonate but is generally related to, but not limited to, levels of bilirubin over 20 mg per 100 ml in full-term neonates.

Jaundice

The most noticeable symptom of hyperbilirubinemia is the appearance of jaundice noted in the skin, sclera of the eye, or oral mucosa. The onset of jaundice is usually on the face, with advancement to the trunk and extremities. Although observations for jaundice may be made by visual inspection, it may be difficult to determine in Orientals or black neonates. In this instance, assessments can be made by blanching the skin on a bony prominence and observing the color return when the pressure is released or by observations of the oral mucous membranes and sclera of the eye. Observations may be altered by artificial lighting and are more accurate when performed in daylight.

When jaundice is observed, the following neonatal and maternal parameters are assessed:

Maternal Parameters

Review of maternal history for determination of blood type with emphasis on Rh negative and O factors

If mother is Rh negative, review results of prenatal indirect Coombs' test and antibody titer

Testing for syphilis

Administration of Rh immune globulin

Antepartal or intrapartal sepsis

Diabetes mellitus

Previous birth with neonatal hyperbilirubinemia

Review of medications taken by mother during prenatal or intrapartal period

Neonatal Parameters

Determination of direct and total serum bilirubin levels, hemoglobin, serum albumin level, platelets, reticulocyte count, glucose levels and serology

Assessment of blood type and Rh factor

Review results of direct Coombs' test on cord blood at time of delivery (measures the number of fetal cells coated with maternal antibodies)

Assessments for cephalhematoma or bruising

Assessments for complications associated with hyperbilirubinemia (hepatosplenomegaly, edema, hypovolemia, cardiac failure)

Breastfeeding

Jaundice is considered pathologic if the following criteria are present:

Jaundice is present within the first 24 hours following birth

Total serum bilirubin levels are above 6 mg per 100 ml in the first 24 hours following birth

Direct serum bilirubin levels over 1 to 2 mg per 100 ml

Increments of total serum bilirubin over 5 mg per 100 mg in a 24-hour period

Total serum bilirubin level over 12 mg per 100 ml in full-term neonate and 15 mg per 100 ml in preterm neonate

Jaundice present for more than one week in a full-term neonate and two weeks in a preterm neonate

Medical and Nursing Interventions

The treatment of hyperbilirubinemia is concentrated on elimination of bilirubin from the body. Early feedings and the use of phototherapy are two methods of treatment that appear to have a significant effect on the resolution of hyperbilirubinemia.

EARLY FEEDINGS

Early feedings are important to stimulate digestive processes in the intestine necessary to establish bacterial flora and to decrease enterohepatic circulation of bilirubin. Until bacterial flora are present in the intestine to change conjugated bilirubin to urobilogen, an enzyme, β-glycuronidase, acts to convert conjugated bilirubin back to unconjugated bilirubin. In this unconjugated form, the bilirubin is recirculated through the enterohepatic circulation, sustaining elevated bilirubin levels. Once normal digestion and elimination are proceeding, this mechanism seems to diminish.

PHOTOTHERAPY

Phototherapy is another important method of treating hyperbilirubinemia. A phototherapy unit containing day fluorescent light tubes is placed over the bed or Isolette of the undressed neonate (see Fig. 31–1). The light, for as yet unknown reasons, breaks down the bilirubin in the skin by photooxidation and/or photoisomerization which reduces total indirect serum bilirubin levels.

During phototherapy the eyes of the neonate must be covered to prevent retinal damage by the continuous bright light. The eyes should be closed when the wrap is put on to avoid damage to the cornea from any abrasive surfaces. Careful assessment of the temperature in the Isolette and of the neonate are done to eliminate the possibility of hyperthermia or hypothermia. Neonatal position is changed frequently during treatment, exposing all surfaces to the light. The neonate is removed from the light and held during feedings. During these periods the eye wraps are removed in an effort to provide visual stimulation and foster socialization. The effects of phototherapy on the genitalia are not fully known and therefore the genital area is covered, but the neonate is not diapered.

Measurement of serum bilirubin levels are assessed every 8 to 12 hours. When blood samples are drawn, the bili light is turned off in order to prevent breakdown of the bilirubin in the sample, which would give a falsely low reading.

Insensible water loss is increased when phototherapy is used, and assessments of intake, output, skin turgor, and daily weights are required during treatment. Glucose water may be given between feedings to compensate for fluid loss.

Although phototherapy is an important adjunct to the treatment of hyperbilirubinemia, it is not without side effects, including changes in the characteristics of the stools and skin changes.

The stools often become loose, with a greenish color characteristic. These loose stools are irritating to the skin in the diaper area and may cause excoriation of the buttocks. They also contribute to increased fluid loss. When diarrhea is severe it may be necessary to use a lactose-free formula.

A bronze discoloration of the skin is frequently observed in neonates receiving phototherapy. This discoloration is usually associated with a coexisting obstructive jaundice and generally disappears within a few weeks following phototherapy. A transient skin rash resembling small flea bites is also often noticed but is not of any clinical significance. Black neonates receiving phototherapy experience a degree of hyperpigmentation, which gradually fades over time, following treatment.

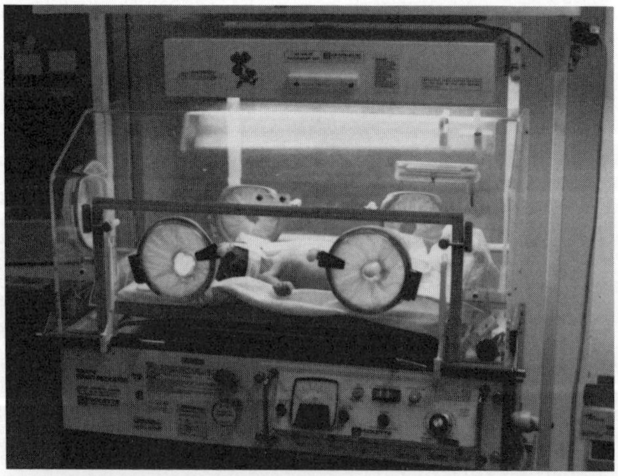

FIGURE 31–1. Phototherapy unit.

ALBUMIN

Treatment of hyperbilirubinemia also includes assessment of factors that may alter the degree of bilirubin-albumin binding. Since bilirubin is transported to the liver for conjugation bound to albumin, any factors that alter this process or affect the level of serum albumin must be considered. This fact is of particular importance, since albumin-bound bilirubin is not able to penetrate the blood-brain barrier, which aids in the prevention of kernicterus.

When serum albumin levels are low, the amount of bilirubin that can be bound is reduced. Preterm neonates and neonates with respiratory distress syndrome are classic examples of neonates with decreased levels of albumin and reduced bilirubin-binding capacity.

Other substances will readily bind with albumin and therefore compete with bilirubin for binding sites. Free fatty acids, produced when neonates are exposed to cold stress, will bind to albumin and eliminate bilirubin binding sites. Acidosis also alters the affinity of albumin for bilirubin by decreasing its binding capacity, and increasing bilirubin levels in neonates with anoxia and asphyxia. Certain drugs, such as sulfa, heparin, and aspirin, taken by the mother in large doses during pregnancy also alter the ability of bilirubin to bind with albumin.

PHENOBARBITAL

Phenobarbital has been used as a pharmacologic agent to reduce bilirubin levels. Its direct action is not clear, but it is thought to enhance activation of glucuronyl transferase. Controversy exists over the use and effectiveness of this mode of treatment, and at present, it is not a widely recommended method of treatment.

EXCHANGE TRANSFUSION

Exchange transfusion of the neonate's blood produces the most direct method of eliminating bilirubin. Since it is not without complications, its use is generally reserved for more severe cases of hyperbilirubinemia, with bilirubin levels exceeding 20 mg per ml in the full-term and 15 mg per ml in the preterm. If other indications of increasing severity of hyperbilirubinemia are present, exchange transfusions may be performed at lower bilirubin levels.

The goal of the transfusion is to exchange the neonate's blood with fresh donor blood, facilitating the removal of bilirubin and antibody-coated red blood cells and to correct anemia. During blood exchange, the umbilical or femoral veins are used to remove small amounts of the neonate's blood, alternating with replacements of equal amounts of compatible donor Rh− blood. The total amount of donor blood given will be twice the amount of neonatal blood volume with replacement of 85 percent of the neonate's red blood cells.

Preliminary preparations include explanations to the parents and parental signature on consent forms, assembly and preparation of equipment using sterile technique, and careful assessment and recording of the neonate's physiologic status to serve as a baseline for assessments during and following the procedure. Feedings are withheld for 4 hours before the procedure, or if necessary, the stomach contents may be aspirated to prevent vomiting and aspiration. Resuscitative equipment is readily available and cardiac and temperature monitors are placed before beginning the procedure.

TABLE 31–1
SAMPLE NURSING CARE PLAN: HYPERBILIRUBINEMIA

Baby girl M. was born on 1-22 at 7:14 am to Lana (gravida 1, para 1) (A-RH^+), age 24, and Mike M., age 28. Lana's prenatal, and labor and delivery history were uneventful and within normal limits. Delivery of Baby M. was spontaneous, LOA, and without anesthesia. At birth, Baby M's Apgar scores were 7 at 1 minute and 9 at 5 minutes. Upon admission to the newborn nursery, the following data was obtained:

Data Base:

Weight 3884 gm
Length 49.4 cm
Gestational age assessment 40 weeks
Vital signs:
- Temperature 36.9°C assessed rectally
- Respirations 40 regular, no increased respiratory efforts or distress
- Bilateral lung sounds—no rales or rhonchi
- Apical pulse 124, heart sounds clear—no murmurs—regular rhythm
- B/P 70/46

Physical examination upon admission to the nursery within normal limits
Dextrostix glucose evaluation 60 mg/100 ml
Cord normal vessels, no staining
Meconium stool passed when rectal temperature assessed
Breastfeeding initiated in the birthing room, bonded with parents
During the following 48-hour period Baby M's physical status, voidings, and stools remained within normal limits. She was receiving 1/2 to 1 ounce at breast every 2 to 4 hours

Assessments on 1-24 at 7:00 am noted a slight amount of jaundice discoloration of the face. The pediatrician was notified, and at 11:00 am a moderate amount of jaundice was assessed on the face and the sclera of the eyes of Baby M.
Laboratory assessments obtained at 12:45 pm revealed the following:
- Blood type and Rh A+
- Total serum bilirubin level 12 mg/100 ml
- Direct serum bilirubin level 1 mg/100 ml
- Hematocrit 52%
- Platelets 150,000/mm^3
- Reticulocytes 4%
- Red blood cells 5,000,000/mm^3
- White blood cells 15,000/mm^3
- Blood sugar 60 mg/100 ml

Based on the physical and laboratory assessments, Dr. W. ordered Baby M. to receive phototherapy and assessment of serum bilirubin levels every 12 hours.
Baby M.'s nursing care plan was revised at 2:00 pm and included the following plan of care.

Nursing Diagnosis	Goals	Nursing Interventions	Rationale	Evaluation
Potential fluid volume deficit: related to fluid loss from effects of phototherapy	The neonate will remain well hydrated during phototherapy treatment	Assess hydration status noting: Skin turgor Moistness of mucous membranes Depressed fontanels Sunken eye orbitals Monitor urinary output	Poor skin turgor and dry mucous membranes denote tissue fluid loss Decreased urinary output less than 30 ml/kg/24 hr indicates dehydration	Assessments of hydration @ 3:00, 5:00, 7:00, 9:00 and 11:00 pm indicated mucous membranes moist, fontanels not depressed, no tenting of skin, or orbital changes Voided at 3:00, 4:30, 7:30, and 10:00 pm, diaper moderately saturated

		Assess specific gravity of urine	Increasing specific gravity over 1.012 denotes decreasing hydration	Specific gravity of urine remains within normal limits, see flow sheet for specific levels
		Assess daily weight	Losses over 5% of total body weight in 24 hour period above normal parameters indicating rapid fluid loss	Daily weights assessed and evaluated every 24 hours at 6:00 am Birth weight, 3884 gm
		Monitor lab values Na+ Serum protein Hematocrit	Abnormal levels indicating dehydration Na+ > 143 mEq/L Serum protein > 7.g/100 ml Hct > 60%	Laboratory evaluations within normal range, see chart for values
		Maintain adequate fluid intake providing 140–200 ml/kg/24 hours	Increasing insensible water loss necessitates adequate fluid intake	Total fluid intake from 3:00 to 11:00 pm, 180 ml, adequate intake
Potential for injury related to impairment of physiologic status secondary to potential increase in bilirubin levels	The neonate will experience no physiologic impairment due to increasing severity of hyperbilirubinemia	Assess degree of jaundice visible on skin, sclera, and mucous membranes of neonate q 2 hours		Jaundice visible on face, trunk and sclera of the eye as assessed at 3:00, 5:00, 7:00, 9:00, & 11:00 pm
		Assess skin by placing pressure on bony prominence & releasing, assess in daylight when possible	Blanched area will appear jaundiced; artificial lighting can distort color, and assessment is inaccurate	
		Monitor laboratory values of serum bilirubin levels	Detects increasing severity of hyperbilirubinemia and effectiveness of phototherapy Total serum bilirubin levels > 12 mg/100 ml and > 1–2 mg/ml of direct serum bilirubin above normal values	Laboratory assessments to be obtained q 12 hours @ 6:00 am and 6:00 pm 1-24, 6:00 pm Total serum bilirubin 12 mg/100 ml Direct serum bilirubin 1 mg/100 ml
		Monitor for decreasing physiologic status Assess cardiac, respiratory, and neurologic parameters	Deterioration in vital functions may be prelude to developing kernicterus	Vital signs and assessments within normal range Normal reflexes and no indications of deteriorating neurologic status, (see chart for record of assessments)

TABLE 31-1 (continued)

Nursing Diagnosis	Goals	Nursing Intervention	Rationale	Evaluations
Potential for injury related to environmental hazards associated with phototherapy treatment	The neonate will exhibit no evidence of injury to the eyes during phototherapy treatment	Place protective coverings securely over the eyes during phototherapy treatment	Eye coverings protect eye from direct, bright light during treatment	Neonate's eyes closed as eye patches were securely placed over eyes at the onset of phototherapy treatment
		Close eyes of neonate before applying coverings	Prevents damage to the retina from possible abrasive surface of eye covers	
		Assess eyes for evidence of conjunctivitis q 8 hrs. Note: Inflammation Irritation Discharge	Irritation of eyes may occur from continued use of eye coverings	Eye coverings removed and eyes examined @ 10:00 pm No evidence of inflammation, irritation or discharge
	The neonate will experience no adverse effects to genitals from phototherapy light	Place small, light covering over genital area during phototherapy	Effects of phototherapy on genitals are not established, although adverse effects more suspect in male neonates	Light covering in place over genitals during treatment
	Maintain temperature in neutral thermal range during phototherapy	Assess temperature of neonate q 4 hrs. Note: Elevations > 37.0°C or temperature below 36.6°C	Neonate may experience hyperthermia from increased warmth of light or hypothermia from heat loss by conduction and radiation	Axillary temperature assessed @ 3:00 pm 37.0°C 7:00 pm 37.2°C 11:00 pm 37.0°C No significant alterations
Skin integrity, potential for impairment related to potential excoriation from loose stools	The neonate will experience no skin impairment in genital, rectal or buttocks area	Assess characteristics of stools Note: Color Consistency Amount Odor	The neonate under phototherapy will have loose, greenish stools as photodegradation of bilirubin occurs These stools may be irritating to the skin	Moderate amount of yellow, soft stool @ 4:30 & 10:30 pm No irritation in genital, rectal or buttocks area

Social isolation, related to separation of neonate from environmental and social stimuli	The neonate will experience periods of visual stimulation	Shut off bili light and remove protective coverings from eyes when: Feeding Parent visitation Physical examinations Laboratory assessments	Prolonged deprivation of visual stimulation can alter sensory development and adaptation to environment	Neonate removed from bili light and eye coverings removed for 15 to 30 minute periods @ 3:00, 5:30, 7:00, 10:00 pm
		Provide tactile stimulation during phototherapy by stroking and touching the neonate	Provides neonate with feelings of reassurance	Neonate stroked and fondled during repositioning q 30 min
		Reposition neonate q 30 minutes	Repositioning of the neonate provides tactile stimulation and exposes all skin areas for breakdown of bilirubin	
	Maintain social interactions during phototherapy treatments	Remove neonate from bili light and hold during each feeding and q 2 hrs	Promotes socialization	Parents present for all feedings 3:00 to 11:00 pm. Held and rocked neonate following each feeding
		Encourage parents to hold and feed neonate	Promotes parental attachment	
		Offer appropriate explanations to parents regarding treatment		

Verification of the correct blood type and Rh factor are noted, as is the age of the blood to be transfused.

During the transfusion, the neonate is positioned on his back, restrained, and placed under a radiant warmer to prevent cold stress. Central venous pressure and cardiac and respiratory status are assessed. Emphasis is placed on observations for apnea, bradycardia, arrhythmias, changes in central venous pressure, and indications of circulatory overload. All blood is warmed before transfusing, to prevent ventricular fibrillation and vasospasms and to decrease the viscosity of the blood. With each blood withdrawal, the time, the amount of blood withdrawn, and the amount transfused are recorded. Following exchange of approximately 100 ml, the physician may choose to give calcium gluconate to prevent cardiac irritability.

Upon completion of the transfusion, neonatal assessments include observations for symptoms of hypocalcemia or hypercalcemia, hypoglycemia, cardiac arrhythmias, sepsis, thrombi, and hemorrhage at the infusion site.

Table 31-1 provides a sample nursing care plan for a neonate with hyperbilirubinemia.

NEONATAL HEMOLYTIC DISEASE

Hemolytic disease of the neonate (erythroblastosis fetalis) occurs when there is a blood incompatibility between fetal and maternal blood that produces isoimmunization and subsequent destruction of fetal red blood cells. Isoimmunization may be the result of blood incompatibilities of the Rh factor or ABO factor (see Chapter 25). When the Rh factor is involved, the mother is Rh negative, and the fetus is Rh positive. In the case of ABO incompatibility, the mother is blood type O and the fetus is generally type A, but incompatibility also occurs with the blood type B fetus.

Rh Incompatibility

Since the circulations of the mother and the fetus are separate, sensitization of the mother's Rh− blood with fetal Rh+ antigens, for the most part, occurs at the time of placental separation. A very small amount of blood interchange may occur in utero, but the amount is insignificant in the first pregnancy. The fetus of the first pregnancy will generally not be affected, since sensitization of the mother does not occur until placental separation at delivery. The fetus of a subsequent pregnancy with an incompatible blood type (Rh positive) will, however, be subjected to maternal antibodies, which have been formed following the first pregnancy and which cross the placenta and destroy the blood cells of the fetus. If the fetus and mother are both Rh negative, no incompatibility exists, and antibodies are not stimulated to react to a foreign antigen. With each ensuing pregnancy involving an Rh positive fetus, the antibody level is increased, placing the fetus at risk for development of erythroblastosis. Fortunately, Rh immune globulin, if given to the mother during pregnancy and after birth, will prevent the development of antibodies and consequently erythroblastosis.

CLINICAL MANIFESTATIONS

Maternal antibodies produced in response to sensitization from the fetal blood cells cross the placenta and destroy fetal red blood cells, causing increased in utero erythropoiesis, anemia, jaundice, and edema. If the in utero anemia has been severe, the neonate may develop cardiac failure and *hydrops fetalis.* This condition is characterized by gross edema of the fetus, imparting a waxy appearance to the skin. Besides being very edematous at birth, these neonates exhibit an extreme pallor and often are in respiratory distress. They are frequently stillborn, but if born alive, do not usually survive.

Most neonates with hemolytic disease will not display such extreme symptoms, although anemia, jaundice, edema, and liver and spleen enlargement are typically noted. The neonate will commonly show signs of jaundice in the first 24 hours following birth. If treatment is not instituted, hyperbilirubinemia may progress to toxic levels, anemia becomes severe, and cardiac decompensation occurs. Eventually, kernicterus ensues and death is imminent.

DIAGNOSIS

The diagnosis should be confirmed as soon as possible so that treatment may be undertaken. Ideally, prenatal assessments have identified the pregnancy at risk for the development of hemolytic disease of the neonate, and administration of Rh immune globulin, amniocentesis, or in utero exchange transfusions have been employed as necessary. Following delivery, a sample of cord blood is obtained from the neonate to determine the blood type, Rh factor, direct Coombs' test, serum bilirubin level, and laboratory evaluations. Rh determinations at this time may not be accurate, however, owing to the influence of the mother's Rh antibodies. When both the Coombs' test and the Rh determination are negative, the neonate is assumed to be Rh negative, since a positive Coombs test depends on the presence of Rh antibodies. Criteria for diagnosis depend on previously mentioned clinical symptoms and the results of laboratory assessments. Elevated cord serum bilirubin levels over 5 mg per 100 ml, a positive direct Coombs' test, an Rh positive factor, decreased hemoglobin, an elevated reticulocyte count (over 3 percent), and the presence of many immature red blood cells are laboratory findings consistent with hemolytic disease.

Treatment depends on the severity of the disease, with consideration given to the use of phototherapy or exchange transfusions. With early treatment, the prognosis is good.

ABO Incompatibility

Incompatibility existing between the blood of the O type mother and an A or B blood type neonate may exist in the first pregnancy as well as following pregnancies. Sensitization of these mothers has occurred naturally by immune stimulation of A and B type substances found in some foods and in gram-negative bacteria. A pregnant woman with O type blood may have produced A and B antibodies long before her first pregnancy, accounting for the increased incidence of ABO incompatibility in first pregnancies. The severity of the incompatibility does not increase with subsequent pregnancies as it does in Rh incompatibility.

Jaundice and enlargement of the spleen may be present, but severe anemia is not usually incurred.

Diagnostic evaluations may reveal a weakly positive or negative Coombs' test, caused by the reduced number of A and B reactive sites present in neonatal red blood cells, as compared with the adult. The indirect Coombs' test, however, will be positive. Peripheral blood smears reveal an increased number of reticulocytes, nucleated red blood cells, and the presence of spherocytes (a form of erythrocyte).

Treatment of ABO incompatibility involves the use of phototherapy for hyperbilirubinemia, but exchange transfusions are seldom necessary.

POLYCYTHEMIA

Neonates with venous hematocrit levels above 65 percent are considered polycythemic, which predisposes them to hyperviscosity of the blood. Blood in the vessels becomes sluggish, obstructing the capillaries and resulting in poor tissue perfusion and damage to the tissues and organs.

Risk factors associated with the development of polycythemia are:

Neonates
Born at high altitudes
With delayed cord clamping and/or milking of the cord at delivery
With intrauterine hypoxia and asphyxia
With decreased placental functioning, such as SGA neonates
Postmature
Of diabetic mothers
Experiencing hypoglycemia or hypothermia
In utero twin-to-twin transfusion (one twin will be anemic and the other will have polycythemia)
With chromosomal abnormalities (Down's syndrome)

Neonates with polycythemia may appear plethoric but will often become cyanotic when crying. Cardiac and respiratory symptoms, including tachycardia, tachypnea, respiratory distress, and congestive heart failure, are related to circulatory problems, resulting from increased viscosity of the blood. Neurologic symptoms caused by decreased cerebral perfusion may be observed as lethargy, tremors, hypotonia, poor reflexes, and seizures. Hyperbilirubinemia is commonly present owing to the hemolysis of the increased volume of red blood cells. Formation of thrombi may occur, resulting in renal vein thrombi and cerebral artery thrombi. Necrotizing enterocolitis is also a complicating factor.

Although venous sampling of blood is more accurate for the diagnosis of polycythemia, a capillary heel stick may be used. When capillary levels are elevated, evaluation of a venous blood sample is necessary to eliminate a possible false elevation caused by poor circulation in the heel.

If hematocrit levels are elevated and the neonate is symptomatic, a partial exchange transfusion may be indicated. Plasmanate or fresh frozen blood is used to lower the hematocrit to 60 percent or lower.

ANEMIA

Although many factors must be considered when evaluating neonatal hemoglobin levels, the lower limit of normal is generally considered 13 gm per 100 ml. Causative factors associated with anemia of the neonate are:

Fetal blood loss
Cord rupture, placenta previa and abruptio placentae
In utero fetomaternal transfusion
In utero twin-to-twin transfusion
Trauma during an amniocentesis
Placental incision during a cesarean delivery

Red blood cell hemolysis
Blood incompatibilities (ABO, Rh factor)
Disseminated intravascular coagulation (DIC)
Effects of maternal drugs
Sepsis cytomegalovirus syphilis, rubella, toxoplasmosis, etc.

Red blood cell defect
Glucose 6 phosphate dehydrogenase deficiency (GGPD) (X-linked recessive enzyme disorder producing abnormal RBCs)
Red blood cell membrane defects

Deficient red blood cell production
Alpha thalassemia (hereditary hemolytic anemia)

Neonatal bleeding
Very large cephalhematoma
Intracranial hemorrhage
Ruptured liver or spleen
Lung hemorrhage

Vitamin E deficiency
Preterm neonate

Frequent blood sampling
Preterm neonate

Careful evaluation of the antepartal and intrapartal history of the neonate with a low hemoglobin level is necessary. Laboratory evaluations include CBC, platelet, serum bilirubin level, direct and indirect Coombs' tests, blood typing and Rh factor, and a peripheral blood smear. Low reticulocyte counts indicate decreased production of red blood cells, while an elevated reticulocyte count is associated with RBC hemolysis and blood loss.

Nursing assessments are important to detect symptoms of anemia. The anemic neonate is pale, with decreased responses. Weight gain is diminished and weight loss beyond that expected of the normal newborn (5 to 10 percent) may be noted. Tachycardia may be present and is pronounced (>160), with acute hemorrhage and impending shock. The neonate with severe hemorrhage and shock is tachypnic and will not respond to oxygen therapy.

Treatment of anemia depends on the cause and severity. If the anemia is not severe, elemental iron may be given (as a supplement in formula). When anemia is severe, transfusions of packed RBCs may be necessary.

NECROTIZING ENTEROCOLITIS

Necrotic deterioration of the bowel, with inflammation and hemorrhagic lesions that precipitate bowel perforation characterize necrotizing enterocolitis (NEC). Within the last decade this condition has become more extensively noted in newborn intensive care units, primarily owing to the increased survival of premature neonates.

ETIOLOGY

The exact etiology of necrotizing enterocolitis is unknown, although it has been associated with hypoxia of birth asphyxia and neonatal shock, resulting in ischemia of the intestinal tract. It is most often seen in the premature neonates with birth weights of 1500 gm or under, however 20 percent of cases are seen in full-term neonates. There is an increased incidence in neonates with umbilical artery or venous catheters.

ASPECTS OF CLINICAL MANIFESTATIONS

Symptoms will generally appear after the onset of feedings and within the first two to three weeks. Characteristic symptoms may be noted as early or late symptoms, developing in the course of the disease. Symptomatology includes the following:

Early symptoms	Lethargy
	Abdominal distention
	Vomiting
	Large amounts of gastric aspirates
	Bile in gastric aspirates
	Positive hematest and clinitest
	Hypothermia
	Apnea
Late Symptoms	Metabolic acidosis
	Shiny, tender abdominal wall
	Advanced sepsis
	DIC
	Vasomotor collapse

Laboratory findings reveal an extremely elevated or decreased WBC count, decreased platelet and granulocyte counts, prolonged prothrombin time and neutropenia. Blood, stool, and spinal cultures may be positive for pathogens.

X-rays reveal distention of the bowel with *pneumatosis intestinalis* (bubbly air appearing in the wall of the intestines).

Treatment

If necrotizing enterocolitis is suspected, oral feedings are discontinued and parenteral hyperalimentation instituted. The results of blood or stool cultures will provide the basis for antibiotic therapy. Nasogastric tubes are passed to allow decompression of the stomach. If acidosis occurs, corrective measures are initiated. Plasma transfusion and vitamin K may be given to treat coagulation disorders, and increased IV fluids are administered to counteract hypotension.

Surgery is indicated when there is progressive deterioration, intestinal perforation, or infarction. Bowel resection with anastomosis may be sufficient when small areas are involved, but in more severe cases a gastrostomy may be necessary for decompression of the bowel.

NURSING INTERVENTIONS

Principles of nursing care involve careful assessments of neonates at risk for necrotizing enterocolitis and astute nursing management of neonates having the disorder. Assessments of neonates at risk include examination of stools for occult blood and measurements of abdominal girth every four to eight hours, with attention to any increases over 1 cm. If necrotizing enterocolitis is suspected, measurements of abdominal girth are performed every two hours.

The characteristics and amount of vomitus, gastric aspirates, and voidings are noted. Electrolyte and fluid balance are monitored and vital signs taken every two to four hours, in order to detect any signs of hypothermia or hyperthermia, respiratory distress, and hypotension. Axillary temperatures are taken to avoid trauma to the bowel.

Efforts are made to prevent pressure or trauma to the abdomen. Diapers are generally not used and handling of the neonate is limited. Bowel sounds are carefully assessed, and the abdomen is observed for a shiny appearance or redness. Careful observation for indications of intestinal perforation includes assessments for decreased blood pressure, pallor, sudden increase in abdominal girth, tachycardia, and widening pulse pressures.

Parents are provided with explanations of their baby's condition and the treatment he is receiving. Nursing efforts are directed toward fostering parent-infant attachment, especially when they are not able to hold the infant. If surgery is necessary, parents will need a full description of the surgical procedure, the care following surgery, and the special needs of the infant as a result of surgery. They are provided with opportunities to ask questions, review explanations, and vent their feelings.

NEONATAL SEPSIS

Neonatal sepsis occurs in about 1 of every 1500 neonates, with a mortality rate of approximately 45 percent. Neonates may acquire infections primarily in one of four ways:

Placental transmission from mother to fetus

Ascending infections following rupture of the membranes

Contact with genitourinary organisms during passage through the birth canal

Nosocomial infection following birth

INTRAUTERINE ENVIRONMENT

The intrauterine environment, in most instances, is germ-free. Nonetheless, transmission of infections through the placenta to the fetus may occur, producing spontaneous abortions, intrauterine death, congenital anomalies, intrauterine growth retardation, and neonatal sepsis. Some of these infections produce few, if any, maternal symptoms. In these cases, the pregnant woman or health care provider may be totally unaware of placental transmission of the infectious organism to the fetus. Table 31–2 provides a list of infectious agents that may be transmitted to the fetus via the placenta.

TABLE 31–2
MATERNAL INFECTIOUS AGENTS THAT MAY BE TRANSMITTED TO THE FETUS VIA THE PLACENTA

TORCH complex
Toxoplasmosis
Rubella
Cytomegalovirus
Herpes virus type 2
Syphilis
Chicken pox
Enterovirus
Tuberculosis
Listeria monocytogens
Measles
Plasmodium
Coccidioidomycosis
Malaria

TABLE 31–3
ORGANISMS THE FETUS MAY ENCOUNTER IN THE BIRTH CANAL

Chlamydia trachomatis
Enterovirus
Group B hemolytic streptococcus
Hepatitis B
Neisseria gonorrhoeae
Herpes virus type 2
Candida albicans

BIRTH CANAL

During passage through the birth canal, the fetus encounters genitourinary bacteria and fungi. In most neonates the skin serves as a protective barrier, but if skin integrity is altered, organisms may find a portal of entry. Oral and nasal passages and umbilical cord stump may also provide a site for the entry of organisms encountered in the birth canal. Table 31–3 provides a list of organisms the fetus may encounter in the birth canal.

RUPTURED MEMBRANES

Prolonged rupture of the membranes will readily expose the neonate to infectious organisms. Some organisms may pass through intact membranes, but the incidence is far greater when the membranes are ruptured. Without the protection of the membranes, infectious agents have direct access to the fetus. The frequency of infection is especially increased when there has been aspiration of contaminated amniotic fluid. If a neonate is born following premature rupture of the membranes (over 24 hours), gastric aspirations, ear, throat, umbilical, blood, and cerebrospinal fluid cultures may be indicated.

TABLE 31–4
NOSOCOMIAL AGENTS ASSOCIATED WITH NEONATAL NURSERY INFECTIONS

Gram-negative bacteria; E. coli, Proteus, Klebsiella, Aerobacter and Pseudomonas
Group B beta hemolytic streptococcus
Group A streptococcus
Coxsackie virus
Echovirus

NOSOCOMIAL INFECTIONS

In the neonatal nursery, infants may be exposed to pathogenic organisms carried on the hands of care givers or by contact with contaminated equipment. Strict aseptic technique is the best preventative measure against this source of infection. Table 31–4 gives examples of agents commonly associated with neonatal nursery infections.

Symptoms of Sepsis

Symptoms of neonatal sepsis vary with the type of infection and its related causative organism. Although many conditions present symptoms similar to those caused by infections, neonates exhibiting any of the following symptoms are assessed for infection:

Temperature instability
Hypothermia or hyperthermia
Abdominal distention
Diarrhea
Respiratory distress
Lethargy

Irritability
Apnea
Poor feeding
Jaundice
CNS irritability
Hypotonia
Petechiae
Hepatosplenomegaly
Cyanosis
Increased amounts of residual associated with gavage feedings

Diagnosis

Neonates with increased risk factors such as premature rupture of the membranes, neonates of the gravida with herpes type 2, and neonates with symptomatology should be evaluated diagnostically. The following diagnostic workup may be indicated:

- Ear, nose, and gastric aspirates cultures
- Suprapubic bladder aspiration for culture of urine and Gram's stain
- Lumbar puncture for culture of spinal fluid, Gram's stain, glucose, and protein
- Rectal swab and culture
- Skin cultures, if irritated areas noted
- Umbilical cord cultures
- Complete blood count with attention to
  - Leukocytosis
  - Neutropenia
  - Abnormal band/neutrophil ratio
  - Platelet count with attention to thrombocytopenia
  - Chest x-ray
  - Antibody titers
  - Serology

Medical and Nursing Interventions

Following the septic workup and identification of the causative organisms, antibiotic therapy may be instituted. Nursing interventions focus on supportive management of the neonate and assessment for increasing severity of infection or resulting complications as evidenced by hypotension, acidosis, hemorrhage, tachycardia, and respiratory distress. Supportive treatment includes management of cardiac and respiratory functions, attention to nutritional needs, fluid and electrolyte balance, provision for a stable thermal environment, and observation for hypoglycemia, hyponatremia, hypocalcemia, hyperbilirubinemia, and hepatosplenomegaly. The infected neonate is isolated from other neonates in the nursery.

Table 31-5 provides a list of clinical manifestations of infectious disease processes seen in the neonatal nursery.

NEONATAL EFFECTS OF MATERNAL DRUG USAGE

Fetal Alcohol Syndrome

The precise amount of alcohol consumed by the pregnant woman that will definitely result in adverse fetal effects is not known. However, it is known that even small amounts of alcohol can cause damage to the developing fetus and have lasting neonatal effects.

Fetal alcohol syndrome occurs in neonates of mothers who abuse alcohol. A typical pattern of abnormalities may be seen:

Microcephaly
Craniofacial abnormalities
Epicanthal folds
Prenatal and postnatal growth defects
Congenital heart defects
Mental retardation
Abnormal palmar creases

Neonates may exhibit alcohol withdrawal symptoms following delivery, characterized by hyperactivity, tremors, and lethargy. These

TABLE 31-5
CLINICAL MANIFESTATIONS OF NEONATAL INFECTIONS

Infection	Causative Organism	Fetal and Neonatal Manifestations	Associated Symptoms
Toxoplasmosis	Protozoan Toxoplasma gondii found in animal feces and rare or raw meat Frequently associated with cat feces Placental transmission	Abortions Stillbirths Prematurity IUGR Microcephaly Hydrocephaly Neurologic impairment Chorioretinitis Immune deficiencies	Thrombocytopenia Petechiae Ecchymosis Lymphadenopathy Convulsions Jaundice
Rubella	Virus Placental transmission Most severe damage in first 10 weeks of gestation	Abortions Prematurity IUGR Congenital heart defects (patent ductus arteriosus) Cataracts Deafness Mental impairment Encephalitis Microcephaly Cerebral palsy Glaucoma Pneumonia	Hepatosplenomegaly Anemia Petechiae Purpura Thrombocytopenia
Cytomegalovirus	Cytomegalovirus Member of the herpesvirus group Transplacental transmission May be acquired during passage through the birth canal	IGUR Microcephaly Deafness Chorioretinitis Encephalitis Pneumonitis	Lethargy Jaundice Purpura Hepatosplenomegaly Petechiae
Herpes Type 2	Herpesvirus hominis type 2 Transplacental transmission possible, but more commonly transmitted during passage through the birth canal	Abortion Microcephaly Hydrocephaly Blindness Neurologic impairment Hepatitis Conjunctivitis IUGR Patent ductus arteriosus	Wide range of symptoms that may be localized or systemic: Skin lesions (vesicular) Opisthotonos Viremia Respiratory symptoms Bulging fontanel May be asymptomatic at birth with symptoms developing within 2 weeks
Syphilis	Spirochete Treponema pallidum Transplacental transmission	Abortion Preterm delivery Central nervous system involvement Nephrotic syndrome Meningitis Myocarditis Pneumonitis	May be asymptomatic at birth Symptoms include: Petechiae Purpura Hepatosplenomegaly Maculopapular rash Rhinitis Seizures

TABLE 31-5 (continued)

Infection	Causative Organism	Fetal and Neonatal Manifestations	Associated Symptoms
Gonorrhea	Neisseria gonorrhoeae contact with organism during passage through birth canal	May be asymptomatic Conjunctivitis with development of ophthalmia neonatorum Prophylactic treatment is required at birth with silver nitrate or antibiotic ointment	
Streptococcal infection	Group B beta hemolytic streptococcus	Septicemia Meningitis Respiratory distress Cellulitis Mental impairment Coma Death Blindness Deafness	May develop early or late symptoms Respiratory distress Apnea Jaundice Abscess
Chlamydia	Chlamydia trachomatis	Conjunctivitis Pneumonitis Otitis media Septicemia	
Listeria	Listeria monocytogens Transplacental transmission	Pneumonia Conjunctivitis Meningitis	Symptoms may be present at birth or delayed in onset: Hepatosplenomegaly Petechiae Respiratory symptoms Poor feeding
E. coli	Escherichia coli	Cellulitis Pneumonia Septicemia Otitis media	
Thrush	Candida albicans Contact in birth canal	White plaques on the roof of the palate, gums, tongue and cheeks Resembles milk curds Treated with mycostatin or gentian violet	

symptoms usually subside within the first 72 hours after onset.

Nursing interventions are centered on supportive management of the neonate experiencing alcohol withdrawal. Because they are often small-for-gestational-age, thermal instability may be a problem and protective thermal measures are necessary. A poor sucking reflex, tremors, irritability, and lethargy may make feeding difficult and necessitate special feeding considerations.

Neonates with fetal alcohol syndrome will generally be impaired in development, both physically and mentally. Even if mental impairment is not severe, many of these children are slow learners and require special education.

Neonates of Drug-Dependent Mothers

The neonate exposed to chronic maternal drug use may be affected in any number of ways depending on: (1) the drug or drugs used; (2) the duration of exposure to the drug; (3) the amount and frequency of drug usage; and (4) the period of fetal development during drug exposure. Some of the teratogenic effects may be readily apparent at birth, while others are more subtle, involving delayed mental and physical development.

The fetus of the drug dependent mother may become addicted while in utero. The mother has a choice when using drugs, but the fetus does not—she becomes his supplier and forces him into an addiction even before his birth. If she withdraws from the drug, he must also withdraw, suffering many of the same symptoms as she does and others which are more devastating.

Neonates of drug-dependent mothers are commonly premature or small-for-gestational-age. Maternal drug dependence has also been associated with placental insufficiency and related intrauterine fetal asphyxia. Since drug-dependent mothers frequently have infections associated with drug use, there is an increased risk of neonatal sepsis. Thus, the neonate at birth may suffer not only possible teratogenic effects but also possible asphyxia and sepsis.

SYMPTOMS

Narcotic withdrawal symptoms will, as a rule, appear within the first or second day following birth and subside within the next four to five days. Symptoms that may indicate drug withdrawal are:

Nasal stuffiness, sneezing, yawning, increased sucking efforts, hiccups

Increased secretions, difficulty feeding, drooling, gagging, vomiting, diarrhea

Increased respiratory rate, shrill-cry, respiratory distress

Irritability, tremors, hyperactivity, hypertonia, hyperreflexia, increased Moro reflex, disturbed sleeping pattern

Seizures (infrequent, but may occur in severe cases or with intrauterine asphyxia)

Fever, flushing, diaphoresis

Dehydration

DIAGNOSIS

Diagnosis is based on the symptoms portrayed by the neonate and a maternal history of drug usage. Diagnostic evaluations are conducted to rule out other causative factors such as hypoglycemia, hyponatremia, hypocalcemia, hypomagnesemia, and sepsis.

MEDICAL AND NURSING INTERVENTIONS

Nursing interventions involve support and monitoring of cardiac, respiratory and neurologic functions, and thermal regulation.

Assessment of the neonate's ability to feed and his response to feedings are necessary because of the excessive amounts of secretions and hyperactivity of the infant. Small frequent feedings may be indicated.

Mucus may be problematic and suctioning should be available. Positioning the neonate on his side with the head of the bed elevated will help to prevent choking from the increased mucus secretions.

Safety precautions include protection of the neonate from injury during periods of hyperactivity. Procedures or activities that are stimulating are kept to a minimum during the withdrawal period. Attempts to pacify the neonate include, gentle handling, using a pacifier, speaking in a soft, soothing voice, swaddling, and a quiet environment.

Parent-infant attachment is encouraged but may not be successful until withdrawal symptoms have diminished. Explanations of neonatal behavior are presented to the parents along with suggestions for comforting him. These infants will often continue to have interrupted sleep patterns and may continue to be poor feeders.

Drugs used for relief of withdrawal symptoms include phenobarbital, chlorpromazine (Thorazine), paregoric, diazepam (Valium), and codeine.

BIRTH TRAUMA

Intracranial Hemorrhage

Intracranial hemorrhage is caused by trauma or anoxia in utero or at the time of birth. It most frequently occurs in preterm neonates but may also be found in full-term babies. Approximately 40 percent of preterm neonates under 1500 gm develop intracranial hemorrhage.

Difficult and very rapid deliveries are often associated with intracranial hemorrhages. These traumatic deliveries result in pressure, lacerations, rupture of cerebral blood vessels, and hypoxia, producing hemorrhage into the subdural, subarachnoid, intracerebral, or intraventricular areas of the brain. Episodes of hypoxia in the full-term neonate result in systemic hypotension and associated cerebral cortex necrosis. They are collectively called *hypoxic ischemic encephalopathy.*

Preterm neonates are more susceptible to intracranial hemorrhage, owing to: (1) pliability of the cranium, which allows pressure to be placed on the blood vessels during delivery and impairs cerebral blood flow; (2) fragility of the blood vessels; (3) a tendency toward coagulation defects; (4) decreased ability to regulate cerebral blood flow; and (5) susceptibility to respiratory and metabolic complications associated with asphyxia.

Intraventricular hemorrhage of preterm neonates is usually the result of bleeding into capillaries of the germinal matrix, most commonly occurring on the second or third day following birth. The germinal matrix is a highly vascular structure present in the immature brain that is very susceptible to increasing arterial pressures. Hemorrhage in this area results in destruction of the tissue and may also lead to extension of the hemorrhage into the intracerebral areas of the brain.

SYMPTOMS

Clinical manifestations of cerebral hemorrhage depend on the area of hemorrhage and the amount and extent of the hemorrhage. These symptoms may be very subtle or pronounced, occurring at birth or within several days following birth. Symptoms that may be assessed include:

- Low Apgar scores
- Lethargy
- Blinking
- Tongue thrusting
- Irregular respirations
- Apneic episodes
- Cold, pale, and clammy skin
- Cyanosis
- Bulging or tense fontanels
- Irritability
- Unequal pupils
- Poor sucking
- Vasomotor instability
- Diminishing Moro reflex (present at birth but decreased or absent in ensuing days)
- Opisthotonos
- Seizures

DIAGNOSIS

Assessments of the labor and delivery history and the gestational age of the neonate are important when intracranial hemorrhage is suspected. Attention is focused on breech deliveries, brow and face presentations, and midforceps deliveries as potentiators of cerebral hemorrhage. Episodes of asphyxia, abruptio placentae, and placenta previa may also contribute to a diagnosis of intracranial hemorrhage. Evaluation of intrapartal distress, Apgar scores, and resuscitative measures are considered along with presenting symptoms.

Ultrasound examinations and computerized transaxial tomography scanning (CAT scan) may be helpful in diagnosing the presence and extent of the hemorrhage. Cerebrospinal fluid examinations may reveal the presence of blood, but its absence does not rule out the possibility of cerebral hemorrhage.

MEDICAL AND NURSING INTERVENTIONS

Nursing responsibilities involved in care include assessments for developing and increasing severity of any symptoms. The neonate should be kept in a quiet environment, most generally in an incubator or Isolette, with avoidance of stressful or stimulating procedures. Supportive management includes monitoring respiratory functions and temperature instability. Feeding ability and tolerance are assessed and appropriate feeding measures employed. Sedation is instituted in some instances with the drug of choice being phenobarbital.

Prognosis depends on the severity of the hemorrhage and the precipitating factors. Some neonates demonstrate mild symptoms with few effects, while others may progress to seizuring and death. Survival after a severe insult increases the risk of permanent cerebral damage, hydrocephalus, mental and neurologic impairment, and cerebral palsy.

Erb-Duchenne Paralysis

Damage of nerves within the upper segment of the brachial plexus results in paralysis of an upper extremity. Assessment reveals an internally rotated shoulder, an arm that hangs limply to the side, and a pronated wrist. The Moro reflex is diminished or absent in the affected arm and the neonate is unable to raise the arm. Movement of the fingers is possible and the grasp reflex is present.

The condition is treated by immobilizing and resting the affected part. The arm is positioned to achieve external rotation and abduction. Stress on the arm is avoided, but range of motion exercises are included in the care plan. Without extensive nerve damage the paralysis is temporary, and the neonate will regain full use of the arm.

Diaphragmatic Paralysis

This condition is often seen in conjunction with Erb's paralysis and should be suspected when Erb's paralysis is noted. Injury occurs to the phrenic nerve, which supplies the diaphragm, resulting in respiratory distress, atelectasis of the lung, and pneumonia. Supportive respiratory care is needed until the paralysis disappears and respiratory functions return to normal.

Facial Paralysis

Damage to the facial nerves may occur after a difficult labor or when forceps have been applied during delivery. The involved side of the face will appear immobile, the eye remains open, and the corner of the mouth appears to droop. Nursing care is focused on attention to the neonate's ability to suck. Soft nipples are used and frequent small feedings given. Protective measures should be undertaken to prevent injury to the eye.

DEVELOPMENTAL ANOMALIES

Congenital Heart Disease

Congenital heart disease occurs in approximately 1 of every 125 live births. Causative factors are primarily related to genetic or environmental influences incurred by the fetus in utero. Defects from environmental influences depend on the period of cardiac development in which the fetus was exposed to the teratogen. Environmental factors include drugs, alcohol, viral diseases, and exposure to other teratogenic agents.

Structural defects fall into one of two classifications: cyanotic and acyanotic lesions. Both types of lesions are associated with alteration in pulmonary blood flow, either increasing, decreasing, or having no effect on it.

CLINICAL MANIFESTATIONS

Symptoms depend on the type of lesion and severity or abnormality. Symptoms may not be noted until fetal circulation changes to neonatal circulation. These symptoms include:

Tachypnea
Dyspnea
Difficulty feeding
Heart murmurs
Tachycardia
Pulmonary edema
Mottled skin
Central cyanosis
Lethargy
Cyanosis
Failure to gain weight
Unequal or absent pulses

Cyanotic Lesions

Cyanotic lesions are related to disorders that allow unoxygenated blood to mix with oxygenated blood within the heart and to be circulated throughout the systemic circulation.

TETRALOGY OF FALLOT

Four primary lesions are involved in tetralogy of Fallot (see Fig. 31-2), including:

Ventricular septal defects
Pulmonary stenosis

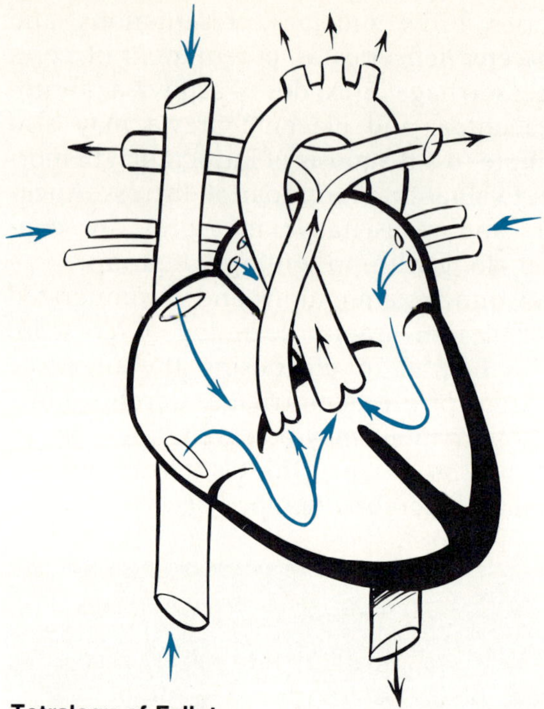

Tetralogy of Fallot

Tetralogy of Fallot is characterized by the combination of four defects: 1) pulmonary stenosis, 2) ventricular septal defect, 3) overriding aorta, and 4) hypertrophy of right ventricle. It is the most common defect causing cyanosis in patients surviving beyond two years of age. The severity of symptoms depends on the degree of pulmonary stenosis, the size of the ventricular septal defect, and the degree to which the aorta overrides the septal defect.

FIGURE 31-2. Congenital heart anomaly: tetralogy of Fallot. Reproduced with permission from Ross Laboratories, Columbus, Ohio. Clinical Education Aid No. 7—Congenital Heart Abnormalities.

Overriding of the aorta
Hypertrophy of the right ventricle

Cyanosis is the result of right-to-left shunting of the blood through the ventricular septal defect into the overriding aorta and left ventricle. Thus, a mixture of unoxygenated and oxygenated blood is delivered into the aorta and throughout the systemic circulation. Hypertrophy of the right ventricle occurs because of the increased pressure within the ventricle from the effects of pulmonary stenosis.

Symptoms may or may not be present at birth; however, they are usually noted within the first month of life. The severity of the symptoms depends on the degree of shunting and pulmonary stenosis. These infants generally do not thrive well, having difficulty with feedings, weight gain, fatigue, anemia, and polycythemia.

A characteristic boot-shaped heart may be noted on x-ray examination. Palliative surgery may create various combinations of shunts until the child is considered old enough for complete corrective surgery.

TRANSPOSITION OF THE GREAT ARTERIES

Transposition of the great arteries (see Fig. 31-3) is most frequently found in male neonates with increased birth weight and often in association with maternal diabetes. The pulmonary artery is transposed with the aorta, thus, the pulmonary artery is positioned in the left ventricle and the aorta arises from the right ventricle. The blood received from the right ventricle will go directly into the aorta, without becoming oxygenated, while oxygenated blood from the left ventricle will go back to the lungs again. During fetal life, this pattern is not consequential, since fetal blood is oxygenated via the placenta. After birth, the effects of the transposition may not be readily noted until the fetal shunts (foramen ovale and ductus arteriosus) close. Then, the blood is not sufficiently oxygenated and the infant becomes cyanotic and hypoxemic. If the condition is not corrected, death will ensue.

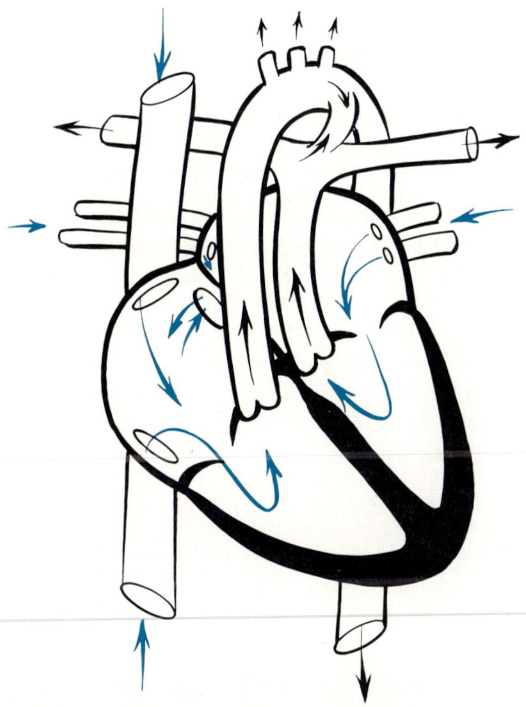

Complete Transposition of Great Vessels

This anomaly is an embryologic defect caused by a straight division of the bulbar trunk without normal spiraling. As a result, the aorta originates from the right ventricle and the pulmonary artery from the left ventricle. An abnormal communication between the two circulations must be present to sustain life.

FIGURE 31-3. Congenital heart anomaly: Complete transposition of the great vessels. Reproduced with permission from Ross Laboratories, Columbus, Ohio. Clinical Education Aid No. 7—Congenital Heart Abnormalities.

Frequently, transposition is accompanied by other septal defects that cause mixing of oxygenated and unoxygenated blood in the systemic circulation. If this is the case, life may be sustained because of the abnormalities which allow mixing of the blood.

Symptoms depend on the presence and type of accompanying lesions. When no other lesions are present, or if the foramen is the only patent shunt, cyanosis with congestive heart failure rapidly occurs. If ventricular septal openings accompany the transposition, cyanosis is not as extreme and the infant will not be in immediate distress.

The x-ray examination displays a characteristic egg-shaped contour of the heart. Echocardiograms reveal an enlarged heart with an increase in pulmonary blood flow.

Palliative procedures may widen the foramen ovale to create an opening that allows mixing of oxygenated and unoxygenated blood at the atrial level. Complete corrective surgery is performed as soon as advisable. (The reader is referred to a pediatric textbook for a complete description of the operative procedure.)

HYPOPLASTIC LEFT HEART SYNDROME

Although this condition is rare, its fatal outcome is devastating to parents. Because of a nonfunctional left ventricle with associated aortic and mitral valve atresia, the right ventricle becomes hypertrophied. The blood flows only from the right ventricle through the pulmonary artery into the ductus arteriosus and out the aorta. Upon closure of the ductus arteriosus, this pathway is eliminated and the neonate develops congestive heart failure followed by death. At present, there is no effective treatment other than a complete heart transplant.

Acyanotic Lesions

PATENT DUCTUS ARTERIOSUS

Failure of the ductus arteriosus to close following birth causes a left-to-right shunt of the blood from the aorta to the pulmonary artery. During fetal life this shunt was right-to-left and functioned to bypass the lungs. At birth, with increasing aortic pressures and decreasing pulmonary pressures, if the ductus arteriosus does not close, the shunt becomes a left-to-right shunt.

This disorder is often seen in preterm neonates and as a complication of respiratory distress syndrome. A complete discussion and description of the disorder is found in Chapter 30 and Figure 30–2.

ATRIAL SEPTAL DEFECTS

These defects are seen as openings between the left and right atria of the heart (see Fig. 31–4). Although abnormal openings may occur in varying sites in the atrial septum, the most frequent defect is shunting through the foramen ovale. Blood is shunted through the defect from the left atrium to the right atrium. It is then directed through the tricuspid valve to the right ventricle and back into the pulmonary artery. Pulmonary blood flow is increased and eventually the right ventricle becomes stressed, owing to the increased volume of blood it is required to pump.

At first, few symptoms may be noted, but as the shunt increases in size, a systolic ejection murmur may be heard on the left upper sternal border, with splitting of the second heart sound. There may also be a diastolic murmur heard at the lower left sternal border.

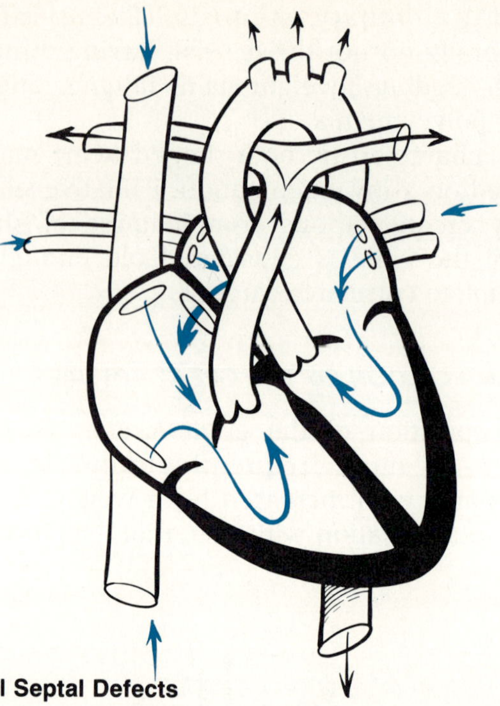

Atrial Septal Defects

An atrial septal defect is an abnormal opening between the right and left atria. Basically, three types of abnormalities result from incorrect development of the atrial septum. An incompetent foramen ovale is the most common defect. The high ostium secundum defect results from abnormal development of the septum secundum. Improper development of the septum primum produces a basal opening known as an ostium primum defect, frequently involving the atrioventricular valves. In general, left to right shunting of blood occurs in all atrial septal defects.

FIGURE 31–4. Congenital heart anomaly: atrial septal defects. Reproduced with permission from Ross Laboratories, Columbus, Ohio. Clinical Education Aid No. 7—Congenital Heart Abnormalities.

This disorder, most commonly found in females, carries a high incidence of infection and requires antibiotic therapy. Corrective surgery is generally necessary.

VENTRICULAR SEPTAL DEFECTS

Ventricular septal defects (see Fig. 31–5) are the most common type of congenital cardiac defects. They often occur in association with and complicating other heart disorders. The defect is characterized by the presence of an

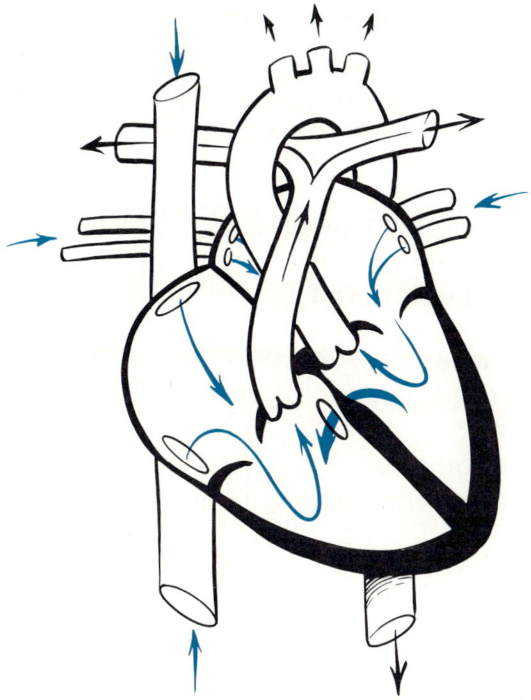

Ventricular Septal Defects

A ventricular septal defect is an abnormal opening between the right and left ventricle. Ventricular septal defects vary in size and may occur in either the membranous or muscular portion of the ventricular septum. Due to higher pressure in the left ventricle, a shunting of blood from the left to right ventricle occurs during systole. If pulmonary vascular resistance produces pulmonary hypertension, the shunt of blood is then reversed from the right to the left ventricle, with cyanosis resulting.

FIGURE 31-5. Congenital heart anomaly: ventricular septal defects. Reproduced with permission from Ross Laboratories, Columbus, Ohio. Clinical Education Aid No. 7—Congenital Heart Abnormalities.

abnormal opening, either in the membranous or muscular portion of the ventricular septum, causing a left-to-right shunt.

When the opening is large, pressures in the right ventricle and pulmonary artery are increased, causing pulmonary hypertension, lung congestion, respiratory infections, and congestive heart failure. If pulmonary hypertension continues, the shunt may reverse to right-to-left, producing cyanosis.

At birth, few symptoms may be noted, owing to increased pulmonary resistance that maintains equal right and left ventricle pressure. As the alveoli of the lungs expand and pulmonary resistance decreases, symptoms may be noted. Generally no murmurs are heard while the neonate is in the hospital, but they are commonly detected at one of the well baby exams within the first three to six weeks. The typical murmur is heard at the left sternal border in the third or fourth interspace.

If the shunt is small, the infant may remain asymptomatic and spontaneous closure occurs. Pulmonary artery banding may be done as a palliative procedure. A tight band placed on the pulmonary artery restricts the flow of the blood through the artery and, in so doing, reduces pulmonary blood volume. Later, when appropriate, the band is removed and closure of the defect is achieved with a heart patch.

ENDOCARDIAL CUSHION DEFECTS

Endocardial cushion defects are a complexity of defects that result from altered development in the embryonic growth centers that form a section of the atrial and ventricular septa and the mitral and tricuspid valves. The combination of left-to-right shunting through the atrial and ventrical defects, and the regurgitation of blood by the defective valves, causes increasing cardiac symptomatology, ranging from murmurs to congestive heart failure. Surgical repair may be initiated but is often unsuccessful. These defects are commonly seen in infants with Down's syndrome.

COARCTATION OF THE AORTA

Narrowing of the aortic arch at a point near or opposite the entry site of the ductus causes coarctation of the aorta (see Fig. 31-6). If the narrowed portion proceeds the ductal site, it is designated as preductal, and if it occurs distal to the ductus, it is postductal. Preductal coarctation often coexists with patent ductus arteriosus and ventricular septal defects.

Effects of the constricting are noted as increased pulses in the upper extremities and absent or weak femoral pulses. Hypertension may be noted in the upper extremities, with a

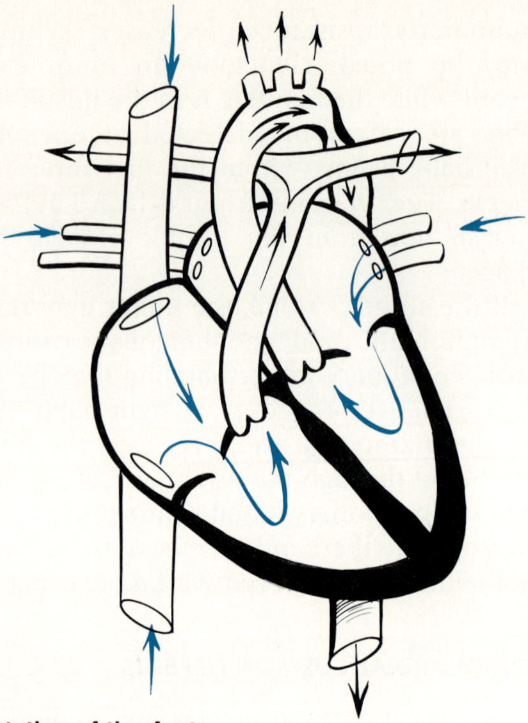

Coarctation of the Aorta

Coarctation of the aorta is characterized by a narrowed aortic lumen. It exists as a preductal or postductal obstruction, depending on the position of the obstruction in relation to the ductus arteriosus. Coarctations exist with great variation in anatomical features. The lesion produces an obstruction to the flow of blood through the aorta, causing an increased left ventricular pressure and work load.

FIGURE 31-6. Congenital heart anomaly: coarctation of the aorta. Reproduced with permission from Ross Laboratories, Columbus, Ohio. Clinical Education Aid No. 7—Congenital Heart Abnormalities.

low systolic blood pressure in the lower extremities. When the defect is located preductally, left ventricular pressure may be increased, resulting in ventricular hypertrophy and congestive heart failure. With postductal constrictions, few symptoms are noted.

Cardiac catheterization is of value when confirming the diagnosis. If coarctation is severe, surgical repair is necessary.

Congestive Heart Failure

Neonates with cardiac complications are often at risk for the development of congestive heart failure. Symptoms that may develop very rapidly and indicate congestive heart failure include:

- Tachypnea
- Tachycardia
- Hepatosplenomegaly
- Cardiomegaly
- Edema (periorbital)
- Dyspnea
- Fatigue
- Poor feeding
- Pallor
- Diaphoresis
- Decreased urinary output

If the heart failure is right-sided, there is ineffective pumping of blood through the right ventricle to the pulmonary artery, and consequently decreased oxygenation of the blood and increased systemic pressures. When the left side of the heart fails, the pumping action of blood from the left ventricle to the aorta is decreased, and pressure increases in the left atrium and pulmonary veins, resulting in pulmonary edema and lung congestion. Since the heart is considered as one pump, failure of either side of the heart will ultimately affect the other side.

The neonate with congestive heart failure needs prompt treatment, focusing on relieving edema, increasing oxygenation, and strengthening cardiac function. Diuretics are used to relieve edema and pulmonary congestion, digitalis preparations to strengthen and decrease heart rate, and oxygen to improve oxygenation.

Nursing interventions include measures to avoid stressing the neonate and to relieve fatigue. Accurate assessments of cardiac and respiratory status, and intake and output evaluations are important. Counseling the parents in the care of the neonate following discharge is important, with special emphasis placed on the administration of drugs, indications of drug toxicity and measures used to prevent fatigue and promote nutrition.

Cleft Lip and Palate

Cleft lip and palate result from alterations in embryonic development occurring between the fourth and tenth week of gestation. The neonate with cleft lip will have a fissure or fissures of varying degrees in the upper lip (see Fig. 31-7). They may appear as a single small notch in the lip or as a bilateral fissure extending to the nostril. Involvement of the palate produces a midline fissure in either the hard or the soft palate or both (see Fig. 31-7). In some instances, both a cleft lip and cleft palate may be noted.

Cleft lip and cleft palate require surgical repair and usually involve several operations. The first operation may be performed within the first two or three weeks following birth.

When providing nursing care to clients with either or both of these anomalies, two care priorities are considered: (1) feeding the neonate, and (2) providing parental support.

Feeding the infant is difficult, owing to the tendency to aspirate the feeding and a decreased ability to suck. Episodes of choking and coughing often occur during the feeding and many times the formula will return through the nose. Feedings must be given very slowly and may be tiring to the neonate. Since large amounts of air are swallowed during the feeding, frequent bubbling is necessary. Large, soft nipples or special cleft-lip nipples may be used to facilitate feeding. When bottle- or breastfeeding is impossible, an aseptosyringe, medicine dropper, or gavage feeding is employed. Breastfeeding mothers may find the use of a nipple shield with a cleft lip nipple helpful.

Position is important with either breast or bottle feeding. Holding the neonate in the

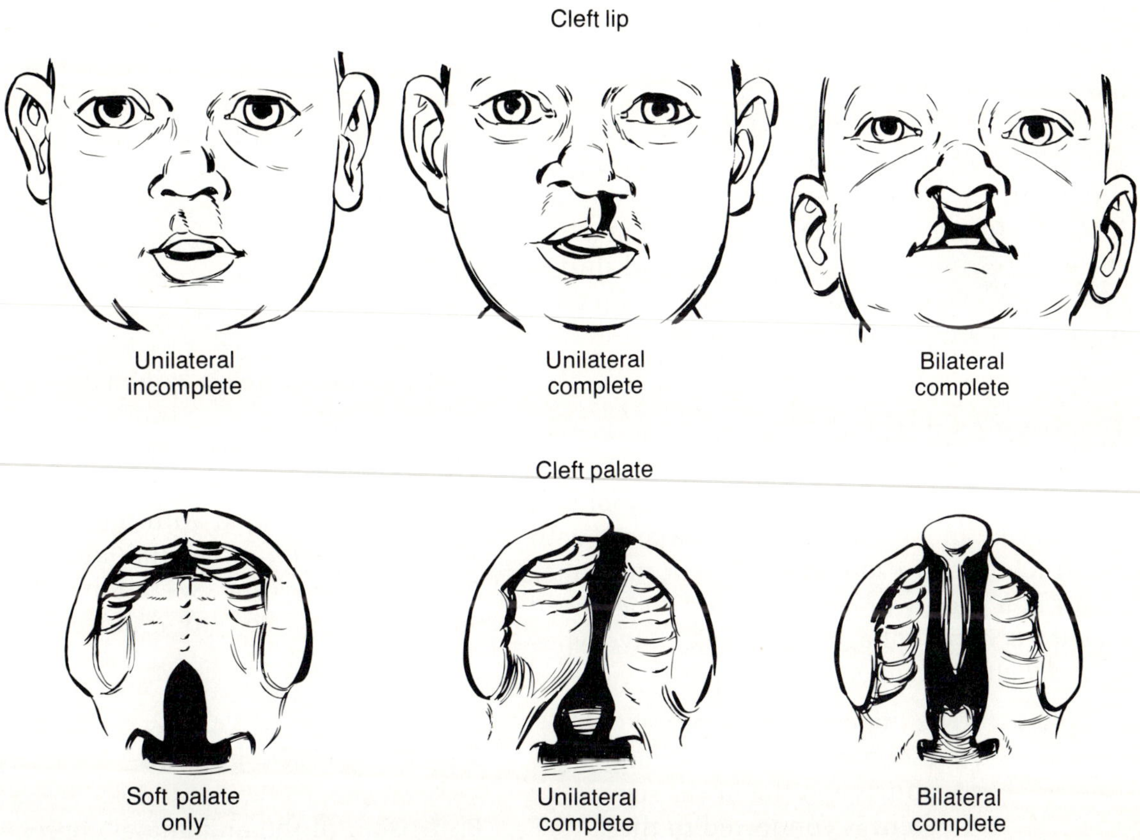

FIGURE 31-7. Cleft lip and palate. Adapted and reproduced with permission from Ross Laboratories, Columbus, Ohio. Clinical Education Aid No. 11—Cleft Lip and Cleft Palate.

upright position facilitates swallowing and helps to prevent aspiration.

The appearance of the neonate with a cleft lip is upsetting to parents. They may find it difficult to look at or establish eye contact with the baby and even be repulsed by his appearance. An understanding and supportive attitude is needed by the nurse to help parents accept the baby and to begin parent-infant attachment. Since their concerns arc initially related to the appearance of the baby, explanations of the measures used for corrective surgery are necessary. Once they have accepted the appearance of the baby, they may then move forward to considerations of his care and nurturing.

Whenever possible, parents are encouraged to feed the baby. The nurse should be present to assist them and to help if he begins to gag or choke. Reassurance is given as the parents are taught to handle the difficulties that arise during feedings. Since the lip may become very dry, the mother is taught how to apply a sterile lubricant to the lip following each feeding.

Parents of infants with this type of anomaly are often very apprehensive about caring for the baby at home. Therefore, they are informed of services available to them and advised of resources that may be helpful in discussing problems or concerns. Follow up care by health care providers is essential.

Tracheoesophageal Fistula

Alterations in early embryonic development may result in abnormalities associated with the trachea and esophagus. These anomalies occur in a variety of forms and are collectively called tracheoesophageal anomalies. Five types of basic abnormalities occur:

- Type I — The upper segment of the esophagus ends in a blind pouch and the lower segment is connected to the trachea via a fistula (see Fig. 31–8, *A*). This type of anomaly is the most common, occurring in about 90 percent of cases
- Type II — The esophagus exist as two separate segments with no communication between them or the trachea (see Fig. 31–8, *B*)
- Type III — The esophagus exist as two separate segments with a fistula between the upper segment and the trachea (see Fig. 31–8, *C*)
- Type IV — A fistula exists between the trachea and an otherwise normal esophagus (see Fig. 31–8, *D*), often called an "H-type" fistula
- Type V — The esophagus is two separate segments with double fistulas, one on the upper segment and one on the lower segment (see Fig. 31–8, *E*)

Tracheoesophageal anomalies often accompany maternal polyhydramnios. Symptoms vary according to the type of abnormality. Assessments of excessive amounts of mucus, drooling and coughing, choking, and cyanosis during the initial feeding are indicative of tracheoesophageal fistulas. When these symptoms are observed, oral feedings are immediately discontinued and withheld until diagnostic evaluations are completed.

The diagnosis is established with x-ray studies, and surgical repair is performed as soon as possible. Until that time, these neonates are positioned with the head of the bed elevated, placed in a humidified environment to help liquify the secretions and frequent suctioning is used to remove excessive secretions.

Diaphragmatic Hernia

Protrusion of the abdominal contents through the diaphragm into the thoracic cavity characterizes diaphragmatic hernia. The weakness or

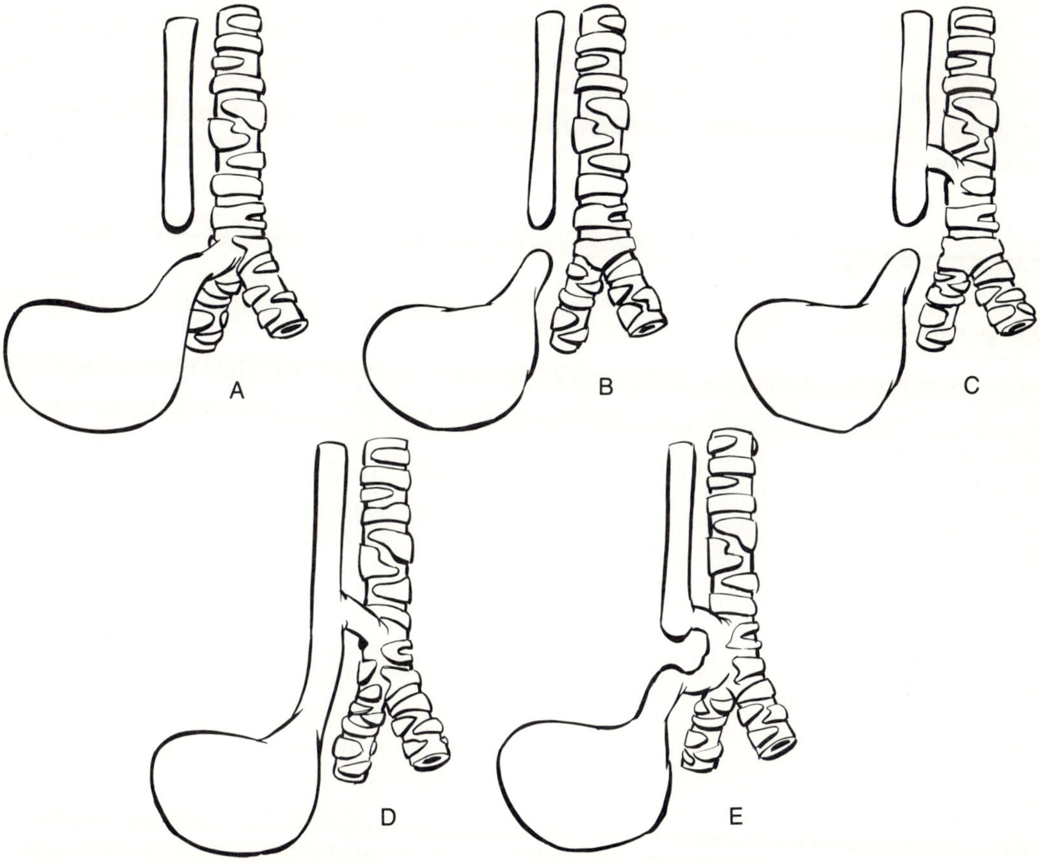

FIGURE 31-8 A. Tracheoesophageal fistula. Upper segment of esophagus ending in blind pouch. Lower segment connected to the trachea via a fistula. B. Two separate esophageal segments—no communication between either. C. Esophagus as two separate segments with a fistula between the upper segment and the trachea. D. A fistula between the trachea and an otherwise normal esophagus, "H-type" fistula. E. Esophagus as two separate segments with a double fistula, one on the upper segment and one on the lower segment.

defect in the diaphragm through which the organs herniate is most frequently located on the left side. The herniated organs place pressure on the lungs, causing lung compression and respiratory distress. Symptoms indicative of diaphragmatic hernia include respiratory difficulties, diminished breath sounds on the affected side, an asymmetrical chest, bowel sounds heard in the chest cavity, heart sounds heard on the right side of the chest, and a scaphoid appearance of the abdomen.

The neonate is placed in a semi-Fowler's position in an attempt to alleviate lung compression. Oxygen is administered to promote respiratory functions and a nasogastric tube is inserted to facilitate gastric decompression.

X-rays confirm the diagnosis and prompt surgical interventions are necessary.

Imperforate Anus

Imperforate anus constitutes surgical emergency, as it is incompatible with life. Abnormalities of embryonic development result in one of three types of anomalies: (1) formation of membranous covering obstructing the rectum, (2) rectal atresia without an anal opening, and (3) rectal atresia with fistulas to the urinary tract, vagina, or perineum. Attempts to assess the neonate's temperature rectally often provide the first indication of imperforate anus. Meconium stools are not present and the neonate becomes increasingly uncomfortable.

Corrective surgery may necessitate a colostomy or removal of the membrane.

Omphalocele

A defect in the abdominal wall at the level of the umbilicus allows herniation of the abdominal contents, within a transparent external sac. Immediately at birth, a gauze strip moistened with warm sterile saline is placed over the sac and kept moist until surgery is performed to return the abdominal contents to the abdomen. Gentle handling of the neonate and protection of the sac are of prime importance to prevent rupture before surgical correction. This rare anomaly often coexists with imperforate anus.

Intestinal Obstructions

Obstructions occurring in the intestinal tract induce symptoms of abdominal distention, vomiting, and abnormal or absent stools within the first 24 to 36 hours of life. The obstruction may be caused by complete atresia or a narrowing of the intestines.

Observations are made of the characteristics and amount of vomitus in an effort to determine the location of the obstruction. Vomiting of unchanged formula indicates an obstruction at the level of the esophagus, while a curdled-milk appearance indicates some action of the gastric secretions. If the vomitus is bile-stained, the obstruction is thought to be beyond the bile duct opening. Vomitus containing fecal material indicates an obstruction found lower in the intestinal tract. Observations also include the type of vomiting, indicating if it is projectile, as seen in pyloric stenosis, or regurgitation from overfeeding. The abdomen is assessed for indications of peristalsis and bowel sounds.

X-ray examination is used to confirm diagnosis, and corrective surgery is performed.

Meningomyelocele (Myelomeningocele)

External herniation of the meninges, cerebrospinal fluid, and spinal cord into a saclike cyst is the result of defective embryonic development of the neural tube. The level of the defect determines the degree of neurologic involvement. Commonly, it is located in the lumbrosacral area, producing symptoms of paralysis of the extremities, poor bowel and bladder control, and sensory defects consistent with or below the level of the lesion. Hydrocephalus is frequently an accompanying complication.

Nursing care focuses on protection of the lesion from trauma and infection. The neonate is placed in a prone position or turned on his side with rolled blankets or towels placed to remove pressure on the site and to maintain positioning. Frequent positional changes are needed to prevent pressure areas from developing on the skin. Sterile coverings may be lightly placed over the sac to prevent infection from urinary or fecal contamination. Observations are made of the extent of neurologic impairment.

Surgical intervention may be undertaken, depending on the severity of the defect. Many cases are inoperable. Support of the parents is essential.

Hydrocephalus

Abnormal increases in cerebrospinal fluid resulting in enlargement of the cerebral ventricles produces hydrocephalus. Neonates with this condition have exceedingly large heads, wide separations of the suture lines, bulging fontanels, a shiny, thin-skinned appearance of the forehead with visable veining, and a setting-sun appearance of the eyes. Soon after birth, the neonate may develop lethargy, a high-pitched cry, irritability, vomiting, and convulsions accompanied by neurologic impairment. Meningomyelocele may accompany the disorder but is not always present.

Supportive nursing care includes protecting the head from injury and providing adequate support. The head is measured every eight hours to determine increases in size. Parents are given explanations of the condition, care, and prognosis of the neonate.

Surgical interventions are necessary to relieve any obstruction in cerebrospinal fluid flow and to provide shunting. Shunts are generally placed in the right atrium (ventriculoarterial shunt) or into the peritoneum (ventriculoperitoneal shunt).

Microcephaly

Microcephaly is a condition in which the head and brain of the neonate are abnormally small. The neonate may or may not be capable of life, depending on the amount of brain development.

Anencephaly

The neonate with anencephaly has absence of a portion of the brain or the entire brain. The skull appears flat and abnormally shaped. This condition is incompatible with life.

BIBLIOGRAPHY

Broune, K. Common hematologic problems of the newborn period. *Journal of Obstetric, Gynecologic & Neonatal Nursing,* 1983, **12,** 19s-26s.

Brown, E. & Sweet, A. Neonatal necrotizing enterocolitis. *Pediatric Clinics of North America,* 1982, **29,** 1149-1170.

Cashore, W.J. & Oh, W. Unbound bilirubin and kernicterus in low birthweight infants. *Pediatrics,* 1982, **69,** 481-485.

Floyd, C. A defective child is born: A study of newborns with spina bifida and hydrocephalus. *Journal of Obstetric, Gynecological & Neonatal Nursing,* 1977, **6,** 56-62.

Gantt, L. & Thompson, C. Short-gut syndrome in the infant. *American Journal of Nursing,* 1985, **85,** 1263-1266.

Haase, G. & Lilly, J. Advances in newborn surgery. *Perinatology-Neonatology,* 1982, **6,** 21-28.

Harrell-Bean, H. & Klell, C. Neonatal ostomies. *Journal of Obstetric, Gynecological & Neonatal Nursing,* 1983, **12,** 69s-73s.

Hazinski, M. Congenital heart disease in the neonate. *Neonatal Network,* 1983, **1,** 29.

Ho, E. Neural tube defects. *Nursing Mirror,* 1983, **2,** 156.

Hodgman, J. Sepsis in the neonate. *Perinatology-Neonatology,* 1981, **5,** 45-49.

Lemons, P. Victims of addiction: The infant born with a habit. *Critical Care Update,* 1983, **10,** 12-20.

Lindor, E., McCarthy, A. & McRae, M. Fetal alcohol syndrome. *Journal of Obstetric, Gynecological & Neonatal Nursing,* 1980, **9,** 222-228.

Lucey, J. Bilirubin and brain damage—a real mess. *Pediatrics,* 1982, **69,** 382.

Miller, G., Black, V. & Lubchenco, L. Intracerebral hemorrhage in a term newborn with hyperviscosity. *American Journal of Diseases of Children,* 1981, **135,** 377-381.

Neches, W. Cardiac catheterization in the newborn. *Perinatology-Neonatology,* 1981, **5,** 37-40.

Philip, A. & Hewitt, J. Early diagnosis of neonatal sepsis. *Pediatrics,* 1980, **75,** 1036–1041.

Sacksteder, S., Gildea, J. & Dassy, C. Common congenital cardiac defects. *American Journal of Nursing,* 1978, **78,** 266-278.

Shor, V. Congenital cardiac defects. *American Journal of Nursing,* 1978, **78,** 256-261.

Stephens, C. The fetal alcohol syndrome: Cause for concern. *MCN,* 1981, **6,** 251-256.

Styer, G. & Freech, K. Feeding infants with cleft lip and/or palate. *Journal of Obstetric, Gynecological & Neonatal Nursing,* 1981, **10,** 329-332.

Volpe, J. *Neurology of the newborn.* Philadelphia: Saunders, 1981.

Whaley, L. & Wong, D. *Essentials of pediatric nursing.* St. Louis: Mosby, 1983.

Wu, P. Phototherapy update. *Perinatology-Neonatology,* 1981, **5,** 45-55.

Waechter, E., Phillips, J. & Holaday, B. *Nursing care of children.* Philadelphia, Lippincott, 1985.

chapter 32

NURSING INTERVENTIONS FOR THE GRIEVING FAMILY

OBJECTIVES

Upon completion of this chapter, the reader will be able to:

1. Describe the stages of the grief process.
2. Identify assessments that predict families needing support to resolve a childbearing crisis.
3. Discuss appropriate nursing interventions in caring for the family that is experiencing a crisis.
4. Identify needs of families in crisis following abortion, preterm delivery, stillbirth, defective neonate, or neonatal death.

KEY TERMS

Crisis
Crisis intervention
Grief
Grief process
Loss
Pathologic mourning

Normal pregnancy and birth are a crisis for the childbearing family requiring psychological adjustment on the part of each person. If an additional burden is imposed on the family by a less-than-perfect neonate, family coping abilities are tested to the fullest. A crisis situation can produce growth or be destructive to the family unit. The way in which a crisis is handled by a family depends on many interrelated factors: individual personality traits, perception of the crisis event, structure of the family unit, problems already present within the family, previous experiences with crisis situations, and the support given by others.

When the normal expectations of birth are replaced by the reality of loss, the role of the nurse is essential to successful resolution of the crisis.

LOSS AND GRIEF

When a crisis interferes with normal psychological functioning during the antepartal, intrapartal, or postpartal periods, both loss and grief are involved in the crisis. *Loss* can be defined as a state of being without something previously owned. Loss can come about through separation or death.

Grief is the characteristic response to the loss of a valued object. The object lost may be a person, possession, job, status, home, or any other item of importance to the individual. The process of grieving runs a fairly predictable course. Kubler-Ross (1969) has identified five steps in the normal grieving process:

1. Denial and isolation . . ."This isn't happening to me."
2. Anger . . ."Why did this happen to me?"
3. Bargaining . . . "If I do this . . ."
4. Depression and anticipatory grief . . . "How can I cope?"
5. Acceptance . . . "I can go on. I have to."

The grief process normally can last up to a year before total acceptance occurs. Each step in the grieving process must be resolved before the next step can be handled. The period immediately following the crisis is one of the most important for appropriate interventions. The family needs to begin mourning shortly after the crisis to progress through the steps in a reasonable amount of time.

Pathologic mourning occurs following some crisis situations. Signs that mourning is pathologic include:

Constant cheerfulness
Avoiding discussion of the topic
Marked, persistent, or inappropriate hostility
Persistent guilt feelings
Insistence that everything is "normal"

GENERAL NURSING INTERVENTIONS DURING CRISIS

In order for the nurse to deal effectively with families in times of crisis, individual coping mechanisms in dealing with crisis situations must be identified. Familiarity with signs of crisis and appropriate interventions is necessary to aid in identification of family crisis situations. In addition to serving as a therapeutic agent for the family, the nurse is often the primary source for referral.

Families at increased risk for crisis should be identified. Accurate and timely assessments are needed. The focus of these assessments is varied, but should include:

Disruption of the normal life pattern of the family unit
Effect on economic status of the family
Ability to handle responsibilities associated with the specific crisis

Emotional status of family members
Presence or absence of immediate support system
Presence or absence of other support systems

An effective crisis intervention plan has the following characteristics (Hoff, 1984):

Focus on the immediate problem
Consideration of the functional level of the family
Cultural and ethnic appropriateness
Includes all family members
Practical
Specifies a time frame for resolution
Renegotiable
Includes followup arrangements

The type of intervention used by the nurse depends on the nurse's knowledge about crisis and individual skills. Referral is appropriate as needed. Therapeutic interventions that may be employed by the nurse include empathetic listening, exploration of family coping mechanisms, using the support system, and encouraging expression of grief in a nondestructive manner. Following any therapeutic interventions, evaluation is needed to modify the interventions to provide support appropriate to the individual family unit.

PRETERM DELIVERIES

Parents are rarely prepared emotionally for a preterm birth and associated neonatal problems. It often creates a crisis for which usual individual coping mechanisms are not adequate.

The mother of a preterm neonate is faced with immediate and prolonged separation and an uncertain neonatal outcome. She may have difficulty in forming an attachment or commitment to the neonate, in developing a sense of confidence in her own abilities as a mother, and in establishing an effective caretaking regimen.

There are certain psychological tasks that parents of a preterm neonate must deal with:

1. Anticipatory grief at the time of delivery
2. Facing and acknowledging failure to give birth to a normal full-term healthy neonate
3. Resumption of the previous process of relating to the fetus that has been interrupted before term
4. An understanding of the specific needs and growth patterns of the preterm neonate

Coping mechanisms of families will vary greatly. Cultural and ethnic norms will often dictate behaviors exhibited by the parents. Healthy coping behaviors exhibited by parents include a willingness to acknowledge the reality of the danger of demise of the neonate and an open concern about the neonate's chances for survival. Judgments about the birth are based on the reality of the situation. Reassurances by health personnel should be based on facts that offer a realistic explanation of the cause of the preterm birth and the neonate's plan of care. Frequent visits to the neonate with efforts to learn about neonatal progress are considered positive healthy coping behaviors.

During the first few months of life, the parents are forced into a supportive position in neonatal care. The staff of the neonatal nursery should make every attempt to keep parents informed of the status of the neonate, whether positive or negative. Parents are encouraged to become involved in caring for the baby as soon as it is feasible. Even when they cannot give direct care because intensive care is needed by the neonate, they should be encouraged to come to the nursery, and to touch and talk to the neonate.

Expectations often must be altered greatly when a preterm neonate is born. Parents may need help in recognizing the neonate as an individual with specific needs. Any discrepancies between expectation and actual neonatal behavior are explained to the parents at a level of understanding that will allow assimilation of information. They should be encouraged to visit frequently with siblings (if appropriate) and telephone for information and questions at any time.

Some specific parental behaviors that may signify future problems in infant care include:

Inability to express feelings of guilt and responsibility for the premature arrival of the neonate

No visible anxiety about survival chances

Constant and continued displacement of anxiety into less threatening matters

Little effort to secure information about neonatal status

Consistent misinterpretation or exaggeration of information about neonatal condition

Inability to share fears with each other

Lack of emotional and practical support systems

Inability to accept and utilize assistance offered

When parental behaviors signify potential problems in caring for the preterm neonate after discharge from the hospital, referral by the nurse to other sources may assist parents in dealing with and altering these behaviors.

NEONATAL DEATH

When a neonate is seriously ill from birth or is born with a congenital anomaly incompatible with extrauterine life, an open discussion of the potential for the neonate should be initiated as soon as possible following delivery. Both parents must be included in this discussion. Parents should be encouraged to visit and touch the neonate in the intensive care nursery. Photographs are taken and given to the parents. If death appears imminent, parents are encouraged to be with the neonate. Holding the neonate is beneficial in accomplishing grief work, but the parents should not be forced to do this.

Certain reactions to neonatal death can be expected in the majority of parents. First, they lose the beautiful baby of their fantasies. This loss may be interwoven with feelings of failure, guilt, and anger. Second, they must deal with the death of a real child. This fact must be assimilated by the parents. Third, the normal grieving process which began at birth is complicated and altered when the neonate dies. Channels of communication between the parents and nursing staff must be open and information given must be clear, concise, and consistent. Repetition of information is usually necessary for comprehension and having parents repeat specific information is helpful to ascertain understanding.

Referral to a support group of parents with similar problems may benefit the parents in working through the grief process. Followup telephone calls or scheduled interviews may identify problems in grief resolution.

DEFECTIVE NEONATE

When a neonate with a defect is born, the family is confronted with a crisis situation. Parental reactions to the defective neonate are based on the severity and location of the deformity, when they are informed of the defect, the amount of energy available at that time, and their past experience with a similar situation.

Their response to the crisis usually follows two separate, yet intertwined stages: (1) disorganization and disequilibrium; and (2) coping and reorganization. In the first stage, parental reaction is shock, followed by denial and disbelief, and then sadness and anger. The shock reaction may be one of hysteria, quiet sobbing, or numbness. This is followed by the desire to flee from the situation and denial of the defect. They may withdraw and verbalize psychosomatic complaints. When sadness and anger occur, they will blame themselves or staff for the defect or may be angry with everyone. They will often keep a distance from the infant, in an effort not to get involved.

In Stage II, the parents exhibit acceptance, followed by adaptation. In the acceptance phase, they search for the cause of the defect.

The normal aspects of the neonate are emphasized in an attempt to relate the child to themselves. They are occasionally depressed, but anxieties are decreased. The future of the child will be a frequent topic of conversation. With adaptation comes a movement toward acceptance of the child as an individual with needs. They will attempt to correct or ameliorate the defect with available resources.

Open communication between the parents and health care personnel is vital to working through these two stages. If the father withdraws in his own personal grief, maternal anxiety will increase. A support system is important to working through the stages.

NURSING RESPONSIBILITIES

Facial expressions of staff in the delivery room are important in acceptance of the neonate by the parents. The parents should be encouraged to see the neonate, but only after they are prepared for the defect that exists. Time for questions is imperative. Accurate information must be given. The parents of a defective neonate need extra support, especially during the initial stage of shock and disbelief. They will need to express their feelings openly, whether these feelings are of guilt or anger. Positive aspects of child development are stressed, but not to the point that negative aspects are ignored. Other nursing responsibilities include:

- Examining individual values
- Accepting grief behaviors
- Empathizing
- Not feeding self-pity
- Establishing a supportive relationship
- Gauging parental readiness for an active role in neonatal care
- Supplying needed information
- Teaching special skills that may be required in daily care
- Planning realistic discharge
- Referral

These parents often will never totally work through the grief process while the infant is alive. They will suffer from chronic guilt that never really resolves itself.

STILLBIRTH

Intrauterine fetal demise is another crisis situation for the childbearing family. If death comes without prior warning, the first stage of grief will usually be lengthy, since there was no preparation for the sudden loss.

When intrauterine death is identified prior to labor, parents have already begun their grief work before admission to labor and delivery. The nurse may need to work with both parents or the mother alone. Getting the client and partner to verbalize feelings will aid in establishment of a therapeutic relationship between nurse and family. Anger and depression are not uncommon responses, and are to be expected. Honesty is the best approach in the majority of cases, without evading questions. Verbal and nonverbal communication is important during the intrapartum period. Parents are encouraged to see and hold their child after delivery.

Many hospitals use a checklist to aid nursing staff in assisting parents who have experienced a stillbirth. This checklist ensures that nursing personnel offer parents all available options, from holding the baby to preparing a "memorial packet" that contains a picture, identification band, footprints, a lock of hair, infant cap, and blanket.

Initial support of the family is also provided by a minister or chaplain, if the parents desire. He or she can also be of benefit in ascertaining the family desires for baptism, funeral arrangements, appropriate religious rites, and so on. Visiting policies are usually modified to allow other significant support persons to aid parents in coping with the loss.

Social service departments can be helpful in providing follow-up support and referral after discharge. Nursing plays a crucial role in aiding families in crisis. The approach should be consistent and organized, but flexible enough to allow individual differences in family units. By recognizing crisis situations and implementing appropriate interventions, the nurse can aid the grieving family to deal with their loss in a constructive manner.

BIBLIOGRAPHY

Borg, S.O. & Lasker, J. *When pregnancy fails: Families coping with miscarriage, stillbirth and infant death.* Boston: Beacon Press, 1981.

Cefalo, R.C. Managing missed abortion and antepartum fetal death. *Contemporary Obstetrics & Gynecology,* 1983, **22,** 17.

Cordell, A. & Apolito, R. Family support in infant death. *Journal of Obstetric, Gynecological & Neonatal Nursing,* 1981, **10,** 281.

Cronenwett, L.R. Network structures, social support, and psychological outcomes of pregnancy. *Nursing Research,* 1985, **34,** 93-99.

Drane, J.F. The defective child; ethical guidelines for painful dilemmas. *Journal of Obstetric, Gynecological & Neonatal Nursing,* 1984, **13,** 42.

Ehrenkranz, R.A. Neonatal death: Caring for parents. *Contemporary Obstetrics & Gynecology,* 1983, **22,** 24.

Hoff, L.A. *People in crisis: Understanding and helping* (2nd ed.). Menlo Park, Calif.: Addison-Wesley, 1984.

Ishida, U. How to deal with grief in childbirth. *Female Patient,* 1980, **5,** 74.

Jackson, P.L. When the baby isn't perfect. *American Journal of Nursing,* 1985, **85,** 396.

Kowalski, K. Managing perinatal loss. *Clinics in Obstetrics & Gynecology,* 1980, **23,** 1113.

Kubler-Ross, E. *On death and dying.* New York: Macmillan, 1969.

Lake, M., et al. The role of a grief support team following stillbirth. *American Journal of Obstetrics & Gynecology,* 1983, **146,** 887.

Lauer, M.E., et al. A comparison study of parental adaptation following a child's death at home or in the hospital. *Pediatrics,* 1983, **71,** 107.

Miles, M.S. Helping adults mourn the death of a child. In H. Wass & C. Corr (Eds.). *Children and death.* New York: Hemisphere, 1984.

———. Emotional symptoms and physical health in bereaved parents. *Nursing Research,* 1985, **34,** 76-81.

Mina, C.F. A program for helping grieving parents, *MCN,* 1985, **10,** 118-121.

Peppers, L.G. & Knapp, R.J. *Motherhood and mourning: Perinatal death.* New York: Praeger, 1980.

Schodt, C.M. Grief in adolescent mothers after an infant death. *Image,* 1982, **14,** 20-25.

Whitfiled, J.M., et al. The application of hospice concepts to neonatal care. *American Journal of Diseases of Children,* 1982, **136,** 421.

appendix A

THE PREGNANT PATIENT'S BILL OF RIGHTS THE PREGNANT PATIENT'S RESPONSIBILITIES*

The International Childbirth Education Association (ICEA) is an interdisciplinary, volunteer organization representing groups and individuals who share a genuine interest in the goals of family-centered maternity care and education for the childbearing year.

ICEA constantly seeks to expand awareness of the rights and responsibilities of pregnant women and expectant parents. Most pregnant women are not aware of their rights or of the obstetrician's legal obligation to obtain their informed consent to treatment. The American College of Obstetricians and Gynecologists has made a commendable effort to clearly set forth the pregnant patient's right of informed consent in the following excerpts from pages 66 and 67 of its *Standards for Obstetric-Gynecologic Services.*

"It is important to note the distinction between 'consent' and 'informed consent'. Many physicians, because they do not realize there is a difference, believe they are free from liability if the patient consents to treatment. This is not true. The physician may still be liable if the patient's consent was not informed. In addition, the usual consent obtained by a hospital does not in any way release the physician from his legal duty of obtaining an informed consent from his patient.

"Most courts consider that the patient is 'informed' if the following information is given:

> The processes contemplated by the physician as treatment, including whether the treatment is new or unusual.
> The risks and hazards of the treatment.
> The chances for recovery after treatment.
> The necessity of the treatment.
> The feasibility of alternative methods of treatment."

"One point on which courts do agree is that explanations must be given in such a way that the patient understands them. A physician cannot claim as a defense that he explained the procedure to the patient when he knew the patient did not understand. The physician has a duty to act with due care under the circumstances; this means he must be sure the patient understands what she is told."

"It should be emphasized that the following reasons are not sufficient to justify failure to inform:

1. That the patient may prefer not to be told the unpleasant possibilities regarding the treatment.
2. That full disclosure might suggest infinite

*"The Pregnant Patient's Bill of Rights/The Pregnant Patient's Responsibilities" written by Doris Haire and members of ICEA, published by the International Childbirth Education Association, P.O. Box 20048, Minneapolis, Minnesota 55420 USA. Reprinted with permission.

dangers to a patient with an active imagination, thereby causing her to refuse treatment.

3. That the patient, on learning the risks involved, might rationally decline treatment. The right to decline is the specific fundamental right protected by the informed consent doctrine."

THE PREGNANT PATIENT'S BILL OF RIGHTS

American parents are becoming increasingly aware that well-intentioned health professionals do not always have scientific data to support common American obstetrical practices and that many of these practices are carried out primarily because they are part of medical and hospital tradition. In the last forty years many artificial practices have been introduced which have changed childbirth from a physiological event to a very complicated medical procedure in which all kinds of drugs are used and procedures carried out, sometimes unnecessarily, and many of them potentially damaging for the baby and even for the mother. A growing body of research makes it alarmingly clear that every aspect of traditional American hospital care during labor and delivery must now be questioned as to its possible effect on the future well-being of both the obstetric patient and her unborn child.

One in every 35 children born in the United States today will eventually be diagnosed as retarded; in 75% of these cases there is no familial or genetic predisposing factor. One in every 10 to 17 children has been found to have some form of brain dysfunction or learning disability requiring special treatment. Such statistics are not confined to the lower socioeconomic group but cut across all segments of American society.

New concerns are being raised by childbearing women because no one knows what degree of oxygen depletion, head compression, or traction by forceps the unborn or newborn infant can tolerate before that child sustains permanent brain damage or dysfunction. The recent findings regarding the cancer-related drug diethylstilbestrol have alerted the public to the fact that neither the approval of a drug by the U.S. Food and Drug Administration nor the fact that a drug is prescribed by a physician serves as a guarantee that a drug or medication is safe for the mother or her unborn child. In fact, the American Academy of Pediatrics' Committee on Drugs has recently stated that there is no drug, whether prescription or over-the-counter remedy, which has been proven safe for the unborn child.

The Pregnant Patient has the right to participate in decisions involving her well-being and that of her unborn child, unless there is a clearcut medical emergency that prevents her participation. In addition to the rights set forth in the American Hospital Association's "Patient's Bill of Rights," (which has also been adopted by the New York City Department of Health) the Pregnant Patient, because she represents TWO patients rather than one, should be recognized as having the additional rights listed below.

1. *The Pregnant Patient has the right,* prior to the administration of any drug or procedure, to be informed by the health professional caring for her of any potential direct or indirect effects, risks or hazards to herself or her unborn or newborn infant which may result from the use of a drug or procedure prescribed for or administered to her during pregnancy, labor, birth or lactation.
2. *The Pregnant Patient has the right,* prior to the proposed therapy, to be informed, not only of the benefits, risks and hazards of the proposed therapy but also of known alternative therapy, such as available childbirth education classes which could help to prepare the Pregnant Patient physically and mentally to cope with the discomfort or stress of pregnancy and the experience of

childbirth, thereby reducing or eliminating her need for drugs and obstetric intervention. She should be offered such information early in her pregnancy in order that she may make a reasoned decision.

3. *The Pregnant Patient has the right,* prior to the administration of any drug, to be informed by the health professional who is prescribing or administering the drug to her that any drug which she receives during pregnancy, labor and birth, no matter how or when the drug is taken or administered, may adversely affect her unborn baby, directly or indirectly, and that there is no drug or chemical which has been proven safe for the unborn child.
4. *The Pregnant Patient has the right* if Cesarean birth is anticipated, to be informed prior to the administration of any drug, and preferably prior to her hospitalization, that minimizing her and, in turn, her baby's intake of nonessential pre-operative medicine will benefit her baby.
5. *The Pregnant Patient has the right,* prior to the administration of a drug or procedure, to be informed of the areas of uncertainty if there is NO properly controlled follow-up research which has established the safety of the drug or procedure with regard to its direct and/or indirect effects on the physiological, mental and neurological development of the child exposed, via the mother, to the drug or procedure during pregnancy, labor, birth or lactation—(this would apply to virtually all drugs and the vast majority of obstetric procedures).
6. *The Pregnant Patient has the right,* prior to the administration of any drug, to be informed of the brand name and generic name of the drug in order that she may advise the health professional of any past adverse reaction to the drug.
7. *The Pregnant Patient has the right* to determine for herself, without pressure from her attendant, whether she will accept the risks inherent in the proposed therapy or refuse a drug or procedure.
8. *The Pregnant Patient has the right* to know the name and qualifications of the individual administering a medication or procedure to her during labor or birth.
9. *The Pregnant Patient has the right* to be informed, prior to the administration of any procedure, whether that procedure is being administered to her for her or her baby's benefit (medically indicated) or as an elective procedure (for convenience, teaching purposes or research).
10. *The Pregnant Patient has the right* to be accompanied during the stress of labor and birth by someone she cares for, and to whom she looks for emotional comfort and encouragement.
11. *The Pregnant Patient has the right* after appropriate medical consultation to choose a position for labor and for birth which is least stressful to her baby and to herself.
12. *The Obstetric Patient has the right* to have her baby cared for at her bedside if her baby is normal, and to feed her baby according to her baby's needs rather than according to the hospital regimen.
13. *The Obstetric Patient has the right* to be informed in writing of the name of the person who actually delivered her baby and the professional qualifications of that person. This information should also be on the birth certificate.
14. *The Obstetric Patient has the right* to be informed if there is any known or indicated aspect of her or her baby's care or condition which may cause her or her baby later difficulty or problems.
15. *The Obstetric Patient has the right* to have her and her baby's hospital medical records complete, accurate and legible and to have their records, including Nurses' Notes, retained by the hospital until the child reaches at least the age of majority, or, alternatively, to have the records offered to her before they are destroyed.
16. *The Obstetric Patient,* both during and after her hospital stay, has the right to have access to her complete hospital medical

records, including Nurses' Notes, and to receive a copy upon payment of a reasonable fee and without incurring the expense of retaining an attorney.

It is the obstetric patient and her baby, not the health professional, who must sustain any trauma or injury resulting from the use of a drug or obstetric procedure. The observation of the rights listed above will not only permit the obstetric patient to participate in the decisions involving her and her baby's health care, but will help to protect the health professional and the hospital against litigation arising from resentment or misunderstanding on the part of the mother.

THE PREGNANT PATIENT'S RESPONSIBILITIES

In addition to understanding her rights the Pregnant Patient should also understand that she too has certain responsibilities. The Pregnant Patient's responsibilities include the following:

1. The Pregnant Patient is responsible for learning about the physical and psychological process of labor, birth and postpartum recovery. The better informed expectant parents are the better they will be able to participate in decisions concerning the planning of their care.
2. The Pregnant Patient is responsible for learning what comprises good prenatal and intranatal care and for making an effort to obtain the best care possible.
3. Expectant parents are responsible for knowing about those hospital policies and regulations which will affect their birth and postpartum experience.
4. The Pregnant Patient is responsible for arranging for a companion or support person (husband, mother, sister, friend, etc.) who will share in her plans for birth and who will accompany her during her labor and birth experience.
5. The Pregnant Patient is responsible for making her preferences known clearly to the health professionals involved in her case in a courteous and cooperative manner and for making mutually agreed-upon arrangements regarding maternity care alternatives with her physician and hospital in advance of labor.
6. Expectant parents are responsible for listening to their chosen physician or midwife with an open mind, just as they expect him or her to listen openly to them.
7. Once they have agreed to a course of health care, expectant parents are responsible, to the best of their ability, for seeing that the program is carried out in consultation with others with whom they have made the agreement.
8. The Pregnant Patient is responsible for obtaining information in advance regarding the approximate cost of her obstetric and hospital care.
9. The Pregnant Patient who intends to change her physician or hospital is responsible for notifying all concerned, well in advance of the birth if possible, and for informing both of her reasons for changing.
10. In all their interactions with medical and nursing personnel, the expectant parents should behave towards those caring for them with the same respect and consideration they themselves would like.
11. During the mother's hospital stay the mother is responsible for learning about her and her baby's continuing care after discharge from the hospital.
12. After birth, the parents should put into writing constructive comments and feelings of satisfaction and/or dissatisfaction with the care (nursing, medical and personal) they received. Good service to families in the future will be facilitated by those parents who take the time and responsibility to write letters expressing their feelings about the maternity care they received.

All the previous statements assume a normal birth and postpartum experience. Expectant parents should realize that, if complications develop in their cases, there will be an increased need to trust the expertise of the physician and hospital staff they have chosen. However, if problems occur, the childbearing woman still retains her responsibility for making informed decisions about her care or treatment and that of her baby. If she is incapable of assuming that responsibility because of her physical condition, her previously authorized companion or support person should assume responsibility for making informed decision on her behalf.

appendix B

RESOURCES, SUPPORT AND PROFESSIONAL ORGANIZATIONS

Alternative Birth Crisis Coalition
PO Box 48731
Chicago, IL 60648

American Academy of Husband-Coached Childbirth
PO Box 5224
Sherman Oaks, CA 91413

American College of Nurse Midwives
Suite 801
1012 14th Street N.W.
Washington, D.C. 20005

American College of Home Obstetrics
P.O. Box 24
River Forest, IL 60305

American Nurses' Association
2420 Pershing Road
Kansas City, MO 64108

American National Red Cross
17th and D Streets, N.W.
Washington, D.C. 20006

American College of Obstetricians and Gynecologists
Suite 300
600 Maryland Avenue S.W.
Washington, D.C. 20024

American Foundation for Maternal and Child Health
30 Beckman Place
New York, N.Y. 10022

American Physical Therapy Association
1111 N. Fairfax Street
Alexandria, VA 22314

American Association for Maternal and Child Health
233 Prospect P-209
LaJolla, CA 92307

American Society for Psychoprophylaxis in Obstetrics
1411 K Street, N.W.
Washington, D.C. 20005

American Academy of Pediatrics
P.O. Box 1034
Evanston, IL 60204

Association for the Advancement of Health Education (AAHE)
1900 Association Drive
Reston, VA 22091

American Public Health Association (APHA)
1015 15th Street, N.W.
Washington, D.C. 20005

Association of Planned Parenthood Professionals (APPP)
810 Seventh Avenue
New York, N.Y. 10019

American Society of Childbirth Educators (ASCE)
P.O. Box 16159
7113 Lynwood Drive
Tampa, FL 33687

Association for Childbirth at Home, International
P.O. Box 1219
Cerritos, CA 90701

Association of Teachers of Maternal and Child Health (ATMCH)
School of Public Health
University of Illinois
2035 W. Taylor Street
Chicago, IL 60680

Boston Women's Health Book Collective, Inc.
Box 192
West Sommerville, MA 02144

Behavior Genetics Association
Box 447
Institute for Behavioral Genetics
University of Colorado
Boulder, CO 80309

BABES, Inc.
52 Berens Drive
Kentfield, CA 94904

Center for Family Growth
555 Highland Avenue
Cotati, CA 94928

Center for Study of Multiple Birth
Suite 463-5
333 E. Superior Street
Chicago, IL 60611

Center for Population Options (CPO)
2031 Florida Avenue, N.W.
Washington, D.C. 20009

Cesarean Birth Council
1402 Nilda Avenue
Mount View, CA 94040

Cesarean/Support Education and Concerns
66 Christopher Road
Waltham, MA 02154

Childbirth Without Pain Education Association
20134 Snowden
Detroit, MI 48235

Childbirth Education Foundation
P.O. Box 37
Apalachin, N.Y. 13732

Child Study Association of America
9 E. 89th Street
New York, N.Y. 10028

Child Welfare League of America, Inc.
44 E. 23rd Street
New York, N.Y. 10010

Cesarean Prevention Movement (CPM)
P.O. Box 152
Syracuse, N.Y. 13210

Childbirth Graphics Ltd.
P.O. Box 17025
Irondequoit Post Office
Rochester, N.Y. 14617

Cooperative Birth Center Network
Box 1, Rt. 1
Perkiomenville, PA 18074

Concerns of Motherhood
P.O. Box 49411
Chicago, IL 60649

Council of Childbirth Education Specialists, Inc.
168 W. 86th Street
New York, N.Y. 10024

Council for Sex Information and Education (CSIE)
Box 23088
Washington, D.C. 20024

Family Service Association of America, Inc.
44 E. 23rd Street
New York, N.Y. 10010

Fertility Research Foundation (FRF)
Suite 103
1430 Second Avenue
New York, N.Y. 10021

Florence Crittenton Association of America
608 S. Dearborn Street
Chicago, IL 60605

Food and Nutrition Board
National Research Council
2102 Constitution Ave, N.W.
Washington, D.C. 20418

Frontier Nursing Services
Wendover, KY 41775

Holistic Chidbirth Institution
1627 Tenth Avenue
San Francisco, CA 94122

Home Oriented Maternity Experience (HOME)
511 New York Avenue
Tokema Park, MD 20012

Informed Homebirth
P.O. Box 788
Boulder, CO 80306

International Association of Parents and Professionals for Safe Alternatives in Childbirth (IAPSAC)
P.O. Box 267
Marble Hill, MO 63764

International Childbirth Education Association
Box 20048
Minneapolis, MN 55420

LaLeche League International, Inc.
9616 Minneapolis Avenue
Franklin Park, IL 60131

Maternity Center Association
48 W. 92nd Street
New York, NY 10028

Nurses' Association of the American College of Obstetricians and Gynecologists (NAACOG)
Suite 200
600 Maryland Avenue
Washington, D.C. 20024

National Association of Parents and Professionals for Safe Alternatives in Childbirth (NAPSAC)
P.O. Box 1307
Chapel Hill, N.C. 27514

National Association of Childbirth Education, Inc. (NACE)
3940 Eleventh Street
Riverside, CA 92501

National Council for Prevention of Child Abuse
Box 2866
Chicago, IL 60690

National Dairy Council
6300 N. River Road
Rosemont, IL 60018

National Foundation—March of Dimes
1275 Mamaroneck Avenue
White Plains, N.Y. 10605

National Genetics Foundation
555 W. 75th Street
New York, N.Y. 10019

National League for Nursing (NLN)
10 Columbus Circle
New York, N.Y. 10019

National Sudden Infant Death Foundation
310 S. Michigan Avenue
Chicago, IL 60604

Nursing Mother's Council
Boston Association for Childbirth Education
726 Washington Street
Whiteman, MA 12382

National Society for Crippled Children and Adults, Inc.
2023 W. Ogden Avenue
Chicago, IL 60612

National Society for the Prevention of Blindness
16 East 40th Street
New York, N.Y. 10016

National Midwives Association (NMA)
1119 East San Antonio
El Paso, TE 79901

Parents of Premature and High Risk Infants International (PPHRII)
Suite 1227
33 W. 42nd Street
New York, N.Y. 10036

Planned Parenthood Federation of America, Inc.
810 Seventh Avenue
New York, N.Y. 10019

Share—Source of Help in Airing and Resolving Experiences
c/o St. John's Hospital
800 Carpenter Street
Springfield, IL 62769

Support Organizatioon for Trisomy 18/13
478 Terrace Lane
Toole, UT 84074

United Cerebral Palsy Association, Inc.
321 West 44th Street
New York, N.Y. 10036

United States Government
Children's Bureau
U.S. Department of Health and Human Services
Washington, D.C. 20402

appendix C

ABREVIATIONS USED IN MATERNITY NURSING

ABC	Alternative birthing center
abo	abortion; miscarriage
AC	abdominal circumference
accel	FHR accelerations
ACTH	adrenocorticotrophic hormone
AFP	alpha-fetoprotein
AFV	amniotic fluid volume
AGA	appropriate for gestational age
AID	artificial insemination by donor
AIH	artificial insemination by husband
AROM	artificial rupture of the membranes
AZ	2 hour pregnancy test
BAT	brown adipose tissue (brown fat)
BBT	basal body temperature
BL	baseline FHR
BMR	basal metabolic rate
BOW	bag of waters
BP	blood pressure
BPD	biparietal diameter of fetal head
BPD	bronchopulmonary dysplasia
BSST	breast self-stimulation test
CAN	cord around the neck
CC	chest circumference
C–H	crown–heel length
CID	cytomegalic inclusion disease
circ	circumcision
cm	centimeter
CMV	cytomegalovirus
CNM	certified nurse-midwife
CNS	central nervous system
CPAP	continuous positive airway pressure
CPD	cephalo-pelvic disproportion
CPR	cardiopulmonary resuscitation
C–R	crown–rump length
CRNA	certified registered nurse anesthetist
CS	cesarean section
CST	contraction stress test
CVA	costovertebral angle
CVP	central venous pressure
DAO	diamine oxidase
D&C	dilation and curettage
dec	FHR deceleration
del	delivery
D/I	dry and intact (dressing)
dil	cervical dilation
DM	diabetes mellitus
DRG	diagnostic related groups
DTR	deep tendon reflexes
EDC	estimated date of confinement
EFM	external fetal monitor
epis	episiotomy
F	fundus
FAD	fetal activity diary
FAS	fetal alcohol syndrome
FBM	fetal breathing movements
FBS	fetal blood scalp sample
FBS	fasting blood sugar
FHR	fetal heart rate
FHT	fetal heart tones
FL	femur length
FM	fetal movement
FSH	follicle-stimulating hormone
FSHRH	follicle-stimulating hormone–releasing hormone
FSI	foam stability index
FTP	full-term pregnancy
GDM	gestational diabetes mellitus

GFR glomerular filtration rate
GI gastrointestinal
GnRF gonadotropin-releasing factor
GnRH gonadotropin-releasing hormone
grav gravida
GTPAL gravida/term/preterm/abortion/living
H&S heat and spray treatment
HAI hemagglutination-inhibition test
HCG human chorionic gonadotropin
HCS human chorionic somatomammotropin
HMD hyaline membrane disease
HPL human placental lactogen
HVH herpesvirus hominis
IDDM insulin dependent diabetes mellitus
IDM infant of a diabetic mother
IPPV intermittent positive pressure ventilation
ISC infant servocontrol
IUD intrauterine device
IUFD intrauterine fetal death
IUGR intrauterine growth retardation
IUP intrauterine pregnancy
LBW low birth weight
LFD low forceps delivery
LGA large for gestational age
LH luteinizing hormone
LHRH luteinizing hormone–releasing hormone
LMA left mentum anterior
LMLE left mediolateral episiotomy
LMP last menstrual period
LMT left mentum transverse
LNMP last normal menstrual period
LOA left occiput anterior
LOF low outlet forceps
LOP left occiput posterior
LOT left occiput transverse
L/S lecithin/sphingomyelin ratio
LSA left sacrum anterior
LSP left sacrum posterior
LST left sacrum transverse
MAS meconium aspiration syndrome
mec meconium
mec st meconium staining
MLE midline episiotomy
multip multipara
NANDA North American Nursing Diagnosis Association
NB newborn
NEC neonatal necrotizing enterocolitis
NGU nongonococcal urethritis
NIDDM non-insulin dependent diabetes mellitus
NP nurse practitioner
NPO nothing by mouth
NSLFD normal single low forceps delivery
NST nonstress test
NSVD normal sterile vaginal delivery
OA occiput anterior
OCT oxytocin challenge test
OF occipitofrontal diameter of fetal head
OM occipitomental diameter
OP occiput posterior
P para
PDA patent ductus arteriosus
PEEP positive end expiratory pressure
PFC persistent fetal circulation
PG phosphatidylglycerol
PG prostaglandin
PI phosphatidyinositol
PID pelvic inflammatory disease
PIH pregnancy induced hypertension
pit pitocin
PKU phenylketonuria
PMI point of maximum impulse
PP postpartum
PPTL postpartum tubal ligation
preemie preterm neonate
preg pregnancy
primip primipara
PROM premature rupture of the membranes

RDA	recommended dietary allowance
RDS	respiratory distress syndrome
REM	rapid eye movements
RIA	radioimmune assay
RLF	retrolental fibroplasia
ROA	right occiput anterior
ROM	rupture of the membranes
ROP	right occiput posterior
ROT	right occiput transverse
RMA	right mentum anterior
RMP	right mentum posterior
RMT	right mentum transverse
RRA	radioreceptor assay
RSA	right sacrum anterior
RSP	right sacrum posterior
RST	right sacrum transverse
SFB	single footling breech
SFD	small for dates
SGA	small for gestational age
SIDS	sudden infant death syndrome
SOAP	subjective data, objective data, assessment, plan
SOB	suboccipitobregmatic diameter
SROM	spontaneous rupture of the membranes
STD	sexually transmitted disease
STH	somatotrophic hormone
SVE	sterile vaginal examination
TCM	transcutaneous monitoring
TNZ	thermal neutral zone
TORCH	toxoplasmosis, other, rubella, cytomegalovirus, herpesvirus hominus type 2
TTN	transient tachypnea of the newborn
UA	urinalysis
UC	uterine contraction
UPI	uteroplacental insufficiency
U/S	ultrasound
UTI	urinary tract infection
vag	vaginal
VBAC	vaginal birth after cesarean birth
VD	venereal disease
VDRL	Venereal Disease Research Laboratories
VE	vaginal examination
WIC	supplemental food program for women, infants, and children

appendix D

MATERNAL LABORATORY VALUES DURING PREGNANCY

	Nonpregnant	Pregnant
Complete blood count		
Hemoglobin, gm/100 ml	12–16	10–14
Hematocrit, %	37–47	32–42
Red cell volume, ml	1600	1900
Plasma volume, ml	2400	3700
Red blood cell indexes	normal	normal
White blood cells, total, mm^3	4500–10,000	5000–15,000
Polymorphonuclear cells, %	54–62	60–85
Lymphocytes, %	38–46	15–40
ESR, mm/hr	<20	30–90
Coagulation studies		
Bleeding time	normal	normal
Clotting time	normal	normal
Platelets, mm^3	175,000–250,000	200,000–350,000
Prothrombin time	Control ± 3 sec	10% decrease
Fibrinogen, mg/100 ml	250	400
Factor VIII	normal	3X normal
Factor V, VII, IX, X	normal	moderate increase
Erythropoietic System		
Serum iron, mcg	75–150	65–120
Total iron-binding capacity, mcg	250–450	300–500
Blood sugar		
Fasting, mg/100 ml	70–80	65
2 hour postprandial, mg/100 ml	60–110	<140 after ingestion of 100 gm CHO meal
Serum proteins		
Total, gm/100 ml	6.7–8.3	5.5–7.5
Albumin, gm/100 ml	3.5–5.5	3.0–5.0
Globulin, total, gm/100 ml	2.3–3.5	3.0–4.0
Protein-bound iodine, μg/100 ml	4.0–8.0	6.5–12.0
Blood pressure, mm Hg	120/80	114/65
Venous pressure, cm H_2O		
Femoral	9	24
Antecubital	8	8
Pulse rate, BPM	70	80
Cardiac output, L/min	4.5	6
Blood volume, ml		
Whole blood	4000	5600
Plasma	2400	3700
Red blood cell	1600	1900

	Nonpregnant	Pregnant
Electrocardiogram	normal	15 degree left axis deviation
V_1, V_2	normal	inverted T wave
V4	normal	low T
III	normal	inverted T wave
aVR	normal	small Q wave
Renal blood flow, ml/min	900	1200
Glomerular filtration rate, ml/min	80–120	110–180
BUN, mg/100 ml	10–18	4–12
Creatinine, mg/100 ml	0.6–1.2	0.4–0.9
Uric acid, mg/100 ml	2.0–6.4	2.0–5.5
Urine glucose	negative	present in 20% of gravidas

appendix E

LABORATORY VALUES OF THE NEONATE

Test	Normal Value in Neonate
Hemoglobin gm/100 ml	15–18
Hematocrit, volume %	45–60
Platelets mm^3	150,000–300,000
Reticulocytes %	3–7
White blood cells mm^3	10,000–35,000
Neutrophils %	46–80
Lymphocytes %	31
Eosinophils %	1–3
Monocytes %	5–10
Red blood cells mm^3	4 to 7 million
Bilirubin, direct mg/100 ml	0.5–1
Bilirubin, total mg/100 ml	5–12
Blood sugar mg/100 ml	40–80
Sodium mEq/L	136–143
Potassium, mEq/L	4.0–7.0
Calcium, mEq/L	4–5
Chloride, mEq/L	95–105
Total protein, gm/100 ml	4.8–7.4
Iron mcg/100 ml	100–200
Urea nitrogen (BUN) mg/100 ml	5–15
Fibrinogen, mg/100 ml	150–300
Prothrombin time (sec)	12–18
Blood Gases	
Arterial	
pH	7.35–7.45
PO_2 mm Hg	50–80
PCO_2 mm Hg	33–45
Plasma bicarbonate mEq/L	20–25
Base excess mEq/L	+4 to −4

appendix F

TEMPERATURE EQUIVALENTS: FAHRENHEIT AND CELSIUS

degrees Fahrenheit	degrees Celsius	degrees Fahrenheit	degrees Celsius
93.2	34	99.1	37.3
93.6	34.2	99.3	37.4
94.3	34.6	99.5	37.5
94.6	34.8	99.6	37.6
95.0	35.0	99.8	37.7
95.4	35.2	100.0	37.8
95.7	35.4	100.2	37.9
95.9	35.5	100.4	38.0
96.1	35.6	100.6	38.1
96.3	35.7	100.8	38.2
96.4	35.8	101.1	38.4
96.6	35.9	101.3	38.5
96.8	36.0	101.5	38.6
96.9	36.1	101.7	38.7
97.2	36.2	101.8	38.8
97.3	36.3	102.0	38.9
97.5	36.4	102.2	39.0
97.7	36.5	102.4	39.1
97.9	36.6	102.6	39.2
98.0	36.7	102.9	39.4
98.2	36.8	103.1	39.5
98.4	36.9	103.3	39.6
98.6	37.0	103.5	39.7
98.8	37.1	103.6	39.8
99.0	37.2	103.8	39.9

appendix G

NEWBORN LENGTH CONVERSION TABLE

Inches	Centimeters
10	25.4
10.5	26.7
11	27.9
11.5	29.2
12	30.5
12.5	31.8
13	33.0
13.5	34.3
14	35.6
14.5	36.8
15	38.1
15.5	39.4
16	40.6
16.5	41.9
17	43.2
17.5	44.5
18	45.7
18.5	47.0
19	48.3
19.5	49.5
20	50.8
20.5	52.1
21	53.3
21.5	54.6
22	55.9
22.5	57.2
23	58.4
23.5	59.7
24	60.9

appendix H

CONVERSION TABLE FOR NEONATAL WEIGHTS: POUNDS TO GRAMS

	Pounds														
Ounces	**0**	**1**	**2**	**3**	**4**	**5**	**6**	**7**	**8**	**9**	**10**	**11**	**12**	**13**	**14**
0	0	454	907	1361	1814	2268	2722	3175	3629	4082	4536	4990	5443	5897	6350
1	28	482	936	1389	1843	2296	2750	3204	3657	4111	4565	5018	5472	5925	6379
2	57	510	964	1418	1871	2325	2778	3232	3686	4139	4593	5046	5500	5954	6407
3	85	539	992	1446	1899	2353	2807	3260	3714	4167	4621	5075	5528	5982	6435
4	113	567	1021	1474	1928	2381	2835	3289	3742	4196	4649	5103	5557	6010	6464
5	142	595	1049	1503	1956	2410	2863	3317	3771	4224	4678	5131	5585	6039	6492
6	170	624	1077	1531	1985	2438	2892	3345	3799	4253	4706	5160	5613	6067	6521
7	198	652	1106	1559	2013	2466	2920	3374	3827	4281	4734	5188	5642	6095	6549
8	227	680	1134	1588	2041	2495	2948	3402	3856	4309	4763	5216	5670	6124	6577
9	255	709	1162	1616	2070	2523	2977	3430	3884	4338	4791	5245	5698	6152	6606
10	284	737	1191	1644	2098	2552	3005	3459	3912	4366	4820	5273	5727	6180	6634
11	312	765	1219	1673	2126	2580	3033	3487	3941	4394	4848	5301	5755	6209	6662
12	340	794	1247	1701	2155	2608	3062	3515	3969	4423	4876	5330	5783	6237	6691
13	369	822	1276	1729	2183	2637	3090	3544	3997	4451	4905	5358	5812	6265	6719
14	397	851	1304	1758	2211	2665	3119	3572	4026	4479	4933	5387	5840	6296	6747
15	425	879	1332	1786	2240	2693	3147	3600	4054	4508	4961	5415	5868	6322	6776

GLOSSARY

Abandonment. In a nurse-client relationship, failure of the nurse to attend to the client, either by absence or failure to notify the proper authority when warranted.

ABO incompatibility. Form of hemolytic disease of the newborn with incompatibility between ABO blood groups of the mother and fetus. Most commonly the mother is type O and the fetus is type A.

Abortion. The interruption of pregnancy and loss of the products of conception before 20 to 24 weeks gestation (when the fetus is considered capable of extrauterine survival—viable).

- **Complete abortion.** All of the products of conception are expelled.
- **Elective abortion.** Pregnancy interruption as a choice of the pregnant woman unrelated to medical reasons.
- **Habitual abortion.** Spontaneous abortion in three or more successive pregnancies.
- **Incomplete abortion.** A portion of the conceptus is expelled from the uterus, while a portion remains within the uterus.
- **Induced abortion.** Voluntary termination of pregnancy
- **Inevitable abortion.** The cervix is dilated and the pregnancy will ultimately be expelled, characterized by uterine cramping, vaginal bleeding, and progressive cervical dilation.
- **Missed abortion.** The fetus dies in utero but is not expelled.
- **Spontaneous abortion.** The products of conception are expelled spontaneously before viability.
- **Therapeutic abortion.** Abortion performed for health reasons.
- **Threatened abortion.** The possibility of abortion exists, but the pregnancy may continue. There is uterine cramping and some vaginal bleeding.

Abruptio placentae. Premature separation of a normally implanted placenta after the 20th week of gestation.

Accelerated/decelerated breathing. During labor when uterine contractions increase in intensity, a shallow, rapid breathing pattern. The rate begins slowly and increases with the intensity of the contraction, reaching a peak at the acme of the contraction and slowly decelerating as the contraction subsides.

Acculturation. Cultural blending of mores between different cultural groups.

Acidosis. A reduced pH level of the blood created by an accumulation of acids or loss of bicarbonates in the body.

Acini cells. The milk-producing cells of the breast.

Acme. The peak and greatest intensity of a uterine contraction.

Acrocyanosis. Bluish discoloration of the hands and feet of the neonate caused by peripheral cyanosis associated with immaturity of circulation or cold stress.

Acrosome. Frontal or head section of the sperm containing enzymes that aid in the penetration of the ovum.

Active transport. Transportation of substances through a semipermeable membrane from an area of lower concentration to one of higher concentration.

Afterbirth. A lay term used to describe the placenta and membranes following birth.

Afterpains. A lay term used to describe uterine cramping following birth.

AGA. Appropriate for gestational age; birth weight of the neonate falling between the tenth and ninetieth percentile.

Agenesis. Lack of formation of an organ.

AID. Artificial insemination using donor semen.

AIDS. Acquired immunodeficiency syndrome; impairment of the body's immune system.

AIH. Artificial insemination using the husband's semen.

Albuminuria. Albumin in the urine in detectable amounts.

Alkalosis. Elevated pH of body fluids, related to an accumulation of bicarbonate or a lack of acid.

Allele. Alternating or contrasting forms of a gene located at the same site on a chromosome.

Alpha-fetoprotein. Protein produced by the fetus, peaking at 14 to 16 weeks gestation, after which it declines. Elevated levels of alpha-fetoprotein in the amniotic fluid are indicative of neural tube defects such as spina bifida, anencephaly, hydrocephalus, or meningomyelocele.

Alveoli. Terminal pulmonary air sacs.

Amenorrhea. Absence of menstruation.

Amniocentesis. Introduction of a needle into the amniotic sac through the abdominal and uterine wall for the purpose of withdrawing amniotic fluid.

Amniography. Injection of a radio-opaque dye into the amniotic fluid followed by x-ray visualization.

Amnion. The inner most membrane of the fetal membranes that form the amniotic sac.

Amnioscopy. Introduction of an amnioscope through the cervix and fetal membranes for visualization of the amniotic fluid and amniotic cavity.

Amniotic fluid. Fluid contained within the amniotic sac that has thermoregulatory functions and provides a protective environment for the fetus.

Amniotic sac. Membranous sac composed of an amniotic and chorionic membrane that contains the fetus and amniotic fluid.

Amniotomy. Rupture of the amniotic sac by artificial means.

Analgesic. Pain relieving substance.

Androgen. Male hormone that potentiates the development of male characteristics.
Android pelvis. A male type of pelvis.
Anencephaly. Congenital malformation of the cranium with absence of the brain.
Anesthesia. Substance which provides relief from pain and partial or complete sensation loss with or without loss of consciousness.
Aneuploidy. Alterations either greater or less in the haploid number of chromosomes.
Anomaly. A malformation.
Anoxia. Absence of oxygen.
Anteflexion. Sharp forward tipping of the uterus at the cervical junction.
Antenatal. Fetal occurrence before birth.
Antepartal. Occurrence before labor and delivery.
Anteversion. Normal position of the uterus with slight forward tipping of the fundus.
Anthropoid pelvis. Pelvis in which there is a wide transverse diameter and a narrow anteroposterior diameter.
Antrum. A fluid-filled space in the center of the targeted primary oocyte containing estrogen produced by the theca cells of the follicle.
Apgar score. Method of assessment of the newborn at birth, developed by Dr. Virginia Apgar, that assesses the heart rate, respiratory effort, muscle tone, reflex response, and color on a scale of 1 to 10 (highest) at 1 and 5 minutes after birth.
Apnea. Cessation of breathing for more than 20 seconds in the neonate, generally associated with bradycardia, pallor, or cyanosis.
Areola. Areas of pigmentation surrounding the nipple.
AROM. Artificial rupture of the amniotic membranes.
Artificial insemination. Placement of semen in the vagina by artificial means for the purpose of conception.
Asphyxia. Decreased oxygen or elevated carbon dioxide levels in the blood.
Aspiration. Inhalation of a substance or substances, such as meconium, mucus, or formula, which causes irritation and pneumonitis or asphyxia.
Atelectasis. Collapse of the alveoli of the lungs.
Atony. Lack of muscle tone.
Atresia. Abnormal absence or closure of an opening or passage.
Attitude, fetal. Relationship of the fetal parts to one another.
Autolysis. The breakdown of body cells by self-digestion, as exemplified in the uterine muscle cells following delivery.
Autosome. Paired chromosomes with the exception of the X and Y chromosomes.
Axis. Either a real or imaginary line running through the center of the body, about which a given part rotates.
Azospermia. An absence of sperm in the semen.
Bag of waters. Lay term used to denote the amniotic sac.
Ballottment. Ability of the fetus to move and rebound when pushed by the examiner's fingers.
Bandl's ring. An area of thickening between the upper and lower uterine segments causing an excessive thinning of the lower uterine segment and a tightly contracted thick upper uterine segment.
Barr bodies. Sex chromatin mass derived from the X chromosome of females, absent in males.
Bartholin's glands. Mucus-secreting vulvovaginal glands located near the vaginal orifice.
Basal body temperature (BBT). Method of determining when ovulation has occurred by recording temperature through the monthly menstrual cycle. Prior to ovulation the record will show the temperature dropping a slight amount and then elevating about 0.4 to 1.0° F. postovulation.
Bicornate uterus. A uterus with two uterine horns.
Bilirubin. A by-product formed by the breakdown of red blood cells, creating a yellowish pigment in the bile.
Bilirubinemia. Abnormal accumulation of bilirubin in the blood.
Biochemical testing, fetal. Assessment of the fetus including human chorionic gonadotropin (HCG) determinations, progesterone evaluation, urinary estriol determinations and maternal plasma tests for estriols, human placental lactogen (HPL), alkaline phosphatase (HRAP), diamine oxidase (DAO), and oxytocinase.
Biophysical assessment, fetal. Assessment of the fetus which uses any of the following methods: ultrasonography, magnetic response, fetoscopy, amnioscopy, roentogenography, chorionic villus sampling.
Biparietal diameter. Transverse diameter of the fetal head, averaging about 9.5 cm at term.
Birth rate. The number of live births per 1000 population.
Blastocele. A cavity during the early development of an embryo.
Blastocyst. Mass of developing cells following the morula stage of cell division characterized by the development of a fluid-filled cavity and an inner cell mass.
Blastomere. Cells produced by early cleavage and cell division of the zygote.
Bloody show. Blood-streaked mucus from the vagina present during labor. It may or may not be present at the onset of labor but often increases as labor progresses.
Bonding. Attachment formed at the onset of a relationship that serves as a uniting factor in the continuation of the relationship; especially significant when applied to maternal-infant attachment following birth.
Brachial palsy. Injury during birth to the fetal brachial plexus, causing varying degrees of paralysis to the arm.
Braxton Hicks' contractions. Painless intermittent uterine contractions present during pregnancy, not characteristic of labor.
Breech birth. Neonate delivered with the buttocks or feet presenting.
- **Complete breech.** Buttocks and feet presenting with the knees and hips flexed.
- **Footling breech.** Extension at the knees and thighs with one or both feet as the presenting part.
- **Frank breech.** Buttocks are presenting, with the hips flexed and the knees on the abdomen.
- **Kneeling breech.** Extension at the thighs and

flexion at the knees with one or both knees presenting.

Bregma. Area of the anterior fontanel of the fetus or neonate.

Bronchopulmonary dysplasia. Condition of the immature lungs of the neonate characterized by damage to the epithelial linings of the alveoli and bronchi with fibrosis and the formation of cystic air lesions.

Brown fat. Type of adipose cell found only in the neonate that provides a readily available source of heat production. Concentrations are found in the axillary region, beneath the scapula, the kidney, and the neck.

Bulbourethral glands. Small pea-shaped bodies found bilaterally near the male urethra. Also known as Cowper's glands.

Candida albicans. A yeastlike fungus causing a vaginal infection characterized by burning and itching; moniliasis.

Capacitation. Process of removal of the protective coating over the acrosomal region of the sperm before fertilization can take place.

Caput succedaneum. Edema occurring under the scalp area of the presenting part of the neonate following a vertex delivery.

Cardinal movements. Changes in position that the fetus undergoes during labor consisting of descent, flexion, internal rotation, extension, restitution, and external rotation.

Carunculae myrtiformes. Hymenal tags, which are remnants of the hymen following intercourse.

Caudal anesthesia. A form of regional anesthesia where the anesthetic agent is injected in the caudal area of the spinal canal.

Cephalhematoma. Accumulation of blood beneath the bone and the periosteum of the newborn skull.

Cephalic. Denoting the head.

Cephalic presentation. The head of the fetus presenting for delivery.

Cephalopelvic disproportion (CPD). Incongruency in the shape or size of the fetal head and the mother's pelvis which prevents passage through the pelvis.

Cervical dilation. Widening of the cervical os during labor from 0 to 10 cm, which allows passage of the fetus.

Cervical os, external. Opening from the cervix to the vagina.

Cervical os, internal. opening from the uterus to the cervix.

Cervix. Lowermost portion of the uterus extending into the vagina.

Cesarean birth. Delivery of the neonate via a surgical abdominal incision into the uterus.

Chadwick's sign. Bluish-violet discoloration of the vaginal mucous during pregnancy caused by increased vascularity.

Chloasma. Increased pigmentation on the face, forming a mask-like appearance over the nose and cheeks during pregnancy; melasma.

Choanal atresia. Obstruction of the nares caused by a membranous or bony growth of tissue.

Chorion. Outermost membrane of the amniotic sac.

Chorionic frondosum. Fetal portion of the placenta.

Chorionic villi. Columns of cytotrophoblastic cells covered with synctiotrophoblast, which comes in contact with the decidua basalis.

Chorionic villi sampling. Placement of a catheter transcervically under ultrasound guidance into the chorion frondosum to obtain samples of the chorionic villi for detection of fetal chromosomal and biochemical defects.

Chromosome. Elongated, rod-shaped, dark-staining bodies contained within the nucleus of the cell that carry genes. They occur in pairs, including 44 autosomes and 2 sex chromosomes.

Chromosome lag. Chromosomes that separate successfully during metaphase but fail to migrate properly during anaphase.

Circumcision. Removal of the foreskin of the penis.

Circumoral cyanosis. Bluish discoloration of the area surrounding the mouth.

Cleavage. Division of the zygote into blastomeres.

Clitoris. Sexually responsive structure located between the folds of the labia minora; female counterpart of the male penis.

Coitus. Act of sexual intercourse.

Coitus interruptus. Withdrawal of the penis from the vagina before ejaculation.

Colostrum. First milklike secretion from the breast before the onset of lactation. Contains increased amounts of proteins and immune bodies.

Colpotomy. Surgical incision made into the wall of the vagina behind the cervix.

Common law. Law based on legal precedent.

Complete abortion. See abortion, complete.

Conceptus. The fetus, placenta, and fetal membranes, and fluid.

Condom. Membranous sheath worn over the penis during sexual intercourse to prevent deposit of sperm into the vagina and to aid in the prevention of transmission of venereal disease.

Conduction, heat. Transfer of heat from one surface to another.

Congenital. Events occurring during intrauterine life.

Contraction stress test. See oxytocin challenge test.

Convection, heat. Heat loss or gain experienced as air or water currents carrying heat toward or away from the body.

Coombs' test

- **Direct.** Test used to detect maternal Rh+ antibodies in the cord blood of the neonate.
- **Indirect.** Detects circulating Rh+ antibodies against red blood cells in maternal blood.

Conscience clause. A statement adopted by some states that allows physicians, nurses, and nonpublic hospitals and clinics to refuse to perform or participate in abortion procedures on moral, religious, or ethical grounds.

Continuous positive airway pressure (CPAP). Method of delivery of continuous distending pressure to the lungs in order to increase functional residual capacity and improve oxygenation; provided by nasopharyngeal tubes, endotracheal tubes, or nasal prongs.

Copulation. The act of sexual intercourse.

Corpus luteum. Developmental stage of the ovarian follicle following ovulation, giving the appearance of a "yellow body" within the follicle. At this stage the follicle is actively secreting progesterone. It will continue to secrete progesterone if pregnancy occurs until the placenta takes over this function. If pregnancy does not occur it will atrophy and slough off shortly before the onset of the next menstrual cycle.

Cotyledon. Lobule of the placenta containing chorionic villi and blood vessels.

Couvade. Physical symptoms normally associated with pregnancy that occur in the father during pregnancy; it also includes the observance of rituals pertinent to fatherhood in certain cultures.

Couvelaire uterus. Condition following abruptio placentae with hemorrhage into the myometrium of the uterus, causing it to become rigid and "boardlike."

Credé prophylaxis. Prevention of ophthalmia neonatorum by instillation of ophthalmic ointment or 1 percent silver nitrate solution into the eyes of the newborn following birth.

Cri-du-chat syndrome. Deletion of a short arm of the chromosome number causing a chromosomal disorder characterized by microcephaly, downward slanted eyes, a cat-like cry, and mental and growth retardation.

Crowning. Fetal head visible at the vaginal orifice.

Cryptorchidism. Undescended testicles.

Cul-de-sac of Douglas. Pouch of peritoneum located between the posterior wall of the uterus and the anterior wall of the rectum.

Culdoscopy. Insertion of a culdoscope into the pelvic cavity via a vaginal incision for visualization of the pelvic contents.

Culture. The general characteristics of a society in regard to belief, values, attitudes, and behaviors that are transmitted from generation to generation.

Curanderos. A native healer.

Cystocele. Bladder herniation into the vagina.

Cytotrophoblast. Innermost layer of cells of the trophoblastic cells of the zygote.

Decidua. Uterine endometrium during pregnancy.

- **Decidua basalis.** Endometrial area located beneath the implantation site.
- **Decidua capsularis.** Area of endometrium that has fused and surrounds the implanted blastocyst.
- **Decidua parietalis (vera).** Remaining endometrial lining of the uterus that is not part of the placenta.

Decrement. Decrease in intensity of a uterine contraction.

Deletion. Breakage of a piece of a chromosome, causing a chromosomal aberration.

Delivery. Expulsion of the products of conception.

Deoxyribonucleic acid (DNA). Major genetic material that carries genetic information.

Descent. Passage of the fetus through the maternal pelvis with onset at the time of engagement and completion at the time of delivery.

Dextrocardia. Position of the heart on the right side of the body.

Diaphragm (contraceptive). Flexible circular ring covered with a cap of latex rubber that is filled with a spermicide and placed over the cervix, providing both a mechanical and chemical form of contraception.

Diaphragmatic hernia. Protrusion of the abdominal contents through a congenital weakness in the diaphragm into the thoracic cavity.

Diastasis recti. Separation of abdominal rectus muscles in the midline.

Diffusion. Transfer of a substance from one area to another.

- **Facilitated diffusion.** Diffusion requiring a carrier system supplied by enzymes; provides a more rapid transfer of substances from an area of higher to lower concentration.
- **Simple (passive) diffusion.** Transfer of substance across a semipermeable membrane such as the placenta from an area of higher concentration to an area of lower concentration.

Dilatation. Gradual opening of the external cervical os during labor from 0 to 10 cm.

Diploid. Two complete sets of homologous chromosomes.

Dipping. When the presenting part of the fetus is entering the inlet of the maternal pelvis but is not yet engaged.

Disseminated intravascular coagulation (DIC). Condition resulting in the rapid utilization of blood clotting factors, leading to occlusion of small blood vessels and a predisposition to hemorrhage. It occurs as a response of the body to a coagulation material such as decidual tissue, amniotic fluid, or an endotoxin entering the circulation.

Dizygotic. Arising from two separate zygotes, as in fraternal (nonidentical) twins.

Doderlein's bacillus (Lactobacillus acidophilus). Gram-positive microorganism normally inhabiting the vagina that contributes to the acidity of the vaginal secretions.

Dominant. A trait expressed when two heterozygous genes are present.

Doppler. Ultrasound sensor used to hear fetal heart tones.

Down's syndrome (trisomy 21). Abnormality of the chromosomes in which there are three number 21 chromosomes instead of two, giving a total of 47 chromosomes.

Dubowitz assessment. Assessment evaluation tool using a set of neurologic and external physical criteria to measure gestational age.

Ductus arteriosus. An anatomic opening normally present in the fetus that serves as a shunt between the pulmonary artery and the aorta; it closes shortly after birth and becomes a ligament.

Ductus venosus. A vessel present in the fetus that acts to bypass the liver, carrying the blood from the umbilical vein directly to the inferior vena cava; it closes shortly after birth and becomes a ligament.

Duncan's mechanism. Delivery of the placenta, with the maternal placental surface presenting first after birth.

Dysmenorrhea. Painful menstruation.

Dyspareunia. Painful sexual intercourse.

Dysplasia. Abnormal alteration in tissue development.

Dyspnea. Labored or difficult breathing.

Dystocia. Difficult labor which may be caused by uterine dysfunction, abnormal presentations and positions, fetopelvic disproportion, or uterine anomalies.

Eclampsia. One form of pregnancy-induced hypertension (PIH); it is characterized by the development of tonic and clonic convulsions.

Ectoderm. Outer germinal layer of the developing embryo, which is responsible for the development of the epidermis, hair, nails, sebaceous glands, inner ear, mammary glands, central nervous system, optic lens, retina, and peripheral nervous system.

Ectopic pregnancy. Implantation of the blastocyst outside of the uterine cavity.

EDC. Expected date of confinement; when the baby is due to be born.

Edema. Abnormal accumulation of fluid in body tissues.

Effacement. Thinning and shortening of the cervix occurring during labor.

Effleurage. Stroking the abdomen gently during labor with the tips of the fingers.

Ejaculation. Emission of semen from the male urethra during sexual stimulation.

Elective abortion. See abortion, elective.

Emancipated minor. Minors who live apart from their parents and have certain rights not normally afforded minors.

Embryo. Developmental stage of the human, from 2 to 8 weeks gestation.

Endocervical. Interior segments of the cervical canal.

Endoderm. Inner germinal layer of the developing embryo responsible for the development of areas such as the bronchi, lungs, liver, gastrointestinal tract, thyroid gland, urinary bladder, pancreas, parathyroid glands, and tonsils.

Endometriosis. Abnormal location of endometrial tissue outside of the uterus in the pelvic cavity, giving rise to symptoms of dysmenorrhea, back pain, pelvic pain, bleeding, and infertility.

Endometrium. Inner uterine lining, shed as the menstrual flow.

En face. Position assumed to facilitate eye to eye contact.

Engagement. The widest diameter of the fetal presenting part has passed through the maternal pelvic inlet; it may occur several weeks before the onset of labor, especially in primigravidas, or it may not occur until the onset of labor or during labor in the multigravida.

Engorgement. Obstetric use refers to the vascular congestion of the breast characterized by swelling of the breast tissue.

Engrossment. The bonding relationship of the father to the newborn.

Epicanthus. Skin fold covering the inner canthus of the eye that extends from the edge of the nose to the median aspect of the eyebrow.

Epididymis. Narrow, tightly coiled tube located on the lateral and anterior aspect of each testis that serves as the passageway for the sperm from the seminiferous tubules to the vas deferens.

Epidural block. Lumbar epidural block involves the injection of an anesthetic solution into the epidural space in the lumbar region of the spine, providing extradural anesthesia.

Episiotomy. Surgical incision of the perineum during the second stage of labor to enlarge the vaginal opening.

Epispadias. Urethral opening located on the dorsum of the penis.

Epstein's pearls. Small, white, raised areas consisting of epithelial cells found on the gums and hard palate.

Erb-Duchenne palsy. See brachial palsy.

Ergot. A drug obtained from fungus that stimulates uterine contractions.

Erythema toxicum. A reddish-pink papular rash with small vesicles and pustules resembling flea bites, appearing on the face, trunk, and genital areas of the neonate.

Erythroblastosis fetalis. Hemolytic disease of the neonate caused by Rh or ABO incompatibility of the mother and fetus; characterized by jaundice, anemia, and hyperbilirubinemia.

Estradiol (E2). The most significant of the estrogens produced by the theca cells of the ovary.

Estriol. The end product from the metabolism of estrone and estradiol.

Estrogen. Name for collective grouping of identified estrogens in the body. They are produced by the ovaries, adrenal cortex, liver, and placenta; classified as female sex hormones.

Estrone. One of the known estrogens produced mainly by the liver.

Ethics. A set of moral principles.

Evaporation, heat. Loss of body heat from moist areas of the body as the water vaporizes.

Exchange transfusion. Replacement of 80 to 85 percent of the neonate's blood with donor blood facilitating the removal of bilirubin and antibody-coated red blood cells and correcting anemia.

Expulsion. Delivery of the shoulders and the remainder of the fetal body at birth.

Extension. Resistance met by the flexed fetal head on the pelvic floor forcing it forward and extending through the vulvar opening.

External rotation. Following the birth of the head at the time of delivery, the external 45 degree turning of the occiput to the right or left in order to maintain alignment with internal shoulder rotation.

Extrauterine. Outside of the uterus.

Fallopian tubes. Oviducts extending from each side of the uterus, terminating at the ovaries.

False labor. Ineffective irregular uterine contractions that do not dilate the cervix or increase in intensity.

False pelvis. Pelvic area above the linea terminalis.

Familial. A trait that occurs in more members of a family than would normally be expected.

Family. The basic unit of society.

- **Extended family.** A group of relatives that form relationships and share a common body of domestic, social, cultural, and economic activities; they may or may not inhabit the same household.
- **Matrifocal family.** Family in which the adult male is a sometime member.
- **Nuclear family.** Family consisting of husband, wife, and children.

Family-centered nursing. Nursing care focusing on the care of the childbearing family as the client.

Fecundation. Occurrence of fertilization.

Ferning. Ferning pattern appearing when dried smears

of cervical or vaginal mucus are viewed under a microscope.

Fern test

Amniotic fluid. A drop of vaginal fluid is obtained and spread on a clean slide and allowed to dry. The dried slide will show a ferning pattern when viewed under a microscope if amniotic fluid is present in the vaginal fluid, indicating rupture of the fetal membranes.

Ovulation. Cervical mucus is placed on a slide and allowed to dry; a ferning pattern will be visible under a microscope if ovulation has occurred, owing to the presence of sodium chloride under the influence of increasing levels of estrogen. As progesterone levels increase following ovulation, the sodium content drops, and ferning is not seen. Because of the high progesterone levels during pregnancy, ferning is not observable.

Fertility. Ability to reproduce.

Fertility rate. The number of births per 1000 women ages 15 to 44 years.

Fertilization. Union of the male spermatozoan and the female ovum.

Fetal. Relating to the fetus.

Fetal alcohol syndrome. Fetal syndrome caused by ingestion of alcohol by the mother during pregnancy; characterized by fetal defects such as microcephaly, intrauterine growth retardation, mental deficiencies, cardiac anomalies, facial defects, and joint defects.

Fetal bradycardia. A sustained fetal heart rate under 120 BPM.

Fetal death. Death of the fetus in utero following the 20th week of gestation; stillbirth.

Fetal distress. Disturbance of fetal physiologic homeostasis, indicated by alterations in the fetal heart rate or activity and/or the presence of meconium-stained amniotic fluid.

Fetal heart rate. The activity of the fetal heart as set by the sinoatrial node when influenced by the parasympathetic and sympathetic nervous system. The normal FHR is between 120 and 160 BPM.

Accelerations. Transitory increase in the fetal heart rate caused by bursts of sympathetic nervous system activity. When noted with fetal movement, uterine contractions, or external stimulation, they are usually considered an indicator of fetal well-being.

Baseline rate. The range in which the fetal heart rate is located during the major portion of a 10 minute interval.

Early deceleration pattern. Onset of decrease in the FHR is early in the uterine contraction with the FHR not falling below 100 BPM and the decrease ending by the completion of the uterine contraction.

Late deceleration pattern. Hypoxic fetal heart rate deceleration pattern associated with a decrease in maternal-fetal oxygen exchange; characterized by onset after the beginning of the uterine contraction and uniformity of shape.

Variable deceleration pattern. Deceleration pattern with a variable onset; the shape of the pattern varies from a V-shape to a wide U-shape; generally caused by umbilical cord compression.

Variability. Fetal heart rate fluctuation around a given FHR level that represents continuous interaction between the fetal sympathetic and parasympathetic nervous system.

Long term variability. Refers to rhythmic fluctuations of the FHR described in terms of frequencies of 2 to 6 BPM with a normal range of 5 to 15 BPM.

Short term variability. Refers to the internal difference in baseline FHR with each successive fetal ECG (beat-to-beat).

Fetal hydrops. Generalized extreme edema of the fetus associated with severe hemolytic disease.

Fetal lie. The relationship of the long axis of the fetus to the long axis of the mother.

Fetal membranes. The amniotic and chorionic membranes of the amniotic sac.

Fetal mortality. See mortality, fetal.

Fetal tachycardia. A sustained fetal heart rate over 160 BPM.

Fetoscope. A stethoscope designed for auscultation of the FHR through the mother's abdomen.

Fetoscopy. Fetal tissue sampling performed by the insertion of a fiberoptic scope through the abdomen into the uterus.

Fetus. The developing conceptus from the 8th week of gestation until birth.

Fibroid. Benign tumorous growth of the uterus.

Fimbria. Fingerlike projections located on the ends of the fallopian tubes.

FiO_2 (fraction of inspired oxygen). Concentration of oxygen when administered.

First stage of labor. From the onset of true contractions to complete dilatation of the cervix.

Flaccid. Lack of muscle tone.

Flexion. The bending of a part, such as the fetal head, which flexes the chin on the chest during labor in order to allow the smallest diameter of the head to enter the birth canal.

Floating. A high fetal presenting part not yet engaged in the maternal pelvis.

Follicle. A saclike structure.

Follicle-stimulating hormone (FSH). Hormone produced by the anterior pituitary gland, which promotes the growth and development of the graafian follicle of the ovary during the follicular phase of the menstrual cycle.

Fontanel. Soft spot on the fetal head where the suture lines intersect, consisting of a band of connective tissue.

Anterior fontanel. Bregma; fontanel between the frontal and parietal bones where the sagittal and coronal sutures intersect; may be felt as a diamond-shaped area.

Posterior fontanel. Lambda; triangular shaped area located between the parietal and occipital bones where the sagittal and lambdoidal sutures intersect; may be felt as a triangular-shaped area.

Food allergies. Hypersensitivity to food substances resulting from immunologic responses.

Food intolerance. Inability to tolerate a specific food substance often associated with an enzyme deficiency but not related to a immunologic response.

Foramen ovale. Opening between the right and left atria of the fetal heart which facilitates fetal circulation and which closes after birth.

Foreskin. Prepuce of the penis.

Fornices, vaginal. Spaces formed in the anterior and posterior areas of the vagina by the extension of the cervix into the vagina.

Fraternal twins. Dizygotic, nonfraternal twins resulting from the simultaneous fertilization of two ova.

Frenulum linguae. Membranous band at the base of the tongue attaching to the floor of the mouth.

Full-term neonate. Neonate delivered between the gestational ages of 38 and 42 weeks.

Functional residual capacity (FRC). The volume of air that remains in the lungs following expiration.

Funic souffle. Soft, blowing sound heard as blood circulates through the umbilical cord; the rate will correspond with the FHR.

Fundus. Uppermost portion of the uterus located between the fallopian tubes.

Galactorrhea. Excessive milk secretion from the breast.

Galactosemia. Inability of the neonate to metabolize the sugar galactose, caused by an autosomal recessive disorder involving a deficiency of the enzyme galactose-1-phosphate uridyl transferase.

Gamete. A mature sperm or ovum.

Gametogenesis. The process through which the primitive female and male germ cells are changed into mature gametes, which includes mitosis and meiosis.

Gastroschisis. An abdominal wall defect not associated with umbilical site which allows herniation of the intestines.

Gastrulation. Process of early development associated with the development of the three germ layers of the embryo.

Gavage. Feeding through a tube inserted into the stomach.

Genes. Areas of molecules of deoxyribonucleic acid (DNA) located in a linear order on chromosomes that carry genetic information determining the characteristics of an individual.

Genetics. The study of heredity.

Genitalia. The organs of reproduction.

Genotype. A description of the genetic constitution of an individual.

Gestation. Entire period of intrauterine development from conception to birth.

Gestational age. The number of completed weeks of embryonic or fetal development from the onset of the mother's last menstrual period.

Gestational hypertension. See pregnancy-induced hypertension.

Glabella. Prominent area above the nose and midway between the eyebrows.

Glans penis. The area designated as the head of the penis that is analogous to the female clitoris

Glomerular filtration rate. The rate at which plasma is filtered through the glomeruli of the kidney.

Glycosuria. Glucose present in the urine.

Gonad. Gamete-producing ovary of the female and testes of the male.

Gonadotropic-releasing factors (GnRF). Hormones produced by the hypothalamus such as follicle-stimulating releasing factor (FSHRF) and luteinizing hormone releasing factor (LHRF) which stimulate the release of FSH and LH from the anterior pituitary gland.

Gonadotropins. Hormones such as FSH and LH which stimulate the gonads.

Goodell's sign. Softening of the cervix during the second month of pregnancy, considered a probable sign of pregnancy.

Good Samaritan Act. A law that exempts individuals from liability of ordinary negligence when rendering care without compensation in emergency situations.

Graafian follicle. The ovarian follicle that has matured and will rupture and release the ovum at the time of ovulation.

Gravid. Pregnant.

Gravida. A pregnant woman.

Gynecoid pelvis. The typical rounded female pelvis that best accommodates childbirth.

Gynecology. The study of health care of the female, focusing on the reproductive organs, urinary organs, and rectum.

Habitual abortion. See abortion.

Harlequin skin change. Skin change that occurs owing to immaturity of the circulatory system which will appear as a sharply demarcated color difference, with the dependent areas appearing red and the superior areas appearing pale when the neonate is placed on his side.

Hegar's sign. Softening of the lower uterine segment assessed during the second and third months of pregnancy; considered a probable sign of pregnancy.

Hematocrit. Volume of red blood cells per 100 ml (deciliter) of circulating blood designated as volume percent.

Hematoma. A swelling caused by accumulation of blood in tissue; often referred to as a "blood tumor."

Hemolysis. Red blood cell destruction.

Hemorrhagic disease of the newborn. A bleeding disorder of the neonate in the first few days of life associated with a vitamin K deficiency.

Hemorrhoids. Varicosities of the rectum.

Hepatosplenomegaly. Enlargement of the liver and spleen.

Herpes genitalis. A sexually transmitted disease caused by the herpes simplex type II virus (HS V-2) characterized by the formation of clusters of genital vesicles.

Heterozygous. Possessing alleles for a trait on each gene of a pair.

Hirsutism. Excessive amount of hair growth.

Homan's sign. Pain experienced in the calf of the leg when the foot is dorsiflexed; diagnostic of thrombophlebitis.

Homeostasis. A state of stability in the physiologic and psychological environment of an individual.

Homozygous. Possessing the same alleles for a trait on each gene of a pair.

Hormone. A substance produced by an organ that regulates the activities of a specific organ.

Human chorionic gonadotropin (HCG). A hormone produced by the synctiotrophoblastic cells of the developing embryo and fetus necessary for the maintenance of the corpus luteum; serves as the basis for pregnancy tests.

Human chorionic somatomammotropin (HCS). Hormone produced by the synctiotrophoblastic cells of the developing embryo and fetus that participates in maternal metabolic activities such as the breakdown of fats for a quick maternal energy source and decreasing the peripheral effectiveness of insulin with a resultant rise in the maternal blood sugar level.

Hyaline membrane disease (HMD). See respiratory distress syndrome.

Hydatidiform mole. Degenerative disorder of the chorionic villi that results in the formation of multiple grapelike cysts. It is characterized by increased maternal levels of HCG, nausea, vomiting, hypertension, and vaginal bleeding. There is no identifiable fetus, and evacuation of the uterus is recommended.

Hydramnios. An abnormally increased amount of amniotic fluid.

Hydrocele. An abnormal accumulation of fluid in a saclike structure such as the testicle.

Hydrocephalus. Abnormal accumulation of cerebrospinal fluid in the cerebral ventricles of the brain, causing enlargement of the ventricles and skull.

Hydrops fetalis. Gross edema of the fetus, caused by increased severity of fetal hemolytic disease from Rh incompatibility; also associated with manifestations of severe anemia and cardiac failure.

Hymenal sheath. Mucous membrane that partially covers the vaginal opening.

Hyperbilirubinemia. An abnormal excess of bilirubin in the blood.

Hypercapnea. An abnormal excess of carbon dioxide in the blood.

Hypercarbia. See hypercapnea.

Hyperemesis gravidarum. Extreme vomiting during pregnancy; also referred to as pernicious vomiting.

Hyperlipidemia. Abnormally increased level of fats in the blood.

Hyperplastic growth. Growth in the embryo and fetus accompanied by an increase in the number of cells.

Hyperreflexia. An abnormally reactive response of a reflex action.

Hypertrophic growth. Growth of the fetus accompanied by an increase in the size of existing cells.

Hyperventilation. Rapid breathing resulting in carbon dioxide deficiency in the blood and a potential alkalosis; characterized by tingling in the extremities, numbness, and a lightheaded sensation.

Hypervitaminosis. Excessive dietary intake of vitamins.

Hypocalcemia. An abnormally low level of calcium in the blood.

Hypocapnia. An abnormally low carbon dioxide content of the blood.

Hypocarbia. An abnormally low carbon dioxide content of the blood.

Hypoglycemia. An abnormally low blood sugar level.

Hypospadias. Urethral opening on the under surface of the penis.

Hypothermia. An abnormally low body temperature.

Hypotonia. A loss of muscle tone.

Hypovolemia. An abnormal decrease in circulating plasma in the body.

Hypoxia. A deficiency of oxygen in body tissues.

Hypoxemia. A low oxygen content of the blood.

Hysterosalpingogram. Injection of a radio-opaque material into the cervix, distending the uterus and fallopian tubes for fluroscope examination of patency of the fallopian tubes.

Hysterotomy. Incision into the uterus made by surgical means.

Iatrogenic. Unintentional adverse effect of medical treatment.

Icterus. See jaundice.

Icterus neonatorum. Jaundice of the newborn that is considered physiologic.

Iliopectineal line. Ridge on the inner surface of the ilium and pubic bones that serves as the landmark for the linea terminalis dividing the true and false pelves.

Ilium. Fan-shaped upper part of the hipbone.

Immunoglobulin. A protein originating within the body that has antibody properties and functions as part of the humoral immune response.

- **IgA.** Immunoglobulin found in colostrum from the breast that offers immunity to the intestinal mucosa of the neonate; it cannot cross the placental barrier.
- **IgD.** Found in low serum concentrations in the neonate but does not cross the placenta; its function is unknown.
- **IgE.** Does not cross the placenta and the neonate has low levels at birth; presents in allergic responses.
- **IgG.** The only immunoglobulin to cross the placenta to the fetus; levels normally fall after birth increasing the sensitivity to infection during three to six months of age.
- **IgM.** Immunoglobulin unable to cross the placental barrier but which is produced in small amounts by the fetus; most important against gram-negative organisms.

Imperforate anus. Embryonic abnormality of anal development, consisting of one of the following anomalies: (1) a membranous covering obstructing the rectum; (2) rectal atresia without an anal opening; or (3) rectal atresia with fistulas to the urinary tract, vagina, or perineum.

Imperforate hymen. A constricted hymen with no opening.

Impetigo. A contagious skin infection caused by streptococcus or staphylococcus and characterized by vesicles and pustules that rupture and form a yellowish crust on the skin.

Implantation. Penetration and embedding of the conceptus in the uterine mucosa.

Impotence. Inability of the male to have or maintain an erection for penetration of the vagina or for ejaculation.

Impregnate. To fertilize or make pregnant.

Inclusion cyst. Small, round grayish cyst found on gums of the newborn that may be mistaken for teeth; they are of no clinical significance; also called retention cysts.

Incompetent cervix. Dilation of the cervix after four months of pregnancy, permitting expulsion of the fetus.

Incomplete abortion. See abortion, incomplete.

Increment. Interval during which the intensity of a uterine contraction increases.

Induced abortion. See abortion, induced.

Induction. A method of artificially stimulating the onset of labor.

Inevitable abortion. See abortion, inevitable.

Infant. Child under one year of age.

Infertility. Inability to conceive after one year of unprotected intercourse.

Informed consent. Consent for treatment given by a client based on an understanding of the nature of the condition, the basis for treatment, the nature of the treatment, the risks and benefits involved in the treatment, and the alternatives to treatment.

Innominate bone. The ilium, ischium, and pubis, which make up the hip bones.

Internal cervical os. Opening located between the cervix and the uterus.

Internal rotation. In utero rotation of the long axis of the fetal head from the transverse or oblique diameter to the anterior-posterior diameter in order to accommodate to the maternal pelvis during labor.

Interstitial cell-stimulating hormone. Male hormone that stimulates the interstitial cells of the testes to secrete testosterone; also referred to as the male luteinizing hormone (LH).

Intervillous spaces. Spaces in the maternal section of the placenta that contain maternal blood and provide areas of maternal-fetal exchange of nutrients, gases, and waste.

Intrapartal. The period of time during labor and delivery.

Intrauterine device (IUD). A piece of inert plastic or metal inserted vaginally through the cervix and into the uterus, used to prevent pregnancy by interferring with implantation of the conceptus.

Intrauterine growth retardation (IUGR). An interruption in the normal pattern of in utero growth, causing a growth deficiency in the fetus; may be of fetal, placental, or maternal origin.

Introitus. An entrance into a canal.

In utero. Within the uterus.

In vitro fertilization. Fertilization of an ovum outside of the body; often referred to as a "test tube" fertilization.

Involution. Return of the female reproductive organs to their normal or near-normal state following pregnancy.

Ischium. The lower part of the hip bone.

Jaundice. yellowish discoloration of body tissues observable in the skin, sclera or eyes, and oral mucous membranes, caused by abnormal accumulation of unconjugated bilirubin.

- **Pathologic jaundice.** Disorder of the neonate observable in the first 24 hours following birth related to Rh or ABO incompatibility.
- **Physiologic jaundice.** Jaundice of the neonate observable after 24 hours most commonly on the second or third day of life; caused by the large number of red blood cells present at birth.

Karotype. Photographic display of systematically arranged chromosomes.

Kegal exercise. Alternately contracting the pubococcygeal muscles of the pelvic floor to improve the muscle tone of the perineal area.

Kernicterus. Damage occurring to brain tissue from deposits of unconjugated bilirubin.

Ketosis. Incomplete oxidation of fatty acids, resulting in the accumulation of ketone bodies.

Labia majora. The outer lips of the vulva, composed of fatty tissue, covered with hair, and extending from the mons pubis to the perineum.

Labia minora. The inner lips of the vulva located between the labia majora; they are thinner than the labia majora and are not covered with hair.

Labor. The series of physiologic events by which the products of conception are expelled from the uterus.

- **Labor phases.** *Latent phase* begins with the onset of labor and lasts until the beginning of the active phase of cervical dilation; it is the longest phase of the first stage of labor. *Active phase* begins with the upswing of the contraction curve (5 cm) and ends with 10 cm cervical dilation.
- **Labor stages.** *First stage* begins with the onset of true contractions through complete dilation of the cervix (10 cm). *Second stage* begins with complete cervical dilation and ends with delivery of the fetus. *Third stage* (placental stage) begins after delivery of the neonate and ends with placental expulsion. *Fourth stage* (recovery stage) begins with placental expulsion and ends with stability of the mother's physiologic status.

Laceration. A cutting or tearing; during childbirth it is used to describe a tear in the perineum. They are classified into four degrees. *First degree* involves only the skin and mucous membranes. *Second degree* involves skin, mucous membranes, and muscles of the perineum. *Third degree* involves skin, mucous membranes, perineal muscles, and the anal sphincter. *Fourth degree* involves skin, mucous membranes, perineal muscles, the anal sphincter, and the lower rectal wall.

Lactation. Secretion of milk from the breast.

Lactiferous duct. Duct conveying milk to the nipple of the breast.

Lactiferous sinus. Dilated portion of the lactiferous duct that serves as a reservoir for milk.

Lactoferrin. Agent in breast milk that prevents bacteria from getting the iron necessary for growth; helps absorb iron into the blood stream and works directly to kill some bacteria.

Lactogenic hormone. See prolactin.

Lactose. A sugar present in milk.

Lactosuria. The sugar lactose present in urine.

Lamaze method. A psychoprophylactic method of childbirth in which mothers and their partners are taught physical and psychological conditioning, including the use of relaxation, breathing techniques, and physical exercises in preparation for childbirth.

Lambda. Area where the lamboidal and sagittal sutures converge.

Lamboidal suture. The suture located between the occipital bone and parietal bone of the skull.

Laminaria. Seaweed that, when processed and dried, is inserted into the cervix, whereby it will absorb moisture, swell, and dilate the cervix; may be used preceding an induced abortion or to dilate the cervix for labor induction.

Lanugo. Fine, soft downy hair found on the fetus during uterine development.

Laparoscopy. Abdominal examination performed by the insertion of a laparoscope (endoscope) into a surgical incision in the abdomen.

Laparotomy. Surgical incision into the abdomen.

Large for gestational age (LGA). Neonates whose birth weight places them above the 90th percentile of normal for their gestational age.

Lecithin/sphingomyelin ratio (L/S ratio). The ratio of phospholipids, lecithin to sphingomyelin, contained in amniotic fluid; fetal lung maturity is indicated by a ratio of 2:1.

Leiomyoma. A benign fibroid tumor of the uterus.

Leopold's maneuvers. A series of four maneuvers used to assess the pregnant abdomen for determination of fetal lie, position, and presentation.

Let down reflex. Reflex that induces the flow of milk from the breasts; initiated by sucking or psychological factors that stimulate the secretion of oxytocin and cause tissue surrounding the alveoli to contract and propel the milk from the alveoli to the ducts of the nipple.

Leukocytosis. An increase in white blood cells.

Leukorrhea. A discharge from the mucous membranes of the vagina or cervix, whitish or yellowish in color; it may be caused by the presence of pathologic organisms or may be a physiologic adaptation of pregnancy.

Libido. Sexual drive.

Lie. See fetal lie.

Lightening. The settling of the fetal presenting part into the lower uterine segment; it may occur two to three weeks before labor in the primigravida, but may not occur until active labor in the multipara.

Linea nigra. Line of pigmentation extending from the pubis to the umbilicus, often seen in pregnant women.

Linea terminalis. Anatomic boundary that divides the true pelvis from the false pelvis.

Lithotomy position. Position of the client on her back with the knees flexed and the thighs brought up toward the chest.

Lobules. Clusters of alveoli in the breast.

Lochia. Vaginal discharge following delivery and during the puerperium.

- **Lochia alba.** Creamy white lochia seen from day eight until approximately three weeks after delivery containing serum, leukocytes, epithelial cells, mucus, and bacteria.
- **Lochia rubra.** Lochia seen in the first few days following delivery that consists of blood and decidual debris that is reddish in color.
- **Lochia serosa.** Pinkish lochia seen from the third to the eighth postpartum day, consisting of erythrocytes, leukocytes, decidua, cervical mucus, and microorganisms.

Locus. Location of a specific gene on a chromosome.

Low birth weight neonate (LBW). A neonate whose weight is less than 2500 gm, regardless of gestational age.

Luke's sign. Calf pain when standing; indicative of possible phlebitis.

Lunar month. A month consisting of 28 days; pregnancy is considered to be 10 lunar months.

Luteal phase. Phase of the menstrual cycle from ovulation until the onset of menstruation; about 14 days in duration.

Luteinization. Transformation of the theca cells of the ovarian follicle following ovulation into the yellow-bodied cells of the corpus luteum.

Luteinizing hormone (LH). Hormone secreted by the anterior pituitary gland that participates in the stimulation of ovulation and the formation of the corpus luteum.

Lymphoadenopathy. Disease process with involvement of the lymph nodes.

Lysozyme. Enzyme found in breast milk, saliva, tears, and sweat that has antiseptic properties.

Macerated fetus. A fetus that has undergone a degenerative process causing breakdown of skin and tissue; may be observed following intrauterine fetal death.

Machismo. A cultural ideal of masculinity that equates maleness with sexual prowess.

Macroglossia. Enlargement of the tongue.

Macrosomia. Enlargement of body size; often associated with neonates of diabetic mothers.

Magnet reflex. Reflex elicited with the neonate in a supine position. The lower limbs are semiflexed and pressure is applied to the soles of both feet. The legs will then extend toward the pressure. If absent in the neonate, indicative of spinal cord injury.

Malpractice. Negligence of a specially trained person when performing his or her job, which results in misconduct or failure to meet the expected and usual standards of care.

Malpresentation. Abnormal presentation of the fetus.

Mammary. Referring to the breast.

Maple syrup urine disease. An inborn error of metabolism resulting in the accumulation of the amino acids leucine, isoleucine, and valine in the plasma and urine secondary to a deficiency of the enzyme decarboxylase; characterized by feeding difficulties, vomiting, lethargy, hypertonicity, and a maple syrup odor to the urine.

Marfan's syndrome. An autosomal dominant disorder characterized by disproportionately long limbs, extremes of height, thin spidery fingers and toes, ocular and skeletal defects, and cardiovascular involvement.

Mask of pregnancy. See chloasma.

Mastalgia. Pain in the breast.

Mastectomy. Surgical removal of breast tissue.

Mastitis. An inflammatory condition of the breast.

Mastodynia. Pain in the breast.

Meconium. The first stool passed by the neonate, formed from swallowed amniotic fluid and epithelial cells in the fetal intestines; it is black, tarry, sticky, and odorless.

Meconium aspiration syndrome. Syndrome produced in utero by the effects of fetal hypoxia. The anal sphincter of the hypoxic neonate relaxes, allowing the passage of meconium into the amniotic fluid. The fetus gasps in utero and inhales amniotic fluid with meconium particles, which block and irritate bronchial passages.

Meiosis. Division and reduction of the germ cells (sperm and ova) which reduces the chromosome number of each in half.

Menarche. The onset of menstruation; generally refers to the first menstrual cycle.

Meningomyelocele. External herniation of the meninges, cerebrospinal fluid, and spinal cord into a saclike cyst, resulting from defective embryonic development of the neural tube.

Menopause. The period during the woman's reproductive years when there is cessation of ovulation and menstruation that heralds the end of reproductive ability and childbearing.

Menorrhagia. Excessive amount of menstrual flow.

Menses. Cyclic vaginal discharge of menstrual blood during the female reproductive years.

Menstruation. The cyclic sloughing of the uterine endometrium that appears monthly as vaginal bleeding.

Mentum. The chin.

Mesoderm. Middle germinal layer of cells of the developing embryo responsible for the development of areas such as muscle, connective tissue, blood, lymph cells, cardiovascular system, skeleton, urogenital system, and spleen.

Metabolic thermogenesis. The production of heat by metabolic processes.

Metacentric. Centrosome located approximately in the center of the chromosome.

Metritis. Inflammatory process of the uterus.

Metrodynia. Uterine pain.

Metrophlebitis. Inflammatory process involving the uterine veins.

Metrorrhagia. Vaginal bleeding between menstrual periods.

Microcephaly. Abnormality of development in which the head and brain of the neonate are abnormally small, resulting in mental retardation.

Midwife. An individual who has training or experience and assists in the childbearing process.

- **Lay midwife.** An individual who performs deliveries but is not a certified nurse midwife (CNM).
- **Nurse Midwife.** A registered nurse with formal specialized training in childbearing and who becomes certified through a national certification process.

Milia. Small white lesions appearing on the face of the neonate, especially the nose, chin, and forehead, owing to unopened sebaceous glands and accumulation of secretions; they are of no clinical significance and disappear spontaneously.

Milk leg. See phlegmasia alba dolens.

Miscarriage. Lay term used to describe a spontaneous abortion.

Missed abortion. See abortion, missed.

Mitosis. The process by which all cells divide, with the exception of cells producing ova and sperm.

Mittelschmerz. Pain experienced in the abdomen at the time of ovulation.

Molding. The ability of the fetal head to change its shape to adapt to the maternal pelvis.

Mongolian spots. Bluish discoloration of the pigment in a given area, usually the back or buttocks of a neonate; it may be mistaken for bruising; of no clinical significance, it disappears by the time the child is five or six years old.

Moniliasis. See candida albicans.

Monosomy. An abnormal number of chromosomes, with one less (45) than the total normal number (46).

Monozygotic. Arising from one fertilized ovum, such as in identical twins.

Mons veneris. Fatty tissue covering over the area of the female symphysis pubis that develops hair at puberty.

Morals. A set of principles involving right or wrong behavior.

Morbidity. The ratio of diseased individuals to a specified population group.

Morbidity temperature. A temperature elevation above 38° C (100.4° F) on any two postpartum days excluding the first 24 hours after delivery.

Moro reflex. "Startle" reflex of the neonate, present at birth.

Morphogenesis. The changes in cells whereby they gain a special form, shape or structure in a series of sequential coordinated changes in fetal development.

Mortality rate. The numbers of death during a select period of time.

- **Fetal mortality rate.** The number of fetal deaths per 1000 live births.
- **Infant mortality rate.** The number of deaths per 1000 children one year of age or younger.
- **Maternal mortality rate.** The number of maternal deaths per 100,000 live births.
- **Neonatal mortality rate.** The number of neonatal deaths per 1000 live births during the first 28 days of life.
- **Perinatal mortality rate.** The number of fetal deaths at 28+ weeks of gestation plus the number of neonatal deaths.
- **Postnatal mortality rate.** The number of deaths per 1000 live births from 28 days of life up to but not including one year of age.

Morula stage. A stage of development at three days after fertilization when a solid mass of blastomeres, shaped like a mulberry, has formed.

Mosaicism. Mitotic nondisjunction occurring during cell division resulting in an individual with two distinctly different chromosomal cell lines.

Mullerian ducts. Structures present in early fetal development that are destined to become the fallopian tubes, uterus, and upper portion of the vagina; also called paramesonephic ducts.

Multigravida. A woman who is pregnant for the second or more time.

Multipara. A woman who has given birth to two or more viable infants.

Mutation. A transmissible change in genetic material that is permanent for that gene.

Myomectomy. Surgical removal of a leiomyoma (fibroid tumor).

Myometrium. The smooth muscle layer of the uterus.

Nagele's rule. Estimation of expected delivery date (EDC) by determining the first day of the last menstrual period, subtracting three months from that month, and adding seven days.

Nalorphine hydrochloride (Nalline). A narcotic antagonist; may be administered to the mother 5 to 10 minutes before delivery if drug-induced depressions of the neonate is expected.

Naloxone hydrochloride (Narcan). A narcotic antagonist; used to reverse narcotic depression in the neonate when a narcotic has been administered to the mother in labor. It has no effect on neonatal depression caused by barbiturates or anesthesia administered to the mother in labor.

Narcosis. A state of stupor that is drug-induced.

Narcotic. A drug that induces narcosis, legally defined as any habit-forming drug; these drugs require a physician's prescription to be purchased.

Natal. Refering to birth.

Navel. The umbilicus.

Necrotizing enterocolitis. Injury to the intestinal mucosa of the neonate, resulting from an ischemic insult from reduction in mesenteric blood flow secondary to fetal hypoxia; it is characterized by necrosis of the bowel with perforation and infection.

Negligence. Failure to exercise the standard of care that is expected of a reasonably prudent person in a specific circumstance.

Neonatal mortality rate. See mortality rate, neonatal.

Neonate. The newborn infant from birth through the first 28 days of life.

Neural tube defect. Embryonic failure of neural tube closure, causing a congenital defect of the spinal column.

Nevus. A congenital area of increased pigmentation; a birthmark.

Nevus flammeus (port wine stain). Capillary angioma with a smooth, reddish surface concentrated in the epidermis of the skin; they do not blanch when pressure is applied; they do not fade and will generally involve a large area on the face or neck.

Nevus vascularis (strawberry mark). Capillary hemangioma formed from dilated capillaries in the dermal and subdermal tissue creating a raised, well-defined area; will regress as the child becomes older.

Nidation. Implantation of the fertilized ovum.

Nitrazine test. A test used to determine if the amniotic membranes have ruptured. A vaginal smear is obtained with a cotton-tipped applicator and applied to a strip of litmus paper. If amniotic fluid is present in the smear, the litmus paper will show an alkaline reaction and turn blue.

Nondisjunction. Failure of a chromosome pair to separate normally with both members of a pair moving into one cell during the first or second meiotic division; one gamete will have two of a particular chromosome and the other will have none.

Nonshivering thermogenesis. A method of increasing metabolic activity to produce heat.

Nonstress test (NST). Evaluation of the relationship of fetal heart rate fluctuations in response to fetal movements with an external fetal monitor.

Normotensive. A blood pressure within the normal range.

Nosocomial. Originating in the hospital.

Nulligravida. A woman who has never been pregnant.

Nullipara. A woman who has never delivered an infant of 20 weeks or more gestation.

Nutrient requirements. The least amount of a particular nutrient that will maintain ideal nutritional health.

Obstetrics. The branch of medicine that deals with the care of the pregnant woman during pregnancy, labor, delivery, and the puerperium.

Occiput. The posterior section of the head.

Ocular hypertelorism. An excessive width between the eyes.

Oligohydramnios. An abnormally decreased amount of amniotic fluid which may be associated with abnormalities of the fetal urinary tract.

Oliguria. A decreased amount of urine secreted by the kidneys.

Oocyte. An immature ovum.

Oogenesis. Development of the ovum.

Oomphalitis. Inflammation and infection of the umbilicus.

Oomphalocele. Herniation of the abdominal contents into the umbilicus.

Oophorectomy. Surgical removal of the ovaries.

Ophthalmia neonatorum. Neonatal infection of the eyes, generally resulting from gonococci present in the birth canal of the parturient with gonorrhea.

Opisthotonos. Arching of the back and backward extension of the head that occurs during a tetanic spasm.

Orchitis. Inflammation of the testes.

Organogenesis. Formation and development of organs during embryonic development.

Orgasm. Sexual climax.

Ortolani's maneuver. Assessment of the movement of the head of the femur on the acetabulum to determine congenital hip dysplasia.

Os. An opening such as the cervical os.

Ova. Eggs produced by the ovary.

Ovary. The female sex gland, which produces ova.

Ovulation. The release of the ovum from the graafian follicle of the ovary, occurring at approximately in the middle of the menstrual cycle.

Ovum. An egg.

Oxytocin. A hormone produced by the posterior pituitary that stimulates uterine contractions and the "let down reflex" of the breast. Also a synthetic agent that will induce uterine contractions.

Oxytocin challenge test (OCT). The stimulation of uterine contractions by the administration of oxytocin and evaluation of the fetal heart rate in an effort to determine the ability of the fetus to withstand the stress of labor; stress test.

$PaCO_2$. The partial pressure of carbon dioxide.

Pallor. Pale appearance of the skin and mucous membranes.

Palpation. Physical examination using the finger and hands to assess by touch.

PaO_2. Partial pressure of oxygen.

Papanicolaou smear (Pap smear). Microscopic examination of cervical scraping to detect the presence of cervical carcinoma.

Para. The number of pregnancies that continued beyond 20 weeks of gestation.

Paracervical block. A method of anesthesia involving

transvaginal injection of a local anesthetic agent into the tissue on either side of the cervix anesthetizing the cervix and upper two-thirds of the vagina.

Paramesonephric duct. See mullerian duct.

Parametritis. Inflammation of the tissue of the parametrium.

Parametrium. Connective tissue located between the two layers of the broad ligament.

Partial pressure. Force exerted by a gas as it moves from one state to another.

Parturient. A woman in labor or childbirth.

Parturition. The birth giving process.

Passage. The rigid bony pelvis and the soft tissues of the cervix, vagina, and introitus.

Passenger. The fetus, who travels through the birth passage during labor.

Patent ductus arteriosus (PDA). An acrocyanotic heart lesion of the neonate with failure of the ductus arteriosus to close following birth, causing a left-to-right shunt of the blood from aorta to the pulmonary artery.

Pathologic retraction ring. See Bandl's ring.

Pelvic inlet. Area of the pelvis bounded by the pubic crest and spine anteriorly, the iliopectineal lines laterally and the sacral promontory posteriorly.

Pelvic outlet. Inferior strait consisting of two triangular planes with a common base of transverse diameters between the ischial tuberosities.

Pelvimetry. Method of measuring the pelvic diameters to determine if the pelvic passage will accommodate the fetus; performed clinically using a pelvimeter or by x-ray pelvimetry.

Pelvis. The bony structure between the moveable vertebrae of the vertebral column and the lower limbs on which the vertebral column rests; made up of two innominate bones, the sacrum, and the coccyx.

Penis. The external male organ of reproduction and urination.

Perinatal mortality rate. See mortality rate, perinatal.

Perinatal period. Time beginning with the 20th week of pregnancy and continuing through the 28th day of postnatal existence.

Perineorrhaphy. Suturing of a laceration in the perineal area.

Perineotomy. Surgical incision of the perineum; episiotomy.

Perineum. Area located between the vulva and the anus in the female or the scrotum and anus in the male; it also includes the muscles and tissues of the lower pelvic area.

Periodic breathing. Neonatal apnea of 5 to 10 seconds followed by an increased respiratory rate of 50 to 60 per minute for 10 to 15 seconds; not associated with cyanosis.

Peripheral vascular resistance. Pressure contained within the arteries.

Peripheral vasoconstriction. A vasomotor response to stress or cold, in which the blood vessels in the skin constrict, reducing their diameter and inhibiting blood flow to the area.

Peritoneum. Membranous lining of the abdominal wall and internal organs.

Petechiae. Areas of pinpoint hemorrhage found on the skin of the neonate, caused by pressure during birth or an infectious process.

pH. Hydrogen ion concentration.

Phenotype. The result of interactions between the genotype and its nongenetic environment seen in the external appearance of an individual.

Phenylketonuria (PKU). Inability of the neonate to metabolize phenylalanine to tyrosine due to a deficiency of the enzyme phenylalanine hydroxylase, causing accumulation of phenylalanine in the blood, which leads to alterations in the development of the brain and mental retardation.

Phimosis. Stricture of the prepuce of the penis, causing it to be tight and nonretractable.

Phlebitis. Inflammation of a vein.

Phlegmasia alba dolens. Phlebitis involving the femoral vein, causing swelling and venous obstruction.

Phocomelia. A congenital anomaly characterized by the absence of the upper part of a limb or limbs, with the hand or foot intact.

Photodegradation. Decompensation caused by light exposure.

Phototherapy. Light therapy used in the treatment of neonatal jaundice to breakdown unconjugated bilirubin to a water-soluble excretable form.

Pica. A craving for a substance not normally considered a food.

Pinna. The exposed portion of the ear.

Placenta. A discoid-shaped vascular structure uniting the fetus to the maternal host and providing nutritive, gas, and waste exchange between the fetal and maternal circulations.

Placenta accreta. Failure of the decidua basalis to develop properly, allowing invasion of the chorionic villi into the uterine musculature, preventing normal placental separation.

Placenta circumvallata. Abnormal configuration of the placenta, in which the chorionic plate is reduced with a double layer of amnion and chorion encasing the decidua.

Placenta previa. Placental attachment and development in the lower uterine segment.

- **Low-lying placenta (marginal previa).** Placenta extending to the margin of the internal cervical os but not over the os.
- **Partial placenta previa.** Placenta partially covering the internal cervical os.
- **Total placenta previa.** Placenta completely covering the internal cervical os.

Placenta succenturiata. Formation of an accessory lobe or lobes connected to the main placenta.

Placental infarct. Localized area of placental necrosis, causing alterations in placental functioning.

Placental souffle. A very soft, blowing sound heard as the blood circulates through the placenta; it will coincide with the heart rate of the mother.

Platypelloid pelvis. A flat pelvis disproportionately wide from side to side, the transverse diameter being wider than normal and with a short diagonal conjugate measurement; frequently associated with cephalopelvic disproportion.

Plethora. A ruddy complexion often associated with polycythemia.

Pneumomediastinum. Collection of air surrounding the mediastinum with a characteristic "halo" effect upon x-ray visualization.

Pneumopericardium. Accumulations of air in the pericardium of the heart.

Pneumoperitoneum. Accumulation of air in the peritoneal cavity.

Pneumothorax. Accumulation of air in the pleural cavity producing decreased breath sounds, a shift in the PMI, and hyperresonance of the chest with abrupt alterations in respiratory status.

Podalic version. See version, podalic.

Polycythemia. An abnormal increase in red blood cells.

Polydactyly. Having an extra finger or toe.

Polygenic inheritance. Two or more independent pairs of genes affect the same characteristics in the same way.

Polyhydramnios. An excessive amount of amniotic fluid; usually considered more than 1500 to 2000 ml.

Polyuria. Excessive secretion of urine.

Position. Relationship of the fetal denominator to the mother's pelvis.

Positive end expiratory pressure (PEEP). End expiratory pressure provided by a mechanical ventilator sustaining pressure during expiration that promotes a extended period for diffusion of inspired air within the lungs.

Positive signs of pregnancy. Absolute confirmation of pregnancy is made when the following signs of pregnancy are present: auscultation of the FHT, fetal movements felt by the examiner, and x-ray/ultrasound visualization of the fetus.

Postcoital test. Sperm analysis test, in which a sample of cervical secretions is obtained following intercourse at the time of ovulation and examined for cervical factors, ferning, and the presence of viable sperm; also called the Sims-Huhner test.

Postnatal. After childbirth.

Postnatal mortality rate. See mortality rate, postnatal.

Postpartal hemorrhage. Hemorrhage of blood involving an amount over 500 ml after delivery.

Delayed hemorrhage. Hemorrhage that occurs after 24 hours following delivery.

Primary hemorrhage. Hemorrage that occurs within 24 hours after delivery.

Postpartum. After delivery.

Postterm neonate. Neonate born after 42 weeks gestation; also referred to as postmature.

Preeclampsia. See pregnancy-induced hypertension.

Pregnancy-induced hypertension. Broad term for hypertensive disorders peculiar to pregnancy; includes preeclampsia, eclampsia, and chronic hypertension; it appears after the 20th week of gestation and is characterized by hypertension, edema, and proteinuria.

Premature neonate. See preterm neonate.

Premature rupture of the membranes (PROM). Rupture of the amniotic sac more than 24 hours before the onset of labor.

Premenstrual syndrome (PMS). A collection of symptoms experienced by a woman preceding her menstrual period characterized by irritability, depression, feelings of fullness, mood swings, breast swelling and tenderness, and tension.

Prenatal. Before birth.

Prepuce. Skin fold over the glans penis.

Presenting part. The part of the fetus lowest in the birth canal.

Presumptive signs of pregnancy. Signs and symptoms suspect of pregnancy that may be present for reasons other than pregnancy; they are not conclusive for pregnancy diagnosis.

Preterm neonate. Neonate born before the 38th week of gestation.

Primary infertility. Infertility in which a pregnancy has never been conceived.

Primary uterine inertia. See uterine inertia, primary.

Primigravida. A first pregnancy; the first time the uterus has been impregnated.

Primipara. A woman who has given birth to her first viable infant.

Probable signs of pregnancy. Signs of pregnancy that, of themselves, are not conclusive for pregnancy but are considered as reliable indicators of pregnancy.

Prodromal. Early signs or symptoms of a disease.

Progesterone. Hormone produced by the corpus luteum of the ovary, the adrenal cortex, and the placenta that influences growth of the uterine endometrium in preparation for implantation, maintains the pregnancy, and participates in the development of breast tissue.

Prolactin. A hormone secreted by the anterior pituitary gland that is responsible for the secretion of milk from the breast following sucking by the neonate; also called lactogenic hormone.

Prolapsed uterus. Loss of uterine support, with the uterus descending into the lower vagina or extending from the vagina.

Prophylactic. A preventive measure.

Prostaglandins. Classification of fatty acids found in bodily tissue but in large concentrations in seminal fluid, ovarian follicles, and in menstrual fluid.

Proteinuria. Protein appearing in the urine.

Pruritis. Itching of the skin.

Pseudocyesis. A false pregnancy.

Ptyalism. Excessive amount of salivation.

Puberty. Stage of human development at which the reproductive organs are mature and reproduction is possible.

Pudendal block. A form of anesthesia in which a local anesthetic agent is injected near the pudendal nerve next to the ischial spines, anesthetizing the lower two-thirds of the vagina and the perineum.

Puerperal sepsis. Infection of the genital tract and reproductive organs associated with childbearing.

Puerperium. The period after the third stage of labor that continues for six weeks, during which the reproductive organs return to near normal states.

Pulmonary embolism. A blood clot that is dislodged and carried to the lungs, blocking the pulmonary circulation.

Pyelonephritis. Inflammation and infection of the renal pelvis and kidney.

Pyrosis. A burning sensation felt in the esophagus, throat, and stomach, accompanied by a sour-tasting eructation; heartburn.

Quickening. Feelings of fetal movement felt by the mother at about 16 to 20 weeks gestation.

Rabbit test (Friedman test). Injection of a woman's urine into unmated mature female rabbit; followed in two days by examination of the rabbit ovaries for the presence of fresh corpus lutea; indicates a positive pregnancy test.

Radiant warmer. A heat-producing unit used to delivery heat to the neonate and promote a neutral thermal range.

Radiation, heat. A method of heat loss that occurs when body heat radiates to cooler environmental air.

Radioimmunoassay (RIA). A pregnancy test on maternal blood that assesses the presence of human chorionic gonadotropin (HCG); may require one to five hours for results.

Rales. Adventitious breath sounds heard in the alveoli and terminal bronchioles; distinguished as interruptive, discrete, crackling sounds that are heard during inspiration.

Recessive trait. A trait that is not dominant; it will be expressed if an individual is homozygous for that particular trait.

Rectocele. Herniation of the rectum into the vagina.

Reflex. Automatic unmediated involuntary response.

Regional anesthesia. Injection of an anesthetic agent into a specified area to block pain impulses and the sensation of pain.

Regurgitation. A reversed flow, such as the spitting up or vomiting of food.

Residual urine. Urine remaining in the bladder following urination.

Respiratory distress syndrome. A severe respiratory disorder of the neonate associated with a deficiency of pulmonary surfactant that is related to immaturity of the lungs; most frequently seen in preterm neonates; also called hyaline membrane disease.

Restitution. Following delivery of the fetal head, the neck untwists and the occiput rotates to its original position to keep the head in alignment with the fetal spine.

Resuscitation. Life supportive mechanism used to revive individuals who have succumbed; employing artificial respiratory assistance and cardiac stimulation.

Retained placenta. Failure of the placenta or a part of the placenta to be expelled from the uterus following delivery of the fetus.

Retractions. Inward drawing of the chest wall with each inspiration.

Retroflexion. Corpus of the uterus bent backward toward the rectum.

Retrolental fibroplasia. Injury to the retina and lens of the eye of the neonate, resulting from the formation of fibroic tissue as a consequence of hyperoxemia; may result in blindness.

Rh factor. Antigen present in the red blood cells of Rh positive individuals and absent in Rh negative individuals.

Rh immune globulin (Rhogam). Agent used for passive immunization of an Rh negative mother to avoid Rh sensitization from an Rh positive fetus.

Rh incompatibility. Incompatibility of the blood cells of the Rh negative mother with the Rh positive blood cells of the fetus.

Rhonchi. Continuous coarse sounds heard in the large bronchioles during both inspiration and expiration.

Rhythm method. A method of natural family planning in which sexual intercourse is avoided during the woman's fertile period.

Ribonucleic acid (RNA). A protein found in the cytoplasm of each cell that functions to organize and coordinate the activities of DNA; it reads the information in DNA, interprets it, takes the message to the ribosomes, and supervises the making of proteins in the proper manner.

Ring formation. A chromosome formation in which the ends are joined together to form a ring.

Ritgen maneuver. Method used to control the delivery of the head of the fetus at birth.

Rollover test. Test used in selected primigravidas at 28 to 32 weeks gestation to predict their risk of developing pregnancy-induced hypertension.

Rooming in. Occupancy of the same hospital room by both the mother and neonate following delivery and during hospitalization following delivery. It serves to enhance maternal-infant relationships and familiarize the mother with care of the neonate.

Rooting reflex. Reflex present in the neonate at birth; observed when the side of the mouth or cheek is stroked. The neonate will turn his head in the direction of the stroking and open his mouth.

Round ligament pain. Discomfort felt in the lower abdomen during pregnancy caused by the stretching of the ligaments.

Rubella. German measles.

Rubin tubal patency test. A test to determine the patency of the fallopian tubes, performed by injecting carbon dioxide into the cervix through the uterus into the fallopian tubes.

Saddle block anesthesia (subarachnoid block). A small amount of an anesthetic agent is injected into the spinal fluid in the area of the subarachnoid space.

Sagittal suture. Connective tissue line separating the two parietal bones.

Scaphoid abdomen. Sunken appearance to the abdomen, somewhat boat-shaped; found in neonates with diaphragmatic hernia.

Scarf sign. With the neonate in a supine position, the arm is extended across the chest toward the opposite shoulder as far as possible. An assessment of the position of the elbow on the chest is made.

Schultz mechanism. Placental delivery with the shiny fetal side presenting.

Sclerema. Large area of thick rigid cold skin seen on the cheeks, buttocks, and eventually all skin areas in neonates with severe infections, malnourished conditions, and severe cold stress.

Scrotum. External rugated sac containing the testes in the male.

Seborrheic dermatitis. Excessive secretion from the sebaceous glands of the scalp, causing a yellowish thick crust to form on the scalp of the neonate; cradle cap.

Secondary infertility. Inability to become pregnant after one year of unprotected intercourse although a pregnancy has been achieved on one or more previous occasions.

Secondary uterine inertia. See uterine inertia.

Second stage of labor. See labor.

Secundines. The afterbirth, consisting of the placenta and membranes.

Semen. Ejaculate of the male, which is a white, thick fluid containing sperm.

Sensory alteration. Increase or decrease in sensory stimulation.

Septic abortion. Uterine infection developing after an abortion performed by unqualified methods or an unqualified individual.

Sexually transmitted disease (STD). Disease transmitted by sexual contact or a sexual relationship with an infected person.

Shake test (foam test). Test used to determine fetal lung maturity by examination for the presence of surfactant in amniotic fluid.

Shunt. A channel or passageway that diverts the flow of blood from one area to another.

Sims' position. Client assumes a left lateral position with the right knee drawn up in the direction of the chest.

Sims-Huhner test. See postcoital test.

Situational crisis. Crisis that occurs in response to a specific circumstance.

Skene's ducts. Ducts located within the vestibule, laterally and somewhat posteriorly to the urinary meatus.

Small-for-gestational-age (SGA). Neonate whose birth weight falls below the 10th percentile.

Smegma. Sebaceous gland secretion, somewhat cheesy in consistency, that is found under the prepuce of the penis.

Somite. Mesoderm on either side of the notochord of the developing embryo that thickens, divides, and segments, forming pairs of cuboidal mesoderm that are destined to be the skeleton of the head and trunk and associated muscles and dermis.

Souffle. See funic souffle; placental souffle.

Spermatozoan (sperm). Mature male sex cell.

Spermatogenesis. Formation of mature sperm, reducing the chromosomal number from 46 to 23 in each spermatozoan.

Spermicide. Sperm-killing agent.

Spider nevi. An area, found on the skin of some pregnant women, consisting of a central arteriole with radiating small blood vessels resembling a spider.

Spina bifida cystica. Congenital anomaly, with failure of the vertebral spaces to fuse, and external herniation of the spinal contents into a sac. If it contains only the meninges it is called a meningocele; if it contains meninges, cerebrospinal fluid, and spinal cord, it is called a meningomyelocele.

Spina bifida occulta. Congenital anomaly occurring during fetal development with failure of the posterior vertebral arches to close.

Spinal anesthesia. Regional anesthesia produced by injection of an anesthetic agent into the cerebrospinal fluid in the spinal canal.

Spinnbarkeit. Term used to describe the stretchability of the cervical mucus at ovulation.

Spiritualist. Native healer of the Puerto Rican culture.

Spontaneous abortion. See abortion, spontaneous.

Startle reflex. See Moro reflex.

Station. Relationship of the presenting part of the fetus to an imaginary line drawn between the maternal ischial spines; expressed in cm.

Statutory laws. Laws such as the Nurse Practice Act that require legislative process and enactment by a city, county, state, or federal legislative body.

Stenosis. Narrowing of a canal.

Sterility. Inability to conceive.

Stillborn. Dead when born.

Stork beak mark. See telangiectatic nevi.

Strabismus. Crossing of the eyes.

Strawberry mark. See nevus vascularis.

Striae albicans. Stretch marks that have faded following pregnancy and appear silvery-white in color.

Striae gravidarum (stretch marks). Reddish or reddish-blue streaks found on the abdomen, thighs, and breasts of the pregnant woman, resulting from separation of the collagen fibers of the connective tissue.

Stridor. High-pitched respiratory sound.

Subculture. Culture that forms as a derivative of another culture.

Subcutaneous fat necrosis. Well-delineated hard masses of varying size found in the subcutaneous tissue as a result of trauma during birth.

Subinvolution. Incomplete involution or failure of the uterus to return to its normal state following pregnancy.

Subluxation. A partial dislocation.

Submetacentric. Centromere located closer to one end of the chromosome than the other.

Superfecundation. During a menstrual cycle, fertilization of two or more ova from separate acts of intercourse.

Supine hypotension syndrome. Obstruction of the vena cava by the weight of the gravid uterus hindering venous return to the heart and causing a drop in the B/P accompanied by dizziness and syncope; relief may be obtained by turning the mother to a left lateral position.

Surfactant. Surface-active phosphoprotein produced by type II epithelial alveolar cells of the lungs, which is responsible for the establishment of alveolar stability by decreasing alveoli surface tension and preventing alveolar collapse.

Symphysis pubis. Area of union of the pubic bones.

Synctiotrophoblast. Outer layer of synctial cells covering the trophoblast of the blastocyst.

Syndactilism. Webbing of the fingers or toes.

Syngamy. The process of fertilization when a sperm unites with an ovum to form a zygote.

Tachodynamometer. External monitor used to assess the pressure of uterine contractions.

Tachycardia. Abnormally fast heart rate; over 160 BPM in the fetus.

Tachypnea. Rapid respirations; greater than 60 per minute in the neonate.

Talipes equinovarus. A congenital deformity in which the heel of the foot is turned inward with the rest of the foot in normal position.

Taking-hold phase. Phase of the puerperium characterized by a more independent attitude of the mother toward self and the neonate; follows the taking-in phase.

Taking-in phase. Phase of the puerperium characterized by dependency needs and passivity of the mother.

Task, maternal. Maternal developmental task that must be completed during the fourth "trimester" of pregnancy.

Telangiectatic nevi (stork-beak mark). Clusters of dilated blood vessels found on the nape of the neck, nose, and eyelids; they disappear within the first year of life.

Teratogen. Any environmental agent capable of causing congenital abnormalities.

Term neonate. A neonate born between 38 and 42 weeks gestation.

Testes. The male sex glands enclosed in the scrotum that produce sperm.

Testosterone. Male hormone secreted by the interstitial cells of the testes that is responsible for the development of secondary male sexual characteristics.

Tetanic contraction. Uterine contraction over 90 seconds in duration.

Tetralogy of Fallot. Congenital heart anomaly characterized by ventricular septal defect, pulmonary stenosis, overriding of the aorta, and hypertrophy of the right ventricle.

Theca cells. Estrogen-producing cells that surround the ovarian follicle.

Therapeutic abortion. See abortion, therapeutic.

Thermogenesis. Production of heat by specific means.

Thermoneutral environment. Environment that enables a neonate to maintain body temperature of 36.5/° C (97.7° F) with normal metabolic and respiratory activity.

Thrombocytopenia. Decreased number of blood platelets.

Thrombophlebitis. Inflammation of a vein with the formation of a blood clot.

Thrombus. Blood clot within and obstructing a vein.

Thrush. An oral fungal infection caused by Candida albicans, that is characterized by formation of white patches on the back of the tongue and membranes.

Tidal volume. Amount of gas inhaled and exhaled during a normal breath.

Tocolytic. Drug agent used to inhibit labor.

Tonic neck reflex. When the neonate's head is turned, the leg and arm of the corresponding side will extend and the leg and arm on the opposite side will flex; fencing position.

TORCH. A group of infections including toxoplasmosis, others such as syphilis and gonorrhea, rubella, cytomegalovirus, and herpes genitalis.

Tort. Any civil wrong committed intentionally or unintentionally.

Torticollis. Inability to move the neck freely as seen in injury to the sternocleidomastoid muscle of the neck.

Toxemia. Term formerly used to describe preeclampsia and eclampsia; currently described as pregnancy-induced hypertension.

Tracheoesophageal fistula. Congenital anomaly with a connection between the trachea and esophagus.

Transient tachypnea of the newborn (Type 2 respiratory distress syndrome). Rapid respirations of the neonate from failure to clear the air passages and/or a delayed absorption or excess of lung fluid, characterized by tachypnea and signs of respiratory distress.

Transitional phase of labor. Period during the first stage of labor when the cervix is dilated from approximately 8 cm to complete dilation.

Translocation. Transfer of a segment of a chromosome to a different site on the same chromosome (reciprocal) or to a different chromosome (centric fusion).

Transposition of the great arteries. Congenital heart abnormality whereby the pulmonary artery is positioned in the left ventricle and the aorta arises from the right ventricle.

Transverse arrest. Arrest of the fetal head in the transverse diameter, usually in the maternal midplane.

Transverse fetal lie. The long axis of the fetus is perpendicular or oblique to the long axis of the mother; the shoulder is usually the presenting part.

Trichomonas vaginalis. A protozoan infection of the vagina characterized by a frothy discharge, burning, and itching of the vulva.

Trimester. Period of time involving three months.

Trisomy. Chromosomal aberration in which an additional chromosome is present in the cell, making three chromosomes instead of two.

Trisomy 21. Down's syndrome; the most common trisomy in which the affected individual has an extra number 21 chromosome for a total of 47 chromosomes.

Trophoblast. Outer layer of cells developing on the blastocyst that will participate in the formation of the placenta.

True pelvis. Pelvic area below the linea terminalis.

Tubercules of Montgomery. Papillae located on the surface of the nipples that secrete a lubricating substance.

Ultrasound. A technique that uses high frequency sound waves directed through a transducer to identify structures; done through the maternal abdomen to identify maternal and fetal tissues, bones, and fluids.

- **Diagnostic ultrasound.** The use of ultrasound to obtain images for diagnosis.
- **Real-time ultrasound.** Using individual B-mode frequencies to obtain a moving display.

Umbilical arteries. Fetal structures that carry primarily deoxygenated blood from the fetus to the placenta.

Umbilical cord. Fetal structure that connects the fetus and the placenta; it normally contains two arteries and one vein, encased in Wharton's jelly.

Umbilical vein. Fetal structure that carries oxygenated blood from the fetus to the placenta.

Umbilicus. Navel; depressed point in the midabdomen that shows the attachment of the umbilical cord during fetal life.

Uniovular. Formed from a single ovum.

Urachus. The urinary canal of the fetus.

Urethra. A canal leading from the bladder to discharge urine externally.

- **Female urethra.** A canal about 4 cm in length passing from the bladder; it lies in close relation to the anterior vaginal wall.
- **Male urethra.** A canal about 20 cm in length that opens in the glans penis; it provides passage for spermatic fluid and urine.

Urethritis. Inflammation of the urethra.

- **Gonococcal urethritis.** Urethral inflammation caused by the gonococcus.
- **Nonspecific urethritis.** Urethral inflammation not caused by the gonococcus.

Urinary meatus. External opening of the urethra.

Uterine. Pertaining to the uterus

Uterine atony. Relaxation of the uterine muscle that may occur following delivery.

Uterine contraction. Muscular contractions of the uterine muscle that aid in expulsion of the products of conception during labor; primary powers of labor. During labor, they are involuntary, rhythmic, intermittent, and increase in intensity. Each has three phases: increment, acme, and decrement. Descriptions of uterine contractions during labor include frequency, duration, and intensity.

Uterine dysfunction. Inability of the uterine muscle to contract efficiently.

Hypertonic uterine dysfunction. A state of greater-than-normal tension of the uterine muscle during labor.

Hypotonic uterine dysfunction. A state of less-than-normal tension of the uterine muscle during labor.

Uterine inertia. Lack of force of the uterine muscle during labor.

Primary uterine inertia. Occurs when the uterus fails to contract with sufficient force to effect labor progress in cervical dilation, cervical effacement, and descent of the presenting part.

Secondary uterine inertia. Occurs when the uterine contractions are vigorous but, as a result of maternal exhaustion or dehydration, are ineffective in labor progress.

Uterine inversion. Turning the uterus inside-out.

Uterine ischemia. Decreased blood supply to the uterus.

Uterine isthmus. Area of the uterus located between the body and the cervix; during pregnancy it becomes soft; during labor, it expands and becomes a part of the lower uterine segment.

Uterine prolapse. Descent of the uterus.

Uterine souffle. Rushing sound of maternal blood entering the placenta that may be identified upon auscultation of the maternal abdomen; it is synchronous with the maternal pulse.

Uterine tetany. Nonrelaxation of the uterine muscle.

Uterus. Hollow muscular organ designed for implantation, growth, and nourishment of the fetus during pregnancy.

Bicornate uterus. Uterus that is divided into two lateral horns as a result of defective embryonic development.

Couvelaire uterus. Purplish-blue uterine discoloration accompanied by rigidity that follows abruptio placentae, with concealed bleeding into the uterine muscle.

Gravid uterus. The state of the uterus during pregnancy.

Retroflexed uterus. The uterine body is bent backward at an angle with the cervix.

Retroverted uterus. Displacement of the uterus by backward tipping of the uterine body.

Vagina. Musculomembranous tube forming the passageway between the uterus and the vaginal introitus.

Vaginal. Pertaining to the vagina.

Vaginal introitus. External opening of the vagina.

Vaginitis. Inflammation of the vagina.

Valsalva maneuver. Forced respiratory effort against a closed airway; sometimes used in second stage pushing.

Variability. See fetal heart rate, variability.

Varicella. Chickenpox.

Varicose veins. Swollen, distended tortuous veins.

Vasa previa. Condition in which one or more fetal blood vessels lies over the internal cervical os during the second half of pregnancy.

Vas deferens. Seminal ducts of the male; bilateral tubes extending from the epididymis to form the ejaculatory ducts.

Vasectomy. Surgical removal of a portion of the vas deferens.

Vasoconstriction. A decrease in the diameter of a blood vessel.

Vasodilatation. An increase in the diameter of a blood vessel.

VDRL test. Abbreviation for Venereal Disease Research Laboratory test; serological test for syphilis.

Vegetarian. One who excludes meat from the diet.

Lacto-ovo-vegetarian. Vegetarian who eats milk products and eggs.

Lacto-vegetarian. Vegetarian who consumes milk products.

Vegan. Pure vegetarian who consumes no foods from animal sources.

Venereal disease (VD; STD). A sexually transmitted disease.

Vernix caseosa. Whitish cheesy material that covers the fetal skin.

Version. Act of turning the fetus to change the presenting part.

External version. Fetal turning by abdominal manipulation during pregnancy under ultrasound guidance to attempt to change the fetal presenting part from breech to cephalic.

Internal version. Fetal turning during labor, done with one hand inserted into the vagina and uterus to change the fetus to a footling breech presentation.

Podalic version. Changing the fetal position by using internal version to a footling breech presentation during labor.

Vertex. The top of the fetal head; area located between the bregma and the lambda.

Verticomental. Relating to the crown of the head and the chin.

Vesicle. Tiny, thin-walled, raised skin lesion that contains clear fluid.

Vestibule, vaginal. Space between the labia minora that contains the urinary meatus and the vaginal orifice.

Viable. Capable of living; usually considered 20 to 24 weeks of fetal development.

Villi. Short vascular processes that appear on some membranes.

Chorionic villi. Tiny vascular projections on the chorionic surface that extend into the maternal uterine blood sinuses.

Vitamin. One of a group of organic substances present in minute amounts in natural foods that are essential to normal metabolism.

Vulva. External female genitalia that consists of the labia majora, labia minora, clitoris, urinary meatus, and vaginal introitus.

Well-baby clinics. Clinics that offer medical and nursing supervision and services to healthy infants.

Wharton's jelly. Gelatinous material that surrounds the umbilical vessels in the umbilical cord.

WIC. Women, Infant, and Children; a supplemental food

program for pregnant, puerperal, and breastfeeding mothers and children up to five years of age.

Witches' milk. Whitish fluid secreted from the neonate's mammary glands for about one week after birth; results from the influence of maternal hormones.

Womb. Lay term for the uterus.

Xanthoma. Yellowish-white plaque on the skin caused by the deposit of lipids.

X chromosome. Female sex chromosome.

X linkage. Genes located on the X chromosome.

Y chromosome. Male sex chromosome.

Y linkage. Genes located on the Y chromosome.

Yolk sac. Highly vascular layer of tissue surrounding the yolk of an embryo.

Zero population growth. Live births are equal to the total number of deaths.

Zona pellucida. Transparent inner layer that surrounds the ovum.

Zygote. Fertilized egg; cell formed by the union of a sperm and an ovum.

INDEX

LABORATORY VALUES OF THE NEONATE

Test	Normal Value in Neonate
Hemoglobin gm/100ml	15–18
Hematocrit, volume %	45–60
Platelets mm3	150,000–300,000
Reticulocytes %	3–7
White blood cells mm3	10,000–35,000
Neutrophils %	46–80
Lymphocytes %	31
Eosinophils %	1–3
Monocytes %	5–10
Red blood cells mm3	4 to 7 million
Bilirubin, direct mg/100ml	0.5–1
Bilirubin, tota mg/100ml	5–12
Blood sugar mg/100ml	40–80
Sodium mEq/L	130–160
Potassium, mEq/L	5.0–7.7
Calcium, mEq/L	4–5
Chloride, mEq/L	95–105
Total protein, gm/100ml	4.8–8.2
Iron mcg/100ml	100–200
Urea nitrogen (BUN) mg/100ml	5–15
Fibrinogen, mg/100ml	150–300
Prothrombin time (sec)	12–18
Blood Gases	
Arterial	
pH	7.35–7.45
P02 mm Hg	50–80
PC02 mmHg	33–45
Plasma bicarbonate mEq/L	20–25
Base excess mEq/L	+4 to −4